P9-AOX-722

PRINCIPLES OF NEUROLOGIC REHABILITATION

NOTICE

Medicine is an ever-changing science. As new research and clinical experience broaden our knowledge, changes in treatment and drug therapy are required. The authors and the publisher of this work have checked with sources believed to be reliable in their efforts to provide information that is complete and generally in accord with the standards accepted at the time of publication. However, in view of the possibility of human error or changes in medical sciences, neither the authors nor the publisher nor any other party who has been involved in the preparation or publication of this work warrants that the information contained herein is in every respect accurate or complete, and they are not responsible for any errors or omissions or for the results obtained from use of such information. Readers are encouraged to confirm the information contained herein with other sources. For example and in particular, readers are advised to check the product information sheet included in the package of each drug they plan to administer to be certain that the information contained in this book is accurate and that changes have not been made in the recommended dose or in the contraindications for administration. This recommendation is of particular importance in connection with new or infrequently used drugs.

PRINCIPLES OF NEUROLOGIC REHABILITATION

EDITOR

Richard B. Lazar, M.D.

Schwab Rehabilitation Hospital and Care Network
Chicago, Illinois
Department of Surgery, Section of Orthopaedic Surgery and
Rehabilitation Medicine and Department of Neurology
Pritzker School of Medicine, University of Chicago
University of Chicago Hospitals
Chicago, Illinois

McGraw-Hill
HEALTH PROFESSIONS DIVISION

New York St. Louis San Francisco Auckland Bogotá
Caracas Lisbon London Madrid Mexico City Milan Montreal
New Delhi San Juan Singapore Sydney Tokyo Toronto

McGraw-Hill

A Division of The *McGraw·Hill* Companies

PRINCIPLES OF NEUROLOGIC REHABILITATION

Copyright © 1998 by The McGraw-Hill Companies, Inc. All rights reserved. Printed in the United States of America. Except as permitted under the United States Copyright Act of 1976, no part of this publication may be reproduced or distributed in any form or by any means, or stored in a data base or retrieval system, without the prior written permission of the publisher.

1234567890   DOC DOC   9987

ISBN 0-07-036794-9

This book was set in Times Roman by Bi-Comp, Inc.
The editors were Joseph A. Hefta and Peter J. Boyle.
The production supervisor was Richard C. Ruzycka.
The cover designer was Robert Freese.
The cover art was rendered by Matthew Dvorozniak.
R. R. Donnelley & Sons Company was printer and binder.

This book is printed on acid-free paper.

Library of Congress Cataloging-in-Publication Data

Principles of neurologic rehabilitation / [edited by] Richard B.
    Lazar.
        p.   cm.
    Includes bibliographical references and index.
    ISBN 0-07-036794-9
    1. Nervous system—Diseases—Patients—Rehabilitation.   I. Lazar,
Richard B.
    [DNLM: 1. Nervous System Diseases—rehabilitation.   2. Nerve
Regeneration.   3. Chronic Disease—rehabilitation.   WL 140 P9575
1997]
RC350.4.P75   1997
616.8′046—dc21
DNLM/DLC
for Library of Congress   97-26656

To Harold Paul Lazar, M.D.
Father, teacher, physician, friend

CONTENTS

PART III   **MANAGEMENT OF CONDITIONS ASSOCIATED WITH CHRONIC**
                      NEUROLOGIC DYSFUNCTION   **287**

CONTRIBUTORS

Mindy Lipson Aisen, M.D.
Cornell University Medical College
Burke Rehabilitation Hospital
White Plains, New York
Chapter 26

Karen L. Andrews, M.D.
Mayo Medical School
Mayo Clinic
Rochester, Minnesota
Chapter 13

Kathleen R. Bell, M.D.
University of Washington
School of Medicine
Seattle, Washington
Chapter 19

David R. Beukelman, Ph.D.
University of Nebraska, Lincoln
Lincoln, Nebraska
Mayer Rehabilitation Institute
Omaha, Nebraska
Chapter 28

Donald R. Bodner, M.D.
Department of Urology
Case Western Reserve University
Cleveland VA Medical Center
University Hospitals of Cleveland
Cleveland, Ohio
Chapter 25

Anjan Chatterjee, M.D.
Department of Neurology
University of Alabama at Birmingham
Birmingham, Alabama
Chapter 35

Jonathan L. Costa, M.D., Ph.D.
Schwab Rehabilitation Hospital
Section of Orthopaedic Surgery and Rehabilitation
Medicine
Pritzker School of Medicine, The University of
Chicago
The University of Chicago Hospitals
Chicago, Illinois
Chapter 14

Bruce H. Dobkin, M.D.
Neurologic Rehabilitation and Research Unit
University of California, Los Angeles
Los Angeles, California
Chapter 6

Mary L. Dombovy, M.D.
St. Mary's Hospital
Rochester, New York
Chapters 7, 12

Susan R. Ehrenthal, M.D.
Harvard Medical School
Department of Physical
Medicine and Rehabilitation
Boston, Massachusetts
Chapter 5

Tanis J. Ferman
Department of Psychiatry
The University of Chicago
Chicago, Illinois
Chapter 33

Hillel M. Finestone, M.D., F.R.C.P.C.
London Health Sciences Centre
University Campus
University of Western Ontario
London, Ontario, Canada
Chapter 24

Kevin M. Frumaga, Pharm.D.
Pharmacology Department
University of Illinois at Chicago
College of Pharmacy
Chicago, Illinois
Chapter 31

Moises Gaviria, M.D.
Pharmacology Department
University of Illinois at Chicago
College of Pharmacy
Chicago, Illinois
Chapter 31

David A. Gelber, M.D.
Southern Illinois University School of Medicine
Memorial Medical Center
Springfield, Illinois
Chapter 18

Monique Gingold, M.D.
Department of Neurology and Pediatrics
West Virginia University Health Science Center
Morgantown, West Virginia
Chapter 11

Michelle S. Gittler, M.D.
Schwab Rehabilitation Hospital and Care Network
Section of Orthopaedic Surgery and Rehabilitation
Medicine
Ptitzker School of Medicine, The University of
Chicago
The University of Chicago Hospitals
Chicago, Illinois
Chapter 16

Mark J. Goddard, M.D.
University of Cincinnati
Cincinnati, Ohio
Chapter 21

Larry Bruce Goldstein, M.D.
Center for Health Policy Research and Education
Duke University
Durham Department of Veterans Affairs Medical
Center
Durham, North Carolina
Chapter 32

David C. Good, M.D.
Department of Neurology
Bowman Gray School of Medicine
Wake Forest University
Winston-Salem, North Carolina
Chapter 2

Jason P. Greenberg, M.D.
Department of Neurology
Bowman Gray School of Medicine
Wake Forest University
Winston-Salem, North Carolina
Chapter 2

Linda S. Greene-Finestone, M.Sc., R.D.
Department of Clinical Nutrition
London Health Sciences Centre
University Campus
University of Western Ontario
London, Ontario, Canada
Chapter 24

Chris Halpin, Ph.D.
Massachusetts Eye and Ear Infirmary
Harvard Medical School
Boston, Massachusetts
Chapter 38

Susan J. Herdman, Ph.D., P.T.
Department of Otolaryngology
University of Miami, School of Medicine
Miami, Florida
Chapter 17

Andrew Hornstein, M.D.
Department of Psychiatry
Helen Hayes Hospital, New York
College of Physicians and Surgeons
Columbia University
New York, New York
Chapter 34

Susan Iannaccone, M.D.
University of Texas Southwestern Medical School
Texas Scottish Rite Hospital for Children
Dallas, Texas
Chapter 11

Robert J. Jaeger
Pritzker Institute of Medical Engineering
Illinois Institute of Technology
Chicago, Illinois
Chapter 36

D. Casey Kerrigan, M.D., M.S.
Harvard Medical School
Division of Physical Medicine and Rehabilitation
Spaulding Rehabilitation Hospital
Boston, Massachusetts
Chapter 5

R. Lee Kirby, M.D., F.R.C.P.C.
Division of Physical Medicine and Rehabilitation
Dalhousie University
Halifax, Nova Scotia, Canada
Chapter 27

Maureen Lacy
Department of Psychiatry
Pritzker School of Medicine
The University of Chicago
The University of Chicago Hospitals
Chicago, Illinois
Chapter 33

Joanne P. Lasker
University of Nebraska
Lincoln, Nebraska
Chapter 28

Richard B. Lazar, M.D.
Schwab Rehabilitation Hospital and Care Network
Department of Surgery
Section of Orthopaedic Surgery and Rehabilitation
Medicine
Department of Neurology
Pritzker School of Medicine, The University of
Chicago
The University of Chicago Hospitals
Chicago, Illinois
Chapter 1

Michael Y. Lee, M.D.
Department of Physical Medicine and Rehabilitation
School of Medicine
University of North Carolina at Chapel Hill
Chapel Hill, North Carolina
Chapter 15

Christine E. Lee, M.D.
University of North Carolina at Chapel Hill
Chapel Hill, North Carolina
Chapter 15

Michael P. McQuillen, M.D., M.A.
Department of Neurology
University of Rochester School of Medicine and
Dentistry
Department of Medicine, Neurology
St. Mary's Hospital
Rochester, New York
Chapter 3

Mark Mennemeier, Ph.D.
Department of Rehabilitation Medicine
University of Alabama at Birmingham
Birmingham, Alabama
Chapter 35

John W. Michael, M.Ed., C.P.O.
Otto Bock
Rochester, Minnesota
Chapter 13

Maureen R. Nelson, M.D.
Baylor College of Medicine
Texas Children's Hospital
Houston, Texas
Chapter 15

John A. Orsini, M.D.
St. Mary's Hospital
Rochester, New York
Chapter 12

Jack H. Petajan, M.D., Ph.D.
School of Medicine, University of Utah
Salt Lake City, Utah
Chapter 23

Michael M. Pfeffer
Cornell University Medical College
Burke Rehabilitation Center
White Plains, New York
Chapter 8

Neil H. Pliskin, Ph.D.
Department of Psychiatry
Pritzker School of Medicine
The University of Chicago
The University of Chicago Hospitals
Chicago, Illinois
Chapter 33

Jochen Quintern, M.D.
Neural Prostheses and Motor Control Laboratory
Neurological Clinic, Klinikum Grosshadern
Department of Neurology
Klinikum Grosshadern
Ludwig-Maximilians University
Munich, Germany
Chapter 36

Michael Reding, M.D.
Cornell University Medical College
Burke Rehabilitation Center
White Plains, New York
Chapter 8

Steven I. Reger, Ph.D.
Department of Physical Medicine and Rehabilitation
The Cleveland Clinic Foundation
Cleveland, Ohio
Chapter 10

Melissa D. Reigle, M.D.
Department of Urology
Case Western Reserve University
Cleveland VA Medical Center
University Hospitals of Cleveland
Cleveland, Ohio
Chapter 25

Vinod Sahgal, M.D.
Department of Physical Medicine and Rehabilitation
The Cleveland Clinic Foundation
Cleveland, Ohio
Chapter 10

Allen D. Seftel, M.D.
Department of Urology
Case Western Reserve University
Cleveland VA Medical Center
University Hospitals of Cleveland
Cleveland, Ohio
Chapter 25

Glenn M. Seliger, M.D.
Department of Neurology
Helen Hayes Hospital, New York
College of Physicians and Surgeons
Columbia University
New York, New York
Chapter 34

Michael E. Selzer, M.D., Ph.D.
Department of Rehabilitation
University of Pennsylvania
Philadelphia, Pennsylvania
Chapter 4

Lynne R. Sheffler, M.D.
Harvard Medical School Department of Physical
Medicine and Rehabilitation
Boston, Massachusetts
Chapter 5

Steven L. Small, M.D.
Department of Neurology
University of Pittsburgh
Philadelphia, Pennsylvania
Chapter 30

Charles R. Smith, M.D.
Medical Rehabilitation Research and Training Center
for Multiple Sclerosis
St. Agnes Hospital
White Plains, New York
Bronx Lebanon Hospital Center
Bronx, New York
Chapter 22

Robin Soffer
Cornell University Medical College
Burke Rehabilitation Hospital
White Plains, New York
Chapter 26

Edythe A. Strand, Ph.D.
Speech and Hearing Sciences
University of Washington
Seattle, Washington
Chapter 37

Guillermo Suarez, M.D.
Mayo Clinic
Rochester, Minnesota
Chapter 13

Sevgi Tetik, M.D.
Department of Physical Medicine
and Rehabilitation
Ankara Hospital
Ankara, Turkey
Chapter 10

Krista Vandeborne, Ph.D.
University of Pennsylvania
Philadelphia, Pennsylvania
Chapter 19

David J. Weiss, M.D.
Schwab Rehabilitation Hospital and Care Network
Section of Orthopaedic Surgery and Rehabilitation
Medicine
Pritzker School of Medicine, The University of
Chicago
The University of Chicago Hospitals
Chicago, Illinois
Chapter 16

F. Todd Wetzel, M.D.
Department of Surgery
Section of Orthopaedic Surgery and
Rehabilitation, and
Anesthesia and Critical Care
Pritzker School of Medicine, University of
Chicago
University of Chicago Hospitals Spine Center
Chicago, Illinois
Chapter 14

Katherine C. Wood
Department of Psychiatry
The University of Chicago
Chicago, Illinois
Chapter 33

Gary M. Yarkony, M.D.

Schwab Rehabilitation Hospital and Care Network
Department of Surgery
Section of Orthopaedic Surgery and Rehabilitation
Medicine
Pritzker School of Medicine
University of Chicago Medical Center
The University of Chicago Hospitals
Chicago, Illinois
Chapters 9, 21

Kathryn M. Yorkston, Ph.D.

Department of Rehabilitation Medicine
University of Washington
Seattle, Washington
Chapter 37

Robert R. Young, M.D.

Department of Neurology
University of California
Irvine, California
Chapter 20

Richard D. Zorowitz, M.D.

UMDNJ–N.J. Medical School
Kessler Institute for Rehabilitation
East Orange, New Jersey
Chapter 29

PREFACE

This text offers a comprehensive discussion of the reha-bilitation of neurologic disease. As editor, I have tried to assemble a set of chapters that represent evidenced-based analysis. As the fields of neuroscience and rehabil-itation continue to expand, the rehabilitation physician will need to refer to more than descriptive discourse in therapeutic decision making. Whenever possible, the rehabilitative approach to the neurologic patient must be based upon principles. The more we know about how the nervous system functions, the more we will know about how to optimize the function of the people we treat.

The quality of information that the authors of this text present is a reflection on neurologic rehabilitation itself. This book is no more and, we hope, no less than a microcosm of our specialty. Weaknesses in evidence-based discussion represent opportunities for investi-gation.

The book is organized into four sections. The first discusses general concepts important to the field of neurologic rehabilitation as a whole. The second part focuses on the rehabilitation of specific neurologic dis-eases. In the third section, we turn to the management of conditions commonly associated with or caused by chronic neurologic dysfunction. Finally, we consider specific therapeutic interventions that have been applied to the rehabilitation of neurologic diseases.

I hope that rehabilitation physicians, residents, and medical students who consult this text will consider it critically. Its real measure of success will be the quality of inquiries the book generates from those who have the ability to ask and answer their own questions.

For helping to complete this endeavor, I especially want to acknowledge my wife Susan, who created space and time for me to work. I owe a special mention of appreciation to Yana Spedale, the master organizer of this project. Finally, well-deserved praise must go to my friends at Schwab Rehabilitation Hospital, including Kathleen C. Yosko, Jo-Ann C. Gruber, Jonathan L. Costa, M.D., Ph.D., Michelle S. Gittler, M.D., Rakesh R. Patel, D.O., Gayle R. Spill, M.D., David J. Weiss, M.D., and Gary M. Yarkony, M.D., all of whom under-stood the importance of this project and created the supportive work environment that allowed it to be suc-cessfully completed.

PRINCIPLES OF NEUROLOGIC REHABILITATION

Part I
GENERAL CONCEPTS

Chapter 1

INTRODUCTION

Richard B. Lazar

A book about principles must, by nature, speak to foundations and cornerstones. Perhaps it is nothing more than the good in all of us that has allowed the process of rehabilitation to become more developed and refined than our understanding of the pathophysiologic principles of recovery. The process of rehabilitation has very few principles. Rehabilitation is a way of approaching the very real, practical, and, in some ways, crucial issues of quality of life. It is team-focused, highly dependent on effective communication skills and leadership, and requires participation of patients and families in nearly every aspect of decision making.

Because it is a process, rehabilitation in and of itself has no diseases of its own. Neurologic rehabilitation is the application of principles of disease to this process in order to restore function. Restoration of function without process and principles of disease has only limited possibilities.

Being kind, empathic advocates for those we serve is simply no longer enough. It is essential that we look closely at principles of disease and wed them to the process of rehabilitation irrevocably. Our social structure and resources will no longer permit us to randomly apply the rehabilitation process to any disease we choose. Trial-and-error rehabilitation will face extinction. Interdisciplinary rehabilitation is too costly to recommend based on intuition alone. We will need to know whom to choose, when, why, and what we plan to offer.

The scientific principles set forth in this volume offer new hope for the neurologically impaired. They begin to add substance and predictability to promise. The most compelling areas for future investigation in neurologic rehabilitation have been set forth recently by Selzer (Table 1-1).[1]

There is reason to be hopeful that anecdotes in neurorehabilitation science will be replaced by hypothe-sis-testing scientific research.[2] This has become increasingly evident in the last decade of the 20th century. An internet query of the National Library of Medicine under "neurologic rehabilitation" and "neurorehabilitation" revealed explosive growth in the past 3 years alone, with science citations during those 3 years exceeding the three previous decades combined, beginning in 1966 (Table 1-2).

The end of the 20th century promises to introduce exciting new technology into the field of neurorehabilitation. A wide range of structural techniques now exist to assess the human brain in health and disease.[3] A sampling of imaging and physiologic technology used for in-vivo study of brain structure and functions is presented in Table 1-3.

Nuclear magnetic resonance imaging promises to revolutionize rehabilitation in a way that will be no less dramatic than what Darwinian theory did for our understanding of evolution and genetics, or histochemistry did for the pathologic basis of disease. This technology is already available in the United States and is widely disseminated throughout the country. By simple, noninvasive imaging, we will be able to detect unique molecular tissue signatures for brain tissue; this has the potential to make the study of anatomic pathology virtually obsolete.

Important scientific insights into the mechanism of secondary neuronal damage are catapulting our capacity to reduce the impact of primary-tissue injury from ischemia and trauma.[4] We now stand ready to understand how the brain destroys itself after it is deprived of critical nutrients and fuel. Only after we fully understand this can we reverse the process of cell death.

More attention must be given to the delivery of rehabilitation care itself. Outcome studies have been encumbered by poor-quality research designs and attri-

Table 1-1

Current and future pathways for enhancing the scientific basis for neurologic rehabilitation

Regeneration of the nervous system

Adaptive mechanisms following nervous-system injury

Computational neural science

Neuromuscular physiology

Neuropharmacology of recovery

Biologic mechanisms for physical retraining

Table 1-3

New technology for in-vivo study of brain structure and function

Positron emission tomography

Single photon emission computed tomography

Magnetic resonance imaging

Computed tomography

Electroencephalography

Magnetoencephalography

Transcranial magnetic stimulation

Intrinsic signal imaging

Electrocorticography

bution bias by therapists.[5] New tools for the assessment of handicap and disability are taking on increasing importance.[6,7] Evaluation of the validity and reliability of outcome measures has also received critical attention.[8] Without clinometric rigor, the effectiveness of specific interventions has been difficult to ascertain.[9]

There is a crucial need to determine the effectiveness of rehabilitation beyond that expected with spontaneous recovery. The optimum duration and intensity of rehabilitation care is a matter of great debate.[10] Furthermore, little is known about the nature of recovery that occurs after the completion of a rehabilitation program.[11] The application of outcome measures must be

Table 1-2

Scientific citations retrieved from the National Library of Medicine[a]

Medline years	Citations retrieved
1966–1974	1
1975–1979	0
1980–1984	2
1985–1989	6
1990–1992	11
1993–1996	29

[a] Through a query using the key words "neurologic rehabilitation" and "neurorehabilitation," 1966–1996—http://igm.nlm.nih.gov (U.S. National Library of Medicine, Bethesda, MD, 1996).

extended to assess the long-term sustaining of goals achieved through the rehabilitation process.[12] The application of critical pathways will be important in creating efficiency in the delivery of comprehensive rehabilitative care.[13]

The natural inclination to conserve health-care resources begs us to try to select carefully those who are likely to benefit from rehabilitative measures. This goal has remained elusive in many forms of rehabilitative care.[14] Substantial efforts are under way to correlate specific neuropathologic diagnoses to functional outcome and patient selection criteria.[15] Rehabilitation interventions are becoming increasingly targeted to specific neurologic deficits.[16] The role of drugs in the enhancement of specific aspects of functional recovery has commanded increasing attention.[17,18]

No doubt, some of the improvements in medical rehabilitation outcomes today represent improvements in general medical care. Surgical treatments required for supportive care are being developed rapidly, and with less risk to the patient.[19] Medical and neurological complications that occur in the rehabilitation setting are no longer legion.[20,21]

Whatever form the rehabilitation process takes, neurorehabilitation requires an understanding of diseases of the nervous system. Continual refining of the process of rehabilitation cannot continue without attention to disease. Right now, we are limited to the most humane of all human endeavors; we provide empathy, support, and patient and family education. Also we provide better general medical care. Just as it is not possible to provide electricity without first understanding the principles of current flow, so rehabilitation specialists are not able to foster functional recovery in the nervous system without bedrock knowledge of the biologic basis of injury and repair. This is our goal.

REFERENCES

1. Selzer ME: Neurological rehabilitation. *Ann Neurol* 1992; 32:695–699.

2. Selzer ME: Neuroscience and neurorehabilitation. *Curr Opin Neurol* 1994; 7(6):510–516.

3. Mazziotta JC: Mapping human brain activity in vivo. *West J Med* 1994; 161(3):273–278.

4. Miller JD: Minor, moderate and severe head injury. *Neurosurg Rev* 1986; 9(1–2):135–139.

5. Macciocchi SN, Eaton B: Decision and attribution bias in neurorehabilitation. *Arch Phys Med Rehab* 1995; 76(6):521–524.

6. Stewart G, Kidd D, Thompson AJ: The assessment of handicap: An evaluation of the Environmental Status Scale. *Disabil Rehab* 1995; 17(6):312–316.

7. Riedmann G, Barolin GS: Evaluation and quality assurance in neurorehabilitation. *Rehabilitation* (Stuttg) 1995; 34(1):28–34.

8. Kidd D, Stewart G, Baldry J, Johnson J, Rossiter D, Petruckevitch A, Thompson AJ: The Functional Independence measure: A comparative validity and reliability study. *Disabil Rehab* 1995; 17(1):10–14.

9. Ottenbacher KJ, Jannell S: The results of clinical trials in stroke rehabilitation research. *Arch Neurol* 1993; 50:37–44.

10. Ernst E: A review of stroke rehabilitation and physiotherapy. *Stroke* 1990; 21:1081–1085.

11. Ferrucci L, et al: Recovery of functional status after stroke: A postrehabilitation followup study. *Stroke* 1993; 24:200–250.

12. Bulau P, Fuger J, Horn H: Validating rehabilitation after stroke. *Nervenartz* 1994; 65(12):836–840.

13. Rossiter D, Thompson, AJ: Introduction of integrated care pathways for patients with multiple sclerosis in an inpatient neurorehabilitation setting. *Disabil Rehab* 1995; 17(8): 443–448.

14. Loewen SC, Anderson BA: Predictors of stroke outcome using measurement scales. *Stroke* 1990; 21:78–81.

15. Katz DI, Alexander MP: Traumatic brain injury: Predicting course of recovery and outcome for patients admitted to rehabilitation. *Arch Neurol* 1994; 51(7):661–670.

16. Hanlon RE, Dobkin BH, Hadler B, Ramirez S, Cheska Y: Neurorehabilitation following right thalamic infarct: Effects of cognitive retraining on functional performance. *J Clin Exp Neuropsychol* 1992; 14(4):433–447.

17. Small SL: Pharmacotherapy of aphasia: A critical review. *Stroke* 1994; 25:1282–1289.

18. Hassid EI: Neuropharmacological therapy and motor recovery after stroke. *Mil Med* 1995; 160(5):223–226.

19. Moore FA, Haenel JB, Moore EE, Read RA: Percutaneous tracheostomy/gastrostomy in brain-injured patients: A minimally invasive alternative. *J Trauma* 1992; 33(3):435–439.

20. Dromerick A, Reding M: Medical and neurological complications during inpatient stroke rehabilitation. *Stroke* 1994; 25:358–361.

21. Kalra L, et al: Medical complications during stroke rehabilitation. *Stroke* 1995; 26:990–994.

Chapter 2

FUNCTIONAL ASSESSMENT IN NEUROLOGIC DISABILITY

Jason P. Greenberg
David C. Good

Rehabilitation physicians, therapists, and nurses are arguably the preeminent assessors of impairment, functional limitations, quality of life, and independence. A carefully selected, scientifically designed measure of function is essential for delineating progress and therapeutic benefits of a rehabilitation program. Such a measure is important for generalizing experience, making comparisons across therapies and scientifically validating results. Reproducible, validated measuring instruments are essential to the evidence-based medicine movement. Reliable, standardized testing instruments are required to provide clear data regarding patients' functional gains and the cost-effectiveness of treatment.

The most fundamental applications of outcome assessment in rehabilitation focus on the individual patient by establishing a baseline clinical description, setting goals, and monitoring the success of interventions. However, outcome measures also have broader applications in rehabilitation medicine, including allocating health care resources, assessing the efficacy of treatment, and determining programmatic quality.

A variety of outcome measures are useful in routine clinical care and research in rehabilitation. These range from easily defined outcomes such as survival or improvement in a specific aspect of neurological impairment (such as strength in an affected extremity), to complex outcomes related to handicap or quality of life. Complex outcomes are more difficult to measure, less medically oriented, and often dependent on multiple independent variables. For example, the assessment of quality of life is multidimensional and depends on functional abilities, general physical health, financial security, and a stable social and family environment. Improvement in one variable may not influence overall well-being if other key variables are not addressed. For example, despite recovering the ability to provide self-care, a stroke patient can be incapacitated by major depression, and hence have a poor quality of life.

SELECTING A MEASURE

Dimensions: Impairment-Disability-Handicap

In selecting a measure, one must first identify the functional attribute of interest. A global outcome measure may be less useful than an assessment of partial function. For example, in treating depression, one is likely to see more change in measures of depressive symptoms than in the ability to perform activities of daily living (ADLs). It is important to select a primary outcome measure closely related to the intervention in question.

When selecting a construct to measure, the World Health Organization's paradigm of impairment, disability, and handicap is particularly useful.[1] Under this rubric, impairment is considered a "loss or abnormality of psychological, physiological, or anatomical structure or function." Disability is the effect of the impairment on one's ability to perform routine activities. Handicap is "a disadvantage . . . resulting from an impairment or a disability, that limits or prevents the fulfillment of a role that is normal (depending on age, sex and social and cultural factors) for the individual." Thus, an amputation or hemiparesis might be one's impairment, and the resulting disability in walking might prevent one from returning to work, thus constituting a handicap. Handicap is highly dependent on expectation, so that a handicap in one society might not be a handicap in another. What would handicap a truck driver might not handicap a physical therapist. Measurements of activities of daily living typically are judged to represent disability. Some have argued that handicap is impossible to measure, but measurements of "extended" or "instrumental" ADLs bridge the gap between disability and handicap, and measurements of health-related quality of life may shed some light on handicap as well.

Impairment measures may be generalizable, such as the Glasgow Coma Scale (GCS), the Fugl-Meyer measure of hemiparesis, or the Galveston Orientation and Amnesia Test, or specific, such as the National Institutes of Health Stroke Scale. Specific scales typically have been developed for a particular disease or for a particular impairment, and they may be inadequate when used for other purposes. In contrast, although the GCS was designed for use in patients with traumatic head injury, it has been successfully used for patients with a variety of other disorders.

Purpose of Comparison

Once the appropriate construct to be measured is chosen, one should consider the purpose of measurement. If the measure is to be used for diagnosis, it is important that it evaluate aspects of the patient that are directly related to the diagnosis in question and the alternatives, and within-subject variation across repeated assessments should be as small as possible and stable. In order to monitor the progress of a patient or a group of patients, the measure should provide reproducible results over time, but also a sufficiently wide range of values with enough sensitivity to detect clinically meaningful differences. Some measures with sensitivity to differences in function may be good for following the progress of a disease but inadequate for diagnosing it. The qualities that make measures useful for diagnosis, prognosis, and evaluation of progress may differ significantly.

Validity

Validity is how well an instrument measures what it purports to measure. Ideally, validity is assessed by comparison to a "gold standard"—this is called "criterion validity." Clinical assessments are often assumed to be valid standards for criterion validity, but upon close inspection commonly used clinical measures often fall short. Unfortunately, validity often must be inferred by indirect evidence. For example, "content validity" represents how completely the instrument covers the range required for measuring the construct in question in a given population. An instrument designed to assess disability in patients with traumatic brain injury would cover a significantly different set of behaviors than an instrument measuring disability in patients with amyotrophic lateral sclerosis. Content validity is often determined by convening a group of experts to define the required scope of the questions for an instrument being developed.

One can test "construct validity" by examining how a measure behaves in regard to the theoretical properties of the construct being measured. Thus, to have good construct validity, a measure should not correlate well with different but related constructs (e.g., an impairment measure should be independent from measures of disability) but should correlate with similar but related constructs (e.g., a measure of gait reasonably might be required to correlate with measures of truncal ataxia). A measure's ability to distinguish between two groups that are known to differ on the construct in question (or who are known to differ on a construct closely related to the one in question) is also an indicator of construct validity.

There are two other types of validity in common use. "Face validity" refers to a primae faciae assessment of the instrument's sensibility. On simple inspection, does it appear to be relevant to the construct to which it claims to relate? "Ecological validity" refers to the relevance of a measure to real-life situations. For example, a measure of attention that is highly reliable and has high content validity and good construct validity when administered in a controlled environment might poorly reflect a subject's attentional abilities in a crowded room. Similarly, the ability to perform a highly structured attentional task may not generalize to the ability to adequately attend in a more natural setting, such as when driving a car.

Reliability

Reliability refers to reproducibility. The value obtained when using a measure represents the sum of the value derived from the underlying state of the construct being measured (the "true" score) and some error introduced by the measurement. A reliable instrument minimizes error, and it will provide the same result for the same underlying state regardless of who does the measurement, when or where it is done, or in which patient. "Inter-rater" reliability is measured when two or more people use the same measure on the same subjects. "Test-retest" reliability is measured when a test is repeated over time by the same examiner. Internal consistency, the correlation between the individual items comprising an instrument, is also an indicator of reliability.

If the items do not covary sufficiently, they may be pointing at different constructs. An instrument with poor internal consistency may not adequately reflect the true state of the construct or may be insufficiently sensitive to change.

Scale and Statistical Considerations

Instruments differ in their scales. Nominal scales simply classify the construct (e.g., the presence or absence of a disease, or different colors of hair). Ordinal scales add hierarchy (e.g., cancer grading schemes, or requiring maximal, moderate, or minimal assistance for ambulation). Interval scales are ordinal scales in which the difference between adjacent levels is constant. Thus, a scale summing scores from a variety of tasks (such as the Barthel Index) typically is ordinal, but commonly used temperature scales are interval. A ratio scale is an interval scale with a meaningful, absolute zero point, such as the time required to complete a task. In ratio scales, the arithmetic ratios between two values makes sense. Completing a task in 10 seconds is twice as fast as completing it in 20 seconds. Interval scales may be subjected to parametric statistics, but ordinal or nominal scales may not (even if the ordinal scale is expressed in a number ranging from 0 to 100). The difference between scores of 20 and 21 on an ordinal scale is not necessarily less than the difference between scores of 30 and 35. Some instrument scores have been derived by adding scores from individual items. If the items measure the same construct, this is valid. The appropriate use of ordinal scales is reviewed elsewhere.[2,3]

Range

The range of possible values on a scale must be adequate to express clinically relevant differences, but not so great as to lose meaning. For example, the Functional Independence Measure uses seven levels for each item measured, ranging from complete independence to complete dependence on assistance to perform an activity. These levels are easily distinguished by most therapists, indicating that they probably represent meaningful differences. Three levels would probably be insufficiently discriminative; 40 levels would provide much more sensitivity, but the differences between levels would become much less clear. Scoring systems can be devised to artificially inflate an instrument's range. The Barthel may be scored from 0 to 20 in 1-point increments or from 0 to 100 in 5-point increments. Either way, there are only 21 levels possible.

Floor/Ceiling Effects

Some instruments lose their discriminative abilities at the extremes. For example, a patient with a significant level of disability might achieve a perfect Barthel score (so-called "ceiling" effect), and there might be important differences between two patients who obtain Barthels of 0 (a "floor" effect). The Barthel is still useful in rehabilitation, however, because it adequately measures disability from the point at which one starts to need assistance in ADLs to when one is completely dependent.

Norms

For some purposes, it is important to have relevant normative data, and the presence and quality of such data may be an important factor in one's choice of an outcome measure. For example, it may be difficult to make conclusions about the effect of stroke on quality of life without referring to the distribution that quality of life measure produces for an age- and sex-matched normal population.

Sensitivity, Specificity, and Predictive Value

These statistics are of concern only for predictive measures, whether they predict future behavior or the presence or absence of a quality that can be measured some other way. Sensitivity refers to the probability that someone who actually has the construct to be predicted (e.g., a certain disease) will be classified appropriately by a given measure; that is, it is a measure's true positive rate. Specificity is the probability that an individual not having the construct is correctly classified; that is, it is the true negative rate. Screening tests generally have high sensitivity, but may lack specificity in comparison with "gold standard" diagnostic tests. The positive predictive value (PPV) is the probability that an individual classified as "positive" (or as having the construct to be predicted) actually is positive; the negative predictive value (NPV) is the probability that someone with a "negative" measure is correctly classified. The PPV and NPV depend on the sensitivity, specificity, and prevalence of the construct.

Sensitivity and specificity should in fact be considered attributes of test thresholds rather than of tests. For example, one could use the Barthel Index to predict whether patients with stroke are discharged to home or to a nursing home. Each possible value of the Index may be used as a cutoff, above which one predicts home discharge and below which one expects institutionaliza-

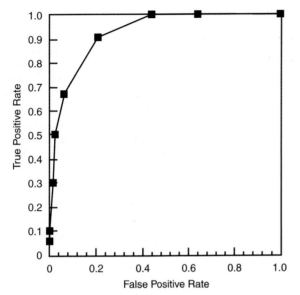

Figure 2-1
Receiver Operating Characteristic Curve. The closer the curve comes to the upper left-hand corner, the greater the area under the curve and the greater the discriminative power. Each point represents a threshold for declaring a "positive" test.

tion. The sensitivity decreases and the specificity increases as the threshold value increases. A graph of the sensitivity (which is the true positive rate) on the y axis versus 1-specificity (which is the false positive rate) on the x axis is called a Receiver Operating Characteristic (ROC) curve. The better the test, the closer the curve comes to the upper left-hand corner (1-specificity = 0, sensitivity = 1), and the larger the area under the curve (see Figure 2-1). ROC curves may be used to select test thresholds depending on the relative needs of sensitivity and specificity. One might be willing to use a threshold with lower specificity in a situation where missing a "positive" individual would be tragic (e.g., predicting who will develop pulmonary embolism) and in which more specific confirmatory tests are available than one would in a situation where one wants to be selective (e.g., screening patients for a drug trial).

Practical Considerations

Practical considerations are equally important. How much training does one need to administer a measure? How much time does it take? Are there cultural or language barriers that pose limitations? How difficult is it to tabulate? How much trouble is it for the respondent? The higher the burden, the less likely one is to get the necessary data.

A good instrument should also be readily interpreted by the intended audience. For this reason, new treatments for multiple sclerosis are often investigated using the widely used Kurtzke Expanded Disability Status Scale (EDSS), in spite of concerns about poor face validity. Including a second measure with better face validity can be useful, but omitting the EDSS would limit the audience's understanding of the results.

Selecting a Measure: An Example

Application of these principles allows us to consider the selection of an optimum measure of ADL functions. There is no agreement on the existence of a widely accepted tool designed to assess ADL status. Literally hundreds of ADL measures exist.[4-7] Of these, the best tested and most widely used are the Barthel Index, the Katz Index of ADL, and the Kenney Self-Care evaluation. Careful consideration should be given to the face validity of each of these. Comprehensiveness and relevance must be carefully assessed. The scope of these three measures is summarized in Table 2-1.

Right from the start, one's choice of an ADL measure depends in part on one's philosophy. If continence is an important ADL goal, using the Kenney scale is clearly advantageous. Grooming skills, on the other hand, are given no consideration by the Katz scale.

The makeup of the study population also is important to consider. The Barthel Index, originally developed to assess function after spinal cord injury, may be less applicable to patients with stroke, in whom aphasia and dementia are prevalent.

Table 2-1
Dimensions of three measures of activities of daily living

Measure	Dressing	Ambulation	Bathing	Feeding	Transfer	Toileting	Grooming	Wheelchair use	Stair climbing	Continence	Bed activities
Katz	+	+	+	+	+	+				+	
Barthel	+	+	+	+	+	+	+	+	+	+	+
Kenney	+	+	+	+	+	+	+	+	+		+

The temptation to develop a new scale is ever-present and should be discouraged. Scale validation and assessment of reliability is time-consuming, and therefore, often overlooked. Using an existing, validated scale, however imperfect, may more clearly define the construct of interest within the boundaries of sound methodological principles.

IMPAIRMENT

Although clinical care focuses on disability and handicap, measures of impairment are equally important in understanding rehabilitation progress. Impairment measures vary widely in simplicity and utility, and should be applicable over a wide range of underlying diseases.

Cognitive Impairment

Cognitive function may be assessed by a myriad of tools. (See Chapter 33 for an in-depth review.) A brief screen for dementia can be obtained using the Folstein Mini-Mental Status Examination (MMSE), which is easily measured at bedside or in the clinic.[8] A score of 24 (out of 30 total) is used to distinguish normal from abnormal. Other simple screens for global cognitive dysfunction are described by Wade.[6]

The Neurobehavioral Cognitive Status Examination is more sensitive than the MMSE, and scores have been shown to correlate with outcome after stroke rehabilitation, as measured by the Barthel Index.[9,10] The Wechsler Adult Intelligence Scale-Revised is often used for a global cognitive assessment by neuropsychologists.[11] Specific scales assess memory, attention, executive functions, and language. These are often used in combination to provide a general survey of the cognitive strengths and weaknesses of neurorehabilitation patients.

For speech and language impairment, the most commonly used instruments are the Boston Diagnostic Aphasia Examination (BDAE), the Porch Index of Communicative Ability (PICA), and the Western Aphasia Battery (WAB).[12-14] The BDAE and WAB take hours to administer, whereas the PICA is more expeditious.

In occasional patients, more detailed, formal neuropsychological testing is useful. Testing may provide clues regarding cognitive strengths and weakness that can alter rehabilitation strategies. In other cases, neuropsychological testing may be useful in determining competency or guiding important decisions, such as returning to work or home. Guidelines for selecting patients for neuropsychological testing have been published and are considered elsewhere in this text.[15,16]

Motor

The most widely used scale of motor impairment is the British Medical Council's scale, which grades muscle power on confrontational clinical testing from 0 to 5.[17] This scale is least sensitive to change at 4, because 4 encompasses all movement that is greater than barely overcoming gravity and less than normal. Grip strength using a dynamometer or the maximal weight that can be lifted on a specified exercise machine have also been used as more quantitative measures of motor impairment. Sophisticated dynamometers can feed information to computers that provide reliable measures of torque, work, and fatigability.

The Fugl-Meyer Scale is a well-validated comprehensive evaluation of motor function in hemiparesis, and includes sections to evaluate upper extremity function, lower extremity function, balance, sensation, and range of motion.[18] Each section may be used separately, or the subscales of all sections summed to give a maximum score of 226. Although the Fugl-Meyer Scale has been widely used as a research assessment tool, it has not achieved widespread clinical usage, since it requires 20 to 30 minutes by a skilled therapist to administer. The Motor Assessment Scale (MAS) also samples a variety of motor activities, and requires half the time as the Fugl-Meyer Scale to administer.[19] Although the MAS is a valid measure of motor function in hemiparesis, the Fugl-Meyer Scale can better discriminate the level of motor recovery in the early stage of recovery or in more disabled subjects.[19]

Spasticity quantification is another common concern of rehabilitation professionals. Although most rehabilitation physicians and therapists easily recognize spasticity, formal measurement is more problematic. The modified Ashworth scale is the only spasticity scale that has been formally evaluated, and shown to be reliable.[20,21] It is widely used, occasionally in conjunction with more technical measurements, such as simultaneous electromyography of agonist and antagonist muscles.

DISABILITY

Rehabilitation goals are primarily focused on disability and handicap, both of which are only partially explained by impairment. This clinometric distinction can be important. For example, a patient with severe neurological impairment can be completely independent in self-care and actively participate in community activities and vocational rehabilitation. Because early treatment focuses on functional activities related to activities of daily living, scales that measure disability have gained widespread popularity in rehabilitation.

Measures of activities of daily living address disability. The Barthel Index (BI) and Functional Independence Measure (FIM) are the most commonly used ADL assessment tools in the United States, and cover a wide range of abilities related to self-care and mobility.[4] The Patient Evaluation Conference System (PECS) may offer sensitivity to change that is superior to that of the FIM while measuring the same underlying construct.[22,23] Furthermore, Rasch analysis allows the PECS and FIM scales to be similarly scaled, so that values from the two systems can be compared.

Barthel (BI)

The gold standard of ADL measurements is the BI, a weighted scale of ten different activities assessing mobility and self-care ability.[24] It can be scored 0–20, or each point can be multiplied by five to yield a 100-point scale (Table 2-2). Changes in score occur in rather predictable patterns. That is, a transition from a score of 75 to 60 usually occurs by losing a similar group of abilities. The BI measures ADL function for those who require some assistance, and it has floor and, importantly, ceiling effects. Thus, a perfect BI score implies continence, independent feeding, bathing, grooming, and dressing, and the ability to transfer and walk independently and ascend and descend stairs. It does not measure personal decision making or safety without supervision.

The BI has limited sensitivity to change, in large part because it has only 21 levels. Nevertheless, it is widely used, valid, and reliable. It has good test-retest and inter-observer reliability, is considered reliable even when the activities are not observed directly, and information is obtained over the telephone.[25–28] The BI has been used to predict the extent of motor loss, mortality, depression, and need for community support in stroke patients.[26,29–31] Some investigators have demonstrated that the BI is superior to the Katz ADL Index and the Kenny Self-Care Evaluation in completeness, sensitivity to change, and ease of statistical manipulation in stroke patients.[32] In an effort to improve sensitivity, the BI has been modified to include five levels rather than three for each activity, and to cover 15 rather than 10 tasks.

Functional Independence Measure

The FIM was introduced in 1986 by the Task Force to Develop a Uniform Data System for Medical Rehabilitation (UDSMR™).[33] It expands the Barthel Index by incorporating additional measures of cognitive and communication skills and social integration and by increasing the number of performance levels for each activity to 7 (see Figure 2-2). This makes the FIM more sensitive to small changes in function than the BI. It has achieved widespread use in the United States in part because it is an integral part of the UDSMR™, which provides training and support materials to subscribing institutions and periodic statistical updates on each institution in comparison to regional and national norms.[34] The total score (range, 18–126 points) is the sum of the individual categories that represent an estimate of overall ability to perform activities of daily living. Rasch analysis indicates the FIM measures two domains, "motor" and "cognitive."[35] Its reliability and validity have been extensively tested.[35,36] There is good agreement between telephone interview and in-person assessment.[37] FIM score on admission to a rehabilitation unit is a good predictor of function at discharge for a wide variety of neurological impairments, and can be used to predict burden of care at home for patients with stroke or multiple sclerosis.[38–40] It does have both ceiling and floor effects, and it does not consider whether the scored ability to perform a task independently translates into a practical benefit (e.g., one may be independent in climbing stairs, but so slow or exhausted afterward that the skill is of no practical importance). The cognitive assessments in particular have important floor and ceiling limitations, and some important functions, such as safety in chewing and swallowing, are not addressed at all.

FIM scores also have been applied for cost-effectiveness and resource allocation analysis. Comparison of mean change in FIM score per hospital day with that of regional and national norms through the UDSMR has been used to establish the efficiency of rehabilitative gains.[41,42] Recently, "Functional Related Groups," based on FIM data, have been proposed to determine reimbursement rates for inpatient rehabilitation.[43,44]

Other ADL Scales

The Katz ADL Index was widely used prior to the introduction of the Barthel.[45] It does not include ambulation, but does rate six activities of daily living. The scoring system is ordinal (a point emphasized by a letter

Table 2-2
The Barthel Index of Activities of Daily Living

Bowels
    0 = Incontinent
    5 = Occasional accident (1×/week), or needs help with enema or suppository
    10 = Continent, able to use enema or suppository if needed

Bladder
    0 = Incontinent, or catheterized and unable to manage
    5 = Occasional accident (maximum 1 ×/24 h)
    10 = Continent (>7 days), or able to manage collecting device if used

Grooming
    0 = Needs help with personal care
    5 = Washes face, combs hair, brushes teeth

Toilet Use
    0 = Dependent
    5 = Needs help, but can do something alone
    10 = Independent (on and off, wiping, dressing)

Feeding
    0 = Unable
    5 = Needs help cutting, spreading butter, etc.
    10 = Independent if food provided

Chair/Bed Transfers
    0 = Completely bedridden, use of chair not possible
    5 = Able to sit, but needs major help (1–2 people) to transfer
    10 = Minor help (verbal or physical) to transfer
    15 = Independent, including locking wheelchair and lifting footrests

Mobility
    0 = Sits on wheelchair, but cannot propel it
    5 = Independent in wheelchair, including corners, etc., for 50 yards
    10 = Walks with help of one person (verbal or physical) for 50 yards
    15 = Independent, but may use any aid

Dressing
    0 = Dependent
    5 = Needs help, but can do about half unaided
    10 = Independent, including buttons, zippers, and laces

Stairs
    0 = Unable
    5 = Needs help (verbal, physical)
    10 = Independent up and down, but may use any aid

Bathing
    0 = Needs help
    5 = Independent (or in shower)

Total (0–100)
Interpretation of Score
    0–20 Very severely disabled
    25–45 Severely disabled
    50–70 Moderately disabled
    75–95 Mildly disabled
    100   Physically independent, but not necessarily normal or socially independent

---

rather than number-based score) and is based on the validated premise that ADLs are lost in a predictable, hierarchical order. The basis for scoring incorporates clinical data, input from the primary caregiver, and direct observation. As such, it is designed to measure independence rather than ability.

The Kenny Self-Care Evaluation rates performance ability in 17 different activities organized into six groups, each on a 0 to 4 scale, depending on the degree of assistance required. It has not been widely used, although it may offer more sensitivity than the Barthel at a cost of reliability.[46]

A number of scales have been designed to test disability in one specific function or body part, termed "focal" disability.[6] For example, timed walking tests are compellingly simple, valid, and reliable measures. The time required to walk a 6.1-meter track, for example, has been used as an outcome measure in a trial of exercise.[47]

Endurance (distance/unit time) has been shown to be more sensitive to change than speed of ambulation in patients undergoing rehabilitation for stroke.[48] The Rivermead Mobility Index (RMI) has been developed specifically to assess mobility. It measures the performance of such specific mobility tasks as turning in bed, managing stairs, and standing without aid for 10 seconds. The RMI has been validated in the stroke population.[49]

Clinometric assessment of upper extremity disability has been challenging. The arm section of some motor impairment scales (e.g., the Motricity Index or Fugl-Meyer) can be used to quantify voluntary motor control, and specific arm functions can be tested with simple measures of single skills. For example, the Nine-hole Peg Test measures the time required to place nine wooden dowels into holes drilled into a wooden base.[50] It is valid and reliable, and continues to be sensitive at high performance levels. There is some floor effect,

L E V E L S	7 Complete Independence (Timely, Safely) 6 Modified Dependence (Device)	No Helper

	Modified Dependence
	  5 Supervision
	  4 Minimal Assist (Subject = 75%+)
	  3 Moderate Assist (Subject = 50%+)
	Complete Dependence
	  2 Maximal Assist (Subject = 25%+)
	  1 Total Assist (Subject = 0%+)
		Helper

	Self-Care	Followup
A.	Eating	☐
B.	Grooming	☐
C.	Bathing	☐
D.	Dressing–Upper Body	☐
E.	Dressing–Lower Body	☐
F.	Toileting	☐
	Sphincter Control	
G.	Bladder Management	☐
H.	Bowl Management	☐
	Mobility	
	Transfer:	
I.	Bed, Chair, Wheelchair	☐
J.	Toilet	☐
K.	Tub, Shower	☐
	Locomotion	
L.	Walk/wheel Chair	ᵂ꜀☐
M.	Stairs	☐
	Communication	
N.	Comprehension	ᵃᵥ☐
O.	Expression	ᵛₙ☐
	Social Cognition	
P.	Social Interaction	☐
Q.	Problem Solving	☐
R.	Memory	☐
	Total FIM	☐
	(maximum 126)	

Note: Leave no blanks; enter 1 if patient not testable due to risk.

Figure 2-2
Functional Independence Measure (FIM). w = walk; c = wheelchair; for Comprehension, a = auditory, v = visual; for Expression, v = vocal, n = nonvocal.

however, and it is in part dependent on sensory loss, ataxia, and neglect. It is relatively insensitive to proximal arm dysfunction. Several batteries of arm skills, such as the Action Research Arm Test and the Frenchay Arm Test, now have been developed. The ARAT assesses strength and dexterity proximally and distally, but may be time-consuming in more disabled patients.[51] The Frenchay is simple, quicker, and focuses on proximal function.[52,53] Both are reliable, valid, and sensitive.

Most ADL assessment instruments are primarily designed for those who have an "intermediate" level of disability. ADL scales usually exhibit a ceiling effect, so that they are less useful at the "high end" of the scale. A "perfect" score on any ADL scale does not necessarily translate into normal neurological function, only independence in all self-care items included on the scale. Furthermore, scored independence in ADLs does not necessarily guarantee a satisfactory quality of life.

HANDICAP

It may be argued that handicap, which depends on an individual's expectations and aspirations, cannot be measured by a standardized instrument. Measures of instrumental activities of daily living and quality of life touch on some aspects of handicap, but no measure directly addresses this important construct.

Instrumental Activities of Daily Living

Instrumental activities of daily living (I-ADLs, or extended activities of daily living, E-ADLs) straddle the divide between disabilities and handicaps. I-ADLs cover activities that are more advanced requirements of social integration such as community mobility (automobile and public transport), domestic tasks (cooking, shopping, laundry, cleaning) financial management, and leisure activities (socializing, gardening, reading). I-ADLs require more cognitive ability than basic self-care skills, and there is evidence that this distinction between I-ADLs and ADLs is an important aspect of successful rehabilitation.[54] I-ADL scales are useful to highlight areas in which a person needs assistance and determine an appropriate living situation. Although most scales provide an aggregate number, more can be learned about a person's capacity for community living by examining subcategory scores. The content of I-ADL scales varies, with some, including the Pfeffer Functional Activities Questionnaire, heavily dependent on cognition.

A number of I-ADL scales are available, but the most commonly used are the Nottingham Extended ADL Index, the Frenchay Activities Index, the Pfeffer Functional Activities Questionnaire, and the Lawton Instrumental Activities of Daily Living Scale.[55–58] The household portion of the Rivermead ADL Index covers I-ADLs, as well.[59,60] The Nottingham is a simple set of questions rating the ease with which certain tasks are done (not at all, with help, alone with difficulty, or alone easily). They form a hierarchical scale in four sections (mobility, kitchen, domestic tasks, and leisure). The Frenchay is a 15-item questionnaire rating the frequency with which a patient has performed specific tasks in the recent past. It covers domestic, leisure, social activities, and work and has been validated by correlation with Barthel Index and Sickness Impact Profile scores.[61] The Lawton I-ADL Scale rates the performance of eight skills necessary for independent living (telephoning, shopping, food preparation, housekeeping, laundry, transportation, medications, and handling finances) and has been shown to be both valid and internally consistent. The Pfeffer expands the Lawton by measuring more cognitively oriented activities (tracking current events; following plots of books, magazines, or television programs; remembering medications and appointments; having hobbies or playing games requiring skill) in addition to domestic activities (shopping, finances, meal preparation, and preparation of coffee or tea). It too has been shown to have good inter-rater reliability, internal consistency, and validity.

Much work recently has been done to shorten functional assessment tools, and some have been modified for patient self-administration or to develop brief check-lists physicians can complete in 1 to 2 minutes. Although simpler, less burdensome measures are generally better, oversimplification also should be avoided. Also, one should note whether a measure scores a subject's ability to perform the task, reported ability, or recent history of performance.[62,63]

Patient reports, caregiver reports, and examiner ratings may not be equivalent. Scores on a subset of FIM items for rehabilitation inpatients scored concurrently by rehabilitation nurses and occupational therapists were different.[64] Studies of scale validity often compare rating scales to a "gold standard" of clinician rating, or to patient reports.

Health-Related Quality of Life

The most important assessment made before, during, and after rehabilitation is that of quality of life. Outcome measures that include quality of life assessments are increasingly expected in the evaluation of drugs and other medical interventions. Quality measures are essential for the illumination of differences between therapies that have marginal differences at the level of impairment.

The major quality domains in chronic neurologic disability are physical status and occupational function, psychological well-being, social interactions, and so-

matic symptoms. Some experts consider economic factors and spiritual status important as well. Health-related quality of life (HRQL) is the multivectoral term that embraces physical, functional, emotional, social, financial, and spiritual factors that impact quality of life. The trend toward using HRQL in medical decision making is truly revolutionary and patient-centered.

As with other functional assessments, HRQL data can be misused and misinterpreted. Individuals asked to estimate quality of life under conditions they have not experienced frequently give much different HRQL ratings than do individuals actually living with that specific disability.[65] Medical personnel tend to rate the quality of life under particular disabilities much lower than do those who actually have such disabilities.[66]

There are two types of HRQL instruments. *Generic* instruments attempt to measure all important aspects of HRQL. They apply to a wide variety of patient types and circumstances, but they are often poorly responsive to change. They are often useful to document the range of disability in a group. For example, such a measure has illustrated the broad-based decrement in HRQL caused by mood disorders.[67] Certain generic instruments attempt to reflect patients' preferences for their quality of life relative to the relatively well-defined qualities of full health and death. Used properly, these HRQL utility measures lend themselves to formal decision analysis.

Specific instruments focus on one aspect of HRQL (such as a specific disease or health-related function) or on a specific population of patients. Some HRQL instruments focus on the elderly, on patients with arthritis, and on HRQL-related aspects of sleep. These measures are more likely than generic instruments to be responsive to change in their narrow field of view. Specific HRQL instruments can be used in combination to cover a wider range of HRQL, or a disease-specific measure may be combined with a global instrument to provide both depth and breadth of coverage.

Because of the complexity of defining quality of life, there is no uniformity of opinion regarding an optimal evaluation instrument.[68] In selecting a suitable measure, there is a trade-off between the level of detail provided and feasibility in terms of patient and staff burden. For example, the Sickness Impact Profile and McMaster Health Index Questionnaire assess a wide range of HRQL domains in depth, but are lengthy to administer and may be difficult for some patients to understand.[69-71] Shorter instruments, such as the Quality of Life Index and Short Form 36 (SF-36) provide less detail, but may not characterize social functioning adequately.[72-76] Given the complexity of HRQL measurement, these instruments may be less relevant to the care of individual patients than to research.[77]

Specific Instruments

One of the most widely used instruments to measure HRQL is the SF-36, a general health status measure that generates a profile of eight "scales" and summary physical and mental health measures.[75] The 36 specific questions are aggregated to provide scores on scales called physical functioning, role-physical, bodily pain, general health, vitality, social functioning, role-emotional, and mental health. The first three scales contribute substantially to the overall physical health summary measure. The last three correlate most highly with the mental health summary measure. Vitality, general health, and social functioning correlate with both summary measures. The SF-36 can be administered by the subjects themselves, by an interviewer in person or over the phone, and generally takes 5 to 10 minutes. It has been adapted to a large number of cultures and languages. It has undergone extensive psychometric testing, and this supports the practices of aggregating individual questions into scale scores without individually weighting each item and analyzing scale values as interval data.[78] The scales and summaries are highly reliable (both test-retest and internal consistency) across a variety of populations. Indirect measures of validity generally are favorable, as well. Perhaps the strongest criticism that can be leveled against the SF-36 is that, while it covers eight concepts generally well-accepted as important to HRQL, it omits several others. These include sleep adequacy, cognitive function, sexual function, health distress, family function, self-esteem, eating, recreation, and communication.

Another widely used measure is the Sickness Impact Profile (SIP).[69] It is substantially longer, with 136 yes-no items. These can be aggregated into 12 categories (ambulation, mobility, body care and movement, communication, alertness behavior, emotional behavior, social interaction, sleeping and rest, eating, work, home management, and recreation and pastimes). Each of the 136 items has a numeric scale value, and the total SIP score is the sum of the scale values for each item endorsed expressed as the percent of the total possible score. The category scores are similarly the percent of the total possible scores for each subset of items. It can be self-administered or given during an interview with fairly high internal consistency. A wide variety of data support its criterion validity and reliability.[79]

Q-TWiST

Q-TWiST (for Quality-adjusted Time Without Symptoms of disease and Toxicity of Treatment) is a method that attempts to integrate measurements of HRQL with measurement of quantity of life for use in comparing treatments.[80,81] Originally designed for cancer chemotherapy trials, Q-TWiST has been used extensively in drug trials for cancer and acquired immune deficiency syndrome. In cancer trials, discrete health states can be identified in which quality of life is relatively uniform: the time before onset of symptoms, a period of initial symptoms and diagnosis, intense therapy with concomitant side effects and toxicities, remission, and a period of further symptoms, diagnosis, and relapse. Each period is assigned a relative utility based on ratings of symptoms, toxicities, and overall quality of life. These include psychosocial morbidity, work disability, and other social costs. The time spent in each health state can be measured, and the Q-TWiST subscore for each state can be calculated as the product of this time and the state-specific utility measure. The sum of these subscores would be a measure of utility-weighted duration of survival. Thus, an individual without significant symptoms or side effects would have the highest possible score, and as the duration of side effects or symptoms increases or the duration of survival decreases the total Q-TWiST score decreases. Such quality-weighted outcome measurements can be used to compare therapeutic options in treatment trials in powerful, patient-centered terms. One can also assess the strength of the Q-TWiST results by calculating the relative utility values at which the treatments would be considered equivalent.

SPECIFIC DISEASES

Stroke

Stroke is the most common neurologic disease requiring rehabilitation, so it is no surprise that the study of outcome assessment for stroke is better developed than for any other disabling condition. Despite the diversity of etiologies and impairments that characterize stroke, the important early rehabilitation goals following stroke can be described by a set of personal care and community living tasks. Whether a person has hemiparesis, sensory loss, speech and language dysfunction, or any of the other protean manifestations of stroke, the initial goal for most is return to community living with the least possible degree of assistance. The fact that most stroke patients are elderly also influences rehabilitation goals. In many cases pre-existent comorbid medical conditions limit functional recovery. Patients with fewer limitations in activities of daily living before stroke generally have fewer limitations after stroke, even after controlling for stroke severity and socio-demographic factors.[82]

The simplest outcome measures related to stroke rehabilitation seek to quantify neurologic impairment. Using motor function as an example, clinicians often grade individual muscle strength on a scale of 0 to 5, using the Medical Research Council Scale, or quantify spasticity with the Modified Ashworth scale.[17,20] More complex scales to assess motor function after stroke include the Fugl-Meyer Scale, and Motor Assessment Scale, discussed earlier.[18,19]

A number of other focused impairment measures are available for specific purposes following stroke. For example, speech and language disorders (aphasia) can be quantified using a number of batteries, including the Boston Diagnostic Aphasia Examination (BDAE), the Porch Index of Communicative Ability (PICA), and the Western Aphasia Battery.[12–14]

Since dementia commonly accompanies stroke and is associated with worse outcome, evidence for dementia may result in changes in the rehabilitation plan.[83–86] The Folstein Mini-Mental State Exam (MMSE) is widely used to screen stroke patients for cognitive problems. A common set of cognitive deficits following stroke is associated primarily with lesions of the nondominant hemisphere. The deficits most likely to result in functional disturbance are neglect and visual-perceptual disturbances. Some studies have suggested worse outcomes in persons with nondominant stroke.[87,88] Visuospatial and tactile neglect often are discovered on the neurological examination, which may reveal failure to attend to the affected side, or extinction on double simultaneous visual or tactile stimulation. A variety of simple bedside tests for visual-spatial neglect include drawing figures, line bisection and line cancellation.[89,90] A somewhat more comprehensive test of neglect is the Behavioral Inattention Test, which is actually a battery of several tests.[91] Since neglect usually has functional consequences, its identification may change rehabilitation strategies. Tests to evaluate other cognitive functions in stroke patients include the Wechsler Memory Scale and attentional tests.[92–95]

A number of more comprehensive impairment scales based on the neurological examination have been developed for stroke.[96–99] Most were designed to monitor neurological status in clinical trials. Various components of the neurological examination are summed to provide an index of neurological status. Because these impairment scales are based on the traditional neurological examination, they are intuitively attractive to physicians. However, critics have argued that the purpose of the neurological examination is diagnosis and localization of abnormalities within the nervous system, and that it cannot logically be adapted for use as a global instrument of neurologic function. These scales are aggregate in nature, with a sum presented as a "degree of impairment." An aggregate score may conceal as much information as it reveals, since different combinations of neurological deficits can result in the same total score. Despite these criticisms, when these scales are administered early after stroke, they correlate with important outcomes, including survival, ability to live at home 3 months after stroke, and functional abilities.[100–102] Patients with multiple neurologic impairments have lower BI scores after stroke and show slower and less complete functional recovery.[103]

Undoubtedly, the Barthel Index is the most extensively studied ADL scale in stroke rehabilitation. The BI score at discharge from the hospital correlates strongly with ability to function independently and return home.[104] A score over 90 (out of total score of 100) ensures functioning at home without major assistance.[104] A score of 60 is generally the cutoff point at which a person can function at home with the reasonable assistance of a spouse or caregiver.[103,105] A BI score of less than 20 correlates with total dependence. Different ADLs present various degrees of difficulty, and stroke patients often become independent in them in a predictable fashion. Thus, the BI has hierarchical characteristics, so that a given BI score quite accurately represents a set of functional activities in which the patient is independent or dependent.[106] Although there are individual exceptions, BI scores at the onset of rehabilitation after stroke correlate with BI scores at discharge, and patients with low BI scores recover more slowly than those with higher scores.[103,105,107] Low BI scores correlate with lower satisfaction with life on long-term follow-up.[106] For younger patients, higher BI scores on admission and discharge from rehabilitation are associated with return to work.[108]

Although a principal advantage of ADL scales is the ability to predict discharge to the community and the amount of assistance needed in self-care after stroke, Granger and colleagues demonstrated that a four-item subscore of the BI consisting of bowel and bladder control, eating, and grooming were almost as accurate as the entire scale in predicting the same outcomes.[106] Nonetheless, because of the practical applicability of all components of ADL scales to clinical rehabilitation, the entire scale is used in clinical practice.

The FIM is also widely used in stroke rehabilitation. For all types of stroke motor impairment, FIM motor functions can be stratified according to degree of difficulty, with feeding the easiest and stair climbing the most difficult.[35] Because of the additional categories and increased sensitivity in comparison to the BI, the FIM is used to follow the clinical progress of stroke patients undergoing rehabilitation and to assist therapists in setting goals.

At times, measurement of limited or focal disabilities is useful in stroke rehabilitation. For example, when ambulation is a major clinical or research focus, a timed walking test (the time required to walk 10 meters), is remarkably simple, reliable, valid and relevant.[6] Other simple measures of ambulation include cadence and stride length. Tests of ability to use the upper extremity in functional tasks include the Frenchay Arm Test, and the Nine-hole Peg Test of finger dexterity, among others.[50,52,53]

Several simple global outcome measures have been applied to stroke. The Rankin scale was first used in 1957.[109] It mixes impairment and disability and is heavily weighted towards mobility (see Table 2-3). Its categories range from no symptoms or disability to severe disability requiring constant attention. The Glasgow Outcome scale is also a well-known global scale designed for head injury assessment which occasionally

has been used in stroke.[110] Global scales are of little practical value for individual patient care, but are useful in population based research studies. They characterize disability in the broadest sense and lack the sensitivity to detect small, but important, changes in function. Global scales have the advantage of being simple to use, making comparative analysis relatively straightforward.[111] The number of categories is relatively few, making retrospective scoring easy.

Independence in the community requires more sophisticated skills than self-care and mobility within the home. Because interaction with society beyond family and caretakers is required, the measurement of these "instrumental" activities of daily living reflects handicap. Successful reintegration at this level is highly dependent on cognitive functioning.

A high degree of dissatisfaction and sense of deterioration of quality of life (HRQL) domains occur after stroke.[112–115] High scores on neurological scales and functional scales usually are correlated with greater satisfaction with life. Those who regain independence frequently do not return to their previous level of wellbeing and social integration.[114–116] The marked change in leisure activity following stroke could be one factor.[117] Studies of HRQL following stroke are complicated by the fact that most stroke patients are elderly, and it is difficult to differentiate physical impairment and disability caused by stroke from the functional decline associated with aging.[68]

Perceived level of social support and depression are clearly associated with HRQL after stroke.[118] The implication for clinicians involved in stroke rehabilitation is that improvement in neurological status and functional abilities is not enough. Emphasis also must be placed on the postdischarge environment, teaching coping skills, and maintaining and strengthening social support systems.

Traumatic Brain Injury

Perhaps the most widely known functional scale developed for brain injury is the Glasgow Coma Scale (GCS) (see Table 2-4).[119] It is a widely used, highly reliable and widely validated global measure of level of neurological functioning.[120–122] Eye opening is rated 1 to 4, motor response to stimuli are rated 1 to 6, and verbal response to stimuli is rated 1 to 5. Thus, a dead person has a GCS of 3, and a neurologically intact patient scores 15. Although the GCS was not designed to provide details of neurological functioning, it has considerable prognostic utility in acute traumatic brain injury. It is highly

Table 2-3
Rankin Scale

Grade	Description
0	No symptoms at all
1	No significant disability, despite symptoms; able to carry out all usual duties and activities
2	Slight disability; unable to carry out all previous activities but able to look after own affairs without assistance
3	Moderate disability; requiring some help, but able to walk without assistance
4	Moderately severe disability; unable to walk without assistance and unable to attend to own bodily needs without assistance
5	Severe disability; bedridden, incontinent, and requiring constant nursing care and attention

Table 2-4
Glasgow Coma Scale

Instructions: *Three sections, each scored separately. Record best response observed to command, voice, or pain.*
Record as: E = _____ , M = _____ , V = _____

Item	Response	Score	Details
Eye Opening	None	1	Even to pain (supraorbital pressure)
	To pain	2	Pain from sternum/limb/supraorbital ridge
	To speech	3	Nonspecific response, not necessarily to command
	Spontaneous	4	Eyes open, not necessarily aware
Motor Response	None	1	To any pain; limbs remain flaccid
	Extension	2	"Decerebrate"; shoulder adducted and internally rotated, forearm pronated
	Abnormal flexion	3	"Decorticate"; shoulder flexes/adducts
	Withdrawal	4	Arm withdraws from pain, shoulder abducts
	Localizes pain	5	Arm attempts to remove supraorbital/chest pain
	Obeys commands	6	Follows simple commands
Verbal Response	None	1	As stated
	Incomprehensible	2	Moans/groans; no words
	Inappropriate	3	Intelligible; no sustained sentences
	Confused	4	Responds with conversation but confused
	Oriented	5	Aware of time, place, person

predictive of both neurobehavioral and global outcome.[123,124]

The duration of posttraumatic amnesia (PTA), measured from the time of injury until the patient has continuous memory, is also a good prognostic indicator.[125] PTA can be difficult to assess from retrospective chart review, but the Galveston Orientation and Amnesia Test (GOAT) is a simple, reliable measure of PTA.[126] It has been shown to correlate with the severity of traumatic brain injury and to help define the end of posttraumatic amnesia.

The Rancho Los Amigos Cognitive Scale also is useful in tracking recovery from TBI.[132] It defines eight levels of cognitive function during recovery after head injury. The Ranchos Los Amigos Cognitive Scale is simple, and easy to use both in monitoring individual recovery and in comparing groups of patients.

Head injury research studies often rely on the Glasgow Outcome Scale.[110] In its original description, it defines five levels of outcome (death, vegetative state, severe disability in conscious patients, moderate disability but independent for ADLs, and good recovery with no more than minor physical or mental deficits or complaints). The eight level version is unreliable. Its simplicity enhances its reliability, but functional classes are so broad that it is poorly sensitive to change and does a poor job of distinguishing between cohorts. The Glasgow Outcome Scale does not clearly delineate cognitive and behavioral deficits. An effort to remedy these limitations led to the development of the Disability Rating Scale.[128] It contains the entire GCS and also includes ratings of ADLs, a global rating of dependence, and a rating of employability. This mixture of impairment, disability, and handicap limits its validity, but it has been shown to be much more sensitive to functional changes over time in brain injury patients and has high interrater reliability.[129–131]

The Neurobehavioral Rating Scale is a modified, structured mental status examination that measures four factors (cognition/energy, metacognition, somatic/anxiety, and language) using 27 questions. It is sensitive to the severity and timing of the injury, and has good interrater reliability.[132] Cognition/energy covers orientation, memory, fatigue, and motor retardation. Metacognition includes agitation, disinhibition, planning, and thought content.

Multiple Sclerosis (MS)

MS is a disease that demands constant vigilance to patient function in neurologic treatment and rehabilitation. The predominant clinical measurement tool for MS is the Kurtzke Expanded Disability Systems Scale (EDSS).[133] The EDSS is based on the Kurtzke Functional Systems Scale, which rates pyramidal, cerebellar, brainstem, sensory, bowel and bladder, visual and mental functions on a 0 to 6 scale (1 to 5 for cerebellar and mental). Zero is normal, 1 implies abnormal signs without disability, 2 usually means minimal disability, and so on to 5 or 6 which is severe dysfunction in the domain in question. The EDSS then combines these individual functional systems scores and provides a EDSS rating of 0 to 10 with increments of 0.5. An EDSS score of 0 implies a normal neurological examination and no Functional Systems (FS) score greater than 0 (although a 1 on mental function, representing mood alterations only, is acceptable). The number of impaired functional systems and the severity of those impairments increases to a score of 4.0, which represents "relatively severe disability" with one FS score of 4, or more than (a) one FS score of 3 and one or two of 2, (b) two FS scores of 3, or (c) five scores of 2. At 4.5 one can walk 300 to 500 meters without aid, and gait distance decreases until at EDSS 7.5 one can take only a few steps. A 9.0 is considered a "helpless bed patient," a 9.5 is a "totally helpless bed patient" who cannot effectively communicate or swallow, and 10.0 is "death due to MS."

Two important clinometric points are evident. First, the definitions of disability for each functional system are arguably more related to impairment than to disability in the WHO sense of the word, as is implied by the names of many of the functional systems. Second, the score is highly dependent on these disability or impairment scores up to a score of 4.0, and then is reflective mainly of ambulatory ability to a score of 7.5 or 8.0. Thus, it can be argued that the EDSS does not measure the same construct throughout its range, and it may not be a true measure of disability. It has also been found to be relatively insensitive to change, and has poor inter-rater reliability that varies across the range of the scale.[134–136] The levels are not evenly spaced, and relatively few patients are given scores of 4 or 5.[137,138] Nonetheless, it continues to be widely used.

Recently, alternatives to the EDSS have been developed. One group has reported preliminary psychometric studies of a six-subscale impairment measure and a disability measure focusing on mobility, hand function, vision, fatigue, cognition, continence, and spasticity.[139] A measure of gait speed and a seven-level mobility rating also have been used, but both focus on mobility.[140] A recent consensus statement outlines the need for further research in appropriate functional assessment instruments for multiple sclerosis and provides excellent guidelines for their development.[141]

Spinal Cord Injury

Functional outcome in complete spinal cord injury is determined by the level of injury and degree of completeness or incompleteness of the injury.[142] The Frankel classification (Table 2-5) of spinal cord injury includes five classes that define various degrees of "completeness" of injury.[143] These range from Class A, complete loss of all motor and sensory function below the level of injury, to Class E, signifying complete return of motor and sensory function. The American Spinal Injury Association (ASIA) system defines the Neurologic Level of Injury as the most caudal segment that tests as normal for both sensory and motor function.[143] Specific dermatomes and muscles define each level. Muscle strength is graded using the Medical Research Council (MRC) Scale. For Frankel Class A, it is easy to clinically determine the level of injury, but for incomplete lesions, this may be much more difficult. There is poor inter-rater reliability for Frankel categories C and D, even when the ratings are done by experts in the field of SCI. It also has poor reliability in cases where

Table 2-5
Spinal Injury: Frankel Scale

Score	Description
A	*Complete injury* No motor or sensory function below the level of injury.
B	*Sensation only* Some preserved sensation below the level of injury; this does not apply to a slight discrepancy between the motor and sensory level, but does apply to sacral sparing.
C	*Motor function useless* Some preserved motor function below the level of injury, but it is of no practical use to the patient.
D	*Motor function useful* Preserved useful motor function below the level of the injury; patients in this group can walk with or without aids.
E	*Recovery* Normal motor and sensory function; abnormal reflexes may be present.

specific dermatomal areas are difficult to assess, or where certain muscles cannot be examined.[144]

Incomplete injuries are often further classified into anatomically localized areas of spinal cord impairment: (1) central cord syndrome; (2) Brown-Séquard syndrome or hemisection of the cord; (3) anterior cord syndrome; and (4) posterior cord syndrome.[150]

Both the Frankel and ASIA classification measure impairment. In complete spinal injury (Frankel A), impairment largely determines disability, the severity of which is defined by the ASIA level of injury. The higher the level of injury, the greater the disability. Disability for incomplete lesions is much more variable, depending on the level of injury, Frankel category, and other factors, including medical comorbidity.

Because disability is so dependent on impairment in SCI, all patients should be classified as accurately as possible, both for clinical and research purposes.[145] Severe early impairment also predicts long-term impairment in SCI. Of patients admitted with Frankel A, 93 percent are still Frankel A at discharge. On the other hand, 52 percent of Frankel C patients will improve to Frankel D or E at discharge.[142] Impairment measured at 72 hours after injury is more accurate than measurement at 24 hours in predicting muscle strength at 3 months.[146]

Because the course of incomplete spinal injuries is variable, more comprehensive aggregate scores of motor function have been devised. Using an aggregate Lower Extremity Motor Score (LEMS), it is possible to demonstrate that the recovery rate following incomplete paraplegia is greatest during the first 3 months after injury, plateauing between 6 and 12 months post-injury.[147]

Measures of limited disability are also important in spinal cord injury. For example, regaining limited ambulation is an important rehabilitation goal for persons with incomplete injury. Motor strength at 1 month is highly predictive of which patients with incomplete paraplegia will develop a reciprocal gait pattern (usually with bracing) and achieve community ambulation at 1 year.[147,148] All patients attaining an MRC grade of >3/5 in at least one quadriceps by 2 months post-injury were able to ambulate at follow-up in one study.[148]

Life expectancy is decreased in traumatic SCI because of a variety of medical causes and external factors. Therefore, survival is a very meaningful outcome measure. In a study of 9,135 persons with traumatic SCI who survived at least 24 hours, the cumulative 12-year survival was 85.1 percent.[149] Positive prognostic factors included age less than 25 years at the time of injury,

incomplete lesions, and paraplegia (vs. quadriplegia). Survivors were better adjusted and more satisfied with many areas of life early after injury.[150]

As in other neurological conditions, other important assessment measures include independence in activities of daily living and community living. For ADLs, assessment instruments such as the BI and FIM are as appropriate for spinal cord injury as other conditions, and predict the need for care but not return to home. About 95 percent of patients with spinal cord injury are able to return to the community, either to their own home or some other residence.[151] Most of the I-ADL measurements discussed elsewhere in this chapter were designed for older persons and may not be valid for the younger population of SCI patients. Special measures of community living skills, largely a reflection of handicap, have been designed for spinal cord injury. Examples include the Craig Handicap Assessment and Reporting Technique (CHART), and the Perceived Handicap Questionnaire (PHQ).[152,153] Both measure physical mobility in the home and community, vocational issues, social integration and economic self-sufficiency. Although their components have face validity, these assessment tools have not undergone rigorous psychometric scrutiny.

Many studies have evaluated dysphoria and depression after SCI, but the results are somewhat confusing.[154] Although almost 20 percent of patients score in the "depressed" range on the Beck Depression Inventory, this likely represents a dysphoric mood rather than organic depression, since most patients improve with time.[155] In another study of newly spinal cord injured patients undergoing rehabilitation, the prevalence of self-reported depressed mood was similar to the general population, and improved with time.[156] In a study of chronic spinal cord injured community residents, the prevalence of depressive symptoms was higher than for the general population.[157] Factors associated with depressive symptoms included female gender, degree of mobility, and low scores on the social integration and occupation sections of CHART, but not impairment (as measured by the ASIA Total Motor Index Score) or disability (measured by the FIM). In another study, dysphoric SCI subjects reported spending fewer days out of the house, receiving more paid personal care assistance, and scored lower on the CHART and the PHQ.[153] Thus, dysphoric symptoms are more strongly associated with measures of handicap than impairment or disability. This suggests that the dysphoria is largely situational, and can be best treated by improving social and community integration.

Measures of life satisfaction in persons with SCI suggest it is lower, on average, than for the general population.[151] However, the majority of people who have been injured for many years rate their quality of life as "good" or "excellent."[158] Adjustment in subjects 15 years after spinal cord injury is stable, and satisfactory adjustment is associated with greater sitting tolerance, more years of education, and greater satisfaction with finances and employment.[159]

Employment is an area of handicap that has received a great deal of attention. Although approximately two thirds of those with spinal cord injury are employed at the time of injury, only one third remain employed 10 years later.[151] Successful employment outcomes are seen in persons who are older at the time of injury, have paraplegia as opposed to quadriplegia, have incomplete injuries, and have completed at least 16 years of education.[160,161]

Parkinson's Disease

The impairments classically associated with Parkinson's disease (bradykinesia, rigidity, and tremor) differ from those of many other neurological conditions requiring rehabilitation. They result in a characteristic set of disabilities that include difficulty turning in bed, going from sit to stand, initiating gait, turning while walking, and unsteady balance. Speech disturbances and difficulty with dressing are other frequent problems. A number of disease-specific scales have been devised to measure these special problems. Assessment in Parkinson's disease is complicated by the frequent variation in symptoms often encountered.[162] However, the overall course is one of progression. Many of the assessment tools used were originally designed to assess the efficacy of specific pharmacologic interventions.

Probably the earliest scale to be widely used was the Hoehn and Yahr scale.[163] It is an ordinal scale that divides Parkinson's disease into five progressive stages. Unfortunately, it is occasionally difficult to accurately to assign an individual patient to a specific grade. The scale also mixes pathology, impairment, and disability.[6] Thus, the scale lacks content validity. Another widely used assessment scale for Parkinson's disease is the Unified Parkinson's Disease Rating Scale.[164] This multifaceted scale measures a variety of impairments and disabilities characteristic of Parkinson's disease. It is weighted towards motor impairment and disability, but also measures traditional ADLs, cognitive function, and "complications of therapy." Although reliable and widely used for research trials, its complexity prevents its use as a clinical outcome tool for individual patients. The McDowell Parkinson's Disease Impairment Index is a simple, weighted scale that includes the most common impairments associated with Parkinson's disease, and may be useful for both clinical and research purposes.[165]

Other less disease-specific measures of outcome are perfectly appropriate for Parkinson's disease, including measures of ADLs and I-ADLs discussed elsewhere in this chapter. Since motor dysfunction is highly characteristic of this condition, "focused" measures of disability, such as timed gait, cadence, stride length, and time required to go from sit to stand, are simple and valid assessment measures. More comprehensive tests of balance, such as the Berg Balance Test and an "obstacle course" could be applicable for research purposes, but are too time-consuming for routine patient care.[166–168]

SUMMARY

Rehabilitation must rely heavily on relatively complex measurements of functional status and progress. There is no parallel in rehabilitation to the Fick-based cardiac output, and there is no quality of life version of the Babinksi sign. This need not make medical care or research in neurological rehabilitation less reliable or scientific. Function must be measured with scientifically sound, reliable outcome measures.

Reliable, validated, patient-centered outcome measures should allow us to begin to understand the real value of rehabilitation, and further refinement of measurement tools will help improve the scientific basis of our efforts to remediate neurologic disability.

REFERENCES

1. World Health Organization: International classification of impairments, disabilities, and handicaps. Geneva: *WHO,* 1980.
2. MacKenzie CR, Charlson ME: Standards for the use of ordinal scales in clinical trials. *Br Med J* 1986; 292:40–43.
3. Merbitz C, Morris J, Grip JC: Ordinal scales and foundations of misinference. *Arch Phys Med Rehab* 1989; 70:308–312.
4. Feinstein AR, Josephy BR, Wells CK: Scientific and clinical problems and indexes of functional disability. *Ann Intern Med* 1986; 105:413–420.
5. Donaldson SW, Wagner CC, Gresham GE: A unified ADL evaluation form. *Arch Phys Med Rehab* 1973; 54:175–179.

6. Wade DT: *Measurement in Neurological Rehabilitation.* Oxford: Oxford University Press, Oxford, 1992.

7. Law M, Letts L: A critical review of scales of activities of daily living. *Am J Occup Ther* 1989; 43:522–528.

8. Folstein MF, Folstein SE, McHugh PR: "Mini-mental state." A practical method for grading the cognitive state of patients for the clinician. *J Psychiatr Res* 1975; 12:189–198.

9. Kiernan RJ, Mueller J, Langston JW, Van Dyke C: The Neurobehavioral Cognitive Status Examination: A brief but quantitative approach to cognitive assessment. *Ann Int Med* 1987; 107:481–485.

10. Mysiw WJ, Beegan JG, Gatens PF: Prospective cognitive assessment of stroke patients before inpatient rehabilitation. The relationship of the Neurobehavioral Cognitive Status Examination to functional improvement. *Am J Phys Med Rehab* 1989; 68:168–171.

11. Wechsler D: *WAIS-R Manual.* New York: Psychological Corporation, New York, 1981.

12. Goodglass H, Kaplan E: *Boston Diagnostic Aphasia Examination.* Philadelphia: Lea & Febiger, 1972.

13. Porch BE: *Porch Index of Communication Ability.* Palo Alto, CA: Consulting Psychologists Press, 1971.

14. Kertesz A: *Western Aphasia Battery.* New York: Grune & Stratton, 1982.

15. Levin HS: A guide to clinical neuropsychological testing. *Arch Neurol* 1994; 51:854–859.

16. Therapeutics and Technology Assessment Subcommittee of the American Academy of Neurology. Assessment: Neuropsychological testing of adults. Considerations for neurologists. *Neurology* 1996; 47:592–599.

17. Medical Research Council, Aids to the Examination of the Peripheral Nervous System: Her Majesty's Stationery Office, London, 1976.

18. Fugl-Meyer AR, Jaasko L, Leyman L, Olsson S, Steglind S: The post-stroke hemiplegic patient. 1. A method for evaluation of physical performance. *Scand J Rehab Med* 1975; 7:13–31.

19. Carr JH, Shepherd RB, Nordholm L, Lynne D: Investigation of a new motor assessment scale for stroke patients. *Phys Ther* 1985; 65:175–180.

20. Ashworth B: Preliminary trial of carisoprodol in multiple sclerosis. *Practitioner* 1964; 192:540–542.

21. Bohannon RW, Smith MB: Inter-rater reliability of a modified Ashworth scale of muscle spasticity. *Phys Ther* 1987; 67:206–207.

22. Harvey RF, Jellinek HM: Functional performance assessment: A program approach. *Arch Phys Med Rehab* 1981; 62:456–460.

23. Fisher WP Jr, Harvey RF, Taylor P, Kilgore KM, Kelly CK: Rehabits: A common language of functional assessment. *Arch Phys Med Rehab* 1995; 76:113–122.

24. Mahoney FI, Barthel DW: Functional evaluation: The Barthel Index. *MD Med J* 1965; 14:61–65.

25. Wade DT, Collin C: The Barthel ADL Index: A standard measure of physical disability? *Int Dis Stud* 1988; 10:64–67.

26. Wade DT, Langton Hewer R: Functional abilities after stroke: Measurement, natural history and prognosis. *J Neurol Neurosurg Psychiatry* 1987; 50:177–182.

27. Granger CV, Dewis LS, Peters NC, Sherwood CC, Barrett JE: Stroke rehabilitation: Analysis of repeated Barthel index measures. *Arch Phys Med Rehab* 1979; 60:14–17.

28. Korner-Bitensky N, Wood-Dauphinee S: Barthel Index information elicited over the telephone. *Am J Phys Med Rehabil* 1995; 74:9–18.

29. Granger CV, Hamilton BB, Gresham GE: The stroke rehabilitation outcome study—Part I: General description. *Arch Phys Med Rehab* 1988; 69:506–509.

30. DeJong G, Branch LG: Predicting the stroke patient's ability to live independently. *Stroke* 1982; 13:648–655.

31. Olsen TS: Arm and leg paresis as outcome predictors in stroke rehabilitation. *Stroke* 1990; 21:247–251.

32. Gresham GE, Phillips TF, Labi ML: ADL status in stroke: Relative merits of three standard indexes. *Arch Phys Med Rehab* 1980; 61:355–358.

33. Guide for the Uniform Data System for Medical Rehabilitation (Adult FIM), version 4.0, Buffalo, NY: State University of New York at Buffalo, 1993.

34. Fiedler RC, Granger CV, Ottenbacher KJ: The Uniform Data System for Medical Rehabilitation: Report of first admissions for 1994. *Am J Phys Med Rehabil* 1996; 75:125–129.

35. Heinemann AW, Linacre JM, Wright BD, Hamilton BB, Granger C: Relationships between impairment and physical disability as measured by the Functional Independence Measure. *Arch Phys Med Rehabil* 1993; 74:566–573.

36. Ottenbacher KJ, Hsu Y, Granger CV, Fiedler RC: The reliability of the Functional Independence Measure: A quantitative review. *Arch Phys Med Rehabil* 1996; 77:1226–1232.

37. Smith PM, Illig SB, Fielder RC, Hamilton BB, Ottenbacher KJ: Intermodal agreement of follow-up telephone functional assessment using the Functional Independence Measure in patients with stroke. *Arch Phys Med Rehabil* 1996; 77:431–435.

38. Heinemann AW, Linacre JM, Wright BD, Hamilton BB, Granger C: Prediction of rehabilitation outcomes with disability measures. *Arch Phys Med Rehab* 1994; 75:133–143.

39. Granger CV, Cotter AC, Hamilton BB, Fiedler RC, Hens MM: Functional assessment scales: a study of persons with multiple sclerosis. *Arch Phys Med Rehab* 1990; 71:870–875.

40. Granger CV, Cotter AC, Hamilton BB, Fiedler RC: Functional assessment scales: a study of persons after stroke. *Arch Phys Med Rehab* 1993; 74:133–138.

41. Carey RG, Posevac EJ: Program evaluation of a physical medicine and rehabilitation unit: A new approach. *Arch Phys Med Rehabil* 1978; 59:330–337.

42. Johnston MV, Keith RA, Hinderer SR: Measurement

standards for interdisciplinary medical rehabilitation. *Arch Phys Med Rehabil* 1992; 73:S12–S23.

43. Stineman MG, Escarce JJ, Goin JE, Hamilton BB, Granger CV, Williams SV: A case-mix classification system for medical rehabilitation. *Med Care* 1994; 32:366–379.

44. Wilkerson DL, Batavia AI, Dejong G: The use of functional status measures for payment of medical rehabilitation services. *Arch Phys Med Rehabil* 1992; 73:111–120.

45. Katz S, Ford AB, Moskowitz RW, Jackson BA, Jaffe MW: Studies of illness in the aged. The index of ADL: A standardised measure of biological and psychosocial function. *JAMA* 1963; 185:914–919.

46. Schoening HA, Anderegg L, Bergstrom D, Fonda M, Steinke N, Ulrich P: Numerical scoring of self-care status of patients. *Arch Phys Med Rehabil* 1965; 46:689–697.

47. Fiatarone MA, O'Neill EF, Ryan ND, Clements KM, Solares GR, Nelson, ME, et al: Exercise training and nutritional supplementation for physical frailty in very elderly people. *N Engl J Med* 1994; 330:1769–1775.

48. Satta NJ, Benson SM, Reding MJ, Sagullo C: Walking endurance is better than speed or functional independence measure walking subscore for documenting ambulation recovery following stroke. *Stroke* 1995; 26:157.

49. Collen FM, Wade DT, Bradshaw CM: Mobility after stroke: Reliability of measures of impairment and disability. *Int Dis Stud* 1990; 12:6–9.

50. Mathiowetz V, Weber K, Kashman N, Volland G: Adult norms for the nine-hole peg test of finger dexterity. *Occup Ther J Res* 1985; 5:24–37.

51. Lyle RC: A performance test for assessment of upper limb function in physical rehabilitation treatment and research. *Int J Rehabil Res* 1981; 4:483–492.

52. DeSouza LH, Langton-Hewer R, Miller S: Assessment of recovery of arm control in hemiplegic stroke patients. Arm function test. *Int Rehabil Med* 1980; 2:3–9.

53. Wade DT, Langton-Hewer R, Wood VA, Skilbeck CE, Ismail IM: The hemiplegic arm after stroke: Measurement and recovery. *J Neurol Neurosurg Psychiatry* 1983; 46:521–524.

54. Norstrom T, Thorslund M: The structure of IADL and ADL measures: Some findings from a Swedish study. *Age Ageing* 1991; 20:23–28.

55. Nouri FM, Lincoln NB: An extended activities of daily living scale for stroke patients. *Clin Rehabil* 1987; 1:301–305.

56. Holbrook M, Skilbeck CE: An activities index for use with stroke patients. *Age Aging* 1983; 12:166–170.

57. Pfeffer RI, Kurosaki MS, Harrah CH, Chance JM, Filos S: Measurement of functional activities in older adults in the community. *J Gerontol* 1982; 37:323–329.

58. Lawton MP, Brody EM: Assessment of older people: Self-maintaining and instrumental activities of daily living. *Gerontologist* 1969; 9:179–186.

59. Whiting S, Lincoln N: An ADL assessment for stroke patients. *Br J Occup Ther* 1980; 43:44–46.

60. Lincoln NB, Edmans JA: A re-validation of the Rivermead ADL scale for elderly patients with stroke. *Age Ageing* 1990; 19:9–24.

61. Schuling J, de Haan R, Limburg M, Groenier KH: The Frenchay Activities Index. Assessment of functional status in stroke patients. *Stroke* 1993; 24:1173–1177.

62. Myers AM: The clinical Swiss army knife: Empirical evidence on the validity of I-ADL functional status measures. *Med Care* 1992; 30:MS96–111.

63. Elam JT, Graney MJ, Beaver T, el Derwi D, Applegate WB, Miller ST: Comparison of subjective ratings of function with observed functional ability of frail older persons. *Am J Pub Health* 1991; 81:1127–1130.

64. Good DC, Pillsbury DC, D'Agostino RB, Peters MS, Redmond SB: Intradisciplinary differences in ADL scoring and goal setting during inpatient rehabilitation. *Arch Phys Med Rehabil* 1995; 76:593.

65. Slevin ML, Plant H, Lynch D, Drinkwater J, Gregory WM: Who should measure quality of life, the doctor or the patient? *Br J Cancer* 1988; 57:109–112.

66. Gerhart KA, Koziol-McLain J, Lowenstein SR, Whiteneck GG: Quality of life following spinal cord injury: Knowledge and attitudes of emergency care providers. *Ann Emerg Med* 1994; 23:807–812.

67. Wells KB, Stewart A, Hays RD, Burnam MA, Rogers W, Daniels M, et al: The functioning and well-being of depressed patients. Results from the Medical Outcomes Study. *JAMA* 1989; 262:914–919.

68. De Haan R, Aaronson N, Limburg M, Langton Hewer R, van Crevel H: Measuring quality of life in stroke. *Stroke* 1993; 24:320–327.

69. Bergner M, Bobbitt RA, Carter WB, Gilson BS: The Sickness Impact Profile: Development and final revision of a health status measure. *Med Care* 1981; 19:787–805.

70. Chambers LW, Sackett DL, Goldsmith CH, MacPherson AS, McAuley RG: Development and application of an index of social function. *Health Serv Res* 1976; 11:430–441.

71. Sackett DL, Chambers LW, MacPherson AS, Goldsmith CH, McAuley RG: The development and application of indices of health: General methods and summary of results. *Am J Public Health* 1977; 67:423–428.

72. Tandon PK, Stander H, Schwarz RP: Analysis of quality of life data from a randomized, placebo-controlled heart-failure trial. *J Clin Epidemiol* 1989; 42:955–962.

73. Spitzer WO, Dobson AJ, Hall J, Chesterman E, Levi J, Shepherd R, et al: Measuring the quality of life in cancer patients: A concise QL-index for use by physicians. *J Chron Dis* 1981; 34:585–597.

74. Ware JE, Brook RH, Williams KN, Stewart AL, Davies-Avery A: Conceptualization and Measurement of Health for Adults in the Health Insurance Study, Vol 1: Model of Health and Methodology. Santa Monica, CA: Rand Corporation, 1980.

75. Ware JE, Snow KK, Kosinski M, Gandek B: *SF-36 Health Survey: Manual and Interpretation Guide.* Boston: Health Institute, New England Medical Center, 1993.

76. Anderson C, Laubscher S, Burns R: Validation of the short form 36 (SF-36) health survey questionnaire among stroke patients. *Stroke* 1996; 27:1812–1816.

77. Ware JE Jr: The status of health assessment 1994. *Ann Rev Public Health* 1995; 16:327–354.

78. Ware JE: The SF-36 health survey, in Spilker B (ed): *Quality of Life and Pharmacoeconomics in Clinical Trials.* Philadelphia: Lippincott-Raven, 1996, pp. 337–345.

79. Damiano AM: The sickness impact profile, in Spilker B (ed): *Quality of Life and Pharmacoeconomics in Clinical Trials.* Philadelphia: Lippincott-Raven, 1996, pp. 347–354.

80. Schwartz CE, Cole BF, Gelber RD: Measuring patient-centered outcomes in neurologic disease. Extending the Q-TWiST method. *Arch Neurol* 1995; 52:754–762.

81. Schwartz CE, Cole BF, Vickrey BG, Gelber RD: The Q-TWiST approach to assessing health-related quality of life in epilepsy. *Qual Life Res* 1995; 4:135–141.

82. Colantonio A, Kasl SV, Ostfeld AD, Berkman LF: Prestroke physical function predicts stroke outcomes in the elderly. *Arch Phys Med Rehabil* 1996; 77:562–566.

83. Tatemichi T, Foulkes M, Mohr J, et al: Dementia in stroke survivors in the stroke data bank cohort. *Stroke* 1990; 21:858–866.

84. Kotila M, Waltimo O, Niemi M, et al: The profile of recovery from stroke and factors influencing outcome. *Stroke* 1984; 15:1039–1044.

85. Lincoln NB, Blackburn M, Ellis S, et al: An investigation of factors affecting progress of patients on a stroke unit. *J Neurol Neurosurg Psychol* 1989; 52:493–496.

86. Pedersen PM, Jørgensen HS, Nakayama H, Raaschou HO, Olsen TS: Orientation in the acute and chronic stroke patient: Impact on ADL and social activities. The Copenhagen Stroke Study. *Arch Phys Med Rehabil* 1996; 77:336–339.

87. Chen Sea M-J, Henderson A, Cermak SA: Patterns of visual spatial inattention and their functional significance in stroke patients. *Arch Phys Med Rehabil* 1993; 74:355–360.

88. Denes G, Semenza C, Stoppa E, et al: Unilateral spatial neglect and recovery from hemiplegia: A follow-up study. *Brain* 1982; 105:543–552.

89. Fullerton KJ, McSherry D, Stout RN: Albert's Test: A neglected test of perceptual neglect. *Lancet* 1986; 1:430–432.

90. Halligan PW, Marshall JC, Wade DT: Visuospatial neglect: Underlying factors and test sensitivity. *Lancet* 1989; 2:908–910.

91. Wilson BA, Cockburn J, Halligan P: Development of a behavioral test of visuospatial neglect. *Arch Phys Med Rehabil* 1987; 68:98–102.

92. Wechsler D: A standardized memory scale for clinical use. *J Psychol* 1945; 19:87–95.

93. Skilbeck CE, Woods RT: The factorial structure of the Wechsler Memory Scale: Samples of neurological and psychogeriatric patients. *J Clin Neuropsychol* 1980; 2:293–300.

94. Raskin SA, Mateer CA: Rehabilitation of cognitive impairments, in Good DC, Couch JR (ed): *Handbook of Neurorehabilitation.* New York: Marcel Dekker, 1994, pp. 243–259.

95. Whyte J: Neurologic disorders of attention and arousal: Assessment and treatment. *Arch Phys Med Rehabil* 1992; 73:1094–1103.

96. Mathew NT, Rivera VM, Meyer JS, Charney JZ, Hartmann A: Double-blind evaluation of glycerol therapy in acute cerebral infarction. *Lancet* 1972; 2:1327–1329.

97. Brott T, Adams HP, Olinger CP, et al: Measurement of acute cerebral infarction: A clinical examination scale. *Stroke* 1989; 20:864–870.

98. Cote R, Hachinski VC, Shurvell BL, Norris JW, Wofson C: The Canadian Neurological Scale: A preliminary study in acute stroke. *Stroke* 1986; 17:731–737.

99. Hanston L, DeWeerdt W, DeKeyser J, Diener HC, Franke C, Palm R, et al: The European Stroke Scale. *Stroke* 1994; 25:225.

100. Muir KW, Weir CJ, Murray GD, Povey C, Lees KR: Comparison of neurological scales and scoring systems for acute stroke prognosis. *Stroke* 1996; 27:1817–1820.

101. D'Olhaberriague L, Litvan I, Mitsias P, Mansbach HH: A reappraisal of reliability and validity studies in stroke. *Stroke* 1996; 27:2331–2336.

102. Jørgensen HS, Nakayama H, Raaschou HO, Vive-Larsen J, Støier M, Olsen TS: Outcome and time course of recovery in stroke. Part I: Outcome. The Copenhagen Stroke Study. *Arch Phys Med Rehabil* 1995; 76:399–405.

103. Reding MJ, Potes E: Rehabilitation outcome following initial unilateral hemispheric stroke. Life table analysis approach. *Stroke* 1988; 19:1354–1358.

104. Granger CV, Sherwood CC, Greer DS: Functional status measures in a comprehensive stroke program. *Arch Phys Med Rehabil* 1977; 58:555–561.

105. Granger CV, Hamilton BB, Gresham GE: The stroke rehabilitation outcome study—Part I: General description. *Arch Phys Med Rehabil* 1988; 69:506–509.

106. Granger CV, Hamilton BB, Gresham GE, Kramer AA: The stroke rehabilitation outcome study: Part II. Relative merits of the total Barthel Index score and a four-item subscore in predicting patient outcomes. *Arch Phys Med Rehabil* 1989; 70:100–103.

107. Skilbeck CE, Wade, DT, Langton Hewer R, Wood VA: Recovery after Stroke. *J Neurol Neurosurg Psychiatry* 1983; 46:5–8.

108. Black-Schaffer RM, Osberg JS: Return to work after stroke: Development of a predictive model. *Arch Phys Med Rehabil* 1990; 71:285–290.

109. Rankin J: Cerebral vascular accidents in patients over the age of 60. 2. Prognosis. *Scot Med J* 1957; 2:200–215.

110. Jennett B, Bond M: Assessment of outcome after severe brain damage. A practical scale. *Lancet* 1975; 1:480–484.

111. Lyden PD, Lau GT: A critical appraisal of stroke evaluation and rating scales. *Stroke* 1991; 22:1345–1352.

112. Viitanen M, Fugl-Meyer KS, Bernspang B, Fugl-Meyer

AR: Life satitsfaction in long-term survivors after stroke. *Scand J Rehab Med* 1988; 20:17–24.

113. Astrom M, Asplund K, Astrom T: Psychosocial function and life satisfaction after stroke. *Stroke* 1992; 23:527–531.

114. Santus G, Rezenigo A, Caregnato R, Inzoli MR: Social and family integration of hemiplegic elderly patients one year after stroke. *Stroke* 1990; 21:1019–1022.

115. Niemi M, Laaksonen, MA, Kotila M, Waltimo O: Quality of life four years after stroke. *Stroke* 1988; 19:1101–1107.

116. Labi MLC, Phillips TF, Gresham GE: Psychosocial disability in physically restored long-term stroke survivors. *Arch Phys Med Rehabil* 1980; 61:561–565.

117. Drummond A: Leisure activity after stroke. *Int Disabil Studies* 1990; 12:157–160.

118. King RB.: Quality of life after stroke. *Stroke* 1996; 27:1467–1472.

119. Teasdale G, Jennett B: Assessment of coma and impaired consciousness. A practical scale. *Lancet* 1974; 2:81–84.

120. Juarez VJ, Lyons M: Interrater reliability of the Glasgow Coma Scale. *J Neurosci Nurs* 1995; 27:283–286.

121. Hartley C, Cozens A, Mendelow AD, Stevenson JC: The Apache II scoring system in neurosurgical patients: A comparison with simple Glasgow coma scoring. *Br J Neurosurg* 1995; 9:179–187.

122. Kennedy F, Gonzalez P, Dang C, Fleming A, Sterling-Scott R: The Glasgow Coma Scale and prognosis in gunshot wounds to the brain. *J Trauma* 1993; 35:75–77.

123. Levin HS, Gary HE Jr, Eisenberg HM, Ruff RM, Barth JT, Kreutzer J, et al: Neurobehavioral outcome 1 year after severe head injury. Experience of the Traumatic Coma Data Bank. *J Neurosurg* 1990; 73:699–709.

124. Choi SC, Narayan RK, Anderson RL, Ward JD: Enhanced specificity of prognosis in severe head injury. *J Neurosurg* 1988; 69:381–385.

125. Ellenberg JH, Levin HS, Saydjari C: Posttraumatic Amnesia as a predictor of outcome after severe closed head injury. Prospective assessment. *Arch Neurol* 1996; 53:782–791.

126. Levin HS, O'Donnell VM, Grossman RG: The Galveston Orientation and Amnesia Test. A practical scale to assess cognition after head injury. *J Nerv Ment Dis* 1979; 167:675–684.

127. Hagen C, Malkmus D, Durham P: Levels of cognition functioning. Downey, CA: Rancho Los Amigos Hospital, 1972.

128. Rappaport M, Hall KM, Hopkins K, Belleza T, Cope DN: Disability rating scale for severe head trauma: Coma to community. *Arch Phys Med Rehab* 1982; 63:118–123.

129. Hall K, Cope DN, Rappaport M: Glasgow Outcome Scale and Disability Rating Scale: Comparative usefulness in following recovery in traumatic head injury. *Arch Phys Med Rehab* 1985; 66:35–37.

130. Gouvier WD, Blanton PD, LaPorte KK, Nepomuceno C: Reliability and validity of the Disability Rating Scale and the Levels of Cognitive Functioning Scale in monitoring recovery from severe head injury. *Arch Phys Med Rehab* 1987; 68:94–97.

131. Giacino JT, Kezmarsky MA, DeLuca J, Cicerone KD: Monitoring rate of recovery to predict outcome in minimally responsive patients. *Arch Phys Med Rehab* 1991; 72:897–901.

132. Levin HS, High WM, Goethe KE, Sisson RA, Overall JE, Rhoades HM, et al: The neurobehavioural rating scale: Assessment of the behavioural sequelae of head injury by the clinician. *J Neurol Neurosurg Psychiatry* 1987; 50:183–193.

133. Kurtzke JF: Rating neurologic impairment in multiple sclerosis: An expanded disability status scale (EDSS). *Neurology* 1983; 33:1444–1452.

134. Goodkin DE, Cookfair D, Wende K, Bourdette D, Pullicino P, Scherokman B, et al: Inter- and intrarater scoring agreement using grades 1.0 to 3.5 of the Kurtzke Expanded Disability Status Scale (EDSS). Multiple Sclerosis Collaborative Research Group. *Neurology* 1992; 42:859–863.

135. Francis DA, Bain P, Swan AV, Hughes RA: An assessment of disability rating scales used in multiple sclerosis. *Arch Neurol* 1991; 48:299–301.

136. Amato MP, Fratiglioni L, Groppi C, Siracusa G, Amaducci L: Interrater reliability in assessing functional systems and disability on the Kurtzke scale in multiple sclerosis. *Arch Neurol* 1988; 45:746–748.

137. Cohen RA, Kessler HR, Fischer M: The Extended Disability Status Scale (EDSS) as a predictor of impairments of functional activities of daily living in multiple sclerosis. *J Neurol Sci* 1993; 115:132–135.

138. Willoughby EW, Paty DW: Scales for rating impairment in multiple sclerosis: A critique. *Neurology* 1988; 38:1793–1798.

139. Schwartz C, Vollmer T, Zeng Q: New outcome measures for multiple sclerosis clinical research: The symptom inventory and the performance scales. *Neurology* 1996; 46:A321.

140. Hohol MJ, Khoury SJ, Hafler DA, Dawson DM, Tourbah A, Lubetzki C, et al: Disease steps in multiple sclerosis: A simple approach to classify patients and evaluate disease progression. *Neurology* 1993; 43:A203.

141. Rudick R, Antel J, Confavreux C, Cutter G, Ellison G, Fischer J, et al: Clinical outcomes assessment in multiple sclerosis. *Ann Neurol* 1996; 40:469–479.

142. Staas WE, Formal CS, Gershkoff AM, Hirschwald JF, Schmidt M, Schultz AR, et al: Rehabilitation of the spinal cord-injured patient, in DeLisa JA (ed): *Rehabilitation Medicine: Principles and Practice*, 2nd ed. Philadelphia: JB Lippincott, pp. 886–915.

143. Donovan WH, Maynard FM, McCluers, Menter RR, et al: Standards for Neurological Classification of Spinal Injury Patients. Atlanta, American Spinal Injury Association, 1990.

144. Donovan WH, Wilkerson MA, Rossi D, et al: A test of the ASIA guidelines for classification of spinal cord injuries. *J Neurol Rehab* 1990; 4:39–53.

145. Closson JB, Toerge JE, Ragnarsson KT, et al: Rehabilitation in spinal cord disorders. 3. Comprehensive management of spinal cord injury. *Arch Phys Med Rehabil* 1991; 72:S298–S308.

146. Brown PJ, Marino RJ, Herbison GJ, Ditunno JF: The 72-hour examination as a predictor of recovery in motor complete quadriplegia. *Arch Phys Med Rehabil* 1991; 72:546–548.

147. Waters RL, Adkins RH, Yakura JS, Sie I: Motor and sensory recovery following incomplete paraplegia. *Arch Phys Med Rehabil* 1994; 75:67–72.

148. Crozier KS, Cheng LL, Graziani V, et al: Spinal cord injury: Prognosis for ambulation based on quadriceps recovery. *Paraplegia* 1992; 30:762–767.

149. DeVivo MJ, Stover SL, Black KJ: Prognostic factors for 12-year survival after spinal cord injury. *Arch Phys Med Rehabil* 1992; 73:156–162.

150. Krause JS, Kjorsvig JM: Mortality after spinal cord injury: A four-year prospective study. *Arch Phys Med Rehabil* 1992; 73:558–563.

151. Ditunno JF, Formal CS: Chronic spinal cord injury. *N Engl J Med* 1994; 330:550–556.

152. Whiteneck GG, Charlifue SW, Gerhart KA, Overholser JD, Richardson GN: Guide for Use of the CHART: Craig Handicap Assessment and Reporting Technique. Craig Hospital, CO, 1988.

153. Tate D, Forchheimer M, Maynard F, Dijkers M: Predicting depression and psychological distress in persons with spinal cord injury based on indicators of handicap. *Am J Phys Med Rehabil* 1994; 73:175–183.

154. Elliott TR, Frank RG: Depression following spinal cord injury. *Arch Phys Med Rehabil* 1996; 77:816–823.

155. Judd FK, Brown DJ, Burrows GD: Depression, disease and disability: Application to patients with traumatic spinal cord injury. *Paraplegia* 1991; 29:91–96.

156. Cushman LA, Dijkers M: Depressed mood during rehabilitation of persons with spinal cord injury. *J Rehabil* 1991; 57:35–38.

157. Fuhrer MJ, Rintala DH, Hart KA, et al: Depressive symptomatology in persons with spinal cord injury who reside in the community. *Arch Phys Med Rehabil* 1993; 74:255–260.

158. Whiteneck GG, Charlifue SW, Frankel HL, et al: Mortality, morbidity and psychosocial outcomes of persons spinal cord injured more than 20 years ago. *Paraplegia* 1992; 30:617–630.

159. Krause JS: Longitudinal changes in adjustment after spinal cord injury: A 15-year study. *Arch Phys Med Rehabil* 1992; 73:564–568.

160. Krause JS, Anson CA: Employment after spinal cord injury: Relation to selected participant characteristics. *Arch Phys Med Rehabil* 1996; 77:737–743.

161. Krause JS: Employment after spinal cord injury. *Arch Phys Med Rehabil* 1992; 73:163–169.

162. Lang AET, Fahn S: Assessment of Parkinson's Disease, in Munsat TL (ed): *Quantification of Neurologic Deficit.* Boston: Butterworths 1989, pp. 285–309.

163. Hoehn MM, Yahr MD: Parkinsonism: Onset, progression and mortality. *Neurology* 1967; 17:427–442.

164. Lang AET, Fahn S: Assessment of Parkinson's Disease, in Munsat TL (ed): *Quantification of Neurologic Deficit.* Boston: Butterworths 1989, pp. 285–309.

165. McDowell F, Lee JE, Swift T, Sweet RD, Ogsbury JS, Kessler JT: Treatment of Parkinson's syndrome with L Dihydroxyphenylalanine (Levodopa). *Ann Int Med* 1970; 72:29–35.

166. Bogle Thorbahn LD, Newton RA: Use of the Berg Balance Test to predict falls in elderly persons. *Phys Ther* 1996; 76:576–585.

167. Berg KO, Wood-Dauphinee SL, Williams JT, Gayton D: Measuring balance in the elderly: Preliminary development of an instrument. *Physiother Can* 1989; 41:304–311.

168. Means KM, Rodell DE, O'Sullivan PS: Use of an obstacle course to assess balance and mobility in the elderly: A validation study. *Am J Phys Med Rehabil* 1996; 75:88–95.

Chapter 3

ETHICAL CONSIDERATIONS IN TREATING NEUROLOGIC DISABILITY

Michael P. McQuillen

In his book *Suffering Presence*—a set of *Theological Reflections on Medicine, the Mentally Handicapped, and the Church*—the philosopher Stanley Hauerwas concluded that "suffering and tragedy are the necessary conditions for (human beings) to be able to act at all," citing Stanley Cavell's observations that

> *if you would avoid tragedy [and suffering], avoid love; if you cannot avoid love, avoid integrity; if you cannot avoid integrity, avoid the world; [and] if you cannot avoid the world, destroy it.*[1]

Hauerwas' primary argument grew to fruition during the time that he spent in a community of mentally handicapped persons and those who cared for them. That argument

> *put in its simplest terms, is that a humane medicine is impossible to sustain in a society which lacks the moral capacity to care for the mentally handicapped.*

It is an argument central to any ethical consideration of whether, why, and how treatment should be rendered to the disabled—especially those with neurologic disabilities, such as those dealt with in this book. To begin that consideration, it is necessary to articulate an approach to the ethical method, and the framework and philosophies upon which that method relies. In the process, it will be important to highlight the differences between *rehabilitation* medicine and the rest of medicine, insofar as those differences affect ethical thought and analysis. Once a grasp of the method is in hand, it can be applied to certain selected neurologic disabilities of particular concern at this time.

THE ETHICAL METHOD

It is an affront to many physicians to suggest that there may be an *ethical* method by means of which they may approach their responsibilities in caring for patients—certainly an affront to suggest that there may be *one* ethical method that is preferable above all others. At the heart of the matter, however, are the conflicting priorities that plague every interaction between human beings. For example, how can the difference between what patients want, and what their physicians feel is best for them, be resolved? Are patients and physicians the only factors in the equation? What about nurses; physical, occupational, speech, and recreational therapists; social workers; psychologists and vocational counselors; and other "health care personnel" so intimately and crucially involved in rehabilitation medicine? Where do the hopes and expectations of families, and the burdens they must bear, enter in? Should cost, and scarcity of resources, be considered; and if so, by whom, and how?

The methodology for a comprehensive, multidisciplinary approach to rehabilitation evolved in this century on a foundation of theoretical and empirical knowledge. That basis permitted persons with functional impairments of diverse origin to make the most of the abilities that remained, after experiencing the insults that led to the impairments. In like manner, a methodology for ethical decision making has developed that permits ranking of priorities and resolution of differences that arise when such priorities and differences come in conflict. Ethical methodology is also based on theoretical and empirical knowledge. An adequate ethical theory is clear, coherent, comprehensive, simple, and practical.[2] It explains and justifies its conclusions and yields new insights, rather than reiterating an intuitive belief or repeating an old conviction—much in the same way as a proposal for managing the persistent vegetative state does.[3]

Types of Ethical Theory

There are several types of ethical theory, each one of which may be more appropriate than another in any given clinical situation (Table 3-1). These include

1. *Utilitarianism.* This theory is the basis of a "burdens-benefits" analysis. According to the theory, the best action is that which produces the most good with the least harm for most people, most of the time. The theory looks at the consequences of acts, rather than at the acts per se. It is a theory that governs the presentation of data by the physician for many decisions, thought to be solely, or at least primarily, medical in nature.

2. *Obligation-based theory.* Actions based on this theory should apply to every person, in all circumstances. Persons acting in accord with this theory do what they *ought* to do. In its original or "pure" form (as articulated by Immanuel Kant), this theory applied only to *rational* persons. In that sense, its application is limited in many neurorehabilitation settings in which significant brain damage interferes with rationality. Such settings call for surrogate decision making, which may be an imperfect substitute for what the once-rational person may have wanted (*vide infra,* advance directives).

3. *Virtue-based theory.* Motive, and the character of the person acting, are the basis of this theory. Many traditional ethical formulations (e.g., the Oath of Hippocrates) are based on the assumption that physicians are ethical persons, who act always and only in the best interests of their patients. This assumption was a foundation source of *paternalism,* an approach that has lost favor in "modern" medical ethical thinking

(*vide infra,* principlism)—although it remains a basis for making ethical sense of much of the decision making in rehabilitation medicine, at least in the early stages of the process.[4]

4. *Rights-based theory.* A concept of *individual justice* weighs heavily in this theory, which determines actions based on the claim that an individual or group is entitled to make on another. Essential to an understanding of the ramifications of this theory is a notion of the obligations that correspond to the rights being invoked, and that devolve on the other on whom the claim is made. That "other" may be another person or group of persons; an entity (such as health or workers' compensation insurance); or even society at large.

5. *Communitarian ethics.* In many ways, this is the obverse of a theory that derives from the rights of an individual—in that the rights, or needs, of the "other" (on whom a claim is made) are paramount in a communitarian ethical theory. To be valid, a communitarian ethic must rely on a deep sense of justice—which can be variably defined (e.g., in the realm of medical vs. the world of business ethics, at war with each other in the battle over "managed care").

6. *The ethics of care.* The basis of this theory is the relationship between persons—one caring for, and attached to, the other; each deriving benefit from that relationship. The theory is often labeled *feminist* ethics, as though the virtue was gender-specific—which it is not.

7. *Casuistry.* Although the term has unfortunate connotations, it really implies the sort of case-based reasoning common to much of medicine. The determinants are the particular circumstances, whereas the judgment is reached by analogy to similar cases. Maxims are derived from such analogies, and help to guide decision making in each new situation.

8. *Four principles approach.* Recent ethical thinking has looked for rules to govern decision making, derived from the principles of so-called "common sense morality"—a theory simply put as "do good and avoid evil." The four such principles that grow out of this theory are the following.

    1. *Autonomy,* or a recognition of the value of persons, and a need to respect and honor their choices for themselves;

    2. *Nonmaleficence,* or the obligation to avoid intentional harm;

    3. *Beneficence,* or the intent to act for the good of another; and

Table 3-1

Types of ethical theory commonly applied in decision theory analysis of neurologic disability

Utilitarianism	Communitarian ethics
Obligation-based theory	Ethics of care
Virtue-based theory	Casuistry
Rights-based theory	Principlism

    4. *Justice,* or the concept of a fair, equitable, and appropriate distribution of goods in society.

The Application of Ethical Theory: Ethics in Acute-Care Practice

The practice of ethics, in many ways, differs not at all from the practice of medicine. To reach a decision in any clinical setting, physicians must first frame the problem in its clinical context, and recognize, identify, and rank the options for dealing with it; in short, conduct an assessment of the problem. Once a decision has been reached, it must be implemented. What happens next is an on-going process of evaluation, with decisions open to change and new decisions implemented as new data permit changes in assessment. John Fletcher and his colleagues have applied this approach to the practice of ethics.[5] In so doing, they have emphasized the process of decision *making* as distinct from the decision per se. This emphasis highlights the conflicts that may arise between physician and patient; between both and society (in particular, the law—and, more recently, the managed care organizations that, in an increasingly pervasive and controlling sense, define and set limits to the clinical setting); and in diverse ethnic, cultural, and religious settings.[6]

In acute-care settings, decision making at one time was a matter of "the doctor knows best"; beneficence ruled supreme at that time. Certainly, the experience, knowledge, and skill of physicians enable them to reach a proper assessment of the medical context in which decisions must be made, but the choice of options is heavily a personal matter, influenced by the values of persons affected by the decision—persons whose values may differ markedly from those of their physician. This dilemma was recognized early in this century in the matter of *Schloendorff v. Society of New York Hospital,* when Justice Benjamin Cardozo proclaimed that "(e)very human being of adult years and sound mind has a right to determine what shall be done with his own body"—thereby settling the dilemma in favor of respect for the autonomy of the patient, no matter what the consequences.[7] It is important to note that respect for autonomy is not an unfettered right; physicians cannot be forced to implement decisions that violate their own consciences; and increasingly, society (through case law and statute) and systems that pay for the costs of health care (especially managed care organizations) are the entities that make medical decisions. Nevertheless, at the heart of the concept of respect for autonomy is

Table 3-2
The four principles approach to ethics

Autonomy	Beneficence
Nonmaleficence	Justice

the requirement that physicians inform patients in great and yet understandable detail of their assessments, of the options for further evaluation and therapy, and of the risks and benefits of each, and not just impose their own choices on their patients. This is the process of informed consent—a process at once simple and yet complex; a process inevitably even if unconsciously burdened with bias; a process fundamentally based on trust.[8] For those reasons, and because of the imbalance between powerful physicians and vulnerable patients, some have suggested that that process be conducted in a "conversation model" according to which physicians, in essence, think "out loud" as they frame their assessments and recommendations, inviting comments and questions from their patients as the process unfolds toward shared decisions to be implemented.[9] This is not a process cast in stone at any point: Physicians alter assessments as new data accumulate, and patients change their minds, even with regard to decisions with life-sustaining implications. Thus, in a study of patient preferences for ventilator support in the context of motor neuron disease, patients regularly opted in favor of such support at one time, rejecting it at another.[10]

But what if the patient is not an adult, or no longer has (perhaps, never did have) the capacity for valid decision making? Who decides, and how, then? There is general agreement that the right to make a decision perdures, even in the absence of capacity. A mechanism to effect that right after capacity is lost—the mechanism of advance directives—has become popular in recent years, even to the point that a federal requirement was imposed, requiring that patients be asked, on admission to the hospital, whether they have executed an advance directive, or wish to do so.[11] Generally, advance directives are of two kinds—a so-called *living will,* which sets forth the patient's preferences for life-sustaining treatments, in greater or lesser detail; and a *durable power of attorney for health care decisions,* by means of which a surrogate is appointed to articulate those preferences. A major disadvantage of living wills is the fact that very rarely can one frame a decision before an event has occurred. Ideally, those who hold durable powers of attorney for health care decisions will know the person in whose stead they decide well enough to make the decision the person would make if he or she were able to do so (by a substituted judgment standard) or—better yet—report faithfully what the patient had to say about the decision he or she would make in such a situation. Often, however, the surrogate acts according to a best interests standard, thereby substituting his or her own judgment for the patient's. In practice, this is what happens when parents decide for children, or any surrogate acts for someone who never had capacity. Surrogates may be selected in accord with a hierarchy spelled out by state law, or even appointed by a court. In practice, it is wise in acute-care settings to seek consensus, and to continue to act in favor of life until consensus has been reached.

"Health care reform" is having a major impact on every aspect of this practice. Whereas heretofore decisions to do something were the rule, now decisions not to do something are in the ascendancy. Unquestionably, "reform" is primarily motivated by concerns about money and other resources: Doing something expends money; not doing something conserves it. A prime motivating factor for the physician under both systems is financial incentive. Formerly, under "fee for service," the more physicians did, the more they were paid. Now, under "managed care"—particularly capitated managed care, a system under which physicians are paid a set amount to render all care to their patients for a set, per-member-per-month fee—the less physicians do, the more they are paid. This raises issues of withdrawing or withholding care, and the ethical implications of such actions—especially when the action will likely, even predictably, result in the death of the patient. In practice, decisions to withdraw or withhold care should be made just as any other medical decision should be made—by the patient; for the patient; in the patient's best interest, as defined by the patient or his or her duly appointed surrogate. As with every other choice, decisions to withdraw or withhold care are made according to a burdens-benefits analysis in most instances, but should include an analysis of intent as well. Thus, when the parents of Karen Ann Quinlan (a young woman in a vegetative state after a cardiac arrest probably brought on in part by sedative ingestion) asked that she be removed from a ventilator, they wanted to eliminate the burden of the ventilator, which was providing no benefit other than sustaining a vegetative life.[12] Even though they recognized that she might die without the support of her ventilator, they did not intend her death—and indeed, she lived for almost a decade after its removal. Contrast

that request with that made by the parents of Nancy Beth Cruzan (another young woman in a vegetative state after an automobile accident) to stop the provision of food and water (described as "artificial nutrition and hydration") through a gastrostomy tube. In this instance, the U.S. Supreme Court—although agreeing that this request was licit if advanced in accord with the stipulations of the jurisdiction in which it was made—recognized that the intent of the request to withdraw artificial nutrition and hydration could only be to "cause her death"; in essence, to eliminate a burdensome life that had no meaning, no benefit for the patient, in the judgment of her parents.[13]

The examples cited emphasize many aspects of decision making, including the ambiguity of clinical intention.[14] It should also be emphasized that withholding therapy before giving it a chance, to see whether it will provide benefit, is more ethically problematic than withdrawing therapy that has been demonstrated to provide no benefit in a given patient.

The Application of Ethical Theory: Ethics in Rehabilitation Medicine

The practice of rehabilitation medicine has long been a team effort, with input from many disciplines. Central to the rehabilitation process is an initial judgment on the likelihood of benefit to the patient from the expenditure of time, effort, and resources to achieve that benefit. Patients do not enter a rehabilitation program at their own request; they do so on invitation, after a sometimes long and usually thoughtful series of evaluations by various team members. Access to rehabilitation services is determined by many factors, including diagnosis and prognosis; age; "vocational potential"; and even ability to pay.[15] It is easy to see how the process of selection for entry into a rehabilitation program can be quite subjective, with real potentials for bias and injustice. Justice demands that people receive that to which they are entitled—but are they entitled only to what they can pay for, or need, or only to what everyone can receive?[16] Should there be an equality of opportunity, or of outcome? Most payors for rehabilitation services demand evidence of movement toward a defined outcome, or else they will deny continued support for those services. Do decisions of this sort place the neurologically disabled—in a certain sense, those most in need of rehabilitation services—in jeopardy simply because of their disabilities?

The experience in Oregon is instructive on this issue. There, the state's Health Services Commission conducted a many-layered process of surveys and public discussions about health care priorities. They did this in order to expand the state's Medicaid coverage to more persons without calling for more public funds for this purpose. Central to their prioritization process was the construction of a *Quality of Well-Being Scale* derived from a telephone survey. The U.S. Department of Health and Human Services turned down the Oregon Plan initially because its prioritization was "based in substantial part on the premise that the value of the life of a person with a disability is less than the value of a person without a disability."[17] How many rehabilitation decisions involve such bias—consciously or unconsciously—not against disability in general, but against one form of disability as opposed to another?

Thus, the process of deciding who shall be offered entry into a rehabilitation program in the first place does not involve patients or their surrogates. Although those affected by the decision may have the capacity to understand and affirm or deny an offer for rehabilitation when made, quite frequently they require time to adjust to the reality of their impairment, and to appreciate, accept, and make the most of their abilities that do remain. This gives rise to what has been termed an educational model for decision making in the rehabilitation setting, as opposed to the contractual model that governs in acute care settings.[18] As the term implies, the educational model describes an evolving relationship in which the team's assessment holds sway at entry, whereas the patient's autonomy becomes more and more informed and respected as the rehabilitation process proceeds. Viewed from one end of the process, the behavior of the team is very paternalistic. From the other end, setting and pursuing plans realistically, sensibly, and collaboratively give witness to respect for the reemerging autonomy of the patient.[19]

All along the way, there is often an implied, unspoken burden on the family of the patient. Families often are drafted by circumstances not of their own choosing into assuming heroic duties that give rise to anger that often generates guilt. Uncertainty of prognosis leads to despair, in trying to cope with a future that promises no relief, no escape. As Callahan has observed, "An action must stem from a free choice . . . to count as moral at all; and morality in general—but self-sacrificial morality in particular—cannot be sustained by will alone."[20] When the language of rights predominates, we forget that "no one of us . . . is independent of the community on which we depend for our moral fulfillment"; as a consequence, one person's misfortune trans-lates into another person's duty.[21] For all such reasons, decision making in rehabilitation medicine must not only take into account the input of the team framing the options for decisions, but also address the needs of everyone—patients, families, society—affected by the decisions.

SELECTED ISSUES IN REHABILITATION

The Vegetative State

Almost a quarter of a century ago, Plum and Jennett described a syndrome of "wakefulness without awareness," which evolves after traumatic brain injury or anoxic encephalopathy.[22] Recently, a Multi-Society Task Force set forth their judgment on what is known about this syndrome—including probabilities of persistence and permanence in persons of diverse age and general health, who remain in this state for varying periods of time; and estimates of the cost of caring for such persons.[23] Such probabilities and estimates are just that—statistical likelihoods that admit of the possibility of exception.[24] Indeed, some feel that they may be self-fulfilling prophecies.[3] Recognizing that the lines that separate the vegetative state from other chronic disorders of consciousness are not as bright as the Multi-Society Task Force would have us believe, some rehabilitation professionals, including physicians, have called for a finer gradation and classification schema.[25] Issues of surrogate decision making, utilization of resources, beneficence, and respect for autonomy pervade the management of persons in the vegetative state. Physicians caring for such patients would be well-advised to be sensitive and honest in recognizing the ethical theory(ies) that guide(s) their judgment in recommending a course of action in any given setting (*vide supra*, Types of Ethical Theory). In view of the paucity of data on outcome of various "coma stimulation" and other therapeutic programs, there is a special mandate to conduct such therapies in a rigorous manner, collecting data and presenting those data before peers for validation before advertising the therapies as proven.[26] Since the *Cruzan* decision made it legal to withhold food and water from such patients in order that they may die, advance directives and surrogates may request that this be done, although not commonly when the patient is in an active rehabilitation program. Physicians should be honest and open in discussing these and other issues in the care of persons in the vegetative state with their surrogates, looking not only at the benefits and burdens of continued therapy, but also at the reasons for choosing one course of action over another.[14]

Quality of Life and "Futile" Treatment

It has been said that

> *people with disabilities have a problem to be medically cured, therapeutically resolved, behaviorally modified, educationally unlearned, socially reconstructed, or spiritually healed, with the intended result that no one should have any problem and thus be like everyone else: normal . . . (i.e.) more or less like everyone else, with little tolerance for exceptions.*[27]

Deeply entwined within that statement—and indeed, within the goals of rehabilitation medicine *in toto*—are implicit (sometimes explicit) judgments about the value and quality of life. Treatments that do not measure up to those judgments, do not achieve a given value or level of quality, are deemed "futile" by some.[28] Futility in its strictest medical sense equates with physiologic futility, or the failure of a given therapy to achieve its indicated physiologic goal. Thus, it would be physiologically futile to continue cardiopulmonary resuscitation for more than (say) 30 minutes, without restoration of a heart beat. All other levels of medical futility beg a value judgment on the desirability and/or probability of a given outcome in the overall context of a particular patient. It is in this sense that some would regard any rehabilitative effort on behalf of a person in the vegetative state to be futile.[29]

A discipline (such as rehabilitation medicine) that functions in accord with the "educational model" (*vide supra*, The Application of Ethical Theory—Ethics in Rehabilitation Medicine) must be exceptionally sensitive to the distinction between objectively validated outcomes and subjective decisions (and the recommendations that flow therefrom), based implicitly or explicitly on quality of life judgments dressed up in the guise of "futility." This dilemma may arise from the other side of the equation, especially when patients (or their families) make demands for care that flow from unrealistic expectations of outcome.[29] Increasingly, managed care systems weight the equation in the direction of limiting care, setting goals by the "critical pathway" process often according to rigid formulae that do not allow for individual differences in rate or extent of improvement.[30] Rehabilitation physicians, used to the team approach to providing care, are accustomed to the role of

dialog and mediation necessary in discerning the proper pathway for a given patient. In applying that approach to the rehabilitation process from assessment to disposition, neurorehabilitation physicians must constantly search for objectivity and fairness on behalf of their individual patients, convince not only the patient but also the system that the course of action recommended is the right one, and remain committed to that course until the patient is satisfied (or at least accepts) the outcome reached. All of this implies a willingness and openness to change, a true and real devotion to the principle of beneficence.[2]

Ethical Issues in Neurologic Rehabilitation Research

Much of present-day clinical research in neurologic rehabilitation concerns itself with outcomes—a necessary focus in an age of limited resources, when third party payors seek to maximize their fiduciary obligations (to their insured as well as their investors) by limiting their expenditures to *proven* therapeutic regimens. More and more, proof in clinical medicine comes from outcomes research—so-called *evidence-based* medicine.[30] Traditionally, rehabilitation was defined "as the process of developing a person with disability to his or her fullest potential."[31] Treatment was "completely individualized, making any comparison of outcomes across individuals suspect." In today's world, improvement must be proportional to cost, with the "best" outcome "the one that imposes the least financial burden on the entity" paying for the care.[31] The problem lies in the number of variables to be addressed by any therapeutic regimen, the gravity of each contributing variable to disability status, and the relationship between a particular measure of a given variable, and overall outcome. In practice, the definition of outcome that rules is not that given by the patient, or even by the rehabilitation physician, but rather its implementation by payors. Outcome studies must be large enough to be credible, comprehensive enough to distinguish the effects of the treatment regimen from other variables, and honest enough to acknowledge the uncertainties of statistical analysis rather than relying on p values to support practically meaningless conclusions. (Real differences in outcome must supercede scored outcomes.) Rehabilitation physicians *must* engage in outcomes research on behalf of their patients, lest insurance providers dictate care on financial grounds alone.

Special obligations obtain in research on vulnerable persons such as those with a neurologic disability.

Hope, a pervading virtue among persons facing a hopeless life, must not be violated in the process of recruiting patients for research studies—especially those that carry a defined and serious risk, with little but speculative benefit to gain. Patients or their surrogates must be full partners in the research, not pawns "gamed" into participating. The collection and use of data that are falsified or manipulated is obviously an error; but conclusions drawn from inadequate data or methodologically flawed studies are equally wrong in a moral sense, especially when they are then used for economically sound but ethically suspect purposes. For example, if outcome measures in a study of traumatic brain injury (TBI) focus on easily stratified motor functions, and ignore or minimize harder-to-quantitate cognitive findings, some insurers might feel justified in their practice of reimbursing physical but not cognitive therapy in such persons. The exhortation that closed a recent review of challenges for research in TBI is particularly apt.

Allied with persons with disabilities and enlightened members of the insurance industry, rehabilitationists can and must inform the direction of rehabilitation's future.

REFERENCES

1. Hauerwas S: *Suffering Presence.* Notre Dame, IN: University of Notre Dame Press, 1986.
2. Beauchamp TL, Childress JF: *Principles of Biomedical Ethics.* New York: Oxford University Press, 1994 (4th ed).
3. Andrews K: Managing the persistent vegetative state. *BMJ* 1995; 310:341–342.
4. Caplan AL, Callahan D, Haas J: Ethical and policy issues in rehabilitation medicine. *Hastings Center Report* 1987; 17(4; spec supp):1–20.
5. Fletcher JC, Hite CA, Lombardo PA, Marshall MF: *Introduction to Clinical Ethics.* Frederick, MD: University Publishing Group, 1995.
6. Iglehart JK: Health policy report. The American health care system. Managed care. *N Engl J Med* 1992; 327:742–747.
7. *Schloendorff v. Society of New York Hospital*, 211 N.Y. 125, 105 N.E. 92, 95 (1914).
8. Faden RR, Beauchamp TL: *A History and Theory of Informed Consent.* New York: Oxford University Press, 1986.
9. Brody H: *The Healer's Power.* New Haven, CT: Yale University Press, 1992.
10. Silverstein MD, Stocking CB, Antel JP, Beckwith J, Roos RP, Siegler M: Amyotrophic lateral sclerosis and life-sustaining therapy: Patients' desires for information, participation in decision making, and life-sustaining therapy. *Mayo Clin Proc* 1991; 66:906–913.
11. Emanuel LL, Emanuel EJ: The medical directive: A new comprehensive advance care document. *JAMA* 1989; 261:3288–3293.
12. *In re Quinlan*, 70 N.J. 10, 355 A2d 647, cert denied sub nom. *Garger v. New Jersey*, 429 U.U. 922 (1976).
13. *Cruzan v. Director*, Missouri Department of Health, 110 S.Ct. 2841 (1990).
14. Quill T: The ambiguity of clinical intentions. *N Engl J Med* 1993; 329:1039–1040.
15. Haas JF: Admission to rehabilitation centers: Selection of patients. *Arch Phys Med Rehab* 1994; 69:329–332.
16. Brody BA: Justice in the allocation of resources to disabled citizens. *Arch Phys Med Rehab* 1994; 69:333–336.
17. Menzel PT: Oregon's denial. Disabilities and quality of life. *Hastings Cent Report* 1992; 22(6):21–25.
18. Caplan AL: Informed consent and provider-patient relationships in rehabilitation medicine. *Arch Phys Med Rehab* 1988; 69:312–317.
19. Scofield JR: Ethical considerations in rehabilitation medicine. *Arch Phys Med Rehab* 1993; 74:341–346.
20. Callahan D: Families as caregivers: The limits of morality. *Arch Phys Med Rehab* 1988; 69:323–328.
21. Will GF: For the handicapped, rights but no welcome. *Hastings Center Report* 1986; 16(3):5–8.
22. Jennett B, Plum F: Persistent vegetative state after brain damage: A syndrome in search of a name. *Lancet* 1972; i:734–737.
23. The Multi-Society Task Force on PVS: Medical aspects of the persistent vegetative state. *N Engl J Med* 1994; 330:1499–1508, 1572–1579.
24. Childs NL, Mercer WN: Brief report: Late improvement in consciousness after post-traumatic vegetative state. *N Engl J Med* 1996; 334:24–25.
25. American Congress of Rehabilitation Medicine: Recommendations for use of uniform nomenclature pertinent to patients with severe alterations in consciousness. *Arch Phys Med Rehab* 1995; 76:205–209.
26. Banja JD: Deception in advertising and marketing: Ethical applications in rehabilitation. *Arch Phys Med Rehab* 1994; 75:1015–1018.
27. Webb-Mitchell B: Disability. II. Philosophical and theological perspectives, in Reich WT (editor-in-chief): *Encyclopedia of Bioethics* (rev ed), New York, Simon & Schuster Macmillan, 1995, pp. 608–615.
28. Solomon MZ: How physicians talk about futility: Making words mean too many things. *J Law Med Eth* 1993; 21:231–237.
29. Miles SH: Informed demand for "non-beneficial" medical treatment. *N Engl J Med* 1991; 235:512–515.
30. Leape LL: Practice guidelines and standards: An overview. *QRB* 1990; 16:42–49.
31. Banja J, Johnston MV: Outcomes in TBI rehabilitation. Part III: Ethical perspectives and social policy. *Arch Phys Med Rehab* 1994; 75:SC-19-26.

Chapter 4

REGENERATION AND PLASTICITY IN NEUROLOGIC DYSFUNCTION

Michael E. Selzer

IMPORTANCE FOR NEUROREHABILITATION

The role of the medical rehabilitation specialist is changing rapidly. In order to maximally restore function, research and clinical practice in rehabilitation medicine have begun to target not only limiting disabilities, but also the reversal of fixed impairments. These efforts require the application of knowledge of the pathophysiology of injury and of the reparative potential of the nervous system.

Following injuries to the central nervous system (CNS), such as those produced by stroke or trauma, some neurons die and others undergo axotomy. The nervous system makes imperfect accommodations for these losses that include behavioral, physiological, and anatomical plasticity. These are not independent of each other, but build on one another. Behavioral adaptations can be optimized by physical and occupational therapists through an understanding of the changes that occur in CNS physiology immediately after injury. Over a longer period, the CNS has a vast and dynamic potential to respond by altering the strength of neural transmission through modifications in the structure and function of neurons and synapses (Figure 4-1). Neurorehabilitation specialists will need to harness this potential in order to achieve even greater functional recovery.

IMMEDIATE ADAPTIVE CONSEQUENCES OF INJURY

Neurophysiological function can be altered rapidly in a way that seems adaptive because of the unmasking of intrinsic connections in the brain. Merzenich and others have demonstrated that following amputation or anesthetization of a finger, its sensory projection cortex rapidly becomes incorporated into the central representation of adjacent spared body parts (Figure 4-2), with a resulting increase in the sensory discrimination of those spared parts.[1] This may be observed virtually as soon as it can be tested (within 1 hour) and does not require prolonged training or stimulation. This suggests that no changes in synaptic efficacy or neuronal morphology are involved in these early plastic alterations.[2]

The most reasonable explanation for such early changes in sensory representation relates to the intrinsic circuitry of the cortex. Individual thalamocortical sensory relay neurons project to cortical neurons in an area with a radius of approximately 1 mm. Recurrent inhibitory connections within somatosensory cortex also have a radius of 1 mm. Elimination of excitatory input to an area of cortex therefore eliminates inhibition to adjacent areas of cortex with a radius of 1 mm, which also is the approximate distance over which early changes in sensory representation are seen following deafferentation or amputation. Reciprocally, injury to the cortical area of representation for one body part may result in rapid compression of the central representation of that part into the adjacent cortex.

The lost functions that accompany CNS injuries often are partially reversible. Optimal recovery would require replacement of lost neurons, regeneration of severed axons, and restoration of all the synaptic contacts that were lost. Strategies to achieve this are under investigation (see Regeneration, below). However, although there is little frank regeneration in the CNS of mammals, surviving neurons may undergo physiological and morphological changes that can con-

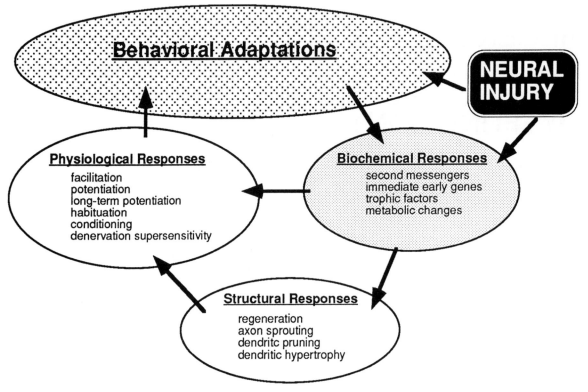

Figure 4-1
Interactions among behavioral, structural, physiological, and biochemical responses of the nervous system to injury. Axotomy results in biochemical changes in the injured neurons by mechanisms that are still not known. The injury also leads to transsynaptic biochemical changes in afferent and efferent neurons. These changes induce expression of genes in a cascade that can lead to structural responses in the injured cell (e.g., axonal regeneration), in its denervated synaptic targets (e.g., dendritic pruning), or in adjacent spared neurons (e.g., collateral sprouting). At the same time, the organism makes behavioral adaptations to the injury, such as overuse of some pathways mediating compensatory behaviors. This overuse leads to other biochemical changes that in turn result in physiological plasticity, such as long-term potentiation. The physiological plasticity in turn leads to more-effective behavioral performance. Some biochemical changes are both structural and physiological in nature since they are visible with the electron microscope (e.g., induction of increased transmitter receptors) and have direct physiological consequences (e.g., denervation supersensitivity).

tribute to spontaneous recovery. Some of these changes are a direct consequence of the altered connectivity, whereas others are owing to the behavioral adaptations employed by the organism. They include changes in the amount of transmitter released, the number and distribution of postsynaptic receptors, the size and complexity of the dendritic trees of spared neurons, and collateral sprouting of spared axons to innervate deafferented neurons.

DELAYED RESPONSES TO INJURY

Synaptic Plasticity

Long-Term Potentiation The behavioral adaptations to injury must necessarily involve changed patterns of use of spared pathways, and this can change the strength of the synapses involved. Several forms

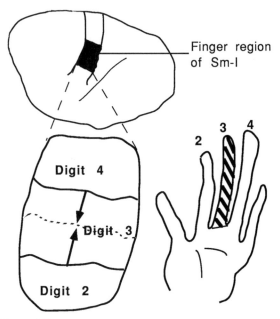

Figure 4-2

Rapid changes in projection maps onto sensorimotor cortex. When the responses of neurons in the monkey's primary somatosensory cortex (Sm-I) are recorded in response to digit stimulation, an orderly somatotopic arrangement is seen, with neurons that respond to stimulation of the third digit located primarily in a region between that representing digit 2 and digit 4. However, following amputation of the third digit, neurons in its former projection area now respond to either digit 2 or digit 4. (Stylized representation of the work of Merzenich MM, Nelson RJ, Stryker MP, et al: Somatosensory cortical map changes following digit amputation in adult monkeys. J Comp Neurol 1984; 224:591–605.)

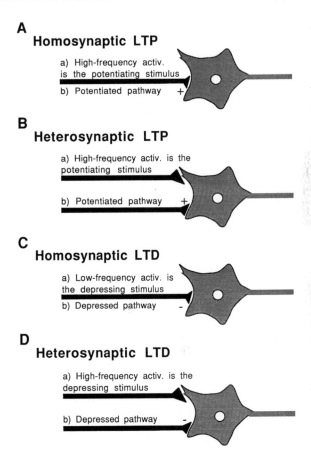

Figure 4-3

Long-term changes in synaptic efficacy. A. Homosynaptic long-term potentiation (LTP). High-frequency stimulation of an afferent pathway leads to long-lasting enhancement of the strength of synaptic transmission of the same pathway. B. Heterosynaptic LTP. High-frequency stimulation of one afferent pathway leads to long-lasting enhancement of the strength of synaptic transmission in another pathway converging on the same postsynaptic neuron. C. Homosynaptic long-term depression (LTD). Low-frequency stimulation of an afferent pathway leads to long-lasting reduction of the strength of synaptic transmission in the same pathway. D. Heterosynaptic LTD. High-frequency stimulation of one afferent pathway leads to long-lasting reduction in the strength of synaptic transmission in another pathway converging on the same postsynaptic neuron.

of long-lasting changes in synaptic efficacy have been described that could contribute to the quality of functional recovery (Figure 4-3). Repeated high-frequency stimulation of excitatory glutamatergic pathways to the pyramidal cells of the CA1 region of the hippocampus results in a large increase in synaptic efficacy of those pathways that lasts for hours or even days.[3] This phenomenon, called long-term potentiation (LTP), is seen in several locations in the brain, and the cellular mechanism may vary from location to location.[4,5] In the CA1 region, LTP appears to result from the binding of glutamate to the N-methyl D-aspartate (NMDA) receptor paired with a large depolarization of the postsynaptic membrane. This permits a large influx of calcium into the postsynaptic cell, resulting

in the activation of an as-yet-unidentified retrograde chemical signal directed back to the presynaptic terminal. The retrograde signal causes an increase in the release of glutamate during subsequent synaptic activations. Some investigators also have suggested that

LTP involves an increased postsynaptic sensitivity to glutamate as well.

An important aspect of LTP is that it can be activated either by homosynaptic or heterosynaptic mechanisms. Homosynaptic activation of LTP (Figure 4-3A) involves stimulation of the potentiated pathway strongly enough that, in addition to binding to the requisite number of NMDA receptors, a large postsynaptic depolarization is produced by the non-NMDA glutamate receptors. Such a mechanism could be relevant to the type of motor learning that occurs when a new skill is practiced. Heterosynaptic LTP (Figure 4-3B) occurs when the potentiated pathway serves as the source of glutamate for NMDA receptor activation while another pathway synapsing on the same postsynaptic neuron

serves to depolarize the postsynaptic membrane. This mechanism could be relevant to associative types of learning, such as classical and operant (trial and error) conditioning.

Long-Term Depression In some circumstances, stimulation of pathways in the brain results in long-term depression (LTD) of synaptic transmission.[6] As with LTP, there are several different mechanisms involved, depending on the location and type of synapse and the pattern of stimulation, and LTD may be either homosynaptic or heterosynaptic. Homosynaptic LTD usually is the result of low-frequency stimulation of the depressed pathway (Figure 4-3C), and involves activation of NMDA receptors. This type of depression could be

Figure 4-4

Denervation supersensitivity at the neuromuscular junction. The innervated portion of the muscle membrane is characterized by postjunctional folds that are located in apposition to the vesicle release sites in the motor axon terminal. Acetylcholine (ACh) released by the presynaptic terminal reacts with receptors (AChR) that are concentrated on the surface of the crests of the postjunctional folds. After a motor axon is cut, the distal stump undergoes Wallerian degeneration and the postjunctional membrane loses its specialized structure. The junctional AChRs disappear and are replaced by a developmentally less mature form of AChR, the extrajunctional AChRs, which are distributed over the entire muscle membrane. Although the portion of membrane previously containing the junctional AChRs is now somewhat less sensitive to the action of ACh, the muscle fiber as a whole is much more sensitive. In the CNS, denervation supersensitivity appears to result from a similar increase in the number of postsynaptic receptors for the various transmitters involved, although they are not necessarily different from the original receptor molecules.

Denervation Supersensitivity at the Neuromuscular Junction

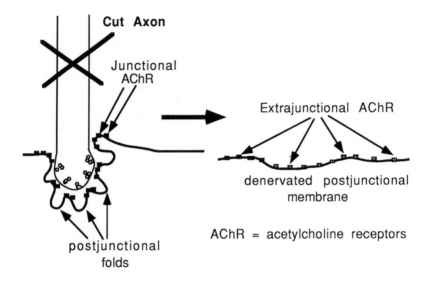

AChR = acetylcholine receptors

involved in a simple form of learning, habituation, in which monotonously repeated stimuli eventually fail to elicit a response. Heterosynaptic LTD occurs when high-frequency activation of one pathway produces a reduction in response of the postsynaptic neuron to stimulation of the second pathway (Figure 4-3D). The mechanism for this type of LTD is unknown, but as with the various forms of LTP, both homosynaptic and heterosynaptic LTD involve an increase in the calcium concentration in the postsynaptic neuron. The differences in the cellular mechanisms relate primarily to the mechanism by which the increase in calcium is achieved; that is, through NMDA receptor activation, voltage-gated membrane calcium channels, intracellular stores, or Na/Ca exchange pumps.

Denervation Supersensitivity When neurons lose a synaptic input, their membranes become more sensitive to the application of the transmitter involved. This process, called denervation supersensitivity, has been studied most extensively at the neuromuscular junction, where it represents an increase in the number of extrajunctional acetylcholine receptors (Figure 4-4) brought about by the loss of electrical activity in the muscle.[7,8] The spread of receptors can be visualized by freeze fracture electron microscopy or by labeling of the acetylcholine receptors with radioisotopic α-bungarotoxin.

Similar processes occur on the surfaces of denervated neurons, including those in the CNS. When the substantia nigra of rats is depleted of dopamine by any of several methods, denervation supersensitivity to dopamine develops in the basal ganglia. This supersensitivity can be demonstrated following intraventricular injection of specific dopamine receptor agonists by behavioral responses, D1 and D2 receptor assays, or ^{14}C-2-deoxyglucose autoradiography.[9,10] Dopamine supersensitivity has been postulated to underlie the dyskinetic toxic reactions to L-dopa in patients with Parkinson's disease. It is reasonable to postulate that, by mediating a compensatory enhancement of responsiveness of neurons that have been partially deafferented by diffuse axonal injury, ischemic neuronal loss, or lacunar infarcts, denervation supersensitivity might participate in the recovery of function that often follows traumatic brain injury or stroke.

Changes in Dendritic Arborizations Loss of innervation can result in altered postsynaptic neuronal morphology. Dendritic spines that have lost their innervation are lost.[11] Dendritic arbors may be simplified, and if insufficient afferent inputs remain, the postsynap-

tic neuron may atrophy. When different inputs to a neuron are segregated on different parts of the dendritic tree, loss of one afferent pathway results in selective reduction in the size of its territory of the dendritic arbor (Figure 4-5).[12] This is termed *dendritic pruning*. How such specificity in the neuron's structural response is achieved has long been a mystery. Electron microscopic observations by Steward and colleagues have

Figure 4-5
Dendritic pruning. Synaptic inputs produce local trophic effects on dendrites. This can be demonstrated in cases where different synaptic inputs are segregated on different parts of the dendritic tree (A). If synaptic pathway A is interrupted, its target dendrites atrophy (B). If afferent pathways A and B were both interrupted, the entire neuron might atrophy.

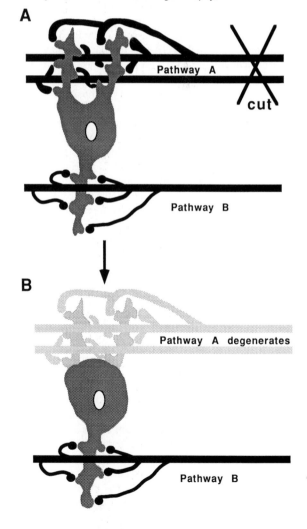

demonstrated clusters of polyribosomes associated with cysternae at the base of dendritic spines. Denervation is associated with loss of these polyribosomes, whereas reinnervation is associated with their return.[13] This suggests that some local trophic influence is transferred across the synapse. Synaptic activity localized to one spine could thus rapidly influence the protein synthesis in that portion of dendrite and thereby affect the size and shape of the dendritic tree.[14]

Collateral Sprouting   Following partial denervation of muscle, neighboring spared axons sprout that reinnervate the denervated muscle fibers.[15,16] The mechanism of this sprouting is not known. Schwann cells of injured axons proliferate in response to contact with degenerating axolemma and increase their expression of nerve growth factor (NGF) receptors.[17,18] The activated Schwann cells also release NGF, probably in response to macrophage-supplied factors such as interleukin-1, but it is unlikely that this is the mechanism for collateral sprouting.[19] Although NGF can stimulate axon elongation of sympathetic and sensory neurons, it does not have this effect on motor neurons. Schwann cells of injured nerve also increase their synthesis of brain-derived neurotrophic factor (BDNF), but this also is likely to affect only sensory and not motor neurons.[20] Schwann cells also make ciliary neurotrophic factor (CNTF), which does have a trophic effect on motor neurons.[21–23] Unlike NGF, CNTF production by Schwann cells decreases in response to nerve injury.[24–26] Nevertheless, it is clear that non-neuronal cells in the vicinity of injured nerves have profoundly altered biologic activities, including expression of many peptides. Some peptides as yet undiscovered, or ones not yet isolated from injured nerve, may be upregulated by axotomy and activate collateral sprouting.

Although initially controversial, it is now established that collateral sprouting also occurs in the CNS. This was first demonstrated by Liu and Chambers in the cat spinal cord by outlining the territory of the central processes of spared dorsal root axons after cutting neighboring dorsal roots.[27] These results were disputed because they were based on degeneration stains, which can give conflicting results. Other methods for detecting dorsal root axons in the cord have upheld the general conclusion that sprouting of dorsal root axons does occur. Similar sprouting of dorsal root axons and corticospinal tract axons was demonstrated autoradiographically in cats and monkeys after a variety of dorsal root and spinal cord lesions.[28,29] Because the time course of the sprouting correlated with the development of hyperreflexia and increased muscle tone following spi-

nal transection, Goldberger and Murray suggested that sprouting might mediate these phenomena, which under some circumstances can be of functional benefit to the CNS-injured organism.

Collateral sprouting also has been demonstrated in the septal nucleus of the brain. Inputs from the fimbria terminate on the dendrites of septal cholinergic neurons, whereas inputs from the median forebrain bundle terminate on both the dendrites and the perikaryon. The synaptic boutons from these two pathways have different appearances in electron micrographs, making it possible to determine the source of synaptic terminals even without the application of anterograde tracing methods. Sectioning of the medial forebrain bundle resulted temporarily in unoccupied postsynaptic sites on the perikarya and dendrites, with a concomitant loss of synaptic spines. These sites became reoccupied over several weeks by synaptic boutons of collateral sprouts from the fimbria (Figure 4-6).[30]

Another example of collateral sprouting in the brain has been described in the hippocampus. The granule cells of the dentate gyrus receive inputs from the ipsilateral entorhinal cortex, the septum, and the contralateral hippocampus. These inputs ordinarily are segregated on different parts of the dendritic tree. Eliminating one of these pathways resulted in loss of synaptic boutons and spines on the predicted portion of the dendrites during the first week.[31] Over the next several weeks, sprouting occurs from fimbrial axons, which form synapses along the denervated portions of dendrites.[32–34] Regardless of location in the CNS, collateral sprouts generally grow no more than 250 μm. An exception is the enlargement of the contralateral projection to the dentate gyrus following ipsilateral entorhinal lesions. In this case, the sprouting fibers may grow as much as 2–3 mm.[34]

The functional effectiveness of sprouting in the brain is not clear. If replacement synapses are from inappropriate sources, the net effect could be malfunctional. However, when there is only partial damage to an afferent pathway, as often occurs with the diffuse axonal injury that occurs with head trauma, the result could be collateral sprouting of spared fibers from the same source as the injured axons. The net effect in this case may be beneficial, as it certainly is at the neuromuscular junction.

REGENERATION

As opposed to collateral sprouting, which involves growth of neurites from spared axons, the term *regenera-*

Figure 4-6

Collateral sprouting in the septal nucleus. A. The cholinergic neurons of the septal nucleus normally receive synaptic input from the fimbria and the medial forebrain bundle (MFB). The fimbrial axons synapse only on the distal dendrites, whereas MFB axons synapse both on the dendrites and perikaryon. The synaptic terminals of these two inputs have different ultrastructural characteristics and can be distinguished from each other on electron micrographs. B. Following lesioning of the MFB, characteristic fimbrial terminals appear on the perikarya of septal neurons and are increased in numbers on the dendrites. This indicates that the axons of the fimbria sprouted collaterals and occupied postsynaptic sites previously occupied by MFB terminals. (After the work of Raisman G: Neuronal plasticity in the septal nuclei of the adult rat. Brain Res 1969; 14:25–48.)

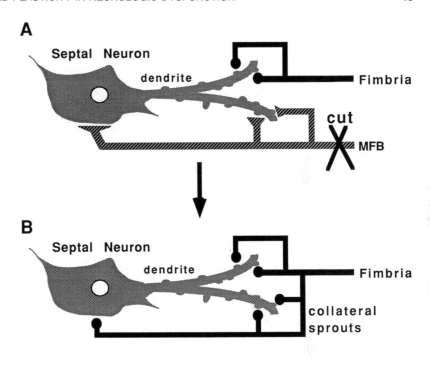

tion generally is applied to regrowth of injured tissue. Regeneration of injured axons does not occur spontaneously to a significant degree within the CNS of mammals, although it may proceed over distances similar to that of collateral sprouting (<1 mm). The failure of regeneration is due to inhibitory influences in the extracellular environment of the growing axon tip. In the early 1980s, Aguayo and colleagues demonstrated that spinal cord neurons of rat could send axons for several cm into sciatic nerve grafts.[35] These observations led to the search for molecules characteristic of CNS, but not PNS, that could block axon growth.

Factors Preventing Regeneration in CNS

Growth Cone Collapsing Factors   Several molecules found in the mature nervous system have been shown to inhibit axon growth in tissue culture by causing collapse of the growth cone. In this type of study, embryonic neurons are grown on various adhesive substrates, such as poly-L-lysine or laminin. Under these circumstances, the leading edge of the growing axon consists of a specialized structure called the *growth cone*, which

is characterized by a flat proximal expanse called a *lamellipodium* and distal fingerlike projections called *filopodia* (Figure 4-7A). The filopodia contain bundles of 1- to 12-actin microfilaments and elongate on the extracellular matrix by a process that probably involves the polymerization and elongation of the actin filaments.[36,37] Microtubules concentrate in the region of actively elongating filopodia, possibly in response to retrograde transport of polymerized actin to the base of the filopodium.[4,5] The lamellipodium spreads forward between adjacent elongating filopodia, thus establishing the direction of forward growth of the axon.[38] This mechanism of axon elongation is specialized for the rapid (1–3 mm/day) growth that characterizes early embryonic development as studied in insects.[39,40] How this relates to the regeneration of mature axons in an injured CNS environment is not known, but work in the lamprey suggests that regeneration in situ may involve quite different mechanisms.

In the lamprey, complete transection of the spinal cord is followed by behavioral recovery and regeneration of 50 to 60 percent of cut axons across the injury site.[41–44] Some of these axons are very large and have been impaled with tracer-containing microelectrodes so

A

Growth Cone in Tissue Culture

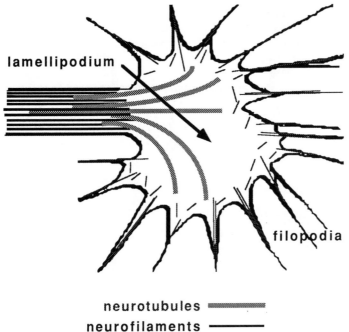

lamellipodium

filopodia

neurotubules
neurofilaments
actin   microfilaments

B

Lamprey Growth Cone Regenerating *In Situ*

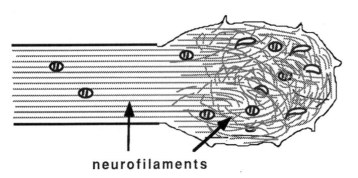

neurofilaments

Figure 4-7
Comparison between growth cones of embryonic neurons grown in tissue culture and growth cones of regenerating axons in the lamprey spinal cord. A. When embryonic neurons are placed on an appropriate adhesive substrate, they send out processes with specialized growing tips called "growth cones." These consist of a flattened broad proximal portion, the lamellipodium, and spikelike projections, the filopodia. The cytoskeleton of the lamellipodium contains microtubules and actin microfilaments. The latter are randomly ordered and may be short or arranged in small bundles of up to 12 long filaments. The filopodia contain only the bundles of long microfilaments. The growth cone contains no neurofilaments, which constitute the most prominent component of the cytoskeleton in the axon proper. B. By contrast, growth cones of regenerating Müller axons in the transected lamprey spinal cord have a simple shape, lacking filopodia and lamellipodia. They contain very little actin and are packed with swirls of neurofilaments. (Lurie DI, Pijak DS, Selzer ME: The structure of reticulospinal axon growth cones and their cellular environment during regeneration in the lamprey spinal cord. J Comp Neurol 1994; 344:559–580.)

that their regenerating tips could be identified in whole-mounted preparations and reconstructed from light and electron microscopic sections.[43,45,46] Unlike growth cones of embryonic neurons, the growth cones of lamprey neurons regenerating in situ are simple in shape, lacking lamellipodia and filopodia (Figure 4-7B). Moreover, although the growth cones of embryonic neurons in tissue culture lack neurofilaments, growth cones of regenerating axons in the lamprey spinal cord contain abundant neurofilaments, which are packed more densely than they are in the proximal axon.[3,46] It has been suggested that in the mature nervous system, in which specific adhesion molecules may be absent from the extracellular environment or their receptors no longer present on neuronal surfaces, transport of neurofilaments into the growth cone may underlie regeneration by pushing the advancing tip forward.

Despite the possible differences between the mechanism of axon elongation as studied in tissue culture and that seen during regeneration in the more mature CNS, most work on the molecular mechanisms involved in growth inhibition have employed tissue culture assays because they permit direct observation of the growth cone. One type of growth-inhibiting effect was described by Schwab and his colleagues, who showed that, although neurons can grow long processes on cultured Schwann cells, they do not do so on CNS myelin.[47] Caroni and Schwab identified two molecules with MW 35,000 and 250,000 on the surfaces of oligodendrocytes that cause growth cones to collapse on contact (Figure 4-8).[48] Both molecules are bound by a single mAb (IN-1), so they are probably structurally related. It has been suggested that the mechanism by which these molecules cause growth cone collapse involves activation of G-proteins and release of calcium from intracellular stores.[49,50] Excess Ca^{2+} can activate disaggregation of cytoskeletal elements, such as microtubules and actin microfilaments, that are thought to be important in growth cone motility. More recently, another myelin surface molecule, myelin associated glycoprotein, has been shown to inhibit axon growth in vitro, but the mechanism and significance of this effect are not known.[51,52]

Similar growth cone collapsing activity is associated with neuronal membranes. Axons from the nasal side of the developing retina grow selectively to the posterior part of the optic tectum, whereas temporal retinal axons grow to the anterior tectum. This effect can be studied in vitro. When neurons from the nasal and temporal retina of the chick were grown on strips of posterior and anterior optic tectum, the posterior tectal membranes caused collapse of temporal but not nasal retinal growth cones.[53] A similar series of collapsing activities was found on neurites of cultured chick CNS and PNS.[54] Growth cones collapsed upon encountering neurites from parts of the nervous system with which they normally did not have contact but continued to advance normally when they encountered neurites from the same part of the nervous system or a normal target. Unlike the myelin-associated collapsing activity of Schwab, the neurite-associated collapsing activity did not involve an increase in growth cone calcium concentration.[55] Raper has extracted a protein from chick brain that causes collapse of dorsal root ganglia growth cones.[56] This factor, which has been called *collapsin*, is an 88 kDa transmembrane protein belonging to the immunoglobulin superfamily.[57] Collapsin has now been shown to be a member of the semaphorin family of transmembrane and secreted proteins, which have been cloned from insects, chicks, mice, and humans.[58–61] In at least some cases, they are expressed by neurons and may represent the collapsing factors that cause neurites to stop growing when they encounter axons of incorrect target neurons. The semaphorins are expressed during early development and appear to be important in guiding the developing axons to their correct targets. Whether semaphorins play a role in inhibiting regeneration in the more mature nervous system remains to be seen.

An important feature of these growth cone collapsing activities is that they require, not only the inhibitory molecule, but also the presence of receptors on the surfaces of susceptible neurons. The same neuron that is unable to regenerate an axon into a myelinated tract following injury in the mature animal may do so readily during development, presumably because the neuron has acquired receptors for myelin-associated growth-inhibiting molecules. This has been convincingly demonstrated by experiments in which embryonic neurons were able to grow long axons when transplanted into various white matter tracts in the adult mouse.[62]

Astrocyte-Derived Extracellular Matrix Molecules   The astrocytic scar is inhibitory to axon growth. It was long assumed that this was related to the scar's hard consistency and other mechanical features, but recent work suggests more-specific molecular mechanisms may be involved. Whereas membrane fractions from gray matter, lacking myelin, support axon growth in vitro, membrane fractions from astrocytic scars do not.[63] This growth-inhibiting activity appears to be associated with an as yet incompletely characterized cell surface

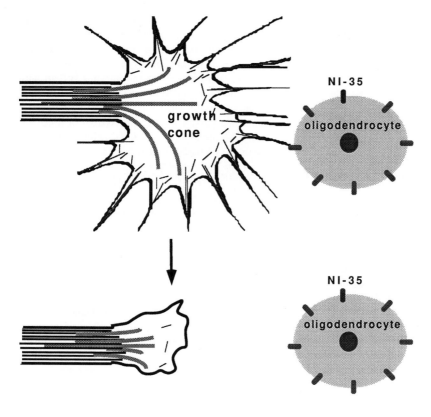

Figure 4-8
Growth cone collapsing molecules associated with CNS myelin. Oligodendrocytes contain two surface molecules, NI-35 and NI-250 that inhibit axon growth by causing collapse of the growth cone on contact. (Caroni P, Schwab ME: Two membrane protein fractions from rat central myelin with inhibitory properties for neurite growth and fibroblast spreading. J Cell Biol 1988; 106:1281–1288.) These molecules appear to interact with receptors that are linked by a G-protein to a release of calcium from intracellular stores. (Igarashi M, Strittmatter SM, Vartanian T, et al: Mediation by G-proteins of signals that cause collapse of growth cones. Science 1993; 259:77–79. Bandtlow CE, Schmidt MF, Hassinger TD, et al: Role of intracellular calcium in NI-35-evoked collapse of neuronal growth cones. Science 1993; 259:80–83.) It is postulated that the excess calcium mediates the dissociation of fibrous actin and microtubules, causing the growth cone to collapse.

glycoprotein of the glycosaminoglycan type. One such molecule, keratan sulfate proteoglycan, is present in the glial roof plate of the developing spinal cord, where it is probably secreted by astrocytes.[64] It may serve as a barrier to abnormal decussation of axons in the dorsal columns.[65] Thus, the secretion of proteoglycans by reactive astrocytes at the site of injury has been proposed as a mechanism by which the glial scar inhibits axonal regeneration in the CNS.[66]

Approaches to Inducing Regeneration in CNS

Peripheral Nerve Bridges The discovery of specific molecular mechanisms by which regeneration is inhibited has suggested interventions that may promote regeneration. However, most approaches to this problem have made use of more-general information about the inhibitory nature of the mature CNS extracellular environment. Aguayo and colleagues have used the ability of CNS axons to regenerate in peripheral nerve grafts to reconnect transected optic nerve to the superior colliculus (Figure 4-9).[67] A few axons reach the tectum and form synapses that mediate electrical responses to illumination of the retina.[68] The nerve grafts appear to be supplying two important components to the axotomized neurons. First they release trophic factors necessary for the survival of the neurons, especially BDNF and neurotrophin 4/5 (NT-4/5).[69–71] Similar nerve grafts have been reported to mediate light-dark discrimination in hamsters.[72] Such techniques have potential for enhancing recovery in cases of complete or near complete interruption of long white matter tracts, as in spinal cord injury. Peripheral nerve grafts might be less useful in those cases of traumatic brain injury in which loss of function

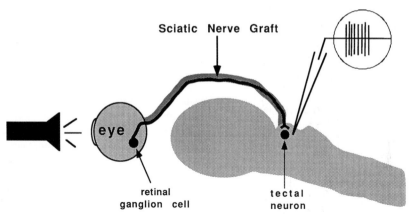

Figure 4-9
Regeneration of retinotectal axons through peripheral nerve bridges. In mammals, cutting the optic nerve is not followed by regeneration but results in death of almost all of the retinal ganglion cells. However, if a graft of sciatic nerve is placed between the proximal cut end of the optic nerve and the tectum, some ganglion cells are rescued and their axons regenerate into the tectum for up to 1 mm. There they form synapses with tectal neurons, which may respond with action potential discharges to stimulation of the retina with light. (Carter DA, Bray GM, Aguayo AJ: Regenerated retinal ganglion cell axons can form well-differentiated synapses in the superior colliculus of adult hamsters. J Neurosci 1989; 9:4042–4050. Aguayo AJ, Bray GM, Rasminsky M, et al: Synaptic connections made by axons regenerating in the central nervous system of adult mammals. J Exp Biol 1990; 153:199–224.)

is attributed to diffuse axonal injury or to neuronal loss secondary to cerebral contusions.

Fetal CNS Transplants   Since axons grow readily in the CNS during early development, fetal CNS transplants have been used not only to replace injured brain or spinal cord neurons, but also to act as bridges for axonal regeneration. This technique was first applied to the problem of replacing transmitter-specific neurons in lesioned animals.

Cholinergic and Dopaminergic Neurons   Transplanted fetal cholinergic neurons restored cholinergic innervation of the hippocampus of rats following bilateral hippocampal deafferentation. This also reversed the learning deficits.[73] Similarly, transplanting dopaminergic neurons into brains of animals restored dopaminergic innervation of the striatum and reversed behavioral deficits in animal models of Parkinson's disease.[74] There is even evidence that transplantation of fetal dopaminergic neurons into human Parkinson's patients is followed by graft survival and symptomatic improvement for periods up to 3 years.[75,76]

Mixed Neuronal Replacement   Functional improvement following transplantation of dopaminergic neurons in experimental animals and humans need not involve establishment of specific synaptic connections, but may be based on a neuroendocrine type of release of dopamine into the brain by the transplanted cells. However, animal models of Huntington's disease have been developed by injection of excitotoxins, such as quinolinic acid, into the neostriatum of rats, resulting in a pattern of neuronal loss that is strikingly similar to that of Huntington's disease, with selective degeneration of the small and medium-sized (GABA- and substance P-containing) spiny neurons.[77–80] The animals develop hyperactivity (not chorea or dystonia) and learning deficits.[81,82] Transplantation of fetal striatum in these animals is followed by survival of the transplants, which become integrated into the host striatum, anatomically connected to appropriate neighboring brain regions, and mediate behavioral recovery.[83,84] A similar model has been developed in primates.[85,86] The successful cloning of the gene for Huntington's disease should permit the development of a transgenic animal model that might mimic the human disease even more closely.[87] A human clinical trial has been initiated, but the outcome has not been reported.[88] Unlike experimental or human Parkinson's disease, the lesions in experimental Huntington's disease are of multiple cell types, and functional recovery is probably based on synaptic reconnection.

Fetal Transplantation in the Spinal Cord Another circumstance that is very likely to require synaptic reconnection for recovery of function is spinal cord injury. Fetal spinal cord tissue has been transplanted into thoracic spinal transections in rats and cats. Although the experience has been disappointing when the transplantation was performed on adult animals, more promising results have been obtained when the recipient was a neonatal animal.[89] As these animals mature, they function better than similarly transected, untransplanted animals.[90,91]

Three mechanisms have been proposed to explain the effectiveness of the transplants (Figure 4-10). First, they may act as sources of target-derived neurotrophic factors and thus rescue axotomized neurons from retrograde cell death.[92,93] The rescued neurons could participate in local reflexes that enhance function, even in the absence of regenerating supraspinal axons (Figure 4-10A). Second, transplants may act as bridges through which axons can regenerate (Figure 4-10B). This has been demonstrated primarily in partially transected neonatal rats with regard to corticospinal neurons, reticulospinal serotonergic neurons, and other brain stem neurons with spinal projections.[94–96] Although some of the axons crossing the transplant represent late-developing pathways, some are regenerating fibers that had been transected.[96] Finally, host neurons may form synapses with neurons in the graft, and these in turn may send axons to the distal cord, making synaptic contacts with target neurons. Thus, the transplant may function as a synaptic relay between neurons located rostral and caudal to the injury. Although tract-tracing studies suggest that few axons from fetal transplants invade adult host spinal cord and vice versa, some adult dorsal root ganglion cell axons have been observed to regenerate into fetal transplants and to form synapses with transplant neurons.[97–99]

Genetically Engineered Cell Lines

Fetal CNS has two significant limitations as a source of transplantable neurons and glia. First, there is limited availability, and second, it is subject to ethical controversy. In recent years, genetically engineered cell lines have been developed that may serve as substitutes for fetal tissue.

Fibroblasts Fibroblasts ordinarily continue to undergo mitosis in vivo and therefore are potentially useful for genetic engineering. These cells have been modified to secrete dopamine and have been implanted into rats made dopamine deficient by injections of 6-OH-dopamine into the substantia nigra. This has resulted in reversal of some of the behavioral deficits.[100] Fibroblasts engineered to express NGF and implanted into the hippocampus of rats enhanced regeneration of cholinergic neurons into the hippocampus.[101] Such cells apparently are able to function in a neuroendocrine fashion, releasing gene product into the surrounding CNS parenchyma. However, they do not send out axons and thus do not have the potential to become incorporated into synaptic circuitry.

Neurons Neural cell lines recently have been developed from human tumors that can be made postmitotic by temperature changes or exposure to retinoic acid.[102,103] When transplanted into the CNS, these cells send out axons and acquire other neuronal phenotypic characteristics.[104] They are now being transfected with genes for desired neuronal products and implanted into the brains and spinal cords of experimental animals. The functional consequences of such implantations are not yet known.

Immortalized Embryonic Precursor Cells Perhaps the most promising transplantable tissues for neural repair are the various neuronal and glial progenitors derived from embryonic CNS. For example, oligodendrocyte progenitor cells have been injected into experimental demyelinating lesions in rat spinal cord and have remyelinated axons.[105] Moreover, when treated with certain neurotrophins—epidermal growth factor (EGF), basic fibroblast growth factor (bFGF), and others—or transfected with immortalizing genes via retroviral vectors, cells of the embryonic nervous system will become immortal in vitro.[106–108] On transplantation into the CNS, these cells become postmitotic after one or two divisions and assume the range of phenotypes for which they were fated at the time of transfection.[109–111] Thus, an immortalized neural precursor cell will give rise to neurons, a glial precursor will give rise to glia, and a stem cell will give rise to a wide range of neuronal and glial phenotypes, depending on the extracellular environment into which it has been placed.[112] These cell lines are now being modified to express a variety of potentially therapeutic molecules, such as trophic factors or transmitter synthesizing enzymes. Enhanced expression of tyrosine hydroxylase by an immortalized

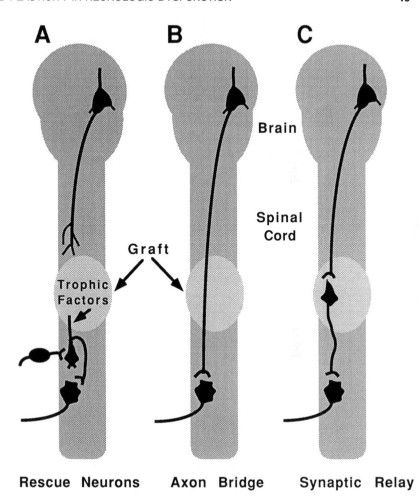

Figure 4-10
Mechanisms by which fetal nerve grafts may enhance function in injured spinal cord. A. They might release trophic factors that rescue axotomized or deafferented neurons from cell death or atrophy. B. They might serve as bridges through which axons can regenerate in order to establish connections with neurons distal to the injury. C. They may permit the reconnection of rostral and caudal stumps of cord indirectly through synaptic relays with neurons in the graft.

substantia nigra–derived cell line has been produced by transfection with tyrosine hydroxylase containing expression vectors. When transplanted into pharmacologically parkinsonian rats and monkeys, these cells produced dopamine and reversed the behavioral deficits.[113] Thus, there is promise that genetically engineered neuronal and glial progenitors may become useful in restoring function to the injured or diseased human nervous system.

Antibodies to Growth Cone–Inhibiting Molecules
Schwab and colleagues have tested the ability of antibodies directed at oligodendrocyte-associated growth cone collapsing factors to promote regeneration.[114] IN-1 secreting hybridomas were transplanted into the parietal lobes of rats, which were then subjected to spi-

nal cord dorsal over-hemisection (Figure 4-11). In rats this interrupts both corticospinal tracts. Regeneration of corticospinal axons was demonstrated by injecting horseradish peroxidase (HRP) into the cortex and waiting for anterograde transport into the growing terminals. In rats with the test hybridomas, corticospinal tract fibers grew up to 15 mm around and beyond the hemisection. Regeneration in control rats was no more than 1 mm. The antibodies presumably enhanced the growth of axons within white matter, since there is no indication that axons were able to grow through the hemisection scar, and these same antibodies neutralize the growth-inhibiting effect of oligodendrocytes in vitro. Recently, it has been reported that the antibody-enhanced regeneration results in behavioral improvement, including the return of contact-placing reflexes in the hindlimbs and

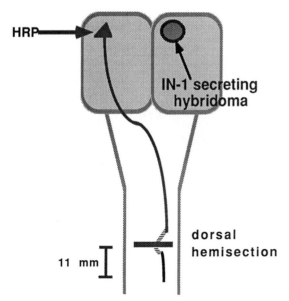

Figure 4-11

Enhancement of regeneration by antibodies to growth-inhibiting molecules. Ordinarily, when the corticospinal tract of a rat is cut by dorsal overhemisection of the spinal cord, the cut axons regenerate no more than 1 mm around the lesion. However, Schnell and Schwab implanted the hybridoma that secretes an antibody (IN-1) directed against two myelin-associated growth cone collapsing proteins into the cortex of rats, and simultaneously performed a dorsal overhemisection of the cord. (Schnell L, Schwab ME: Axonal regeneration in the rat spinal cord produced by an antibody against myelin-associated neurite growth inhibitors. Nature 1990; 343:269–272.) After 2–3 weeks, they injected horseradish peroxidase into the contralateral motor cortex in order to label the regenerating axon terminals by anterograde transport. Corticospinal axons had regenerated as much as 11 mm beyond the lesion.

normalization of stride length.[91] It is possible that similar techniques could be used to overcome other growth inhibitory molecules, such as proteoglycans that are associated with reactive astrocytes, and that this could enhance growth through a scar.

Combination Treatments Since there are multiple regeneration-inhibiting factors at work in the mature CNS, it is likely that optimal recovery will require a combination of approaches. Schnell and Schwab repeated their experiments on dorsal over-hemisections and IN-1 secreting hybridomas, but with the insertion of fetal spinal cord tissue into the lesion.[115] This resulted in a similar increase in distance of axonal regeneration

as was seen with antibody treatment alone. However, there was also an increase in the number of axon sprouts emanating from the lesioned corticospinal tracts. This was attributed to soluble factors released from the transplants because axons grew around the fetal spinal cord transplants and not through them. Fetal spinal cord transplants contain several trophic factors, including NT-3. When local NT-3 injections were substituted for the fetal transplants, the same effect on sprouting and regeneration of corticospinal tract axons was seen.[116] Other neurotrophins did not have the same effect.

Specificity of Regeneration

If quantitatively substantial regeneration in mammalian CNS is achieved, it will be important to determine whether the connections made by regenerating axons are appropriate to their function. Misguided regeneration could be worse than no regeneration if it leads to chaotic useless neuronal activity. It is clear from work on several species of invertebrates and vertebrates that the development of connections between neurons is highly specific, involving both attractive and repulsive molecular interactions.[117–119] A fundamental question for work in regeneration is whether the same or similar molecular cues are present in the mature CNS, so that regenerating axons can be guided in their correct paths and make synapses with their correct target neurons. Several models of regeneration in the CNS of lower vertebrates have suggested that this is so. Following lesions of the optic nerves of fish and frogs, axons regenerate to the optic tectum in a retinotopically correct way, and accurate vision is restored.[120,121] In the frog spinal cord, dorsal roots that have been cut or crushed can regenerate and form synaptic contacts selectively with appropriate agonist motoneurons.[122]

A striking example of specificity in CNS regeneration has been described in the lamprey spinal cord. Following spinal cord transection, axons tend to regrow in their original paths in a manner that suggests that they may be following guidance cues in their local environment.[44,123,124] Regenerating axons form functioning synapses selectively with correct neurons distal to the lesion.[125,126]

The molecular mechanisms underlying the specificity shown by regenerating axons in the CNS of lower vertebrates are still unknown. However, in the lamprey, glial cells may be important in determining the ease and correctness of regeneration, since 80 percent of the growth cone surfaces of regenerating spinal axons are in contact with glial processes.[46] These glial cells differ from mammalian astrocytes in being interconnected by desmosomes and in having intermediate filaments that are heteropolymers of keratin subunits rather than glial fibrillary acidic protein.[127] This type of glial cell also has been found in other lower vertebrates, particularly in parts of the CNS that show axonal regeneration.[128-132] Perhaps the desmosomes serve to stabilize the glial architecture at the site of injury, thus preserving correctly "labeled" pathways for axons to grow along.

It would seem from work in these lower vertebrate models that some recognition molecules must persist or be reexpressed following injury in the mature nervous system. If this is also true of mammals, then therapeutic strategies aimed at increasing the quantity of axonal regeneration may result in functional improvement.

CONCLUSIONS

A variety of mechanisms are available to the central nervous system to compensate for traumatic or ischemic damage. These methods include physiological plasticity in spared synaptic circuits, denervation supersensitivity, dendritic pruning in deafferented neurons, and collateral sprouting of spared axons. In the mammal, there is little evidence that lost neurons can be replaced spontaneously by mitosis or that injured axons can regenerate across a lesion. However, new discoveries concerning the molecular mechanisms underlying this failure of regeneration, technological advances in fetal tissue transplantation, and the revolution in gene transfer technology have brought us close to being able to induce quantitatively significant regeneration in mammalian CNS. The specific trophic factors needed by axotomized neurons in order to forestall their atrophy or death are being discovered and may eventually be supplied through implanted synthetic polymer capsules, appropriate fetal tissue, or genetically engineered cell lines. Lost neurons might be replaced, as in the case of animal models of Huntington's disease. Interrupted axon pathways could be induced to regrow via implanted nerve bridges or synthetic guides. When this is achieved, it will still be necessary for regenerated neurites to form appropriate connections. Evidence primarily from lower vertebrates suggests that some specificity cues that serve to order the embryonic development of neuronal circuitry may persist or become reexpressed in the mature nervous system. If so, then the regeneration encouraged by the application of new technology may result in real functional improvement.

REFERENCES

1. Merzenich MM, Nelson RJ, Stryker MP, et al: Somatosensory cortical map changes following digit amputation in adult monkeys. *J Comp Neurol* 1984; 224:591–605.
2. Merzenich MM, Jenkins WM: Reorganization of cortical representations of the hand following alterations of skin inputs induced by nerve injury, skin island transfers, and experience. *J Hand Ther* 1993; 6:89–104.
3. Bliss TVP, Collingridge GL: A synaptic model of memory: Long-term potentiation in the hippocampus. *Nature* 1993; 361:31–39.
4. Nicoll RA, Malenka RC: Contrasting properties of two forms of long-term potentiation in the hippocampus. *Nature* 1995; 377:115–118.
5. Gozlan H, Khazipov R, Ben AY: Multiple forms of long-term potentiation and multiple regulatory sites of N-methyl-D-aspartate receptors: Role of the redox site. *J Neurobiol* 1995; 26:360–369.
6. Linden DJ, Connor JA: Long-term synaptic depression. [Review.] *Annu Rev Neurosci* 1995; 18:319–357.
7. Lømø T, Rosenthal J: Control of acetylcholine sensitivity by muscle activity in the rat. *J Physiol* (London) 1972; 221:493–513.
8. Eken T, Gundersen K: Chronic electrical stimulation resembling normal motor-unit activity: Effects on denervated fast and slow rat muscles. *J Physiol* (London) 1988; 402:651–669.
9. Rioux L, Gaudin DP, Gagnon C, et al: Decrease of behavioral and biochemical denervation supersensitivity of rat striatum by nigral transplants. *Neuroscience* 1991; 44:75–83.
10. Trugman JM, James CL: Rapid development of dopaminergic supersensitivity in reserpine-treated rats demonstrated with 14C-2-deoxyglucose autoradiography. *J Neurosci* 1992; 12:2875–2879.
11. Caceres AO, Steward O: Dendritic reorganization in the denervated dentate gyrus of the rat following entorhinal cortical lesions: A Golgi and electron microscopic analysis. *J Comp Neurol* 1983; 214:387–403.
12. Deitch JS, Rubel EW: Afferent influences on the brain stem auditory nuclei of the chicken: The course and specificity of dendritic atrophy following deafferentation. *J Comp Neurol* 1984; 229:66–79.
13. Steward O: Alterations in polyribosomes associated with dendritic spines during the reinnervation of the dentate gyrus of the adult rat. *J Neurosci* 1983; 3:177–188.
14. Steward O, Davis L, Dotti C, et al: Protein synthesis and processing in cytoplasmic microdomains beneath postsynaptic sites on CNS neurons. *Mol Neurobiol* 1988; 2:227–261.
15. Edds MV Jr: Collateral regeneration of residual motor axons in partially denervated muscles. *J Exp Zool* 1950; 113:517–552.
16. Brown MC, Holland RL, Hopkins WG: Motor nerve sprouting. *Ann Rev Neurosci* 1981; 4:17–42.

17. Salzer JL, Bunge RP, Glaser L: Studies of Schwann cell proliferation. III. Evidence for the surface localization of the neurite mitogen. *J Cell Biol* 1980; 84:767–778.

18. Tanuichi M, Clark HB, Schweitzer JB, et al: Expression of nerve growth factor receptors by Schwann cells of axotomized peripheral nerves: Ultrastructural location, suppression by axonal contact, and binding properties. *J Neurosci* 1988; 10:664–681.

19. Heumann R, Korsching S, Bandtlow C, et al: Changes of nerve growth factor synthesis in nonneuronal cells in response to sciatic nerve transection. *J Cell Biol* 1987; 104:1623–1631.

20. Meyer M, Matsuoka I, Wetmore C, et al: Enhanced synthesis of brain-derived neurotrophic factor in the lesioned peripheral nerve: Different mechanisms are responsible for the regulation of BDNF and NGF mRNA. *J Cell Biol* 1992; 119:45–54.

21. Dobrea GM, Unnerstall JR, Rao MS: The expression of CNTF message and immunoreactivity in the central and peripheral nervous system of the rat. *Brain Res Dev Brain Res* 1992; 66:209–219.

22. Sendtner M, Arakawa Y, Stockli KA, et al: Effect of ciliary neurotrophic factor (CNTF) on motoneuron survival. *J Cell Sci Suppl* 1991; 15:103–109.

23. Masu Y, Wolf E, Holtmann B, et al: Disruption of the CNTF gene results in motor neuron degeneration. *Nature* 1993; 365:27–32.

24. Sendtner M, Stockli KA, Thoenen H: Synthesis and localization of ciliary neurotrophic factor in the sciatic nerve of the adult rat after lesion and during regeneration. *J Cell Biol* 1992; 118:139–148.

25. Friedman B, Scherer SS, Rudge JS, et al: Regulation of ciliary neurotrophic factor expression in myelin-related Schwann cells in vivo. *Neuron* 1992; 9:295–305.

26. Smith GM, Rabinovsky ED, McManaman JL, et al: Temporal and spatial expression of ciliary neurotrophic factor after peripheral nerve injury. *Exp Neurol* 1993; 121:239–247.

27. Liu CN, Chambers WW: Intraspinal sprouting of dorsal root axons. *Arch Neurol Psychiatr* 1958; 79:46–61.

28. Goldberger ME, Murray M: Restitution of function and collateral sprouting in the cat spinal cord: The deafferented animal. *J Comp Neurol* 1974; 158:37–54.

29. Murray M, Goldberger ME: Restitution of function and collateral sprouting in the cat spinal cord: The partially hemisected animal. *J Comp Neurol* 1974; 158:19–36.

30. Raisman G: Neuronal plasticity in the septal nuclei of the adult rat. *Brain Res* 1969; 14:25–48.

31. Parnavelas JG, Lynch G, Brecha N, et al: Spine loss and regrowth in hippocampus following deafferentation. *Nature* 1974; 248:71–73.

32. Lynch G, Mosko S, Parks T, et al: Relocation and hyperdevelopment of the dentate gyrus commissural system after entorhinal lesions in immature rats. *Brain Res* 1973; 50:174–178.

33. Lynch G, Stanfield B, Parks T, et al: Evidence for selective postlesion axonal growth in the hippocampus. *Brain Res* 1974; 69:1–11.

34. Steward O, Cotman CW, Lynch GS: Growth of a new fiber projection in the brain of adult rats: Re-innervation of the dentate gyrus by contralateral entorhinal cortex following ipsilateral entorhinal lesions. *Exp Brain Res* 1974; 20:45–66.

35. David S, Aguayo AJ: Axonal elongation into peripheral nervous system "bridges" after central nervous system injury in adult rats. *Science* 1981; 214:931–933.

36. Lewis AK, Bridgman PC: Nerve growth cone lamellipodia contain two populations of actin filaments that differ in organization and polarity. *J Cell Biol* 1992; 119:1219–1243.

37. Fan J, Mansfield SG, Redmond T, et al: The organization of F-actin and microtubules in growth cones exposed to a brain-derived collapsing factor. *J Cell Biol* 1993; 121:867–878.

38. Fan J, Raper JA: Localized collapsing cues can steer growth cones without inducing their full collapse. *Neuron* 1995; 14:263–274.

39. Placzek M, Yamada T, Tessier-Lavigne M, et al: Control of dorsoventral pattern in vertebrate neural development: Induction and polarizing properties of the floor plate. *Development* 1991; 2:105–122.

40. Keshishian H, Bentley D: Embryogenesis of peripheral nerve pathways in grasshopper legs. I. The initial pathway to the CNS. *Dev Biol* 1983; 96:89–102.

41. Rovainen CM: Regeneration of Müller and Mauthner axons after spinal transection in larval lampreys. *J Comp Neurol* 1976; 168:5 545–554.

42. Selzer ME: Mechanisms of functional recovery and regeneration after spinal cord transection in larval sea lamprey. *J Physiol* (London) 1978; 277:395–408.

43. Yin HS, Selzer ME: Axonal regeneration in lamprey spinal cord. *J Neurosci* 1983; 3:1135–1144.

44. Lurie DI, Selzer ME: Axonal regeneration in the adult lamprey spinal cord. *J Comp Neurol* 1991; 306:409–416.

45. Wood MR, Cohen MJ: Synaptic regeneration in identified neurons of the lamprey spinal cords. *Science* 1979; 206:344–347.

46. Lurie DI, Pijak DS, Selzer ME: The structure of reticulospinal axon growth cones and their cellular environment during regeneration in the lamprey spinal cord. *J Comp Neurol* 1994; 344:559–580.

47. Caroni P, Savio T, Schwab ME: Central nervous system regeneration: Oligodendrocytes and myelin as non-permissive substrates for neurite growth. *Prog Brain Res* 1988; 78:363–370.

48. Caroni P, Schwab ME: Two membrane protein fractions from rat central myelin with inhibitory properties for neurite growth and fibroblast spreading. *J Cell Biol* 1988; 106:1281–1288.

49. Igarashi M, Strittmatter SM, Vartanian T, et al: Mediation by G proteins of signals that cause collapse of growth cones. *Science* 1993; 259:77–79.

50. Bandtlow CE, Schmidt MF, Hassinger TD, et al: Role of intracellular calcium in NI-35-evoked collapse of neuronal growth cones. *Science* 1993; 259:80–83.

51. McKerracher L, David S, Jackson DL, et al: Identification of myelin-associated glycoprotein as a major myelin-derived inhibitor of neurite growth. *Neuron* 1994; 13:805–811.

52. Mukhopadhyay G, Doherty P, Walsh FS, et al: A novel role for myelin-associated glycoprotein as an inhibitor of axonal regeneration. *Neuron* 1994; 13:757–767.

53. Cox EC, Müller B, Bonhoeffer F: Axonal guidance in the chick visual system: Posterior tectal membranes induce collapse of growth cones from the temporal retina. *Neuron* 1990; 4:31–37.

54. Kapfhammer JP, Raper JA: Interactions between growth cones and neurites growing from different neural tissues in culture. *J Neurosci* 1987; 7:1595–1600.

55. Ivins JK, Raper JA, Pittman RN: Intracellular calcium levels do not change during contact-mediated collapse of chick DRG growth cone structure. *J Neurosci* 1991; 11:1597–1608.

56. Raper JA, Kapfhammer JP: The enrichment of a neuronal growth cone collapsing activity from embryonic chick brain. *Neuron* 1990; 4:21–29.

57. Luo Y, Raper JA: The cloning and expression of collapsin, a protein that induces the collapse of dorsal root ganglia growth cones. *Soc Neurosci Abst* 1993; 23:236.

58. Kolodkin AL, Matthes DJ, Goodman CS: The semaphorin genes encode a family of transmembrane and secreted growth cone guidance molecules. *Cell* 1993; 75:1389–1399.

59. Puschel AW, Adams RH, Betz H: Murine semaphorin D/collapsin is a member of a diverse gene family and creates domains inhibitory for axonal extension. *Neuron* 1995; 14:941–948.

60. Luo Y, Shepherd I, Li J, et al: A family of molecules related to collapsin in the embryonic chick nervous system. *Neuron* 1995; 14:1131–1140.

61. Inagaki S, Furuyama T, Iwahashi Y: Identification of a member of mouse semaphorin family. *Febs Lett* 1995; 370:269–272.

62. Davies SJ, Field PM, Raisman G: Long interfascicular axon growth from embryonic neurons transplanted into adult myelinated tracts. *J Neurosci* 1994; 14:1596–1612.

63. Bovolenta P, Wandosell F, Nieto SM: Characterization of a neurite outgrowth inhibitor expressed after CNS injury. *Eur J Neurosci* 1993; 5:454–465.

64. Snow DM, Steindler DA, Silver J: Molecular and cellular characterization of the glial roof plate of the spinal cord and optic tectum: A possible role for a proteoglycan in the development of an axon barrier. *Dev Biol* 1990; 138:359–376.

65. Snow DM, Lemmon V, Carrino DA, et al: Sulfated proteoglycans in astroglial barriers inhibit neurite outgrowth in vitro. *Exp Neurol* 1990; 109:111–130.

66. McKeon RJ, Schreiber RC, Rudge JS, et al: Reduction of neurite outgrowth in a model of glial scarring following CNS injury is correlated with the expression of inhibitory molecules on reactive astrocytes. *J Neurosci* 1991; 11:3398–3411.

67. Carter DA, Bray GM, Aguayo AJ: Regenerated retinal ganglion cell axons can form well-differentiated synapses in the superior colliculus of adult hamsters. *J Neurosci* 1989; 9:4042–4050.

68. Aguayo AJ, Bray GM, Rasminsky M, et al: Synaptic connections made by axons regenerating in the central nervous system of adult mammals. *J Exp Biol* 1990; 153:199–224.

69. Jelsma TN, Friedman HH, Berkelaar M, et al: Different forms of the neurotrophin receptor *trk*b messenger-RNA predominate in rat retina and optic nerve. *J Neurobiol* 1993; 24:1207–1214.

70. Mansour-Robaey S, Clarke DB, Wang YC, et al: Effects of ocular injury and administration of brain-derived neurotrophic factor on survival and regrowth of axotomized retinal ganglion-cells. *Proc Natl Acad Sci USA* 1994; 91:1632–1636.

71. Cohen A, Bray GM, Aguayo AJ: Neurotrophin-4/5 (nt-4/5) increases adult-rat retinal ganglion-cell survival and neurite outgrowth in vitro. *J Neurobiol* 1994; 25:953–959.

72. Sasaki H, Inoue T, Iso H, et al: Light-dark discrimination after sciatic nerve transplantation to the sectioned optic nerve in adult hamsters. *Vision Res* 1993; 33:877–880.

73. Dunnett SB, Low WC, Iversen SD, et al: Septal transplants restore maze learning in rats with fornix-fimbria lesions. *Brain Res* 1982; 251:335–348.

74. Björklund A, Stenevi U: Reconstruction of the nigrostriatal dopamine pathway by intracerebral nigral transplants. *Brain Res* 1979; 177:555–560.

75. Lindvall O, Widner H, Rehncrona S, et al: Transplantation of fetal dopamine neurons in Parkinson's disease: One-year clinical and neurophysiological observations in two patients with putaminal implants. *Ann Neurol* 1992; 31:155–165.

76. Lindvall O, Sawle G, Widner H, et al: Evidence for long-term survival and function of dopaminergic grafts in progressive Parkinson's disease. *Ann Neurol* 1994; 35:172–180.

77. Davies SW, Roberts PJ: Model of Huntington's disease. *Science* 1988; 241:474–475.

78. Beal MF, Ferrante RJ, Swartz KJ, et al: Chronic quinolinic acid lesions in rats closely resemble Huntington's disease. *J Neurosci* 1991; 11:1 649–1659.

79. Dunnett SB, Svendsen CN: Huntington's disease: Animal models and transplantation repair. *Curr Opin Neurobiol* 1993; 3:790–796.

80. Ferrante RJ, Kowall NW, Cipolloni PB, et al: Excitotoxin lesions in primates as a model for Huntington's disease: Histopathologic and neurochemical characterization. *Exp Neurol* 1993; 119:46–71.

81. Sanberg PR, Calderon SF, Giordano M, et al: The quino-

linic acid model of Huntington's disease: Locomotor abnormalities. *Exp Neurol* 1989; 105:45–53.

82. Block F, Kunkel M, Schwarz M: Quinolinic acid lesion of the striatum induces impairment in spatial-learning and motor-performance in rats. *Neurosci Lett* 1993; 149:126–128.

83. Wictorin K: Anatomy and connectivity of intrastriatal striatal transplants. *Prog Neurobiol* 1992; 38:611–639.

84. Mayer E, Brown VJ, Dunnett SB, et al: Striatal graft-associated recovery of a lesion-induced performance deficit in the rat requires learning to use the transplant. *Eur J Neurosci* 1992; 4:119–126.

85. Hantraye P, Riche D, Maziere M, et al: Intrastriatal transplantation of cross-species fetal striatal cells reduces abnormal movements in a primate model of Huntington disease. *Proc Natl Acad Sci USA* 1992; 89:4187–4191.

86. Helm GA, Palmer PE, Simmons NE, et al: Descriptive morphology of developing fetal neostriatal allografts in the rhesus monkey: A correlated light and electron microscopic Golgi study. *Neuroscience* 1992; 50:163–179.

87. Macdonald ME, Ambrose CM, Duyao MP, et al: A novel gene containing a trinucleotide repeat that is expanded and unstable on Huntington's disease chromosomes. *Cell* 1993; 72:971–983.

88. Sramka M, Rattaj M, Molina H, et al: Stereotactic technique and pathophysiological mechanisms of neurotransplantation in Huntington's chorea. *Stereotact Funct Neurosurg* 1992; 58:79–83.

89. Tessler A: Intraspinal transplants. *Ann Neurol* 1991; 29:115–123.

90. Kunkel-Bagden E, Bregman BS: Spinal cord transplants enhance the recovery of locomotor function after spinal cord injury at birth. *Exp Brain Res* 1990; 81:25–34.

91. Bregman BS, Kunkel-Bagden E, Schnell L, et al: Recovery from spinal cord injury mediated by antibodies to neurite growth inhibitors. *Nature* 1995; 378: 498–501.

92. Bregman BS, Reier PJ: Neural tissue transplants rescue axotomized rubrospinal cells from retrograde death. *J Comp Neurol* 1986; 244:86–95.

93. Himes BT, Goldberger ME, Tessler A: Grafts of fetal central-nervous-system tissue rescue axotomized Clarke nucleus neurons in adult and neonatal operates. *J Comp Neurol* 1994; 339:117–131.

94. Bregman BS, Kunkel-Bagden E, McAtee M, et al: Extension of the critical period for developmental plasticity of the corticospinal pathway. *J Comp Neurol* 1989; 282:355–370.

95. Bregman BS: Spinal cord transplants permit the growth of serotonergic axons across the site of neonatal spinal cord transection. *Dev Brain Res* 1987; 34:265–279.

96. Bregman BS, Bernstein-Goral H: Both regenerating and late developing pathways contribute to transplant-induced anatomical plasticity after spinal cord transection. *Exp Neurol* 1991; 112:49–63.

97. Jakeman LB, Reier PJ: Axonal projections between fetal spinal cord transplants and the adult spinal cord. *J Comp Neurol* 1991; 307:311–334.

98. Itoh Y, Tessler A: Regeneration of adult dorsal root axons into transplants of fetal spinal cord and brain: A comparison of growth and synapse formation in appropriate and inappropriate targets. *J Comp Neurol* 1990; 302:272–293.

99. Itoh Y, Tessler A: Ultrastructural organization of regenerated adult dorsal root axons within transplants of fetal spinal cord. *J Comp Neurol* 1990; 292:396–411.

100. Gage FH, Kawaja MD, Fisher LJ: Genetically modified cells: Applications for intracerebral grafting. *Trends Neurosci* 1991; 14:328–333.

101. Kawaja MD, Rosenberg MB, Yoshida K, et al: Somatic gene transfer of nerve growth factor promotes the survival of axotomized septal neurons and the regeneration of their axons in adult rats. *J Neurosci* 1992; 12:2849–2864.

102. McBurney MW, Reuhl KR, Ally AI, et al: Differentiation and maturation of embryonal carcinoma-derived neurons in cell culture. *J Neurosci* 1988; 8:1063–1073.

103. Pleasure SJ, Page C, Lee VM: Pure, postmitotic, polarized human neurons derived from NTera 2 cells provide a system for expressing exogenous proteins in terminally differentiated neurons. *J Neurosci* 1992; 12:1802–1815.

104. Trojanowski JQ, Mantione JR, Lee JH, et al: Neurons derived from a human teratocarcinoma cell line establish molecular and structural polarity following transplantation into the rodent brain. *Exp Neurol* 1993; 122:283–294.

105. Groves AK, Barnett SC, Franklin RJ, et al: Repair of demyelinated lesions by transplantation of purified O-2A progenitor cells. *Nature* 1993; 362:453–455.

106. Reynolds BA, Weiss S: Generation of neurons and astrocytes from isolated cells of the adult mammalian central nervous system [see comments]. *Science* 1992; 255:1707–1710.

107. Reynolds BA, Tetzlaff W, Weiss S: A multipotent EGF-responsive striatal embryonic progenitor cell produces neurons and astrocytes. *J Neurosci* 1992; 12:4565–4574.

108. Gage FH, Ray J, Fisher LJ: Isolation, characterization, and use of stem cells from the CNS. *Annu Rev Neurosci* 1995; 18:159–192.

109. Renfranz PJ, Cunningham MG, McKay RD: Region-specific differentiation of the hippocampal stem cell line HiB5 upon implantation into the developing mammalian brain. *Cell* 1991; 66:713–729.

110. Snyder EY, Deitcher DL, Walsh C, et al: Multipotent neural cell lines can engraft and participate in development of mouse cerebellum. *Cell* 1992; 68:33–51.

111. Onifer SM, Whittemore SR, Holets VR: Variable morphological differentiation of a raphe-derived neuronal cell line following transplantation into the adult rat CNS. *Exp Neurol* 1993; 122:130–142.

112. Snyder EY: Grafting immortalized neurons to the CNS. [Review.] *Curr Opin Neurobiol* 1994; 4:742–751.

113. Anton R, Kordower JH, Maidment NT, et al: Neural-targeted gene therapy for rodent and primate hemiparkinsonism. *Exp Neurol* 1994; 127:207–218.

114. Schnell L, Schwab ME: Axonal regeneration in the rat spinal cord produced by an antibody against myelin-associated neurite growth inhibitors. *Nature* 1990; 343:269–272.

115. Schnell L, Schwab ME: Sprouting and regeneration of lesioned corticospinal tract fibers in the adult rat spinal cord. *Eur J Neurosci* 1993; 5:1156–1171.

116. Schnell L, Schneider R, Kolbeck R, et al: Neurotrophin-3 enhances sprouting of corticospinal tract during development and after adult spinal-cord lesion. *Nature* 1994; 367:170–173.

117. Tessier-Lavigne M: Axon guidance by molecular gradients. *Curr Opin Neurobiol* 1992; 2:60–65.

118. Kennedy TE, Serafini T, de la Torre JR, et al: Netrins are diffusible chemotropic factors for commissural axons in the embryonic spinal cord. *Cell* 1994; 78:425–435.

119. Keynes RJ, Cook GMW: Repellent cues in axon guidance. *Curr Opin Neurobiol* 1992; 2:55–59.

120. Sperry RW: Orderly patterning of synaptic associations in regeneration of intracentral fiber tracts mediating visuomotor coordination. *Anat Rec* 1948; 102:63–75.

121. Gaze RM, Jacobson M: A study of the retino-tectal projection during regeneration of the optic nerve in the frog. *Proc Roy Soc* (London) 1963; 157:420–448.

122. Sah DWY, Frank E: Regeneration of sensory-motor synapses in the spinal cord of the bullfrog. *J Neurosci* 1984; 4:2784–2791.

123. Yin HS, Mackler SA, Selzer ME: Directional specificity in the regeneration of lamprey spinal axons. *Science* 1984; 224:894–896.

124. Mackler SA, Yin HS, Selzer ME: Determinants of directional specificity in the regeneration of lamprey spinal axons. *J Neurosci* 1986; 6:1814–1821.

125. Mackler SA, Selzer ME: Regeneration of functional synapses between individual recognizable neurons in the lamprey spinal cord. *Science* 1985; 229:774–776.

126. Mackler SA, Selzer ME: Specificity of synaptic regeneration in the spinal cord of the larval sea lamprey. *J Physiol* (London.) 1987; 388:183–198.

127. Merrick SE, Pleasure SJ, Lurie DI, et al: Glial cells of the lamprey central nervous system contain keratin-like proteins. *J Comp Neurol* 1995; 355:199–210.

128. Godsave SF, Anderton BH, Wylie CC: The appearance and distribution of intermediate filament proteins during differentiation of the central nervous system, skin and notochord of *Xenopus laevis*. *J Embryol Exp Morph* 1986; 97:201–223.

129. Fouquet B, Herrmann H, Franz JD, et al: Expression of intermediate filament proteins during development of *Xenopus laevis*. III. Identification of mRNAs encoding cytokeratins typical of complex epithelia. *Development* 1988; 104:533–548.

130. Markl J, Franke WW: Localization of cytokeratins in tissues of the rainbow trout: Fundamental differences in expression pattern between fish and higher vertebrates. *Differentiation* 1988; 39:97–122.

131. Giordano S, Glasgow E, Tesser P, et al: A type II keratin is expressed in glial cells of the goldfish visual pathway. *Neuron* 1989; 2:1507–1516.

132. Rungger-Brändle E, Achtstätter T, Franke WW: An epithelium-type cytoskeleton in a glial cell: Astrocytes of amphibian optic nerves contain cytokeratin filaments and are connected by desmosomes. *J Cell Biol* 1989; 109:705–716.

Chapter 5

ANALYSIS OF GAIT

D. Casey Kerrigan
Lynne R. Sheffler
Susan R. Ehrenthal

Although a number of stereotypical gait patterns have been described in patients with neurologic diagnoses, each patient presents with a unique set of impairments, disabilities, and compensations. *Hemiplegic gait* or *hemiparetic gait* broadly refers to a gait pattern common in patients with stroke, brain injury, or cerebral palsy. *Diplegic gait* is used to describe a stereotypical gait pattern observed exclusively in patients with spastic diplegic cerebral palsy. The term *paraparetic gait* often describes gait in patients with spinal-cord injury or brain injury affecting bilateral lower extremities. Other common descriptions for gait specify the abnormal motion observed during walking. For instance, reduced knee flexion (stiff-legged gait), excessive knee flexion (crouched gait), or excessive ankle plantarflexion (equinus gait) are common descriptions of motion abnormalities observed in patients with neurologically based disability.

The first step in evaluating the patient with a neurologically associated gait disability is to describe the stereotypical motion abnormalities, such as stiff-legged, crouched, or equinus. The next step, assuming the abnormality is functionally significant, is to determine the most likely impairments causing the abnormality in that particular patient. For this step, all information that can be obtained from a standard clinical evaluation and a quantitative gait laboratory analysis are useful. From these findings, a rational individualized treatment plan aimed at these impairments can be prescribed.

GAIT TERMINOLOGY

Gait refers to any particular way of moving on foot, which in bipedal humans includes both walking and running. *Walking* is defined as a gait in which the feet are lifted alternately, with one foot always on the ground. In general, two-legged (bipedal) gait is less stable than four-legged (quadrupedal) gait, for the main reason that a biped's center of mass is located above its base of support rather than within its base of support. Thus, the goal of bipedal gait is to progress the body forward while maintaining stability. This requires coordinated movements of multiple limb segments and joints within the lower extremities.

The functional unit of gait, a *gait cycle,* also referred to as a *stride,* is defined as the events occurring between sequential corresponding points of contact of a single limb. Various gait cycle events have been investigated since the late 1800s. Jules Marey, a French physiologist, used chronophotographic equipment to record the time each foot spends on the ground when running, and photographer Eadward Muybridge sequentially triggered a series of cameras to record patterns of gait, in both animals and humans.[1,2] The biomechanical understanding of gait was greatly enhanced after World War II by Saunders and Inman, who studied normal and amputee gait.[3,4] Modern-day gait laboratory analysis, including kinematics (measurement of joint and limb segment motion), kinetics (moments and powers about joints), and/or dynamic electromyography, have been used for studying both nondisabled and disabled gait. Recent computer technology has allowed for easy analysis of massive amounts of information obtained from a variety of sources, including optoelectronic motion analysis systems, force transducers, and electromyography. From the data collected using these devices, a number of parameters during the gait cycle can be measured routinely. Analysis of these parameters, along with information from a standard clinical assessment, can be extremely useful in evaluating a neurologically based

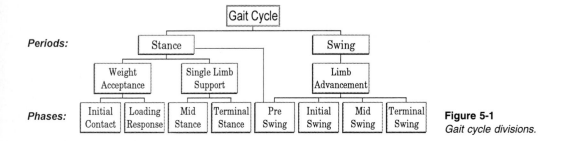

Figure 5-1
Gait cycle divisions.

Nomenclature of Gait Cycle Events

In evaluating a patient with gait disability, it is useful to become familiar with the currently accepted nomenclature of gait events. A new system for describing gait events recently has been developed (see Figure 5-1).[5] In this classification, the gait cycle is divided into three functional tasks: weight acceptance, limb support, and limb advancement. Weight acceptance and limb support comprise the *stance period,* whereas limb advancement comprises the *swing period.* The stance period is subdivided into the following phases: initial contact, which includes the point in the gait cycle when the foot makes initial contact with the ground; loading response, beginning with initial contact and continuing until the other foot is lifted for swing; mid-stance, beginning as the other foot is lifted for swing and continuing until the heel rises from the ground; terminal stance, beginning with heel rise and continuing until the other foot makes contact with the ground; and pre-swing, beginning with initial contact of the opposite limb and ending with ipsilateral toe-off. The swing period consists of initial swing, mid-swing, and terminal swing, each phase comprising one-third of the swing period.

The stance period also can be subdivided into three phases according to foot-floor contact patterns: initial double support, when both feet are in contact with the ground, corresponding to the loading response phase; single support, when only one foot is in contact with the ground, corresponding to both the mid- and terminal stance phases; and final double support, when both feet are in contact with the ground again, corresponding to the pre-swing phase. At average walking speeds, approximately 60 percent of the gait cycle time is spent in the stance period, with each double support phase accounting for 10 percent and the single limb support phase accounting for 40 percent. The relative amount of time during the stance period decreases as the speed of walking increases. Also, as the speed of walking increases, the relative amount of time in double support decreases, whereas the relative amount of time in single support increases. Walking becomes running when there is no longer a double support phase. Running is comprised of two periods, single limb support, when one foot is on the ground, and flight, when neither foot is on the ground.

A particular person's gait may be described according to speed, distance traversed with each gait cycle, or cadence, the rhythm of gait cycles. *Stride length* is defined as the distance traversed during gait from initial contact of one foot to initial contact of the same foot. *Step length* is the distance from initial contact of one foot to initial contact of the other foot. *Stride cadence* refers to the number of strides per unit time, whereas *step cadence* is the steps per unit time. The relative amount of time during the single-support phase and double-support phase are reported as single-support time and double-support time.

ENERGY DEMANDS OF GAIT

Often the energy demand of walking for patients with disabled gait exceeds that for nondisabled subjects. To better understand the mechanisms typically responsible for this increased energy demand, it is useful to appreciate the energetics of gait in nondisabled gait. First, even nondisabled bipedal gait is more costly in energy terms than locomotion on wheels. The best evidence for this fact is that wheelchair marathoners finish the race well before the runners. One reason for this may be that the body's center of gravity must rise and fall with each step during gait, whereas in wheeled locomotion the center of gravity does not rise and fall. Energy is expended with each vertical displacement of the body's center of gravity during the gait cycle. The work needed to lift the body with each step can be roughly estimated by multiplying the overall vertical displacement of the center of gravity during that step by the body weight.

The overall events that occur in each gait cycle with respect to center-of-gravity motion have been defined classically as the six determinants of gait: pelvic rotation, pelvic tilt, knee flexion in mid-stance, foot and knee motion, and lateral displacement of the pelvis.[4] If flexibility is maintained only about the hip joints, and the pelvis, knee, and ankle joints are fixed, walking can occur only in a compass-like motion. Under these hypothetical circumstances, at an average walking speed, the center of gravity has been calculated to go up and down 4 inches with each step.[4] These six determinants are mechanisms or events that bipedal humans utilize to reduce and smooth out the path of the center of gravity. Under these conditions, the rise and fall of the center of gravity actually is 2 inches at an average walking speed or roughly one-half the calculated compass gait value at any speed of walking.[6] The first five determinants of gait effectively either raise the center of gravity at its would-be lowest point at double support, or lower the center of gravity at its would-be highest point at mid-stance.

The first determinant of gait is pelvic rotation. With four degrees of pelvic rotation in either direction during double support, the limbs essentially are lengthened. This determinant effectively raises the center of gravity's would-be lowest point.

The second determinant is pelvic tilt, which occurs in mid-stance. During this phase, the pelvis tilts four degrees on the swing side and carries the center of gravity with it. This determinant essentially lowers the center of gravity's would-be highest point. The third determinant is knee flexion in mid-stance, which also effectively lowers the center of gravity's would-be highest point. The fourth and fifth determinants are foot and knee motion. The ankle pivots on the posterior heel at initial contact. The pivot point progresses to the forefoot by terminal stance, at which time plantarflexion occurs. These combined actions heighten the center of gravity's would-be lowest point. Both knee and foot motion also act to smooth the motion to a sinusoidal curve.

The last determinant of gait concerns the lateral displacement of the pelvis. The hip joints are displaced in the horizontal plane by the pelvic width. Valgus align-

ment at the knees combined with hip adduction allow the feet to approximate one another in the horizontal plane. This anatomic alignment allows less excursion of the center of gravity in the horizontal plane.

In summary, the determinants of gait are biomechanical strategies used in nondisabled gait to reduce the overall motion of the body's center of gravity throughout the gait cycle, thereby reducing the energy required to walk. Theoretically, any neurologic impairment that interferes with one or more of these determinants may result in an energy-inefficient gait. For instance, the lack of knee flexion (or knee hyperextension) during stance interferes with the third determinant of gait, and thus, theoretically, increases the energy requirement of walking. Classically, this concept has been accepted in rehabilitation practice and serves as the basis for evaluating an impairment from the perspective of energetics. Although regularly applied in practice, the gait determinant theories may predict the energetic requirements of gait only partially. The forces generated by internal muscular work also must be considered during gait analysis. Unfortunately, these have proven difficult to measure directly, even with modern-day sophisticated gait-analysis equipment. Although undoubtedly there is a balance between the forces needed to move the center of gravity during gait and internal muscular work, more research is needed to evaluate their quantitative relationship in normal and pathologic gait.

INITIAL APPROACH TO A PATIENT WITH A NEUROLOGICALLY BASED GAIT DISABILITY

Each patient with a gait disorder presents with a unique set of impairments, disabilities, and compensations. Even nondisabled subjects with the same basic anatomic and physiologic makeup have unique gait patterns. Informal observational gait analysis is performed routinely by clinicians and should be the first step in evaluating a patient with a neurologically based gait disability.

Abnormal gait motion can be observed even from bedside observational analysis, such as reduced knee flexion during the swing period, excessive knee flexion during the stance period, or excessive ankle plantarflexion during the swing period.

The next step is to determine whether the abnormality is functionally significant. In order to do this, each specific gait deviation should be evaluated with respect to four criteria: (1) energy requirement; (2) risk of falling; (3) biomechanical injury; and (4) cosmesis.

A gait disability can be evaluated with respect to energy requirement directly by measuring oxygen consumption per unit distance. In a clinical setting, however, comfortable walking speed can serve as a reasonable indicator of the energy required to walk. People with disabilities utilize the same amount of oxygen per unit time as nondisabled subjects during walking.[7] In order to compensate, subjects with disability reduce their comfortable walking speeds, so they are inversely correlated with the energy required to walk a given distance.

Although a gait abnormality can be assessed as having an increased energy requirement, it is more important from a diagnostic and treatment standpoint to determine the mechanism of this increased requirement. For instance, a specific gait disability may affect one or more determinants of gait, thereby increasing the center of gravity's vertical displacement with each step.

Gait deviations must be evaluated with respect to risk for falling. For instance, excessive plantarflexion (equinus) or reduced knee flexion (stiff-legged gait) could predispose to tripping and subsequent fall injury. A gait abnormality also can predispose to biomechanical injury about a specific joint. For example, knee hyperextension or genu recurvatum during stance period may cause progressive posterior capsule and ligament injury about the knee. Gait analysis also can be useful in helping to assess excessive biomechanical forces that may produce soft tissue injury. Finally, gait abnormality should be evaluated for appearance and impact on the self-esteem of the individual.

Observational Gait Analysis

Observational gait analysis consists of observing the patient walking, without the use of sophisticated electronic devices. Often it is difficult to appreciate all the joint and limb segment motions through the phases of gait because of the difficulty in simultaneously observing multiple body segments and limb motions.[8] Videotaping the patient and observing the tape several times in slow motion, or even frame by frame, may be valuable in evaluating various motion abnormalities present in a patient with neurologic disability.[9] In some instances, however, neither observational nor video analysis may pick up subtle motion abnormalities that are revealed later with sophisticated quantitative gait-analysis methods.

Excessive anterior pelvic tilt associated with hip flexor tightness, for example, may be apparent only with quantitative gait-analysis techniques and not with obser-

vational or video analysis. Highly sophisticated techniques and procedures to assist in objective, normative-based gait analysis are available now.[5,10]

Normal Joint Motions During Gait

Kinematics is the term used to describe the spatial motion of joints and limb segments, and *kinetics* is the term used to describe the torques or forces that generate the joint and limb segment motion. Although multiple studies in the literature describe the normal kinematics during gait, the data from these studies vary depending on the methods used to measure the kinematics, the speed of walking, and the age of the subjects studied.[4,11,12] In the gait laboratory of the Spaulding Rehabilitation Hospital, the average speed of walking is approximately 0.80 meters per second in young, healthy adults.

The average kinematics of the pelvis and right lower extremity from one stride of 40 adult nondisabled subjects, measured in our laboratory, are demonstrated in Figure 5-2. On average, the pelvis moves approximately 4 degrees in the sagittal plane, with a relative increase in anterior pelvic tilt during midstance and initial swing. In the coronal plane, the ipsilateral side of the pelvis rises from mid-swing to loading response and then drops again from midstance to initial swing. The pelvis rotates on average 8 degrees in the transverse plane. The pelvis is rotated internally at initial contact by 4 degrees, externally rotates throughout stance, and then internally rotates again in swing.

The hip is maximally flexed to 35 degrees at initial contact, and extends throughout stance to reach maximal extension of 10 degrees at terminal stance. Flexion begins in pre-swing and continues throughout the swing phase. Knee motion is characterized by two waves of flexion/extension motion occurring in stance and in swing. Although the knee is fully extended at initial contact, it flexes approximately 20 degrees in loading response, and then extends in mid-stance. It begins flexing again in pre-swing, achieving 35 degrees of flexion at toe-off. The knee continues flexing in initial swing, reaching a maximum 65 degrees between initial and mid-swing. The knee extends again from mid- to terminal swing.

The ankle also moves through two waves of motion. The ankle is in a neutral position at initial contact, rapidly plantarflexes in loading response, and then dorsiflexes gradually to approximately 10 degrees at terminal stance. The ankle then plantarflexes and reaches a

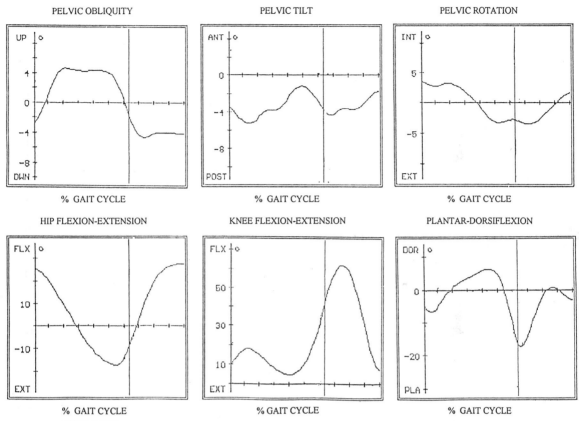

Figure 5-2

Average kinematic data from nondisabled subjects about the pelvis and the right hip, knee, and ankle for one gait cycle. For each graph, the horizontal axis represents the percent of one gait cycle from 0 to 100 percent, with marks at 10 percent intervals. The numbers on the vertical axis represent degrees of motion. The vertical lines represent the division between the stance and swing period.

peak plantarflexion angle of 15 to 20 degrees in initial swing.

LIMITATIONS OF A STATIC EVALUATION IN ASSESSING A PATIENT WITH GAIT DISABILITY

After evaluating the patient walk, the next step is to perform a static assessment including strength, tone, and range-of-motion evaluations. The static evaluation alone, however, is very limited in determining which muscles are truly weak, spastic, or tight during walking.

Quantitative gait laboratory analysis probably is much more helpful in assessing these variables.

Strength and Tone Evaluation

Static strength is of limited use in a patient with spastic paretic gait for whom, unlike a patient with lower motor-neuron pathology, weakness may not be the primary problem. The patient with spastic paresis may have impaired voluntary-muscle control and may not be able to selectively activate a certain muscle while simultaneously relaxing its antagonist. The relationship between static strength performance and dynamic strength associated with gait can be highly variable and inconsistent.

There is credible documentation of some patients with hemiplegic gait who were unable to dorsiflex the foot during a static evaluation but appropriately dorsiflexed the foot during the swing period when walking.[13,14] Conversely, some patients with full voluntary control and normal dorsiflexion strength of the ankle during a static evaluation have demonstrated equinus dynamically during the swing phase of gait.[13,14] A high degree of variability between tone present on static and dynamic evaluations during gait has been demonstrated.[14]

Joint Range of Motion

Determining the passive range of motion of each joint is the traditional method to assess tissue contracture. Recent studies demonstrated that ranging of joints and differentiating between contracture of a one- or two-joint muscle is difficult in patients with upper motor-neuron pathology, presumably because of impaired selective control of these muscles.[15,16] For instance, the Duncan-Ely test traditionally is used to differentiate rectus femoris from iliopsoas contracture by utilizing the fact that the rectus femoris acts as both a hip *flexor* and knee *extensor*. For this test, the patient is placed in a prone position and the knee is flexed rapidly. If a contracture of the rectus femoris exists, the hip will flex and the buttocks will rise off the table. Although theoretically useful, fine-wire electromyographic recordings have shown that the Duncan-Ely test in patients with cerebral palsy induced electromyographic activation of both the rectus femoris and iliopsoas muscle.[15]

Similarly, the Silverskiold test for differentiating contracture of the gastrocnemius from contracture of the soleus may not be reliable.[17] In this test, the knee is flexed at 90 degrees, and the foot is brought to the position of maximum dorsiflexion. The knee then is extended. If the gastrocnemius is contracted, some of the dorsiflexion will be lost. Although theoretically useful, some investigators have demonstrated that in patients with cerebral palsy, electromyographic activation of the soleus still occurs with the knee extended.[16] This suggests that the Silverskiold test is not clinically reliable in patients with upper motor-neuron pathology.

QUANTITATIVE GAIT LABORATORY ANALYSIS

Quantitative gait analysis, including kinematic, kinetic, and dynamic electromyography assessment, appears to be a promising clinical tool in evaluating gait disability of neurologic origin. Already it has been reported to be an essential tool in providing an effective treatment plan for orthopedic decision making in patients with spastic paretic gait from cerebral palsy.[20–23] Children with cerebral palsy often undergo tendon-lengthening procedures to improve range of motion in the lower extremities, in an effort to improve gait disability. Perhaps the most systematic study to date demonstrating the effectiveness of a quantitative gait evaluation was in a sample of 23 patients showing that surgery performed based on gait analysis resulted in better outcomes than surgery performed without formal quantitative gait analysis.[21]

For the same reasons that it has been found useful in orthopedic decision making, quantitative gait analysis should be useful for directing the rehabilitation plan for a patient with spastic paretic gait.[24] Intuitively, proper rehabilitation, like orthopedic planning, relies on the correct determination of specific underlying impairments causing gait disability.

Overall Description of Quantitative Gait Laboratory Analysis

Measurements of kinematics, kinetics, and muscle activity for multiple muscles during gait typically are made in a specialized gait laboratory environment, with optoelectronic equipment to measure kinematics, force plates to help measure kinetics, and a multi-channel dynamic electromyographic (EMG) apparatus to measure electrical muscle activity in multiple muscles during gait. Our clinical experience is that quantitative gait laboratory analysis routinely provides information that differs from what might have been expected from static and observational evaluations. Our rehabilitation plans thus commonly are modified, often resulting in improved outcome.

Kinematics

Electrogoniometers Electrogoniometers basically are computerized versions of the simple goniometer commonly used in clinical practice to assess joint range of motion. One or more potentiometers are placed between two bars with one bar strapped to the proximal limb segment and the other strapped to the distal limb segment. The potentiometer, placed over the joint, provides a varying output depending on the instantaneous angle between the two limb segments. The information from the potentiometer then can be interfaced to an A-to-D convertor and a personal computer for data acquisition. A combination of three potentiometers allows for measuring three rotations between limb segments.[25] Some disadvantages of current electrogoniometers are that they need to be tethered to a data recorder and may be difficult to apply, particularly at the hip and ankle, where they have relatively poor accuracy. A modified electrogoniometer that utilizes a double parallelogram design about the knee joint has been described and may be useful for measuring the relative joint angle about this joint. Unfortunately, even with good repeatability of measurements, the results obtained from electrogoniometers provide only relative joint-angle information, and not absolute positions of the joints or limb segments. Thus, the results cannot be correlated with force-plate data to generate joint kinetics.

Cinematography with Manual Digitization   Historically, gait analysis was performed using sequential photographs or motion pictures. Markers mounted on various anatomic landmarks were used to help identify the location of limb segments and joints. The location of markers then would be manually digitized, frame by frame, so that the marker position in two dimensions could be determined. In both cinematographic and optoelectronic systems, a single camera provides two-dimensional information. By using two cameras, triangulation could be performed to determine the three-dimensional position of the marker. Although this cinematographic system may be as accurate as what can be obtained with modern optoelectronic systems, the time necessary to manually digitize and process the data was so great that it made this procedure impractical for clinical assessment.

Modern-Day Automated Optoelectronic Motion Analysis Systems   Current optoelectronic systems can measure the three-dimensional location of an individual marker with greater ease than manual digitization methods. Multiple markers are affixed to the skin of the pelvis and the lower extremities in relationship to bony landmarks. Two systems are used commonly: (1) active marker systems, where the markers are actively illuminated by a computer; and (2) passive marker systems.

An advantage of the active optoelectronic marker system is that computer software programs are not needed for marker identification, since the computer knows which marker it is illuminating at any given point.

Currently the main disadvantages of an active marker system, however, are the need for wires attached to the patient and that the patient or someone else needs to carry power packs for the illuminators. In contrast, passive marker systems do not require attachment of wires to the markers or power packs. Passive markers, however, do require computer software to automate the digitization process. Fortunately, software has improved considerably in recent years, making passive marker systems easier to use in routine clinical practice.

The general layout of our laboratory, utilizing a passive marker system with four cameras positioned posteriorly, is demonstrated in Figure 5-3. Both active and passive marker systems allow measurement of the three-dimensional position of each of the markers affixed to various landmarks. The optoelectronic camera system, the size of the markers, and the laboratory environment are factors in determining the accuracy of the system in determining the marker position. Typically, the resolution of a marker position is within a few millimeters.

If markers were placed only near the joints, then it would be difficult to differentiate motion in each plane. Imagine if markers were only placed over the hip, knee, and ankle and the knee angle was defined as the angle between the longitudinal axes of the thigh and shank. In this case, although true knee flexion in the sagittal plane would affect the measured angle, so could varus and valgus motion.

To differentiate joint angle positions in the sagittal, coronal, and transverse planes, three markers must be placed on each limb segment, define a three-dimensional coordinate system for that segment. Euler angles, used to describe orientation of one coordinate system relative to another, are commonly used to determine joint angles.[26] There are several potential errors associated with measuring kinematics, including error from skin and soft-tissue motion and error from the marker potentially becoming lost from the view of one of the cameras.[27]

Kinetics

Kinetics about any particular joint are in a state of equilibrium when the externally applied forces are countered by internal joint forces and moments generated by muscle activity and/or soft tissue. *Joint power* refers to the net rate of generating or absorbing energy and is the mathematical product of the joint moment and the joint angular velocity. A positive joint power implies that the net muscle contraction is concentric, since the

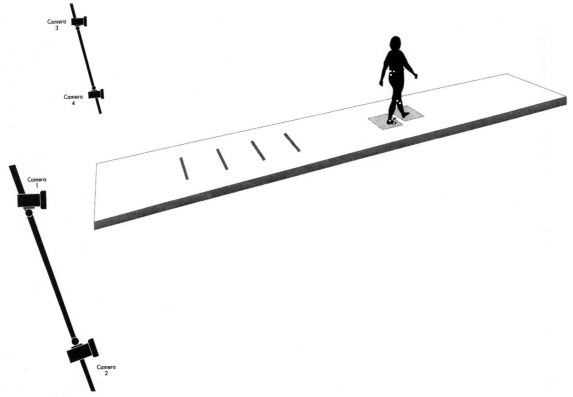

Figure 5-3
General layout of a gait laboratory. The multiple cameras capture the three-dimensional images of markers placed on the body. The patient walks over force plates that simultaneously provide ground reaction force information necessary to calculate kinetics.

joint angular velocity and moment are in the same direction. A negative power implies that the net muscle contraction is eccentric, as angular velocity and joint moment are in opposite directions.

Joint kinetics are calculated using inverse dynamic techniques, according to Newton's Second Law of Motion. This calculation requires (1) knowledge of the position of the joint in relation to the ground reaction force; (2) estimates of body segment masses and moments of inertia; and (3) knowledge of the body segment positions, velocities, and accelerations.[28-30] Ground reaction forces are measured using force plates, which comprise piezoelectric or strain-gauge transducers. One or more force plates are embedded at ground level in the walkway, in the hopes that the patient naturally will step onto the force plate with one foot.

In order to measure joint kinetics, kinematic measurement must be collected synchronously with force-plate data. The locations of the force plates are predetermined within a calibrated volume where the kinematic data are measured. The positions of two force plates are shown in Figure 5-3. A combination of measurements taken on a patient then can be juxtaposed with normative tables based on cadaver data, to estimate body segment masses and moments of inertia.[31,32]

Clinical gait laboratories report joint moments or torques as either external or internal. An external torque or moment refers to the net external load applied to the joint measured directly with inverse dynamic techniques. The internal torque, which is equal and opposite in sign to the external torque, is the presumed torque owing to the sum of muscle activity and soft-tissue forces that maintains the joint in equilibrium. For example, an external dorsiflexion moment or torque about the ankle during the stance period of a gait cycle implies that the ground reaction force is anterior to the ankle and that

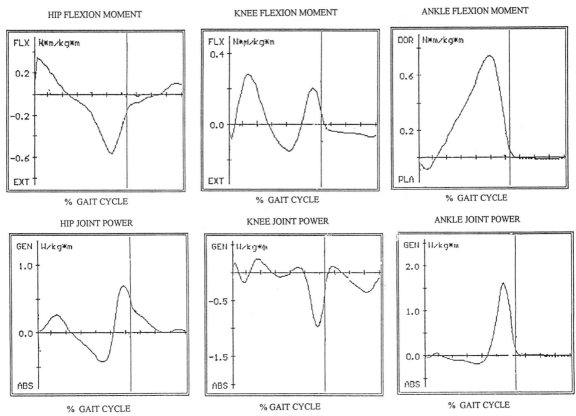

Figure 5-4

Average moments and powers for nondisabled subjects. The units of moment in the vertical axis are in newton-meters/kilogram-meters and the units of power are in watts/kilogram-meter.

an equal and opposite internal torque provided by the ankle plantarflexors or heel cord is present to maintain joint stability. Similarly, an external flexor torque about the hip implies that the ground reaction force is anterior to the hip and that this external torque must be restrained by hip extensors.

The average external moments, normalized for mass and height (newton-meters/kilogram-meters), in the sagittal plane about the hip, knee, and ankle, for 40 nondisabled subjects are demonstrated in Figure 5-4. At the hip there is a flexor moment and then an extensor moment during stance followed by another flexor moment in swing. At initial contact there is an extensor moment at the knee, followed by a flexor, extensor, and flexor moment during stance and then an extensor moment throughout swing. The ankle has a plantarflexor moment at initial contact, followed by a dorsi-flexor moment throughout stance. Average powers normalized for mass and height (watts/kilogram-meter) in the sagittal plane about the hip, knee, and ankle are also represented in Figure 5-4. Generation of power implies that a concentric contraction is occurring, whereas absorption of power implies that an eccentric contraction is occurring.

Dynamic Electromyography (EMG)

Quantitative gait analysis also includes measurements of muscle activity during walking obtained using dynamic EMG. Dynamic EMG provides useful information about whether or not a muscle is firing appropriately and, if not, how this nonphasic activity impacts on gait, particularly in patients with spastic paretic gait. Unfortunately, quantification of muscle activity in terms of the magnitude of force generated is not practical in patients. However, relative normalization of muscle activity over the gait cycle to the peak level of activity whether it occurs during strength testing or during walking has been described and shown to increase the clinical usefulness of the EMG data.[5]

Muscle activity is measured using either surface electrodes attached to the skin or fine-wire electrodes that are inserted through a needle directly into the muscle. Surface electrodes are adequate to study activity in large superficial muscle groups. Data from surface electrodes are replicated more easily. Also, fine-wire electrodes may induce spasticity in some patients with upper motor-neuron injury or may cause cramping that can lead to false representation of muscle activity during walking. On the other hand, fine-wire electrodes are not as prone to cross-talk from nearby muscles and thus are necessary for analysis of smaller muscles, as well as for deeper muscles such as the iliopsoas and posterior tibialis.[33,34]

Muscle timing errors in patients with upper motor-neuron lesions and spastic paretic gait traditionally are classified into seven categories: premature onset, delayed onset, curtailed period, prolonged, absent, out of phase, or continuous.[35] Although these categorizations are useful in describing activity in each muscle, it is important to note that they do not necessarily imply pathology about that particular muscle. In some instances, muscle activity differs from that of a nondisabled subject because of compensation. As an example, prolongation of quadriceps activity into the mid- and terminal stance phases would be compensatory in a patient with an excessive external knee flexor torque. Thus, muscle firing patterns are assessed optimally in conjunction with kinetic data, to help differentiate inherent pathology from compensatory action.

Overall Gait Laboratory Analysis Procedure

The overall gait analysis procedure takes approximately 2 hours of time for data acquisition and an additional 2 hours for analysis and interpretation. The majority of the acquisition time is spent applying and confirming placement of the multiple markers and EMG electrodes. The patient is typically evaluated barefoot, with shoes, and with and without an orthosis.

Interpretation of Gait Laboratory Information

The combined kinematic, kinetic, and dynamic EMG information can be very useful in localizing specific weakness, tightness, or spasticity of individual muscles groups. In turn, the valuable information can be used to optimize the medical, surgical, and rehabilitation management in patients with upper motor-neuron pathology. The gait laboratory data can provide critical information about the activation state of any particular muscle at any particular point during the gait cycle.

Inappropriate quadriceps activity during the preswing or initial swing phases of gait may be observed with dynamic electromyographic assessment and implicated as a cause for reduced knee flexion or stiff-legged gait. Again, it is important to analyze the dynamic electromyographic activity in conjunction with the kinetics to determine if the quadriceps activity is compensatory or truly inappropriate. For instance, if the quadriceps is activated in the pre-swing of the gait cycle, and there is an external flexor moment about the knee at the same time, the quadriceps activity should be considered compensatory. Inappropriate activity may be limited to only one or two heads of the quadriceps. In this case, therapeutic intramuscular neurolysis to one or two heads of the quadriceps may effectively treat the reduced knee flexion.

In the case of excessive equinus, the diagnostic considerations should include pathologic soleus, gastrocnemius, or posterior tibialis activity. This is observed and measured readily with electromyographic assessment. A tight heel cord present on static evaluation may not be functionally significant if good dynamic range of motion is observed with the kinematic evaluation. A varus foot may be owing to inappropriate activation of either or both the anterior or posterior tibialis, which would be readily evident and quantifiable by dynamic electromyographic assessment.

The combination of joint kinematics and kinetics are useful in determining if a particular muscle group is weak. For instance, reduced hip-power generation in pre-swing might imply dynamically weak hip flexors. Reduced hip power also could be a result of inappropriate hamstring activity keeping the hip from flexing. Dynamic electromyographic information obtained from the hamstrings would help differentiate between these two possibilities. A poor external flexor moment about the knee during mid-stance may imply weakness of the quadriceps. A reduced external ankle dorsiflexion moment in conjunction with reduced ankle power generation may imply weakness of the ankle plantarflexors. In this latter case, the effect of an ankle-foot-orthosis can be evaluated to assess if it allows for an increased ankle dorsiflexion moment, which implies that the brace provides adequate resistance into dorsiflexion.

There are no simple algorithms to evaluate the vast amount of data that are obtained from a quantitative gait analysis. The kinematic, kinetic, and dynamic electromyographic presentations are complex, and each patient presents with unique problems and findings. For this reason, the interpretation process probably is the most time-consuming phase of a gait laboratory evaluation.

SUMMARY

A neurologically based gait disorder may be functionally significant on the basis of energy requirement, risk for fall, risk for biomechanical injury, or poor cosmesis. Although many gait deviations appear stereotypical, in fact each patient presents with a unique set of underlying impairments. Quantitative gait analysis including kinematic, kinetic, and dynamic electromyographic measurement, together with a standard clinical assessment, provides crucial information about the nature and physiology of aberrant gait, and new hopes for more rational therapy.

REFERENCES

1. Marey EJ: *Animal Mechanism: A Treatise on Terrestrial and Aerial Locomotion*. New York: Appleton, 1874.
2. Muybridge E: *The Human Figure in Motion*. New York: Dover, 1955.
3. Inman VT, Ralston HJ, Todd S: *Human Walking*. Baltimore: Williams & Wilkins, 1981.
4. Saunders JB, Inman VT, Eberhart HD: Major determinants in normal and pathologic gaits. *Am J Bone Joint Surg* 1953; 35A:543–558.
5. Perry J: *Gait Analysis: Normal and Pathological Function*. Thorofare, NJ: Slack, Inc., 1992.
6. Kerrigan DC, Viramontes BE, Corcoran PJ, LaRaia P: Measured versus predicted vertical displacement. *Am J Phys Med Rehab* 1995; 76:3–7.
7. Gonzalez EG, Corcoran PJ: Energy expenditure during ambulation, in Downey JA, Myers SJ, Gonzalez EG, Lieberman JS (eds): *The Physiologic Basis of Rehabilitation Medicine,* 3rd ed. Stoneham, UK: Butterworth-Heineman, 1994, pp. 413–446.
8. Saleh M, Murdoch G: In defense of gait analysis. *Am J Bone Joint Surg* 1985; 67B:237–241.
9. Krebs DE, Edelstein JE, Fishman S: Reliability of observational kinematic gait analysis. *Phys Ther* 1985; 65:1027–1033.
10. Winter DA: Concerning the scientific basis for the diagnosis of pathological gait and for rehabilitation protocols. *Physiother Can* 1985; 37(4):245–252.
11. Murray MP, Drought AB, Kory RC: Walking patterns of normal men. *Am J Joint Bone Surg* 1964; 46A:335–360.
12. Kadaba MP, Ramakrishnan HK, Wooten ME: Measurement of lower extremity kinetics during level walking. *J Orthop Res* 1990; 8:383–392.
13. Perry J, Giovan P, Harris LJ, Montgomery J, Azaria M: The determinants of muscle action in the hemiparetic lower extremity and their effects on the examination procedure. *Clin Orthop* 1978; 131:71–89.
14. Perry J: Determinants of muscle function in a spastic lower extremity. *Clin Orthop* 1993; 288:10–26.
15. Perry J, Hoffer MM, Antonelli D, Plut J, Lewis G, Greenberg R: Electromyography before and after surgery for hip deformity in children with cerebral palsy. *Am J Bone Joint Surg* 1976; 58A:201–208.
16. Perry J, Hoffer Giovan P, Antonelli D, Greenberg R: Gait analysis of the triceps surae in cerebral palsy. *Am J Bone Joint Surg* 1974; 56A:511–520.
17. Silverskiold N: Reduction of the uncrossed two-joint muscles of the leg to one-joint muscles in spastic conditions. *Acta Chir Scand* 1923; 56:315.
18. Lee EH, Mather A, Goh JC, Teng B, Bose K: Gait analysis in cerebral palsy. *Ann Acad Med Singapore* 1985; 14(1):37–43.
19. Gage JR: Gait analysis for decision-making in cerebral palsy. *Bull Hosp Joint Dis Orthop Inst* 1983; 43(2):147–163.
20. Gage JR: Gait analysis: An essential tool in the treatment of cerebral palsy. *Clin Orthop* 1993; 288:126–134.
21. Lee EH, Goh JC, Bose K: Value of gait analysis in the assessment of surgery in cerebral palsy. *Arch Phys Med Rehabil* 1992; 73(7):642–646.
22. DeLuca PA: Gait analysis and the treatment of the ambulatory child with cerebral palsy. *Clin Orthop* 1991; 264:65–75.
23. Lee EH, Mather A, Goh JC, Teng B, Bose K: Gait analysis and cerebral palsy. *Ann Acad Med Singapore* 1985; 14(1):37–43.
24. Kerrigan DC, Glenn M: An illustration of clinical gait laboratory use to improve rehabilitation management. *Am J Phys Med Rehab* 1994; 73:421–427.
25. Chao EYS: Justification of triaxial goniometer for the measurement of joint rotation. *J Biomechan* 1980; 13:989–1006.
26. Grood ES, Suntay WJ: A joint coordinate system for the clinical description of three-dimensional motions: Applications to the knee. *J Biomech Eng* 1983; 105:136–144.
27. Kadaba MP, Ramakrishnan HK, Wooten ME, Gainey J, Gorton G, Cochran GVB: Repeatability of kinematic, kinetic, and electromyographic data in normal adult gait. *J Orthop Res* 1989; 7:849–860.
28. Winter DA: *Biomechanics and Motor Control of Human Movement*. New York: Wiley and Sons, 1990.
29. Yack HJ: Techniques for clinical assessment of gait. *Phys Ther* 1984; 64(12):1821–1829.

30. Vaughn CL, Davis BL, O'Connor JC: *Dynamics of Human Gait.* Champaign, IL: Human Kinetics, 1992.

31. Dempster WT: Space requirements of the seated operator. Dissertation, Ann Arbor, MI: University of Michigan, 1955.

32. Zatsiorsky VM, Seluyanov VN: The mass and inertia characteristics of the main segments of the human body, in Matsui H, Kobayashi K (eds): *Human Kinetics,* Champaign, IL: Raven, 1983, pp. 1152–1159.

33. Perry J, Easterday CS, Antonelli DJ: Surface versus intramuscular electrodes for electromyography of superficial and deep muscles. *Phys Ther* 1981; 61(1):7–15.

34. DeLuca CJ, Merletti R: Surface myoelectric signal crosstalk among muscles of the leg. *Electroenceph Clin Neurophysiol* 1988; 69:568–575.

35. Bekey GA, Chang C, Perry J, Hoffer MM: Pattern recognition of multiple EMG signals applied to the description of human gait. *Proc IEEE* 1977; 65(5):674–691.

Chapter 6

FUNCTIONAL NEUROIMAGING IN NEUROLOGIC RECOVERY

Bruce H. Dobkin

Neuroimaging techniques, such as computer tomography (CT) and magnetic resonance imaging (MRI), offer remarkable anatomic detail of the structural injuries incurred from stroke, traumatic brain injury (TBI), spinal cord injury, multiple sclerosis, and other diseases. Many correlative studies have been attempted to predict outcomes for impairments and disabilities based on the size and location of an area of infarction, hemorrhage, or encephalomalacia. Recently, imaging studies of the neuronal uptake of glucose and oxygen, cerebral blood flow, neurotransmitter localization, and electrophysiologic activity have been used to gain insight into the neuronal and synaptic adaptations associated with brain injury and restitution of function.

The techniques that are most likely to be of interest in neurorehabilitation are listed in Table 6-1. These techniques can reveal mechanisms of restitution and substitution by neuronal assemblies and pathways that allow gains after a central or peripheral nervous system injury.[1] In particular, positron emission tomography (PET) and functional magnetic resonance imaging (fMRI), especially when aligned with the anatomic landmarks provided by MRI, have provided maps of the distributed systems of the brain that carry out movement and cognition under normal conditions and after focal injuries. Imaging also has confirmed the representational adaptability of neuronal assemblies that participate in specific tasks. Activation studies that induce task-related changes in neuronal function over milliseconds to seconds will offer insights into some of the mechanisms of recovery and failure of recovery from impairments. They may also allow neurorehabilitation specialists to explore the efficacy of specific interventions.

FUNCTIONAL NEUROIMAGING TECHNIQUES

Techniques vary widely in their spatial and temporal resolution, in the volume of tissue sampled, and the minimal time interval required between consecutive tests. Some techniques demonstrate real-time representations of thoughts and movements better than others. Some are more practical than others in terms of expense, special equipment requirements, and the constraints on patient participation. All techniques are quite new in their potential applications for studies in neurorehabilitation.

Many functional imaging techniques require no radiologic or nuclear medicine support. Quantitative electroencephalography (EEG) with frequency analysis and topographical displays, sometimes referred to as EEG brain mapping, uses signal averaging and statistical approaches to assess EEG and evoked potential signals. The technique reflects the activity of a few square centimeters of cortical surface dipoles and has far greater temporal than spatial sensitivity. Greater numbers of electrodes in various configurations over the scalp may improve spatial sensitivity. Also, EEG and MRI data have been combined to provide a three-dimensional map in experiments that seek greater temporal and spatial resolution for functional imaging.[2] In special circumstances, such as preoperative evaluations for epilepsy, tumor, or arteriovenous malformation surgery, cortical electrode grids and electrodes placed deep into cerebral tissue achieve spatial resolution of about 100 microns[3] over a small region of interest.

Magnetoencephalography (MEG) reveals changes in weak electrical fields associated with neuronal activity

Table 6-1
Functional Neuroimaging Techniques

Individual methods
  Positron emission tomography (PET)
  Functional magnetic resonance imaging (fMRI)
  Single photon emission computerized tomography
    (SPECT)
  Magnetic resonance spectroscopy (MRS)
  Transcranial electrical and magnetic stimulation
  Quantitative electroencephalography (EEG)
  Magnetoencephalography (MEG)
  Transcranial doppler (TCD)
  Optical imaging
Integrated methods
  PET, SPECT, or fMRI superimposed upon MRI
  EEG or MEG superimposed on MRI

that occurs, like the EEG signal, over milliseconds. The MEG signal is less distorted by the skull than an EEG signal.[3] The procedure takes considerable time to sample the entire brain and requires rooms that are isolated from external magnetic interferences and devices that are expensive. However, this technique has detected cortical plasticity in human studies.[4]

Magnetic and electrical scalp stimulation techniques apply a transient clockwise current from a stimulating coil placed on the scalp in an optimal position to induce a counterclockwise current in the brain. This painlessly activates cortical neurons that, for example, will excite single bulbar and spinal motorneurons. Maps of cognitive and sensorimotor activity have been made.[5,6] Another technique, transcranial doppler ultrasonography, can map gross changes in cerebral blood flow associated with hemispheric motor activity.[7] Finally, high resolution optical imaging of human cortex at the time of a craniotomy may aid investigations of the cortical organization of sensorimotor and cognitive processes.[8] These signals are related to neuronal activity, ionic currents, oxygen delivery, changes in blood volume, or other metabolic processes.

Single photon emission tomography (SPECT) is performed with radiopharmaceuticals that are given intravenously or by inhalation. Radioisotopes that emit gamma rays include xenon-133, iodine-123, and technetium-99m. SPECT does not directly assess neuronal function, but cerebral perfusion, blood volume, and the distribution of several receptors, which are readily measured by SPECT, may indirectly reflect metabolism and

neuronal network activity. Early after stroke, SPECT tends not to differentiate between viable and irreversibly ischemic tissue, because the uptake of the radiotracer is not linearly related to perfusion. For post–acute ischemia studies that might be applicable to rehabilitation interventions, SPECT's spatial resolution is just under 1 cm^3.

PET measures the concentration of radioactivity in a volume of tissue after injection of a specifically labeled substrate such as water or glucose. Positron-emitting isotopes, which must be made at the time of a study, include fluorine-18, oxygen-15, nitrogen-13, and carbon-11. More biologically important radiopharmaceuticals are available for PET compared to SPECT. Future PET labeling techniques may allow studies of enzymatic reactions, protein synthesis, and neurotransmitter receptors in addition to the dopamine receptor that is already available. Spatial resolution for PET is about 125 mm^3. Whole brain samples and isotopes that have half-lives of seconds allow repeated studies every 10 minutes in some instances. PET studies are expensive and not generally available. Scanning equipment and cyclotrons to manufacture the radiotracers are becoming less cumbersome, but still require a dedicated team of physicists and other scientists.

PET has had its greatest impact on our understanding of some of the specific operations within the distributed neural systems for movement, language, attention, memory, perception, and other aspects of cognition.[9,10] Activation studies can reveal the location of important parallel, component computations that are orchestrated to complete a cognitive task. To get at these components, subtraction studies have come into common use. For example, the subject is given two or more behavioral tasks that are related, but differ by a defined process. Each differentially activates cerebral regions. By subtracting the activation produced by one from the other, the anatomical basis for one process is isolated. Movement paradigms might include a rest period, one or more variations on an upper limb movement, and imagining the movement. This allows a subtraction of the resting state of metabolic activity from the activity during willed movement and allows the resting state or movement state to be related to certain cognitive aspects of the movement, which are manifested by having a subject imagine doing the task. Imagery may play an important role in subtraction studies that are relevant to rehabilitation.[11]

Scanning during the rest or active periods must be done for about 45 seconds when using an oxygen tracer to detect a change in perfusion of as little as 5 percent. Repeated studies during the same session are limited by the total radiation exposure and the time it takes the radiotracer to no longer be detectable in the structures of interest. For example, studies with F-18-fluorodeoxyglucose require considerably longer times to carry out, up to 30 minutes after injection, due to the metabolic properties of the radioisotope, which takes a few minutes to be cleared from the cerebral circulation.

Functional MRI can be carried out less expensively than PET, without pharmaceutical preparation and exposure to radiation. The signal arises when neuronal activity increases local blood flow and volume with little or no change in oxygen consumption. This increases the oxygen content of local venous blood, which increases the intensity of the magnetic resonance signal.[12] A variety of modifications are in use, such as head coils, high field magnets, intravenous agents such as the paramagnetic chelate of gadolinium (Gd-DPTA), and a variety of pulse sequences. fMRI signals peak within several seconds and have a resolution that approaches 1 to 2 mm during visual, motor, sensory, and cognitive activation studies.[13] The results reflect differences between the baseline MR image intensity and one or more activation conditions. Any head movement may seriously compromise the images, although reregistration and realignment techniques for acquired data are available. Thus, this imaging technique could become a key method for evaluating the topographic reorganization of the brain after stroke and TBI.

MRI is based on the nuclear magnetic resonance (NMR) signal from water protons. Magnetic resonance spectroscopy (MRS) uses high field magnets to detect NMR signals in brain tissue from carbon-13, phosphorus-31, sodium-23, and fluorine-19.[14] This biochemical assay, which compares regions of interest, has a spatial resolution of 1 to 2 cm^3 and requires rather long imaging times.

Just what the activity represents that is quantified with any of the techniques in Table 6-1 is open to some controversy. Indeed, changes in functional activity, perhaps within the first week or two after a stroke or first month after TBI, may reflect a range of local metabolic activities that are not directly related to neuronal function. It is not yet clear when resting local and transynaptic neuronal activity and perfusion are stable postinjury. Further research with these tools, however, offers the possibility that we will have measures of regional brain activity that reflect the fine details in time and space of local neural activity and connectivity.

POTENTIAL APPLICATIONS OF FUNCTIONAL NEUROIMAGING

Neuroimaging indices of synaptic and neuronal activity could play an important role in the rehabilitation of motor and higher cognitive functions. For example, in patients with stroke, PET and fMRI could detect the evolution of functional reorganization throughout the involved network. The techniques reveal what are presumably critical parts of the circuits that reverberate during a learning task. They show the increase in synchrony along the parts of a distributed pathway as a subject performs. The uses of functional neuroimaging in rehabilitation are limited more by experimental designs and analytical techniques than by the need for major advances in technology. Many issues can at least begin to be addressed.

Functional neuroimaging might be used to examine the natural history of resting metabolic and rCBF patterns at clinically important milestones from onset of injury to time of maximal degree of recovery. This might lead to predictors of restitution of impairments and disabilities. Certain patterns might be related to the readiness of patients for rehabilitation, especially after TBI and hemispheric stroke. Task-related activation paradigms have great potential. By comparing a brain-injured patient's response to that of a normal subject in an activation paradigm for a cognitive or motor activity, therapists might offer interventional strategies that put less demand on processes that appear defunct in their patients. They might also use the patient's pattern of activation to predict whether or not an intervention is likely to be of benefit. If the training technique does not elicit the predicted activations, perhaps it could be modified to do so. This approach might reduce the number of subjects needed to study the efficacy of a new intervention.

Activation patterns and functional outcomes or changes in impairments might also be correlated with variations in the type, duration, and intensity of physical and cognitive therapies. Studies might assess the effects of medications on levels of activation and changes in patterns of engaged regions. In the near future, functional imaging could be used to monitor the effects of implants that replace neurons, produce neurotransmitters, and provide trophic factors. Such imaging has provided insight into the actions of dopamine-producing transplants in recipients who have Parkinson's disease.[15] As metabolic maps of cognitive and sensorimotor functions are defined for tasks carried out by normal subjects and by those who suffer a focal injury, rehabilitation specialists will better understand the pathways that subserve recovery and the effects of physical and pharmacologic interventions on plasticity.

STUDIES OF FUNCTIONAL OUTCOMES

Global correlations between the amount of ischemia and outcome have been made with most of the techniques in Table 6-1. In the near future, diffusion-weighted MRI and related techniques might distinguish between viable and nonviable tissue within 1 hour after stroke. PET studies that combine imaging of regional cerebral blood flow (rCBF) and oxygen consumption reveal early patterns that correlate with the presence of viable tissue and with clinical outcome.[16] The absence of cerebral perfusion and oxygen uptake has the poorest prognosis for a good functional outcome after cerebral ischemia. Hyperemia with some oxygen uptake points to tissue recovery and has the best prognosis. Low rCBF with higher oxygen uptake suggests misery perfusion in which cells grab as much oxygen as is available. This pattern has an intermediate, variable prognosis.

PET studies performed within 1 to 2 weeks of an acute stroke have also suggested that a higher ipsilateral global and contralateral cerebral metabolic rate for glucose correlates with better functional outcome in survivors at a mean of 3 and 50 months.[17,18] Low glucose consumption within the unaffected hemisphere in hypertensive patients was associated with poorer activities of daily living, perhaps because of a subclinical hypertensive arteriopathy producing tissue damage that limited compensation.[18] Predictive imaging information could aid the rehabilitation specialist who must make decisions about the appropriateness of the use of therapy resources.

SPECT, performed with technetium-99m-labeled hexamethyl-propyleneamine oxime or other tracers in the first 6 hours after stroke, has predicted poor outcomes at 1 month in some studies of large hemispheric infarction.[19] At 72 hours poststroke, a larger volume of regional hypoperfusion after a middle cerebral artery distribution infarction correlated with a poorer Barthel Index and Canadian Neurological Score.[20] Since SPECT studies are far more available compared to PET, investigators are likely to try to improve the spatial resolution and number of radiotracers available for studies in a clinical setting.

STUDIES OF SENSORIMOTOR RECOVERY

Transcranial magnetic and electrical stimulation studies have occasionally demonstrated residual activity in the corticospinal tract after a brain or spinal injury, which has predicted better recovery about as well as the clinical examination anticipated. Stimulation studies have also suggested activity in the undecussated corticospinal pathway.[21,22] Magnetic stimulation of the motor cortex ipsilateral to the affected side of subjects with hemiplegic cerebral palsy has produced bilateral hand movements in some subjects.[23] This flexion and extension correlated with a prenatal injury prior to about 32 weeks' gestation and with intense mirror movements of the hands. Other studies that included PET suggested to the investigators that such subjects had an aberrant cortical motor organization, as well as corticospinal pathways with prominent ipsilateral and contralateral actions.[24] Functional imaging has revealed other instances of reorganization. Overactivity of multiple contralateral and bilateral motor areas was found during a PET study when patients with hemidystonia that followed TBI used their affected upper extremity.[25] Thalamo-frontal disinhibition appeared to follow disruption of the usual inhibitory action of the basal ganglia in these patients. The physiologic explanations of behaviors provided by neuroimaging could lead to more theory-based interventions.

MRI and PET can also reveal spared tissue that accounts for subsequent partial recovery. For example, some patients with blindsight have been shown to have an island of spared striate cortex.[26] Functional imaging holds the greatest promise for identifying spared architecture in the neural networks for specific tasks.

PET and SPECT may reveal the phenomenon of diaschisis and transneuronal hypometabolism. Tissue remote from the ischemic injury can be hypometabolic owing to loss of afferent input from the damaged neural network or from disconnection from the input of one of the several diffuse neurotransmitter systems, such as noradrenergic or serotonergic modulation from the brain stem. For example, beyond 3 months after a left-sided striatocapsular infarction in patients who had recovered contralateral hand function, resting rCBF by PET was significantly lower in the left basal ganglia, thalamus, and the primary sensorimotor, insular, and dorsolateral prefrontal cortices; in the left cerebral peduncle; and in the ipsilateral right cerebellum compared to normal subjects.[27] This pattern corresponds to the circuit between the basal ganglia, thalamus, and cortical projections. The remote effects of the striatocapsular lesion were postulated to be related to either a transsynaptic functional deactivation or to structural changes from transsynaptic or retrograde degeneration. Also, rCBF was increased in the left posterior cingulate and premotor cortices and ipsilateral caudate. The investigators speculated that a loss of the functional inhibition of these areas by homotopic regions of the opposite hemisphere had developed. It is unclear whether or not these changes in activity have a clinical consequence. Functional imaging studies after stroke and TBI have not clearly shown that the presence of transneuronal hypometabolism limits functional recovery or that some level of restitution accompanies the resolution of apparent diaschisis.[28,29] Such clinical correlations would have a potential impact on the timing and duration of rehabilitation efforts.

Restitution of movements might result from adaptive changes in the coupling of the cortical and subcortical neuronal assemblies that represent a movement.[30,31] Cortical representational expansion has been observed in a study of patients after stroke. Patients with lesions limited to the posterior limb of the internal capsule who recovered the ability to oppose the thumb and fingers of the affected hand showed a 1-cm extension of activation within the contralateral primary sensorimotor cortex.[32] This corresponded to a spread from the hand area into the cortex that represented the face. This metabolically visualized enlargement of the contiguous cortical sensorimotor field is consistent with the multiple representations of muscles and movements within the motor cortex and with the mutability of neuronal representational maps.[1] Activated sites have differed in relationship to the precise location of the subcortical lesion.

Functional imaging studies have begun to map the regions of the brain that participate in the distributed parallel processing and hierarchical control of cognitive and motor functions. The capacity for functional reorganization has been especially apparent in the brains of infants and children after hemispherectomy for epilepsy and after early stroke.[33] Ipsilateral cortical efferent pathways can come to subserve, for example, hand activity.[34] This correlates with the maturational changes of human sensorimotor cortex through age 15, prior to the natural, perhaps activity-dependent regression of neurons and synapses in the developing brain.[35]

Bihemispheric reorganization has also been mapped after stroke in adults. Hemiparetic adults who were able to repeatedly squeeze a ball about 4 weeks after a cortical stroke were found, compared to normal

subjects, to activate their bilateral inferior parietal regions (Brodmann's areas 3, 1, and 2) when tested during a xenon-133 study of rCBF.[36] It has been postulated that undecussated corticospinal fibers from the ipsilateral hemisphere were involved in this restitution of function.[36]

Regional CBF studies by PET demonstrated considerable functional adaptation in a group of patients who recovered from a motor stroke. At least 3 months after a striatocapsular infarction, patients were tested under the conditions of rest, repeated thumb-to-finger opposition of the recovered right hand, and the same movement for the left hand.[27] During the motor task with either hand, the contralateral motor cortices and ipsilateral cerebellum were activated to the same degree as in normals. However, for the patients with recovered hand function, rCBF was greater than in normal subjects in the bilateral ventral premotor, supplementary motor, anterior insula, and parietal cortices, as well as in the ipsilateral premotor cortex, basal ganglia, and contralateral cerebellum. These nonprimary cortical motor areas appear to have served a compensatory function.

The bilateral recruitment may also explain the associated or mirror movements in the left hand that often accompanied a right-handed task. In a related study of individual cases with lesions of variable location within the striatocapsular complex, the ipsilateral primary sensorimotor cortex was activated more than in normal subjects only in those who exhibited associated movements of the unaffected hand during the finger opposition task by the recovered hand.[32] These PET studies of recovery offer other insights. Opposition of the fingers of the normal left hand activated the right insula, anterior cingulate, striatum, and the lateral prefrontal, premotor, and inferior parietal cortices more than normal. This might reflect the need for a greater effort by the patients. The experiments also showed that the lateral prefrontal and cingulate cortices and the angular gyrus were activated by a simple task after the stroke, suggesting that these interconnected areas related to selective attention and intention must come into play, at least when an automatic or previously learned movement recovers.

Another group of patients with subcortical strokes showed common patterns of activation, as well as individual variations. During a PET study, they made discriminations about the length of rectangular objects that they manipulated in the recovering hand without visual input.[37] Poor task performance correlated with low rCBF in the contralateral sensorimotor cortex at rest and bilateral activation during the task. The ipsilateral premotor cortex and contralateral anterolateral cerebellum were usually activated. The contralateral premotor cortex, supplementary motor area, and the bilateral posterior cingulate cortices were variably activated. The intact hemisphere appeared to participate in the initiation and maintenance of exploratory finger movements. Indeed, multiple functional regions of the neural system were activated during the recovering behavior.

Metabolic imaging studies are yielding many instances of compensatory shifts in neuronal systems, especially in primary sensory and association cortex. These shifts are evident as the paretic subject carries out and monitors difficult motor activities.[38] Activation paradigms during rehabilitation could serve as probes to learn whether or not a particular training approach will successfully engage areas that must be brought into play.

In normal subjects, transcranial magnetic stimulation also reveals motor plasticity during skill acquisition. Subjects who practiced a five-finger piano exercise for 2 hours a day for 5 days showed an enlarging motor cortical area targeting the long finger flexors and extensors, followed by a decreased threshold for activation as they learned the skill.[39]

Additional evidence suggests that cortical output maps to the muscles involved in a serial reaction time task, in which subjects had to learn from ongoing experience which buttons to push, enlarge as subjects learn the task.[40] Up to that point, they had implicit or unconscious knowledge of the task. When they achieved explicit or verbalizable knowledge of how to do the task, the map of cortical output returned to baseline. These examples of rapid motor learning with enlarging maps suggest that synaptic connections are unmasked and the motoneurons form new movement associations. Once the procedure is overlearned and automatic, cortical excitation related to learning is no longer needed and knowledge about the movement is at least partly stored elsewhere. Similar observations have been made with PET.[41] These imaging techniques could reveal whether or not a particular rehabilitative intervention affects representational plasticity in association with changes in impairments and disabilities.

PET studies of normal subjects, performed with fluorodeoxyglucose, have shown increased activity in the cerebellar vermis and the bilateral occipital and paramedian motor cortices during normal walking.[42] Subtraction images were made between supine position at rest and treadmill walking. Increases in activation

were also observed in Brodmann's areas 4, 18, 22, 40, and 43 in the left hemisphere and the superior vermis. This activity presumably reflects the integration of visual, auditory, and somatosensory information with motor activity in the leg region for motor control during rhythmic stepping. SPECT data obtained during treadmill walking and compared to standing reveal similar activations.[43] Bilateral primary sensorimotor and supplementary motor cortices were especially active during walking, along with cingulate and prefrontal cortices that may be needed for rhythmic movement and attention in the setting of treadmill locomotion. Functional imaging studies of the activations associated with hemiparetic gait are in progress at several centers.

STUDIES OF LANGUAGE AND COGNITIVE RECOVERY

PET studies of a cognitive task can be revealing. They may also be misleading.[44] Unrecognized processes that are below the resolution of PET might be at work. On the other hand, automatic, subconscious processing that is not neccessary for the task might activate regions. For example, anterior language areas can be activated by preparation for speech, in the absence of articulation. Instructions, practice, habituation, level of difficulty, attentional demands, emotional state, rate and order of stimulation, and other features of experimental design all affect metabolic localization. Both PET and fMRI reveal how the nature of a task, such as its degree of difficulty, whether it is internally or externally cued, and how it is learned, will alter what cerebral regions come into play.[45,46] Other limitations for the assessment of cognitive processes include the relative slowness of SPECT, PET, and fMRI scanning, measured in seconds rather than in the milliseconds in which cognitive processing transpires. In addition, studies within and across subjects may be confounded by the adequacy of statistical methods used to compare two or more activation states and errors in mapping. Such errors may occur when a PET image is transposed onto an MR image to combine exact anatomy with physiological activity.

Despite these potential limitations, functional imaging will increasingly allow the generation and testing of hypotheses about motor and cognitive processes and about adaptive functional changes after a cerebral injury. Patients with aphasia of all types who can speak spontaneously have a higher left hemisphere regional metabolic rate for glucose by PET during speech activation 2 weeks after onset compared to those who are not fluent.[47] These observations have strengthened predictions for a better recovery at 4 months.[47]

In patients who recovered from Wernicke's aphasia despite destruction of the left posterior perisylvian language area, increased rCBF by PET was found in the left frontal and right perisylvian areas.[48] This dual activation suggests the existence of a bilateral network for the distributed, parallel processing of language that may serve as a mechanism for restitution of language function. More metabolic-clinical correlation studies are needed.

Activation paradigms have the potential to assume increasing importance for speech therapists in assessing the intactness of areas that may enhance the likelihood of gains in specific language functions. For example, a noninvasive method to test for hemispheric specialization for language has been suggested using fMRI.[49] Distributed, unilateral signal increases have been found for a linguistic task that involved processing single words based on their semantic content. In contrast, a nonlinguistic task activated the temporal lobe auditory areas and the bilateral dorsolateral frontal lobes as subjects processed pure tones.

PET and fMRI studies have also begun to reveal the functional anatomy of other cognitive functions that are often impaired by TBI and stroke. Examples include the association between depression and metabolic activity in a left limbic-thalamo-prefrontal cortical circuit that includes the amygdala, the lexical processing of language within the left frontal and temporal lobes, the functional architecture of various types of memory, and the regional localization of learning for a variety of motor tasks.[44,50-54]

PET, fMRI, and other functional neuroimaging techniques can become the tools of rehabilitation specialists for studying hypotheses about training and recovery. The functional organization associated with learning and task-oriented skills training are especially likely to be imaged. Carefully designed experiments and clinical trials that incorporate these tools continue to pave a scientific approach to neurorehabilitation.

REFERENCES

1. Dobkin BH: *Contemporary Neurology Series: Neurologic Rehabilitation.* Philadelphia: FA Davis, 1996.
2. Crease R: Biomedicine in the age of imaging. *Science* 1993; 261:554.
3. Cohen D, Cuffin B, Yunokuchi K, et al: MEG vs EEG localization test using implanted sources in the human brain. *Ann Neurol* 1990; 28:811.
4. Mogilner A, Grossman J, Ribary U, et al: Somatosensory cortical plasticity in adult human revealed by magnetoencephalography. *Proc Natl Acad Sci USA* 1993; 90: 3593.
5. Perrine K, Uysal S, Dogali M, Devinsky O: Functional mapping of memory and other nonlinguistic cognitive abilities in adults, in Devinsky O, Beric A, Dogali M (eds): *Electrical and Magnetic Stimulation of the Brain and Spinal Cord.* New York: Raven Press, 1993, pp. 165–177.
6. Cohen L, Brasil-Neto J, Pascual-Leone A, Hallett M: Plasticity of cortical motor output organization following deafferentation, cerebral lesions, and skill acquisition, in Devinsky O, Beric A, Dogali M (eds): *Electrical and Magnetic Stimulation of the Brain and Spinal Cord.* New York: Raven Press, 1993, pp. 187–200.
7. Silvestrini M, Caltagirone C, Cupini L, et al: Activation of healthy hemisphere in poststroke recovery: A transcranial doppler study. *Stroke* 1993; 24:1673.
8. Haglund M, Ojemann G, Hochman D: Optical imaging of epileptiform and functional activity in human cerebral cortex. *Nature* 1992; 358:668.
9. Mazziotta J, Gilman S: *Contemporary Neurology Series: Clinical Brain Imaging: Principles and Applications.* Philadelphia: FA Davis, 1992.
10. Posner M, Petersen S, Fox P, Raichle M: Localization of cognitive operations in the human mind. *Science* 1988; 240:1627.
11. Decety J: Can motor imagery be used as a form of therapy? *J NIH Res* 1995; 7:47.
12. Turner R: Magnetic resonance imaging of brain function. *Ann Neurol* 1994; 35:637.
13. Cohen M, Bookheimer S: Localization of brain function using magnetic resonance imaging. *Trends Neurosci* 1994; 17:268.
14. Prichard J, Rosen B: Functional study of the brain by NMR. *J Cereb Blood Flow Metab* 1994; 14:365.
15. Freed C, Breeze R, Mazziotta J, et al: Survival of implanted fetal dopamine cells and neurologic improvement 12 to 48 months after transplantation for Parkinson's disease. *N Engl J Med* 1992; 327:1549.
16. Marchal G, Serrati C, Baron J, et al: PET imaging of cerebral perfusion and oxygen consumption in acute ischaemic stroke: Relation to outcome. *Lancet* 1993; 341:925.
17. Kushner M, Reivich M, Fieschi C, et al: Metabolic and clinical correlates of acute ischemic infarction. *Neurology* 1987; 37:1103.
18. Heiss W-D, Emunds H-G, Herbolz K: Cerebral glucose metabolism as a predictor of rehabilitation after ischemic stroke. *Stroke* 1993; 24:1784.
19. Giubilei F, Lenzi G, DiPiero V, et al: Predictive value of brain perfusion single-photon emission computed tomography in acute ischemic stroke. *Stroke* 1990; 21:895.
20. Davis S, Chua M, Lichtenstein M, et al: Cerebral hypoperfusion in stroke prognosis and brain recovery. *Stroke* 1993; 24:1691.
21. Wasserman E, Fuhr P, Cohen L, Hallett M: Effects of

transcranial magnetic stimulation on ipsilateral muscles. *Neurology* 1991; 41:1795.

22. Palmer E, Ashby P, Hajek V: Ipsilateral fast corticospinal pathways do not account for recovery in stroke. *Ann Neurol* 1992; 32:519.

23. Carr L, Harrison L, Evans A, Stephans J: Patterns of central motor reorganization in hemiplegic cerebral palsy. *Brain* 1993; 116:1223.

24. Cohen L, Meer J, Tarkka I, Hallett M, et al: Congenital mirror movements. *Brain* 1991; 114:381.

25. Ceballos-Baumann A, Passingham R, Marsden C, Brooks D: Motor reorganization in acquired hemidystonia. *Ann Neurol* 1995; 37:746.

26. Fendrich R, Wessinger C, Gazzaniga M: Technical Notes: Sources of blindsight. *Science* 1993; 261:493.

27. Weiller C, Chollet F, Friston K, Wise R, Frackowiak R: Functional reorganization of the brain in recovery from striatocapsular infarction in man. *Ann Neurol* 1992; 31:463.

28. Bowler J, Wade J, Jones B, et al: Contribution of diaschisis to the clinical deficit in human cerebral infarction. *Stroke* 1995; 26:1000.

29. Bergsneider M, Kelly D, Shalmon E, et al: Remote metabolic depression following human traumatic brain injury: A PET study. *J Neurotrauma* 1994; 12:110.

30. Merzenich M, Recanzone G, Jenkins W, Nudo R: How the brain functionally rewires itself, in Arbib M, Robinson J (eds): *Natural and Artificial Parallel Computations.* Cambridge, MA: MIT Press, 1990, pp. 170–198.

31. Dobkin BH: Neuroplasticity: Key to recovery after central nervous system injury. *West J Med* 1993; 159:56.

32. Weiller C, Ramsay S, Wise R, Frackowiak R: Individual patterns of functional reorganization in the human cerebral cortex after capsular infarction. *Ann Neurol* 1993; 33:181.

33. Chugani H, Shewmon D, Peacock W, Mazziotta J, et al: Surgical treatment of intractable neonatal-onset seizures: The role of PET. *Neurology* 1988; 38:1178.

34. Sabatini U, Toni D, Pantano P, et al: Motor recovery after early brain damage. *Stroke* 1994; 25:514.

35. Chugani H, Phelps M, Mazziotta J: Positron emission tomography study of human brain functional development. *Ann Neurol* 1987; 22:487.

36. Brion J-P, Demeurisse G, Capon A: Evidence of cortical reorganization in hemiparetic patients. *Stroke* 1989; 20:1079.

37. Weder B, Herzog H, Seitz R, et al: Tactile exploration of shape after subcortical ischaemic infarction studied with PET. *Brain* 1994; 117:593.

38. Blood K, Perlman S, Bailliet R, et al: Visual cortex hyperactivity during arm movements in brain injured individuals: Evidence of compensatory shifts in functional neural systems. *J Neurol Rehab* 1991; 5:211.

39. Pascual-Leone A, Cohen L, Dang N, Hallett M, et al: Acquisition of fine motor skills in humans is associated with the modulation of cortical motor outputs. *Neurology* 1993; 43(suppl):A157.

40. Pascual-Leone A, Grafman J, Hallett M: Modulation of cortical output maps during development of implicit and explicit knowledge. *Science* 1994; 263:1287.

41. Grafton S, Mazziotta J, Presty S, et al: Functional anatomy of human procedural learning determined with regional cerebral blood flow and PET. *J Neurosci* 1992; 12:2542.

42. Ishii K, Senda M, Toyama H, et al: Brain function in bipedal gait: A PET study. *Human Brain Mapping* 1995; 2(suppl 1):321.

43. Greenstein J, Bastineau E, Siegel B, et al: Cerebral hemisphere activation during human bipedal locomotion. *Human Brain Mapping* 1995; 2(suppl 1):320.

44. Frackowiak R: Functional mapping of verbal memory and language. *Trends Neurosci* 1994; 17:109.

45. Rao S, Binder J, Bandettini P: Functional magnetic resonance imaging of complex human movements. *Neurology* 1993; 43:2311.

46. Remy P, Zilbovicius M, Leroy-Willig A, et al: Movement- and task-related activations of motor cortical areas: A positron emission tomographic study. *Ann Neurol* 1994; 36:19.

47. Heiss W-D, Kessler J, Karbe H, et al: Cerebral glucose metabolism as a predictor of recovery from aphasia in ischemic stroke. *Arch Neurol* 1993; 50:958.

48. Weiller C, Isensee C, Rijntjes M, et al: Recovery from Wernicke's aphasia: A positron emission tomographic study. *Ann Neurol* 1995; 37:723.

49. Binder J, Rao S, Hammeke T, et al: Lateralized human brain language systems demonstrated by task subtraction functional magnetic resonance imaging. *Arch Neurol* 1995; 52:593.

50. Drevets W, Videen T, Price J, et al: A functional anatomical study of unipolar depression. *J Neurosci* 1992; 12:3628.

51. Damasio A, Tranel D: Nouns and verbs are retrieved with differently distributed neural systems. *Neurobiology* 1993; 90:4957.

52. Perani D, Bressi S, Cappa F, et al: Evidence of multiple memory systems in the human brain: A PET metabolic study. *Brain* 1993; 116:903.

53. Kawashima R, Roland P, O'Sullivan B: Fields in human motor areas involved in preparation for reaching, actual reaching, and visuomotor learning: A PET study. *J Neurosci* 1994; 14:3462.

54. Jenkins I, Brooks J, Frackowiak R, et al: Motor sequence learning: A study with positron emission tomography. *J Neurosci* 1994; 14:3775.

Part II

REHABILITATION OF DISEASES OF THE NERVOUS SYSTEM

Chapter 7

TRAUMATIC BRAIN INJURY

Mary L. Dombovy

EPIDEMIOLOGY

Traumatic brain injury (TBI) can be defined as the delivery of force to the brain, by any means, that leads to transient or permanent alteration in neurologic function. TBI occurs at a rate of 200 per 100,000 population and has its peak incidence in the second and third decade.[1] The majority of these cases are classified as "mild" (130/100,000) and generally will not require rehabilitation.[2] However, many patients with "mild TBI" do have symptoms, and some will have lasting cognitive and behavioral changes that require neurologic assessment and rehabilitation in order to achieve optimal functional recovery.[2]

Ten percent of TBI are fatal.[2] An additional 20 to 30 percent of all persons with TBI sustain moderate to severe brain injuries that necessitate extensive hospital-based rehabilitation. Severe head injury is less common in children, and mortality from severe brain injury is also less compared to adults.[3] Based on available statistics, it is estimated that in a community of 1 million people, each year 313 people will be discharged alive following a TBI that results in some degree of neurological or neuropsychological impairment.[1] The prevalence of TBI survivors with some degree of related disability is estimated at 400 per 100,000 population. The most common cause of TBI in adults is motor vehicle accidents, and in young children, falls.[4]

Severity of brain injury is commonly determined from the Glasgow Coma Scale (GCS, Table 7-1) at the time of admission; the length of coma (the duration that the patient is <9 on the GCS); or the duration of post-traumatic amnesia (PTA, considered to be a score of <75 on the Galveston Orientation and Amnesia Test [GOAT, Table 7-2]).[6] Patients with an admission GCS of <9, a duration of coma greater than 8 hours, or a PTA of greater than 24 hours may be considered to have a severe TBI. Patients with admission GCS of 9–12 are considered to have a moderate injury, and those with GCS 13–15 or a PTA of <1 hour, a mild injury.

Inherent weaknesses of the GCS include its difficult administration to young children, patients with significant swelling owing to facial trauma, patients who are intoxicated, and those affected by language impairments. Immediate intubation and sedation also obviously will affect the score. Accurately determining the time at which any patient emerges from post-traumatic amnesia also is challenging and highly variable. Delayed intracranial hemorrhage, the effects of somatic physical injury, and systemic metabolic responses may confound the accurate assessment of primary central nervous system injury. Approximately 10 percent of adults initially talk following TBI and then deteriorate.[7] Fifty percent of these patients die or have a very poor outcome. Hence, the determination of severity of brain injury is an estimate at best.

PATHOPHYSIOLOGY

Two distinct components contribute to the pathophysiology of brain injury: the immediate trauma (primary injury) resulting from the forces applied to the brain, and the secondary injury that develops from subsequent metabolic responses, delayed injury, and systemic complications (Table 7-3). Two separate forces often combine to produce the initial injury: impact, leading to skull deformation and fracture with underlying focal brain injury; and inertial loading, including both linear and rotational acceleration-deceleration forces that re-

Table 7-1
Glasgow Coma Scale

	Examiner's test	Patient's responses	Assigned score
Eye opening	Spontaneous	Opens eyes on own	B4
	Speech	Opens eyes when asked to in a loud voice	3
	Pain	Opens eyes on pressure	2
	Pain	Does not open eyes	1
Best motor response	Commands	Follows simple commands	M6
	Pain	Pulls examiner's hand away on pressure	5
	Pain	Pulls a part of body away on pressure	4
	Pain	Flexes body inappropriately to pain (decorticate posturing)	3
	Pain	Body becomes rigid in an extended position on pressure (decerebrate posturing)	2
	Pain	Has no motor responses to pressure	1
Verbal response (talking)	Speech	Carries on a conversation correctly and tells examiner where he/she is, who he/she is, and the month and year	V5
	Speech	Seems confused or disoriented	4
	Speech	Talks so examiner can understand patient but makes no sense	3
	Speech	Makes sounds that examiner cannot understand	2
	Speech	Makes no noise	1

sult in both focal and diffuse injury. When brain injury occurs as a result of a motor vehicle accident (acceleration), the resultant damage is likely to be greater than that produced by crushing injuries to the stationary head.

The pathology that is produced by acceleration is owing to the differential rates that propel the skull and the brain. Initially, the displacement of bone with respect to brain causes abrasive frictional forces that damage the outer surface of the brain. Once the forward movement of the skull is stopped abruptly by contact with an immovable object, the brain continues forward until it collides with the skull opposite the point of initial impact. The elasticity of the cranial contents allows this process to be repeated through several oscillations during deceleration, exposing the friable cortical surface to repeated impacts.

Contusional injury is seen commonly in brain tissues that interface with unyielding edges and ridges of the skull: the orbital surface of the frontal bone, the sphenoid ridge, the petrous portion of the temporal bone, and the sharp edges of the falces. Therefore, the basal and polar portions of the frontal and temporal lobes are most vulnerable to contusional injury.[8]

However, not all contusions are confined to these areas. Cavitation phenomena contribute to the contrecoup injury, basal frontal contusions, and microvascular hemorrhage. Cavitation theory predicts that fluid molecules will translocate to the impact pole, creating a negative pressure gradient that causes an explosive liquid to gas phase shift in the region of the opposite pole and in the microvasculature.[9]

Diffuse axonal injury (DAI) can be produced either mechanically or biochemically by metabolic responses to injury. The shearing forces between brain tissues of different densities physically damages cellular structure during acceleration–deceleration. Cytotoxic neurochemicals are released at the time of impact, initiating a cascade of metabolic events that lead to neuronal death. These devastating injuries often escape detection even with modern imaging techniques.

Deep brain lesions are thought to result from rotational forces that produce shearing between structures of varying density and different mobility.[10] These effects are most pronounced at the junctions between grey and white matter. Areas most susceptible to this type of injury include the reticular formation, superior cerebellar peduncles, basal ganglia, fornices, hypothalamus, and corpus callosum. Widespread tissue destruction may occur, accompanied by microhemorrhage and eventually axonal degeneration.

The clinical expression of these lesions includes disturbances of consciousness and attention, vestibular dysfunction, and a variety of motor impairments and

Table 7-2
Galveston Orientation and Amnesia Test

Name: _____ Age: _____ Sex: M   F

Date of Test: _____ Day of the Week: _____

Diagnosis: _____ Date of Injury: _____

Galveston Orientation and Amnesia Test (GOAT)   Error Points

1. What is your name? (2) _____   When were you born? (4) _____   _____
    Where do you live? (4) _____

2. Where are you now? (5) city _____   (5) Hospital _____   _____
    (unnecessary to state name of hospital)

3. On what date were you admitted to this hospital? (5) _____   _____
    How did you get here? (5) _____

4. What is the first event you can remember after your injury? (5) _____ _____   _____
    Can you describe in detail (e.g., date, time, companions) the first event you can recall
    after injury? (5) _____

5. Can you describe the last event you recall before the accident? (5) _____   _____
    Can you describe in detail (e.g., date, time, companions) the first event you can recall
    before the injury? (5) _____

6. What time is it now? _____ (-1 for each $\frac{1}{2}$ hour removed from correct time to   _____
    maximum of -5).

7. What day of the week is it? _____ (-1 for each day removed from correct one).   _____

8. What day of the month is it? _____ (-1 for each day removed from correct date   _____
    to maximum of -5).

9. What is the month? _____ (-5 for each month removed from correct one   _____
    to a maximum of -15).

10. What is the year? _____ (-10 for each year removed from correct one to   _____
    maximum of -30).

                                                        Total Error Points   _____
                            Total GOAT score ($100 =$ total error points)   _____

movement disorders. In addition, devastating long-term consequences may arise from the resultant disconnection syndromes leading to considerable psychobehavioral morbidity.

Delayed cell degeneration may also occur after DAI. Pathologically, there is a lag time between the occurrence of the injury and the development of the full array of pathological markers of DAI.[11] Some have hypothesized that TBI focally alters the axonal cytoskeleton, impairing axonal transport, leading to axonal swelling and detachment as early as 6–12 hours after the injury.[12] The proximal axonal segment then undergoes Wallerian degeneration.

Following TBI there is a tremendous outpouring of excitatory neurotransmitters that results in a self-perpetuating cascade of metabolic events in response

Table 7-3

Mechanisms of injury in TBI

Primary injury	Secondary injury
Diffuse axonal injury/multiple petechial hemorrhages	Increased intracranial pressure
Contusions	Hypoxia-ischemia/ hypotension
Subdural, epidural, intracerebral hemorrhage (may be secondary)	Cerebral infarction
Subarachnoid hemorrhage	Hydrocephalus Autodestructive cellular processes Delayed hemorrage Infection Hyponatremia Hypoglycemia

to CNS injury. This may lead to changes in ion gradients across cell membranes with uncontrolled calcium influx, activation of lipases and proteases, and the eventual destruction of the cell membrane. Calcium interacts with free radicals to produce arachidonic acid that is converted to vasoactive metabolites that may further compromise blood flow.[13]

Traumatic hematomas result from lacerations to or shear stress applied to the vasculature supplying the brain. Traumatic hematomas generally are named after the space they occupy. They can occur shortly after impact, or accumulate after a delay of minutes to hours. About 90 percent of epidural hematomas are associated with skull fractures, or with bleeding originating from lacerated dural vessels, ruptured dural sinuses, or torn meningeal arteries.[14] Subdural hematomas result from laceration or shearing of cortical veins that bleed into the subdural space. Vascular injury usually is associated with underlying cortical contusion and, in general, indicates more severe DAI.[15] Subdural hematomas occurring in the elderly often are associated with trivial trauma. Intracerebral hematomas are produced by cortical lacerations and deep shearing injuries. Within a few days of the initial trauma, these small deep lesions may coalesce into a large hematoma that can lead to rapid herniation. Often this is precipitated by renewed bleeding as vessels previously tamponaded by edema and vasospasm rebleed and vessels injured by ischemia and trauma leak.[16]

Cerebral edema can also lead to secondary injury following TBI.[17] Vasogenic edema is the accumulation of excess water in the extracellular space owing to the disruption of the blood-brain barrier. This process begins in the first several hours following TBI and usually peaks within days. In cytotoxic edema, impairment of cell membrane metabolism leads to the diffusion of water from the extracellular into the intracellular space. As cells swell, capillary lumina are blocked, setting up a pernicious and sometimes lethal cycle of edema and ischemia. Vasogenic edema can be reduced partially by the use of hyperosmolar agents. Cytotoxic edema, as a rule, cannot.

Hydrocephalus, either communicating or noncommunicating, can develop nearly any time following TBI. Acute hydrocephalus usually is related to obstruction of the foramina of the ventricular system by compression from edema, expanding mass lesions, or by intraventricular hemorrhage. Subacute or chronic hydrocephalus is more commonly the communicating type, owing to either obstruction of cerebrospinal fluid (CSF) absorption in the dural sinuses or foramenal/aqueductal obstruction of CSF circulation by blood products or protein.

Hematomas, edema, and hydrocephalus, alone or in combination, may increase intracranial pressure. Increases in intracranial pressure ultimately decrease cerebral blood flow, and may lead to cerebral ischemia. Following TBI, autoregulation is impaired. Even small elevations in intracranial blood pressure may result in significant reductions in cerebral blood flow. When increases in intracranial pressure are accompanied by decreases in systemic blood pressure, cerebral blood flow is critically reduced, and ischemic encephalopathy is likely to result.[18]

In addition to causing ischemia, increases in intracranial pressure can cause physical shifts of brain tissue from one compartment to another, referred to as herniations.[9] The most common of these is the Subfalcine herniation, when an asymmetric mass lesion forces the cingulate gyrus under the falx. This herniation is visible on CT scanning, and may be asymptomatic or, in more extreme cases, result in entrapment of the anterior cerebral artery leading to frontal lobe infarction. Transtentorial herniation occurs when the temporal lobe is displaced medially and caudally between the midbrain and tentorium. Early clinical signs include pupillary dilation and vomiting. Progressive herniation leads to ocular paresis, decerebrate rigidity, coma, and death. The posterior cerebral arteries may be entrapped, resulting in occipital and mesial temporal lobe infarction. Because the hippocampal formation is damaged by this process, memory difficulties are common in those who survive.

Tonsilar herniation results from extrusion of the cerebellar tonsils and medulla through the foramen magnum, crushing the lower brainstem and upper spinal cord. Death may result from damage to vasomotor and respiratory control centers.

Intracranial infections such as meningitis and abscess may develop in the days to weeks following TBI.[19] Depressed skull fractures, facial, sinus, and basilar skull fractures predispose to their development. Persistent CSF leaks related to dural tears create an ongoing risk of infection.

Systemic toxic and metabolic factors that may lead to secondary CNS injury include hypoxemia, hypotension, hypercapnia, anemia, hyponatremia, hypoglycemia, and sepsis.[15] Sixty percent of severe and 40 percent of moderate brain injuries are accompanied by one or more systemic complications.[9] Hypoxemia occurs in more than 30 percent of severe TBI.[15] The hippocampal structures involved in learning and memory are particularly vulnerable to hypoxemic damage. In addition, hypotension may lead to arterial border zone infarction. Twenty percent of patients with TBI sustain thoracic and abdominal trauma that may contribute to hypotension.[7]

The nature of deficits following TBI and the time course of recovery are related chiefly to three major pathologic processes: (1) diffuse axonal injury (DAI); (2) focal injury (focal hemorrhage, focal ischemia); and (3) diffuse hypoxic–ischemic injury (HII).

CLINICAL-PATHOLOGICAL DIAGNOSIS AND TREATMENT PLANNING

To facilitate rehabilitation treatment planning, several pieces of information must be pulled together to formulate a patient profile and estimate injury severity (Table 7-4).

Consequences of Focal Lesions

As with focal lesions of any cause, the profile of impairments from focal TBI corresponds to their location and size. Table 7-5 displays the typical locations of focal lesions in TBI. The commonly occurring anterior and inferior frontal and temporal lobe lesions often result in impairments of the following functions.

Table 7-4

Clinical-pathological diagnosis and treatment planning

Cause of injury

History of patient condition when first discovered

Depth of coma (GCS) immediately after stabilization

Duration of coma (time to GCS >8, or time to purposeful movement)

Duration of PTA

Presence of focal lesions; neuroimaging data

Early signs of herniation and increased intracranial pressure (e.g., third nerve palsy)

Signs of brainstem injury or compression

History of hypoxemia, hypotension, cardiac arrest

History of other injuries and medical complications

1. *Processing functions* (manipulating, organizing, and sequencing multimodal information);

2. *Executive functions* (anticipating, planning, selecting, modifying, and experimenting during environmental interaction);

3. *Monitoring functions* (self-awareness, self-control, insight into impairments); and

4. *Drive* (initiating, modulating, and inhibiting behavior).

These portions of the brain contain paralimbic and multi-modal or heteromodal association areas highly connected to limbic structures and motor and sensory association areas.[20] The size of the lesion(s), particularly the depth of subcortical involvement, is an important determinant of long-term effects. Contusions with greater subcortical involvement will result in greater and more widespread deafferentation and deefferentation of these critical frontal and temporal multi-modal association areas. The effects of focal cortical injury usually are masked initially and complicated by the presence of DAI and/or HII.

The frontal lobe can be divided into four neurobehavioral sections, based on anatomic physiologic and behavioral data from animal and human studies: superior mesial, inferior mesial, dorsolateral, and orbital. The specific clinical and cognitive impairments that are associated with damage to these regions are summarized in Table 7-6. The superior mesial frontal lobe is connected with motor and diverse limbic structures, and indirectly to the diencephalon and other cortical association areas, thus influencing motor, endocrine, and auto-

Table 7-5

Focal lesions in TBI: location and consequences

Lesions	Location	Consequences
Focal cortical contusion	Frontal polar and orbital frontal	Alterations in affect and behavior (higher-level intellectual abilities, e.g., executive functions, self-awareness)
	Anterior-inferior temporal	Alterations in affect and behavior, agnosias
Deep hemorrhages	Basal ganglia area	Hemiparesis, incoordination, hypertonia, movement disorders, tremor, aphasia (left), neglect, and visual disorder (right)
Focal hypoxic-ischemic injury	Posterior cerebral artery infarct	Hemianopia, cortical blindness (bilaterally), amnesia, aphasia (alexia, anomia, mesial temporal occipital, agraphia, posterior parietal; left), neglect, topographical disorientation (right), other complex visual disturbances

Modified from Katz and Alexander, 1992.

nomic functions. Bilateral injury to this area results in profound akinesia and mutism, with absence of spontaneity. In most instances, patients are not confused, and may briefly speak or otherwise respond normally. Treatment with a dopamine agonist such as bromocriptine appears to improve this deficit.[21] Unilateral lesions result in less severe impairments, but include apraxias, reduced spontaneity and initiation, and impaired affective expression. The superior mesial frontal lobe contributes a prominent activation component to internal states and behavior, as well as motor programming, self-regulation, and mental flexibility.[22,23]

The inferior mesial frontal region contains the structures of the basal forebrain. Damage to this area causes amnesia, particularly for the temporal-spatial aspects of recent memory, confabulations, disinhibition, inattentiveness, lack of motivation, and utilization behavior.[24–27] In TBI, bilateral injury to this area is the rule.

Table 7-6

Neurobehavioral impairments associated with damage to specific lobe regions

Superior mesial	Inferior mesial	Dorsolateral	Orbital
Akinesia	Amnesia	Poor integration and synthesis	Personality change
Mutism	Confabulations	Disorganized thinking and behavior	Impulsive actions
Apathy	Disinhibition	Perseveration	Poor social judgment
	Lack of motivation	Cognitive rigidity	Reduced empathy
	Inattention	Poor planning	Lack of goal-directed behavior
	Utilization behavior	Impulsive responding	
		Stimulus-boundedness	
		Lack of empathy	
		Impaired self-regulation	
		Right: left hemispatial neglect, poor spatial cognition	
		Left: nonfluent aphasias	

Modified from Eslinger et al., 1995.

The dorsolateral frontal region encompasses large areas of the prefrontal cortex, including the frontal pole, and mediates cognitive processes that are to some degree lateralized to left or right. The cognitive and behavioral systems operating in this area are multi-modal and supra-modal. This region is strongly interconnected with posterior cortical association regions that provide highly processed visual, auditory, and somatosensory information.[28,29] There are also strong connections with subcortical structures, including the thalamus, hypothalamus, amygdala, and septum. The dorsolateral frontal lobe contributes to the converging corticostriate pathways to the head of the caudate nucleus that form functional circuits linked to cognitive flexibility and the capacity for set-shifting responses.[30] The dorsolateral region also is highly connected with the orbital region, providing for mediation of internal states and autonomic functions with perception and decisions related to external circumstances. Characteristic impairments associated with focal injury to this region include poor integration and synthesis of information, disorganization in thinking and behavior, perseveration, rigidity, concrete thinking, poor planning, impulsivity, irritability, and lack of empathy.[21] Left-sided lesions have been associated with transcortical motor aphasia and to other executive–cognitive functions that require verbal mediation. Damage to the right dorsolateral frontal region is associated with spatial cognitive impairments, including left hemispatial neglect and spatially disorganized thought and behavior. Dorsolateral frontal damage also may lead to poor self-monitoring, and limit self-recognition of the nature and extent of the disability.

The orbital frontal region has rich connections to limbic regions, the dorsolateral frontal region, and diencephalon. Orbital frontal damage without involvement of the basal forebrain region has been associated with significant change in personality and social behavior, as well as impulsivity, lack of sustained goal-directed behavior, and reduced empathy.[31,32] Damage to this region may lead to recovery to the point of normal measured intelligence, language abilities, learning and short-term memory, structured problem-solving, and perception.[21] The profound cognitive impairments associated with dorsolateral frontal damage, the akinesia associated with superior mesial damage, or the amnesia associated with inferior mesial damage are the exception rather than the rule. Orbital frontal injury may lead to marked difficulties in adjustment and adaptation, out of proportion to any degree of cognitive or neurologic disability. These problems may become apparent only later in rehabilitation when high-level judgment of social and other complex situations is required. Such patients may appear to be malingering, because their neurological examination is normal.

Traumatic temporal lobe lesions also may involve connections between tertiary sensory association areas and limbic structures. The typical anterior–inferior location of temporal contusions causes damage to the paralimbic temporal neocortex that is highly connected to frontal areas. These regions may function as a unit involved in the emotional regulation of behavior.[20] Medial temporal and more posterior inferior temporal regions occasionally may be directly damaged or compressed by local mass effect and herniation. If this occurs, prominent memory problems result. Bilateral anterior–medial temporal lesions damaging the amygdala and sensory–limbic connections lead to a severe defect in the attribution of significance to environmental stimuli.[20] At the extreme is the Kluver-Bucy syndrome.[33] Fragments of this syndrome have been described in humans after traumatic anterior temporal injury and include placidity, compulsive exploratory behavior, bulimia, and altered sexual behavior.[34] Delusional thinking and paranoid psychoses are also seen following temporal lobe injury.[35] The mechanism does not appear to be based on memory impairment alone. Temporal–spatial disorientation may occur with right temporal lesions, and Wernicke's aphasia, transcortical sensory aphasia, or anomia occur with posterior left temporal lesions.

Prefrontal and temporal lobe damage directly affect mechanisms underlying human adjustment and adaptation.[36] These include coping and compensatory strategies, problem solving, and goal setting and attainment. Frontal lobe damage may lead to the inability to use available information to guide behavior. Curiously, this may occur even when the ability to verbalize the steps or guidelines that should be followed is intact. There is a "disconnection" between knowing required information and actually using that information to guide behavior.[21] There is an appearance of normalcy on informed questioning, yet extreme safety risks become apparent when required to perform.

Difficulties with social self-regulation most commonly are expressed as reduced initiation and volition in social settings; impaired social discourse; limited appreciation for social boundaries; and difficulty in inhibiting impulsive responses in social contexts. A lack of ability to appreciate other points of view or the emotional experiences of others may become apparent.[37]

The general content of rehabilitation must address acquired deficits in self-regulation and the executive control of cognition and social behavior. The following approaches are helpful: (1) providing structure to the daily schedule; (2) consistent and immediate feedback on inappropriate behaviors; (3) identifying specific and concrete goals; (4) making the component steps of a task explicit, and delivering immediate feedback on completion of each step; (5) providing organizational strategies; (6) emphasizing verbal mediation and external cuing during problem solving and daily tasks; (7) focusing on alternate thinking, perspective taking, and cognitive flexibility skills; (8) improving self-awareness and self-monitoring of behavior; and (9) the incorporation of behavioral management techniques to extinguish unacceptable behaviors and shape positive ones.

Focal hypoxic–ischemic injury (HII) also may contribute specific problems to the deficits seen after focal TBI. The most common are watershed infarctions related to hypoperfusion. These may lead to aphasia, visuospatial disorientation, severe memory impairment, hemianopsia, or cortical blindness.

Consequences of Diffuse Injury

Clinical presentations attributable to frontal and temporal lobe injury also can arise as a consequence of DAI, even in the absence of focal pathology, owing to a disconnection of projections to and from these areas. The immediate effect of DAI is loss of consciousness without a lucid interval.[38] Emergence from coma is followed by a period of confusion and amnesia. Depending on the severity, multiple behavioral, cognitive, and physical impairments will persist for varying periods of time.

Beyond the issues of arousal, the principal cognitive deficits of DAI affect attention, memory, and higher-level processes such as organizational skills and planning. The aspects of attention most affected by TBI (probably combined effects of DAI and frontal lesions) are divided attention and the ability to shift attention.[39] Susceptibility to distractibility and interference in the middle of a mental operation also is demonstrated.[40] These may all relate to decreased information processing speed and/or cumulative "noise" in neural transmission owing to widespread axonal disruption and disconnection.[41]

Memory impairment is a feature of both early and late recovery from diffuse TBI.[42] Early memory loss may be a reflection, in part, of attentional impairments. However, learning remains inefficient for several reasons after PTA has cleared. Attentional deficits and reduced speed of information processing play important roles, as do inefficiencies in problem solving and learning. Procedural memory (the ability to learn new motor

and other skills) usually is preserved out of proportion to declarative memory.[43] Preserved procedural memory has been successfully used to teach simple routines to some amnestic patients.[43]

Performance scores on intelligence tests are slower to improve than verbal scores; this is likely due to the sensitivity of performance tasks to attention and speed of information processing.[44] As recovery progresses, general intelligence tests may become normal, despite the persistence of disabling "executive" dysfunction. In monitoring recovery from TBI, tests that tap into executive abilities, such as the Wisconsin Card Sorting Test, will better capture some of the long-term cognitive deficits.[45,46] Although complex verbal skills frequently are affected by TBI, specific language disorders are relatively uncommon absent a focal injury.[47]

In general, personality changes associated with diffuse injury distribute along the same lines as that described for focal frontal brain lesions, but they are related to disruption of frontal projections by DAI.[48] Personality changes commonly seen include apathy and motivational loss, as well as disinhibited, aggressive behavior.[49] Behavioral problems and personality changes always must be managed in the context of the clinical stage of recovery. Persistent behavioral problems imply the presence of temporal and frontal contusions.

Disintegration of social skills and interpersonal relationships are common consequences of pathologic behaviors and cognitive impairment. These are the major contributors to long-term family stress after TBI. The severity of personality and behavioral alteration is an even better predictor of family dysfunction than is severity of injury.[50] Family malfunctioning often is delayed until the patient is discharged home. The degree of perceived burden and stress appears to intensify with time.

Physical problems following moderate to severe DAI are less consistent and predictable than the characteristic cognitive and behavioral problems. DAI generally is associated with a mix of motor impairments attributable to diffuse, bilateral disruption of multiple motor systems. The usual patterns of distribution of DAI (parasaggital frontal and dorsolateral midbrain) and the varying density of preserved versus destroyed axons in affected areas differentiate the characteristic motor dysfunctions of DAI from more focal motor system lesions. There is no clear relationship between the severity of cognitive and behavioral impairments and motor deficits, but the more severe injuries are associated with more severe and lasting motor deficits.[48]

Several common patterns of motor dysfunction

may be observed. Deficits usually are bilateral, but asymmetrical. Head, trunk, balance, and gait control problems are common. Poorly coordinated limb movements and loss of fine motor control are also common. Limb weakness and spasticity may occur in a hemiplegic or quadriplegic pattern. Movement disorders, including tremor, dystonia, and torticollis occur also, but are less frequent. Dense, unilateral focal deficits are less common than bilateral deficits.[48] Motor behavior also may be disrupted by apraxia, abulia, and other cognitive–behavioral disorders.

Dysphagia is common after TBI, but usually resolves by the time that cognitive and behavioral disturbances clear.[51] Dysarthria is very common, especially with ataxic and spastic components. In severe injuries, dysarthria persists.

Diffuse HII leads to profound memory impairment owing to damage to the hippocampus. If anoxia is prolonged, Parkinsonian features, cerebellar ataxia, globally impaired cognition, spasticity, and quadriparesis are noted.

General Treatment Strategies for Diffuse Injury

As DAI is the overriding pathology influencing early recovery from TBI, it is helpful to organize treatment strategies based on the stages of recovery of DAI. These stages are outlined by the Rancho Los Amigos Scale (Table 7-7) and generally are more appropriate for moderate to severe injuries.[52]

Coma is defined by absent cerebral response to any environmental stimulation. Typically, the eyes remain closed. Spinal and brainstem reflexes may occur. The Glasgow Coma Score is <9. Treatment and evaluation strategies in the coma stage include managing acute surgical and medical problems; preventing secondary complications such as infection, skin breakdown, venous thromboembolism, and contractures; ensuring adequate hydration and nutrition; and frequent reassessment of responsiveness.

The unresponsive vigilance/vegetative state occurs with the restoration of spontaneous eye opening and the resumption of sleep–wake cycles. Transition to this stage usually occurs within 4 weeks of injury. There is still no apparent cerebral responsiveness to stimuli. Visual fixation and tracking often herald the transition to the next stage. Appropriate interventions at this stage include all of those noted previously, in addition to institution of a scheduled stimulation and monitoring program. Although there is no solid evidence in humans that structured stimulation programs hasten emergence from coma, there is evidence from animal models that providing an "enriched environment," which includes increased handling and social contact, improves recovery from cerebral injury.[54]

Data tracking response to external stimulation must be accurately recorded, so that emergence from

Table 7-7
Rancho Los Amigos Scale

1. No response: Unresponsive to any stimulus

2. Generalized response: Limited, inconsistent, nonpurposeful responses; often to pain only

3. Localized response: Purposeful responses; may follow simple commands; may focus on presented object

4. Confused, agitated: Heightened state of activity; confusion, disorientation, aggressive behavior; unable to do self care; unaware of present events; agitation appears related to internal confusion

5. Confused, inappropriate: Nonagitated; appears alert; responds to commands, distractable; does not concentrate on task; agitated responses to external stimuli; verbally inappropriate; does not learn new information

6. Confused, appropriate: Good directed behavior, needs cueing; can relearn old skills as activities of daily living (ADLs); serious memory problems; some awareness of self and others

7. Automatic, appropriate: Appears appropriate, oriented; frequently robot-like in daily routine; minimal or absent confusion; shallow recall; increased awareness of self, interaction in environment; lacks insight into condition; decreased judgment and problem solving; lacks realistic planning for future

8. Purposeful, appropriate: Alert, oriented, recalls and integrates past events; learns new activities and can continue without supervision; independent in home and living skills; capable of driving; defects in stress tolerance, judgment, abstract reasoning persist; many functions at reduced levels in society

coma can be monitored. Responses initially may be intermittent, highly variable, have a latency of onset, and be extremely fatiguable. It is important to capitalize on the patient's periods of wakefulness. Family or nurses often are the first to detect responsiveness. Secondary neurosurgical and medical complications such as hydrocephalus, infection, and medication toxicity may decrease responsiveness.

The mute/low-level responsiveness stage occurs when the patient demonstrates cognitive responsiveness. The ability to follow simple commands usually occurs before spontaneous speech. Muteness tends to last longer in young children, and also may be prolonged in those with extensive parasaggital DAI or focal left frontal lesions.[55,56] The main goal of this stage is the establishment of a simple reliable means of communication. If more than 3 or 4 weeks have elapsed since the time of injury before the emergence of this phase, a trial of CNS stimulant may be beneficial. Dopaminergic agents also may be helpful.[21]

The confusional state occurs when verbal communication is established but behavioral operations are degraded significantly by severe attention deficits. Agitation, undirected aggression, or fluctuation between minimal responsiveness and agitation often is present. A state of dense anterograde amnesia (PTA) persists, and virtually no encoding of new events or new learning occurs. Disorientation, with little or no insight, is the rule. The end of this stage is marked by the resumption of continuous day-to-day memories (emergence from PTA, GOAT > 75). Appropriate levels of stimulation and adequate structure are most important at this stage. Treatment sessions may need to be shortened and take place in a quiet environment. Familiar persons, objects, and pictures may help with orientation. Interactions with staff, family, and friends should be short and simple, avoiding argument. Fatigue may add to confusion. Regulation of sleep–wake cycles, pacing of activities, and rest periods during the day are helpful. The goal is to gradually increase orientation and attention. Immediate-reward behavior-management programs may work with some patients to gain increasing periods of cooperation. Stimulants and dopamine agonists also may prove to be helpful in this stage, and are considered first-line treatment for agitation.[57] Increasing attention may reduce confusion and agitation. A triad of psychostimulants has been recommended for 2 to 5 days.[57] Sedatives and tranquilizers should be avoided if possible. If a stimulant improves attention, but is only minimally effective in decreasing agitation, the addition of buspirone or one of the selective serotonergic antidepressants may be helpful (see below).

The stage of evolving independence occurs with the resolution of PTA and marked improvements in attentional skills. Interactions with therapists become more appropriate. Continence often follows, responsibility for daily living skills emerges. Family involvement is critical. Structured treatment remains important, but patient involvement in goal setting contributes to empowerment and independence.

The attainment of intellectual and social competence occurs over a proportionally longer span of time, taking months to years. Many severely injured patients never achieve this level. Persistent disturbances in executive and organizational skills, information-processing speed, and behavioral disturbances are the usual impediments to successful community and family reintegration. Residual physical impairments and mental fatigue may be limiting also. Premorbid drug and alcohol abuse may reemerge, and family instability may become apparent. Neuropsychological assessment should be repeated periodically after major TBI to track recovery and aid in goal setting. Hasty, premature return to work and school can have disastrous consequences. Return to driving often is an issue at this stage. Referral to a driver's testing and training program that specializes in assessment of persons with disabilities is recommended if the capacity to drive is at all in question.

OUTCOME

Predicting and assessing outcome following TBI is a difficult task. The heterogeneity of TBI and the multiplicity of factors affecting outcome defy straightforward study. The studies that have been used suffer from a number of methodological inconsistencies, including differences in the population studied, definitions of coma and PTA, the outcome measures used, and the timing of assessments. Global outcome studies generally have used the Glasgow Outcome Scale (GOS) (Table 7-8).[58] The major difficulty with the GOS (aside from its very gross categorization) is the inability to properly classify patients because of lack of specific criteria that separate severe from moderate or moderate from good recovery. Good recovery does not mean, nor was it intended to mean, complete recovery. Other outcome measures used in the study of TBI include the Disability Rating Scale (DRS) and the Functional Independence Measure (FIM).[59,60] The use of the FIM is increasing in rehabilitation facilities and despite its limited ability to

Table 7-8
Glasgow Outcome Scale

1. Good Recovery	Resumption of "normal" life, may have "minor" neurologic or psychologic deficits
2. Moderate Disability	Disabled, but independent in ADL and community
3. Severe Disability	Dependent on others for all or part of care/supervision
4. Vegetative	Unresponsive and speechless
5. Death	

Modified from Jennett and Bond, 1975.

take into account cognitive and behavioral deficits, it provides functional outcome information that can be generalized.

Although a number of pre-injury, injury, and post-injury factors affect outcome, global outcome following TBI is predicted best by the length of coma or length of PTA, modified by the patient's age (the best prognosis is in the 5- to 15-year-old group). Depth and duration of coma and duration of PTA are markers of the severity of DAI.[48] Of those still comatose 1 month after injury (all ages), approximately 50 percent will later regain consciousness, but over 60 percent of those will remain severely disabled by 1 year after injury.[61] The prognosis for children is better. Children between the ages of 5 and 15 may be in coma for 3 months and have the same prognosis for recovery as adults in coma for 1 month. Mortality and morbidity increase with advancing age after the second decade.[62,63] For those in coma less than 1 week, more than half will achieve a good recovery and approximately one-third will be moderately disabled.[61]

If measured accurately, the duration of PTA has an even stronger relation to recovery than length of coma. In a series of 114 TBI patients admitted to a rehabilitation facility, PTA of <2 weeks was compatible with 80 percent good recovery and 13 percent moderate disability. For patients with PTA between 4 and 6 weeks, 46 percent achieved good recovery and 54 percent moderate disability.[61] None with PTA of over 12 weeks achieved a good recovery (Table 7-9).

In comparison, for the same length of coma, outcome following hypoxic–ischemic injury (HII) is much poorer, with little chance of recovery for patients still in coma at 1 week.[64] The presence of HII can be inferred from any history of periods of prolonged hypotension, hypoxia, or need for cardiopulmonary resuscitation.

Recovery from DAI proceeds from coma to a confusional state, followed by a prolonged period of recovery lasting months to a few years. The Rancho Los Amigos Scale (Table 7-7) tracks this recovery process in its early stages.[52] The pervasive attentional and information-processing deficits following TBI largely result from DAI. In general, at 1 year after injury, 10 percent of patients initially classified as mild TBI will have some neurological limitation, 65 percent of those with moderate injury, and 100 percent of those surviving a severe injury will have some residual disability.[1]

The impact of focal pathology on outcome is difficult to study in large groups of patients with TBI because important clinical distinctions based on anatomical location are lost in large group studies. Neurologic consequences of focal injury may be embedded in clinical phenomena associated with diffuse pathology. The location and size of the lesion, as well as mass effect are the main factors determining outcome from focal brain injury. Recovery from focal lesions evolves and plateaus more rapidly than that of DAI. Bilateral focal lesions in homologous areas produce more severe and enduring effects than unilateral lesions. Small differences in lesion location and depth can make large differences in the characteristics of residual deficits and in the prognosis.

The most enduring and disabling deficits are neurobehavioral and cognitive. The pattern of persisting behavioral and cognitive deficits can be similar, the most significant of which involve memory, insight, attention, information processing, alertness, irritability, and blunted affect. The choice of neuropsychological measures will profoundly affect outcome. Many patients with mild to moderate injuries may achieve normal or near-normal scores on composite intelligence tests, but continue to suffer from organizational, information-processing, and behavioral-control deficits that impair their performance. Premorbid intelligence also must be taken into account, as a normal IQ likely represents a decline for a professional, where even small impairments may preclude returning to their former occupation.

These cognitive and behavioral deficits overshadow physical impairments, disrupting the family, limiting social interaction, and prohibiting return to work. Return to work is a frequently used outcome measure. Pre-injury factors, such as age, previous occupational and educational level, and social support combine with injury factors to determine vocational outcome.[65] The higher the educational or work level before injury, the greater the chance of returning to any type of work.

Table 7-9
Glasgow Outcome Scores 1 year after injury

PTA duration (weeks)	Severe disability	Moderate disability	Good recovery	Number of patients
>24	88	12	0	8
16–24	20	80	0	5
12–16	27	73	0	11
8–12	18	64	18	11
4–8	0	54	46	24
2–4	0	40	60	25
0–2	7	13	80	30
TOTAL = 114				

Modified from Katz et al., 1992.

Return to work diminishes considerably after age 40.[65] Fewer than 10% of those with moderate or severe injuries will return to their previous occupation.[65]

COGNITIVE DYSFUNCTION

Cognitive deficits and their rehabilitation are covered in detail elsewhere in this volume. Nevertheless, information pertinent to TBI bears some special mention. Cognitive changes will impact on every area of function, from basic self-care to vocational pursuits and leisure activities.

Recognition and identification of cognitive changes are needed to design the rehabilitation program, as specific goals and treatment approaches will be developed based on the patient's ability to understand, learn, and apply various skills, strategies, and adaptations.

Neuropsychological Assessment

It is important to understand that many of the persistent cognitive deficits following brain injury will not be detected by tests of general cognition, such as the Wechsler Adult Intelligence Scale—Revised (WAIS-R).[66] In many cases of even mild to moderate TBI, deficits in "executive functions" will escape detection by conventional intelligence testing. The WAIS-R may be normal in cases where function at work or in the classroom remains significantly impaired. In addition, excessive reliance on scores from test batteries may obscure a

pattern of strengths and weaknesses. Scores from tests evaluating different cognitive domains must be given and the results explained in relation to their functional impact. Test results must always be interpreted with reference to the person's premorbid level of function and education.

Standardized assessments of mood, motivation, and personality are important components of the complete neuropsychological evaluation. Suggested management, treatment, and remediation strategies are essential to a complete evaluation and should be shared with the treatment team.

Cognitive Rehabilitation

The effectiveness of cognitive rehabilitation is controversial.[67,68] Well-developed studies of cognitive rehabilitation efficacy are few, chiefly because of consumer demand for services and complex methodological issues.

There are many models of cognitive rehabilitation, most of which can be broadly classified into either functional skills training or process-oriented rehabilitation.

Functional skills training involves the retraining of specific activities of daily living or work in the particular environment they will be performed in. Each task must be analyzed in relation to a constellation of skills and deficits, the environment, and a list of potential compensatory strategies. Generalization to other skills is not expected, nor is it necessarily considered a goal of treatment. Although the targeting of specific tasks relevant to the activities of daily living has obvious functional value, the narrow focus and sheer intensity and time involved will limit application to a few essential living skills.

The process approach involves focused remediation of specific cognitive deficits. The areas frequently targeted include attention, concentration, motor planning, visual–spatial processing, neglect, memory, and executive functions. The process approach proceeds in a hierarchical fashion, invoking techniques based in cognitive, experimental, and educational psychology. Therapy exercises are performed repeatedly until predetermined goals are met in each cognitive area.

In process-oriented rehabilitation, both restoration of cognitive dysfunction and compensation are emphasized. In many instances generalization of the cognitive retraining to a wide variety of situations is not achieved.[68]

Within process training, the noetic method has been used successfully to train the individual to recognize and regulate his own behavior.[69] This approach is particularly useful in patients with frontal lobe dysfunction. Through a procedure of diminished cuing, often beginning with external monitoring, the individual learns to internalize specific self-monitoring skills and apply them to a variety of situations. This approach is most successful when cognitive function is relatively preserved, but also has been effective in the face of global cognitive impairments.

In practice, a combination of the preceding approaches based on the patient's cognitive and behavioral profile and the functional demands works best.

Attentional skills are essential to many other cognitive functions, and therefore often a first step in cognitive rehabilitation. One method of attentional retraining is based on the hierarchical conceptualization of attention as defined by Sohlberg and Mateer. Treatment tasks specific to each of these levels have been developed. Memory has been observed to improve solely as a consequence of improved attention.

Memory loss can be a major challenge to rehabilitation specialists. Mnemonics and exercises do not in general aid those with amnesia.[72] In addition to external memory aids, Glisky and Schacter have made use of preserved procedural memory to teach subjects with severe memory loss a complicated computer task using vanishing cues.[73] Retention of the gains were solidified over several weeks.[74] This approach has been applied successfully to other daily living and work activities.

Pharmacologic enhancement of cognitive function is promising. The use of dopaminergic and noradrenergic drugs in the treatment of attentional disorders is common.[51] Success has been reported with methylphenidate, amantadine, pemoline, and others. Response patterns to different drugs is highly variable. Most of these medications are well tolerated. There are no double-blind, placebo-controlled studies to prove efficacy, and the characteristics of responders versus nonresponders are not defined. Clonidine, a centrally acting alpha-blocker, has been used in the sustained release forum to treat attention deficit in children, and also may be useful in the brain-injured population. Likewise, cholinergic therapy for memory dysfunction also remains in an experimental stage.[75]

NEGLECT AND VISUAL–PERCEPTUAL DISORDERS

Neglect

Unilateral spatial neglect is one of the most striking and disabling disorders after TBI. Whole regions of space contralateral to their lesions may vanish. The head and eyes may be deviated ipsilaterally, even in the absense of oculomotor paresis. Sound emanating from contralateral space may lead to an incessant search ipsilaterally for its source. Walking or wheeling a wheelchair may prove difficult. Repeatedly striking contralateral objects, or only making ipsilateral turns are common. In the early stages, neglect of body parts is dramatic. Failure to shave one side of the face or to dress contralaterally are common. At times denial of ownership of the affected body part can be elicited, often accompanied by an intense disregard.

Neglect is more common and severe after right than left hemisphere damage, and is a frequent consequence of TBI.[76] Brain injuries producing neglect also may result in other neurologic deficits, such as visual field defects, hemisensory, or hemiparesis. However, primary sensory or motor abnormalities do not produce neglect, and these deficits occur because of the proximity of sensory and motor cortices to structures critical for spatial awareness.

Since most patients with neglect have relatively intact language ability, they may be able to carry on appropriate conversations and solve verbal reasoning problems, giving the impression that they can function safely. When placed in an actual or contrived situation, they seldom execute activities of daily living skills commensurate with their verbal reasoning ability.

Neglect may not be a unitary neuropsychological entity, but rather a family of symptoms, analogous to

Table 7-10
Behavioral manifestations of underlying mechanisms in unilateral spatial neglect

Attentional deficits	Intentional deficits	Representational deficits
Extinction to double simultaneous stimulation	Akinesia	Anterograde contralateral memory deficits
Ipsilateral orientation bias	Directional hypokinesia	Retrograde contralateral memory deficits
Limited attentional capacity	Motor extinction	Contralateral confabulation
	Motor impersistence	

the concept of "aphasia" as a group of related language disorders.[77] The Behavioral Inattention Test is a published neuropsychological test that incorporates several measures of neglect, and can be used to quantify the severity of the deficit and follow recovery and response to treatment.[78]

The phenomenology of neglect is puzzling and disturbing. Contemporary theories of neglect focus on underlying attentional, intentional, and representational mechanisms.[77] Table 7-10 lists the behavioral manifestations that occur as a result of the disruption of these mechanisms.

The severity of neglect and patterns of recovery are highly variable. If neglect persists, it can be a major impediment to functional recovery. Persistent neglect can be as functionally incapacitating as severe language deficits. Unfortunately, no treatment protocols have been shown to be unequivocally effective in neglect. A number of early reports show considerable promise for new rehabilitation strategies, including scanning, cuing, eye patching, vestibular stimulation, prisms, and treatment with dopaminergic agents or stimulants.[77]

Cortical Visual Dysfunction

Damage to the human cerebral cortex can result in a number of distinct visual perceptual impairments, including visual field defects, oculomotor dysfunction, visual agnosias, visuospatial disorders, impaired binocular fusion, visual hallucinations, defective discrimination, and achromatopsia. Damage to any of several cortical regions, including the primary visual cortex (area 17), extra-striate occipital association cortex (areas 18 and 19), visual and polymodal association cortex of the parietal and temporal lobes (areas 37 and 39), and the frontal eye fields (area 8) can be seen after TBI. Some form of visual dysfunction occurs in over 50 percent of TBI patients.[79]

Visual perceptual deficits are common in rehabilitation settings and have been shown repeatedly to be associated with poorer functional outcome.

Success has been limited in restoration of visual fields. Efforts in rehabilitation have been directed at training in scanning strategies, which have shown the most promise.[80]

BEHAVIORAL AND MOOD DISORDERS

Behavioral and mood disorders are common following TBI. They are poorly understood, often under- or overtreated, and yet may be one of the most disabling features of the injury. Polypharmacy is common, but rarely appropriate. Subtherapeutic dosing or inadequate trials often are erroneously considered medication failures.

Depression

Depression also occurs in 40 percent of patients with TBI, and is difficult to diagnose because of confounding neurologic abnormalities.[81]

Treatment of depression is covered elsewhere in this text, and pharmacologic therapy is effective.[81]

Mania

Mania is estimated to occur in approximately 10 percent of TBI patients.[82] If one includes patients with symptoms suggestive of hypomania, the incidence is much higher. It appears to be associated with temporal basopolar lesions, particularly on the right. There is no association with severity of cognitive or physical deficits, nor is there any association with the development of post-traumatic epilepsy. Unlike depression, the incidence of TBI-induced mania has no association with a history of prior psychiatric disorder. Aggression and agitation are more frequent in patients with mania.

There have been no systematic studies of the treatment of TBI-induced mania or hypomania. Carbamazepine, valproate, and clonidine all have been reported to be effective in some cases.[81] Lithium appears to have been the most successful in controlling symptoms, and if not contraindicated, remains a reasonable first choice.[81] Neuroleptics may need to be added in refractory cases. Behavioral management approaches should be used in conjunction with pharmacologic therapy.

Anxiety and Related Disorders

Anxiety is common following TBI, particularly in patients with aphasia and severe cortical visual deficits. Post-traumatic stress disorder occurs in 20 to 30 percent of TBI patients. Obsessive–compulsive disorders occur in approximately 5 percent of TBI patients and may relate to the rigidity in thinking and perseveration that can occur following frontal lobe injuries.[83] Generalized anxiety and panic states appear to occur more frequently in subjects with left hemisphere lesions, whereas obsessive–compulsive symptoms are associated more frequently with right orbito-frontal injury. Anxiety also may be associated with seizures as an aura or a part of ictal phenomena.

In many cases a psychotherapeutic and/or behavioral approach may suffice. If this approach fails, and the patient continues to exhibit symptoms that interfere with functioning, pharmacologic treatment should be considered. The agent used should be chosen to minimize the chances of side effects. Any drug with the potential to diminish arousal in patients with TBI may cause increased confusion, leading paradoxically to anxiety and agitation.

Buspirone appears to be a promising agent for the treatment of anxiety and agitation in TBI patients because it causes relatively little cognitive impairment.[83] Dosage should be gradually increased from a starting dose of 5 mg tid to a maximum of 20 mg tid. Response to treatment may take several weeks. Some symptoms of anxiety, particularly the physical or overt symptoms may respond to propranolol.[84] Benzodiazepines, commonly used to treat anxiety, generally should not be used in TBI patients unless agitation or aggression pose a significant safety risk. Neuroleptics also should be avoided generally. If pharmacotherapy is necessary for obsessive–compulsive symptoms, fluoxitine, buspar, or a combination of the two are recommended.[83] Clomi-

pramine also may be used, but has a greater tendency to provoke memory problems owing to anticholinergic side effects, and may lower the seizure threshold. Post-traumatic stress disorder symptoms may respond to Buspirone or other antidepressants.[85] Trazodone, beginning at 50 mg qhs, is particularly helpful for treating sleep disturbance.[85]

Agitation and Aggression

Agitation and aggression are perhaps the most dramatic behavioral consequences of brain injury. The development of effective management strategies has been hampered in part by the lack of consensus definitions and reliable measurement scales. Agitation and aggression often are used synonymously. Although agitated patients may display aggression, they do not always, and aggression may occur randomly, with or without provocation in nonagitated persons with TBI. Additionally, the distinction between the agitation and aggression occurring early and that appearing late after injury is essential to proper assessment and management.

Agitation can be defined as an emotional state associated with severe anxiety, fear, or uncertainty, and motor restlessness. Aggression describes explosive, violent behaviors that occur with or without provocation. They may be verbal and/or physical, and may be undirected (nonpurposeful) or directed at self, others, or inanimate objects.

The Agitated Behavior Scale (ABS) (Table 7-11) recently has been shown to be a valid and reliable scale for monitoring the severity of agitation as well as differentiating confusion and inattention from agitation.[86] The Overt Aggression Scale (OAS) (Table 7-12) likewise has been shown to be a valid and reliable instrument for monitoring the occurrence of aggression.[87]

Patients in the coma-emergent state after TBI are in a confusional state appropriately referred to as delirium.[88] The approach to management of this state involves a thorough search for a treatable underlying cause, treatment of the underlying etiology where possible, environmental modification, and medication. Table 7-13 lists the more common underlying causes of delirium and agitation following TBI.

Environmental changes are directed at providing familiarity and structure to compensate for cognitive disorganization. Approaches often include setting family pictures nearby, a clock and calendar with the days marked off in full view, frequent reorientation by staff, providing structured periods of therapy in a quiet environment, limiting exposure to crowds, and ensuring the

Table 7-11
The Agitated Behavior Scale

Patient: _____ Date: _____

Observ. Environ.: _____

Rater/Disc.: _____ Time: _____

1 = Absent: The behavior is not present
2 = Present to a slight degree: The behavior is present but does not prevent the conduct of other, contextually appropriate behavior. (This individual may redirect spontaneously, or the continuation of the agitated behavior does not disrupt appropriate behavior.)
3 = Present to a moderate degree: The individual needs to be redirected from an agitated to an appropriate behavior, but benefits from such cueing.
4 = Present to an extreme degree: The individual is not able to engage in appropriate behavior owing to the interference of the agitated behavior, even when external cueing or redirection is provided.

____ 1. Short attention span, easy distractibility, inability to concentrate
____ 2. Impulsive, impatient, low tolerance for pain or frustration
____ 3. Uncooperative, resistant to care, demanding
____ 4. Violent and/or threatening violence toward people or property
____ 5. Explosive and/or unpredictable anger
____ 6. Rocking, rubbing, moaning, or other self-stimulating behavior
____ 7. Pulling at tubes, restraints, and so on
____ 8. Wandering from treatment areas
____ 9. Restlessness, pacing, excessive movement
____ 10. Repetitive behaviors, motor and/or verbal
____ 11. Rapid, loud, or excessive talking
____ 12. Sudden changes of mood
____ 13. Easily initiated or excessive crying and/or laughter
____ 14. Self-abusiveness, physical and/or verbal

____ Total Score

Modified from Corrigen JD, Bogner JA: Assessment of agitation following brain injury. *Neurorehabilitation* 1995; 5:205–20.

staff and family approach the patient in a consistent fashion. Therapists often structure tasks to include frequent breaks as well as activities that allow the patient some choice and a reasonable chance of success. Assuring patient safety often can be accomplished without the use of restraints by padding bed rails, using a bed alarm, placing the patient in a floor bed, or providing 1-to-1 supervision. When restraints are used, a properly secured lap belt in a chair, or in combination with a bed alarm, often works quite well. Posey vests are a more restraining alternative. Soft single-limb restraints may be needed to prevent the pulling out of intravenous tubing, tracheostomies, or gastrostomy tubes. Padded hand mitts also are effective, and allow free movement of the arms.

Pharmacologic management of aggression and ag-

itation is reserved for special situations of danger or in order to preserve the therapeutic mileu. Nursing, therapy staff, and family need to be educated about agitation, and develop a tolerance for motor restlessness and calling out. Medication always is a therapy of last resort.

Neuroleptics, because of their quick and predictable onset of action, often are a first choice.[89] The clearest indication for neuroleptics after TBI is agitation owing to or accompanied by psychotic symptoms, such as delusions, paranoia, or hallucinations. Haloperidol is most often used because of its safety profile in medically ill patients, lower potential for sedation, and ease of route of administration. Haloperidol, however, is a potent dopaminergic blocker and may be more likely to cause movement disorders. The akithisia that often develops as a result of the use of haloperidol may be

Table 7-12

The Overt Aggression Scale

Patient: _____   Date: _____

Rater: _____   Time: _____

Verbal aggression	Physical aggression against self	Physical aggression against objects	Physical aggression against others	Intervention (check all that apply)
Makes loud noises, shouts angrily	Picks or scratches skin, hits self, pulls hair (with no or minor injury only)	Slams doors, scatters clothing, makes a mess	Makes threatening gestures, swings at people, grabs at clothes	None
Yells mildly personal insults, e.g., "you're stupid"	Bangs head, hits fist into objects, throws self onto floor or into objects (hurts self without serious injury)	Throws objects down, kicks furniture without breaking it, marks the wall	Strikes, kicks, pushes, pulls hair (without injury to them)	Talking to patient
Curses viciously, uses foul language in anger, makes moderate threats to others or self	Small cuts or bruises, minor burns	Breaks objects, smashes windows	Attacks others causing mild-moderate physical injury (bruises, sprains, welts)	Closer observation
Makes clear threats of violence toward others or self ("I'm going to kill you") or requests to help control self	Mutilates self, makes deep cuts, bites that bleed, internal injury fracture, loss of consciousness, loss of teeth	Sets fires, throws objects dangerously	Attacks others causing severe physical injury (broken bones, deep lacerations, internal injury)	Immediate medication given by mouth Immediate medication given by injection Isolation without seclusion (time out) Seclusion Use of restraints Injury requires immediate medical treatment for patient Injury requires immediate treatment for other person

Comments: _____

Modified from Yodufsky SC, Silver JM, Jackson W, et al: The overt aggression scale for the objective rating of verbal and physical aggression. *Am J Psychiatr* 1986; 143:35–39.

Table 7-13

Potential etiology of delerium in patients with brain injury

General	Specific consideration in brain injury
Drug intoxication/withdrawal	Seizures (ictal and post-ictal stares)
Metabolic/electrolyte/vitamin deficiency	Hydrocephalus
Infection (system/CNS)	Hygromas
Endocrine	Delayed hemorrhage
Toxis/environmental exposure	Medication side effect/interaction
Vascular (e.g., arrhythmias, pulmonary embolus)	Endocrine (hypothalamic or pituitary dysfunction)

misinterpreted as heightened agitation and lead to increasing doses and further motor restlessness. Benzodiazepines, particularly lorazepam, also are often useful. However, they often increase the level of confusion, paradoxically leading to agitation.[89] Both neuroleptics and benzodiazepines have been shown in some studies to delay or impair recovery from TBI, and they should be used cautiously with careful monitoring as an interim measure while other agents are started.[90]

Buspirone often is quite helpful for agitation and aggression.[91] Because of its latency of onset of action, haloperidol or lorazepam may need to be used on an interim basis until a therapeutic dose is reached. Likewise, propranolol may also be useful in decreasing agitation, but also may take several weeks to reach a therapeutic level.[92] Hypotension and bradycardia may occur, and limit its use. Lithium has a relatively quick onset of action (days to a week), and has been useful in agitated patients with and without other symptoms of mania.[89]

A more recent approach involves the use of stimulants in treating agitation that occurs in the setting of confusion and severely impaired attention.[91] By improving awareness and attention, confusion may decrease, resulting in a concomitant decrease in agitation. Most of these CNS stimulants have noradrenergic and dopaminergic properties that may hasten the recovery process. Examples include amantadine, methylphenidate, bromocriptine, l-dopa, and pemoline. Methylphenidate has a quick onset of action, with improvements occurring in 1 to 3 days. Amantadine is well tolerated even by the elderly. Effective doses range from 50 to 150 mg bid, with onset of effects in 3 to 7 days. Use of these medications currently is a trial and error process, and patients may respond to one and not another. Studies underway now should further define relative efficacy and determine the characteristics of those that are likely to respond.

Late onset aggression after TBI is a major source of disability, occurring in about 40 percent of TBI patients who receive acute inpatient rehabilitation.[92] Low frustration tolerance and explosive behavior may develop, with little or no provocation or warning. These episodes may range in severity from simple irritability to outbursts that result in damage to property or assaults. Neurotransmitters thought to be involved in the mediation of aggression include serotonin, norepinephrine, dopamine, acetylcholine, and GABA.[91] Areas of the brain that play a role include the hypothalamus, amygdala, temporal, and frontal lobes.

Treatment often involves an interdisciplinary approach. Medication may be combined with a variety of behavioral approaches, depending on the nature of the aggression, the cognitive ability of the patient, and the social constraints. The use of neuroleptics to treat chronic aggression usually fails unless the aggression is associated with psychotic features.[93]. The anticonvulsants carbamazepine and valproate have been shown to have beneficial effects and may be a reasonable first choice.[89] Lithium is likewise effective in some, especially those with features of mania or euphoria with lack of insight.[89] The serotonergic antidepressants are useful, particularly in patients with underlying depression or lability.[91] Buspirone also may be helpful in cases of persistent depression or anxiety.[91] Propranolol also has been shown to benefit some.[92] Trial and error, guided by the co-occurring symptomology, accompanied by behavioral management techniques and family education, summarizes the current approach to treatment of chronic aggression.

Psychosis

Transient, intermittent, or chronic psychosis occurs in up to 20 percent of TBI patients.[93] Different types of delusions have been associated in the literature with differing lesion locations (Table 7-14). There also is an association of psychosis with post-traumatic temporal lobe epilepsy.

Treatment consists of first ruling out delirium and searching for all of the possible causes of delirium, particularly medication toxicity (Table 7-13). As in the treatment of other behavioral disorders after TBI, there is a paucity of research to guide pharmacologic treatment. It is here that the use of neuroleptics makes the

Table 7-14
Relationship between neuroanatomy and types of associated delusions

Site of lesion(s)	Clinical characteristics of delusions
Diffuse lesions in cortical association areas and hippocampus associated with dementia of Alzheimer type or multi-infarct dementia	Simple, loosely held persecutory beliefs that often are transient and that respond moderately well to treatment with neuroleptics.
Subcortical (basal ganglia, thalamus, and rostral brain stem) and limbic lesions	Complex delusions that tend to be chronic and resistant to treatment
Left-sided temporal lobe lesions	Chronic schizophrenia-like delusional syndromes
Right-sided parieto temporal lesions	Short-lived hallucinatory delusional syndromes
Right-hemisphere lesions	Capgras syndrome and reduplicative paramnesia

Adapted from Cummings, 1985.

most sense. Several other medications also may be helpful, including anticonvulsants, lithium, and clonazepam.

POST-TRAUMATIC SEIZURES

In a population study of over 2,700 patients with closed head injury, 5 percent had a seizure in the first 2 weeks post-injury.[94] Only 1 percent develop seizures if no seizure occurs in the first week after injury; however, if a seizure occurs during the first week, the lifetime incidence increases to 25 percent. Those with brain contusions, hematomas, and depressed skull fractures or open injuries are at greater risk. When the dura has been penetrated, 30 to 50 percent of the patients develop post-traumatic seizures. Given the same severity of injury, the incidence of early post-traumatic seizures is higher in children than adults.[95] The long-term prognosis for post-traumatic seizures is good. Fifty percent of patients with post-traumatic seizures will no longer experience seizures 5 to 10 years after injury, 25 percent will have good seizure control on medication, and 25 percent will continue to have seizures.[96]

Seizure prophylaxis appears to have little benefit beyond the first few weeks after injury, and can be tapered and discontinued in those who have not had a seizure.[97] Discontinuing anticonvulsants at a later time in patients who have had early seizures requires a careful clinical evaluation and judgement. An EEG may be helpful if it shows persistent interictal spikes, suggesting that an epileptogenic focus remains. Valproic acid or carbamazepine has been recommended as the first-line drug for treatment of seizures in patients with TBI.[98]

Seizure disorders are associated with an increase in psychopathology, including mood disorders, psychoses, personality disorders, irritable-impulsive traits, and anxiety. It is unclear whether or not the same pathology results in both the psychologic disturbance and the seizures, or if the seizures contribute in some way to the development of these specific psychological characteristics or traits.

MILD TRAUMATIC BRAIN INJURY

Mild TBI often is treated in textbooks as though it is an entirely different disorder from severe TBI. However, DAI is the common pathology underlying all acceleration-deceleration trauma. Animal studies have demonstrated the pathological changes at even the mildest end of the spectrum.[55] Even the secondary effects of

excitatory neurotransmitter release are qualitatively similar.[99] At the very mildest level, there may be no actual disruption of axons, only transient shifts in neurotransmitter release and membrane depolarization. At more severe, but still mild levels, there is scattered axonal disruption and loss, following the same time course and topography as that of severe TBI.

At the clinical level, the stages of evolution of DAI as described for severe injury still occur in modal TBI, but in a condensed fashion. Coma lasts seconds to minutes, mute responsiveness for minutes, PTA for minutes to hours, and recovery over days to a few months. The American Congress of Rehabilitation Medicine has adopted a definition of mild TBI; coma for <1 hour, and/or PTA of <1 day.[100] Other definitions based on the initial GCS have been proposed, but are only useful if the GCS is administered at the same time after injury and there is no associated focal injury. DAI should be viewed as a continuum, with guidelines for expected outcomes based on all measures of severity: initial GCS, length of coma and PTA, and CT/MRI data.

Recovery from mild DAI is quick, and the injury may be trivialized. Minor TBI is best viewed as the interaction of three components: (1) neurological, including problems with arousal, attention, memory, and behavior; (2) psychological, with depression, anxiety, post-traumatic stress disorder; and (3) peripheral, consisting of headache, cervical pain, and vestibular dysfunction.

Regarding arousal and attention, excessive time sleeping or restless, shallow sleep is common. Poor concentration or distractibility is seen early. Complex attentional skills must be examined thoroughly. Memory loss is common, and may reflect diminished efficiency of learning (poor strategies). This may be due to a combination of decreased information-processing speed and executive dysfunction. The efficiency of learning a 10-word list over five trials, and then recalling the list in 5 minutes often is an informative test, as are other tests of executive function. Behavior abnormalities are protean after mild TBI and include irritability, sensitivity to noise and crowds, withdrawal, nightmares, anxiety and depression. The time course of recovery of these deficits may span 1 to 6 months.[101] A small number of patients may have long-term cognitive and behavioral deficits following a seemingly minor TBI.

The psychological injuries after mild TBI arise from having to deal with "soft" impairments, the trauma of the injury, and are compounded by the expectations of others that they are well and should return to their usual activities. Commonly, no one has performed the appropriate tests to detect higher-level cognitive dysfunction. Return to work may be characterized by marginal performance. Depression often ensues and continues, lengthening the time of recovery. Underestimation of severity may be owing to the failure to diagnose a focal contusion that may not be accompanied by prolonged PTA.[48]

Severe migraine headaches and a persistent balance disorder can emerge out of a seemingly trivial TBI. The usual course of resolution of the headache, neck pain, and dizziness is in less than 1 year.[102]

Antidepressants often are helpful adjuncts to treatment, not only of depression, but also posttraumatic headaches.

Detailed neuropsychological assessment can be useful in distinguishing those with persistent abnormalities of cognitive–behavioral dysfunction, from those seeking conscious or unconscious secondary gain. Referral to a neuropsychologist with expertise in TBI is essential to obtaining the appropriate tests and interpretation. In cases where cognitive and/or behavioral problems persist, cognitive therapy, and counseling, often including the family, are sometimes useful.

CHILDREN AND ADOLESCENTS

Epidemiology and Pathology

Accidents are the leading cause of death in children, and TBI accounts for a large proportion of these.[103] It is estimated that more than one million children sustain a TBI each year in the United States, and approximately one-sixth of these are admitted to the hospital. The overall incidence of pediatric TBI per 100,000 population is 270 in males and 116 in females, with the highest incidence in the 15-to-24 year age range.[104] TBI is more common in families who are exposed to psychosocial adversity and who live in congested areas of the city. In addition, TBI is more likely to occur in children who exhibit behavioral disturbances before the accident, have a low IQ, or have a history of previous head injury.

Falls are the major cause of TBI in children under 5 years of age.[4] Pedestrian–motor vehicle accidents, bicycle accidents, and non-organized sports and recreational injuries predominate in the 5-to-14 year age range. Motor vehicle accidents predominate in those over 15. Child abuse is an important cause of TBI, especially in children under the age of 2 years.[105] It is extremely uncommon for a fall from a table onto a carpeted floor to produce significant brain damage, and a

history of such in a child with significant brain injury should prompt a suspicion of abuse.

A change in the shape of the brain without a change in its volume is the most common type of TBI in children because their skulls are more easily deformed than that of adults. The most common brain lesions seen by MRI are small oval lesions in white matter tracts close to the cortical grey mater, or at times in the splenium of the corpus callosum. In general, brain damage following TBI is less severe in infants and children than adults, but it depends on the extent of vascular injury and edema.[3] Children under the age of 5 years are more prone to the development of significant brain edema following acceleration–deceleration injuries.

Subdural hematoma is a relatively frequent complication of TBI in children. It can be either acute or chronic, and in both, symptoms of increased intracranial pressure predominate. Chronic subdural hematomas are rare in small children and more frequent in adolescents. Clinical manifestations include a gradual change in personality and alertness, headaches, and seizures. A history of antecedent trauma need not be present. The prognosis for recovery from subdural hematoma owing to child abuse is poor.[95]

Neuropsychologic Sequelae

When assessed on the bases of both a teacher's questionnaire and a psychiatric interview, children of normal intelligence with a history of TBI are twice as likely as children with other physical handicaps to show nonspecific behavioral disturbances.[106] The incidence of persistent behavioral abnormalities parallels the severity of the injury, and is uncommon in children with a PTA of <1 week. However, since persistent neurologic findings tend to occur only with more severe injuries, behavioral abnormalities commonly occur in children without persistent neurologic signs. The most characteristic behavioral abnormalities are social disinhibition and moodiness. Multiple premorbid and post-injury factors, as well as lesion load, contribute to the development of behavior and cognitive abnormalities after brain injury in children (Table 7-15).

In a study following school-age children with TBI for over 2 years, nine of 10 with a PTA of over 3 weeks showed persistent cognitive impairment.[107] In contrast, when PTA was less than 2 weeks, no child showed permanent deficits and three showed transient deficits. In the first year following injury, visual–motor and visual–spatial functions were more impaired than verbal functions, but this difference had disappeared at 2 years.

Table 7-15
Factors contributing to the development of behavioral and cognitive deficits in children with TBI

Severity of trauma

Extent of lesion: bilateral greater than unilateral; deeper greater than superficial

Localization of lesion: right versus left hemisphere; subcortical versus cortical

Secondary complications such as seizures, subdural hematoma, infection, anoxia

Premorbid IQ

Premorbid history of psychiatric disturbance

Family psychosocial or economic disadvantage

Family reaction to the trauma

Parental psychiatric disorder

Lack of community support systems

The effects of mild TBI on cognitive function in children are not clear. The literature contains conflicting information, some of which is undoubtedly owing to differences in the definition of mild TBI and the tests chosen for assessment.[108] Since children''s cognitive functions are still emerging, it is difficult also to determine if a mild TBI reduces future potential. Some studies show decreased IQ in children sustaining a mild TBI when compared to controls, but some of this difference may be owing to premorbid differences, as there were no changes in the TBI group over a 1-year period.[109] Others have shown persistent and transient deficits in performance IQ and executive functions in children with mild TBI. A history of mild head injury is ten times more common in high-school adolescents with learning disabilities and hyperactivity.[110]

Follow-up assessments are recommended for those children with a loss of consciousness of greater than a few minutes PTA of greater than 1 hour, and any abnormality on CT or MRI.

Prognosis

As in adults, prognosis bears a direct relationship with the severity of TBI. CT and MRI also are useful in predicting outcome. In children in coma for more than 90 days after TBI, a CT scan showing minimal atrophy at 2 months predicted a good outcome (IQ > 70) with 89 percent accuracy.[111] Deep lesions on MRI at 18 months after injury are associated with poor neuropsychological test performance.[112]

In a recent cohort study of 72 children with TBI over 3 years of follow-up, those with moderate (initial GCS of 9–12 or GCS = 15 not achieved within 3 days) and severe (initial GCS of 3–8) TBI had persistent neuropsychological deficits throughout the 3 years of follow-up.[113] Among those with mild injury (GCS of 13–15), some had transient deficits, but none had deficits that persisted. In those with moderate and severe injuries, improvement was greatest over the first year, and plateaued after 2 years.

TREATMENT APPROACHES

For many of the impairments and disabilities that follow TBI in children, treatment approaches are similar. Important differences and areas of emphasis deserve special comment.

Pharmacologic considerations for the treatment of cognitive and behavioral disorders is similar to that of adults. Use of neuroleptics in children, however, should be avoided, unless there are documented symptoms of a frank psychosis. Stimulants (methylphenidate, pemoline) are recommended for those with symptoms of attention deficit hyperactivity disorder (ADHD).[108] Carbamazepine and propranolol have both been used with some success in children for treatment of posttraumatic agitation and aggression. More research is needed in the area of pharmacologic management of behavior after TBI in children.

The Benefits of Rehabilitation for TBI

A persistent and troublesome question for insurers, health-care professionals, patients, and families is whether the benefits of rehabilitation for individuals with TBI outweigh the costs of care. Most studies suffer from common methodological problems: the heterogeneity of brain injury and the difficulties in accurately determining its initial severity; the effects of spontaneous recovery; lack of control for preinjury characteristics; choice of appropriate outcome measures, and lack of controlled studies. More recent studies strongly suggest improved outcomes for patients with similar severities of TBI who received rehabilitation earlier, and who received more intensive therapies than those who did not.[114,115] Improved outcome has also been shown in patients who are beyond the period of spontaneous recovery and have received additional rehabilitation.[115]

Experimental studies in animals, much of it in primates, supports the conclusion that proper environment and training, and the early initiation of training after brain injury improve both the speed of recovery and the final outcome.[54] Recent animal research has suggested that there are "critical periods" during which interventions must occur to produce the maximum benefit.[116] These "critical periods" may vary with the type of deficit, as well as with the severity and location of injury.

SUMMARY

Traumatic brain injury produces an array of impairments and disabilities, the most significant of which often are cognitive and behavioral. Although the neuropathology of TBI now is better understood, we are just beginning to understand the recovery process and how we might limit secondary damage and best facilitate recovery. Recovery from TBI occurs in predictable stages, and general rehabilitation strategies are developed based on the stage of recovery. The pharmacologic treatment of TBI-induced behavioral and cognitive deficits is in its infancy, although reasonable recommendations for treatment strategies can be made. Overall treatment for significant TBI involves an interdisciplinary approach. Rehabilitation appears to have a beneficial effect on outcome following TBI. More research is needed to determine specific effects, and to obtain information on the cost-effectiveness of various interventions.

REFERENCES

1. Kraus JF, Sorenson FB: Epidemiology, in Silver JM, Yudofsky SC, Hales RE (eds): *Neuropsychiatry of Traumatic Brain Injury.* Washington, DC: American Psychiatric Press, 1994, pp. 3–41.
2. Kraus JF, Black MA, Hessol N, et al: The incidence of acute brain injury and serious impairment in a defined population. *Am J Epidemiol* 1984; 119:186–201.
3. Stalhammar D: Experimental models of head injury. *Acta Neurochir Suppl* (Wien) 1986; 36:33–40.
4. Annegers JF, Grabow JD, Kurland LT, et al: The incidence, causes and secular trends of head trauma in Olmsted County, Minnesota, 1935–1974. *Neurology* 1980; 30:912–919.
5. Teasdale G, Jenette B: Assessment of coma and impaired consciousness: A practical scale. *Lancet* 1974; 2:81–84.
6. Levin HS, O'Donnell VM, Grossman RG: The Galveston Orientation and Amnesia Test: a practical scale to assess cognition after head injury. *J Merv Ment Dis* 1979; 167:675–686.

7. Cassident JW: Neuropathology, in Silver JM, Yudofsky SC, and Hales RE (eds): *Neuropsychiatry of Traumatic Brain Injury.* Washington, DC: American Psychiatric Press, 1994, pp. 43–79.
8. Courville CG: Pathology of the central nervous system, part IV. Mountain View, CA: Pacific, 1937.
9. Pang D: Physics and pathophysiology of closed head injury, in Lezak MD (ed): *Assessment of the Behavioral Consequences of Head Trauma.* New York: Alan R. Liss, Inc., 1989, pp. 1–17.
10. Alexander MP: Traumatic brain injury, in Benson DF, Blumer E (eds): *Psychiatric Aspects of Neurologic Disease,* vol 2. New York: Grune & Stratton, 1982, pp. 219–248.
11. Povlishock J: Current concepts on axonal damage due to head injury. *Proceedings of the XIth International Congress of Neuropathy* 1991; 4 (suppl):749–753.
12. Povlishock J: Traumatically induced axonal injury: Pathogenesis and pathobiological implications. *Brain Pathol* 1992; 2:1–12.
13. Faden A, Demediuk P, Panter S, et al: The role of excitatory amino acids and NMDA receptors in traumatic brain injury. *Science* 1989; 244:798–800.
14. Ford LE, McLaurin RL: Mechanisms of extradural hematomas. *J Neurosurg* 1963; 20:760–769.
15. Miller JD, Pentland B, Berol S: Early evaluation and management, in Rosenthal M, Griffen ER, Bond MR, et al (eds): *Rehabilitation of the Adult and Child with Traumatic Brain Injury,* 2nd ed. Philadelphia, PA: F.A. Davis Co., 1990, pp. 21–25.
16. Teasdale G, Mendelow D: Pathophysiology of head injuries, in Brooks N (ed): *Closed Head Injury: Psychological, Social, and Family Consequences.* Oxford: Oxford University Press, 1984, pp. 4–36.
17. Miler JD: Clinical management of cerebral oedema. *BR J Hosp Med* 1979; 21:152–166.
18. Miller JD, Adams JH: The pathophysiology of raised intracranial pressure, in Adams JH, Corsellis JAN, Duchen LW (eds): *Greenfield's Neuropathology,* 4th ed. London: Edward Arnold, 1984, pp. 53–84.
19. Miller JD: Infection in head injury, in Braakman R (ed): *Handbook of Neurology,* vol 24. *Injuries of the Brain and Skull, part II.* Amsterdam: North-Holland, 1976, pp. 215–230.
20. Mesulum MM: *Principles of Behavioral Neurology.* Philadelphia: F.A. Davis, 1985, pp. 1–70.
21. Eslinger PJ, Grattan LM, Geder L: Impact of frontal lobe lesions on rehabilitation and recovery from acute brain injury. *Neurorehabilitation* 1995; 5:161–182.
22. Damasio AR, Van Hoesen GW: Emotional disturbances associated with focal lesions of the limbic frontal lobe, in Heilman KM, Satz P (eds): *Neuropsychology of Human Emotion.* New York: Guilford, 1983, pp. 86–110.
23. Heilman KM, Watson RT: Intentional motor disorders, in Levin HS, Eisenberg HM, Benton AL (eds): *Frontal*

Lobe Function and Dysfunction. New York: Oxford University Press, 1991, pp. 199–213.

24. Lindquist G, Norlen G: Korsakoff's syndrome after operation on ruptured aneurysm of the anterior communicating artery. *Acta Psychiatr Scand* 1966; 42:24–36.

25. Eslinger PJ, Damasio AR: Behavioral disturbances associated with rupture of anterior communicating artery aneurysms. *Sem Neurol* 1984; 4:385–389.

26. DeLuca J, Cicerone KD: Confabulation following aneurysm of the anterior communicating artery. *Cortex* 1991; 27:417–423.

27. Lhermitte F: Utilization behavior and its relation to lesions of the frontal lobes. *Brain* 1983; 106:237–255.

28. Pandya DN, Barnes CL: Architecture and connections of the frontal lobe, in Perecman E (ed): *The Frontal Lobes Revisited.* New York: IRBN Press, 1987, pp. 41–72.

29. Pandya DN, Yeterian EH: Prefrontal cortex in relation to other cortical areas in rhesus monkey: Architecture and connections. *Prog Brain Res* 1990; 85:63–94.

30. Eslinger PJ, Grattan LM: Frontal lobe and frontal-striatal substrates for different forms of human cognitive flexibility. *Neuropsychologia* 1993; 31:17–28.

31. Eslinger PJ, Damasio AR: Severe disturbance of higher cognition after bilateral frontal lobe ablation: Patient EVR. *Neurology* 1985; 35:1731–1741.

32. Grattan LM, Bloomer RH, Archambault FX, Eslinger PJ: Cognitive flexibility and empathy after frontal lobe lesion. *Neuropsychiatr Neuropsychol Behav Neurol* 1994; 7:251–259.

33. Kluver H, Bucy PC: *Arch Neurol Psychiatr* 1939; 42:979–1000.

34. Lilly R, Cummings JL, Benson DF, Frankel M: The human Kluver-Bucy syndrome. *Neurology* 1983; 33(9):1141–1145.

35. Lishman WA: Organic Psychiatry: *The Psychological Consequences of Cerebral Disorder.* Oxford: Blackwell Scientific Publications, 1978.

36. Grattan LM, Eslinger PJ: Frontal lobe damage in children and adults: A comparative review. *Dev Neuropsychol* 1991; 7:283–326.

37. Damasio AR, Tranel D, Damasio HC: Somatic makers and the guidance of behavior: Theory and preliminary testing, in Levin HS, Eisenberg HM, Benton AL (eds): *Frontal Lobe Function and Dysfunction.* New York: Oxford University Press, 1991, pp. 217–229.

38. Adams JH, Graham DI, Gennarelli TA, Maxwell WL: *J Neurol Neurosurg Psychiatr* 1991; 54:481–483.

39. Stuss DT, Ely P, Hugenholtz H, Richard MT, LaRochelle S, Poirier CA, Bell I: Subtle neuropsychological deficits in patients with good recovery after closed head injury. *Neurosurgery* 1985; 17(1):41–47.

40. Stuss DT, Stethem LL, Hugenholtz H, Picton T, Pivik J, Richard MT: Reaction time after head injury: Fatigue, divided and focused attention, and consistency of performance. *J Neurol Neurosurg Psychiatr* 1989; 52(6):742–748.

41. Gronwall D, Wrightson P: Memory and information processing capacity after closed head injury. *J Neurol Neurosurg Psychiatry* 1981; 44(10):889–895.

42. Oddy M, Coughlan T, Tyerman A, Jenkins D: Social adjustment after closed head injury: A further follow-up seven years after injury. *J Neurol Neurosurg Psychiatr* 1985; 48(6):564–568.

43. Ewart J, Levin HS, Watson MG, Kalisky Z: Procedural memory during post traumatic amnesia in survivors of severe closed head injury: Implications for rehabilitation. *Arch Neurol* 1989; 46:911–916.

44. Mandelberg IA: Cognitive recovery after severe head injury. *J Neurol Neurosurg Psychiatr* 1976; 39:1001–1007.

45. Berg EA: *J Gen Psychol* 1948; 39:15–22.

46. Stuss DT, Buckle L: Cognitive recovery after severe head injury. *J Head Trauma Rehab* 1992; 7:40–49.

47. Sarno MT: The nature of verbal impairment after closed head injury. *J Nerv Ment Dis* 1980; 168:685–692.

48. Katz DI, Alexander MP: Traumatic brain injury, in Good DC, Couch JR (eds): *Handbook of Neurorehabilitation.* New York: Marcel Dekker, 1994, pp. 493–549.

49. Eames P: *J Head Trauma Rehab* 1988; 3:1–6.

50. Livingston MG, Brooks DN, Bond MR: Patient outcome in the year following severe head injury and relatives' psychiatric and social functioning. *J Neurol Neurosurg Psychiatr* 1985; 48:876–881.

51. Yorkston KM, Honsinger MJ, Mitsuda PM, Hammen V: *J Head Trauma Rehab* 1989; 4:1–16.

52. Hagen C, Malkmus D, Durham P: *Levels of Cognitive Functioning.* Downey, CA: Ranchos Los Amigos Hospital, 1972.

53. Alexander MP: *Psychiatric Aspects of Neurologic Disease* (Benson DF, Blumer D, eds), New York: McGraw-Hill, 1982, pp. 251–278.

54. Dombovy ML, Bach-y-Rita P: Clinical observations on recovery from stroke, in Waxman SG (ed): *Physiologic Basis for Functional Recovery in Neurologic Disease.* New York: Raven, 1988.

55. Gennarelli TA, Thibault LE, Adams JH, Graham DI, Thompson CJ, Marcincin RP: *Ann Neurol* 1982; 12:564–574.

56. Alexander MP, Benson DF, Stuss DT: Frontal lobes and language. *Brain Lang* 1989; 37(4):656–691.

57. Gualtieri CT, Evans RW: Stimulant treatment for the neurobehavioral sequelae of traumatic brain injury. *Brain Inj* 1988; 2:273–290.

58. Jennett B, Bond M: Assessment of outcome after severe brain damage: Practical scale. *Lancet* 1975; 1:48–484.

59. Rappaport M, Hall K, Hopkins HK, Belleza T, Cope N: Disability rating scale for severe head trauma patient: Coma to community. *Arch Phys Med Rehab* 1982; 63:118–123.

60. Keith R, Granger C, Hamilton B, Sherwin F: The functional independence measure: A new tool for rehabilitation, in Eisenburg MG, Grzesiak RC (eds): *Advances in*

Clinical Rehabilitation. New York: Springer Publishing Co., Inc., 1987, pp. 6–18.

61. Katz DI: *J Head Trauma Rehab* 1992; 7:1–15.

62. Vollmer DG, Torner JC, Jane JA, et al: *Neurosurgery* 1991; 75(suppl):37–49.

63. Katz DI, Kehs GJ, Alexander MP: *Neurology* 1990; 40(suppl):276.

64. Levy DE, Caronna JJ, Singer BH, Lapinski RH, Frydman H, Plum F: Predicting outcome from hypoxic-ischemic coma. *JAMA* 1985; 253(10):1420–1426.

65. Brooks N, McKinlay W, Symington C, Beattie A, Campsie L: Return to work within the first seven years of severe head injury. *Brain Inj* 1987; 1:5–19.

66. Wechsler D: Wechsler Adult Intelligence Scale. New York: Psychologic Corporation, 1955.

67. Mazmanian PE: Cognitive rehabilitation: Theory and informal practice. *Neurorehabilitation* 1991; 1:86–89.

68. Gordan WA: Cognitive rehabilitation, in Zasker ND, Dreutzer JS (eds): *Neurorehabilitation* 1992; 2:1–67.

69. Ben-Yishay Y, Prigatano GP: Cognitive remediation, in Rosenthal M, Griffith ER, Bond MR, Miller JD (eds): *Rehabilitation of the Adult and Child with Traumatic Brain Injury,* 2nd ed. Philadelphia: F.A. Davis, 1990.

70. Sholberg MM, Sprunk H, Metzelaar K: Efficacy of an external cuing system in an individual with severe frontal lobe damage. *Cog Rehab* 1988; 6:36–41.

71. Sohlberg MM, Mateer CA: Effectiveness of an attention training program. *J Clin Exp Neuropsychol* 1987; 9:117–130.

72. Sohlberg MM, Mateer CA: *Introduction to Cognitive Rehabilitation: Theory and Practice.* New York: Guilford, 1989.

73. Schacter DL, Glisky EL: Memory remediation, restoration, alleviation, and the acquisition of domain-specific knowledge, in Uzzel B, Gross Y (eds): *Clinical Neuropsychology of Intervention.* Boston: Martinus Nijoff, 1986.

74. Glisky E, Schacter D, Tulving E: Learning and retention of computer-related vocabulary in memory-impaired patients: Method of vanishing cues. *J Clin Exp Neuropsychol* 1986; 3:292–312.

75. Glisky E, Schacter D: Long-term memory retention of computer learning by patients with memory disorders. *Neuropsychologia* 1988; 26:173–178.

76. D'Esposito M, Alexander MP: The clinical profiles, recovery and rehabilitation of memory disorders. *Neurorehabilitation* 1995; 5:141–159.

77. Gainotti G, Messerli P, Tissot R: Qualitative analysis of unilateral and spatial neglect in relation to laterality of cerebral lesions. *J Neurol Neurosurg Psychiatr* 1972; 35:545–550.

78. Chatterjee A: Unilateral spatial neglect: Assessment and rehabilitation strategies. *Neurorehabilitation* 1995; 5:115–128.

79. Wilson B, Cockburn J, Halligan PW: *Behavioral Inattention Test.* Titchfield, Hants: Thames Valley Test Co., 1987.

80. Schlageter K, Gray B, Hall K, Shaw R, Sammet R: Incidence and treatment of visual dysfunction in traumatic brain injury. *Brain Injury* 1993; 7:439–448.

81. Anderson SW, Rizzo M: Recovery and rehabilitation of visual cortical dysfunction. *Neurorehabilitation* 1995; 5:129–140.

82. Robinson RG, Jorge R: Mood disorders, in Silver JM, Yudofsky SC, Hales RE (eds): *Neuropsychiatry of Traumatic Brain Injury.* Washington, DC: American Psychiatric Press, 1994, pp. 219–250.

83. Jorge RE, Robinson RG, Starkstein SE, et al: Manic syndromes following traumatic brain injury. *Am J Psychiatr* 1993; 150:916–921.

84. Epstein RS, Ursano RJ: Anxiety disorders, in Silver JM, Yudofsky SC, Hales RE (eds): *Neuropsychiatry of Traumatic Brain Injury.* Washington, DC: American Psychiatric Press, 1994, pp. 285–311.

85. Rose M: The pace of drugs in the management of behavior disorders after traumatic brain injury. *J Head Trauma Rehab* 1988; 3(3):7–13.

86. Silver JM, Sanberg DP, Hales RE: New approaches in the pharmacotherapy of posttraumatic stress disorder. *J Clin Psychiatr* 1990; 5(suppl):33–38.

87. Corrigan JD: Development of a scale for assessment of agitation following traumatic brain injury. *J Clin Exp Neuropsychol* 1989; 11:261–277.

88. Yudofsky SC, Silver JM, Jackson W, et al: The overt aggression scale for the objective rating of verbal and physical aggression. *Am J Psychiatr* 1986; 143:35–39.

89. Trzepacz PT: Delirium in: *Neuropsychiatry of Traumatic Brain Injury.* Washington, DC: American Psychiatric Press, 1994, pp. 43–79.

90. Rowland T, DePalma L: Current neuropharmologic interventions for the management of brain injury rehabilitation. *Neurorehabilitation* 1995; 5:219–232.

91. Goldstein LB: Basic and clinical studies of pharmacologic effects on recovery from brain injury. *J Neural Transplant Plast* 1993; 4:175–192.

92. Bell KR, Cardenas DC: New frontiers of neuropharmologic treatment of brain injury agitation. *Neurorehabilitation* 1995; 5:223–244.

93. Brooke MM, Patterson D, Questad K, et al: The treatment of agitation during initial hospitalization after traumatic brain injury. *Arch Phys Med Rehab* 1992; 73:917–921.

94. Smelzer DJ, Nasrallah HA, Miller SC: *Psychoses: Neuropsychiatry of Traumatic Brain Injury.* Washington, DC: American Psychiatric Press, 1994, pp. 251–283.

95. Jennett WB: *Epilepsy after Non-missile Head Injuries.* Chicago: Yearbook Medical Publishers, 1975, pp. 35–49.

96. Menkes JH, Till K: Postnatal trauma and injuries by physical agents, in *Textbook of Child Neurology,* 4th ed. Philadelphia, PA: Lea & Febiger, 1990, pp. 462–496.

97. Salazar AM, Jabbari B, Vance SC, et al: Epilepsy after penetrating head injury: I. Clinical correlates: A report of the Vietnam head injury study. *Neurology* 1985; 35:1406–1414.

98. Hauser WA: Prevention of post-traumatic epilepsy. *N Engl J Med* 1990; 323(8):540–541.

99. Dugan EM, Harwell JM: Postraumatic seizures. *Emer Med Clin N Am* 1994; 12:1081–1086.

100. Povlischock JT, Coburn TH: *Mild Head Injury* (HS Levin, HM Eisenberg, and AL Benton, eds), Oxford University Press, New York, 1989, pp. 37–53.

101. American Congress of Rehabilitation Medicine, Mild Traumatic Brain Inury and Committee: *Definition of Mild Traumatic Brain Injury.* Head Injury Interdisciplinary Special Interest Group Publications, 1991.

102. Barth JT, Alves TV, Ryan SN, et al: *Mild Head Injury* (HS Levin, HM Eisenberg, and AL Benton, eds), Oxford University Press, New York, 1989, pp. 257–275.

103. Dikmen SS, McLean A, Temkin N, et al: *J Neurol Neurosurg Psychiatry* 1986; 49:1227–1232.

104. Silver JM, Hales RE, Yudofsky SC: Neuropsychiatric aspects of traumatic brain injury, in Hales RE, Yudofsky SC (eds): *The American Psychiatric Press Textbook of Neuropsychiatry,* 2nd ed. Washington, DC: American Psychiatric Press, 1992.

105. Goldstein F, Levin HS: Epidemiology of pediatric closed head injury: Incidence, clinical characteristics and risk factors. *J Learning Disab* 1987; 20:518–525.

106. Billmire ME, Myers PA: Serious head injury in infants: Accident or abuse. *Pediatrics* 1985; 75:340–342.

107. Rutter M, Graham P, Yule W: A neuropsychiatric study in childhood, in *Clinics in Development Medicine,* 35/36. London: William Heinemann Medical Books/SIMP, 1970.

108. Brown GL, Chadwick O, Shaffer D, et al: A prospective study of children with head injuries, III: Psychiatric sequelae. *Psychol Med* 1981; 11:63–78.

109. Birmaker B, Williams DT: *Children and Adolescents: Neuropsychiatry of Traumatic Brain Injury.* Washington, DC: American Psychiatric Press, 1994, pp. 393–412.

110. Chadwick O, Rutter M, Brown G, et al: A prospective study of children with head injuries, II: cognitive sequelae. *Psychol Med* 1981; 11:49–61.

111. Segalowitz SJ, Brown D: Mild head injury as a source of developmental disabilities. *J Learning Disabil* 1991; 24:551–558.

112. Kriel RL, Kranch LE, Shean M: Pediatric closed head injury: Outcome following prolonged unconsciousness. *Arch Phys Med Rehab* 1988; 69:678–681.

113. Wilson JT, Weidman KD, Hadley DM, et al: Early and late magnetic resonance imaging and neuropsychological outcome after head injury. *J Neurol Neurosurg Psychiatr* 1988; 51:391–396.

114. Jaffe KM, Polissar NL, Gay GC, Liao S: Recovery trends over three years following pediatric traumatic brain injury. *Arch Phys Med Rehab* 1995; 76:17–26.

115. Hall KM, Cope DN: The benefit of traumatic brain injury rehabilitation: A literature review. *J Head Trauma Rehab* 1995; 10:1–13.

116. High WM, Boake C, Lehmkuhl LD: Critical analysis of studies evaluating the effectiveness of rehabilitation after traumatic brain injury. *J Head Trauma Rehab* 1995, 10:14–26.

117. Feeney DM, Sutton RL: Pharmacotherapy for recovery of function after brain injury. *CDC Crit Rev Neurobiol* 1987; 3(2):135–197.

Chapter 8

STROKE REHABILITATION

Michael M. Pfeffer
Michael J. Reding

STROKE DIAGNOSIS, EPIDEMIOLOGY, TREATMENT

Stroke is defined as a focal abnormality of brain function, lasting longer than 24 hours, caused by altered cerebral circulation. If neurologic signs or symptoms last for less than 24 hours the event is defined as a transient ischemic attack (TIA). Strokes are categorized as either ischemic (caused by blockage of cerebral blood flow) or hemorrhagic (caused by rupture of a cerebral vessel). Ischemic strokes are further divided into thrombotic (thrombus develops at the site of blockage), or embolic (thrombus develops proximally then travels downstream to the site of blockage).

In the United States 550,000 people suffer from stroke each year. It is the third leading cause of mortality, accounting for 150,000 deaths per year. There are 3 million stroke survivors with varying degrees of neurological impairment, making it the most common cause of disability requiring rehabilitation.[1] It has been estimated that the cost of acute and chronic stroke care, plus loss of income, amounts to 30 billion dollars per year.[2]

The frequency of stroke increases with age, doubling every decade after age 55. Strokes occur more frequently in men than women, and more frequently among African Americans than whites.[3]

Ischemic strokes account for 80 percent of first strokes, intracerebral hemorrhages for 16 percent, and subarachnoid hemorrhages for 4 percent.[4–7] The diagnosis of stroke type and etiology is important for appropriate acute treatment and for prophylaxis against recurrence. Strokes caused by embolization from the heart are treated with coumadin, whereas those caused by embolization from the carotid artery are treated with

endarterectomy, aspirin, or ticlopidine. Progressive thrombosis within the cerebral circulation is treated with intravenous heparin. Intracerebral hemorrhage is usually due to hypertension, arterial-venous malformation, or congophilic angiopathy. Subarachnoid hemorrhage is usually due to congenital aneurysms, which require craniotomy and surgical clipping.

The 30-day mortality for ischemic stroke is 15 percent, and 30 percent for hemorrhagic stroke. Some studies suggest that if patients survive the initial 30 days, functional recovery may be better for those with hemorrhagic lesions.[8]

Risk factors for stroke may be seen as either modifiable or nonmodifiable.[9] Modifiable risk factors are hypertension, diabetes, atrial fibrillation, and cigarette smoking. Nonmodifiable risk factors include age, sex, race, prior stroke, and family history.

Stroke is often associated with age and atherosclerosis-related comorbid medical problems. Stroke survivors have a higher prevalence of arthritis, obesity, ischemic heart disease, left ventricular hypertrophy, congestive heart failure, and diabetes mellitus than age-matched controls.[10]

Stroke-related immobility predisposes patients to a number of medical complications: deep venous thrombosis, pulmonary embolization, aspiration pneumonia, urinary retention, incontinence and shoulder–hand pain syndrome. Stroke, although focal in nature, is often associated with neuropsychiatric complications, indicating diffuse cerebral dysfunction: depression, delirium, dementia, and seizures. The recovery phase following stroke requires management of comorbid medical problems, and ongoing surveillance and prophylaxis for the development of secondary complications.

NEUROLOGIC AND FUNCTIONAL RECOVERY

Recovery of neurologic impairments following stroke is due to a combination of factors: (1) recovery of dysfunctional cells in the ischemic penumbra around the area of actual infarction; (2) recovery from diaschisis; and (3) unmasking of secondary neural circuits.[11] Patients with lesions that are too extensive or strategically located will not fully recover from their neurologic impairment, but may show improvement in function by learning adaptive techniques such as shifting hand dominance and one-handed dressing techniques. Assistive devices such as canes and braces allow patients to show improvement in walking safety and endurance without change in strength, balance, or somatosensory scores.

Stroke may impair all activities of daily living. The functional consequences of neurologic impairments span the gamut of human activities. Addressing this diversity of functional deficits has given rise to an interdisciplinary team approach to rehabilitation following stroke.

THE REHABILITATION-TEAM APPROACH TO RECOVERY

The stroke-rehabilitation team consists of many specialists, whose focus is to achieve the best level of function for each patient. Physical therapists assist in the recovery of standing, ambulation, transfers, balance, and endurance. They also provide support, training, assistive devices, and bracing to improve lower extremity function. Occupational therapists address difficulties with feeding, dressing, grooming, bathing, toileting, and other essential daily-living skills. Speech-language pathologists target problems with language, speech articulation, and feeding. Social workers evaluate the patient's coping mechanisms and social support systems, and help organize the patient's transition back into the community. Psychologists evaluate the patient to help the rehabilitation team optimize therapy for patients with cognitive or behavioral deficits. Recreational therapists use leisure activities to enhance and solidify physical, occupational, speech, and nursing rehabilitation gains.

Team concepts have evolved from the multidisciplinary approach described above to a more dynamic interdisciplinary model. The interdisciplinary team attempts to transcend therapy roles and address patient goals more holistically. In such a team, the physical and occupational therapists might also address speech goals while working on self-care and ambulation activities. The occupational therapist might address physical therapy goals by having the patient stand at a stand-table while working on upper-limb activities.

Table 8-1

Stroke rehabilitation units improve outcome: randomized controlled trials

Reference	Size	Benefits
Feigenson *Stroke*, 1979	$n = 667$	Ambulation Disch. Home
Garraway *BMJ*, 1980	$n = 307$	Ambulation Self-care
Smith *BMJ*, 1981	$n = 133$	Ambulation Self-care
Strand *Stroke*, 1985	$n = 293$	Ambulation Self-care
Indredavik *Stroke*, 1991	$n = 206$	Ambulation Self-care Disch. Home
Kalra *Stroke*, 1993	$n = 245$	Ambulation Self-care Disch. Home
Kaste *Stroke*, 1995	$n = 243$	Self-care Disch. Home
Jorgensen *Stroke*, 1995	$n = 1241$	Mortality Disch. Home Self-care Cost

VALIDATION OF THE FOCUSED STROKE-REHABILITATION TEAM APPROACH

The benefits of focused stroke-rehabilitation units have been documented by eight controlled trials conducted in five countries.[12–19] These studies show that focused stroke-rehabilitation programs improve functional outcome, decrease length of stay, and reduce the need for nursing-home care (see Table 8-1).

In Feigenson's study, 589 of 667 stroke patients were admitted to a focused stroke unit.[12] The remainder were admitted to general rehabilitation wards. Despite the fact that the patients in the stroke unit were initially weaker, had longer onset–admission intervals, greater neurological deficits, and more comorbidity, at discharge these patients had greater mobility and were more frequently discharged home. Similarly, Garraway studied stroke patients on a specialized stroke unit compared with those placed on a general medical floor and found significant differences in both ambulation and self-care in favor of the group that had been on the stroke unit.[13] Smith studied 133 stroke patients and randomized them to one of three groups: (1) intensive outpatient rehabilitation 3 days/week for 6 hours/day; (2) conventional rehabilitation 3 days/week for 3 hours/day; and (3) home visits by a nurse without rehabilitation.[14] Improvements in ambulation and self-care were greatest for patients receiving the most intensive rehabilitation. Strand compared the outcome of 110 stroke patients on a stroke unit with 183 stroke patients on a general medical ward. Self-care recovery and ambulation were greatest for patients on the stroke unit.[15] Indredavik compared stroke patients on a stroke unit to those on a general medical ward and found functional levels to be higher for those patients on the stroke unit after both 6 and 52 weeks.[16] Kalra and Kaste in independent studies randomized patients with stroke to stroke units or general medical units. Both found improved functional outcome for patients randomized to the stroke unit.[17,18] Kaste's study also showed that patients discharged from the stroke unit were more likely to go home rather than to a nursing home. Jorgensen compared the outcome of patients from two different medical districts in Copenhagen.[19] One district had a focused stroke-rehabilitation unit, the other did not. The two groups were demographically similar with respect to age, race, income, educational level, and initial stroke severity. At discharge, patients from the focused stroke rehabilitation unit had significantly lower mortality, better functional outcome, decreased length of stay, and higher prevalence of returning to home.

These studies reflect an international consensus that focused stroke rehabilitation units improve functional outcome, increase the percentage of patients returning home, and decrease the length of acute-care hospitalization.

REHABILITATION OPTIONS AND SCREENING CRITERIA

Rehabilitation issues are an integral part of stroke management and should be addressed from the time of entry into the emergency room. The more severe the patient's functional deficits, the greater the need for early attention to proper positioning and protection of flaccid limbs. Within 24 to 48 hours a passive range-of-motion program should be in place if needed. Those who are more alert can begin bed mobility training and bridging exercises to help with pressure relief, dressing, and toileting. The ideal stroke unit is one that cares for the patient from emergency room to home, in a seamless continuum of care. Such systems have been established, usually within socialized medical care systems such as in Great Britain and Scandinavia. In the United States, medical evaluation and treatment are provided by acute-care hospitals, where rehabilitation services may be limited. Patients deemed appropriate for more intensive rehabilitation are referred either to a separate ward within the same institution, or to an independent rehabilitation facility. Those needing rehabilitation but who do not require inpatient care are referred for outpatient or home-care services. The more discontinuous the rehabilitation process, the greater the need for screening evaluations to match patients to the appropriate level of care available within the community.

Screening patients for rehabilitation should address the following issues: (1) Will rehabilitation in any form or intensity significantly improve the patient's quality of life or reduce the cost or burden of care on caregivers? (2) If so, what level of medical, nursing, and rehabilitative care is appropriate?

Approximately 20 percent of stroke survivors recover full functional independence by 2 weeks following stroke.[20] Such spontaneous recovery occurs without rehabilitation intervention. Another 20 percent have such severe functional deficits that they are expected to remain nonambulatory and continue to require assistance with all activities of daily living (ADLs) irrespective of rehabilitation efforts. The remaining 60 percent of stroke survivors will benefit from some level of rehabilitation intervention. Occasionally, devoted families will resolve to care for the most dependent and burdensome patients at home. Such families can often benefit from intensive rehabilitation efforts directed not at improving the patient's function, but at training family members in patient-care skills, including bathing, skin-bowel-bladder care, and hemiplegic dressing and transfer techniques. Attempting to teach such skills once the patient has been discharged to home can be overwhelming for the family and unsafe for the patient.

Rehabilitation admission criteria usually state that the patient should be medically stable. This means that the diagnosis has been established, treatment has begun, and the patient is not at significant risk for cardiopulmonary decompensation. One of the roles of the physician on the rehabilitation team is to provide medical supervision as the patient evolves from being bed-bound to recovering optimal mobility function. Medicare guidelines for intensive rehabilitation require that patients be able to tolerate, participate, and benefit from at least 3 hours of therapy per day. The 3 hours need not be continuous. Program schedules can be modified for low-level patients so that they are given rest periods between activities.

Screening criteria concerning the patient's medical stability should be institution-specific. The availability of respiratory care, intravenous management, non-oral alimentation, and monitoring services differs widely among rehabilitation settings. Rehabilitation units physically connected to acute-care hospitals are able to accept patients requiring more active medical management. Transportation of patients back to the acute-care hospital for diagnostic or monitoring studies limits acceptance of such patients to freestanding rehabilitation hospitals.

Triage of patients to the appropriate level of rehabilitation care is based on the patient's functional status. Those who are ambulatory without assistance, are continent and require only minimal assistance with ADL functions are appropriate for home or outpatient care. Those who are wheelchair-dependent, incontinent, or require assistance with walking and other ADL activities are appropriate for inpatient care.

Patients requiring inpatient care who are expected to benefit from rehabilitation but cannot tolerate 3 hours of rehabilitation per day can be referred to subacute rehabilitation units able to provide 3 to 5 hours of therapy per week. Such patients with limited physical endurance may improve sufficiently to permit reevaluation for more intense therapy at a later date.

MEASURING SELF-CARE FUNCTIONS, COMMUNITY SKILLS, AND QUALITY OF LIFE

Activity-of-daily-living (ADL) scales are important to determine the functional impact of neurologic impairments, establish goals, and monitor progress. Most ADL scales measure several activities including feeding, dressing, grooming, bathing, toileting, and mobility. Some also include measures of cognition, social behavior, and communication. The most commonly used ADL scales are the Barthel Index and the Functional Independence Measure (FIM).[21–23] These scales are accurate and reproducible across different observers but show

limited sensitivity to change in patient function. Both scales have a ceiling effect that limits their use in patients with mild disability. They do not adequately score the speed or quality of self-care functions.

Newer assessments called Instrumental ADL scales contain the basic self-care components mentioned previously, but include more complex tasks such as using public transportation, balancing a checkbook, shopping, laundering, and housekeeping.[24]

Rehabilitation goals have traditionally focused on maximizing patient function. It has traditionally been assumed that increased function leads to improved quality of life. The development of quality-of-life scales has shown such assumptions to be only partially correct, and have advanced the scope of rehabilitation efforts. Such scales help identify family, community, work, or leisure-time limitations on the patient's recovery that can then be improved in therapy.

SETTING REHABILITATION GOALS

Outcome expectations are constrained by a number of patient-specific parameters: (1) functional level prior to the stroke, (2) stroke severity; and (3) presence of family members or others able and willing to assist with home care. Patients needing a cane prior to stroke will need some device following stroke. Stroke severity ranges from full recovery after 24 hours to needing maximal assistance for self-care. If the patient does not regain independence and continues to require assistance with self-care, the discharge disposition will depend on the availability of supportive family and friends.

Setting rehabilitation outcome goals assumes that patients can be grouped into clinically relevant groups that have predictable recoveries. The groups should be as homogeneous as possible with respect to premorbid independence, stroke etiology, and location. One approach to outcome prediction is applicable to patients who were previously independent who suffered an initial unilateral ischemic hemispheric stroke. This group is conveniently divided according to the extent of associated neurologic impairments. The presence of pure motor weakness indicates a lacunar subcortical stroke and good functional recovery. Motor weakness *and* hemihypesthesia signals either a larger subcortical lesion or a cortical stroke affecting the motor and sensory cortex, with more protracted and incomplete recovery. Motor weakness, hemihypesthesia, and homonymous hemianopia indicate an extensive subcortical lesion or a cortical lesion extending into the subcortical geniculocalcarine

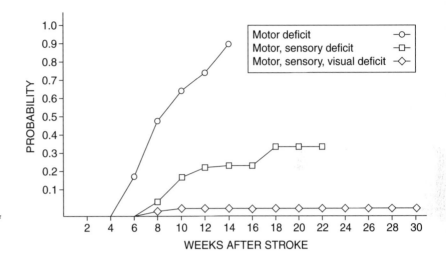

Figure 8-1
Life Table Analysis. Probability of walking ≥150 ft without assistance.

tracts with the lowest outcome expectations. Other combinations of motor, sensory, and visual deficits occur but are infrequently seen on an inpatient stroke service. Further subdivision of these groups according to the presence or absence of aphasia or cognitive impairment adds complexity without significantly improving prediction of recovery.

Figure 8-1 shows the probability of recovering the ability to walk 150 feet independently for patients with initial unilateral hemispheric stroke. These patients were all living independently in the community prior to their stroke. Comparison of patients with isolated motor deficits to those having motor, somatic sensory, and hemianopic visual deficits reveals highly significant differences. Patients with pure motor hemiparesis have greater than a 90 percent probability of recovering independent ambulation by 14 weeks post-stroke. Those with motor, somatosensory, and visual deficits are unlikely to achieve this goal even after 30 weeks post-stroke. For these patients, a more realistic goal is to be able to walk 150 feet with assistance, as shown in Figure 8-2. They have a 95 percent probability of reaching this goal by 30 weeks post-stroke. Figure 8-3 presents the probability of achieving a Barthel score of 60 or higher for patients with motor deficits with and without somatosensory and hemianopic visual deficits. Even those with the most extensive deficits had a 50 percent probability of reaching this goal by 16 weeks post-stroke. This is the Barthel level at which an aged spouse can assist with the patient's home care without need for nursing-home placement.

Similar outcome probabilities can be estimated for patients categorized according to the severity of their functional deficits as indicated by their rehabilitation hospital admission Barthel scores. Figure 8-4 presents the probability of walking 150 feet with assistance for patients previously independent in the community with initial unilateral ischemic hemispheric strokes. Even those with admission Barthel scores of 40 or less have a 60 percent probability of reaching this ambulation goal.

MEDICAL MANAGEMENT: ACUTE PHASE

In the acute phase, post-stroke medical attention is directed at identifying and controlling stroke-related comorbidity, and initiating prophylactic intervention to prevent stroke-related complications. The most common medical comorbitities are hypertension, diabetes, ischemic heart disease, osteoarthritis, and congestive heart failure. The most common complications in the stroke-rehabilitation setting are: problems with deglutition, pneumonia, dehydration, malnutrition, venous thromboembolism, pressure sores, falls, constipation, and neuropsychiatric complications including delirium, depression, and dementia.

Following stroke there is often an acute, reflex increase in blood pressure to overcome the effects of focal cerebral hypoperfusion. Although it is accepted that chronic hypertension is a major risk factor for accelerated atherosclerosis and stroke, this chronic process has limited relevance for the acute, reflex increase in blood pressure after stroke. Hypertensive encephalopathy is a rare occurrence associated with papilledema,

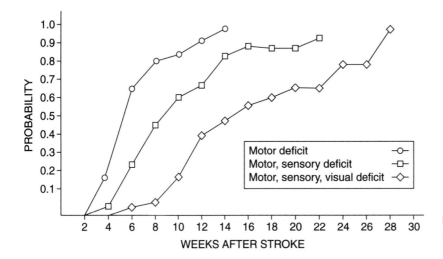

Figure 8-2
Life Table Analysis. Probability of walking ≥150 ft with assistance.

focal neurological signs, systolic blood pressures above 220 mmHg, and diastolic pressures above 130 mmHg. Such hypertensive crises require emergent reduction in systolic pressures below 180 mmHg and may require intraarterial blood-pressure monitoring and intravenous nitroprusside infusion. Except for acute hypertensive encephalopathy, there is no advantage to rapidly reducing the stroke patient's blood pressure when it is noted to be elevated in the stroke-rehabilitation setting. Reduction of mean arterial pressure may only further compromise blood flow in the ischemic penumbra. Recent studies of patient blood-pressure management after stroke indicate that overly aggressive control of blood

pressure leads to reductions in cerebral perfusion, activities of daily living, and neuropsychological function.[25] The risks of relative hypotension usually far outweigh the risks of hypertension in the early management of blood pressure after acute stroke. Gradual reduction in pressure over several days is the safest alternative.

Hyperglycemia with associated lactate accumulation in the ischemic penumbra has been shown to be associated with worsened stroke outcome.[25–27] Intravenous glucose infusion during the acute stroke phase of recovery should be avoided. It is now accepted that all microvascular complications of diabetes can be minimized by tight control of blood glucose with multiple

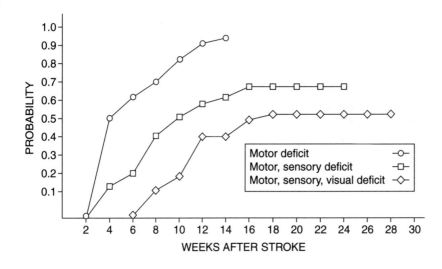

Figure 8-3
Life Table Analysis. Probability of reaching a Barthel score ≥60.

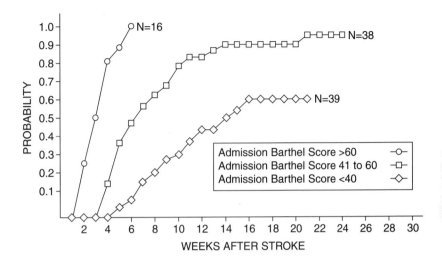

Figure 8-4
Probability of walking 150 ft with assistance.

daily insulin injections guided by fingerstick blood-sugar determinations.

That notwithstanding, it is important to acknowledge the unique predicament of the diabetic following stroke. Patients may lose awareness of impending hypoglycemia, have variable exercise demands, and may have tremendous dietary fluctuations due to dysphagia or suppressed sensorium. For these reasons, diabetic regulation following stroke is expected to require close medical and nursing supervision. The blood glucose target may have to be readjusted from euglycemia to a less ideal but safer goal of between 100 to 200 mg%.

Approximately 60 percent of patients with stroke will have a history of either ischemic heart disease or congestive heart failure. A past history of such diagnoses is not as clinically useful as a functional classification of heart disease. What is needed is some understanding of the limitations imposed by cardiac function on exercise tolerance. The New York Heart Association classification has been widely studied and used.[28] Class 1 means that the patient has had symptoms in the past but no functional limitations. Class 2 means that symptoms have produced mild functional limitations. Class 3 means that the patient's activities have been restricted to household level ambulation. Class 4 means that the patient is bedridden or limited to sitting in a chair.

Hemiplegic wheelchair propulsion and assisted ambulation using a cane and brace are not more physically demanding than walking prior to stroke, as long as the patient is able to self-select the pace of movement. The exercise expenditure per unit of time will be the same, although the expenditure per foot of distance

moved will be increased.[29,30] Rehabilitation for stroke following acute myocardial infarction, coronary artery bypass graft, or heart-valve surgery is not different than for such patients who would otherwise have returned home to resume their usual level of household ambulation and stair-climbing activities. The caveat is that patients select their own wheelchair and walking speed.

The patient's ability to swallow must be assessed soon after admission. The incidence of dysphagia after stroke may be as high as 50 percent and may be seen during any phase of swallowing. During the oral phase of swallowing, dysphagia may be observed owing to altered control of the lips, mouth, tongue, or soft palate.[31] During the pharyngeal phase there may be altered control of the pharynx or larynx. The esophageal phase of swallowing is rarely affected following stroke. The most common problem noted following stroke is a delayed swallowing reflex.[31] Early evaluation and treatment intervention can decrease the possibility of aspiration, and improve nutrition and oral intake of liquids.

Oral feedings should be initiated as soon as the patient can swallow without significant risk of aspiration. A bedside swallowing evaluation may reveal poor lip closure, difficulty with bolus control, pocketing of food on one side of the mouth, coughing when swallowing, or the presence of a hoarse, gurgling voice after swallowing.[32] Although obviously important, such bedside observation techniques still underdiagnose the presence of pharyngeal-phase dysfunction and aspiration.[33] A videofluoroscopic modified barium swallow (MBS) evaluation is the definitive test of swallowing function.[34] Videofluoroscopy as defined by Logemann using small volumes of barium ($\frac{1}{3}$ teaspoon) can assess how the patient handles various bolus consistencies. Larger bolus volumes of 20 to 30 mL can assess the patient's response to more normal stimulation. The MBS evaluation allows the therapist to test the effect of different bolus consistencies and volumes, and compensatory swallowing strategies on treating dysphagia.

The goal of dysphagia management in the stroke rehabilitation setting is to prevent complications and restore the patient's ability to chew and swallow safely. Swallowing therapies include exercises to improve oral strength and control. Compensatory treatments involve changes in posture, such as head turn toward the paretic side, and chin-tuck maneuvers. Swallowing techniques such as decreasing bolus size and using thickened consistencies also can be helpful. At least one large case series has shown that 89 percent of dysphagic patients were able to resume oral feeding following stroke. None developed aspiration pneumonia after beginning a compensatory feeding program.[31]

Close monitoring of nutritional status is essential following stroke. The patient's weight, blood urea nitrogen, serum sodium, and albumen levels provide objective measures of state of hydration and nitrogen balance. The presence of urinary ketones without glycosuria is a sensitive indicator of inadequate calorie intake, but may take several days to develop. If oral intake is not safe or effective, tube feedings either by nasogastric or gastrostomy routes can be initiated. Patients still requiring nasogastric feedings 2 weeks post-stroke are considered candidates for percutaneous gastrostomy. Surgically placed gastrostomy tubes are used only when there is a contraindication for percutaneous gastrostomy, or a permanent ostomy site is needed.

Decreased mobility predisposes to a number of medical complications. The patient who is unable to roll in bed is at high risk for development of pressure sores. The National Survey of Stroke found that 14.5 percent of stroke patients develop pressure sores.[35] Frequent turning of the patient on a 2-hour schedule with attention to proper support and positioning of plegic limbs is required. Heel protectors, gel mattresses, and wheelchair seat cushions help redistribute pressure over bony prominences and reduce the risk of pressure-sore formation. Air-flotation beds are useful if wounds develop or progress during the use of less expensive pressure-relief systems. Skin breakdown over the sacrum or over the greater trochanter of the femur is often caused by pressure from the mattress. Breakdown over the ischial tuberosities usually is caused by pressure from the chair. Treatment of pressure sores requires that pres-

sure, friction, and maceration due to incontinence be eliminated. Stage I and II decubiti will respond to local treatment with hydrocolloid dressings. Some stage III and all stage IV lesions require costly surgical intervention with debridement of necrotic tissue and closure with myocutaneous flaps.

Decreased mobility also predisposes to deep vein thrombosis and pulmonary embolism, an important cause of mortality after stroke, accounting for 10 percent of all deaths.[36] Other studies have shown that up to 75 percent of hemiplegic patients have venous thrombosis in their first week post-stroke.[37] Prophylaxis using low-dose heparin yields a 45 percent risk reduction.[37] Low-molecular-weight heparin has been reported to result in a 79 percent reduction in thromboembolic complications. Warfarin, elastic stockings, and intermittent pneumatic compression have also been shown to be of benefit.[38] Appropriate management of the nonambulatory patient with stroke includes early mobilization, elastic stockings, and prophylaxis with one of the above agents, if no contraindication exists. Heparin can be discontinued once the patient is ambulatory for a distance of 150 feet irrespective of the amount of therapist assistance required.[39]

Urinary retention and incontinence are common following stroke. Regular bladder emptying without distention must be assured, reducing the risk of urinary tract infection, hydronephrosis, and renal insufficiency. With urinary retention, scheduled bladder catheterization should be initiated until spontaneous voiding has begun. Computerized ultrasound bladder scanners are easy for nursing staff to use, help document retention, and can indicate the need for intermittent catheterization. Indwelling bladder catheters carry an increased risk of symptomatic bladder infection and are best avoided, except in older males with prostatic hypertrophy. Trauma associated with recurrent intermittent catheterizations can be problematic for such patients. Urinary incontinence with pressure-sore formation is another possible indication for use of an indwelling catheter. By the end of the first month after stroke, patients may develop a small-capacity irritable bladder with urinary frequency and urge-incontinence. Witholding fluids after supper and initiating a program of timed prompted voiding one half hour after meals and every 2 hours while awake provides symptomatic management.

Management of constipation consists of assuring adequate fluid intake, providing a high-fiber diet containing at least 35 grams of fiber, and use of stool softeners. The bowel regimen should be started early in the patient's course before constipation and impaction become a problem. When possible, patients should be placed on a bedside commode or taken to the bathroom. Timed evacuations can be achieved using bisacodyl suppositories. These provide mechanical stimulation of the colon reflex when inserted, and subsequent contact with the rectal mucosa produces pharmacologic stimulation of colonic smooth muscle. The suppository form produces evacuation half an hour after administration. Oral bisacodyl tablets given at night induce a bowel movement the following morning.

MEDICAL MANAGEMENT: SUBACUTE PHASE

As patients spend more time out of bed, they are at increased risk of falling. Falls are the most frequent cause of injury in patients who are hospitalized with stroke. The risk of falls is increased by hemianopia, somatosensory deficits, imbalance, confusion, and aphasia. The head and paretic limbs usually receive most of the trauma. Care must be taken by the staff to prevent these injuries. Bed siderails and lap-belts in the wheelchair are helpful, and are easily tolerated by patients. Posey vest restraints and padded enclosed beds may be necessary for selected high-risk patients who have fallen using less restrictive safety devices. Family or sitters at bedside may be needed to help assure patient safety.

Even patients who were previously cardiovascularly stable while in bed or in a chair often will have difficulty with orthostatic hypotension, fatigue, or even syncope once they are more active on the rehabilitation unit. Cardiovascular or diabetic medications that were adequate for the sedentary patient may now require adjustment as the patient begins to perform more active transfer and ambulation tasks. Rest periods between programs help manage fatigue caused by deconditioning.

Depression is a significant problem following stroke. It is probably due to downregulation of noradrenalin and serotonin neurotransmitter systems following brain injury. As many as 40 percent of patients with stroke develop clinical depression. Decreased motivation for self care, and lower self-care and mobility scores may be early signs of depression. Depression should be considered when patients either appear depressed or express feelings of depression, show evidence of diminished interest in their own progress, or have signs or symptoms of anorexia, insomnia, loss of energy, agitation, or impaired concentration. Family members may note depressive changes in the patient's personality before they are evident to the rehabilitation staff. When depression develops and interferes with progress toward rehabilitation goals, pharmacologic treatment is warranted.[40] Psychotherapy for depression following stroke may be limited by blunting of insight, memory, and attention. Nortriptyline, desipramine, trazadone, and fluoxetine have been suggested as best suited for patients with depression following stroke. Initial doses should be small and side-effects should be monitored closely. Electroconvulsive therapy has been shown effective in some selected stroke patients with severe depression.[41,42]

Spasticity and resultant contractures restrict movement and can limit functional recovery. The best treatment for contractures is prevention: controlling spasticity, providing daily range-of-motion exercises, and judicious use of spasticity-reduction splints. Systemic therapy for post-stroke spasticity rarely is effective, and should be attempted only when the spasticity interferes with the patient's self-care or mobility function. One controlled trial of dantrolene sodium found no effect on impaired limbs and decreased strength in the unaffected limbs.[43] Use of dantrolene requires periodic monitoring for liver toxicity. Oral baclofen is rarely helpful. Trials of intrathecal baclofen for intractable spasticity after stroke have not been undertaken. Motor-point nerve blocks aimed at permanent neurolysis using phenol injections can be selectively used for focal spasticity, but are associated with undesirable sensory dysesthesias in 10 percent of patients.[44] Botulinum toxin injection leads to selective, temporary neurolysis, and may be a more acceptable means of controlling focal spasticity. It has no known sensory effects, is considered safe, and lasts for approximately three months.[45]

Pain is a frequent complaint in the subacute phase post-stroke. Shoulder and hand pain may develop on the paretic side despite early protection, mobilization, and splinting. Pain may be due to biceps, supraspinatus or subscapularis tendonitis, or subdeltoid or subachromium bursitis. Oral nonsteroidal anti-inflammatory agents should be beneficial as initial treatment.

Chronic pain from any of the preceding may lead to immobilization of the shoulder with resultant adhesive capsulitis. Intra-articular steroid injection is the treatment of choice. If persistent, chronic inflammatory pain after stroke in an affected limb may develop into a causalgic pain syndrome, often involving both the shoulder and hand. The presence of causalgic shoulder-hand pain, hand edema, and evidence of altered vasomotor tone fulfill the diagnostic criteria for shoulder-hand pain syndrome, a form of reflex sympathetic dystrophy. Radiologic confirmation of this condition can be accomplished by plain radiogram or radionuclide bone scan. Treatment consists of a course of prednisone 40 to 60 mg/day tapered over one month. If this fails, stellate ganglion blockade is a more invasive diagnostic and treatment option.

Pain in the back and in the paretic leg are also commonly encountered. Back pain may be due to immobility and poor sitting posture in the wheelchair. Use of a wheelchair backboard, a lumbar roll, or alternative seat cushion should be tried. Customized wheelchair seating systems may improve posture and function, while reducing pain. Pain in the paretic hip may be due to external rotation of the affected limb while lying in bed. This may be relieved by use of a foam calf support to place the knee in mild flexion. Pain in the hip or knee associated with hemiplegic ambulation may be due to weight bearing on an externally rotated hip or to hyperextension of the knee during stance phase of gait. Gait training may serve to reduce pain in the hip. An ankle brace set in several degrees of dorsiflexion can reduce knee hyperextension.

Patients discharged from the stroke rehabilitation unit usually require continued medical and rehabilitation care. Arrangements must be made prior to discharge for all applicable services, with medical and rehabilitative histories and recommendations passed on to subsequent providers after discharge. A single provider must take responsibility for continuity of medical and other services after discharge. The patient's progress toward rehabilitation goals should be reevaluated by interdisciplinary team conferences at monthly intervals following discharge from the stroke-rehabilitation unit. The rehabilitation physician should monitor the patient's condition and equipment regularly to optimize functional outcome.

NURSING CARE

Nursing staff on the stroke unit are skilled in dealing with aphasic, apraxic, and confused patients. They work closely with the patient and are often first to note any deterioration in the patient's accustomed level of function. Prompt efforts to define the cause of declining function may uncover an adverse medication effect, an intercurrent medical problem, depression, or stroke progression. Rehabilitation nurses are responsible for evaluating the patient's response to bowel and bladder management, skin care, and fall and safety protection protocols.

Rehabilitation nurses reinforce hemiplegic self-care techniques taught by therapists in individual sessions: feeding, dressing, grooming, bathing, toileting, transfers, and assisted ambulation. They assure implementation of therapy goals, use of splints, and paretic limb-protection protocols outside of therapy time at night and on weekends. Rehabilitation nurses are educators teaching patients and their families about diabetes, skin care, incontinence, catheters, and optimum diet and nutrition.

PHYSICAL THERAPY

In the acute stage of recovery, the physical therapist assures adequate range of motion, and begins teaching bed mobility, rolling, bridging, and sitting techniques, as tolerated. Mobility goals are hierarchical, progressing from rolling to sitting to standing, and then to walking. Therapy is advanced from bedside to the therapy gym as soon as the patient's level of arousal and endurance permits.

A variety of therapy techniques exist for increasing muscle tone in the flaccid patient or for inhibiting spasticity in the spastic patient. The Brunnstrom approach uses mass flexion or extension-reflex patterns to elicit movement of paretic limbs.[46] Brunnstrom techniques rely heavily on the use of tonic neck reflexes, the head extension reflex, and upper- and lower-limb crossed flexion and extension reflexes to initiate mass flexion or extension movements of upper- and lower-limb muscle groups. Neurodevelopmental techniques described by Bobath use reflex inhibitory movement patterns and postural balance reactions to inhibit spasticity and normalize muscle tone.[47] The Rood technique facilitates muscular contraction by using mildly noxious cutaneous stimulation over the dermatome appropriate to the target muscle group.[48] Proprioceptive neuromuscular facilitation exercises rehearse functional movement patterns with superimposition of quick stretch to augment voluntary movement.[49]

Individual therapists, depending on their training, usually have their own treatment preferences. Treatment responses may vary across patients to different therapeutic techniques, and even for the same patient at different times following stroke. A number of controlled studies have failed to show that any one physical therapy approach is superior to the others.[50–51]

Functional electrical stimulation (FES) is another method used to promote muscle function, prevent atrophy, increase strength, and decrease shoulder subluxation.[55] In selected patients where some voluntary control is present, FES can improve function.[56] In one study, FES has been shown to improve ankle dorsiflexion strength and benefit gait.[57]

Electromyographic (EMG) biofeedback is another method designed to promote recovery. Patients with keen cognitive function may use this technique to learn how to suppress dystonic postures. One study has shown that use of both FES and EMG biofeedback resulted in greater improvement than either therapy alone.[58]

Ambulation can begin once the patient is able to sit unsupported. A rigid hemibar allows the patient to stand, weight shift, and begin ambulation. The weaker the patient, the greater the need for therapist assistance. The patient stands holding onto the hemibar with his unaffected hand with his paretic side away from the hemibar. The therapist stands on the patient's paretic side and stabilizes the patient at the hip and knee, advancing the paretic leg with his own knee or foot from behind, if needed.

With improved ambulation, the patient can be advanced from the hemibar to other assistive devices, such as hemiwalker, quadruped cane, or standard cane. Stair-climbing activities are initiated once the patient has enough balance and endurance to walk with a quadruped cane. When patients are able to ambulate with minimal assistance families can be trained to walk with them, thereby reenforcing goals.

Up to 60 percent of patients discharged from an inpatient stroke rehabilitation unit require an ankle-foot orthosis (AFO).[59] The brace prescribed for the hemiparetic patient should provide medial-lateral stabilization of the ankle, toe clearance during the swing phase of gait, and knee control during stance phase. Bracing after stroke is a dynamic process requiring more supportive bracing early, with the brace assuming a more dynamic movement and less restrictive structure as the patient recovers tone and voluntary motion. Most inpatient physical therapy departments have the ability to apply temporary bracing from a supply of stock braces. The bracing prescription can be deferred as long as possible if substantial, rapid recovery is anticipated. On the other hand, modifiable bracing systems may permit early bracing and mobilization and reduce complications of immobility, such as venous thromboembolism.

A variety of different AFOs are available for the stroke patient. Articulating AFOs provide a more normal gait, allowing the ankle to dorsiflex as the foot travels from single-stance to toe-thrust phase of the gait cycle. Rigid AFOs can control the knee during stance phase, inhibiting buckling or preventing hyperextension. Both types will provide ankle stability in the medial–lateral planes and both can be constructed either from plastic or metal and leather.[60]

OCCUPATIONAL THERAPY

Occupational therapy focuses on functional use of the upper extremities for vocational, recreational, and self-care activities including feeding, dressing, grooming, bathing, toileting, transfers, and home-management skills. Cognitive and perceptual deficits also are identified and treated.

Upper-extremity dressing can be taught once the patient can sit unsupported. Once able to sit and bend forward, lower-extremity dressing can be taught. Hemiplegic dressing techniques start with the paretic arm, and differ for front buttoning versus pullover shirts. Dressing modifications such as shoes with Velcro closures, pants with elastic waistbands, and use of suspenders make dressing easier. Many other personal-care devices also are available: clothing hooks, button hooks, stocking aids, long-handled shoe horns, and rocker knives, for example.

The occupational therapist also oversees support and range of motion for the paretic upper extremity. Support of the hand and shoulder in the subacute phase post-stroke is best accomplished with either a wheelchair-based lap board or arm trough. Other shoulder support systems include the Bobath axillary roll, Bobath hemiplegic-cuff sling, and figure-of-eight clavicular strap. These methods all attempt to prevent shoulder subluxation, but there is little proof they work. Therapist and patient preferences usually determine the choice of system prescribed.

Edema in the paretic hand often can be reduced by use of a foam wedge on the lap board or the arm trough. This enhances drainage of interstitial fluid from the paretic limb. Edema that does not respond to elevation may respond to additional use of Isotoner gloves that apply local pressure to the hand and wrist. Massage of the paretic limb as well as continuous passive range-of-motion machines can also help to reduce edema.

Wheelchair evaluations usually are performed by either the occupational therapist or the physical therapist. A proper fit is essential for patients expected to spend most of their day in a wheelchair.[61] Hemiparetic patients have special needs: a low seat (17 inches off the floor) to allow the patient to use his or her spared leg for wheelchair propulsion and guidance; a brake extension on the paretic side; elevating legrests with heel loops. Patients with poor trunk balance, as with posterior fossa stroke, may benefit from a reclining backrest or a high-back extension with headrest.

A variety of wheelchair cushions are available to help with pressure-sore prevention or treatment. Patients who require special protection may benefit from a Roho cushion composed of either one- or three-inch multiple, air-filled balloons, a Jay cushion with molded plastic base and gel-filled detachable cover, or a temperature-sensitive cushion that uses body heat to allow it to mold to body contours. Motorized wheelchairs are not recommended for hemiparetic patients with visual neglect, distractibility, cognitive impairment, or slowed reaction time.

Transfer techniques are an important facet of occupational therapy. The patient learns to get from the wheelchair to bed, tub, or toilet and back again. The stand–pivot transfer technique uses body mechanics and can allow an aged spouse to assist with safe transfers. As the patient improves, ambulatory transfers can be taught, extending progress made in physical therapy. At this point, the occupational therapist may begin assessing the patient's home environment for accessibility and safety. Environmental factors such as home setup, floor plan, presence of stairs, and bathroom layout are considered. Modifications are suggested to maximize the patient's independence and safety. This usually includes provision of bathing and toileting assistive devices, such as a raised toilet seat with armrests, a shower or bath seat, or grab bars for the tub. Entryways may require widening and ramps may need to be installed to improve wheelchair accessibility.

The occupational therapist also assesses and treats cognitive impairment, visual-field deficits, visual and somatic neglect, and dyspraxia. Cognitive or perceptual deficits increase the severity of functional disability. They also interfere with personal, family, and environmental adaptation after the patient returns home. A number of strategies are available for the occupational therapist to deal with these impairments. The treatments emphasize retraining, substitution of intact abilities, and compensatory approaches. In treating apraxia the goal is to restore the patient's ability to perform appropriate habitual or novel movements. Treatments emphasize manually guided movement, mental imagery, and backward chaining. A number of studies have been published in support of the effectiveness of these treatments.[62–64]

SPEECH THERAPY

Speech-language pathologists work with patients with aphasia, dysarthria, and dysphagia. Early intervention in the acute phase after stroke can help treat dysphagia (as discussed previously) and improve basic communication problems. This requires that the therapist be able to establish some form of verbal or gestural communication with the patient.

The treatment goal for aphasic patients is to improve comprehension and verbal expression. Difficulties with reading and writing also are addressed. Coping and compensatory strategies to help manage the frustration and isolation associated with aphasia also are taught. Speech therapists teach families about the patients' language deficits and about how to circumvent them.

Many aphasia treatment techniques are now available, and deficit-specific approaches are now emerging. Language Oriented Treatment, Melodic Intonation Therapy, and direct stimulus-response treatment are among the traditional stimulus-response modality-specific treatments.[65–67] The Treatment of Aphasic Perseveration and Visual Action Therapy are techniques that work on underlying language disorders.[68,69] Methods that teach compensatory strategies include Conversational Coaching and Promoting Aphasic Communicative Effectiveness.[70,71] Programmatic techniques combine elements of all of the preceding.[72] These techniques also are useful for patients with language deficits owing to cognitive impairment. Treatment techniques found useful for a particular patient are taught to the patient's family or caregiver, enabling them to assist with treatment, and to improve their communication with the patient.

For the patient who is dysarthric or has speech apraxia, the goal is to improve the intelligibility of speech. Direct methods of treatment for dysarthria are based on production of speech under carefully controlled conditions. Indirect methods include sensory stimulation, exercises to strengthen speech musculature, modification of position or posture, and improving respiratory efficiency. Articulation is the major focus of treatment in the patient with speech apraxia. A programmatic approach based on learning to intone speech has been successful in apraxic speech.[73]

In many cases, aphasia, dysarthria, and apraxia of speech coexist. In these cases, the contribution of each deficit to problems in functional communication must be assessed and an integrated treatment plan developed. Severely impaired speakers may benefit from devices such as communication boards, metronomes, and electronic communication devices.

Patients with nondominant hemispheric stroke may have problems with interpretation of humor, emotional expression, and concentration. These patients may benefit from a right-hemisphere conversational skills group-training program. Here treatment focuses on organization of language, its use in context, and learning to interpret figurative language. The group setting allows for more efficient use of therapy time for patients with higher-level language deficits.

Large prospective controlled trials have shown speech therapy to be beneficial.[67,74,75] Individual therapy may be better than group therapy. Treatment by a speech and language pathologist is more effective than treatment by a trained therapist-aide. There is general agreement that the speech therapist can educate the family and teach them how to interact more effectively with the patient.

RECREATION THERAPY

Recreation therapy allows patients to work toward cognitive, speech, physical, and occupational therapy goals in a nonconfrontational teaching paradigm that utilizes leisure time activities to facilitate recovery of function. In developing a treatment plan the recreation therapist assesses the patient's previous leisure lifestyle, educational level, and social and emotional functioning. Crafts and games then can be offered based on the patient's interests that focus on important rehabilitation issues such as memory, visual scanning, language, upper-extremity movement, balance, and walking. Family members are encouraged to participate, especially in cases where patient comprehension or attention span is limited. Recreational therapy groups can be organized to stimulate socialization, while addressing important functional skills. For example, horseback riding can be used to remediate difficulties with sitting balance, while building self-confidence. Recreational activities help patients cope with boredom, frustration, depression, and poor self-image. If not addressed, these problems can impede recovery.

SOCIAL WORK AND DISCHARGE PLANNING

Social workers meet with the patient and their families to evaluate community and family resources, obtain community services, and implement discharge plans. Social workers also provide counseling and education.

Discharge planning begins at the time of admission. Information about the patient's financial and social support systems is obtained. The discharge plan should assure a safe residence with caregivers who are adequately trained, arrange for necessary community services, and provide for continued medical and rehabilitative care, if needed.

A safe discharge plan balances patients' disabilities with their caregivers' abilities. Assessment of the caregivers' support is of the utmost importance. One cannot assume that a spouse who lived with the patient prior to the stroke will be able to tolerate the physical and emotional demands of caregiving. Adult children also may be unable to provide support. A home visit by one or more of the patient's treatment team with the patient and primary caregiver can help solve important questions concerning architectural barriers in the living environment. When this is not possible, a careful review of the home environment must be conducted with the patient and caregivers.

Counseling and education are important aspects of the social worker's role on the rehabilitation team. Coping with disability is always difficult for the patient and family, and can lead to psychosocial stress that hinders rehabilitation. If such problems are identified, counseling can help the patient and/or family approach problems with objectivity. The social worker also assesses concerns that the patient and his or her spouse may have concerning sexuality following stroke. Further counseling and evaluation can be arranged to target specific factors in sexual dysfunction after stroke.

REFERENCES

1. Prescott. Survey shows stroke to be one of the most expensive medical illnesses in the United States. *Int Med World Rept* 1994; 9(12):1–5.
2. Matchar DB, McCrory DC, et al: Medical treatment for stroke prevention. *Ann Int Med* 1994; 121(1):41–53.
3. Gillum RF: Strokes in blacks. *Stroke* 1988; 19:1–6.
4. Broderick JP, Phillips SJ, Whisnant JP, O'Fallon WM, Bergstralh EJ: Incidence rates of stroke in the eighties: The end of the decline in stroke. *Stroke* 1989; 20:577–582.
5. Kiyohara Y, Ueda K, Hasuo Y, et al: Incidence and prognosis of subarachnoid hemorrhagge in a Japanese rural community. *Stroke* 1989; 20:1150–1155.
6. Oxfordshire Community Stroke Project: Incidence of stroke in Oxforshire: First year's experience in a stroke register. *BMJ* 1983; 287:713–717.

7. Ward G, Jamrozik K, Stewart-Wynn E: Incidence and outcome of cerbrovascular disease in Perth, Western Australia. *Stroke* 1988; 19:1501–1506.

8. Bonita R, Steward A, Beaglehole R: International trends in stroke mortality: 1970–1985. *Stroke* 1990; 21:989–992.

9. Dyken ML, Wolf PA, et al: Risk factors in stroke: A statement for physicians by the subcommittee on risk factors and stroke council. *Stroke* 1984; 15:1105–1111.

10. Gresham GE, Phillips TF, Wolf PA, et al: Epidemiologic profile of long-term stroke disability: The Framingham study. *Arch Phys Med Rehab* 1979; 60(11):487–491.

11. Bach-y-Rita P: Process of recovery from stroke, in Brandstater ME, Basmajian JV (eds): *Motor Deficits Following Stroke.* Chicago, Year Book, 1987, pp. 79–107.

12. Feigenson JS, Gitlow HS, Greenberg SD: The disability oriented rehabilitation unit: A major factor influencing stroke outcome. *Stroke* 1979; 10(1):5–8.

13. Garraway WM, Akhtar AJ, et al: Management of acute stroke in the elderly: preliminary results of a controlled trial. *BMJ* 1980; 281:827–829.

14. Smith DS, Goldeberg E, et al: Remedial therapy after stroke: A randomised controlled trial. *BMJ (Clin Res)* 1981; 282(6263):517–520.

15. Strand T, Asplund K, et al: A non-intensive stroke unit reduces functional disability and the need for long-term hospitalization. *Stroke* 1985; 16(1):29–34.

16. Indredavik B, Bakke F, et al: Benefit of a stroke unit: A randomized controlled trial. *Stroke* 1991; 22:1026–1031.

17. Kalra L, Dale P, Crome P: Improving stroke rehabilitation. *Stroke* 1993; 24:1462–1467.

18. Kaste M, Palomaki H, Sarna S: Where and how should elderly stroke patients be treated? *Stroke* 1995; 26:249–253.

19. Jorgensen HS, Hirofumi N, et al: The effect of a stroke unit: Reductions in mortality, discharge rate to nursing home, length of hospital stay, and cost: A community-based study. *Stroke* 1995; 26:1178–1182.

20. Kelley-Hayes M, Wolf P, et al: Factors influencing survival and need for institutionalization following stroke: The Framingham study. *Arch Phys Med Rehab* 1988; 69:415–418.

21. Wade DT, Collin C: The Barthel ADL index: A standard measure of physical disability? *Int Disabil Stud* 1988; 10(2):64–67.

22. Mahoney FI, Barthel DW: Functional evaluation: The Barthel index. *Md State Med J* 1965; 14:61–65.

23. Guide for the uniform data set for medical rehabilitation (Adult FIM), version 4.0. Buffalo, NY: State University of New York at Buffalo, 1993.

24. Lawton MP: Instrumental activities of daily living (IADL) scale: Original observer-rated version. *Psychopharmacol Bull* 1988a; 24(4):785–787.

25. Meyer JS, Judd BW, Tawakha T, Rogers RL, Moctel KF: Improved cognition after control of risk factors for multiinfarct dementia. *JAMA* 1986; 256:2203–2209.

26. Siesjo BK: Pathophysiology and treatment of focal cerebral ischemia: Mechanisms of damage and treatment. *J Neurosurg* 1992; 77:337–354.

27. De Couten-Meyers GM, Meyers RE, Schoolfield L: Hyperglycemia enlarges infarct size in cerebrovascular occlusion in cats. *Stroke* 1988; 19:623–630.

28. The Criteria Committee of the New York Heart Association: *Diseases of the Heart and Blood Vessels: Nomenclature and Criteria for Diagnosis,* 6th ed. New York: New York Heart Association/Little, Brown and Company, 1964.

29. Hash D: Energetics of wheelchair propulsion and walking in stroke patients. *Orthop Clin No Am* 1978; 9:372–374.

30. Olney SJ, Trilok NM, et al: Mechanical energy of walking stroke patients. *Arch Phys Med Rehab* 1986; 67:92–98.

31. Horner J, Massey E, et al: Aspiration following stroke: Clinical correlated and outcome. *Neurology* 1988; 38:1359–1362.

32. Emick-Herring B, Wood P: A team approach to neurologically based swallowing disorders. *Rehab Nurs* 1990; 15(3):126–132.

33. Logemann J: *Diagnosis and Treatment of Swallowing Disorders.* San Diego: College Hill, 1983.

34. Logemann J: *A Manual for the Videofluoroscopic Evaluation of Swallowing.* San Diego: College Hill, 1986.

35. Roth EJ: Medical complications encountered in stroke rehabilitation. *Phys Med Rehab Clin No Am* 1991; 2(3):563–578.

36. Silver FL, Norris JW, Lewis AJ, Hachinski VC: Early mortality following stroke: A prospective study. *Stroke* 1984; 25:666.

37. McCarthy S, Turner J, Robertson D, et al: Low-dose heparin as a prophylaxis against deep-vein thrombosis after acute stroke. *Lancet* 1977; 2:800–801.

38. Clagget GP, Anderson FA, Levine MN, et al: Prevention of venous thromboembolism. *Chest* 1992; 102(4):(suppl)391S–407S.

39. Bromfield EB, Reding MJ: Relative risk of deep vein thrombosis or pulmonary embolism post-stroke based on ambulatory status. *J Neurol Rehab* 1988; 2:51–57.

40. Reding MJ, Orto LA, et al: Antidepressant therapy after stroke: A double-blind trial. *Arch Neurol* 1986; 43(8):763–765.

41. Currier MB, Murray GB, Welch CC: Electroconvulsive therapy for post-stroke depressed geriatric patients. *J Neuropsych Clin Neurosci* 1992; 4:140–144.

42. Murray GB, Shea V, Conn DK: Electroconvulsive therapy for poststroke depression. *J Clin Psychiatr* 1986; 47:258–260.

43. Katrak PH, Cole AMD, et al: Objective assessment of spasticity, strength, and function with early exhibition of dantrolene sodium after cerebrovascular accident: A randomized double-blind study. *Arch Phys Med Rehabil* 1992; 73:4–9.

44. Katz RT: Management of spasticity, in Braddom RL, et al. (eds): *Physical Medicine and Rehabilitation.* Philadelphia: WB Saunders, 1996, p. 597.

45. Awad EA, Dykstra D: Treatment of spasticity by neurolysis, in Kotke FJ, Lehman JF (eds): *Krusen's Handbook of Physical Medicine and Rehabilitation,* 4th ed. Philadelphia: WB Saunders, 1990, pp. 1154–1161.
46. Brunnstrom S: *Movement Therapy in Hemiplegia: A Neurophysiological Approach.* Philadelphia: Harper & Row, 1970.
47. Bobath B: *Adult Hemiplegia: Evaluation and Treatment,* 2nd ed. London: Heineman, 1984.
48. Flanagan EM: Methods for facilitation and inhibition of motor activity. *Am J Phys Med* 1967; 46(1):1006–1011.
49. Knott M, Voss D: *Proprioceptive Neuromuscular Facilitation,* 2nd ed. New York: Harper & Row, 1968.
50. Dickstein R, Hocherman S, et al: Stroke rehabilitation: Three exercise therapy approaches. *Phys Ther* 1986; 66(8):1233–1238.
51. Jongbloed L, Stacy S, Brighton C: Stroke rehabilitation: Sensorimotor integrative treatment versus functional treatment. *Am J Occup Ther* 1989; 43(6):391–397.
52. Logigan MK, Samuels M, et al: Clinical exercise trial for stroke patients. *Arch Phys Med Rehab* 1983; 64(8):364–367.
53. Lord JP, Hall K: Neuromuscular reeducation versus traditional programs for stroke rehabilitation. *Arch Phys Med Rehab* 1986; 67(2):88–91.
54. Stern PH, McDowell F, et al: Effects of facilitation exercise techniques in stroke rehabilitation. *Arch Phys Med Rehab* 1970; 51(9):526–531.
55. Kralj A, Acimovic R, Stanic U: Enhancement of hemiplegic patient rehabilitation by means of functional electrical stimulation. *Prosthet Orthot Int* 1993; 17:107–114.
56. Benton L, Baker L, Bowman R, et al: *Functional Electrical Stimulation: A Practical Guide,* 2nd ed. Downey, CA: Rancho Los Amigos Rehabilitation Engineering Center, 1981.
57. Merletti R, Zelaschi F, et al: A control study of muscle force recovery in hemiparetic patients during treatment with functional electrical stimulation. *Scand J Rehab Med* 1978; 10(3):147–154.
58. Cozean CD, Pease WS, Hubbel SL: Biofeedback and functional electrical stimulation in stroke rehabilitation. *Arch Phys Med Rehab* 1988; 69:401–405.
59. Reding MJ, McDowell F: Stroke rehabilitation. *Neurol Clin* 1987; 5(4):601–630.
60. Aisen ML: *Orthotics in Neurologic Rehabilitation.* New York: Demos Publications, 1992.
61. Lobley S, Freed MM, et al: Wheelchair prescription and design for the patient with neurologic impairment. *Semin Neurol* 1983; (3):171–179.
62. Sodderback I: The effectiveness of training intellectual functions in adults with acquired brain damage: An evaluation of occupational therapy methods. *Scand J Rehab Med* 1988; 20(2):47–56.
63. Gordon WA, Hibbard MR, et al: Perceptual remediation in patients with right brain damage: A comprehensive program. *Arch Phys Med Rehab* 1985; 66(6):353–394.
64. Carter LT, Howard BE, O'Neil WA: Effectiveness of cognitive skill remediation in acute stroke patients. *Am J Occup Ther* 1983; 37(5):32–36.
65. Shewan C, Bandur D: *Treatment of Aphasia: A Language-Oriented Approach.* San Diego, CA: College Hill, 1982.
66. Therapeutics and Technology Assessment Subcommittee of the American Academy of Neurology: Assessment: Melodic intonation therapy. *Neurology* 1994; (44):566–568.
67. Wertz RT, Weiss DG, et al: Comparison of clinic, home, and deferred language treatment for aphasia: A Veterans Administration Cooperative Study. *Arch Neurol* 1986; 43(7):653–658.
68. Helm-Estabrooks N, Emery P, Albert ML: Treatment of aphasic perseveration (TAP) program: A new approach to aphasia therapy. *Arch Neurol* 1987; 44:1253–1255.
69. Helm-Estabrooks N, Fitzpatrick P, Barresi B: Visual action therapy for global aphasia. *J Speech Hear Dis* 1982; 44:385–389.
70. Holland AL: The usefulness of treatment for aphasia: a serendipitous study, in Brookshire RH (ed): *Proceedings of the Conference of Clinical Aphasiology.* Minneapolis: BRK Publishers, 1980, pp. 240–247.
71. Davis G, Wilcox J: *Adult Aphasia Rehabilitation: Applied Pragmatics.* San Diego, CA: College Hill, 1985.
72. Springer L, Glinderman R, et al: How efficacious is PACE therapy when language systematic therapy is incorporated? *Aphasiology* 1991; 5:391–399.
73. Rosenbeck D: The dysarthrias, in Johns D (ed): *Clinical Management of Neurogenic Communicative Disorders.* Boston: Little, Brown, 1985.
74. Poeck K, Huber W, Willmes K: Outcome of intensive language treatment in aphasia. *J Speech Hear Dis* 1989; 54:471–479.
75. Shewan CM, Kertesz A: Effects of speech and language treatment on recovery from aphasia. *Brain Lang* 1984; 23(2):272–299.

Chapter 9

SPINAL CORD INJURY REHABILITATION

Gary M. Yarkony

Spinal cord injury has been known as a medical ailment since 1700 B.C. An Egyptian physician first described traumatic spinal cord injury in a text now known as the Edwin Smith Surgical Papyrus.[1] For centuries the life span of persons with spinal cord injuries was limited and the quality of their lives was poor. Death often occurred within weeks after injury. Specialized centers for the care of persons with spinal cord injuries were pioneered in the middle of this century by Munro in Boston and Guttmann in England.[2,3] These centers, through research, teaching, and clinical experience, have resulted in improved life expectancy and enhanced quality of life with diminished complications.

Spinal cord injury remains an uncommon condition. Injured persons are described as being young, active, and educated.[4] The majority of people injured are less than 30 years old and involved in the work force. The incidence has been estimated to be between 29.4 and 50 cases per million.[5–8] The prevalence of spinal cord injury or the number of persons in the United States who live with a spinal cord injury is not exactly known. The most recent estimate is 721 per million, or 176,965 persons. Other estimates range from 525 to 1,124 cases per million.

Persons with a spinal cord injury are generally male (2.4 : 1), white (8 : 1), and have a median age at time of injury of 26. Most people are in the 25 to 44 age range. They are less likely to be married and are more likely to have a high school diploma or some college than the noninjured population.

Motor vehicle crashes are the most common cause (45.4 percent) of injury, followed by falls (16.8 percent) and violence. In urban centers there is a trend toward and increasing incidence of spinal cord injury caused by violence, with violence being the leading cause of injury in some ethnic groups.[9]

DESCRIPTION OF SPINAL CORD INJURIES

The International Standards for Neurological and Functional Classification of Spinal Cord Injury are the current standard for neurological classification.[10] The basis of this system, described herein, is a systematic neurological examination with detailed evaluation of sensory and motor function.

The term quadriplegia has been replaced by tetraplegia, which is consistently derived from Greek roots. Injury within the cervical region of the spinal canal results in tetraplegia. This results in varying degrees of loss of sensory, motor, bowel, bladder, or sexual function. Injury to the thoracic, lumbar, or sacral segments, or to the conus medullaris or cauda equina results in paraplegia. The terms quadriparesis and paraparesis are not used, because they are imprecise and the extent of injury is better described using the ASIA Impairment Scale. This terminology does not describe injuries that may mimic spinal cord injury, such as injuries to the lumbar or brachial plexuses, as all injury must be within the spinal canal.

The sensory and motor level on each side of the body is used to described the neurological level of injury, and motor level is the most caudal level with normal sensory and motor function. Figure 9-1 indicates the key areas of each dermatome. Table 9-1 indicates the key muscles to be tested for each myotome. Muscles are examined from the most rostral to the most caudal segments and graded with the standard 0, which is absent, to 5, which is normal. If a muscle has at least antigravity (3/5) strength and next most rostral muscles in the classification is 4/5, that muscle is considered to have intact innervation. There is a commonly used motor score that sums up the muscle grades of the ten key muscles and a

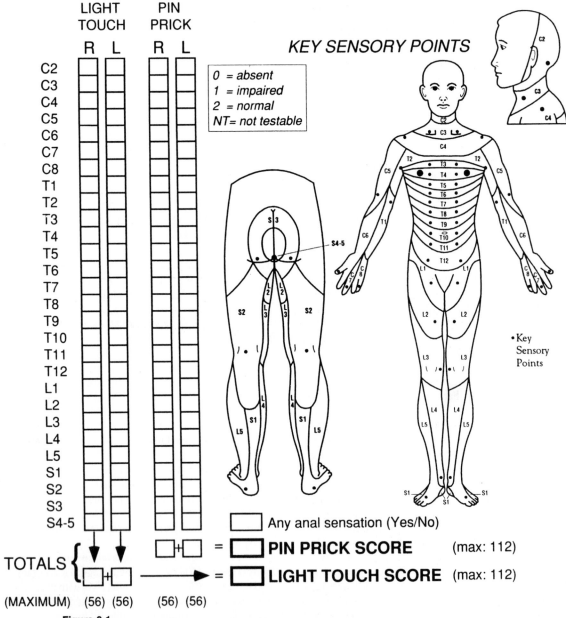

Figure 9-1

Dermatomes with key areas for testing sensation and sensory scores. (Reproduced with permission from the American Spinal Injury Association: International Standards for Neurological Classification of Spinal Cord Injury. Chicago: American Spinal Injury Association, 1992.)

Table 9-1

Key muscles for determining the level of injury

C5	Elbow flexors (biceps, brachialis)
C6	Wrist extensors (extensor carpi radialis longus and brevis)
C7	Elbow extensors (triceps)
C8	Finger flexors (flexor digitorum profundus) to the middle finger
T1	Small finger abductors (abductor digiti minimi)
L2	Hip flexors (iliopsoas)
L3	Knee extensors (quadriceps)
L4	Ankle dorsiflexors (tibialis anterior)
L5	Long toe extensors (extensor hallucis longus)
S1	Ankle plantarflexors (gastrocnemius, soleus)

Table 9-2

American Spinal Injury Association Impairment Scale

A	*Complete:* No motor or sensory function is preserved in the sacral segments S4–S5.
B	*Incomplete:* Sensory but not motor function is preserved below the neurological level and extends through the sacral segments S4–S5.
C	*Incomplete:* Motor function is preserved below the neurological level, and the majority of key muscles below the neurological level have a muscle grade less than 3.
D	*Incomplete:* Motor function is preserved below the neurological level, and the majority of key muscles below the neurological level have a muscle grade greater than or equal to 3.
E	*Normal:* Motor and sensory function is normal.

less commonly used and more tedious sensory score is contained within the classification system.

The definitions of complete and incomplete are based on physical examination, using the sacral sparring definition described by Waters.[11] This definition is preferred because persons with a spinal cord injury do not generally change from incomplete to complete and the use of the term incomplete more closely correlates with return of neurological function. A complete lesion lacks sensory or motor function at the rectum, the lowest sacral segment. Sensation is considered to be present if found on either rectal digital exam or at the anal mucocutaneous junction. Motor function is considered to be present if there is voluntary contraction of the external anal sphincter on digital exam. The Frankel Scale has been modified to better describe the extent of injury.[12] Now known as the ASIA Impairment Scale (Table 9-2), it allows for differentiation of the extent of the lesion based on neurological examination.

Injuries to the spinal cord may follow several commonly recognized patterns. The Brown-Sequard Syndrome initially was described as hemisection of the spinal cord.[13] It is now described as a lesion that produces greater ipsilateral proprioceptive and motor loss, with contralateral loss of sensation to pin and temperature. Since the lesion is partial, the prognosis for bowel and bladder recovery is excellent.[14]

The Central Cord Syndrome initially was described by Schneider.[15] Injury occurs within the central part of the cervical area and there is greater weakness in the upper than lower limbs. There are varying degrees of bowel and bladder impairment. A common mechanism resulting in this injury is hyperextension injury in an older person with pre-existing degenerative changes, following a fall.[16,17]

An injury that primarily affects the anterior cord and preserves the posterior columns is known as the Anterior Cord Syndrome. Proprioception is spared, but there is a variable loss of motor, pinprick, and temperature loss.[8] Generally, it results from trauma to the anterior spinal artery or direct trauma to the anterior aspect of the cervical spine.

Injuries to the conus medullaris usually result in areflexic bowel and bladder, with flaccid lower extremity paralysis. If the lesion is more proximal to the distal terminus of the conus, the bulbocavernous or micturition reflexes may be preserved.[19] Cauda Equina syndrome results in a lower motor-neuron-type syndrome characterized by bowel and bladder incontinence and lower-limb flaccid paralysis.[10]

REHABILITATION DURING ACUTE CARE

Rehabilitation efforts must begin at the roadside. From the initial contact the injured person has with emergency medical personnel, all efforts are directed toward minimizing further damage to the spinal cord, and preventing secondary complications of spinal cord injury. Management of the spine and spinal fractures has been reviewed extensively by others, and is beyond the scope of this chapter.[18,20,21]

Methylprednisolone, a synthetic steroid, acts to diminish secondary damage to the spinal cord if given in appropriate dosages within 8 hours.[22,23] It acts as a free-radical scavenger. Gangliosides are complex acidic glycolipids that are present in central nervous system cells that may stimulate the repair of damaged nerve cells. G_{M1} ganglioside is currently under investigation during the acute-care phase after spinal cord trauma.[24]

Bladder management during acute care is as important as the need to monitor fluid intake and output. Generally, an indwelling catheter is inserted and intermittent catheterization begun every 4 hours, when feasible. Intermittent catheterization is only of value if done consistently, with urine volumes maintained below 450 cc. This approach may not result in any long-term advantages in terms of reduction of upper-tract pathology, infection rate, or the ultimate method of bladder drainage.[25] A suprapubic catheter may be required, with trauma to the penis. Indwelling catheters used for more than 3 months may result in an increased incidence of urethral complications.

Bowel management is aimed at avoiding fecal impactions.[26] A high-fiber diet with maximized fluid intake will assist in establishing a satisfactory bowel regimen. Enemas and strong cathartics should be avoided, whereas stool softeners such as docusate are often helpful. Impactions are best removed manually if low, or softened with mineral oil enemas if high.

Prevention of pressure ulcers is essential, and continues to be a major challenge for persons with spinal-cord injury.[27,28] The areas at greatest risk initially after injury are the sacrum, heels, ischium, and trochanter. Sacral ulcers often occur in persons immobilized in the supine position on a spine board, and can begin as early as during or while awaiting transport. Turning and positioning methods remain the basis for pressure ulcer prevention. Specialized beds, including minimal-air-loss beds, may supplement pillows and wedges for positioning.[29,30] The need to provide life-saving medical and nursing care often interferes with the prevention of pressure ulcers. One example of this is the need to stop rotating beds for suctioning and other medical procedures. Nonblanchable erythema is considered a Grade I pressure ulcer, the heralding lesion of pressure ulceration. When a Grade I lesion is present, a reassessment of the skin-care program to prevent further complications should be undertaken.

Prevention of joint contractures is another area of concern during acute care.[31] A multifaceted approach includes orthotics, positioning, and range of motion.[32] If necessary the ankle is splinted at 90 degrees. The wrist is maintained in the functional position with the web space of the thumb maintained, the thumb opposed, and the fingers positioned to prevent flexion. Particular attention should be paid to the shoulder joints and if feasible they should be abducted to 90 degrees while at rest.[33] The best guide as to the effectiveness of a range of motion program is goniometry. Although flaccid joints may require daily range of motion, a spastic joint may require ranging several times per day.

The rehabilitation physician should be involved in the care of the injured person as soon as possible during the acute-care phase. Counseling should be available to the patient and family, as these injuries have a devastating emotional impact.[34] A balance must be maintained between the injured person's hope for the future and the need for participation in a rehabilitation program. The team must recognize associated injuries, such as brain trauma, that will have a significant impact on long-term outcomes. Brain injury commonly occurs in traffic accidents and has been reported to occur in 50 to 60 percent of injuries.[35,36] A careful mental-status exam is followed by appropriate neurological evaluation and neuropsychological testing as the clinical situation warrants. Staff communication and instructional methods during therapy may be impacted by a concurrent brain injury.

FUNCTIONAL OUTCOMES BY LEVEL

Motor function has generally served as the basis for outcome analysis.[37,38] The individual's guideline for functional outcome will vary with age, motivation, and physical characteristics, such as weight. Aging diminishes functional abilities. Many highly motivated individuals will exceed the guidelines. Rehabilitation efforts should include caregiver instruction as well. The overall program should include teaching of the injured person, caregivers, and relevant family members methods to prevent secondary complications of spinal cord injury. The injured person should be taught to direct others in performing activities for which he or she requires assistance. The entire rehabilitation treatment program should be individualized, with an ultimate goal of community reintegration. This requires evolving access to the community's restaurants, stores, public transportation, airports, and other facilities.

HIGH TETRAPLEGIA

Injuries from C_1 through C_4 are considered to be high tetraplegia. Functional goals and technologic interventions are the same for persons at this level irrespective of the need for ventilatory support. Individuals at this level learn to direct others in the proper techniques for positioning, transfers, range of motion, and other self-care activities. Environmental controls, computers, and other technical aids are key components of the rehabilitation process if funding is available. Page turners, door openers, emergency call systems, and speakerphones are commonly used devices. Occupational therapists and rehabilitation engineers are essential to assist in adapting these devices for each individual's particular needs. Methods of access include breath (sip and puff) mouth sticks, tongue switches, and chin control. Mobility is accomplished with a power wheelchair. A manual chair serves as a backup for the power chair for times when it is being repaired, recharged, or for times when the heavy power chair is not practical.[39]

C_5 TETRAPLEGIA

Persons who are tetraplegic at the C_5 level have functional biceps. When this motor function is facilitated by orthotic management, significant functional advances occur. Arm placement is often facilitated by a balanced forearm orthosis (BFO). The BFO also is used in C_4 tetraplegics with partial elbow flexion. Feeding and writing are accomplished using static splints, such as the long opponens orthosis. The long opponens orthosis maintains wrist stability, as well as being an attachment for utensils. Other devices that are not commonly used include ratchet, cable-driven, or electrically powered tenodesis splints.

The person injured at C_5 generally is able to feed him- or herself with the food provided and cut up.[40] Oral facial hygiene, table-top communication, and leisure skills are also performed with setup. He or she can assist with upper-body dressing and is dependent with lower-extremity dressing. A power wheelchair is propelled by a hand control. Pressure reliefs may be assisted by a power recline mechanism if needed. Oblique hand-rim projections will assist with manual wheelchair propulsion, which is most successful on flat surfaces and indoors.

C_6 TETRAPLEGIA

At the C_6 level the presence of radial wrist extension allows for improved functional abilities, as it results in the ability to employ tenodesis.[31,41] Tenodesis occurs during wrist extension as the thumb and index fingers oppose with active wrist extension. Orthotics are available to assist this function, although they are not often used after discharge because of poor cosmesis and skill development. The Rancho Los Amigos design of the tenodesis orthosis of metal and Plastizote is heavy, expensive, cosmetically unappealing, and requires an orthotist. The fabrication in occupational therapy of simpler designs made of orthoplast therefore is encouraged. Most persons prefer to use a short opponens orthosis with a utensil slot, or utensil cuffs with D-ring velcro closures for writing, hygiene, and feeding.

When food is provided and cut, these individuals generally feed themselves. They can perform oral facial hygiene with splints. Upper-extremity dressing and some aspects of lower-extremity dressing are possible. Motivated individuals may perform their own catheterizations and bowel programs.

Although many individuals rely solely on a manual wheelchair, a power chair may be required for long distances. Power chairs are especially valuable for long-distance travel, and for vocational or educational purposes. Manual wheelchair propulsion often is assisted by coated rims or vertical projections. Transfers generally require a sliding board, but some individuals will require a lift. Independent driving is possible, with a van with hand controls and a lift.

C_7–C_8 TETRAPLEGIA

At the C_7 level, triceps function results in the opportunity for greater independence in mobility and transfers. Innervation at finger extensors and wrist flexors improves performance of activities of daily living as well. At this level most persons are able to perform bowel and bladder management and upper-extremity dressing within a reasonable time period. Many individuals perform lower-extremity dressing, including shoes and socks, although performance in this area can be variable.

The presence of flexor digitorum profundus at the level of C_8 provides for a marked improvement in hand function, although it is not normal because of the lack of innervation of the intrinsic musculature by T_1. Many individuals injured at C_8 are independent from the wheelchair level. Some individuals may transfer from a lightweight wheelchair into a car, and therefore may not need a van for transportation, although this skill is difficult and will diminish with age.

THORACIC AND LUMBAR PARAPLEGIA

Independence from the wheelchair level is possible at all levels of thoracic paraplegia.[43] The outcome generally does not vary by specific thoracic level of injury, although the ability to ambulate does improve the more distal the level of injury. Persons with thoracic paraplegia and more distal injuries can live independently in the community. Many factors may interfere with this expectation. These include weight, spasticity, spinal orthoses, motivation, and other medical complications. Older complete paraplegics will have greater difficulty with more complex self-care skills such as dressing, bathing, bowel, and bladder as well as complex mobility skills such as toilet, bath, and chair transfers.

Several authors have attempted to develop predictive measures of ambulation potential in persons with a spinal cord injury. Initial studies indicate that pelvic control, hip flexors, one quadriceps, ankle proprioception, and hip proprioception are required for community ambulation.[45] An ankle-foot orthosis can be used to compensate for distal weakness, and canes and/or crutches can compensate for the lack of hip extension and hip abduction. The ambulatory motor index (AMI) is another predictive measure. This technique tests five muscle groups in each leg; hip flexion, hip abduction, hip extension, knee extension, and knee flexion. Muscle grades used are 0 = absent, 1 = trace or poor, 2 = fair, and 3 = good or normal. The AMI is a percentage of the maximum score of 30. For scores greater than 79 percent, community ambulation is possible with no assistive devices. With a score greater than 60 percent, one knee-ankle-foot orthosis (KAFO) generally is required, and with scores less than 40 percent two KAFOs usually are required.

The American Spinal Injury Association Motor Score can be used to predict ambulation potential.[47] Predictions can be made as early as 1 month. At that time, if the score is greater than 10 and there is hip or knee extension of at least 2/5, the prognosis for community ambulation at 1 year is favorable. If the neurologic level of injury is used as a guide, incomplete paraplegics below T12 have a good chance of becoming community ambulators. The presence of quadriceps function also has been used as a predictive guide for ambulation.[48]

There are numerous designs of orthotic devices to assist ambulation with spinal cord injury. Because of the substantial energy required to use bilateral long leg braces, they are not frequently used in the community.[49–51]

Energy expenditure can be as high as six to twelve times per unit distance. Many injured persons will use these devices for exercise or standing, although there is often an intense period of usage shortly after injury. Rejection rates of these devices are reported to be as high as 75 percent.[52,53] Definitive KAFOs should be prescribed to highly motivated individuals who are successful with training orthoses in therapy.[54]

Long leg braces (KAFOs) are based on the original design of standard metal uprights with drop-lock knee joints, a double-action ankle, and upper and lower thigh bonds. They can be attached directly to the shoes with a stirrup and extended steal shank or a shoe insert. Pelvic bands and hip joints were used in the past, but they increase weight and energy requirements, and are not needed.[55] A significant improvement on the standard KAFO is the Scott Craig variant.[56] It is lighter, and donning and doffing is easier, since the calf band and lower thigh band are eliminated. It has a patellar tendon strap, a rigid ankle support, and a bale lock at the knee that releases when sitting.

There are numerous designs of orthoses that allow for a reciprocal gait pattern. These include the Reciprocal Gait Orthoses developed at Louisiana State University and often known as the LSU RGO.[57] Other similar devices include the Hip Guidance Orthoses (HGO or Parawalker) and the Advanced Reciprocator Gait Orthoses (ARGO).[58,59] These braces have been combined with electrical stimulation that offers an advantage in that energy consumption is reduced.[60] These designs do not appear to have a better long-term acceptance rate than standard brace designs.

WHEELCHAIR SEATING AND POSTURE

Wheelchair posture and positioning have a significant impact on numerous aspects of self-care and mobility, and therefore must be addressed early.[61] The overall goal is to provide a chair that facilitates functional activities and mobility while preventing pressure ulcers, pain, and deformity.

The traditional wheelchair design, with a sling seat, can result in pelvic obliquity and spinal kyphosis, and should be avoided. As the need for proper positioning has become generally recognized, proper seating often can be accomplished with commercially available equipment. Manufacturers now provide numerous solid backs and seats, as well as arm rests, trunk supports, and cushions. High tetraplegics often require custom seating systems. These systems must integrate technology for power controls, mobility, pressure relief, and use of environmental controls. Prevention and accommodation of deformity must also be considered. The technology employed must consider the support available in the home and community environment to maintain and repair the equipment.

Wheelchair designs and options have improved significantly during the past 20 years.[61] Lightweight materials such as titanium, Kevlar, and composites are now available. Chairs may have standing features or special features for sports. Funding for wheelchairs unfortunately continues to be a problem, and cost often has a major bearing when design features are prioritized.

RECOVERY OF MOTOR AND SENSORY FUNCTION

During the initial rehabilitation phase and outpatient follow-up, motor and sensory function is re-evaluated. Changes will have a significant impact on rehabilitation potential. Recovery of motor function in complete paraplegics is highly dependent on the level of injury.[63] Persons with injuries above T_9 are not likely to regain motor function. This correlates with the poor vascular supply at the midthoracic cord, known as the watershed zone. Recovery is more likely below T_9, and 20 percent of persons at T_{12} and below may regain hip flexor and knee extensor function to ambulate with crutches and orthotic devices. Ninety-six percent of persons will remain complete at 2 year follow-up. Incomplete paraplegics have a better potential for neurological recovery.[64] The majority of recovery occurs during the first 6 months. The amount of recovery does not depend on the specific neurological level. Incomplete paraplegic patients with a lower, extremity motor score greater than 10 at 1 month are generally able to become community ambulators.

Complete tetraplegics are most likely to experience the majority of motor recovery with the first 6 months.[65] Between the C_4 and C_8 levels, motor recovery is not dependent on the lesion level. Muscles that have trace or poor strength 1 month after injury are likely to be fairly strong by 1 year. Most injuries remain complete, and conversion to incomplete does not substantially increase the chance of motor recovery. In incomplete tetraplegia, motor and sensory recovery again occurs predominantly within the first 6 months.[66] A lower-extremity motor score of 10 or more at 1 month indicates a good potential for ambulation at 1 year using crutches and orthotic devices. Muscles that are trace or poor at 1 month are more likely to gain fair strength at

1 year than zero-grade muscles. Sensory recovery begins to decline at 3 months. Wrist extensory recovery in tetraplegics has been studied extensively.[65,67] The use of electrical stimulation and biofeedback does not seem to enhance wrist extensor recovery during the acute-care phase.[68] In one study, motor recovery continued for up to 2 years.[69] The strength of the elbow flexors can be a guide to motor recovery. If elbow flexion is zero out of five at 1 month, wrist extension will not return. However, if elbow flexion is trace or poor, fair wrist extension is likely to return. Elbow extensors that are trace or poor at 1 month will likely have fair strength at 1 year.

MEDICAL COMPLICATIONS OF SPINAL CORD INJURY

Autonomic Dysreflexia

Autonomic dysreflexia is also commonly know as autonomic hyperreflexia. A noxious stimulus below the lesion level in persons with injuries generally above T_6 results in a sympathetic discharge from the splanchnic outflow, resulting in hypertension, sweating, pounding headache, nasal congestion, piloerection, and facial flushing. Although a reflex bradycardia has been reported classically, the pulse may be normal or tachycardia may be present. Autonomic dysreflexia generally does not occur until 2 months after injury and the incidence has been reported to be from 43 to 83 percent. There have been cases reported below T_6.[74]

Autonomic dysreflexia occurs because of the inability of supraspinal inhibitory signals to modulate the exaggerated sympathetic response that is brought on by a noxious stimulus applied to the ascending spinothalamic and dorsal columns. The most common causes are bladder and bowel distension. Tight clothing or leg bag straps, pressure ulcers, ingrown toenails, and urinary tract infections are other inciting causes. Uterine contractions brought on by pregnancy are another common cause that often goes unrecognized.[75] Iatrogenic causes include catheterization, rectal stimulation, cystometrograms, and extracorporeal shock wave lithotripsy.[76,77]

For the most part, morbidity and mortality from AHR is a consequence of uncontrolled hypertension. Hypertensive encephalopathy, loss of consciousness, seizures, intracerebral hemorrhage, and death have been reported.[74,78,79] Visual disturbances, atrial fibrillation, acute myocardial failure, and pulmonary edema also are known to occur.[80–82]

When AHR is first identified, the first measure to be taken is to sit the person up or raise the head of the bed. The inciting cause should be sought immediately. Generally, this includes bladder catheterization, and unkinking or changing a slowly draining or blocked indwelling catheter. If a fecal impaction is suspected, a rectal examination may exacerbate the problem. An anesthetic ointment should be inserted into the rectum. Dysreflexia from fecal impaction is often self-limited.

Pharmacologic management varies depending on the clinical situation.[83] During the acute phase, medications that rapidly drop the blood pressure are necessary. These include nitrates, prazosin, hydralazine, mecamylamine, and diazoxide. Prophylactic medications most commonly used are terazosin and phenoxybenzamine. The best long-term prophylaxis is proper medical management with particular attention to bowel bladder and skin care.

Pulmonary Complications

Pulmonary complications diminish the lower the level of the lesion. Above the C_4 level, ventilators or phrenic-nerve pacemakers are provided.[84,85] To use a phrenic pacemaker, the nerve must be intact. Many patients prefer this technique to mechanical ventilation, as it is quieter and less obtrusive. Pneumobelts and other similar devices inflate over the abdominal wall, causing a forced expiration and passive inspiration.[86] These devices provide useful ventilatory support in cases of high tetraplegia.

With paralysis of the chest wall during the acute phase of spinal cord injury, abnormal breathing patterns occur. The chest wall retracts during inspiration, as opposed to physiologic expansion. The abdomen rises as the diaphragm contracts. After injury, pulmonary function improves.[87] The vital capacity, inspiratory capacity, and total lung capacity increase. There is a decrease in the functional residual capacity. Inspiratory capacity can increase by almost 50 percent during the first year after injury.

Because persons with spinal cord injury have restrictive pulmonary disease, they may take shallow and more rapids breaths. Vital capacity may be diminished, and late-onset ventilatory failure may supervene.[88] A pattern similar to sleep apnea may occur. Nocturnal oxyhemoglobin desaturation and an increase in end-tidal carbon dioxide tension have been observed.[89]

Methods to prevent complications include: position changes, incentive, spirometry, and breathing exercises with increased resistance (Pflex).[90,91] Cough assist by providing manual pressure against the upper abdominal or lower chest wall can assist in clearing lung secretions. Caution must be exercised in persons with vena cava filters, as these maneuvers can lead to deformation or migration of the device.[93] Electrical stimulation is being studied as a means to assist cough by abdominal muscle stimulation.[94]

The clavicular portion of the pectoralis major muscle has been identified as a muscle of expiration.[95] Strengthening of this muscle may assist with active expiration. Another technique that may assist high tetraplegics is glossopharyngeal breathing, by allowing these individuals to be off a ventilator for a short time and providing an alternative method of breathing in case of emergency.[96] The lips, soft palate, mouth, tongue, and pharynx are used to force air into the lungs (often referred to as frog breathing).

Spasticity

Spasticity is characterized by a velocity-dependent increase in muscle tone and an increase in muscle stretch reflexes. It is a component of the upper motor neuron syndrome.[97,98] After the injured person emerges from spinal shock there is a gradual increase in spasticity. Flexor spasticity occurs, but with time extensor spasticity predominates.

In spinal cord injury, some special consideration is given to the management of spasticity.[99] Avoidance of urinary tract infections, an adequate bowel program, and proper skin care will all help to diminish noxious stimuli that can exacerbate spasticity. Range of motion may decrease spasticity for several hours. This may be because of mechanical changes in the musculotendinous unit with a decrease in spindle sensitivity and gamma activity. Standing on a tilt table may aid in reducing extensor spasticity.[100] Many spinal-cord-injured persons find that a range of motion program consisting of prolonged stretch on awakening and/or prior to sleep greatly diminishes spasticity and increases comfort at night.

Medical intervention is recommended when spasticity interferes with activities of daily living, comfort, functional activities, or provision of care. It may be necessary to prevent or relieve deformity or to improve sleep. A detailed discussion of the pharmacologic management of spasticity is found elsewhere in this text. Nevertheless, some pharmacologic information has specific relevance to spasticity arising from spinal cord injury.

Baclofen is generally considered to be the first-line drug in management of spasticity in spinal cord injury. It is a centrally acting γ-aminobutyric acid agonist (GABA). GABA is a central nervous system inhibitory neurotransmitter. It activates GABA-B receptors in primary sensory afferents and enhances Renshaw cell activity and depresses fusimotor responses.[101]

Baclofen is considered safe for chronic administration.[102] It is given initially in a low dose and titrated upward from 5 mg po bid or tid to 20 mg qid. Although 80 mg is the upper limit, many physicians prescribe higher dosages. If the drug is discontinued, it must be tapered. Abrupt withdrawal can induce seizures, hallucinations, and psychosis.

Diazepam is a benzodiazepine that is commonly used to treat spasticity. Problems often occur because of its potential for abuse. It may confer special benefit to individuals with continuous painful spasms.[105] It acts by penetrating the postsynaptic effects of GABA, with a resultant increase in presynaptic inhibition. Although dosages as high as 60 mg daily have been reported, the potential for sedation and abuse generally limits the maximum daily dosage to 15 to 20 mg.[97] Intellectual impairment, lightheadedness, decreased coordination, vertigo, dizziness, and ataxia are all possible side effects. Long-term use can result in insomnia, anxiety, hostility, hallucinations, and a paradoxical increase in spasticity. Diazepam should be avoided in individuals with a history of substance abuse, alcoholism, and depression.

Dantrolene sodium has a different mechanism of action than the more commonly used drugs. It acts directly at the muscular level to reduce the release of calcium from the sarcoplasmic reticulum.[101] It is considered a second line agent in the management of spasticity after spinal cord injury.

Recently clonidine, originally used to treat hypertension, has been utilized to treat spasticity.[106,107] It can be given orally or topically.[108] Dosages are generally low enough that there is not a risk of rebound hypertension. Average dosage is in the range of 0.4 to 0.5 mg/day. Clonidine is a centrally acting α-2-adrenergic agent.

Tizanidine is the latest medication to enter the market in the United States.[109] It is an α-2-adrenergic agonist that can be used in dosages up to 36 mg/day. Side effects include somnolence, xerostomia, and fatigue. It can be used in combination with baclofen and diazepam, and its efficacy compares favorably to existing drugs. Casting and orthotic management can assist with positioning and increase range of motion.[111,112] In the past, destructive surgical procedures were performed, including rhizotomy, intraneurolytic phenol, and myelo-tomy.[113–117] Two newer techniques have largely removed the need for these destructive procedures. Botulinum toxin can now be injected directly into muscles to decrease spasticity. Dosage varies by the size of the muscle targeted. Its effect generally lasts from 3 to 4 months and can be repeated. Muscles can be injected by anatomical localization or by electromyography. Side effects are minimal, but the cost of the medication is considerable.

Baclofen can now be administered intrathecally by a programmable pump.[120–122] It is most useful for generalized spasticity after spinal cord injury, and has a greater benefit in the lower than upper extremities. An implantable pump is placed in the abdominal wall and the intrathecal catheter inserted in the lumbar area. Intrathecal baclofen should be used when conventional measures fail. The daily dose generally ranges from 180 to 900 μ/day. Dosage may increase with time. Prior to pump implantation, testing is done through a standard lumbar puncture. Pharmacologic tolerance is common after 2 to 5 years. If drug tolerance occurs, intrathecal morphine can provide a drug holiday.[123] Intrathecal baclofen has largely supplanted the use of ablative procedures in the management of spasticity after spinal cord injury.

VENOUS THROMBOEMBOLISM

The immediate period of immobilization that follows a spinal cord injury puts the injured person at high risk for development of deep venous thrombosis (DVT).[124] The incidence has been reported to be as high as 100 percent in some series.[125–129] Virchow's Triad, the classic description of risk factors for deep venous thrombosis, explains this risk. A hypercoagulable state occurs owing to the increase in thrombogenic factors. Venous stasis develops owing to immobility and muscle paralysis. Endothelial or vessel wall damage can occur owing to associated trauma or external pressure on the paralyzed extremity.

Diagnosis of deep venous thrombosis by clinical means is not reliable, and, in fact, there may be no findings on physical examination.[123,130] Duplex ultrasound has been found to be a highly accurate method to evaluate for deep venous thrombosis, and has supplanted other noninvasive methods, such as doppler ultrasonography and impedance plethysmography.[132,134] It is not entirely accurate because of limitations in evaluating calf veins, iliac veins, and the femoral vein in the adductor canal. Heterotopic ossification and hematomas can cause false-positive studies because of external compression of the veins.[76] Venography still remains the gold standard for diagnosis.[130]

Prevention is the key to decreasing the morbidity and mortality from deep venous thrombosis and pulmonary embolism. Although external pneumatic compression boots and rotating beds are helpful, pharmacologic management is necessary.[136] Standard heparin at doses of 5,000 u sq bid or tid will decrease the incidence of deep venous thrombosis.[122] If the dose of heparin is adjusted to prolong the activated partial thromboplastin time to 1.5 times control, the incidence of deep venous thrombosis is further diminished. Unfortunately, the risk of complications owing to hemorrhage increases. Low-molecular-weight heparin is currently the most effective means of preventing deep venous thrombosis.[137–139] It can be combined with external pneumatic compression and continued for 12 weeks.[140] There is a decreased incidence of bleeding complications with low-molecular heparin, as it does not inhibit platelet function or bind to thrombin.

If deep venous thrombosis occurs after spinal cord injury, treatment is similar to traditional management. Intravenous heparin is initiated with warfarin at 3 days, unless contraindicated. The international normalized ratio (INR) should be maintained at 2 to 3 for 3 to 6 months.[141] Repeat venous flow studies should be obtained before discontinuing Coumadin, as venous recanalization may be delayed.[142] If anticoagulation is contraindicated, a Greenfield filter should be placed to prevent pulmonary embolism.

Pulmonary embolism is 46.9 times more likely to occur in a patient after spinal cord injury than in an age-matched control cohort in the general population.[143] It may present as autonomic hyperreflexia or arrythmias.[96] Pleuritic chest pain in the absence of other symptoms is a classic presentation, as is dyspnea, unexplained tachycardia, low-grade fever, and hemoptysis. Although a lung scan may be helpful in diagnosis, there is a high risk of false-negative studies. Pulmonary angiography remains the method of definitive diagnosis.

Heterotopic Ossification

Heterotopic ossification (HO) is also known as paraosteoarthropathy, myositis ossifications, neurogenic heterotopic ossification, and ectopic bone.[146] HO is a diverse process whereby extraskeletal bone matrix is deposited in abnormal soft-tissue locations in spinal cord injury. The etiology of HO after spinal cord injury remains unknown. The incidence in spinal cord injury varies

from center to center and year to year, and has been reported to be in the range of 5 to 53 percent.[147]

HO begins as an immature inflammatory mass that is hypervascular. It develops into cancellous bone with blood vessels, haversian canals, and cortex. The initial immature calcium phosphate is replaced by hydroxy apatite crystals. The appearance of mature bone begins at 6 months. Although bone morrow is present, hematopoieses is minimal. After 6 months of growth, the bone begins to mature.

The clinical presentation of HO varies. It may be seen as an incidental finding on x-ray or present as localized swelling, warmth, redness, fever, or loss of range of motion. Joint effusion may be present. HO must be differentiated from fracture, soft-tissue trauma, deep venous thrombosis, hematoma, and septic arthritis. Onset is generally 1 to 4 months after injury and rarely after 1 year. Although serum alkaline phosphatase is elevated and may reflect extraaxial skeletal matrix formation, this is a common finding after spinal cord injury. If bone is not seen on plain x-ray, a triple-phase bone scan may confirm the diagnosis. The first two phases are the most sensitive for early detection, as they show the dynamic blood flow and static blood pool.[150]

The joints most commonly affected are the hips and knees.[151] The shoulder, elbows, and paravertebral area may also be affected, and occurrence in the hands and feet is rare.[152] HO is more common after complete spinal-cord injury.[153]

HO must be distinguished from DVT (see Figure 9-2).[154,155] HO can lead to false-positive noninvasive studies for deep venous thrombosis. When HO is present and DVT is suspected, the venogram will be the definitive test to avoid unnecessary anticoagulation.

Etidronate disodium is useful for both prevention and treatment of HO.[156] It inhibits crystalline growth of hydroxyapatite crystals. Prophylactically, it decreases the amount, but not the incidence, of HO.[157] Prophylaxis begins about 3 weeks after injury, and continues for 12 weeks. The initial dose is 20 mg/kg for 2 weeks, followed by 10 mg/kg for 10 weeks.[158] Although radiation therapy and indomethacin have been useful in preventing HO after total hip arthoplasty, they have not been studied in spinal cord injury. Range of motion exercises are established for the preservation of joint function.

When range of motion and medical management fail, surgery may be considered for bone that interferes with function or causes pressure ulcers.[159,160] The bone should be mature when resected to prevent recurrence. Serial bone scans may be helpful.[161] Etidronate diso-

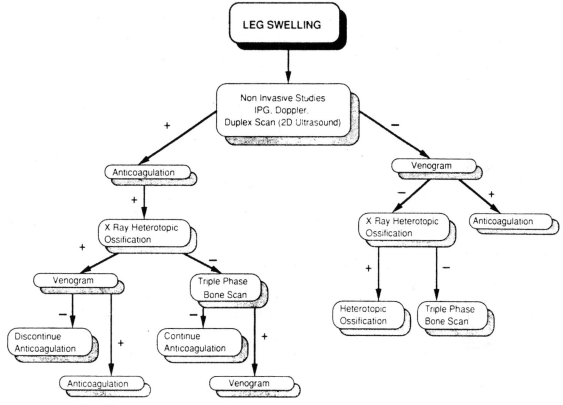

Figure 9-2
Differentiating deep venous thrombosis and heterotopic ossification. (Reproduced with permission from Yarkony et al.[135])

dium is restarted, and range of motion exercises begins when drains are removed.[158] Etidronate disodium should be continued for up to 1 year. Postoperative complications include infection, bleeding, and recurrence of HO. A wedge resection to restore range of motion and limit complications is suggested for that reason by some surgeons.

Posttraumatic Syringomyelia

Posttraumatic syringomyelia or cystic myelopathy is an uncommon, yet often devastating, complication of spinal cord injury. Although the prevalence ranges from 0.3 to 3.2 percent, in those individuals in which it occurs, it can result in serious functional loss.[162,163] Several theories have evolved to explain the etiopathogenesis of syringomyelia.[164,165] Several cystic cavities in areas of infarction and necrosis may merge to form a larger syr-

inx. Cavities may occur from increased venous pressure or the release of cellular lysosomes following trauma. These cavities develop in the area between the dorsal and ventral blood supply of the spinal cord where flow is diminished.

Clinical presentation can occur anywhere between 2 months and 34 years after injury.[166] The predominant picture is weakness, sensory loss, or pain. The pain is described as a dull, aching pain in the upper arms that may be aggravated by coughing, sneezing, or straining. The sensory loss can be caudal or rostral. Facial numbness can occur, if the descending tract of the fifth cranial nerve is affected. If syringobulbia occurs, symptoms of recurrent laryngeal nerve palsy, tongue atrophy, hiccups, and nystagmus may develop.

Syrinxes developing in the thoracic segments can extend cranially and cause symptoms in the cervical segments. Other reported symptoms include excessive sweating, orthostatics, hypotension, and Horner's Syndrome.[167-169]

When there is a clinical suspicion, diagnosis is confirmed by magnetic resonance imaging.[170] Myelography with computerized tomographic imaging can show a widened cord with subarachnoid block and contrast material within the syrinx, if MRI is not available. Treatment is surgical, but results are variable. A shunt to the subarachnoid space or peritoneal cavity can drain the syrinx, decrease pain, and improve strength.[171,172]

DYSESTHETIC PAIN SYNDROME

Pain occurs in all persons in some form after a spinal cord injury. It can be owing to peripheral nerve injury or visceral, psychogenic, musculoskeletal, or central cord pain, commonly referred to as the dysesthetic pain syndrome. This section will concentrate on dysesthetic pain syndrome. A careful history and physical exam is required to rule out other causes before treating this condition.

Onset is generally within the first year after injury and pain generally diminishes over time.[28,38] It is most often described as burning, but other common complaints include stinging, pressure, tightness, aching, tingling, or shooting. It is often distal to the lesion, in the legs, buttocks, rectum, abdomen, or in the arms of the tetraplegic.[176,177] It can be exacerbated by urinary-tract infections and bowel impactions. Persons with spinal cord injury caused by gunshot wound commonly complain of this type of pain. The impact of the pain varies from a minor nuisance to so severe that it limits functional activities and sleep.

In the mild cases, the only treatment that may be necessary is to reassure the individual and make him or her aware of the availability of treatment if requested in the future. A small group of patients will benefit from nonsteroidal anti-inflammatory drugs or acetaminophen. Most will require a centrally acting medication. Narcotic analgesics should be avoided. They rarely help, and may interfere with bowel management and have disabling central side effects.

The most commonly effective drugs are anticonvulsants and antidepressants. Unfortunately, controlled studies are limited.[178-180] These drugs act by diminishing the presynaptic uptake of serotonin. Clinical experience with tricyclic antidepressants, such as amitriptyline and doxepin, appear to be the most efficacious. Anticonvulsants, such as clonazepam and phenytoin, often are helpful and may be used in combination with anti-

depressants.[181] Psychological counseling and pain-management techniques may assist a number of patients in conjunction with medical management. Transcutaneous electrical-nerve stimulation rarely is beneficial.[182]

When interdisciplinary measures have failed and pain is refractory, with significant functional or psychological consequences, surgical intervention should be considered. In the past, destructive procedures such as cordotomy were advocated.[183] Dorsal column stimulators have been used with limited success.[184,185]

Currently, the dorsal-root entry zone procedure (DREZ) is the most effective surgical procedure.[103] Results are variable, with approximately 50 percent of persons obtaining some benefit. Results are poor in persons with diffuse, distal pain. The procedure includes placing destructive lesions in the dorsal root, and the entry zone above and around the area of trauma. There is a risk of increased sensory and motor loss and cerebrospinal fluid leak.

CALCIUM METABOLISM

There are significant changes in bone metabolism after spinal cord injury. During the initial weeks after injury, there is increased bone turnover, resulting in hypercalciuria and hydroxyprolinuria. This turnover continues for as long as 18 months, but usually reaches its peak at 3 months.[187] In spite of this, clinically significant hypercalcemia is uncommon, except in children and adolescents,[188,189] particularly white males under age 21 and those with higher neurological levels of injury, complete injuries, and prolonged immobilization.[188,189]

Symptoms of hypercalcemia most commonly develop at 4 to 8 weeks, although elevated serum calcemia has been seen anywhere between 1 to 16 weeks. Symptoms included anorexia, nausea, lightheadedness, headache, malaise, listlessness, and depression. In more severe cases there is nausea and vomiting, fecal impaction, acute gastric dilatation, abdominal pain, polyuria, polydipsia, and cardiac arrhythmias.

Treatment of hypercalcemia involves vigorous hydration, including intravenous saline and furosemide. If this is not effective, calcitonin alone or in combination with glucocorticoids may be necessary.[188,191] Etidronate disodium may be used. Dietary measures are not helpful.

Osteoporosis below the level of injury is a consistent long-term sequela of the increased calcium resorption from bone. The risk of lower extremity fractures is increased.[192,193] Bone loss is not a generalized pattern as pelvic bone loss is greater than that in the lumbar spine.[194] Although ambulation will help prevent hypercalciuria, it is not clear if osteoporosis is reversed. Functional electrical stimulation provided by bicycle ergometry does not reverse osteoporosis, but may reduce the rate of bone loss.[195,196] Passive weight bearing in the initial phases of injury will decrease hypercalciuria.[197]

BOWEL AND BLADDER MANAGEMENT

Bowel and bladder management must be considered in relation to level of injury, social situation, personal goals and desires, assistance available, housing, and work circumstances. These factors may impede as well as promote certain forms of management. Although many methods are preferred, no method is ideal if it impedes reintegration into society or other personal goals of the injured individual. An open discussion should take place when consideration is given to any new management strategy.

The most desirable urological outcome is a catheter-free state. The detrusor reflex generally returns within 6 months after injury in most upper motor neuron lesions. Voiding with a low residual urine volume will decrease the risk of urinary tract complications, including infection and stones.[198,199] An intermittent catheterization program is initiated to facilitate voiding. The frequency of catheterizations is diminished as voiding occurs and is discontinued with residual urine less than 50 cc. If bacteruria develops, it is treated initially in an attempt to sterilize the urine. Asymptomatic bacteruria is not treated, to avoid development of antibiotic resistance.[200]

If fever, spasticity, leukocytosis, or increased spasticity develop, the infection is treated. The concept of the "safe emptying interval" is used to decrease residual urine by increasing catheterization frequency, thereby decreasing bacterial growth.[201] In a small group of individuals, reflex voiding with a balanced bladder and low residuals is achievable. This occurs in about 15 percent of men, who then must be able to use an external catheter.[202] There is a danger of vesicoureteral reflux and hydronephrosis in these individuals. Annual urologic follow-up with renal ultrasound is required. Unfortunately, there is no practical external catheter for women. Other problems include difficulty in fitting external catheters, and an improperly placed condom catheter that is too tight can result in obstructive symptomatology.

In highly motivated individuals, long-term intermittent catheterization is an option. This may be supple-

mented by medications to decrease bladder contractility such as oxybutynin. External catheters may still be necessary between catheterizations.[203] Clean technique can be used on outpatients.[162,206] This technique may be facilitated by self-contained catheters with urinary collection bags.[206]

Many injured persons will prefer an indwelling catheter. This is common in persons who are high tetraplegics and women. They should be made aware of the increased risk of developing bladder carcinoma.[207] A suprapubic catheter is a valuable elective surgical procedure in many individuals. It decreases the risk of penile damage and a larger bore catheter can be used.

There are numerous surgical options to promote bladder drainage. In the past, sphincterotomy, with or without transurethral resection of the bladder neck, was common.[208] Bladder drainage is constant, requiring an external catheter, and reflex activity is needed to assist with voiding. There is a risk of impotence and retrograde ejaculation. Because of the destructive nature of this procedure, it is becoming more uncommon. Continent diversion procedures particularly for injured women have been described. The bladder is emptied from a urostomy site, such as the umbilicus.[209,210] Further long-term studies are needed in this area.

Bowel management begins on admission to the rehabilitation facility.[211,212] It is common for the person to present with constipation or diarrhea on admission. Although diarrhea is often owing to a fecal impaction, infection causes such as clostridia difficile should be investigated. Impactions should be relieved manually, since the lack of sphincter tone makes enemas difficult. If an abdominal x-ray reveals stool throughout the ascending and transverse colon, this may be relieved by several days of mineral oil, followed by magnesium citrate. Mineral oil is not recommended as a long-term management technique.

Long-term management is based on a proper diet with adequate fiber and fluid intake. Although stool softeners, such as docusate, are used initially, they may be abandoned with time. A convenient bowel program should be arrived at that avoids impaction or accidents. This is often determined by personal wishes and attendant care availability. Generally, this consists of a suppository every other day.

Newer water-based suppositories or "mini-enemas" are now available. They appear to have a decreased response time. Many people prefer these over the standard bisacodyl suppository. Persons with distal lesions, unfortunately, will often require manual removal.

Gastrointestinal complications include hemorrhoids and gallstones. The incidence of gallstones is increased, and they are often an incidental finding on renal ultrasound.[213] Hemorrhoids are also common, and often related to a sedentary lifestyle, laxative abuse, obesity, chronically increased intra-abdominal pressure, and rectal manipulation during the bowel program. Superior mesenteric artery syndrome occurs in individuals with severe weight loss.[214] The artery compresses the third portion of the duodenum, resulting in postprandial nausea, emesis, abdominal pain, and bloating. It is exacerbated by the supine position and the abdominal orthosis. Treatment methods include small frequent meals, with the person positioned on his or her side, and metaclopromide.

LONG-TERM OUTLOOK AND REINTEGRATION INTO SOCIETY

The ultimate goal of rehabilitation after spinal cord injury is for the injured person to be reintegrated into society. As almost every sphere of life is affected by these injuries, adjustment is challenging, no matter how well adjusted the injured person was premorbidly.[215,219] Psychological counseling should be provided, if needed, and is generally required after most injuries. Acceptance of adjustment to disability, and family impact, sexuality, and vocational issues should all be addressed.

The psychologist also has an important role in dealing with the rehabilitation team as they provide suggestions in dealing with issues of behavior and learning. Acting out is common, and can be disruptive to rehabilitation efforts. Neuropsychological assessment and feedback to the patient, family, and team in regard to cognitive deficits owing to concurrent brain injury and other factors is critical.[217,218] Psychological adaptation can take several years and be challenged throughout the life cycle as the impact of the injury changes through the aging process.[29] Substance abuse is a problem that can predate a spinal cord injury or develop subsequent to rehabilitation.[220,221] Fully 50 percent of persons with SCI develop chemical dependency at some time after injury, and treatment should begin during rehabilitation.

Vocational rehabilitation generally continues well beyond discharge from the rehabilitation facility.[219] Issues related to work and school are important for successful community reintegration. Often, financial disincentives to return to work preclude successful reemployment. The majority of persons with a spinal cord injury do not work.[9]

Factors associated with successful return to work are a younger age, preinjury vocational status, and completion of a vocational rehabilitation program. Those who are less likely to return to work are the least educated, minority members, and those whose preinjury work demands cannot be performed by a paraplegic or tetraplegic. Persons with paraplegia and an incomplete injury have a slightly better chance of returning to work.[4]

Spinal cord injury is occurring in older persons more frequently and people are living longer than was expected in the past.[224] Most people with paraplegia can have a normal life expectancy with proper medical care, equipment, and supplies. Life expectancy in tetraplegia is improving, but not normal. The poor prognosis for persons with a spinal cord injury has improved with specialized centers of care and medical advances.[225] Although in the past urological complications were the leading cause of death, pneumonia and pulmonary embolism are now the major causes of mortality.

As the person with a spinal cord injury ages, functions may decline. Increased reliance on the assistance of others and the need for more equipment and supplies are common.[226,227] Most persons with spinal cord injury rely a great deal on their arms for mobility and care needs. As a result, degenerative arthritis, tendonitis, and nerve entrapments, such as carpal-tunnel syndrome, are common. As skin constitution changes, susceptibility to the development of pressure ulcers increases.[228] Glucose intolerance is common, and is felt to result from insulin resistance.[229,230] Inactivity can result in an increased risk of cardiovascular disease, because of a decrease in high-density lipoprotein concentration. However, the cardiovascular risk profile after SCI may not be any greater than in the population at large.[231] Diagnosis of coronary artery disease can be obscured by the spinal deafferentiation. Exercise results in an increased high-density lipoprotein level and decrease in the risk of cardiovascular disease.

The rehabilitation physician specializing in spinal cord injury must coordinate the lifelong follow-up of the spinal-cord-injured person. Ongoing assessment is needed to insure the prescription of proper equipment and supplies and monitoring of areas of particular concern, such as skin, genitourinary, gastrointestinal, and cardiovascular systems. Hopefully, progress will be made in the area of aging to decrease its long-term impact on functional abilities and quality of life.

REFERENCES

1. Hughes JT: The Edwin Smith surgical papyrus: An analysis of the first case reports of spinal cord injuries. *Paraplegia* 1988; 26:71–82.

2. Bedbrook GM, Sedgley GI: The management of spinal injuries: Past and present. *Int Rehab Med* 1980; 2:45–61.

3. Guttman L: *Spinal Cord Injuries: Comprehensive Management and Research,* 2nd. ed. Boston: Blackwell Scientific, 1976.

4. Berkowitz M, Harvey C, Greene CG, et al: *The Economic Consequences of Traumatic Spinal Cord Injury.* New York: Demos, 1992.

5. Bracken MG, Freeman DH Jr, Hellenbrand K: Incidence of acute traumatic hospitalized SCI in the United States, 1970–1977. *Am J Epidemiol* 1981; 113:615–622.

6. Fine PR, DeVivo MJ, McEachran AB: Incidence of acute traumatic hospitalized spinal cord injury in the United States, 1970–1977. *Am J Epidemiol* 1982; 15:475–477.

7. Kalsbeek WD, McLaurin RL, Harris BSH, et al: The national head and spinal cord injury survey: Major findings. *J Neurosurg* 1980; 53:S19–S43.

8. Kraus JF, Franti CE, Riggins RS, et al: Incidence of traumatic spinal cord lesions. *J Chron Dis* 1975; 28:471–492.

9. Go BK, Devivo MJ, Richards JS: The epidemiology of spinal cord injury, in Stover SL, DeLisa JA, Whiteneck GG (eds): *Spinal Cord Injury: Clinical Outcomes from the Model Systems.* Gaithersburg, MD: Aspen, 1995, 21–55.

10. American Spinal Injury Association: *International Standards for Neurological Classification of Spinal Cord Injury.* Chicago: American Spinal Injury Association, 1992.

11. Waters RL, Adkins RH, Yakura JS: Definition of complete spinal cord injury. *Paraplegia* 1991; 9:573–581.

12. Frankel HL, Hancock DO, Hyslop G, et al: The value of postural reduction in the initial management of closed injuries of the spine with paraplegia and tetraplegia. *Paraplegia* 1969; 7:179–192.

13. Roth EJ, Park T, Pang T, et al: Traumatic cervical Brown-Sequard and Brown-Sequard-plus syndromes: The spectrum of presentations and outcomes. *Paraplegia* 1991; 29:582–589.

14. Koehler PJ, Endtz LJ: The Brown-Sequard syndrome: True or false? *Arch Neurol* 1986; 43:921–924.

15. Schneider RC, Cherry G, Pantek H: Central cervical spinal cord injury with special reference to the mechanics involved in hyperextension injuries of cervical spine. *J Neurosur* 1954; 11:546–577.

16. Hardy AG: Cervical spinal cord injury without bony injury. *Paraplegia* 1977; 14:296–305.

17. Roth EJ, Lawler MH, Yarkony GM: Traumatic central cord syndrome: Clinical features and functional outcomes. *Arch Phys Med Rehab* 1990; 71:18–23.

18. Bauer RD, Errico TJ: Cervical spine injuries, in Errico TJ, Bauer RD, Waugh T (eds): *Spinal Trauma.* Philadelphia: JB Lippincott, 1991, 71–121.

19. Paulakis AJ, Siroky MG, Goldstein I, et al: Neurologic findings in conus medullaris and cauda equina injury. *Arch Neurol* 1983; 40:570–573.

20. Cotler JM, Cotler HB (eds): *Spinal Fusion: Science and Technique.* New York: Springer-Verlag, 1990.

21. Meyer PR Jr: *Surgery of Spine Trauma.* New York: Churchill Livingstone, 1989.

22. Bracken MG, Shephard MJ, Collins WF, et al: A randomized, controlled trial of methylprednisolone or naloxone in the treatment of acute spinal-cord injury. *N Engl J Med* 1990; 322:1405–1411.

23. Bracken MG, Shepard MJ, Collins WF Jr, et al: Methylprednisolone or naloxone treatment after acute spinal cord injury: 1-year follow-up data. *J Neurosurg* 1992; 76:23–31.

24. Geisler FH, Dorsey FC, Coleman WP: Recovery of motor function after spinal cord injury: A randomized, placebo-controlled trial with GM-1 ganglioside. *N Engl J Med* 1991; 324:1829–1838.

25. Lloyd LK, Kuhlemeier KV, Fine PR: Initial bladder management in spinal cord injury: Does it make a difference? *J Urol* 1986; 135:523.

26. Zejklik CM: *Management of Spinal Cord Injury.* Belmont, CA: Wodsworth, 1983.

27. Panel for the prediction and prevention of pressure ulcers in adults: *Pressure Ulcers in Adults: Prediction and Prevention.* Clinical practice guideline No. 3 AHCPR Publication No. 92–0047. Rockville, MD: Agency for Health Care Policy and Research, Public Health Service, U.S. Department of Health and Human Services, 1992.

28. Yarkony GM, Heinemann AW: Pressure ulcers, in Stover SL, DeLisa TA, Whiteneck GG: *Spinal Cord Injury: Clinical Outcomes from the Model Systems.* Gaithersburg, MD: Aspen, 1995, 100–119.

29. Ferrell BA, Osterueil D, Christenson P: A randomized trail of low-air-loss beds for treatment of pressure ulcers. *JAMA* 1993; 269:494–497.

30. Inman KJ, Sibbald WJ, Rutledge FS, et al: Clinical utility and cost-effectiveness of an air suspension bed in the prevention of pressure ulcers. *JAMA* 1993; 269:1139–1143.

31. Yarkony GM, Bass LM, Keenan VIII, et al: Contractures complicating spinal cord injury: Incidence and comparison between spinal cord centre and general hospital acute care. *Paraplegia* 1985; 23:265.

32. Hill JP: *Spinal Cord Injury: A Guide to Functional Outcomes in Occupational Therapy.* Rockville, MD: Aspen, 1986.

33. Scott JA, Donovan WH: The prevention of shoulder pain and contracture in the acute tetraplegic patient. *Paraplegia* 1981; 19:313–319.

34. Guttman L: New hope for spinal cord sufferers. *Paraplegia* 1979; 17:6–15.

35. Davidoff G, Morris J, Roth E, et al: Cognitive dysfunction and mild closed head injury in traumatic spinal cord injury. *Arch Phys Med Rehab* 1985; 66:489–491.

36. Morris J, Roth E, Davidoff G: Mild closed head injury and cognitive deficits in spinal cord injured patients: Incidence and impact. *J Head Trauma Rehab* 1986; 1:31–42.

37. Bergstrom EMK, Frankel HR, Galer IAR, et al: Physical ability in relation to anthropometric measurements in persons with complete spinal cord lesion below the sixth cervical segment. *Int Rehab Med* 1985; 7:51–55.

38. Yarkony GM, Roth EJ, Heinemann AW, et al: Benefits of rehabilitation for traumatic spinal cord injury: Multivariate analysis in 711 patients. *Arch Neurol* 1987; 44:93.

39. Nixon V: *Spinal Cord Injury: A Guide to Functional Outcomes in Physical Therapy Management*. Rockville, MD: Aspen, 1985.

40. Yarkony GM, Roth E, Lovell L, et al: Rehabilitation outcomes in complete C5 quadriplegia. *Am J Phys Med Rehab* 1988; 67:73–76.

41. Yarkony GM, Roth EJ, Heinemann AW, et al: Rehabilitation outcomes in C6 tetraplegia. *Paraplegia* 1988; 26:177–185.

42. Welch RD, Lobley SJ, O'Sullivan SB, et al: Functional independence in quadriplegia: Critical levels. *Arch Phys Med Rehab* 1986; 676:235–240.

43. Yarkony GM, Roth EJ, Meyer PR, et al: Rehabilitation outcomes in complete thoracic spinal cord injury. *Am J Phys Med Rehab* 1990; 69:23–27.

44. Yarkony GM, Roth EJ, Heinemann AW, et al: Spinal cord injury rehabilitation outcome: the impact of age. *J Clin Epidemiol* 1988; 41:173–177.

45. Hussey RW, Stauffer ES: Spinal cord injury: Requirements for ambulation. *Arch Phys Med Rehab* 1973; 54:544–547.

46. Waters RL, Yakura JS, Adkins R, et al: Determinants of gait performance following spinal cord injury. *Arch Phys Med Rehab* 1989; 70:811–818.

47. Waters RL, Adkins RH, Yarkur JS, et al: Motor and sensory recovery following incomplete paraplegia. *Arch Phys Med Rehab* 1994; 75:67–72.

48. Crozier KS, Cheng LL, Graziani V, et al: Spinal cord injury: Prognosis for ambulation based on quadriceps recovery. *Paraplegia* 1992; 30:762–767.

49. Coughlan JK, Robinson CE, Newmarch B, et al: Lower extremity bracing in paraplegia: a follow-up study. *Paraplegia* 1980; 18:25–32.

50. Heinemann AW, Magier-Planey R, Schiro-Geist C, et al: Mobility for person with spinal cord injury: An evaluation of two systems. *Arch Phys Med Rehab* 1987; 68:90–93.

51. O'Daniel WE, Hahn HR: Follow-up usage of the Scott-Craig orthosis in paraplegia. *Paraplegia* 1981; 19:373–378.

52. Merkel KD, Miller NE, Westbrook PR, et al: Energy expenditure of paraplegic patients standing and walking with two knee-ankle-foot orthoses. *Arch Phys Med Rehab* 1984; 65:121–124.

53. Miller NE, Merritt JL, Merkel KD, et al: Paraplegic energy expenditure during negotiation of architectural barriers. *Arch Phys Med Rehab* 1984; 65:778–779.

54. Waters RL, Miller L: A physiological rationale for orthotic prescription in paraplegia. *Clin Prosthet Orth* 1987; 2:66–73.

55. Warren CG, Lehmann JF, deLateur BJ: Pelvic band use in orthotics for adult paraplegic patients. *Arch Phys Med Rehab* 1975; 56:221–223.

56. Rosman N, Spira E: Paraplegic use of walking braces: Survey. *Arch Phys Med Rehab* 1974; 55:310–314.

57. Douglas R, Larson PF, D'Ambrosia R, et al: The LSU reciprocation gait orthosis. *Orthopedics* 1983; 6:834–839.

58. Patrick JH, McClelland MR: Low energy reciprocal walking for the adult paraplegic. *Paraplegia* 1985; 23:113–117.

59. Liberty Mutual Research Center: *Steeper A.R.G.O.* Hoplinton, MA: Liberty Mutual Research Center, 1991, 1–4.

60. Hirokawa S, Grimm M, Le T, et al: Energy consumption in paraplegic ambulation using the reciprocating gait orthosis and electrical stimulation of the thigh muscle. *Arch Phys Med Rehabil* 1990; 71:687–694.

61. Zacharkow D: *Wheelchair Posture and Pressure Sores*. Springfield, IL: CC Thomas, 1984, 12–53.

62. Cooper RA: *Rehabilitation Issues Related to Mobility and Integrated Controls*. Proceeding at the Spinal Cord Research Symposium, Spinal Cord Research Foundation Washington, D.C., December 12–14, 1996, 12.

63. Waters RL, Yakura JS, Adkins RH, et al: Recovery following complete paraplegia. *Arch Phys Med Rehab* 1992; 73:784–789.

64. Waters RL, Adkins RH, Yakura JS, et al: Motor and sensory recovery following incomplete paraplegia. *Arch Phys Med Rehab* 1994; 75:67–72.

65. Waters RL, Adkins RH, Yakura JS, et al: Motor and sensory recovery following complete tetraplegia. *Arch Phys Med Rehab* 1993; 74:242–247.

66. Waters RL, Adkins RH, Yakura JS, Sie I: Motor and sensory recovery following incomplete tetraplegia. *Arch Phys Med Rehab* 1994; 75:306–311.

67. Ditunno JF, Sipski MJ, Posuniak E, et al: Wrist extensor recovery in traumatic quadriplegia. *Arch Phys Med Rehab* 1987; 68:287–290.

68. Kohlmeyer KM, Hill JP, Yarkony GM, Jaeger RJ: Electrical stimulation and biofeedback effect on recovery of tenodesis grasp: A controlled study. *Arch Phys Med Rehab* 1996; 77:702–706.

69. Ditunno JF Jr, Stover SL, Freed MM, et al: Motor recovery of the upper extremities in traumatic quadriplegia: A multicenter study. *Arch Phys Med Rehab* 1992; 73:431–436.

70. Colachis SC III: Autonomic hyperreflexia with spinal cord injury. *J Am Paraplegia Soc* 1992; 15:171–186.

71. Kurnick NB: Autonomic hyperreflexia and its control in patients with spinal cord lesions. *Ann Int Med* 1956; 44:678–686.

72. Erickson RP: Autonomic hyperreflexia: Pathophysiology and medical management. *Arch Phys Med Rehab* 1980; 61:431–440.

73. Lindan R, Joiner E, Freehafer AA, et al: Incidence and

clinical features of autonomic dysreflexia in patients with spinal cord injuries. *Paraplegia* 1980; 18:285–292.

74. Gimovsky ML, Ojecda A, Ozaki R, et al: Management of autonomic hyperreflexia associated with a low thoracic spinal cord lesion. *Obstet Gynecol* 1985; 153:223–224.

75. McGregor JA, Meeuswen J: Autonomic hyperreflexia: A mortal danger for spinal cord-damaged women in labor. *Am J Obstet Gynecol* 1985; 151:330–333.

76. DeVivo MJ, Fine PR, Maetz HM, et al: Prevalence of spinal cord injury: A re-estimation employing life table techniques. *Arch Neurol* 1980; 37:707–708.

77. Kabalin JN, Lennon S, Grill HS, et al: Incidence and management of autonomic dysreflexia and other intraoperative problems encountered in spinal cord injury patients undergoing extracorporeal shock wave lithotripsy without anesthesia on a second generation lithotriptor. *J Urol* 1993; 149:1064–1067.

78. Abouleish E: Hypertension in a paraplegic parturient. *Anesthesiology* 1980; 53:348.

79. Yarkony GM, Katz RT, Wu YC: Seizures secondary to autonomic dysreflexia. *Arch Phys Med Rehab* 1986; 67:345–349.

80. Johnson B, Thomason R, Pallares V, et al: Autonomic hyperreflexia: Review. *Milit Med* 1975; 140:345–349.

81. Nieder RM, O'Higgins JW, Aldrete JA: Autonomic hyperreflexia in urologic surgery. *JAMA* 1970; 213:867–869.

82. Pine ZM, Miller SD, Alonso JA: Atrial fibrillation associated with autonomic dysreflexia. *Am J Phys Med Rehab* 1991; 70:271–273.

83. Sutin JA, del Greco F: Blood pressure disorders in the disabled, in Green D (ed): *Medical Management of Long-term Disability*. Gaithersburg MD: Aspen, 1990, 155–180.

84. Lee MY, Kirk PM, Yarkony GM: Rehabilitation of quadriplegic patients with phrenic nerve pacers. *Arch Phys Med Rehab* 1989; 70:549–552.

85. Yarkony GM, Jaeger RJ: Phrenic nerve pacemakers for tetraplegia. *Top Spinal Cord Inj Rehab* 1995; 1:80–85.

86. Whiteneck G (ed): *The Management of High Quadriplegia*. New York: Demos, 1989.

87. Haas F, Axen K, Pineda H, et al: Temporal pulmonary function changes in cervical cord injury. *Arch Phys Med Rehab* 1985; 66:139–144.

88. Bach JR: Inappropriate weaning and late onset ventilatory failure of individuals with traumatic quadriplegia. *Paraplegia* 1993; 31:430–438.

89. Jackson AB, Groomes TE: Incidence of respiratory complications following spinal cord injury. *Arch Phys Med Rehab* 1994; 75:270–275.

90. McMichan JC, Micheal L, Westbrook P: Pulmonary dysfunction following traumatic quadriplegia. *JAMA* 1980; 243:528–531.

91. Gross D, Ladd HW, Riley EJ, Maclem PT, Grassino A: The effect of training on strength and endurance of the diaphragm in quadriplegia. *Am J Med* 1980; 68:275.

92. Jaeger R, Yarkony GM: Cough in tetraplegia. *Top Spinal Cord Inj Rehab,* in press.

93. Balshi JD, Cantelmo NL, Menzoian JO: Complications of caval interruption by greenfield filter in quadriplegics. *J Vasc Surg* 1989; 9:553–562.

94. Jaeger RJ, Turba RM, Yarkony GM, Roth EJ: Cough in spinal cord injured patients: Comparison of three methods of cough production. *Arch Phys Med Rehab* 1993; 74:1358–1361.

95. DeTroyer A, Estene M, Heilporn A: Mechanism of active expiration in tetraplegic subjects. *N Engl J Med* 1986; 314:740–744.

96. Clough P: Glossopharyngeal breathing: Its application with a traumatic quadriplegic patients. *Arch Phys Med Rehab* 1983; 64:384–385.

97. Katz RT: Management of spasticity. *Am J Phys Med Rehab* 1988; 67:108–116.

98. Katz RT, Rymer WZ: Spastic hypertonia: mechanisms and measurement. *Arch Phys Med Rehab* 1989; 70: 144–155.

99. Merritt JL: Management of spasticity in spinal cord injury. *Mayo Clin Proc* 1981; 56:614–622.

100. Bohannon RW: Tilt table standing for reducing spasticity after spinal cord injury. *Arch Phys Med Rehab* 1993; 74:1121–1122.

101. Davidoff RA: Antispasticity drugs: Mechanisms of action. *Neurology* 1985; 17:107–116.

102. Roussan M, Terence C, Gromm G: Baclofen versus diazepam for the treatment of spasticity and long-term follow-up of baclofen therapy. *Pharmatherapuetica* 1985; 4:278–284.

103. Rivas DA, Chancellor MB, Hill K, et al: Neurological manifestations of baclofen withdrawal. *J Urol* 1993; 150:1903–1905.

104. Terrance CG, Fromm GH: Complications of baclofen withdrawal. *Arch Neurol* 1981; 38:588–589.

105. Young RR, Delwaide PJ: Drug therapy: Spasticity. *N Engl J Med* 1981; 304:96–99.

106. Donovan WH, Carter RE, Rossi D, et al: Clonidine effect on spasticity: A clinical trial. *Arch Phys Med Rehab* 1988; 69:193–194.

107. Maynard FM: Early clinical experiences with clonidine in spinal spasticity. *Paraplegia* 1986; 24:175–182.

108. Weingarden SI, Belen JG: Clonidine transdermal system for treatment of spasticity in spinal cord injury. *Arch Phys Med Rehab* 1992; 73:876–877.

109. Nance PW, Bagaresti J, Shellenberger K, Sheremata W, et al: Efficacy and safety of tizanidine in the treatment of spasticity. *Neurology* 1994; 44(suppl 19):544–552.

110. LaTaste X, Emre M, Davis C, Groves L: Comparative profile of tizanidine in the management of spasticity. *Neurology* 1994; 44(Suppl 9):553–559.

111. Booth BJ, Doyle M, Montgomery J: Serial casting for the management of spasticity in the head-injured adult. *Phys Ther* 1983; 63:1960–1966.

112. Genard JM, Arias A, Berlan M, et al: Pharmacological evidence of alpha 1- and 2-adrenergic supersensitivity in

orthostatic hypotension due to spinal cord injury: A case report. *Eur J Clin Pharm* 1991; 41:593–596.

113. Dimitrijeric MR, Sherwood AM: Spasticity: Medical and surgical treatment. *Neurology* 1980; 30:19–27.

114. Gibson JC, White LE: Denervation hyperpathia: A convulsive syndrome of the spinal cord responsible to carbamazepine therapy. *J Neurosurg* 1971; 35:285–290.

115. Putty TK, Shapiro SA: Efficacy of dorsal longitudinal myelotomy in treating spinal spasticity: A review of 20 cases. *J Neurosurg* 1991; 75:397–401.

116. Scott BA, Weinstein Z, Chiteman R, et al: Intrathecal phenol and glycerin in metrizamide for treatment of intractable spasms in paraplegia. *J Neurosurg* 1985; 63:125–127.

117. Wood KM: The use of phenol as a neurolytic agent: A review. *Pain* 1978; 5:205–229.

118. Grafco MA, Polo KB, Jasper B: Botulinum toxin A for spasticity, muscle spasms and rigidity. *Neurology* 1995; 45:712–717.

119. Piersol SH, Katz DI, Tarsi D: Botulinum toxin A in the treatment of spasticity: Functional implications and patient selection. *Arch Phys Med Rehab* 1996; 77:717–721.

120. Abel NA, Smith RA: Intrathecal baclofen for treatment of intractable spinal spasticity. *Arch Phys Med Rehab* 1994; 75:54–58.

121. Coffey RJ, Cavil D, Steers W, et al: Intrathecal baclofen for intractable spasticity of spinal origin: Results of a long-term multicenter study. *J Neurosurg* 1993; 78:226–232.

122. Penn RD: Intrathecal baclofen for spasticity of spinal origin: Seven years of experience. *J Neurosurg* 1992; 77:236–240.

123. Erickson DL, Blacklock JB, Michaelson M, et al: Control of spasticity by implantable continuous flow morphine pump. *Neurosurgery* 1985; 16:215–217.

124. Green D, Rossi E, Yao J, et al: Deep vein thrombosis in spinal cord injury: Effect of prophylaxis with calf compression, aspirin and dipyridamole. *Paraplegia* 1982; 20:227–234.

125. Brach B, Moser K, Cedar L, et al: Venous thrombosis in acute spinal cord paralysis. *J Trauma* 1977; 17:289–292.

126. Merli G, Herbison G, Ditunno J, et al: Deep vein thrombosis in acute spinal cord injured patients. *Arch Phys Med Rehab* 1988; 69:661–664.

127. Myllynen P, Kammonen M, Rokkanen P, et al: DVT and pulmonary embolism in patients with acute spinal cord injury: A comparison with non-paralyzed patients immobilized due to spine fractures. *J Trauma* 1985; 25:541–543.

128. Rossi E, Green D, Rosen J, et al: Sequential changes in factor VIII and platelets preceding deep vein thrombosis in patients with spinal cord injury. *Br J Hematol* 1980; 45:143–151.

129. Todd J, Frisbie J, Rossier A, et al: Deep venous thrombosis in acute spinal cord injury: A comparison of 125 I fibrinogen leg scanning, impedance plethysmography and venography. *Paraplegia* 1976; 14:50–57.

130. Hall R, Hirsch J, Sackett DL, et al: Combined use of leg scanning and impedance plethysmography in suspected deep venous thrombosis: An alternative to venography. *N Engl J Med* 1977; 296:1497–1500.

131. Hall R, Hirsch J, Sackett DL, et al: Cost effectiveness of clinical diagnosis, venography, and noninvasive testing in patients with symptomatic deep-vein thrombosis. *N Engl J Med* 1981; 304:1561–1567.

132. Lensing A, Prandoni P, Brandjes D, et al: Detection of deep-vein thrombosis by real-time B-mode ultrasonography. *N Engl J Med* 1989; 320:342–345.

133. White RH, McGahan JP, Dashbuch MM, et al: Diagnosis of deep-vein thrombosis using duplex ultrasound. *Ann Int Med* 1989; 11:1297–1304.

134. Longsfield M: Duplex B-mode imaging for the diagnosis of deep venous thrombosis. *Arch Surg* 1987; 122:587–591.

135. Yarkony GM, Lee MY, Green D, et al: Heterotopic ossification pseudophlebitis. *Am J Med* 1989; 87:342–344.

136. Becker D, Gonzalez M, Gentil A, et al: Prevention of deep vein thrombosis in patients with acute spinal cord injuries: Use of rotating treatment tables. *Neurosurgery* 1987; 20:675–677.

137. Harris S, Chen D, Green D: Enoxaparin for thromboembolism prophylaxis in spinal injury. *Am J Phys Med Rehab* 1996; 75:326–327.

138. Green D, Lee M, Lim A, et al: Prevention of thromboembolism after spinal cord injury using low-molecular weight heparin. *Ann Int Med* 1990; 113:571–574.

139. Green D, Chen D, Chmiel JS, et al: Prevention of thromboembolism in spinal cord injury: Role of low molecular weight heparin. *Arch Phys Med Rehab* 1994; 75:290–292.

140. Green D: Prophylaxis of thromboembolism in spinal cord injured patients. *Chest* 1992; 102:6495–6515.

141. Merli G: Management of deep vein thrombosis in spinal cord injury. *Chest* 1992; 102(6):652S–657S.

142. Lim AC, Roth EJ, Green D: Lower limb paralysis: Its effect on the recanalization of deep-vein thrombosis. *Arch Phys Med Rehab* 1992; 73:331–333.

143. DeVivo M, Black K, Stover S: Causes of death during the first 12 years after spinal cord injury. *Arch Phys Med Rehab* 1993; 74:248–254.

144. Fluter GC: Pulmonary embolism presenting as a supraventricular tachycardia in paraplegia: A case report. *Arch Phys Med Rehab* 1993; 74:1208–1210.

145. Kelley MA, Carson JL, Palevsky HI, et al: Diagnosing pulmonary embolism: New facts and strategies. *Ann Int Med* 1991; 114:300–306.

146. Jensen LL, Halar E, Little JW, et al: Neurogenic heterotopic ossification. *Am J Phys Med* 1988; 66:351–363.

147. Venier LH, Ditunno JF: Heterotopic ossification in the paraplegic patient. *Arch Phys Med Rehab* 1971; 52:475–479.

148. Hernandez AM, Forner JV, de la Furent T, Gonzalez C, Miro R: Para-articular ossification in our paraplegics and tetraplegics. *Paraplegia* 1978–1979; 16:272–275.

149. Orzel JA, Rudd TG: Heterotopic bone formation: Clini-

cal, laboratory and imaging correlation. *J Nucl Med* 1985; 26:125–132.

150. Freed JH, Hahn H, Menter MD, et al: The use of the three-phase bone scan in the early diagnosis of heterotopic ossification (HO) and in the evaluation of Didronel therapy. *Paraplegia* 1982; 20:208–216.

151. Tibone J, Sakimura I, Nickel VL, et al: Heterotopic ossification around hip in spinal cord injured patients. *JBJS* 1978; 60A:769–775.

152. Lynch C, Pont A, Weingarden SI: Heterotopic ossification in the hand of a patient with a spinal cord injury. *Arch Phys Med Rehab* 1981; 62:291–292.

153. Nicholas JJ: Ectopic bone formation in patients with spinal cord injury. *Arch Phys Med Rehab* 1973; 54:354–359.

154. Orzel J, Rudd T, Will B: Heterotopic bone formation (myositis ossification) and lower extremity swelling mimicking deep venous disease. *J Nucl Med* 1984; 25:1105–1107.

155. Knudsen L, Lundberg D, Ericsson G: Myositis ossificans circumscripta in para-tetraplegics. *Scand J Rheumatol* 1982; 11:27–31.

156. Finerman GAM, Stover SL: Heterotopic ossification following hip replacement or spinal cord injury. Two clinical studies with EHDP. *Metab Bone Dis Relat Res* 1981; 4 & 5:337–342.

157. Stover SL, Hahn HR, Miller JM: Disodium etidronate in the prevention of heterotopic ossification following spinal cord injury (preliminary report). *Paraplegia* 1976; 14:146–156.

158. Stover SL: Heterotopic ossification after spinal cord injury, in Black RF, Bagbaum M (eds): *Management of Spinal Cord Injuries*. Baltimore: Williams & Wilkins, 1986, 284–301.

159. Garland DE: Clinical observations on fractures and heterotopic ossification in the spinal cord and traumatic brain injured populations. *Clin Orthop* 1988; 233:86–101.

160. Garland DE, Orwin JF: Resection of heterotopic ossification in patients with spinal cord injuries. *Clin Orthop* 1989; 242:169–176.

161. Tanaka T, Rossier AB, Hussey RW, Ahnberg DS, Treces S: Quantitative Assessment of pain-osteo-arthopathy and its maturation on serial radionuclide bone images. *Radiology* 1977; 123:217–221.

162. Rossier AB, Foo D, Shillito J, et al: Posttraumatic cervical syringomyelia: Incidence, clinical presentation, electrophysiological studies, syrinx, protein and results of conservative and operative treatment. *Brain* 1985; 108:439–461.

163. Umback I, Heilport A: Review articles: Post-spinal cord injury syringomyelia. *Paraplegia* 1991; 29:219–221.

164. Kao CC, Chang LW: The mechanism of spinal cord cavitation following spinal cord transection. *J Neurosurg* 1977; 46:192–209.

165. Williams B: On the pathogenesis of syringomyelia: A review: *J Roy Soc Med* 1980; 73:798–806.

166. Yarkony GM, Sheffler LR, Smith J, et al: Early onset posttraumatic cystic myelopathy complicating spinal cord injury. *Arch Phys Med Rehab* 1994; 75:102–105.

167. Stanworth PA: The significance of hyperhydrosis in patients with post-traumatic syringomyelia. *Paraplegia* 1982; 20:282–287.

168. Maynard F: Posttraumatic cystic myelopathy in motor incomplete quadriplegia presenting as progressive orthostatis. *Arch Phys Med Rehab* 1984; 65:30–32.

169. Ben Zur PH: Intermittent Horner's syndrome: Recurrent, alternate Horner's syndrome in cervical cord injury. *Ann Ophthalmol* 1975; 7:955–962.

170. Wilberger JE, Marron JC, Prostko ER, et al: Magnetic resonance imaging and intraoperative neurosonography in syringomyelia. *Neurosurgery* 1987; 20:599–605.

171. Dworkin G, Staas W: Posttraumatic syringomyelia. *Arch Phys Med Rehab* 1985; 66:329–331.

172. Vernon J, Silver J, Symon L: Post-traumatic syringomyelia: The results of surgery. *Paraplegia* 1983; 21:37–46.

173. Donovan WH, Dimitrijevic MR, Dahm L, et al: Neurophysiological approaches to chronic pain following spinal cord injury. *Paraplegia* 1982; 20:135–146.

174. Botterell EH, Callaghan JC, Joussi AT: Pain in paraplegia: Clinical management and surgical treatment. *Proc Roy Soc Med* 1953; 47:281–288.

175. Burke DC: Pain in paraplegia. *Paraplegia* 1973; 10: 297–313.

176. Rossier AB: *Rehabilitation of the Spinal Cord Injury Patient*. Documenta Geigy Acta Clinica No. 3 North American Series, 1964, 80–82.

177. Nepomuceno C, Fine PR, Richards JS, et al: Pain in patients with spinal cord injury. *Arch Phys Med Rehab* 1979; 60:605–609.

178. Davidoff G, Guarracini M, Roth E, et al: Trazodone hydrochloride in the treatment of dysesthetic pain in traumatic myelopathy: A randomized, double-blind placebo-controlled study. *Pain* 1987; 29:151–163.

179. Heilporn A: Two therapeutic experiments on stubborn pain in spinal cord lesions: Coupling melitracen-flupenthixen and the transcutaneous nerve stimulation. *Paraplegia* 1977; 15:368–372.

180. Maury M: About pain and its treatment in paraplegics. *Paraplegia* 1977; 15:349–352.

181. Gibson JC, White LE: Denervation hyperpathia: A convulsive syndrome of the spinal cord responsive to carbamazepine therapy. *J Neurosurg* 1971; 35:287–290.

182. Davis R, Lentini R: Transcutaneous nerve stimulation for treatment of pain in patients with spinal cord injury. *Surg Neurol* 1975; 4:100–101.

183. White J, Kjellberg R: Posterior spinal rhizotomy: A substitute for cordotomy in the relief of localized pain in patients with normal life-expectancy. *Neurochirurgia* 1973; 16:141.

184. Long DM, Erickson DE: Stimulation of the posterior columns of the spinal cord for relief of intractable pain. *Surg Neurol* 1975; 4:134–141.

185. Nashold BS, Friedman H: Dorsal column stimulation for

control of pain: Preliminary report on 30 patients. *J Neurosurg* 1972; 36:590–597.

186. Friedman A, Nashold BS: Dorsal root entry zone lesions for relief of pain related to spinal cord injury. *J Neurosurg* 1986; 65:465–469.

187. Claus-Walker J, Spencer WA, Carter RE, et al: Bone metabolism in quadriplegia: Dissociation between calciuria and hydroxyprolinuria. *Arch Phys Med Rehab* 1975; 56:327–332.

188. Maynard FM: Immobilization hypercalcemia following spinal cord injury. *Arch Phys Med Rehab* 1986; 67:41–44.

189. Tori JA, Hill LL: Hypercalcemia in children with spinal cord injury. *Arch Phys Med Rehab* 1978; 59:443–447.

190. Maynard FM, Imai K: Immobilization hypercalcemia in spinal cord injury. *Arch Phys Med Rehab* 1977; 58:16–24.

191. Carey DE, Raisz LG: Calcitonin therapy in prolonged immobilization hypercalcemia. *Arch Phys Med Rehab* 1985; 66:640–644.

192. Ingram RR, Suman RK, Freeman PA: Lower limb fractures in the chronic spinal cord injured patients. *Paraplegia* 1989; 28:133–139.

193. Ragnarsson KT, Seli H: Lower extremity fractures after spinal cord injury: A retrospective study. *Arch Phys Med Rehab* 1981; 62:418–423.

194. Leslie WD, Nance PW: Dissociated hip and spine demineralization: A specific finding in spinal cord injury. *Arch Phys Med Rehab* 1993; 74:960–964.

195. Leeds EM, Klose SK, Ganz W, et al: Bone mineral density after bicycle ergometry training. *Arch Phys Med Rehab* 1990; 71:207–279.

196. Hangartner TN, Rodgers MM, Glaser RM, et al: Tibial bone density loss in spinal cord injured patients: Effects of FES exercise. *J Rehab Res Dev* 1994; 31:50–61.

197. Kaplan PE, Rodin W, Gilbert E, et al: Reduction of hypercalciuria in tetraplegia after weight-bearing and strengthening exercises. *Paraplegia* 1981; 19:289–293.

198. Guttman L, Frankel H: The value of intermittent catheterization in the early management of traumatic paraplegia and tetraplegia. *Paraplegia* 1966; 4:63–82.

199. Merritt JL: Residual urine volume: Correlate of urinary tract infection in patients with spinal cord injury. *Arch Phys Med Rehab* 1981; 62:558–561.

200. Stover SL, Lloyd LK, Waites KB, et al: Urinary tract infection in spinal cord injury. *Arch Phys Med Rehab* 1989; 70:47–54.

201. Wu Y: Total bladder care for the spinal cord injured patient. *Ann Acad Med* 1983; 12:387–399.

202. Cardenas DD, Mayo ME, Kina JC: Urinary tract and bowel management in the rehabilitation setting, in Braddom RL (ed): *Physical Medicine and Rehabilitation*. Philadelphia: WB Saunders, 1995, 555–579.

203. Thüroff JW, Bunke B, Ebner A, et al: Randomized, double-blind, multicenter trial on treatment of frequency, urgency and incontinence related to detrusor hyperactivity: Oxybutynin versus propantheline versus placebo. *J Urol* 1991; 145:813–817.

204. King RB, Carlson CE, Mervine J, et al: Clean and sterile intermittent catheterization methods in hospitalized patients with spinal cord injury. *Arch Phys Med Rehab* 1992; 73:798–802.

205. Maynard FM, Glass J: Management of the neuropathic bladder by clean intermittent catheterization: 5 year outcomes. *Paraplegia* 1987; 25:106–110.

206. Wu Y, King RB, Hamilton BB, et al: RIC–Wu catheter kit: New device for an old problem. *Arch Phys Med Rehab* 1980; 61:455–459.

207. Locke JR, Hill DE, Walzer Y: Incidence of squamous cell carcinoma in patients with long-term catheter drainage. *J Urol* 1985; 133:1034–1035.

208. Fam BA, Rossier AB, Blunt K, et al: Experience in the urologic management of 120 early spinal cord injury patients. *J Urol* 1978; 119:485–487.

209. Goldwasser B, Webster GD: Continent urinary diversion. *J Urol* 1985; 134:227–236.

210. Moreno JG, Lofti MA, Rivas DA, et al: Continent urinary diversion using an umbilical stoma in quadriplegic patients. *J Am Para Soc* 1994; 17:125 (abstract).

211. Stone JM, NinoMurcia M, Wolfe UA: Chronic gastrointestinal problems in spinal cord injury patients: A prospective analysis. *Am J Gastroenterol* 1990; 85:1114–1119.

212. Frost FS: Gastrointestinal dysfunction in spinal cord injury. In Yarkony GM (ed): *Spinal Cord Injury Medical Management and Rehabilitation*. Gaithersburg, MD: Aspen, 1994.

213. Arrowood JA, Mohanty PK, Thames MD: Cardiovascular problems in the spinal cord injured patients. *Phys Med Rehab State Art Rev* 1987; 1:448–456.

214. Roth EJ, Fenton LL, Gaebler–Spira DJ, et al: Superior mesenteric artery syndrome in acute traumatic quadriplegia: Case reports and literature review. *Arch Phys Med Rehab* 1991; 72:417–420.

215. Guttman L: *Spinal Cord Injuries: Comprehensive Management and Research*, 2nd ed. Boston: Blackwell, 1976.

216. Morris J: Spinal injury and psychotherapy: A treatment philosophy. In Yarkony GM (ed): *Spinal Cord Injury: Medical Management and Rehabilitation*. Gaithersburg, MD: Aspen, 1994.

217. Morris J, Roth E, Davidoff G: Mild closed head injury and cognitive deficits in spinal cord injured patients: Incidence and impact. *J Head Trauma Rehab* 1986; 1:31–42.

218. Richards JS, Brown L, Hagglund K, et al: Spinal cord injury and concomitant traumatic brain injury: Results of a longitudinal investigation. *Am J Phys Med Rehab* 1988; 67:211–216.

219. Trieschmann RB (ed): *Spinal Cord Injuries: Psychological, Social and Vocational Adjustment*. Elmsford, NY: Pergamon Press, 1976.

220. Heinemann AW, Doll MD, Armstrong KJ, et al: Substance abuse and receipt of treatment by persons with long-term spinal cord injuries. *Arch Phys Med Rehab* 1991; 72:482–487.

221. Heinemann AW, Donohue R, Keen M, et al: Alcohol use

by persons with recent spinal cord injury. *Arch Phys Med Rehab* 1988; 69:619–624.

222. Walker BC, Holstein S: Vocational rehabilitation and spinal cord injury, in Yarkony GM (ed): *Spinal Cord Injury Medical Management and Rehabilitation.* Gaithersburg, MD: Aspen, 1994.

223. Deyoe FS Jr: Spinal cord injury: Long-term follow-up of veterans. *Arch Phys Med Rehab* 1972; 53:523–529.

224. DeVivo MJ, Rutt RD, Black KJ, et al: Trends in spinal cord injury demographics and treatment outcomes between 1973 and 1986. *Arch Phys Med Rehab* 1992; 73:424–430.

225. Whiteneck GG, Charlifue SW, Frankel HL: Mortality, morbidity and psychosocial outcomes of persons spinal cord injured more than 20 years. *Paraplegia* 1992; 30:617–630.

226. Yarkony GM: Aging after traumatic spinal cord injury, in Felsenthal G, Garrison SJ, Steinberg FU (eds): *Rehabilitation of the Aging and Elderly Patient.* Baltimore: Williams & Wilkins, 1993.

227. Gerhart KA, Bergstrom E, Charlifue SW, et al: Long-term spinal cord injury: Functional changes over time. *Arch Phys Med Rehab* 1993; 74:1030–1034.

228. Yarkony GM: Aging skin, pressure ulcerations, and spinal cord injury, in Whitelock GG (ed): *Aging with Spinal Cord Injury.* New York: Demos, 1993, 39–92.

229. Duckworth WC, Jallepalli P, Solomon SS: Glucose intolerance in spinal cord injury. *Arch Phys Med Rehab* 1983; 64:107–110.

230. Duckworth WC, Solomon SS, Jallepalli P, et al: Glucose intolerance due to insulin resistance in patients with spinal cord injuries. *Diabetes* 1980; 29:906–910.

231. Cardus D, Ribas-Cardus F, McTaggart WG: Coronary risk in spinal cord injury: Assessment following a multivariate approach. *Arch Phys Med Rehab* 1992; 73: 930–933.

232. Brenes G, Dearwater S, Shaper R, et al: High density lipoprotein cholesterol concentrations in physically active and sedentary spinal cord injured patients. *Arch Phys Med Rehab* 1986; 67:445–450.

Chapter 10

REHABILITATION FOR MUSCULAR DYSTROPHIES AND PROGRESSIVE MYOPATHIC DYSFUNCTION

Vinod Sahgal
Sevgi Tetik
Steven I. Reger

Skeletal muscles make up about 40 percent of the human body weight and produce voluntary movements, maintain posture, and provide dynamic stability to the articulations. The vital functions of dexterous skills, mobility, respiration, defecation, and emotional expression, as well as characteristic body forms, are dependent on the skeletal muscles. Muscle function requires the integrity of the circulatory, respiratory, digestive, central, and peripheral nervous systems, as well as the metabolic system.

STRUCTURE

Skeletal muscle consists of two parts, namely, belly and tendons. The belly consists of muscle fibers covered with sheaths of connective tissue, the endomysium. The endomysium is formed of reticular fibers, fibroblasts, and macrophages. Muscle fibers are collected into bundles, termed fascicles, which are covered by a thick connective tissue layer called the perimysium. The perimysium sends trabeculae into the bundles. The fascicles, in turn, are covered by epimysium, which is again made up of connective tissue and is continuous with the perimysium.[1-3]

Muscle fiber is formed of myofibrils, consisting of an outer membrane called the sarcolemma, which is formed by the plasma and basement membrane.[4] The cytoplasm of the muscle cell is called the sarcoplasm. The sarcoplasm consists of myofibrils striated by dark and light bands, as well as the sub-sarcolemma nuclei. At the ultrastructural level, the contractile unit of the myofibril is known as the sarcomere, which is the segment between the dark lines, called the Z bands. It repeats at a periodicity of 2–3 μm. The sarcomere includes isotropic I bands formed of actin and an isotropic A band of myosin. The A band has an area of isotropy called the H zone, which has an anisotropic region known as the M line.[5]

The interfibrillary cytoplasm is known as the sarcoplasm, consisting of a sarcoplasmic reticulum formed by anastomotic tubules dispersed horizontally. This is known as the transverse tubular system, which is dilated at the Z band into sacs. The density of the tubular system is a function of the speed of contraction of the muscle fibers. The fast-contracting fibers have a dense tubular system. The muscle fibers have numerous peripheral ovoid sub-sarcolemmal nuclei that arise from the fusion of many myoblasts.

Mitochrondria form another significant part of the muscle structure. This sarcoplasmic organelle contains the respiratory enzymes and is the principal site of synthesis of high-energy phosphate compounds necessary for the contraction of the fibers. The density of mitochondria is a function of the speed of muscle contraction—the fast fibers have few and the slow fibers have abundant mitochondria.[6]

DEVELOPMENT

The development of the musculoskeletal system occurs in two steps—myogenesis and morphogenesis. The former refers to the development of muscle tissue, whereas the latter refers to the organs. In myogenesis, the muscle tissue forms at two sites, one coming from the paired somites and the other from the mesenchyme around the branchial arches. The somite consists of medial sclerotome, intermediate myotome, and lateral sclerotome. Myogenesis begins with myoblasts becoming myotubes that mature into muscle fibers. These, in turn, subsequently differentiate into various fiber types.[7]

The differentiation of the myotome into the muscle organ begins in the fifth week of gestation in humans. By the eighth week, definitive muscles of the fetus are well defined. The process of morphogenesis also occurs in two steps. The first is migration of the myotome from their original dorsal position to midline, forming the epiaxial mass that is innervated by the dorsal branch of the spinal nerves. The ventral migration forms the hypaxial mass innervated by the ventral branches. The next process is the fusion of the myotomes to form individual muscles, as well as longitudinal and transverse splitting to form subdivision and layers.[7]

BLOOD AND LYMPH SUPPLY

The connective tissue lattice of the belly of the muscle supports the blood and lymph vessels. These vessels enter the muscle together along the connective tissue trabeculae where they break into capillaries, which form networks in the endomysium. This arrangement provides the muscles with nutrients needed for contraction.[8] The nerve supply of the muscle has a motor and a sensory component. The sensory component is provided by the muscle spindle and the Golgi tendon organs, whereas the motor innervation is by the dorsal and the ventral branches of the spinal, as well as cranial nerves. The motor innervation consists of the axon and the number of muscle fibers it innervates, constituting a motor unit. Each muscle has many motor units.[9]

The muscle fibers come in contact with the nerve axon at the neuromuscular junction, also known as the motor endplate. The motor endplate is a specialized region designed for rapid transmission of nerve impulse to muscle. It consists of a presynaptic, unmyelinated portion with mitochondria and synaptic vesicles, as well as a postsynaptic portion, which is thrown into folds. The

two regions are separated by the basement membrane of the muscle fiber.[9]

MUSCLE-FIBER TYPES

As far back as the seventeenth century, the different types of skeletal muscle were recognized. It was Ranvier who correlated the color of the muscle (red and white) with its speed of contraction (red-slow; white-fast).[10] However, it was not until 1919 that Bullard and then Denny-Brown (in 1929) noted that light fibers had low and dark fibers had high fat content (Sudan III stain).[11–12] With the advent of histochemical reactions, skeletal muscle fibers were divided into the red oxidative fibers, which were rich in myoglobin, fat droplets, oxidative enzymes (succinate dehydrogenase, lactic dehydrogenase, cytochrome oxidase), and demonstrated alkali-labile and acid-stable adenosine triphosphatase (ATPase), low phosphorylase activity, and glycogen content. The white fibers, on the other hand, demonstrated high glycogen content, phosphorylase, as well as alkali-stable, acid-labile ATPase activity. The fat content and oxidative enzyme activity in these fibers are low. These characteristics led to the classification of the two broad fiber types—Type I and Type II. A more careful examination of the muscle-fiber types resulted in the subclassification of Type II fibers into the Type II A, B, and C (see Table 10-1). The Type II C fiber is also called the fetal type.[13]

Table 10-1
Muscle-fiber type

	Type I	Type II A	Type II B	Type II C
ATPase pH 9.4	+1	+3	+3	+3
pH 4.6	+3	0	+3	+3
pH 4.3	+3	0	0	+2
NADHTR	+3	+2	+1	+2
SDH	+3	+2	+1	+2
PAS	+1			
Phosphorylase	+1	+3	+3	+3
Menadione-linked α-glycophosphate	0	+2	+2	+1

0 = No reaction.
+1 = Faintly positive.
+2 = Intermediate.
+3 = Intense.
ATPase = Adenosine triphosphatase.
NADHTR = Nicotinamide adenine dinucleotide tetrazolium reductase.
SDH = Succinyl dehydrogenase.
PAS = Periodic acid-Schiff.

Table 10-2
Histochemical and physiological properties of muscle-fiber types

Histochemical type		Physiologic nomenclature	
Type I	slow twitch[14]	slow twitch[15] oxidative	slow twitch[16,17]
Type II A	Fast twitch (red)	Fast twitch oxidative glycolytic	Fast twitch fatigue-resistant
Type II B	Fast twitch (white)	Fast twitch glycolytic	Fast twitch fatiguing
Type II C			

Fiber-type differentiation is complete at about 30 weeks gestation, at which time the checker-board pattern is distinct. At 18 weeks gestation, however, the muscle fibers show uniform ATPase reaction that is acid stable (C II). At 20–28 weeks some strong oxidative and weak phosphorylase-reacting fibers can be recognized. At birth (full term or premature), the fiber-type differentiation always is complete. Correlative physiological and histochemical studies have demonstrated that motor units are histochemically uniform. Motor units are of the three physiologic types—fast, intermediate, and slow (Table 10-2).

The composition of the motor-unit type is dependent on its innervation, speed of nerve stimulation, and pattern of use. However, the specific fiber-type composition of muscle is genetically determined, although it can be altered by either cross innervation or electrical stimulation.[18] These studies demonstrate that muscle fiber can undergo reprogramming, and can switch from the synthesis of fast myosin to slow myosin. Eisenberg and Salmons, using electrical stimulation, also demonstrated reorganization of the subcellular structure, namely, the T system and the mitochondria during fast to slow transformation.[19]

EXERCISE, MUSCLE STRENGTH, AND FIBER TYPE

Lack of muscle activity results in deconditioning and decline in physical capacity, as measured by strength and endurance.[20–22] Normal strength is preserved by muscle contraction. Kottke emphasized the relationship between the decline in muscle strength and endurance to loss of activity.[23] This decline is a function not only of lack of strength, but also of cardiovascular reserve. Decline in muscle strength occurs at the rate of 3 percent per day and is affected by volume loss of the muscle owing to decrease in the cross-sectional area of both fiber types.[23] Type I fibers are relatively more vulnerable than Type II.[24] Disuse atrophy in experimental animals is preceded by loss of mitochondrial respiratory control as early as 24 hours from onset of inactivity.[24] This is followed by cardiovascular deconditioning.[25] This decrement in myopathic function is dependent on the premorbid physical state. Sedentary individuals decondition much more rapidly than those who are active.[26] If inactivity results in muscle weakness and deconditioning, then the logical method for the maintenance of strength and conditioning would be exercise. Some exercises build endurance preferentially over strength. These typically consist of lower-resistance and high-repetition activities, such as walking, swimming, and long-distance running. High-resistance, low-repetition exercises, on the other hand, such as weight lifting, contribute more to strength than to endurance.

Although a host of literature exists on the effects of high- and low-intensity exercise on muscle-fiber type and metabolic activity in animals similar studies in humans are relatively recent. Gollnick et al., in 1972, studying the fiber-type composition of the vastus lateralis and deltoid muscles in young adults (trained and untrained), found a preponderance of Type I fibers in trained compared to untrained adults.[27] Studying the effects of intensive endurance training, investigators have described an increase in oxygen uptake of 13 percent, and a 95–113 percent increase in succinate dehydrogenase (SDH) and phosphofructokinase (PFK) activity, respectively.[28] Oxidative potential increases in both fiber types, whereas glycogen capacity increases only in the Type II fibers.

The myosin ATPase profile of muscle remains constant, whereas the area occupied by Type I fibers increases because of an increase in fiber size. Thorstensson, however, found no effect of strength training in fiber type or area of the vastus lateralis muscle.[29] Sequential metabolic changes studied following bicycle ergometry reveal that glycogen depletion is directly related to the intensity of the exercise.[30] Type I fibers preceded Type II fibers in low-intensity exercise, whereas Type II fibers precede Type I after high-intensity exercise. Endurance training further decreases the ratio of Type II B to A, whereas immobilization increases this ratio and decreases the fiber size.[31]

A comprehensive classification of muscle disorders is beyond the scope of this chapter. The end result of progressive myopathic dysfunction leads to a specific functional and musculoskeletal system complex. Targeted pathophysiologically based treatment by rehabilitation professionals may lead to improved function and quality of life.

Most disorders of muscle function cause considerable disability and physical, social, and psychological handicap. Weakness, postural abnormalities, and cardiovascular decompensation results in physical decline, loss of mobility, wheelchair confinement, and attendant complications. The common goal in management of these disorders is to maintain strength and mobility, avoid contractures, and provide proper equipment, such as seating to prevent scoliosis. Psychosocial support for patients and families, education, and vocational training and placement are essential elements of any effective care plan. To effect all of these, a multidisciplinary approach is necessary.

Rehabilitation thus forms the cornerstone of management.

GENERAL PRINCIPLES OF MUSCLE TRAINING

Since muscle strength and endurance, as well as posture and physical capacity, are dependent on activity, physical therapy is an essential part of the therapeutic regimen. The goal of physical therapy is to maintain posture, prevent contractures, and improve mobility, strength, and endurance through the use of exercise.

Disuse results in the impairment of muscle function as well as a loss in functional capacity. The *maintenance* of muscle strength requires regular maximum tension exerted each day of at least 20 percent of capacity or more.[23] Anything less leads to a decrease in strength

at a rate of about 3 percent of total exercise capacity per day.[23] Disuse atrophy affects both fiber types, and correlates with duration of inactivity. In addition, a significant decline in cardiovascular function and reserve contributes independently to exercise intolerance.[23] The role of exercise is to maintain muscle strength and endurance, and to enhance physical capacity by increasing cardiovascular reserve. The optimum exercise prescription must be pathophysiologically based.

Training for strength utilizes resistance exercises with high intensity and low repetition. Increased muscle-fiber size and some increase in the number of fibers should be anticipated. Performance is enhanced because of the efficient use of agonist muscles, as well as incremental motor unit recruitment. When applied to patients with muscle disease, no negative effects owing to overwork weakness have been demonstrated.[32] Pre-exercise strength determines the extent of gains, with most investigators advocating early intervention.[33] Even slowly progressive myopathic disease can respond favorably to exercise.[34]

The role of resistive exercises is controversial. Although Abramson and Rogoff found resistive exercise effective, Hoberman showed no increase in strength, but did not observe any decline in strength.[36,37] Low-resistance high-repetition exercises may not increase strength, but prevention of disuse atrophy has been demonstrated clearly. The negative effect of overwork on muscle strength, first observed by Bennett and Knowlton, has been attributed to severe lengthening of diseased muscle fibers.[32]

Endurance training relies on low-resistance, high-repetition exercises.[33,34] The goal of this type of exercise is to enhance the work capacity of muscle and maximize oxygen-carrying capacity. Endurance training is most effective in metabolic, inflammatory, and congenital myopathies, since these disorders are nonprogressive. Exercise prescriptions often combine endurance and strength features for maximum effectiveness.[35] Controlled studies detailing the comparative effectiveness of different exercise programs for specific muscle diseases have not been performed.

PRINCIPLES OF SEATING AND MOBILITY

The overall objective of the support and mobility system for individuals with progressive muscular disease is to improve the quality of life. This is accomplished effectively by reducing energy consumption, sparing inherent muscle activity for essential functions of daily living, and substituting external power and support for other activities.[39] The key to success is to match external assistive devices to the patient's needs. The prescription and application of support and mobility aids varies with the stage and type of the disease. In the early, ambulatory stage of progressive myopathic disorders, mobility aids and assistive devices are temporary, but later they take on a permanent function, with life-support characteristics.

Ambulatory Stage

The use of a lightweight wheelchair with a firm seat and back and a foam cushion, even at the ambulatory stage of illness, can be extremely beneficial. Access to wheelchair mobility in this stage will increase range of mobility without taxing energy reserves needed to perform essential activities of daily living.

"Tilt in space" wheelchair systems with a padded, firm back, lumbar cushion, with or without lateral trunk supports, may be needed even in the transitional phase between ambulatory and wheelchair-dependent stages. Tilting of the entire seat provides more effective pressure relief than reclining of the backrest only.[40] The tilting maneuver also produces temporary extension of the spine and stretching of the anterior spinal ligaments, and may lead to improvement of the ventilatory function.[41] An absolute requirement of the "tilt in space" support is the attachment of a head support to control neck hyperextension and provide protection for the cervical spine in the tilted position.

Wheelchair Mobility Stage

The use of powered wheelchairs and other assistive devices will be essential when ambulation is no longer feasible. Early in this stage surgical stabilization of the spine may be required to arrest the progression of kyphoscoliosis, while the patient's physiologic strength is optimally suited to tolerate the metabolic stress of surgery. The use of custom-molded seating and back supports, with or without spinal orthotic body jacket, may be recommended to preserve spinal alignment.[42] Molded body supports usually are fitted as removable or permanently attached inserts in the wheelchair frame. In manual wheelchairs a removable insert is important to preserve the folding ability of the frame for convenient transportation in the car. When a powered wheelchair is used, the folding ability is usually excluded by the more complex heavy construction of the frame, which must accommodate the batteries, motors and controllers. The removability of molded seat inserts, therefore, is no longer essential. For community mobility, a van equipped with a lift becomes an important consideration. The use of securements and restraints for the wheelchair and the user is necessary to insure the safety of all passengers in the vehicle.[43]

Custom-contoured supports can be prescribed to include a molded seat and back, or a molded back with "off the shelf" gel or pneumatic seat cushions on a level, firm base. When a powered wheelchair is planned, a valuable option to consider is the inclusion of a powered tilt mechanism with head support that enables the patient to independently change posture, tilt the seat and back, and gain pressure relief and comfort. Control of the powered wheelchair should be placed in a centralized location. A laterally placed "joystick" may lead to poor seating posture and position. As disability advances, a chin, head, or "sip and puff" control may be needed. Currently available sip and puff wheelchair controls may be used even in the presence of ventilatory support devices. The exact location of the controls with respect to the patient's range of motion and function is critical. Often seemingly minor changes in control location can determine the ability for independent wheelchair control.

Computer-Aided Fabrication of Custom-Contoured Supports

The clinical need for custom-contoured body supports in the rehabilitation of patients with progressive muscular diseases has been increasing. The popularity of these supports arises from simultaneous improvement in postural control, pressure relief, and comfort. The individualized application of contoured supports adjusted for corrective support force distribution have been restricted in the past by the cost of prescription, accuracy of fit, and time-consuming hand-fabrication methods.

Computer-aided prescription and a computer-aided manufacturing technology (CAD/CAM) have been developed and introduced recently for the fabrication of custom-contoured wheelchair inserts.[44,45] Using commercially available technology (Signature 2000™, Akron-Cleveland Home Medical Services, Inc.) the reliability of the prescription and the accuracy of the fit is enhanced by simulation of the desirable sitting posture in a dilatant casting chair (bead bag and vacuum) (Figure 10-1).[46] To obtain a weight-bearing tissue contour in the desired posture, the partially evacuated bead bag is molded to the wheelchair user. Tissue contours then are modified by the molding clinician to enhance or

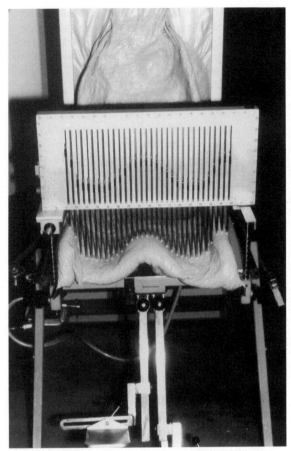

Figure 10-1
Dilatancy casting chair with shape sensor scanning the seat contour for digitized reproduction.

relieve support pressure at the desired anatomic locations of the patient–bead bag interface. Under full vacuum, the bead bag is made rigid, the patient transferred, and the remaining molded shape in the bead bag digitized by scanning an electromechanical sensor over the contoured surfaces. The digitized shape information is displayed in wire-mesh format on a computer monitor (Figure 10-2).

On-screen shape modification is accomplished through mouse and menu-driven software and the three-dimensional-like graphic display. The shape data is transferred electronically to a computer-controlled milling machine, and the contours are cut from foam blocks and lined with soft, high-resiliency foam for fitting to the patient and mounting in the wheelchair frame (Fig-

ure 10-3). The dilatancy molding and the CAD/CAM support system results in effective control of posture and interface pressure for the wheelchair-using patient.

Contractures

A contracture is defined as the condition in which articular and periarticular muscle and tissues around the joint are shortened, which prevents full range of motion at that joint.

In myopathies, contractures develop at the major weight-bearing joints because of proximal muscle weakness. The joints most commonly affected are the hips and knees. Walking may be affected by loss of range of motion, further aggravating muscle weakness through disuse. This creates a vicious cycle of disuse weakness and lack of mobility, resulting in worsening contractures. The restriction in the range of motion results in loss of flexibility of connective tissue, impeding its mobility. This weakens the muscle acting across the joint, enhancing muscle fatiguability.[47]

Contractures at the hips and knees lead to constant postural adjustment in order to maintain standing equilibrium and efficient ambulation. The habitual position of the knee and hip results in flexion contractures.[48] Muscle imbalance in the early ambulatory stage shortens the Achilles tendon, causing equinovarus deformity. This accounts for the characteristic posture of lumbar lordosis, hip flexion and abduction, knee flexion, and equinus of the foot. This deformity creates a small weight-bearing area, leading to frequent falls and collapse of the standing stance. Likewise, shoulder girdle weakness causes elbow-flexion weakness, contractures of the upper extremity, and impaired function.

The first step in contracture management is aggressive range of motion, using passive stretching of the involved muscles. The muscles targeted are the gastrocnemius, soleus, hamstrings, tensor fasciae latae, and the iliotibial band. The parameters of frequency and duration for stretching exercises remains empirical, but there is evidence to suggest that twice daily is optimal.[49,50] However, a program of daily stretching and standing has been shown to delay heel-cord tightening and prolong ambulation.[51,52]

When intrinsic muscle disease results in weakness that makes standing no longer possible, orthotic intervention should be considered. The ideal orthotic prescription is a knee-ankle-foot orthosis that extends the knee and brings the ankle to a neutral position, as opposed to an ankle-foot-orthosis. The orthotic prescription does not replace the need for stretching or proper

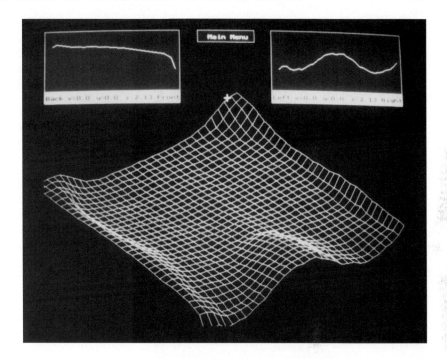

Figure 10-2
Wire-mesh display of digitized seat contour data.

wheelchair prescription. Early surgical intervention has not been found to be effective.[53,54] The combination of surgical release and knee-ankle-foot orthosis may prolong ambulation by 1–2 years.[55,56]

SCOLIOSIS

Scoliosis is a well-established complication of muscular disorders that results from paraspinal muscular weakness, postural instability, and poor seating and positioning.[57] Axial musculature weakness in myopathic disorders during skeletal growth results in pelvic obliquity, owing to contractures of the hip and asymmetric positioning of the torso.[58] As a result, a posture of lumbar lordosis develops that shifts the center of gravity backward. This position locks the lumbosacral facet joints and prevents lateral spinal deformity, and is advantageous for ambulation.[59] Any attempt to correct these deformities either orthotically or surgically (by tendon lengthening or hamstring release) may impair ambulation and accelerate the need for a wheelchair.[60] Wheelchair-bound patients during the skeletal-growth phase invariably end up with progressive scoliosis. The rate of progression is typically 1 degree per month until the age of 13 years, after which a very rapid progression occurs until the age of 14–16 years.

However, if ambulation is maintained until skeletal maturity, scoliosis can be avoided. Nevertheless, the demands of posture and station control may be so high that upper-extremity function can be limited. Wheelchair use may in fact be more practical. While in the wheelchair, weakness in the arms makes maneuvering of the chair difficult. Patients then resort to using forward thrust of the body to propel the wheelchair, thus exaggerating the curvature. Progressive scoliosis leads to restrictive ventilation and cardiopulmonary decompensation.

Nonsurgical treatment options begin with the use of a contoured seating system to help maintain spinal posture and retard the progression of scoliosis. Optimum positioning should attempt to control pelvic tilt, provide lateral and head support, and provide foot placement to avoid equinous deformity.[61] Bracing, once widely used in the past, has fallen from favor because it is uncomfortable, confining, and limits independence.

SPINAL FUSION

The devastating cardiopulmonary effects of scoliosis and poor experience with bracing prompted the aggressive approach of spinal fusion. Since maximum increase in the curve occurs after 13 years of age, it is customary

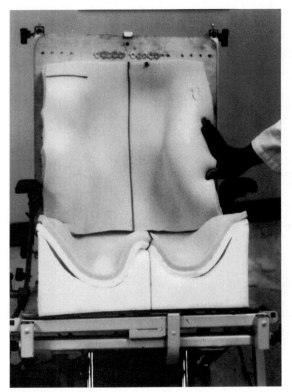

Figure 10-3
Custom-contoured foam support. Foam-lined seat and back at the time of trial fit to the patient before upholstery and installation to the wheelchair frame.

to offer fusion when the curve reaches 30 degrees at or before 13 years of age. Another parameter used is vital capacity less than 35 percent of the predicted maximum. These criteria have stayed fairly constant over the last 10 years. The techniques have changed from the use of Harrington rods to Luque L-shaped rods buried to the facets.[62] The immobilization should traverse from the upper thoracic spine to the sacrum. A review of data from the Toronto Sick Children Hospital indicates that over 70 percent of children with Duchenne muscular dystrophy without fusion became bedridden, whereas none of the operated patients were bedridden[63] These observations as well as improved techniques of anesthesia and surgery have made this a more acceptable option.

VENTILATOR SUPPORT

When the patient reaches the stage of ventilatory compromise, physical assistance with airway clearance and/

or ventilator support should be considered.[64] The most common system currently in use is positive-pressure ventilation. A portable system that can be mounted on a wheelchair frame is used. Volume flow rate, humidity, and fraction of inspired oxygen can be controlled easily. These devices can be used with or without intubation. Since patients with progressive muscle disease generally maintain consciousness and oral pharyngeal control, this method is an ideal ventilatory support.[65]

HOME ENVIRONMENT

In order to maintain maximum independence, the home should be converted to a wheelchair-accessible environment, with ramps and wide spaces for easy maneuvering. A 12 : 1 slope is ideal, and doors should be at least 30 inches wide, with hallways having a 4-foot clearance. Floors should be constructed of hard surfaces with tight pile carpet.

Psychological support should be provided to the patient and the family, and it should be tailored by individual therapeutic intervention and group programs. Organized camps and recreational activities are available, and improve and maintain quality of life for many.

REFERENCES

1. Borg TK, Caulfield JB: Morphology of connective tissue in skeletal muscle. *Tissue Cell* 1980; 12:197–207.
2. Bowman W: On the minute structure and movement of voluntary muscle. *Phil Trans R Soc Lond (Biol)* 1860; 130:457–501.
3. Trotter JA, Corbett K, Avner BP: Structure and function of murine muscle-tendon junction. *Anat Rec* 1981; 201:293–302.
4. Horwitz AF, Schofland DL: The plasma membrane of muscle fiber, in Engel A, Banker BQ (eds): *Myology*. Philadelphia, McGraw Hill, 1986, pp. 177–209.
5. Hanson J, Huxley HE: Structural basis of the cross striation in muscle. *Nature* 1953; 172:532.
6. Eisenberg BR: Quantitative ultrastructure of mammalian skeletal muscle, in Peachy LD, Adrian RH (eds): *Hand Book of Physiology Skeletal Muscle*. Baltimore, American Physiological Society, Williams & Wilkins, 1980, pp. 73–112.
7. Konigoberg IR: The embryonic origin of muscle, in Engel A, Banker BQ (eds): *Myology*. Philadelphia, McGraw-Hill, 1986, pp. 39–71.
8. Bloomfield LB: Intramuscular vascular pattern in man. *Proc R Soc Med* 1965; 38:617.
9. Santa T, Engel AG: Histometric analysis of neuromuscular

junction ultra structure in rat red, white, and intermediate muscle fibers, in DeSmedt JE (ed): *New Development in Electromyography and Clinical Neurophysiology,* vol 1. Basel, Karger, 1973, pp. 41–54.

10. Ranvier L: De quelques faits relatifs a l'histologie et a la physiologie des muscles stries. *Arch Physiol* 1874; 6:1.

11. Bullard HH: Histological as relating to physiological and chemical differences in certain muscles of cat. *Johns Hopkins Hosp Rep* 1919; 18:328.

12. Denny-Brown D: The histological features of striped muscle in relation to its functional activity. *Proc R Soc* 1929; B104:371.

13. Brooke MH, Engel WK: The histographic analysis of human biopsies with regard of fiber types. 1. Adult male and female. *Neurology* 1969; 19:221–233.

14. Barnard RJ, Edgerton VR, Frukawa T, et al: Histochemical, biochemical, and contractile properties of red, white, and intermediate fibers. *Am J Phys* 1971; 220:410–414.

15. Peter JB, Barnard VR, Edgerton VR, et al: Metabolic profiles of three fiber types of skeletal muscles in guinea pigs and rabbits. *Biochemistry* 1972; 11:2627–2633.

16. Burke RE, Levine DM, Zajac FE, et al: Mammalian motor units: Physiological-histochemical correlation in three types of cat gastrocnemius. *Science* 1971; 174:709–712.

17. Burke RE, Levine DN, Tsairis P, et al: Physiological types and histochemical profiles in motor units of cat gastrocnemius. *J Physiol* 1973; 234:723–748.

18. Buller AJ, Eccles JC, Ecles RM: Interactions between motor neurons and muscles in respect of the characteristic speeds of their responses. *J Physiol* 1960; 150:417–439.

19. Eisenberg BR, Salmons S: The reorganization of subcellular structure in muscle undergoing fast-to-slow type transformation: A stereological study. *Cell Tissue Res* 1981; 220(3):449–471.

20. Lamb LE, Stevens PM, Johnson RL: Hypokinesia secondary to chair rest from 4 to 10 days. *Aerospace Med* 1965; 36:755–763.

21. Cooper KH: *Aerobics.* New York, Bantam Books, 1968.

22. Katz DR, Kumar VN: Effects of prolonged bed rest on cardiopulmonary conditioning. *Orthop Rev* 1982; 11: 89–93.

23. Kottke FJ: The effects of limitation of activity upon the human body. *JAMA* 1966; 196:825–830.

24. Edstrom L: Selective atrophy of red muscle fibres in the quadriceps in long-standing knee-joint dysfunction following injuries to the anterior cruciate ligament. *J Neurol Sci* 1970; 11:551–558.

25. Taylor HL, Henschel A, Brozek J, et al: Effects of bed rest on cardiovascular function and work performance. *J Appl Physiol* 1949; 2:223–239.

26. Saltin B, Blomqvist G, Mitchell JH, et al: Response to exercise after bed rest and after training. A longitudinal study of adaptive changes in oxygen transport and body composition. *Circulation* 1968; 38:111–178.

27. Gollnick PD, Armstrong RB, Saubert CW, et al: Enzyme activity and fiber composition in skeletal muscle of un-

trained and trained man. *J Appl Physiol* 1972; 33:312–319.

28. Gollnick PD, Armstrong RB, Saltin B, et al: Effect of training on enzyme activity and fiber composition of human skeletal muscle. *J Appl Physiol* 1973; 34:107–111.

29. Thorstensson A, Hulten B, Von Dobeln W, et al: Effect of strength training on enzyme activities and fiber characteristics in human skeletal muscle. *Acta Physiol Scand* 1976; 96:392–398.

30. Gollnick PD, Karlsson J, Piehl K, et al: Selective glycogen depletion in skeletal muscle fibers of man following sustained contractions. *J Physiol* 1974; 241:59–67.

31. Gollnick PD, Piehl K, Saltin B: Selective glycogen depletion pattern in human muscle fibers after exercise of varying intensity and at varying pedaling rates. *J Physiol* 1974; 241:45–57.

32. Bennett RL, Knowlton GC: Overwork weakness in partially denervated skeletal muscle. *Clin Orthop* 1958; 12: 22–29.

33. Milner-Brown HS, Miller RG: Muscle strengthening through electric stimulation combined with low resistance weights in patients with neuromuscular disorders. *Arch Phys Med Rehabil* 1988; 69:20–24.

34. Milner-Brown HS, Miller RG: Muscle strengthening through high-resistance weight training in patients with neuromuscular disorders. *Arch Phys Med Rehabil* 1988; 69:14–19.

35. De Lateur BJ, Giaconi RM: Effect on maximal strength of submaximal exercise in Duchenne muscular dystrophy. *Am J Phys Med* 1979; 58:26–36.

36. Abramson AS, Rogoff J: An approach to rehabilitation of children with muscular dystrophy. *Proceedings of the First and Second Medical Conferences of the MDAA, Inc.* New York, Muscular Dystrophy Association of America, Inc, 1953, pp. 123–124.

37. Hoberman M: Physical medicine and rehabilitation: Its value and limitations in progressive muscular dystrophy. *Am J Phy Med* 1955; 34:109–115.

38. Wratney MJ: Physical therapy for muscular dystrophy children. *Phys Ther Rev* 1958; 38:26–32.

39. Bleck EE: Mobility of patients with Duchenne muscular dystrophy. *Dev Med Child Neurol* 1979; 21:823–824.

40. Reger SI, Chung KC: Posture, contour and pressure distribution in wheelchair seating. *38th ACEMB,* Chicago, IL, 1985, p. 137.

41. Henderson B: *Seating in Review: Current Trends for the Disabled.* Winnipeg. Otto Bock Orthopedic Industry of Canada, 1989.

42. Letts RM: *Principles of Seating the Disabled.* Boca Raton, CRC Press, 1991.

43. Adams TC, Reger SI, Sahgal V: Guidelines for wheelchair securement and personal restraint. *Proceedings of the RESNA '94 Annual Conference.* Nashville, RESNA Press, 1994.

44. Reger SI, Neth DC, McGovern TF: Computer aided prescription of specialized seats for wheelchairs, in Popovic

D (ed): *Advances in External Control of Human Extremities*, 9th ed. Belgrade, Tanjug, 1987, pp. 559–562.

45. Reger SI, Neth DC, Jenkins D, Lewis D: The use of CAD-CAM methods for custom contoured wheelchair seat fabrication. *Proceedings, Seventh World Congress of the International Society for Prosthetics and Orthotics*, Chicago, IL, 1992.

46. Bhasin CA: CAD-CAM seating technology: The clinical perspective on Signature 2000 rehabilitation seating system. *Eleventh International Seating Symposium*. Pittsburgh, University of Pittsburgh, 1995, pp. 239–242.

47. Krusen FH, Kottke FJ, Ellwood PM: *Handbook of Physical Medicine and Rehabilitation,* 2nd ed. Philadelphia, W.B. Saunders, 1971.

48. Lovett RW: The treatment of infantile paralysis *JAMA* 1915; 64:2118.

49. Vignos PJ Jr, Archibald KC: Maintenance of ambulation in childhood muscular dystrophy. *J Chronic Dis* 1960; 12:273–290.

50. Vignos PJ Jr, Spencer GE, Archibald KC: Management of progressive muscular dystrophy in childhood. *JAMA* 1963; 184:89–96.

51. Harris SE, Cherry DB: Childhood progressive muscular dystrophy and the role of physical therapy. *Phys Ther* 1974; 54:4–12.

52. Scott OM, Hyde SA, Goddard C, et al: Prevention of deformity in Duchenne muscular dystrophy: a prospective study of passive stretching and splintage. *Physiotherapy* 1981; 67(6):177–180.

53. Eyring EJ, Johnson EW, Burnett C: Surgery in muscular dystrophy. *JAMA* 1972; 222:1056–1057.

54. Johnson EW: Pathokinesiology of Duchenne muscular dystrophy: Implications of management. *Arch Phys Med Rehabil* 1977; 58:4–7.

55. Roy L, Gibson DA: Pseudohypertrophic muscular dystrophy. *Can J Surg* 1970; 13(1):13–21.

56. Bach JR, McKeon J: Orthopedic surgery and rehabilitation for the prolongation of brace-free ambulation of patients with Duchenne muscular dystrophy. *Am J Phys Med Rehabil* 1991; 70(6):323–331.

57. Sahgal V, Shah A, Flanagan N, et al: Morphologic and morphometric studies of muscle in idiopathic scoliosis. *Acta Orthopaedica Scand* 1983; 54:242–251.

58. Kaplan PE, Sahgal V, Hughes RL, et al: Neuropathy in thoracic scoliosis. *Acta Orthopaedica Scand* 1980; 51: 263–266.

59. Rideau Y, Glorion B, Delaubiber A, et al: The treatment of scoliosis in Duchenne muscular dystrophy. *Am J Phys Med Rehabil* 1979; 58(1):26–36.

60. Siegel IM, Silverman O, Silverman M: The Chicago insert: An approach to wheelchair seating for the maintenance of spinal posture in Duchenne muscular dystrophy. *Orthot Prosthet* 1981; 35(4):27–29.

61. Siegel IM: Equinocavovarus in muscular dystrophy. *Arch Surg* 1972; 104:644–646.

62. Luque ER: Segmental spinal instrumentation for correction of scoliosis. *Clin Orthop* 1982; 163:192–198.

63. Moseley CF: Natural history and management of scoliosis in Duchenne muscular dystrophy, in Serratric G, Cros D, et al (eds): *Neuromuscular Diseases.* New York, Raven, 1984, pp. 545–556.

64. Bach J, O'Brien J, Krotenberg R, et al: Respiratory management of patients with Duchenne muscular dystrophy. *Arch Phys Med Rehabil* 1985; 66:524.

65. Bach JR, Campagnolo DI, Hoeman S: Life satisfaction of individuals with Duchenne muscular dystrophy using long-term mechanical ventilatory support. *Am J Phys Rehabil* 1991; 70:129–135.

Chapter 11

CEREBRAL PALSY AND DEVELOPMENTAL DISABILITIES

Monique Gingold
Susan T. Iannaccone

HABILITATION

Rehabilitation implies regaining function that was once present. Children with congenital delays have never had the abilities they are attempting to acquire. Hence, the term habilitation is particularly applicable to children with both acquired developmental delays and/or congenital neurological disabilities.[1] Habilitation has a demonstrable effect on the functional outcome of children with cerebral palsy and developmental disabilities.[2] Habilitation involves a wide range of activities, interactions, processes, and approaches that enable neurologically impaired children to develop new abilities and optimize their level of function. In a broader sense, habilitation is a comprehensive team-oriented intervention strategy that has as its goal enhanced capability to participate in society and culture.[3]

PLASTICITY

Brain plasticity can be defined as the adaptive and nonadaptive changes in structure and function produced by endogenous or exogenous influences.[9]

Several reports have provided examples of infants diagnosed with motor deficits who later "outgrew" them.[4–8] Some were only followed until 6–14 months of age.[5,6] However, a small number of infants diagnosed with cerebral palsy (CP) apparently have experienced spontaneous resolution of their motor deficits.[4,7,8] These observations suggest the brain has plasticity.

In humans, the hand and tongue have large areas of functionally related cortex compared to other body parts.[10] This differential cortical representation has been attributed to frequent use and requirement for fine motor control. For example, training a kitten to develop forelimb dominance causes the contralateral motor cortical representation of the trained limb to be four times larger than that of the untrained forelimb.[11] Maximal ability to reorganize the primary somatosensory cortex in humans occurs prior to age 12 years.

This age-dependent limitation has been demonstrated in a study of stringed-instrument musicians who had begun playing at various ages.[12] The thumb and fifth finger of the left hand received somatosensory stimulation. Resulting cortical current dipoles were recorded and superimposed onto a magnetic resonance imaging (MRI) reconstruction of the cerebral cortex. The area of cortical representation of the left hand was enlarged only when musical study had been initiated prior to age 12 years.

Such plasticity research in animals and humans has demonstrated the ability of experience to effect cortical growth and specialization and has direct implications for early therapeutic interventions in neurologically impaired infants and children.

In a study of hemiplegic children with marked mirror movements, the corticospinal tract from the undamaged cerebral hemisphere has been shown to innervate ipsilateral as well as contralateral hand motor neurons.[13] Two explanations have been proposed for this observation.[13] First, in response to injury during postnatal development, corticospinal tract branching in the spinal cord may occur so that bilateral motor neuron pools are innervated. Such corticospinal tract branching has been shown to occur in hamsters.[14] Alternatively, during normal fetal development, corticospinal tract axons project bilaterally to motor neuron pools. Normally, corticospinal projections to ipsilateral spinal motor neurons degenerate. Following damage to motor pathways in the fetal or neonatal period, degeneration of corticospinal projections to ipsilateral spinal motor neurons may be attenuated.

EARLY IDENTIFICATION

The capacity for plasticity in the immature brain implies that early identification of children at high risk for neonatal central nervous system injury is important. Habilitation services have been shown to enhance children's academic achievement, language, growth, and social skills.[15] The potential benefits to society include ultimately reduced need for special education, decreased societal dependence, and increased family integrity. The economic reward for society has been reviewed and discussed extensively.[2,16,17]

Hence, the provision of free early intervention (EI) services for children under 3 years of age who have or are at risk for developmental disabilities is required by statutory mandate. The child is evaluated and an individual's rehabilitation program is established. Once the child is preschool-aged (3 years) and has disabilities that may affect school performance, physical therapy (PT) and occupational therapy (OT) services are required by federal statute. Each state has policies specifically addressing mandatory special education for exceptional students. Individualized educational planning meetings with school representatives and parents occur annually and result in a program itemizing detailed educational goals and therapies to be offered each child. Specific therapeutic interventions must be implemented in a timely manner according to the recommendations set forth in the individualized educational program.

IDENTIFICATION OF CHILDREN WITH CEREBRAL PALSY AND DEVELOPMENTAL DISABILITY

Early identification of infants at high risk for CP and developmental disabilities is not easy. Such infants often are selected based on a history of low birth weight, prolonged stay in neonatal units, birth asphyxia, developmental delay, congenital infections, neonatal meningitis or seizures, ultrasonic abnormalities of fetal brain, intraventricular hemorrhage, spina bifida, and hypoto-

nia (see Table 11-1).[15,18–24] Attempts to develop prognostic criteria with high predictive value have been made.[15,23]

Clinical clues in the history and physical examination can alert the physician to the possibility of CP or developmental disability (see Table 11-2). Infants with feeding problems, such as difficulty coordinating suck with swallow or tongue thrust interfering with feedings, have an increased risk of becoming developmentally delayed and should be considered for early referral and evaluation.[1,25] Infants with unusual posturing, poor head control, asymmetric movements, or early hand dominance (prior to 18 months) also deserve early evaluation.[1]

Infantile reflex abnormalities can signify injury to the central nervous system early in development: persistence of primitive reflexes beyond their normal time (extensor plantar response, Moro, crossed adductor, asymmetrical tonic neck) (Figure 11-1) or delay or lack of acquisition of normal reflexes (parachute, Landau, neck righting, positive supporting) should prompt the physician to consider the possibility of CP or developmental disability (see Figure 11-2).[26–28]

With more severe neurologic impairment, easier and earlier identification is possible. In 43 percent of cases, a high-risk infant is identified by 6 months of age, and 70 percent are established by 1 year.[29] Parents commonly identify a problem with their child by 5 months of age, whereas the physician may require an additional several months of observation.[1]

A substantial group of patients with develop-

Table 11-1

Commonly used criteria for selection of infants at high risk for cerebral palsy and developmental disability

---

Low birth weight

Prolonged stay in neonatal intensive care unit

Asphyxia at birth

Developmental delay

Congenital infection

Neonatal seizures

Neonatal meningitis

Fetal brain ultrasound abnormalities

Intraventricular hemorrhage

Spina bifida

Hypotonia

Table 11-2
Clinical clues suggesting possible cerebral palsy or developmental delay

Feeding difficulties

Poor suck and swallow coordination

Tongue thrusting

Unusual posturing

Poor head control

Asymmetric movements

Hand dominance established before 18 months

Persistence of primative reflexes

Delay in acquisition of normal reflexes

WHEN TO INITIATE TREATMENT

Therapies should begin once the high-risk infant is identified. Goals and objectives will depend on the age of the child. Certain needs, such as adaptive equipment, will depend on the developmental level of the child. However, involvement of the family or caregivers in the process of habilitation is crucial in all phases.[1,2] Improvement has been shown to be positively influenced by family involvement, both parent and sibling.[32,33] In addition to treating the child, the habilitation team must educate and counsel the family in the care and support of the child's achievements and attempts to be independent. Anticipatory guidance is important for the family.

mental delay initially are hypotonic. In a sizable group, tone may change with time, and choreoathetosis and/or spasticity may become more evident, and a diagnosis of CP made.[30] Another cluster of infants remains hypotonic and ultimately may be diagnosed with a congenital myopathy, genetic disorder, or central nervous system structural anomaly.[31] These diagnostic categories and spina bifida will be discussed later in this chapter. Other less common etiologies of hypotonia and developmental disabilities such as hypothyroidism, neurodegenerative disorders, lesions of the spinal cord, and inborn errors of metabolism are beyond the scope of this text.

GOALS

In the early phases of treating an infant, a major component of therapy focuses on educating the parents so that everyday activities become therapeutic in nature.[2,34] The goal is not to make therapists out of parents. However, once caregivers understand the basic tenets and goals of therapy, they will easily understand how feeding, holding, diapering, and bathing can be beneficial physically and cognitively. For example, a baby with increased tone moves in a sagittal plane and lacks trunk rotation. If the parent gently rotates the baby's pelvis to slip the

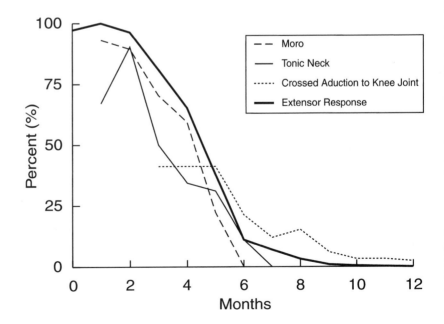

Figure 11-1
Disappearance of primitive reflexes.

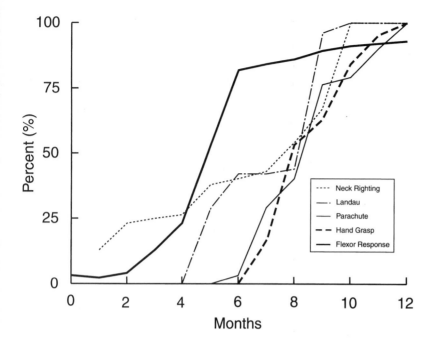

Figure 11-2
Reflexes that develop with increasing maturity.

diaper on and off, hypertonia will be decreased by this therapeutic maneuver. Likewise, babies with truncal hypotonia should be encouraged to use their trunk musculature. Keeping this in mind, parents holding a child can strive to provide support as low on the trunk as tolerated, encouraging the child to use trunk muscles.

Goals will change with time according to the child's developmental stages, both physical and cognitive. Physiological recovery and normal development continue to occur during habilitation.

TREATMENT MODALITIES IN CP AND DEVELOPMENTAL DISABILITY

Physical Therapy

The evaluation and treatment of developmental and gross motor disabilities is the domain of physical therapy. Physical therapists also fit and modify wheelchairs, walkers, and seating and positioning devices. Various therapeutic intervention theories and methods abound. However, neurodevelopmental therapy (NDT), as developed by the Bobaths, is the most widely used method in the treatment of CP and developmental disability.

The Bobath model is based on the premise that brain damage interferes with the development of normal postural control against gravity, resulting in abnormal patterns of coordination.[35] In addition, difficulty with motor development interferes with normal exploratory behavior, causing decreased sensory and perceptual input and secondary developmental delay.[35] Parental training is crucial in NDT. The family must be regarded as a member of the team. If the family understands the rationale for therapy, they can assure that the principles are applied to everyday life and activities.

The treatment program uses tactile stimulation to facilitate movement and proprioceptive stimulation to enhance tone in cases of hypotonia. Key points of control (shoulder or pelvic girdle, head, or hand) are used by the therapist to inhibit abnormal movement while facilitating desired movement. An NDT therapist provides guidance and facilitates normal movement and postural reactions (Figure 11-3). If hypertonicity is a problem, treatment will attempt to inhibit the abnormal patterns of postural reflex activity and facilitate normal postural reactions. In cases of hypotonicity, other techniques, such as proprioceptive input and compression, are employed to augment cocontraction and increase tone. NDT does not adhere to a strict developmental movement sequence, recognizing the fact that a child is perfecting multiple skills simultaneously during normal development. For example, a 9-month-old child normally is crawling on hands and knees, pulling to stand,

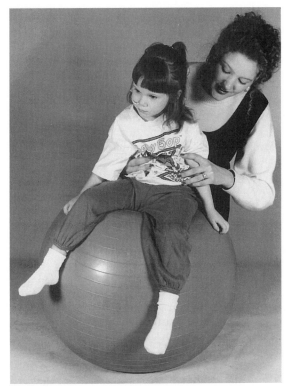

Figure 11-3
NDT therapy facilitating postural reactions.

and cruising. Treatment incorporates such functional tasks as exploration, play, and dressing, with the idea that the sensorimotor input during these activities will carry over into other functional skills. The child is continually reevaluated from a developmental standpoint, and the treatment plan modified accordingly.

Another treatment approach used by physical therapists is sensorimotor integration (SMI), which advocates tactile and vestibular stimulation.[36] SMI originally was designed for learning-disabled children, but its elements have been utilized for other developmental disabilities with the goal of enhancing sensori-motor function and automatic postural responses.[37]

Doman and Delacato formulated a very intense, around-the-clock treatment regimen, requiring four to five individuals per patient to passively move each extremity through a set of patterns in an attempt to train cerebral dominance and normalize function.[38] Doman and Delacato also recommended periods of carbon dioxide rebreathing and occasional fluid restriction. There is no scientific basis for these theories, nor any evidence

that this treatment method is effective.[39] The Doman–Delacato system is not recommended by the American Academy of Pediatrics.

Functional electrical stimulation of peripheral nerves is being utilized to stimulate the agonist muscles and facilitate desired movements.[40] Research is ongoing to evaluate the degree of effectiveness of these methods as well as their long-term benefits.

Other therapeutic modalities that show promise include pool therapy, biofeedback, behavioral programming, equestrian therapy, and music and dance therapy.[41,42]

Occupational Therapy (OT)

OT focuses on fine motor control, oral motor function, visual-perceptual skills, and activities of daily living (ADL). Occupational therapists can be instrumental in feeding programs. In children under 3 years of age, either a PT or an OT will conduct NDT sessions. In early intervention programs, therapists work closely together, and with the teacher. Once the child is over 3 years old, there is increased specificity in therapeutic goals and a separation of PT and OT. The OT may provide adaptive devices to aid with feeding, writing, and dressing, and, where appropriate, fabricates upper extremity splints. There are programs in OT that address attentional disorders and learning disabilities, both of which may be seen with increasing frequency in the cerebral palsy/developmental disability population.[43,44]

Speech Therapy (ST)

Speech therapists address issues of dysphagia, articulation, and receptive and expressive language. During the initial evaluation, a determination should be made whether speech and language delays are owing to poor motor control or an accompanying cognitive deficit.[45] The speech therapist may be called on to evaluate the child's language and cognition to determine readiness for use of augmentative/alternative communication systems such as communication boards, sign language, gestures, communication devices, and adaptive use of computers.[45] They play a very important role in establishing effective communication between caregivers and team members at an age-appropriate level with the child. A feeding program led by a speech therapist may be necessary to facilitate swallowing, stimulate tongue movements, decrease drooling, and desensitize the perioral region. Hypersensitivity of the oral and perioral region often is present in children who are neurologically impaired and have had experiences with feeding that resulted in gagging and choking. This may substantially interfere with feeding. Densensitization entails gradually introducing various stimuli, of differing intensities and structures, in and around the mouth area, often a lengthy process.

Recreation Therapy (RT)

The pursuit of leisure activities affords children a sense of accomplishment that is empowering as they pursue therapeutic goals. Participation by disabled children in arts and crafts, sports, and community integration activities should be directed by a recreation therapist. For example, handicapped horseback riding, something children greatly enjoy, has therapeutic value for improving balance. Specialty camps for children allow children with special needs to enjoy independence from parents, outdoor activities, and the comradeship of peers in a nonthreatening environment, building confidence and self-esteem.

Interdisciplinary Physician Care in Cerebral Palsy and Developmental Disability

Neurosurgery Neurosurgeons are crucial participants in the care of spina bifida patients, initially with closure of the myelomeningocele, subsequently with ventriculo-peritoneal shunt placement and monitoring and, lastly, with management of spasticity. Selective dorsal rhizotomy (SDR) is a procedure during which the posterior roots from the second lumbar to first sacral spinal nerves are isolated, selectively electrically stimulated, and muscular responses observed by electromyography.[46] The rootlets that elicit a sustained or incremental motor response to repetitive stimulation, have a very low threshold for stimulation, or demonstrate evidence of spreading motor responses to distant myotomes are identified and cut. The success of this operation is dependent on the selection of the right candidate patient.[47]

It appears that two types of individuals can best benefit from this procedure. The first is a child with spasticity but no contractures, who ambulates independently or with assistive devices, and has an equinovarus gait with hip adduction (scissoring). The second is an individual with severe spastic quadriplegia that interferes with perineal care, seating, dressing, and toileting.[47,48] Benefits of surgery in the former include decreased spasticity, improved ambulation and function,

and, in the latter, prevention of hip subluxation and facilitation of daily care routines. Caution must be exercised in recommending a severely involved child for surgery. The child may be using the spasticity to facilitate standing and transferring. SDR has been documented to improve upper extremity function in 50 percent of cases.[48,49] Carefully controlled studies still are needed to clarify which patients will benefit from this procedure. Prospective studies are warranted to separate the benefits of increased physical therapy following surgery from the benefits of SDR.[46,48,50]

Cervical cord and cerebellar stimulation have not been demonstrated to cause significant improvement in spasticity. These procedures currently are not recommended.[51,52]

Intrathecal injection of local anesthetic agents has been attempted to decrease spasticity and rigidity.[50,53] Intrathecal baclofen has undergone clinical trials and currently an open study is evaluating reduction of spasticity in children.[53] The amount of baclofen required is significantly smaller than the oral dosage needed to effect a reduction in spasticity. Therefore, the adverse sedative effects are avoided. Baclofen is not indicated for rigidity or athetosis.

Orthopedic Surgery Orthopedic care for children with developmental disabilities is essential. They are at risk for scoliosis and contractures, especially children with cerebral palsy who have spastic quadriplegia.[55] Scoliosis, if significant, can impair pulmonary function, make positioning difficult, and cause pain.[56] Children with myelodysplasia often require extensive scoliosis surgery. As with most surgery, early weight-bearing improves recovery time and prevents loss of function owing to deconditioning.

Restorative orthopedic surgery can be helpful in managing the musculoskeletal consequences of longstanding spastic hypertonia. Spasticity is not cured by surgery, nor is limb deformity, which may recur at any time. A teamwork approach including neurology, neurosurgery, orthopedics, and physiatry is most effective in determining appropriate treatment of spasticity as long as the patient and family do not have unrealistic goals and expectations.

Surgery for contractures or hip dislocation/subluxation may become necessary in children with severe spastic quadriplegia.[47,57] Surgically lengthening a contractured muscle tendon has variable results.[57] Proper supported seating and the use of assisted standing devices are important in preventing hip subluxation and the associated intractable pain. Soft-tissue release may prevent dislocation. Children frequently develop severe joint pain on motion or difficulty in positioning when a dislocated hip is present. Femoral head surgical resection may be necessary to relieve the pain. Customized wheelchair support enables severely involved children to sit properly, diminishing the need for more involved orthopedic care.[57]

Pediatric Neurology and Physiatry Pediatric neurologists and physiatrists frequently function as the coordinating physician or team leader for children with developmental disabilities and CP. It is usually they who are called on to make referrals for early intervention and therapy, and to provide prescriptions for braces, wheelchairs, prone standers, and other adaptive equipment. The rehabilitation physician provides prescriptions for school-based therapies, if the need for therapy is educationally related. They facilitate and encourage the families to become advocates for their children. Pediatric neurologists and physiatrists may participate in the treatment of spasticity by injecting alcohol or botulinum toxin to weaken certain muscles and improve function. Pediatric neurologists treat seizures and investigate the etiology of the developmental disability.

Nutrition and Feeding Rapid infant growth makes adequate nutrition essential for growth and cognitive development.[25,59] Feeding difficulties or inadequate weight gain warrants thorough investigation. Feeding difficulty may herald the diagnosis of pseudobulbar palsy and/or bulbar palsy accompanying CP, or severe congenital myopathy.[30,31]

Difficulty achieving adequate nutritional intake in children with cerebral palsy has been attributed to various factors. Communication difficulties may interfere with requests for food. Impaired self-feeding skills, inability to forage, and oral-motor dysfunction all have been reported to undermine nutritional balance.[25] Many abnormalities of oral-motor control, alone or in combination, may lead to nutritional deficiency in cerebral palsy (see Table 11-3). A child may exhibit a poor suck, difficulty coordinating suck and swallow, a hyperactive gag reflex, tongue thrust, a tonic bite reflex, poor lip closure, limited or absent lateral tongue movements, persistence of infantile oral reflexes interfering with sucking, and/or frequent coughing and choking with meals leading to refusal to eat.[1] Parents report that up to 59 percent of the time spent caring for their children with special needs is used in feeding.[60] Nurses have noted that hospitalized children with cerebral palsy take up to 15 times longer to feed, and mothers of such

Table 11-3

Abnormalities in oral motor control that impair nutrition in children with cerebral palsy

Poor suck reflex

Poor swallow reflex

Difficulty coordinating suck and swallow

Hyperactive gag reflex

Tongue thrusting

Tonic bite reflex

Poor lip closure

Tongue weakness

Persistent infantile reflexes

children report spending up to 7 hours a day engaged in feeding.[25]

As a result, malnutrition is common in neurologically impaired children.[25,61] Children normally gain height and weight continuously until the late teens. Should this rate of growth slow, a feeding and swallowing evaluation may be necessary, even before weight loss occurs. Poor growth may result from poor oral intake owing to dysphagia and associated gastroesophageal (GE) reflux. Abnormal posturing in an infant after meals may signify abdominal pain or esophagitis from reflux. GE reflux may lead to pulmonary complications (aspiration pneumonia), irritability, and poor weight gain.[61]

The feeding evaluation usually is performed by a speech therapist, although in some institutions, an interdisciplinary feeding clinic is available.[25] A swallow evaluation initially will be conducted by observation and will consider whether various factors are interfering with feeding. Ordinarily, the physician or therapist must evaluate positioning of the child, feeding technique, the presence of perioral hypersensitivity and interfering reflexes, and tongue motility.[25] Caregivers can be instructed in facilitating lip closure, swallowing, and tongue movements during meals.[25,59] Therapeutic intervention may include caloric supplementation, improved seating and positioning, thickening liquids, and oral desensitization.

Presence of gastroesophageal reflux can be documented properly with a barium swallow series of radiographs and/or a pH probe. Conservative treatment options include medication (metoclopromide and cimetidine) along with proper positioning following meals. When medical management fails, Nissan fundoplication and pyloroplasty may be necessary to prevent reflux.[61]

Dysphagia may be evaluated with a modified barium swallow. Aspiration in children with moderate to severe CP is reported in up to 60 percent of cases, depending on food consistencies being fed.[59] Since coughing is often not present, one must have a high index of suspicion for silent aspiration. A modified barium swallow examines the oral control of solid and liquid boluses in the oral cavity as they transit through the pharynx to the stomach during swallowing. Poor bolus formation, delayed swallow initiation, and inefficient food transfer through the pharynx are common.[59,62] False negative swallow examinations in children suspected of aspiration may occur because proper positioning is utilized during the study.[62] This only serves to emphasize the importance of correct positioning during meals.

A gastrostomy feeding tube should be considered when there is evidence of aspiration or inadequate growth rate from malnutrition.[25,59–61,62] Studies have documented improved seizure control once a feeding tube is placed.[61] Prior to the placement of a feeding tube, GE reflux should be ruled out. Both a feeding tube placement and a Nissan fundoplication may be performed together.[61]

Dental Because of decreased lateral tongue movements and prominent tongue thrusting, the palate frequently is high and very arched. Good dental hygiene is important, especially if the child is on phenytoin, which causes gingival hyperplasia. Bruxism may contribute to poor dental hygiene. A pedodontist comfortable with children with special needs should be available for routine management.

Drooling Drooling is a stigmatizing affliction and may be particularly troubling for children and families. Poor lip closure, oral hypersensitivity, and inefficient swallowing may contribute to a significant problem with drooling. A bandana, instead of a bib, tied around the neck may help and be socially acceptable for some children. Biofeedback with electromyography has been shown to be effective under some circumstances.[63] Pharmacologic management may include benzhexol hydrochloride, atropine sulfate, scopolamine patches, and other anticholinergic agents. Surgical divergence of the salivary duct has not been clearly shown to be beneficial.[66]

Seizures The incidence of seizures depends upon the underlying etiology of the developmental disability and the nature of the disorder. Evaluation and treatment should be managed by the pediatric neurologist.

Behavior Cognitive impairments may be present and depend on the extent and nature of the disability. Major behavior problems are more frequently encountered in children with neurological disorders such as cerebral palsy, seizures, and hydrocephalus.[43,44] Behavioral problems are strongly linked to concomitant mental retardation. Studies have found a significantly increased incidence of adverse psychological effects on siblings of handicapped children.[67] Psychosocial stressors for families of children with chronic neurologic disorders must be recognized.[3] Counseling may be crucial in maintaining family integrity and balance.

Incontinence Incontinence of bowel and bladder frequently is encountered in neurologically impaired children. Several factors contribute to the difficulty in toilet training: The child may not be able to communicate his or her needs effectively. Mobility difficulties may make it difficult or impossible for a child to get to a toilet in a timely manner. A conventional toilet may not provide adequate trunk support for a child to void or defecate properly. It is important to identify and correct such factors when considering a child for toilet training. Unless a child has specific neurologic deficits affecting sphincter control or severe cognitive deficits, toilet training should be considered as an important part of the comprehensive rehabilitation of a child with developmental delay.

Equipment An occupational therapist can provide invaluable insight into adaptive devices that facilitate activities of daily living. The range of possibilities includes items useful for feeding, dressing and undressing, writing, and bathing.[68] The need for adaptive equipment will vary with developmental level, physical involvement, and age of the child. A home evaluation can be arranged, if need be, and is often especially useful. Bathing needs should be investigated so that devices for support and safety in a bathtub can be provided.[68] For an older child, a bath or shower seat may be useful. For heavier and more involved children, a bath lift may be required. Toileting may be facilitated with trunk support devices that either attach to the toilet seat or are free-standing.

Aids to ambulation, such as walkers and crutches, may be especially useful. The child's physical therapist often can determine the most appropriate device for optimizing function by hands-on trial and error. Frequently, a child with spasticity may walk better with a reverse walker that is turned around and behind the child. This posterior-faced walker facilitates trunk extension, increases walking speed, and decreases double stance time (time in gait spent weight-bearing on both feet simultaneously).[69] Numerous types of walkers with various adaptable grips also are available. Forearm crutches provide greater mobility than a walker, but require near-normal balance. Forearm crutches are often used with hip-knee-ankle-foot-orthoses (HKAFO) or knee-ankle-foot-orthoses (KAFO), such as in myelodysplasia.

Static positioning devices are very important in compensating for abnormal skeletal alignment, improving functional use of extremities, and maintaining musculoskeletal integrity.[1] They consist of sidelyers, adapted seats for home use and travel, and prone and supine standers (see Figure 11-4). These standing devices are essential. A non-weight–bearing individual is prone to develop osteoporosis. Weight-bearing in a properly supported position may prevent the occurrence of contractures. Orthotics often are required to maintain joint alignment and assist with weight-bearing in a prone stander. Prone standers can "grow" with the child and usually are available with attached tables that enable a child to participate in school work during standing time. It is important that children use these prone standers on a daily basis while attending school, especially if one is not available in the home.

Tone in the lower extremities is the essential determinant for proper leg bracing. There is a vast difference in the bracing needs of a child with hypotonia, as in myelodysplasia, compared to a child with CP. A flaccid child needs a device that provides stability and improves joint alignment. If the device crosses the knee joint, it should allow flexion in sitting, but will be locked in extension during stance. With a HKAFO, the patient's body is braced from mid-trunk to feet. Myelodysplasia patients requiring this level of support will usually require a thoracolumbosacral orthosis (TLSO), a molded polypropylene "jacket" to control scoliosis that can attach to the HKAFOs.

When standing is appropriate developmentally, around age one in a young child with thoracolumbar myelodysplasia, a parapodium often is introduced. This type of device combines a TLSO and bilateral HKAFOs with the benefits of a prone stander (see Figure 11-5). With a parapodium, the young child is weight-bearing, and, when ready, may use a walker to start shifting weight in preparation for ambulation. Weight bearing and ambulation provide the opportunity for trunk, and upper and lower extremity strengthening. At the same time, balance-training activities can be facilitated while providing prolonged weight-bearing for the prevention of osteoporosis and contractures. Other options for standing and ambulation include a swivel walker, conventional long-leg braces, and reciprocating gait orthosis.[1]

An ankle-foot-orthosis (AFO) is frequently used in both hypotonic and hypertonic children (see Figure 11-6). A child with spasticity usually requires an AFO to allow ankle stability while maintaining a 90-degree (neutral) position for gait and standing. The ankle joint can be built to allow for active dorsiflexion. In some cases, braces crossing the ankle and knee joints may be designed that allow for a gradual change of joint angles in order to stretch contractures. In the hypotonic patient, the AFO prevents genu recurvatum or back-kneeing by not allowing plantar flexion during the stance phase of gait.

Figure 11-4
Child in prone stander.

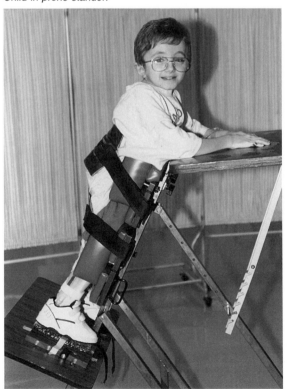

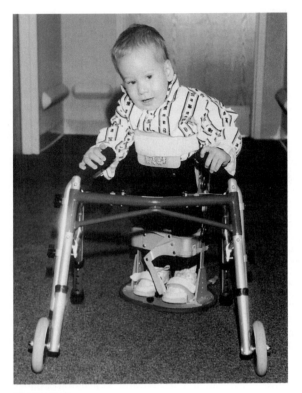

Figure 11-5
Child with myelodysplasia in parapodium, shifting weight to ambulate with walker.

"Inhibitive" or serial casting is useful for immobilization, weight bearing, and management of spasticity by causing a prolonged, passive stretch. The casts are applied serially to gradually increase the range of motion when contractures are present. Once maximal position and optimum range of motion have been attained, the cast may be bivalved. The cast is simply cut in half and Velcro straps attached so that it can be worn intermittently to maintain range of motion.

Wheelchair fitting usually is accomplished by a physical therapist, with or without the input of various members of the interdisciplinary team. Functional positioning and access to communication devices are major issues in determining appropriate fit. Wheelchairs may be self-propelled, attendant-controlled, or power-operated. Safety is most important. The wheelchair must provide appropriate support and stability. Useful adjuncts to the basic wheelchair frame might include lateral supports for trunk stability, seat belt, trunk harness, hip abduction orthosis, lumbar roll, head support, and foot rests with appropriate straps. Proper positioning may slow the progression of neurogenic scoliosis.[55,70]

A lumbar roll will facilitate good posture by keeping the pelvis anteriorly rotated, allowing the child to develop a more upright posture.[1] Children with spastic quadriplegia often have extremity hypertonicity and truncal hypotonicity, providing a challenging task in fitting a wheelchair. If a child is well supported in his or her chair, upper extremity function is enhanced.[71–74] If a child has the capability for self-propulsion, it is important that an appropriate chair be chosen. Large, anteriorly situated and readily accessible wheels and brakes are vital. For young children, small chairs not only enhance independence, but allow the child to transfer independently. The chair, ideally, should be situated low to the ground, so that the child is at the same table level as other seated children (see Figure 11-7). Most children, families, and schools prefer these small wheelchairs. However, the family must be aware that the smaller wheelchair with smaller wheels will be more difficult to manipulate and propel on uneven terrain.

Figure 11-6
Hemiparetic child with AFO.

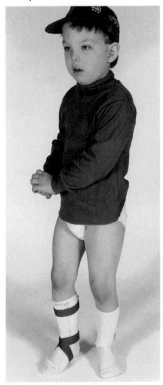

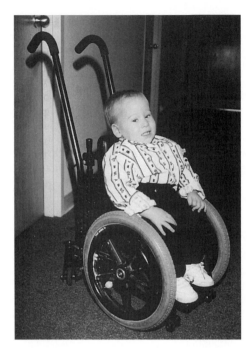

Figure 11-7
Small, table-height wheelchair.

Frequently, a physician is presented with a request for a power chair. The decision to obtain a power wheelchair should not be taken lightly. First, a child must have the cognitive capability not just to be able to operate the chair, but to understand safety issues. Adequate attention span and visuospatial reasoning skills are important. Second, physical ability to manipulate the control panel in a coordinated fashion must be present. Third, cost is an issue. Fourth, a power chair's base weight of close to 150 pounds requires a special van with a lift. The availability of two chairs—a power chair for school and a manual one for home is useful. Power three-wheeled scooters, although less expensive, afford limited trunk and head support, and may be inadequate for some children who need powered mobility.

Management of Spasticity Several oral medications have been used to decrease spasticity in children, the most widely used being diazepam and baclofen. Baclofen should not be prescribed in children under 5 years of age. A dose that significantly reduces spasticity often results in marked sedation and increased oral secretions. The endpoints of treatment (decrease in scissoring, facilitated dressing, improved wheelchair seating) should be determined beforehand, and the dose carefully titrated toward reaching these goals. This way adverse effects often can be avoided.

In deciding to treat spasticity, whether surgically or medically, careful consideration must be given to the individual's functional use of the spasticity. Some children utilize their spasticity to weight-bear during transfers and ambulation. Decreasing spasticity could adversely affect function.

The starting dose of diazepam for infants is 1 mg orally every 12 hours. This can be increased in frequency, as needed and as tolerated, to every 4 to 6 hours. In children over 5 years of age, baclofen should be initiated at low dosages, such as 10 mg orally, twice daily.

For certain patients, reversible motor nerve blocking agents such as alcohol, phenol, or botulinum toxin have been used successfully as an adjunct treatment for spasticity.[47,75–77] Nerve blocks may be useful prior to casting or splinting, in order to improve positioning, or to improve ambulation in patients with an equinovarus gait.

Alcohol injections may relieve spasticity, but they often are accompanied by severe pain owing to local irritation, necessitating the use of sedation. Other side effects include dysesthesias, excessive weakness, and long-term permanent denervation.[78,79] Motor nerves can be injected proximally, distally, or at motor points.

Botulinum toxin causes only transient pain, and functions by blocking the release of acetylcholine at the presynaptic nerve terminals.[80] The blocking effect lasts until new neuromuscular junctions are generated by terminal sprouting, generally in the range of 2 to 6 months. The duration of the toxin effect is dose-dependent, and also may vary with the magnitude and frequency of use for a spastic muscle. Theoretically, longitudinal muscle growth is allowed, reducing the incidence or degree of fixed contractures, and increasing range of motion and motor function.[75,77] A multi-center, randomized, double-blinded study using botulinum toxin for weakening plantar flexors and adductor muscles in ambulatory children without fixed contractures is currently underway.[47]

Toddlers grow rapidly and consequently, when heel-cord lengthening surgery is performed at age 2 to 3 years, the deformity frequently recurs, necessitating a repeat surgery at age 7 to 8 years. Preliminary results indicate that botulinum toxin injection therapy may lead to deferral of early heel-cord lengthening surgery in toddlers until school age, eliminating a surgical procedure and its attendant risks and complications.[47,76] Studies now are underway to identify which patients are benefited by botulinum toxin injections and optimal dosing.

Surgical management of spasticity, including selective dorsal rhizotomy and intrathecal baclofen, is discussed in the neurosurgery section.

Long-Term Planning

Once a child is in elementary school, cognition should be formally evaluated every 2 years to enable long-range planning. In a preschool child, intelligence is difficult to predict and may be affected by the nature of the disability and genetic, social, and environmental factors. Language development correlates relatively well with intelligence.

As soon as possible, academic goals should be determined, to decide if college or vocational school are realistic options. In high school, vocational counseling should be obtained from county, state, or private agencies. The evaluating agency will conduct a comprehensive evaluation of the individual's cognitive, neurological, social, and medical status, and make recommendations for vocational training and residential living arrangements.[17] The Americans with Disabilities Act of 1990 was passed to assist with full inclusion of persons with disabilities within their communities. This act prohibits discrimination on the basis of disability in the areas of employment, transportation, public accommodations, telecommunications, and state and local government agencies.[16] Supported employment often is found to be effective for individuals with CP.[17] Cognitive ability is more important than physical functioning in predicting success in the workplace and independent living.

CEREBRAL PALSY

Definition

CP results from an injury occurring to a normally forming brain that results in a chronic, nonprogressive disorder of movement or posture. A spectrum of deficits may be present. CP, like mental retardation (MR), is a condition with numerous causes and protean manifestations.[23]

Epidemiology

The prevalence of CP has risen since the 1980's.[81] The prevalence of CP in infants weighing greater than 2500 grams at birth is unchanged.[80] However, the prevalence of CP in very low birth weight (VLBW) infants (birth weight < 1500 g) has increased. Survival of VLBW infants in the United States has increased from 6.5 to 461.2 per 1000 live births from the 1960s to the 1980s.[81] VLBW infants accounted for 12.2 percent of those with CP in 1960 and for 27.2 percent in 1986.[82] The incidence of CP in infant survivors with a birth weight over 2500 grams is 1.3 : 1000, 8.5 : 1000 in infant survivors weighing between 1501 and 2499 grams, and 77 : 1000 in neonatal survivors with a birth weight less than 1500 grams.[82] The United Cerebral Palsy Association estimates that more than 500,000 Americans have CP.

Etiology

In 1862, a London orthopedic surgeon, William J. Little, speculated that motor deficits occurring in young children resulted from a lack of oxygen during difficult births.[83] His critics were many and included Sigmund Freud, who criticized this theory in 1897, speculating that preexisting abnormalities in the fetus caused perinatal difficulties.[84]

It appears now that Freud was more correct. A known cause of CP, perinatal hypoxic ischemic injury, accounts for only 4.5 percent of CP cases.[20,23] The etiology of the majority of cases of CP is unknown.[19] Fifty-five percent of children diagnosed with CP have Apgar scores of 7 or greater at 1 minute, and 73 percent have such a score at 5 minutes.[85] Only in infants receiving an Apgar score of <3 at 20 minutes could cerebral damage be expected.[85] Factors that increase the risk of CP include low birth weight, prolonged neonatal hospitalization, maternal mental retardation, maternal epilepsy, poor prenatal care, maternal age younger than 16, the administration of estrogen or thyroid hormones during pregnancy, multiple births, and severe proteinuria in the third trimester.[15,21,22] Known causes of CP include pre- or postnatal infections such as encephalitis or meningitis, kernicterus, and pre- or postnatal stroke.[18,86,87] In spite of advancements in monitoring for fetal distress in labor and delivery, and an increasing number of cesarean section deliveries, perinatal morbidity and mortality have not decreased.

Very often, the term CP is used inappropriately to denote children with genetic syndromes, chromosomal anomalies, cerebral malformations, nerve and muscle disorders, and inborn errors of metabolism. The term CP is easily understood by the lay public, as well as schools and government agencies and may facilitate qualification for special services in the educational, financial, and therapeutic arenas. For clarity and accuracy in medical records, the correct medical diagnosis and terminology always should be used.

Classification

CP can be classified in many ways, one of which is according to cause. Therefore, categories could include hypoxic/ischemic encephalopathy, intraventricular hemorrhage, intrauterine viral infection, and perinatal ischemic infarction, for example. An alternative CP nosology can be based on the location and type of motor deficit, such as hemiparesis, diparesis (legs more involved than arms), or quadriparesis. A descriptive prefix for the type of muscle tone predominating (hypotonia, dystonia, rigidity, or spasticity) often is used. When there is an associated movement disorder, such as chorea or athetosis, an additional adjectival prefix is used. Mixed tone frequently occurs, one example being children with spastic quadriparesis who exhibit truncal hypotonia.

Issues and Management

Nutrition and Feeding   Feeding difficulties may be the presenting complaint in children with CP and should be evaluated carefully. Secondary difficulties include drooling, aspiration, and gastroesophageal reflux. Children do not outgrow these feeding difficulties so growth must be monitored carefully to ensure medical intervention occurs in a timely manner.[25,59,61] Constipation is not infrequent and usually responds to a high-fiber diet, stool softeners, and laxatives.

Growth   Besides nutritional factors contributing to a disturbance in growth, differential growth may be evident in hemiplegic individuals, with the presence of asymmetry in the size of limbs and face.

Speech and Language   Motor deficits and/or central processing problems may be responsible for the gamut of speech and language problems seen with CP.

Seizures   In aggregate, seizures are present in one third of all children with CP.[30] The incidence of epilepsy varies with the type of CP. Between 55 and 72 percent of children with hemiplegic CP experience seizures, compared to only 23 percent of children with choreoathetosic CP. Seizures usually manifest by 2 years of age. Should a child's condition or developmental

functioning appear to deteriorate, the possibility of epilepsy should be considered. In a child with CP and known seizures, break through seizures may be a cause for functional deterioration.

Cognition and School Placement   Two thirds of children with CP have mental retardation.[28,88] In cases where intelligence is normal, a learning disability often is present. As in seizures, the incidence of MR varies depending on the type of CP. Nearly 60 percent of individuals with hemiplegic CP have normal intelligence compared to 30 percent of those with spastic quadriparesis or mixed CP. Psychometric testing should be performed prior to starting school, at around 3 to 4 years of age, by a trained psychometrician in conjunction with a child psychologist. Neuropsychological testing may be indicated, especially if behavioral issues and learning disability are a concern. Annual educational planning meetings with the family, specialists, and school representatives will rely on testing and achievement to devise an optimal educational and therapeutic plan for each child.

Behavior   Behavioral concerns are not uncommon in children with CP. Behavioral issues may include attentional deficits, impulsivity, aggressive/violent behavior, depression, and sleep disorders. Children with severe retardation may exhibit stereotypic or self-mutilating behaviors, as well as autistic tendencies.[43] In milder cases of CP, emotional disorders such as anxiety states, depression, lack of self-confidence, a tendency to worry, fearfulness, and temper tantrums are more common.[43] Asperger Syndrome, a disorder similar to autism albeit with normal language development, has been reported in children with mild hemiparetic CP. This association may provide clues to the underlying brain dysfunction in Asperger Syndrome.[43]

Children with cerebral palsy and normal intelligence exhibit three times higher rates of personality disorders than controls matched for age, sex, intelligence quotient, and socioeconomic class.[43] Children with CP also may exhibit normal childhood behavior that may be difficult for parents to recognize. A language deficit, for example, may mask the expression of normal childhood fears and anxieties. Examples include school phobia, fear of sleeping alone, and night terrors. Adolescents may have low self-esteem and concerns regarding sexuality. Some workers point out that adolescent rebelliousness in a handicapped teenager may be a positive prognostic sign.[3]

Consideration should be given to the fact that certain medications, notably anticonvulsants, may aggravate behavioral disorders. Behavioral symptoms may also be exacerbated by psychosocial stressors such as marital discord, financial hardship, and codependency between mother and child. The family of a child with CP often has crisis points at various stages of their child's development, and should be made aware of counseling options.[3,43] Problematic behaviors in family members usually will respond to a comprehensive program that includes parent education, behavior modification, counseling, or medication.[43,54]

Vision   Visual concerns are varied and may include refractive errors, amblyopia, nystagmus, and abnormal visual pursuits. Premature infants may have retinopathy of prematurity. Likewise, individuals with hemiplegic CP may have a homonymous hemianopia. Periodic evaluation by an ophthalmologist is indicated.

Hearing   Hearing impairment, if present, usually results from complications of neonatal meningitis or kernicterus.

Motor Disturbances   By definition, motor deficits are present in CP. The nature of these disturbances is predicated by the location and the extent of the brain injury. In the first few months after birth, most infants are hypotonic. If spasticity is to supervene, usually it is evident by 18 months of age. Secondary sequelae of spasticity include kyphoscoliosis, contractures, hip subluxation, and acetabular dysplasia.[55]

CP is a static encephalopathy and by definition, not subject to deterioration. An apparent deterioration in gait or other functional ability may result from various causes. In an older ambulating child, obesity may cause a decline in gait by increasing workload on already weak muscles.[89] Alternatively, there may be a worsening in function because of the formation of flexion contractures, either from poor compliance with therapy or worsening rigidity or spasticity. Adverse effects of medication also may account for inexplicable changes in function, as can new onset or breakthrough seizures.

Therapies   Neurodevelopmental therapy (NDT) is the most widely used therapeutic intervention strategy for CP in both the United States and England.[90] An integrative approach using NDT principles through co-treatment often is useful.[90]

A recent survey of NDT therapists revealed that, in actuality, NDT therapy sessions integrate elements of developmental skill training, sensory integration, resistive exercises, mobilization, and computer technology.[91] NDT handling techniques were used in 75 percent of the therapy sessions. The importance of this eclectic approach by therapists is highlighted by the fact that resistive exercise have been shown to be beneficial and improve quadriceps strength.[89] Therefore, by utilizing resistive exercises with a cooperative school-aged child, a crouch gait pattern (flexion of hips and knees), commonly seen in hemiparetic patients, may be ameliorated.

Benefits of Early Physical Therapy

Studies performed to evaluate and document the relative benefits of PT compared to EI have not consistently shown the advantages of one over the other.[92–94] Overlap between the two methods may explain most of the picture. NDT therapists work on developmental skills during NDT sessions.[91,92] PT teaches social interactions, language development, and sensory stimulation. The EI approach includes cognitive, sensory, language, and motor activities. It is difficult to separate PT from EI, much less compare their benefits. Parents involved with intervention gain a better understanding of their infant's development, improving their ability to interact.[92] Infants involved with intervention gain motivation to explore their environment, thereby having a positive influence on their motor development.[92] Thus, any intervention, whether EI or PT, is better than no intervention at all.

There are several problems with studies of intervention in CP, including: (1) use of descriptive study design; (2) lack of controls; (3) suboptimal statistical analysis; (4) small sample sizes; (5) lack of long-term follow-up; and (6) lack of sensitive instrumentation to measure motor function.[34,92–96] In addition, it is inherently difficult to match groups of patients with CP.[97] The clinical manifestations of CP are protean. Differences in tone, intelligence, degree of impairment, psychosocial support, therapy intensity and type—all have the potential to impact outcome. Future investigations must address these concerns. A large, multicentered, randomized, controlled trial using sensitive and reliable outcome measurements may provide a more accurate appraisal of therapeutic efficacy.[95]

With growing evidence that the cortical regions can be shaped by current needs and experiences, and evidence that infants can "outgrow" CP or at least diminish its impact, there is reason to believe that early intervention, regardless of therapy type, is extremely beneficial.[11,12]

Prognosis

When first confronted with the fact that their child has CP, parents frequently focus on future expectations. At the time of initial diagnosis, a clear forecast for future growth, development, and care needs may not be possible. However, no one but a well-informed, compassionate physician is in a better position to understand and give guidance about this condition. Patients and families need to clearly understand that CP is not a disease, but rather a static, nonprogressive injury. The importance of early intervention and therapy should be stressed. The 30-year survival rate for individuals with CP is 87 percent, with significantly lower survival if spastic quadriparesis, seizures, and severe to profound MR are present.[98]

Despite the early difficulty predicting functional outcome, some rules of thumb, none of them absolute, can be successful. If a child with CP does not sit alone by 2.5 to 3 years of age, it is unlikely the child will walk independently. If ambulation is not achieved by age 6, independent ambulation is unlikely to occur.[28] Hemiparetic and athetotic children generally achieve independent ambulation. In spite of the fact that cerebral palsy can causes lifelong disabilities, patients, parents, and professionals should realize that many individuals with CP can have long, well-adjusted, and productive lives.

HYPOTONIC SYNDROMES

The introduction of histochemistry and electron microscopy in the 1950s and 1960s heralded the discovery of specific disorders causing hypotonia, the congenital myopathies. The development of chromosomal analysis and further advances in the field improved our capabilities of diagnosing hypotonic infants with entities such as Prader-Willi (PWS) and Down syndrome (DS). More recently, the fine detail available with magnetic resonance imaging has enabled us to identify other disorders associated with hypotonia such as a delay in myelination and structural abnormalities such as cerebellar hypoplasia and cerebellar hyperplasia.[99,100]

Prader-Willi Syndrome

The two most common genetic entities presenting with hypotonia are PWS and DS.[31] PWS was initially recognized in 1956. Associated gene deletions or translocations were not identified until the late 1970s. Infants present with marked hypotonia, mild dysmorphic features, and associated feeding difficulties. The hypotonia gradually improves and ambulation is achieved after 2 years of age. In the newborn period, the feeding difficulty is such that a feeding tube may be necessary. Ironically, after age 2, the infant develops hyperphagia and morbid obesity. Other complications include obstructive apnea, seizures, behavioral problems, and scoliosis, usually manageable without surgery.[31]

Down Syndrome

Trisomy 21 is the most common cause of mental retardation. Pronounced hypotonia, developmental delay, seizures, strokes, mental retardation, and atlantoaxial instability constitute the major features. Ambulation usually does not occur until after age 2, but the possibility of joint laxity resulting in atlantoaxial instability can not be fully evaluated until age 5. Therefore, caution with physical activities must be exercised. Instability occurs in up to 31 percent of individuals but subluxation and dislocation in only 1 to 2 percent of cases.[101]

Congenital Myopathies

The congenital myopathies are a diverse group of disorders in both pathology and onset of symptomatology.[31] Some cases clearly are congenital, but others do not present until childhood. Inheritance pattern varies. Nonprogression is the rule.

Presentation is often in the newborn period as a floppy infant lying with "frog" legs. Alternatively, the weakness may not be noted until early childhood, when either proximal girdle weakness becomes apparent or generalized body and face weakness predominates.

A complete discussion of congenital myopathies is beyond the scope of this text. Myotubular myopathy frequently involves ocular and facial muscles. Individuals with nemaline rod myopathy have an increased likelihood of associated dysmorphic features (kyphoscoliosis, pes cavus, high arched palate, long facies) and diaphragmatic weakness causing respiratory embarrassment. Central core disease causes a mild, nonprogressive muscle weakness and is associated with malignant hyperthermia. Congenital fiber type disproportion (CFTD) is a poorly defined entity and may be confused with spinal muscular atrophy and congenital myotonic dystrophy. Establishment and confirmation of the correct diagnosis is important for prognostication as CFTD presents with variable weakness neonatally but rarely progresses after 2 years of age.

Rehabilitation of the Hypotonic Child

Numerous rehabilitation issues are unique to hypotonic, developmentally delayed children. Early identification and therapy remain important, although cognitive development may be normal. Intervention is important in order to prevent nutritional, respiratory, and orthopedic complications of hypotonia.

Nutrition and Feeding

Failure to thrive may be the initial presentation because facial and naso-pharyngeal weakness may interfere with feedings. Severely hypotonic infants may require gavage feeds and the placement of a gastrostomy. Gastroesophageal reflux should be ruled out. After infancy, children with PWS may require behavioral or pharmacologic management for hyperphagia.

Therapies

Therapeutic goals include stimulating tone, improving gross and fine motor skills, and advancing developmental skills with proprioceptive stimulation NDT techniques. EI classes are often held for toddlers with DS. The occurrence of contractures caused by weakness can be prevented by teaching the family correct positioning and range-of-motion exercises. With onset of ambulation, gait should be evaluated for genu recurvatum caused by quadriceps femoris weakness. Genu recurvatum may lead to knee-joint deformity and pain. The use of ankle-foot orthoses to decrease ankle plantar flexion during ambulation can prevent knee hyperextension effectively. A spinal brace may prevent or stabilize scoliosis. Should contractures develop, surgical intervention may be needed.

Respiratory Dysfunction

Nocturnal hypoventilation may be under-diagnosed with congenital myopathies and PWS. Nocturnal hypoventilation may be evaluated with a sleep study. If pulmonary function is abnormal, the caregiver should be taught to perform chest physical therapy to promote bronchopulmonary hygiene.

SPINAL DYSRAPHIC SYNDROMES

Spinal dysraphism refers to the group of syndromes with spinal abnormalities caused by imperfect fusion of the midline mesenchymal, bony, and neural structures. Meningocele is the most common manifestation, with incomplete closure of the spinal canal and midline bony abnormalities, without nervous-system involvement. If the defect is repaired surgically, no neurological deficits remain.

Myelomeningocele (MMC) involves the spinal cord. The overall incidence of MMC in the United States has declined from 2.0 per 1000 births in 1968 to 0.2–0.4 per 1000 births in 1989.[102] The administration of folate prior to conception and during pregnancy has been instrumental in the decline.[103] Numerous anomalies and clinical deficits accompany MMC.

The incidence of hydrocephalus, a major complication of MMC, varies depending on the location of the lesion. It is as high as 90 percent with lesions above S1, and 60 percent in lesions located at or below S2.[104]

A Chiari II malformation accounts for many of the clinical deficits associated with MMC including hydrocephalus. A Chiari II malformation consists of an abnormally shaped and small fourth ventricle, caudal displacement of the lower cerebellum and medulla into the cervical canal, and tectal beaking. The malformation is noted in almost every case of thoracolumbar, lumbar, and lumbosacral myelomeningocele.[30]

Other clinical features in MMC are attributable to lower brain-stem anomalies involving cranial nerve nuclei, or compression and traction. One third of infants demonstrate feeding disturbances with dysphagia, laryngeal stridor, and abnormalities of ventilation (obstructive and central) with frank apnea and cyanosis.[105]

Bowel and bladder involvement is the rule with MMC. Careful urologic evaluation yields useful information as to the neurological function of the bladder. Both lower and upper motor neuron neurogenic bladders are common. Neonatal renal ultrasonography may detect the presence of renal and bladder malformations. A voiding cystourethrogram can demonstrate bladder function.

Significant post-void residual urine volume can lead to cystitis, ascending pylonephritis, nephrolithiasis, hydronephritis, and chronic renal failure. To prevent renal damage, regularly scheduled catheterization is important. Once children with MMC reach the age of 5, they should be instructed in self-catheterization. Regularly scheduled genitourinary ultrasonography, blood urea nitrogen, creatinine, and urinalysis are essential components of safe monitoring. Chronic constipation occurs frequently and is managed by a high-fiber diet, stool softeners, and enemas.

Major causes of death in this population include

pneumonia, shunt infections, sudden death, and urosepsis if the individual is prone to frequent urinary-tract infections. End-stage renal disease, decubitus ulceration, and osteomyelitis are also important causes of morbidity and mortality.

Rehabilitation

Early and continued intervention in MMC is important for stimulating development. Home exercises administered under therapists' guidance prevent contractures and optimize upper-body strength. Adaptive equipment for activities of daily living and gait are essential. Ambulation may be a goal if quadriceps femoris and hip adductor strength are present and adequate, corresponding to an L3–L4 level or below. Depending on the degree and extent of weakness, braces may be required in conjunction with forearm crutches.

Most MMC patients require use of a wheelchair. Sensation is diminished in the lower extremities, increasing the likelihood of decubitus ulcer formation. Selection of the seat cushion is crucial in prevention of decubitus ulcer formation. Training in periodic weight shifting while sitting may decrease the likelihood of developing decubiti.

Scoliosis is a major complication of myelomeningocele. The incidence depends on the level of the lesion. Children with lesions above L2 typically have scoliosis significant enough to require surgical intervention. Those with lesions below S1 rarely encounter this complication.[30] Once a curve reaches 50 degrees, the rate of progression increases. Bracing and adequate sitting support may assist in stabilizing the degree of curvature.

Behavior

With the current use of selective, aggressive, early surgical intervention, more than 80 percent of children with MMC have an IQ over 80.[30] Yet, behavioral problems, low self-esteem, and hyperactivity are common. Various language disorders occur in children with MMC, such as echolalia, "cocktail party syndrome," and deficits in the use and understanding of language, even in children with normal intelligence.[106]

REFERENCES

1. Kurtz L, Scull S: Rehabilitation for developmental disabilities. *Ped Clin No Am* 1993; 40(3):629.

2. Russman BS: Are infant stimulation programs useful? *Arch Neurol* 1986; 43:282.

3. Pellegrino L: Cerebral palsy: A paradigm for developmental disabilities. *Dev Med Child Neurol* 1995; 37:834.

4. Fujimoto S, Yokochi K, Togari H, Nishimura Y, et al: Neonatal cerebral infarction: Symptoms, CT findings and prognosis. *Brain Dev* 1992; 14:48.

5. Wulfeck BB, Trauner DA, Tallal PA: Neurologic, cognitive, and linguistic features of infants after early stroke. *Pediatr Neurol* 1991; 7:266.

6. Ment LR, Duncan CC, Ehrenkranz RA: Perinatal cerebral infarction. *Ann Neurol* 1984; 16:559.

7. Piper MC, Mazer B, Silver KM, et al: Resolution of neurological symptoms in high-risk infants during the first two years of life. *Dev Med Child Neurol* 1988; 30:26.

8. Nelson KB, Ellenberg JH: Children who "outgrew" cerebral palsy. *Pediatrics* 1982; 69:539.

9. Buchwald JS: Comparison of plasticity in sensory and cognitive processing systems. *Clin Perinatol* 1990; 17(1):57.

10. Carpenter MD: *The Cerebral Cortex: Core Text of Neuroanatomy* 4th ed. Baltimore: Williams & Wilkins, 1991, Chap 13, pp. 404–422.

11. Spinelli DN: Plasticity triggering experiences, nature, and the dual genesis of brain structure and function. *Clin Perinatol* 1990; 17(1):77.

12. Elbert T, Pantev C, Wienbruch C, et al: Increased cortical representation of the fingers of the left hand in string players. *Science* 1995; 270:305.

13. Farmer SF, Harison LM, Ingram DA, et al: Plasticity of central motor pathways in children with hemiplegic cerebral palsy. *Neurology* 1991; 41:1505.

14. Merline, K: Cell death of corticospinal neurons is induced by axotomy before but not after innervation of spinal targets. *J Comp Neurol* 1990; 296:506.

15. Kirby RS, Swanson ME, Kelleher KJ, et al: Identifying at-risk children for early intervention services: Lesson from the infant health and development program. *J Pediatr* 1993; 122(5):680.

16. Schelly C, Sample P, Spencer K: The Americans with Disabilities Act of 1990 expands employment opportunities for persons with developmental disabilities. *Am J Occup Ther* 1992; 46(5):457.

17. Wehman P, Revell G, Kregel J, et al: Supported employment: An alternative model for vocational rehabilitation of persons with severe neurologic, psychiatric, or physical disability. *Arch Phys Med Rehabil* 1991; 72:101.

18. Scher MS, Belfar H, Martin J, et al: Destructive brain lesions of presumed fetal onset: Antepartum causes of cerebral palsy. *Pediatrics* 1991; 88(5):898.

19. Freeman JM, Avery G, Brann AW, et al: Special article: National institutes of health report on causes of mental retardation and cerebral palsy. *Pediatrics* 1985; 76(3):457.

20. Freeman JM, Nelson K: Special articles: Intrapartum asphyxia and cerebral palsy. *Pediatrics* 1988; 82(2)240.

21. Nelson KB, Ellenberg JH: Antecedents of cerebral palsy. *AJDC* 1985; 139:1031.

22. Nelson KB, Ellenberg JH: Antecedents of cerebral palsy. *N Engl J Med* 986; 315:81.

23. Nelson KB: What proportion of cerebral palsy is related to birth asphyxia? *J Pediatr* 1988; 112(4):572.

24. Nelson KB: Prenatal origin of hemiparetic cerebral palsy: How often and why? *Pediatrics* 1991; 88:1059.

25. Reilly S, Skuse D: Characteristics and management of feeding problems of young children with cerebral palsy. *Dev Med Child Neurol* 1992; 34:379.

26. Gingold M, Jaynes M, Bodensteiner JB: The evolution of the plantar response in infancy. *Neurology* 1996; 46:A15.

27. Paine RS, Oppé TE: *Reflexes, Responses and Infantile Automatisms. Neurological Examination of Children.* Lavenham, UK: Lavenham Press Ltd., 1966, Chap XII, pp. 171–195.

28. Eicher PS, Batshaw ML: Cerebral palsy. *Pediatr Clin No Am* 1993; 40(3):537.

29. Nelson KB, Ellenberg JH: Neonatal signs as predictors of cerebral palsy. *Pediatrics* 1979; 64:225.

30. Volpe JJ: *Neurology of the Newborn*, 3rd ed. Philadelphia: W.B. Saunders Co., 1995, Chap 9, pp. 338–366.

31. Dubowitz V: *The Floppy Infant Syndrome: Muscle Disorders in Childhood,* 2nd ed. London: W.B. Saunders Co Ltd., 1995, Chap 12, pp. 457–472.

32. Clydesdale TT, Fahs IJ, Kilgore KM, et al: Social dimensions to functional gain in pediatric patients. *Arch Phys Med Rehabil* 1990; 71:469

33. Craft MJ, Lakin JA, Oppliger RA, et al: Siblings as change agents for promoting the functional status of children with cerebral palsy. *Dev Med Child Neurol* 1990; 32:1049.

34. Ferry PC: Infant stimulation programs: A neurologic shell game? *Arch Neurol* 1986; 43:281.

35. Bobath K: A neurophysiological basis for the treatment of cerebral palsy, in *Clinics in Developmental Medicine.* Philadelphia: J.B. Lippincott, 1980.

36. Ayres AJ: *Sensory Integration and Learning Disorders.* Los Angeles: Western Psychological Services, 1972.

37. Matthews DJ: Controversial therapies in the management of cerebral palsy. *Pediatr Annals* 1988; 17(12):762.

38. Doman RJ, Spitz EB, Zueman E, et al: Children with severe brain injuries. *JAMA* 1960; 174:257.

39. Sparrow S, Zigler E: Evaluation of a patterning treatment for retarded children. *Pediatrics* 1978; 62(2):137.

40. Merletti R, Andina A, Galante M, et al: Clinical experience of electronic peroneal stimulations in 50 hemiparetic patients. *Scand J Rehab Med* 1979; 11:111.

41. Finley WW, Niman CA, Standley J, et al: Electrophysiologic behavior modifications of frontal EMG in cerebral palsied children. *Biofeedback Self Reg* 1977; 2:59.

42. Horn EM, Warren ST, Jones HA: An experimental analysis of a neurobehavioral motor intervention. *Dev Med Child Neurol* 1995; 37:697.

43. Gillberg C: *Clinical Child Neuropsychiatry.* New York: Cambridge University Press, 1995.

44. Lovell RW, Reiss AL: Dual diagnoses: Psychiatric disorders in developmental disabilities. *Pediatr Clin No Am* 1993; 40(3):579.

45. Jolleff N, McConachie H, Winyard S, et al: Communication aids for children: Procedures and problems. *Dev Med Child Neurol* 1992; 34:719.

46. Peacock WJ, Arens LJ, Berman B: Cerebral palsy spasticity: Select posterior rhizotomy. *Pediatr Neurosci* 1987; 13:61.

47. Koman LA, Mooney JF, Smith BP, et al: Management of spasticity in cerebral palsy with botulinum-A toxin: Report of a preliminary, randomized, double-blind trial. *J Pediatr Orthop* 1994; 14(3):299.

48. Dudgeon BJ, Libby AK, McLaughlin JF, et al: Prospective measurement of functional changes after selective dorsal rhizotomy. *Arch Phys Med Rehabil* 1994; 75:46.

49. Kinghorn J: Upper extremity functional changes following selective posterior rhizotomy in children with cerebral palsy. *Am J Occup Ther* 1992; 46(6):502.

50. Landau W, Weaver R, Hornbein T: Fusimotor nerve function in man. *Arch Neurol* 1960; 3:32.

51. Hugenholtz H, Humphreys P, McIntyre W, et al: Cervical spinal cord stimulation for spasticity in cerebral palsy. *Neurosurgery* 1988; 22(4):707.

52. Pen RD, Myklebust BM, Gottlieb GL, et al: Chronic cerebellar stimulation for cerebral palsy: Prospective and double-blind studies. *J Neurosurg* 1980; 53:160.

53. Albright AL, Cervi A, Singletary J: Intrathecal baclofen for spasticity in cerebral palsy. *JAMA* 1991; 265(11):1418.

54. Koop SE, Lonstein JE, Winter RB, Denis F: The natural history of spine deformity in cerebral palsy. *Dev Med Child Neurol* 1990; 33:19.

55. Mallory Jr G, Stillwell P: The ventilator-dependent child: Issues in diagnosis and management. *Arch Phys Med Rehab* 1991; 72:43.

56. Iannaccone ST: Cerebral palsy, in Good DC, Couch FR (eds): *Handbook of Neurorehabilitation.* New York: Marcel Dekker, 1994, pp. 619–635.

57. Rang M, Wright J: What have 30 years of medical progress done for cerebral palsy? *Clin Ortho Rel Res* 1989; 247:55.

58. Turner S, Sloper P: Paediatricians' practice in disclosure and follow-up of severe physical disability in young children. *Dev Med Child Neurol* 1992; 34:348.

59. Gisel E, Applegate-Ferante T, Benson J, et al: Effect of oral sensorimotor treatment on measures of growth, eating efficiency and aspiration in the dysphagic child with cerebral palsy. *Dev Med Child Neurol* 1995; 37:528.

60. Barabas G, Matthews W, Zumoff P: Care-load for children and young adults with severe cerebral palsy. *Dev Med Child Neurol* 1992; 34:979.

61. Stringel G, Delgado M, Guertin L, et al: Gastrostomy and Nissen fundoplication in neurologically impaired children. *J Pediatr Surg* 1989; 24(10):1044.

62. Gisel E, Applegate-Ferante T, Benson J, et al: Oral senso-

rimotor treatment on measures of growth, eating efficiency and aspiration in the dysphagic child with cerebral palsy. *Dev Med Child Neurol* 1995; 37:528.

63. Koheil R, Sochaniwskyj A, Bablich K, et al: Biofeedback techniques and behavior modification in the conservative remediation of drooling by children with cerebral palsy. *Dev Med Child Neurol* 1987; 29:19.

64. Reddihough D, Johnson H, Staples M, et al: Use of benzhexol hydrochloride to control drooling of children with cerebral palsy. *Dev Med Child Neurol* 1990; 32:985.

65. Siegel LK, Klingbeil MA: Control of drooling with transdermal scopolamine in a child with cerebral palsy. *Dev Med Child Neurol* 1991; 33:1010.

66. Webb K, Reddihough DS, Johnson H, et al: Long-term outcome of saliva-control surgery. *Dev Med Child Neurol* 1995; 37:755.

67. Coleby M: The School-aged siblings of children with disabilities. *Dev Med Child Neurol* 1995; 37:415.

68. Korpela R, Seppanen RL, Koivikko M: Technical aids for daily activities: A regional survey of 204 disabled children. *Dev Med Child Neurol* 1992; 34:985.

69. Greiner BM, Czerniecki JM, Deitz JC: Gait parameters of children with spastic diplegia: A comparison of effects of posterior and anterior walkers. *Arch Phys Med Rehab* 1993(Apr); 74(4):381.

70. Katz K, Liebertal M, Erken EHW: Seat insert for cerebral-palsied children with total body involvement. *Dev Med Child Neurol* 1988; 30:222.

71. Myhr U, Vendt LV, Norrlin S, et al: Five-year follow-up of functional sitting position in children with cerebral palsy. *Dev Med Child Neurol* 1995; 37:587.

72. Myhr U, Wendt LV: Improvement of functional sitting position for children with cerebral palsy. *Dev Med Child Neurol* 1991; 33:246.

73. Noronha J, Bundy A, Groll J: The effect of positioning on the hand function of boys with cerebral palsy. *Am J Occup Ther* 1989; 43(8):507.

74. Pope PM, Bowes CE, Booth E: Postural control in sitting: The Sam system: Evaluation of use over three years. *Dev Med Child Neurol* 1994; 36:241.

75. Cosgrove AP, Corry IS, Graham HK: Botulinum toxin in the management of the lower limb in cerebral palsy. *Dev Med Child Neurol* 1994; 36:386.

76. Chutorian A, Root L: Management of spasticity in children with botulinum-A toxin. *Int Pediatr* 1994; 9(Suppl 1):35.

77. Calderon-Gonzalez R, Calderon-Sepulveda R, Rincon-Reyes M, et al: Botulinum toxin A in management of cerebral palsy. *Pediatr Neurol* 1994; 10(4):284.

78. Carpenter EB: Role of nerve blocks in the foot and ankle in cerebral palsy: Therapeutic and diagnostic. *Foot Ankle* 1983; 4:164.

79. Carpenter EB, Seitz DG: Intra-muscular alcohol as an aid in management of spastic cerebral palsy. *Dev Med Child Neurol* 1980; 22:497.

80. Duchen LW, Strich SJ: The effect of botulinum toxin on the pattern of innervation of skeletal muscle in the mouse. *Quart J Exp Physiol* 1968; 53:84.

81. Bhushan V, Paneth N, Kiely J: Impact of improved survival of very low birth weight infants on recent secular trends in the prevalence of cerebral palsy. *Pediatrics* 1993; 91(6):1094.

82. Kleinman JC, Fowler MG, Kessel SS: Comparison of infant mortality among twin and singletons: United States, 1960 and 1983. *Am J Epidemiol* 1991; 133:133.

83. Little WJ: On the influence of abnormal parturition, difficult labors, premature birth, and physical condition of the child, especially in relation to deformities. *Trans Obstetr Soc Lond* 1861–1862; 3:293–344.

84. Freud S: *Infantile Cerebral Paralysis* (1897) (L. Russian, Trans.). Coral Gables, FL: Univ of Miami Press, 1968.

85. Nelson KB, Ellenberg JH: Apgar scores as predictors of chronic neurologic disability. *Pediatrics* 1981; 68:36.

86. Burke C, Tannenberg A: Prenatal brain damage and placental infarction: An autopsy. *Dev Med Child Neurol* 1995; 37:555.

87. Painter MJ: Animal model of perinatal asphyxia: Contributions, contradictions, clinical relevance. *Semi Peds Neurol* 1995; 2(1):37.

88. Pharoah PO, Cooke T, Rosenbloom L, et al: Effects of birth weight, gestational age, and maternal obstetric history on birth prevalence of cerebral palsy. *Arch Dis Child* 1987; 62:1035.

89. Damino D, Vaughan C, Abel M: Muscle response to heavy resistance exercise in children with spastic cerebral palsy. *Dev Med Child Neurol* 1995; 37:731.

90. Partridge C, Cornall CA, Lynch ME, et al: *Physical Therapies: Neurological Rehabilitation*. Edinburgh: Churchill Livingstone, 1993, Chap 17, pp. 189–198.

91. DeGangi G, Royeen CB: Current practice among neurodevelopmental treatment association members. *Am J Occup Ther* 1994; 48(9):803.

92. Palmer FB, Shapiro BK, Wachtel RC, et al: The effects of physical therapy on cerebral palsy. *N Engl J Med* 1988; 318:803.

93. Parette H, Hourcade JJ: A review of therapeutic intervention research on gross and fine motor progress in young children with cerebral palsy. *Am J Occup Ther* 1984; 38(7):462.

94. Piper MC, Kunos VI, Willis DM, et al: Early physical therapy effects on the high-risk infant: A randomized controlled trial. *Pediatrics* 1986; 78(2):216.

95. Tirosh E, Rabino S: Physiotherapy for children with cerebral palsy. *AJDC* 1989; 143:552.

96. Bower E, McLellan DL: Evaluating therapy in cerebral palsy and child care. *Health Dev* 1994; 20:409.

97. Brown JK: Editorial: Too few cooks: Too many cooks. *Dev Med Child Neurol* 1992; 34:565.

98. Crichton JU, Mackinnon M, White CP: The life-expectancy of persons with cerebral palsy. *Dev Med Child Neurol* 1995; 567.

99. Shevell M, Majnemer A: Clinical features of develop-

mental disability associated with cerebellar hypoplasia. *Ann Neurol* 1995; 38:528.

100. Bodensteiner JB, Schaefer GB, Keller GM, et al: Cerebellar hyperplasia: Clinical features of a newly recognized anomaly, presented at the CNS/Society for Pediatric Pathology Joint Poster Session (24th Annual Meeting of the CNS), October 28th 1995, Baltimore, MD.

101. Pueschel SM: Atlanto-axial instability and Down Syndrome. *Pediatrics* 1981; 81:879.

102. Yen IH, Khoury MJ, Erickson JD, et al: The changing epiderm of neural tube defects: The United States, 1968–1989. *Am J Dis Child* 1992; 146:857.

103. Milunsky A, Jick H, Jick S, et al: Multivitamin/folic acid supplements in early pregnancy reduces the prevalence of neural tube defects. *JAMA* 1989; 262:2847.

104. Lorber J: Systematic ventriculographic studies in infants born with meningomyelocele and encephalocele. *Arch Dis Child* 1961; 36:381.

105. McLone DG, Dias L, Kaplan WE, et al: Concepts in the management of spina bifida. In Marlin, AE (ed): *Concept in Pediatric Neurosurgery*, vol 5. Basel: Karger, 97, 1989, p. 97.

106. Dennis M, Barnes MA: Oral discourse after early-onset hydrocephalus linguistic ambiguity, figurative language, speech acts and script-based references. *J Pediatr Psychol* 1993; 18:639.

Chapter 12

MULTIPLE SCLEROSIS AND PARKINSON'S DISEASE REHABILITATION

John A. Orsini
Mary L. Dombovy

MULTIPLE SCLEROSIS REHABILITATION

Multiple sclerosis (MS) is the third leading cause of disablility in adults from 20 to 50 years of age. In this respect it trails only trauma and arthritis.

MS is an aquired disease of the central nervous system characterized by destruction of the myelin sheaths of the nerve fibers, a relative sparing of other elements of nervous tissue, an infiltration of inflammatory cells in a perivascular distribution, and a distribution of lesions that is often periventricular. These scattered inflammatory and demyelinating central nervous system lesions result in combinations of motor, sensory, coordination, and cognitive impairments. The prognosis is quite difficult to predict. The course can range from occasional mild relapses resulting in minimal to no disability to total disability within a few months.[1]

Neurologic dysfunction is primarily the result of partial, complete, or intermittent block of nerve conduction through demylinated areas, and in the case of acute excerbation, through areas of acute inflamation. Recovery of function may be due to a number of circumstances, including the following: resolution of inflammation, decrease in edema, removal of various theoretical humoral factors, partial remyelination, conduction through demyelinated axons, and rerouting of nerve transmission through alternative pathways.[2–5]

Incidence

The incidence of MS in the United States is at least 8000 cases per year. It is higher in women than men at a 1.7:1 ratio. Aproximately two out of three cases of MS present between the ages of 20 and 40. In the smaller number of people in whom the disease develops late in adult life, the early symptoms may have been forgotten or never declared themselves. In contrast the incidence

of MS in children is very low; only 0.3 to 0.4 percent of all cases occur during the first decade.[1]

Prevalence

Multiple sclerosis is one of the most prevalent neurologic diseases. Up to 350,000 persons in the United States are diagnosed with MS. The disease has a geographically variable prevalence of less than 1 per 100,000 in equatorial areas; 6 to 14 per 100,000 in the southern United States and southern Europe; and 30 to 80 per 100,000 in Canada, northern Europe, and the northern United States. Similar geographic gradients are seen in other parts of the globe. In the United States African Americans have a lower risk than whites but the geographic gradient is similar for both races. The work of Dean and Kurtzke indicate that persons who migrate from an area of high risk to one of lower risk bring with them at least part of the risk of their place of origin. For instance the prevalence in native white South Africans was 3 to 11 per 100,000, whereas the prevalence in immigrants from northern Europe was about 50 per 100,000, similar to that in their country of origin. Also, persons who immigrated before 15 years of age had a risk similar to that of native South Africans, whereas those who immigrated after this age had a risk more similar to that of their place of birth.[6]

A Leading Cause of Disability

Multiple sclerosis is the most commonly diagnosed disabling neurologic disorder of young to middle-aged adults and the third leading cause of significant disability in this age group, after trauma and arthritis. More severely disabled patients are more likely to be seen by health care professionals. As a result the prognosis for function is better than what may be generally assumed.

Eighty-five percent of MS patients have a normal life expectancy and more than 65 percent will continue to ambulate for 20 or more years after diagnosis.[2,7–9]

The National Center for Health Statistics conducts a periodic study in which they interview people throughout the United States to identify illnesses that they might have and functional limitations that they experience as a result of these illnesses. The condition that causes limitation in the highest proportion of cases is mental retardation. Eighty-five percent of people with mental retardation have some functional limitation. MS is a close second, with 77 percent reporting that MS produces some functional limitation in their everyday lives.[10]

Presentation

The diagnosis of MS requires that symptoms be disseminated throughout the central nervous system (CNS) and over a period of time. This fact is reflected in its varied temporal and symptomatic presentation and course. In half of the patients the initial symptoms are weakness or numbness in one or more limbs. In perhaps as many as 40 percent, symptoms may initially evolve over a matter of hours; over days in another 30 percent; and over weeks to months in 20 percent. A slow and insidious onset with steady progression may be seen in another 10 percent, who are also those most likely to be over 45 years of age. Posterior column involvement may result in tingling of the extremities and band-like paresthesias about the trunk or limbs. Weakness or ataxia often present as a spastic or ataxic paraparesis. Upper tract signs of hyperreflexia and extensor plantor responses may appear later, whereas abdominal reflexes may disappear early. Lhermitte's sign (electric-like tingling down the back with passive neck flexion) may be seen as well. Optic neuritis, often evolving to partial or total vision loss in one eye over hours or days, is the initial manifestation in about one quarter of all patients. A myriad of other neurologic symptoms and signs may less often signal the onset of MS. Included in this list are (in descending order of frequency): unsteadiness in walking, nystagmus, diplopia, vertigo, vomiting, disorders of micturition, overt hemiplegia, trigeminal neuralgia or other pain syndromes, facial paralysis, deafness, or seizures (Table 12-1).[1]

Certain clinical syndromes are noted in established cases. One-half of these will be that of a mixed picture, with signs pointing to involvement of the optic nerves, brainstem, cerebellum, and spinal cord. Primarily spinal disease is seen in 30 to 40 percent, and a

Table 12-1

Common signs and associated symptoms in the presentation of multiple sclerosis (by system)[a]

System symptoms	Signs
Motor/Cerebellar	
Feeling weak in specific distribution	Weakness on manual muscle test
Feeling uncoordinated/ clumsy	Ataxia, dysmetria, spasticity
Speech difficulties	Dysarthia
Coughing during or after meals	Dysphagia
Sensory	
Numbness/Paresthesias/ Pain	Altered sensory testing or exam
	Lhermitte sign
	Trigeminal neuralgia
Bladder	
Urgency/Hesitancy	Frequency/Incontinence
Sexual/Herniatal	
Decreased libido	Impotence
Impaired sensation	Decreased vaginal lubrication
Visual	
Diplopia/Dizziness	Nystagmus/Dysconjugate gaze
Cognitive/Affective	
Foregetfulness	Impaired memory on cognitive testing
Feelings of inability to focus or pay attention	Impaired attention and concentration on mental status testing
Unusual emotional status	Lability/Euphoria/Depression altered affect
Other	
Complaints of low energy level/Feeling tired	Easy fatigibility
Heat intolerance	Impaired strength/Function with elevated body temperature (e.g., fever, bathtub)

[a]Adapted from Cobble.[2]

predominantly cerebellar or pontobulbar-cerebellar form will be seen in about five percent of cases.[1] Multiple sclerosis is progressive in the vast majority of patients, but the course varies considerably. Within 15 years of onset, approximately 50 percent of persons reach a

Kurtzke Expanded Disability Status Scale of 6.[11] Life expectancy is definitely, but not largely, reduced in the general MS population. Approximately 75 percent of patients with the diagnosis will be alive 25 years after onset. One study showed that among patients seen in MS clinics, the overall life expectancy for a cohort under the age of 60 (excluding suicide) is approximately six to seven years less than for the non-MS population.[12]

The pathophysiology of MS consists of inflammatory white matter lesions that continuously appear, resolve, and recur, even during periods of apparent quiesence. Immunocompetent lymphocytes and macrophages enter the CNS, initially, as a result of disruption of the blood-brain barrier secondary to antigenic stimulation. Edema characterizes acute and active lesions. Early discrete areas of periventricular white matter inflammation enlarge by outward extension and coalescence. Myelin lamellae are stripped away by activated macrophages. Axons eventually are left bare, but they most often remain fairly well preserved even in chronic lesions. Eventually, residual gliotic areas or plaques accumulate, scattered throughout the CNS. Older plaques are progressively less inflammatory. The firm sclerotic texture of the older plaque comes about as oligodendrocytes are destroyed and astrocytes proliferate, producing glial fibers.[2,13,14] Studies of serial magnetic resonance imaging (MRI) in patients with relapsing-remitting disease have shown that relapse rate significantly underestimates disease activity as detected by MRI.

In two separate studies the degree of disease activity in relapsing patients as detected by MRI was shown to be as high as five times the clinical relapse rate.[4,15–17] Partial, complete, or intermittent block of nerve conduction through demyelinated areas is the cause of the characteristic neurologic dysfunction. A nerve impulse reaching a demyelinated area is unable to continue by either saltatory or sequential conduction. Electrical current may "leak out" of the demyelinated segments, preventing the buildup of sufficient electrical potential to depolarize the next internode for saltatory conduction. The demyelinated region also cannot conduct current sequentially, because the internode axon membrane lacks the necessary sodium–potassium channels.[2–5]

Etiology

The etiology of MS is unknown, but characteristics of people at higher risk for MS have been identified (Table 12-2). The best evidence for etiology suggests exposure to a common environmental agent that triggers a dysreg-

Table 12-2
Risk factors for developing multiple sclerosis[a]

Gender	Women are two times more likely than men to have multiple sclerosis.
Family history	Risk is greatest in those with siblings with the disease.
Age	Midlife. People between 20 and 40 years of age.
Race	European ancestry has a greater risk than African ancestry. Asians have the lowest risk.
Location	Residence before age 15 in a temperate climate.

[a]Adapted from Cobble.[2]

ulated immune response in genetically susceptible people.[2,18] The agent has not been identified, but a virus is most often suspected. A virus theoretically could persist in the CNS with intermittent reactivation or it could induce a dysregulated autoimmune response.[2,19]

Diagnosis (Table 12-3)

Multiple sclerosis is only one among several diseases and syndromes that may present with neurologic signs and symptoms of dissemination in time and space. For all patients seen in a comprehensive care setting, there should be a reconfirmation of diagnosis by review of history, laboratory studies, and currrent neurologic exam. The differential diagnosis in this setting includes, but is not limited to, neoplastic disease of primary or metastatic nature, vascular disease, vasculitic and connective tissue diseases, spirochetal and other chronic infections, HIV, HTLV-1, Vitamin B_{12} deficiency, chronic immune disseminated polyneuropathy (CIDP), and cervical spondylopathy.[2,20,21,22] Historical, clinical, and or laboratory findings must demonstrate that lesions of the white matter have occurred in multiple areas on more than one occasion. Primarily, diagnosis is based on history and clinical signs with laboratory and paraclinical studies (e.g., electrophysiologic studies) offering supportive evidence.[2,23] Most commonly, laboratory evidence consists of the demonstration of cerebrospinal fluid (CSF) immunologic abnormalities and includes increased CNS immunoglobulin production and CSF oligoclonal bands in the absence of serum bands. Cerebrospinal fluid oligoclonal bands are present in 90 to 98 percent of patients with clinically definite MS but are

Table 12-3
Diagnostic testing in multiple sclerosis[a]

Clinical test (by type)	Findings/interpretations
Cerebrospinal fluid analysis	Increased proteins or cells; oligoclonal bands; indicative of immune activation. Myelin basic protein/indicative of myelin breakdown.
Electrophysiologic Testing VER BAER SSEP Blink Reflex	Prolonged latency may expose clinically silent lesions.
EMG/NCS	May rule out myopathy/periphal neuropathy.
EEG	Rule out seizure disorder.
Imaging MRI	Most sensitive to multiple lesions of various size. Useful to rule out other CNS pathology (e.g., tumor, CSF obstruction).
CT with contrast	May demonstrate active lesions with breakdown of blood–brain barrier (also may be useful to rule out other CNS pathology).

[a]Adapted from Cobble.[2]

also found in other neurologic diseases of immunologic or viral origin. Other CSF findings in MS include elevated myelin basic protein, representing active but nonspecific demyelination during exacerbations.[2,24,25] Evoked responses (visual, auditory, somatosensory) may be helpful in identifying disseminated disease when only one lesion is evident clinically but MS is suspected by history and other clinical evidence.[8,25] CNS imaging can offer supportive evidence also. MRI is more sensitive than CT, yet may still be negative in early, mild MS, when supportive evidence would be most helpful. Although MRI cannot specifically differentiate MS lesions from other etiologies, it is helpful to note that MS lesions tend to localize to periventricular white matter, the corpus collosum, or infratentorially to the cerebellar peduncles. When active inflammation is present, the lesions will enhance with gadolinium.[2,26–29] The clinical course is the most important factor in the diagnosis of MS, since all laboratory related evidence is nonspecific.

Medical Treatment of Multiple Sclerosis

The primary goal of medical treatment of MS is to decrease the severity, number, and length of exacerbations. Inversely, this may be looked at as decreasing the time to recovery from an exacerbation. Most medical therapies are immune-modulating in nature. Many have shown modest positive effects, but not without toxicity. There is no single appropriate treatment. This fact is owing to a rapidly changing field in which none of the treatments has gained universal acceptance. A specialist in the medical treatment of MS should be consulted before initiating any of these therapies. Betaseron has recently been approved for the treatment of relapsing-remitting MS in ambulatory patients. One of the most common treatments for severe exacerbations and for progressive MS is high-dose intravenous methylprednisolone given at 1 gram a day for no more than 10 days in single or divided doses. A 10- to 30-day taper with oral prednisone or dexamethasone usually follows. ACTH and oral steroids may reduce recovery time, but prednisone has been associated with an increased risk of recurrence of optic neuritis. Cyclophosphamide has significant toxic potential (leukopenia, hematuria, and infection especially), although it may diminish the progression of disease in some patients. Studies have shown mixed results using azathioprine (Imuran) for chronic progressive disease. Again toxicity (hepatotoxicity and leukopenia) can be a significant problem. Total lymphoid irradiation, once a promising treatment, has become less appealing because of toxicity. Although not approved by the Food and Drug Administration (FDA), cyclosporine has shown some benefit in chronic progressive disease. There have been reports, both positive and negative, regarding plasmapheresis. Neither of these are widely accepted treatments at this time. In addition to beta interferon, other interferons have been evaluated. Gamma interferon increases the risk of exacerbation. Alpha interferon has shown several positive results and has recently received FDA approval. Copolymer 1 (cop-1) and oral myelin basic protein are other potential treatments under study.[30]

Results of a physician survey indicated that most clinicians regularly use high-dose intravenous pulse methylprednisolone therapy for the treatment of acute exacerbations.[31] Oral prednisone still is used regularly by a majority of those sampled, despite the fact that patients with optic neuritis have a higher relapse rate when treated with oral corticosteroid, than when treated with either high-dose intravenous methylprednisolone therapy or placebo. A slight majority report the use of an oral prednisone taper following pulse intravenous steroids. Approximately one third of clinicians regularly administer the IV treatment at home, whereas the same proportion never does so.[31]

MEASUREMENT OF DISABILITY, PROGRESSION, AND OUTCOMES

Evaluation of measures of function in MS has been a consistent topic of discussion in medical literature. Areas of interest have included comparisons of functional assessment scales and assessment of disability rating scales.[32,33] Disagreement in rating neurologic impairment has led to discussions of the significance of the disability status scale, the importance of inclusion of tool inter- and intrarater reliability when using the Expanded Disability Status Scale (EDSS) as well as recent comparison of the EDSS and graded exercise performance.[33–37]

Historically the biggest difficulty in designing and carrying out therapeutic trials in MS rehabilitation has been the the absence of an ideal or uniform measurement of outcome. The Kurtzke EDSS has the advantage of wide familiarity and easy application, but it has many flaws. It is not a very sensitive measure of disease activity or progression. Even among progressing patients, the EDSS changes at a mean of only 0.5 points per year. The scale places excessive emphasis on ambulation and is nonlinear.[38] Interpretation of scores tends to be bimodal, and increments of progression are not measured evenly. For example, MS is progressive in the vast majority of patients, but the course varies considerably. Approximately 15 percent of persons with MS reach a Kurtzke EDSS score of 6 (requiring a unilateral aide to walk) by 15 years after onset of symptoms. Expressed differently, the median time to EDSS 6.0 is 15 years.[31] Perhaps most importantly, Kurtzke scores do not correlate well with other measures of clinical or functional status.[39]

The Minimal Record of Disability (MRD) for MS incorporates several physician and paramedical administered rating scales for evaluating MS disease status (including the widely used EDSS) and its effects on the patient's life. There is now general consensus in the use of this assessment tool as a rating scale for MS.[10] The best known and most frequently used scales incorporated in the MRD are the Kurtzke Expanded Disability Status Scale (EDSS) and the Kurtzke Functional Systems Score (FS), both administered by a physician.[10]

Also included is the Incapacity Status Scale (ISS), an activities of daily living scale typically administered by a nonphysician examiner.[10] The ISS has not been fully tested in a clinical trial in MS. Other rating instruments have been developed for MS but are not widely implemented.[40–46] The Functional Independence Measure (FIM) has been shown to accurately predict the burden of care in MS patients.

STUDIES OF REHABILITATION EFFECTIVENESS IN MS

Efficacy of Rehabilitation in MS

As economic pressures come to bear on our methodology of care for years to come, proof of the value of rehabilitation will be required. Which interventions are most beneficial and which are cost effective will need to be carefully considered.

One early study of MS rehabilitation evaluated the benefits of inpatient rehabilitation and the cost/benefits ratio.[47] Feigenson studied 20 inpatients with MS who received a comprehensive array of inpatient rehabilitative services, including medical care, nursing, physical therapy, occupational therapy, social work, psychology, and others. The average age was 44.8 years and average duration was 12.9 years. The average length of stay (with two outliers removed) was 39.6 ± 10.9 days. There was little or no change in impairment, that is, in the neurological dysfunction of the patients. However, improvement was seen in functional areas, such as self-care, transfers, ambulation, ability to manage a wheelchair, and homemaking. Of 20 measures, nine showed statistically significant improvement at $p < .05$.[47]

Reding et al. published a small study that considered whether MS patients who had been admitted to an acute care hospital for nonemergent problems could have been handled just as well in a rehabilitation hospital.[48] All patients were recruited from the MS center at a large university hospital, where the acute hospital group were inpatients. Using a retrospective chart review, the investigators found that 56 percent of 168 consecutive admissions to the acute hospital would have met standard criteria for admission to the involved rehabilitation facility. A comparison of outcome and costs was complete for 14 pairs of patients matched for sex and severity of MS who were hospitalized either at the acute hospital or at the rehabilitation facility. All 28 patients would have met the criteria for admission to the rehabilitation unit. Although those admitted for acute hospitalization had a higher per diem cost ($625 vs $364 in the rehabilitation facility), the shorter stay at the acute care facility (14 vs 35 days) made the inpatient rehabilitation more expensive. Outcomes were comparable. With inpatient rehabilitation stay shortening over the last few years for MS, inpatient MS rehabilitation cost effectivenesss has improved recently.[48]

Francabandera et al. studied 67 MS patients in order to compare the cost effectiveness of inpatient and outpatient MS rehabilitation.[49] Following informed consent, patients were randomized to either an inpatient or an outpatient setting. The services provided were similar to those in the Feigenson et al. study.[47] Outpatient treatment was provided by visiting nurse services and consisted mainly of nursing, physical therapy, and occupational therapy. The sample was 78 percent female, with an average age of 49 ± 11.6 and an average Expanded Disability Status Scale score (Kurtzke, 1983) of 7 ± 0.8. Although some of the patients were still ambulators, most were confined to wheelchairs.[49]

Evaluations were performed prior to admission and at 3, 6, 9, and 12 months following discharge. Length of stay for the inpatients was approximately three weeks, significantly less than in the Feigenson et al. study. The shorter length of stay probably reflected the evolution of MS rehabilitation and economic pressure of third-party payers. The measures included the Incapacity Status Scale (ISS), part of the MRD.[50] The ISS is very similar to the Barthel Index and covers activites of daily living, such as mobility and self-care ability. The second outcome measure was the number of hours paid assistance was required by each patient.[10] Three months following discharge, the inpatient group showed less disability on the ISS than the outpatient group. Over the next 9 months, both groups showed a gradual worsening of their disability. By 12 months, both groups were back where they had started and there was no difference between the two of them.[10] These results suggest an early advantage to inpatient rehabilitation that is lost in the long run, implying that MS patients may require periodic rehabilitation to most effectively maintain gains in function.[10] Carey et al. published their multicenter study that used the Revised Level of Rehabilitation Scale (LORS-II).[51] It looked at over 6,000 patients, fewer than 200 of which had MS. The result was a 16-point gain on the LORS-II for MS patients versus 24 for all other conditions, suggesting that MS patients do benefit from rehabilitation, but they differ substantially from other rehabilitation populations and may require a different approach.[51]

Greenspun et al. examined the impact of inpatient rehabilitation on mobility and ADL as measured by the Computerized Rehabilitation Data System (CRDS).[52] The average age of the patients was 42 years, and the average duration of their MS was 12.2 years. The inpatient stay ranged from 5 to 57 days, with an average of 28 days. Assessments were completed at admission, discharge, and 3 months following discharge in an uncontrolled study. "Dramatic" improvement in independence in most areas was observed. For example, at admission, 18 percent of patients were independent in ambulation, whereas at discharge, 75 percent were. Independence in transfers went from 58 to 82 percent, and in bathing from 39 to 70 percent. Most of these gains were sustained at 3-month follow up. Unfortunately, longer follow-up was not performed.[52]

Gehlsen et al. also studied rehabilitation effects looking specifically at gait in greater detail.[53] They looked at the effects, of a single form of treatment on a number of gait parameters. Their sample consisted of 11 MS patients. Their average score on Kurtzke's DSS was 4 ± 1. Treatment consisted of an aquatic exercise program three times per week for 10 weeks. This study also had no controls. Assessments were made just prior to the treatment, at mid-treatment, and immediately post-treatment. The lack of statistically significant improvements in the measured parameters in this study may relate to the small sample size. It was found that DSS scores were positively associated with step length and with hip and ankle joint excursion so that overall disability seemed to be correlated with with measurable deficits in specific parameters of gait.[53]

The question of the value of comprehensive rehabilitation in MS at the individual patient and at the community level remains only partially answered. It is difficult to draw firm conclusions concerning rehabilitation in MS because of the small number of studies and the methodological limitations of those that do exist. Future studies in this area might move in several directions. Many of the studies cited in this review used small samples out of convenience drawn from a single institution. To facilitate analysis and enhance statistical power, samples need to be larger. More multicentered studies are needed. Consistency of treatment protocols across facilities would provide for ease of comparison and generalization. Controlled studies are desperately needed. Objective measures should be used whenever possible.[10]

Although only a small number of studies have been completed, there is significant evidence that medical rehabilitation in many forms does have usefulness in the MS population. Medical rehabilitation of MS or any progressive neurologic disorder can be a costly intervention. However, regardless of progressiveness of the disease most patients decline slowly enough that rehabilitation intervention is warranted.[10]

GENERAL PRINCIPLES IN REHABILITATION OF MS

Rehabilitation of the MS patient is unique in several ways. It is a progressive disease and in this sense, patient care differs from the classic rehabilitation model of the static single event lesion such as seen in stroke, spinal cord injury, or brain injury. Its relapsing and remitting nature offers the rehabilitation team a complex moving target to aim at in setting treatment goals. Areas affected can involve a wide variety of functional systems in the CNS, including strength, mobility, cognition, and language ability. Deficits in these areas may impact on self-care, hygiene, bladder and bowel dysfunction, social roles, and self-image. It is the unpredictable nature of the progression and distribution of the lesion load that makes caring for these patients all the more challenging.

The theory behind rehabilitation of the MS patient is not much different from that of other neurologic injuries. There are still pre-lesion, lesion, and post-lesion factors. Much of the rehabilitation process is directed toward functional training through appropriately timed stimulation, with pharmacologic augmentation. Facilitation of new compensatory behavior through personal training and counseling aimed at community reintegration are emphasized. Symptomatic management of the various complications of the disease is a third target of rehabilitation intervention.

In approaching the rehabilitation evaluation for the MS patient, the physician and team must see the patient in the context of his or her disease. The pattern and pace of illness and response must be taken into consideration on an individualized basis. Rehabilitation goals should be keyed on the pattern of disease. The goals for one patient with slow progression of disease may differ considerably from another with more aggressive disease.[54] Functional status may vary during different times of the day or with medication effects, so that many patients can benefit from learning a range of skills, as well as appropriate timing of daily activities.

Most patients with longstanding MS know their disease well. Therefore, goal setting must be done with the patient as an active participant. Fatigue and weakness can be remediated through energy conservation techniques and simplification of tasks, as well as through the use of lightweight equipment of proper design.

Some rehabilitation treatment issues derive from the fact that MS is an illness that is likely to progress. The team is likely to work with a given patient more than once. It is important to try to treat into the future, predicting needs down the road when setting goals and prescribing equipment.[54]

The care of MS patients can be particularly intense. Because MS can be so multifaceted, the team will have a tendency to think that they must do everything. That is not possible, nor effective. The team must become comfortable with selecting, prioritizing, and focusing. It is also important for the team to appropriately define success. Over time, rehabilitation interventions help people regain or maintain some function in spite of overall disease progression. Multiple sclerosis can affect nearly every facet of existence, and it is therefore only natural for a compassionate team to be tempted to address every deficit for the patient. This is neither efficacious nor realistic. The team and especially its leader (the rehabilitation physician) must be able to prioritize and keep the team focused on the most important goals. Part of setting goals is defining success.[55] Defining success for an individual patient, as well as for the program as a whole, is important in maintaining team morale, in what may otherwise be perceived as a constantly losing battle against a disease that nearly always progresses.

Mobility and Strength

The physical therapist is, with appropriate physician guidance, the primary allied health professional concerned with mobility and strength. Mobility is intricately related to disability, function, and to predictions of the quality of life in MS.[34,55] Mobility includes ambulation (both conventional and wheelchair), transfers, coordination, sitting and standing balance, and bed mobility, among other skills.

Although MS-specific data on strength training is sparse, there is some evidence to indicate treatment benefit. A few MS-specific progressive resistive exercise studies have shown that gains in strength are possible.[56–58] Kraft et al. looked at eight MS patients. Four subjects had mild disease defined by EDSS less than or equal to 3.0 and four had more severe disease with EDSS greater than or equal to 6. Strength training was performed with each subject for 12 weeks in a classic progressive resistive fashion three times per week for 12 weeks. Quadriceps, hamstrings, biceps, and triceps were the muscle groups trained in all subjects. Significant increases in strength were observed in all muscle groups of the mildly involved subjects and in all but the quadriceps group of the more severely involved group.[56] The same subjects were evaluated for functional benefits from training. Mobility outcome measures were a self-selected ambulation velocity, stair climbing, and a sit to stand evaluation. Both mild and severe groups showed improvement in these measures, although significant changes were seen only in the mild group and only in the ambulation velocity. There were significant improvements in both groups in self-reported disability, as measured by the sickness impact profile (SIP).[59]

Although more work is needed in this area, strength training should be considered in appropriate patients. Different types of exercise, including balance treatments, coordination, and conditioning, all may have important places in the treatment of MS patients. Exercise prescriptions should be complete and precise, safe, and efficacious. Rest periods should be interspersed with exercise. Exercise programs need to be reassessed frequently, because progression is slow for many patients. Feedback is important for reasonable goal-setting. Reassessment also may serve as an opportunity to monitor for safety and efficacy.[54] Strengthening exercises in muscles supplied by severely demyelinated axons may have little usefulness. However, strengthening unaffected or mildly affected muscle groups may be helpful and may compensate for severely affected muscle groups.[30]

Drug Treatment for Weakness   There are currently no available medications to treat weakness, although 4-aminopyridine and 3,4-diaminopepidine are promising. These potassium channel blockers increase the transmission of impulses along demyelinated axons. In fact, they may be useful for many nonmotoric symptoms of MS. However, they do not affect the course of the disease.[30]

Incoordination, Ataxia, and Tremor

Incoordination, ataxia, and tremor may result from lesions of the cerebellum and its connections, the brain stem or dorsal columns. Associated impairments may include an ataxic gait, truncal ataxia, head or trunk titubation, intention tremor, dysmetria, dysarthria, and dysphagia. Propranolol, clonazepam, primidone glutethemide, and isoniazid are worth considering if the tremors are functionally disabling.[30] Compensatory strategies are emphasized in the physical therapeutic

interventions. These include balance and coordination retraining and relaxation, as well as weighted cuffs and mobility equipment. Ease of fatiguability and weakness may limit the usefulness of some forms of exercise.[2,60]

Paroxysmal Activity

Paroxysmal activity is often underdiagnosed. However, intermittent ataxia, intermittent pain, dysarthria, or "clonic spinal cord seizures" often are easily treated with anticonvulsants such as carbamazepine.[30]

Balance

Balance too may be affected by cerebellar and associated lesions, brain stem, and posterior column involvement. Because balance is a response of the body to outside forces, the weakness of pyramidal tract lesions may also affect it. The practitioner survey by Chan et al. found a wide variety of assessment and treatment strategies used clinically with MS patients.[61] Four of 15 used equipment to assess balance deficits. Four used the Clinical Test for Sensory Interaction in Balance (CTSIB).[61,62] Two used the Tannate Gait and Balance Tool.[63,64] Four practitioners used habituation exercises for treatment of balance deficits. Other therapists surveyed indicated other unique treatment regimens to treat balance deficits.[61]

Although specific interventions to treat impaired balance are not clear-cut, it should not be forgotten that many of the medications used to treat spasticity, ataxia, and tremor may also impair the body's ability to respond to external perturbations.

Prett et al. performed platform postureography on 10 ambulatory MS patients with Kurtzke scores of 1 to 4 in an effort to determine if different postural responses result from lesions in different areas of the CNS and if they are similar to the postural responses of people with cerebellar lesions.[65] They concluded that postural dyscontrol in subjects with MS is distinctly different than cerebellar subjects, even though balance deficits in MS often are described as cerebellar-like.[61]

Fatigue

Lassitude or classic MS fatigue has been described frequently.[68,69] MS fatigue is unlike the fatigue of non-MS adults. It can occur at a specific time of day, usually in the afternoon. Fatigue can occur with minimal activity, and lead to a sense of continuous exhaustion. Slightly different from this generalized fatigue is loss of function after repetitive movement. Even during reading, extra-ocular muscle fatigue can lead to symptoms of blurred vision. Some patients have normal ankle strength when they begin to walk, but have a marked foot drop by the time they reach the end of a hallway. Fatigue may be related to inefficient nerve transmission in demyelinated pathways, with slowing or dispersing of nerve signal. Many MS patients have poor sleep patterns that may contribute to a sense of fatigue. Others have fatigue as part of depression, which must be identified and treated.[36,70]

Copperman et al. found that fatigue has been described extensively in relation to physical activities.[36,70,71] More specifically, fatigue can be viewed as either an inability to maintain a determined force output or as an increased sense of effort to maintain a given force output.[70]

Treatment of Fatigue   Regular exercise has long been known to diminish the impact of the fatigue associated with deconditioning. Aerobic exercise has recently been accepted as appropriate when properly prescribed for patients with MS.[71,72] Exercise may also have an important role to play in research design to answer questions specific to fatigue in MS.[73]

Pharmacologic interventions with amantadine and Pemoline have proven somewhat effective in the symptom-oriented management of fatigue.[74–78] Instruments such as the fatigue severity scale have been developed to quantify this type of MS fatigue.[78]

Fatigue management includes moderate conditioning exercise, normalizing movement, decreasing spasticity, rest periods, decreasing the relative excess work by using adaptive equipment, and energy conservation for mental as well as physical effort. Adequate nighttime sleep should also be insured by treating nighttime spasms, nocturia, and other conditions that interfere with sleep. Medications for fatigue, including amantadine and pemoline, help approximately 50 percent of people. Neural transmission enhancers also are under study, including 4-aminiopyridine (see the preceding).[36,70]

Cooperman et al. have reported that generalized fatigue is a major problem for most persons with MS, with 60 percent of responding neurologists giving a range of 40 to 80 percent of their patients suffering from generalized fatigue.[36] Occupational therapists can teach energy conservation techniques that can be useful to successfully manage fatigue. Instruction in energy conservation usually takes two to three sessions, and includes goal setting, daily activity diaries, work simplification, and written materials. Specific interventions that have been used successfully include cool showers, ice packs, and cooling vests.[36]

Heat Sensitivity   Heat sensitivity is particularly important for MS patients, and frequently leads to fatigue. Heat intolerance can increase both the number and intensity of signs and symptoms, in nearly 50 percent of MS patients.[2,54,55] An increase in core body temperature can lead to a significant loss of function, whether it is brought on by fever, environment, or physical activity. Air conditioning is a legitimate medical need for these patients. Pools, baths, and showers should be around 29°C (84°F).[2]

SPASTICITY

Spasticity is usually a result of corticospinal tract demyelination. The most effective treatment plan is a combination of physical therapy and medication. However, spasticity may be useful to some patients for a more stable stance and gait. In these patients, treatment of spasticity may actually increase the effect of existing weakness. Stretching exercises are commonly instituted, although the degree of their benefit is not clear. Passive range of motion in patients with severe spasticity also can be helpful. A number of medications are used for treating spasticity, but the mainstay of treatment is baclofen. Diazepam, sodium dantrolene, and clonazepam are second-line medications. Intrathecal baclofen is now available and is extremely helpful in selected patients. Motor point blocks and botulinum toxin are also therapeutic approaches that should be considered.[30]

Measurement of Spasticity

A variety of measurement tools for spasticity have been cited in recent literature, including the Ashworth Scale, electrogoniometer, Cybex II, electromyography, Minimal Record of Disability, and Fugl-Meyer Motor Assessment.[57,59,79–89] Bohannon reported high interrater reliability for the Ashworth Scale.[81] Katz examined the correlation between the various tools and reported that the Modified Ashworth Scale and the Fugl-Meyer Motor Assessment Scale are reliable clinical measures of spasticity.[80] Brar reported a significant correlation between Cybex II and the Ashworth Scale.[61,89] Although, there are several pieces of equipment used in the laboratory setting for objective measurement of spasticity, the Ashworth Scale is the only clinical tool validated by research and utilized by clinicians.[61] For a discussion of specific pharmacologic and surgical therapeutic interventions used in spasticity management see Chapter 20.

Spasticity: Physical Therapy Treatment

Stretching Several investigators have reported short-term reduction of spasticity after stretching of finger flexors, use of air splint, weight bearing, use of hand orthoses, and stretching programs.[90–96] However, well-documented controlled evidence of the effectiveness of stretching exercises is sparse.

One controlled study has compared the effects of baclofen and stretching exercises in patients with an EDSS score of 5.5. Three approaches to the measurement of spasticity were used. First, they used the Ashworth scale. Additionally, the investigators utilized a questionnaire on functional abilities derived from the ISS. Finally, objective instrumented measures were obtained in the form of Cybex flexion scores. This study used double-blind, placebo-controlled, crossover design lasting 10 weeks. Assessments were done at 2-week intervals. Four possible treatment combinations were offered, baclofen alone, placebo alone, baclofen plus stretching exercises, and placebo plus stretching exercises. Low-dose baclofen was used (20 mg or less per day). Improvement in spasticity was only seen in the baclofen only and baclofen plus exercise group, and there was no significant difference between the two. The results indicate that stretching exercises add little or nothing to the beneficial effects of baclofen in treatment of spasticity. Improvements were seen in the Cybex flexion scores and the Ashworth scale, but no improvement in the patient self-reported functional status was observed.[96]

Inhibitive or Serial Casting/Splinting

Many investigators have reported positive results with the use of splinting, inhibitive casting, or serial casting for relief of spasticity, particularly when the goal is improving joint range of motion and/or voluntary muscle contraction of the antagonist.[97–108] Most studies unfortunately were case reports, with a bias toward subjects with lower extremity spasticity. The perceived effectiveness in one study was moderate, and the frequency of use of this technique was low.[61]

Biofeedback

Nash reported three cases of reduced reflex sensitivity after visual biofeedback in children.[109] A contemporaneous study by Wissel et al. reported improved function and strength in the 10 of 11 adults with spasticity by using EMG audio feedback.[110] In spite of these encouraging preliminary studies, the use of biofeedback in the management of MS spasticity is not widespread.

Electrical Stimulation The use of electrical stimulation to reduce spasticity in MS has been investigated extensively. Functional electrical stimulation (FES), transcutaneous electrical stimulation, and electrical stimulation by placing surface electrodes over spastic muscles or over peripheral nerves have all garnered special interest.[82,83,88,111–113] Fredrickson et al. stimulated the skin over the dorsal column and reported increased control of bladder and knee flexion in 18 out 27 subjects with MS.[61,113] Dimitrijevic et al. reported inhibition of ankle clonus and improved ambulation after surface stimulation of the peroneal nerve in MS patients.[61,112] Walker has demonstrated inhibition of contralateral ankle clonus after subcutaneous stimulation of the median, radial, and sural nerves in MS patients.[61,114]

PAIN IN MS

Pain in multiple sclerosis is relatively common. Mechanical factors related to weakness, spasticity, and incoordination may produce secondary musculoskeletal dysfunction and pain. Pain symptoms are best treated by minimizing the factors producing musculoskeletal dysfunction and treating the pain symptomatically. Physiatric management includes improvement in posture, altered activity patterns, reduction in muscle spasticity, and treatment of trigger points.[2]

Central nervous system pain is often dysesthetic in quality. Distortions of sensation may include tightness, tingling, itching, swelling, stabbing, burning, and electrical sensations, particularly down the neck and back with neck flexion (Lhermitte's sign). Discomfort may vary from mildly distracting to significantly distressful.[2] Carbamazepine, phenytoin, clonazepam, and trycyclic antidepressants can be helpful in minimizing this discomfort.[30] Corticosteroids may be beneficial in pain syndromes associated with acute MS exacerbation. Dysesthesias and other sensory symptoms often resolve within several weeks or months, and medication can be discontinued.[2]

BOWEL AND BLADDER MANAGEMENT

Bladder Dysfunction

Bladder symptoms effect nearly 80 percent of individuals with MS. They are part of the initial symptom complex in about 10 percent, and the sole presenting complaint in another 2 percent. We have come to understand the pathophysiology of the neurogenic bladder in MS and have classified bladder dysfunction into three categories:

1. Failure to store due to uninhibited detrusor contractions, small bladder capacity, or sphincter dysfunction;

2. Failure to empty due to detrusor dysfunction or outlet obstruction; and

3. Combinations of failure to store or failure to empty commonly called detrusor-sphincter dyssynergia.[115]

The bladder dysfunction of greatest concern is retention of urine. Recurrent urinary tract infections may result from urinary retention and are cited as a major health risk for persons with MS. The strategies for management have been borrowed from other neurologic disorders, primarily spinal cord injury.

Intermittent catheterization is the most important management technique, but has not totally eliminated the urinary tract infections. Intermittent catheterization was introduced in 1972, to manage neurogenic bladder retention in persons with a spinal cord injury. Numerous studies between 1976 and 1988 supported intermittent catheterization as safe and effective in managing urinary retention.[115] The reuse of straight catheters with clean technique has become the standard for this process. At present, there are no studies that have assessed the impact of intermittent clean self-catheterization on the incidence of urinary tract infections in MS.[115]

Sterile catheters may contribute to lower infection rates when compared with clean catheters, but definitive scientific proof is lacking. Rinsing catheters after each use and proper storage in an antiseptic, antimicrobial solution is important. The need for serious attention to bladder dysfunction management is illustrated in one recent study where nearly one fourth of 162 MS cases identified by the Mayo Clinic had frequent urinary incontinence, a need for almost constant catheterization, or a long-term need for assistive measures to evacuate stool.[115]

Post-void residual urine (PVR) volume is essential to identify underlying urinary retention. Volumes post-void in excess of 100 to 200 cc generally signify voiding dysfunction. Urodynamic studies that measure intravesicular pressures with filling, voiding flow rates, sphincter electromyography and bladder ultrasound are considered standard noninvasive methods for assessing bladder function.

Although medications and intermittent self-catheterization remain the mainstays of management, suprapubic tapping, double voiding, the Crede maneuver, and foley or condom catheters are necessary in some patients.[115]

When the bladder of an MS patient fails to store urine, the anticholinergic agent propantheline can be particularly useful in promoting vesicle relaxation. Urgency owing to sphincter dyssynergy should be treated with oxybutyrin. External sphincter relaxation can also be treated with the peripheral alpha antagonist phenoxybenzamine. Urinary retention caused by bladder wall relaxation should be treated with thanechol. Methenamine mandelate can be used to inhibit bacterial growth in acidified urine of a large spastic bladder, reducing bladder wall irritability.[2]

Immediately after treatment for an acute exacerbation with corticosteroids, a period of diuresis lasting 7 to 10 days often follows. This diuretic challenge to a neurogenic bladder can lead to severe frequency, urgency, and incontinence. Some patients with subclinical bladder dysfunction can precipitously go into acute urinary retention. Diuresis during or immediately after steroid treatment leads to rapid bladder filling and overdistention. Therefore, bladder function should be carefully evaluated before steroid treatment. Measurement of the PVR by catheterization or bedside ultrasound is optimal.

Management requires careful monitoring of residuals, increased frequency of timed voids and, sometimes, short-term indwelling catheterization, to reduce voiding frequency and bladder overdistension. Diuresis usually resolves within 7 to 10 days. Patients discharged directly after corticosteroid treatment must be educated about steroid-induced diuresis.[54]

Bowel Dysfunction

The most common bowel symptom in MS is constipation. Reduction in bowel motility has been attributed to poor dietary habits, relative physical inactivity, medication side-effects, depression, weakness of abdominal muscles, postponement of defecation due to immobility, and restriction of fluid intake to control bladder symptoms.[2] Effective management of constipation can nearly always be accomplished with proper nutrition, fluid intake, and medications.[30]

Diarrhea and incontinence are uncommon, but may be caused by antibiotic therapy for urinary tract infections. When fecal incontinence is present, a scheduled daily or every other day suppository-induced evacuation can be implemented by a rehabilitation nurse, the patient, or caregivers.[2]

SEXUAL DYSFUNCTION

Sexual dysfunction is much more commonly recognized in men with MS than women. If women are questioned in detail, this discrepancy appears to diminish. Despite evidence that sexual dysfunction is prevalent in MS, specific prospective data delineating the natural history of sexual dysfunction in MS is sparse.[31]

The most common complaint among men is erectile dysfunction (63–80 percent), but impaired ejaculation and loss of libido also are noted. Erectile dysfunction in MS has been postulated to be caused by spinal lesions proximal to the sacral spinal cord.[116] Women often experience difficulty achieving orgasm (57–58 percent), loss of libido, diminished genital sensitivity (49–68 percent), and impaired genital lubrication. Both men and women often have difficulty with arousal. Symptoms of sexual dysfunction may fluctuate, especially during acute exacerbations.[31]

Motor deficits, ataxia, tremor, spasticity, and fatigue also interfere with sexual function.[11] Medications often interfere with normal sexual function, especially tricyclic antidepressants, anticholinergic agents, beta adrenergic blockers, and benzodiazepines.

Treatment

Effective treatment always begins with counseling and education of both patient and partner. A variety of therapeutic interventions are available for both men and women.[30]

For men, intra-corporeal penile injection of papaverine, phentolamine, and prostaglandins, can improve erectile dysfunction.[31,117] The extent of long-term acceptance and effectiveness is uncertain. Vacuum penile tumescence and constriction therapy have proven to yield long-term results.[118]

In contrast, specific therapies to remedy sexual dysfunction in women with MS are lacking. However, when women with MS encounter difficulties with sexual intercourse, they can respond positively to alternative sexual activities such as masturbation, petting, oral sex, and the use of stimulating devices.[31]

Sexual counseling can be useful in coping with physical changes that lead to alteration of body image and sexual identity, as well as concomitant emotional stress. Patient and partner education is essential so that both understand the diverse ways in which MS can interfere with sexual feelings and performance. Adaptive strategies must emphasize clear communication about self-image, self-esteem, and feelings about sexual identity.[119]

COGNITIVE

Until the last decade, cognitive impairment was believed to be rare in MS. More recent evidence indicates that MS-related cognitive impairment is quite common. Prevalence estimates adjusted for rates of impairment and healthy control range from 43 percent for a large community-based sample to 59 percent for a large clinic based sample.[120,121] The prevalence of MS-related cognitive impairment generally tends to be underestimated. Fischer has shown that the level of recognition of impaired cognitive performance among MS patients treated in MS centers varies with the level of experience of the examiner.[122] Rao reported that 16 percent of a group of cognitively impaired MS patients were employed, compared to 44 percent of a group of cognitively intact MS patients matched for physical ability.[123] Several case reports and group studies have shown that even patients with minimal physical disabilities (less than 4 on Kurtzske's Expanded Disability Status Scale) have cognitive impairment sufficient to limit or preclude employment or adversely impact social functioning.[124–128] Using criteria set forth by formal neuropsychological testing, 54 to 65 percent of patients with MS exhibit measurable cognitive impairment, 5 to 20 percent of which are rated as severe.[129] These rates are appreciably higher than estimates of cognitive impairment based on bedside neurologic examination alone or performance on mental status tests, such as the Mini-Mental Status Examination.[129–134]

Mild to moderate deficits can have a significant impact. Cognitive deficits are more often associated with a chronic progressive course of MS and with cerebral lesion load. MS-induced cognitive deficits can occur in the absence of physical disability. Clinical features include slowed information processing, impaired attention, and impaired short-term and working memory.

Frontal lobe plaques can lead to disturbances in the executive functions, abulia, behavioral disinhibition, and mental.[2,30,131]

Defining Cognitive Dysfunction in MS

Rao suggested that the pattern of cognitive and behavioral changes in MS is similar to that observed in the subcortical dementias associated with Huntington's disease, Parkinson's disease, and progressive supranuclear palsy.[135] This pattern is often characterized by personality and mood disturbances, impaired abstraction and problem solving, poor visual-spatial skills, slowed information processing, attentional disturbances, and memory deficits that improve with cuing. Aphasia, agnosia, acalculia, and true dementia typical of Alzheimer's disease occur quite infrequently.[131]

Cross-sectional studies generally find only slight differences between controls and MS patients on measures of verbal intelligence quotient (IQ), such as those dervied from the Wechsler intelligence battery.[135] Patients with MS generally score 7 to 14 points lower on the performance IQ scales than on verbal IQ scales. Although cross-sectional studies indicate a negligible influence of MS on verbal IQ, longitudinal studies suggest a more pronounced effect. Canter obtained premorbid IQ scores on the Army General Classification Test for 23 males healthy at the time that they entered military service.[137] When retested 4 years later, after developing MS, IQ scores had dropped an average of 13.5 points. Canter observed a 3.7 point drop in verbal IQ and a 7.8 point drop in performance IQ in MS patients retested after a 6-month interval.[137] Over the same period, controls improved 4.1 and 7.8 points on the verbal performance IQs, respectively.[131]

Using the National Adult Reading Test to estimate premorbid IQ and the Wechsler Adult Intelligence Scale, Revised (WAIS-R) to measure current IQ, an IQ drop of 6.8 points was observed for MS patients compared to controls, whose scores improved an average of 0.7 points.[138] A modest decline of verbal IQ and a larger deficit in performance IQ from estimated premorbid levels can occur early in the course of MS. In one large, controlled study, MS patients averaged 6.3 points lower than controls on the WAIS-R verbal IQ.[134] One longitudinal study has shown enlargement of this gap after 3 years followup.[131]

Clear patterns of neuropsychological functioning appear to be emerging. Measures of visual and auditory attention, indicate impairment, including the oral version of the Symbol Digit Modalities Test, the Paced Auditory Serial Attention Test, the Stroop Interference Test, and various tasks that require vigilance or divided attention to auditory and visual tasks presented simultaneously.[126,133,134,138,139] Studies using the Sternberg Memory Scanning Test provide the most direct evidence for slowed information processing speed in MS.[131]

Approximately 22 to 25 percent of community-based samples of MS patients demonstrate impairment on measures of complex attention and information processing speed.[120] This has been observed in both auditory and visual modalities.[122,140–142]

Memory

We know that MS-related cognitive dysfunction is generally circumscribed, not global, and that recent memory and information processing are affected most often. Depending on the sample selection methods and criteria used to define impairment, approximately 20 to 42 percent of MS patients are impaired in their free recall of recently learned verbal and visual material.[120,143,144] Recognition of recently learned information also can be impaired, although to a much lesser extent than free recall.[143,145] Impairments of verbal fluency and, to a lesser extent, confrontation naming are often associated with memory impairment.[141,143,146] This has led some investigators to suggest that MS primarily produces deficits in memory retrieval, rather than acquisition.[36] Although memory deficits are common in MS, some specific memory processes appear to be resistant to degradation.[140,147] The rate of learning and semantic ability are preserved in all but the most impaired MS patients.[120,125,130,140,141,147] Implicit memory, the ability to learn new information or skills without explicitly focusing also usually is preserved.[122]

The status of immediate memory in MS remains controversial. On the most common measure, Digit Span, from the WAIS, mild deficits have been reported in some studies, but not in others.[131,134,148,149]

Deficits in executive functions, such as problem solving, also are relatively common. Thirteen to 19 percent of the community-based sample have deficits in this aspect of cognitive function.[120] Multiple sclerosis patients make an inordinate number of errors on problem solving tasks, primarily because of difficulty using feedback to modify incorrect problem-solving strategies.[121,150]

In relation to disease course, patients with chronic progressive or relapsing progressive MS consistently perform more poorly as a group on neuropsychological testing than those with relapsing-remitting disease. However, even relapsing-remitting MS patients tested during remission show deficits compared to healthy controls.[122]

Cognitive deficits in MS can not be explained by extraneous factors, such as fatigue, depression, or medications.[121,123,141,143] Recent studies using quantitative magnetic resonance imaging have established that neuropsychological test performances is moderately correlated with total lesion burden.[123] More extensive cognitive impairment has been associated with confluent pariventricular lesions and a thinning of the corpus callosum.[123,151] Positron emission tomography studies of cerebral metabolism and event related potentials (ERP) provide additional evidence of an association between cognitive impairment and cereberal involvement.[124,152,153]

Failure to recognize subtle cognitive impairment may create unreasonable expectations on the part of the patients, families, rehabilitation professionals, and employers. Failure to appreciate cognitive impairment may also be confused by family and caregivers for lack of motivation or secondary gain.[131]

The fact that significant cognitive deficits may occur early in the course of MS suggests that neuropsychological assessment should be conducted soon after diagnosis, and at regular intervals thereafter. A core battery of tests has been proposed by the cognitive function study group of the National Multiple Sclerosis Society.[154] Evidence of moderate to severe lesion load in the periventricular white matter or corpus callosum is a good predictor of cognitive impairment, and should prompt a consideration of the need for comprehensive neuropsychological evaluation.[131]

A variety of methods can be used to assess cognitive function clinically in patients with MS. A thorough mental status examination is the first step. The Mini-Mental Status Examination (MMSE) has been shown to be insensitive to MS-related cognitive dysfunction. Patients and caregiver reports correlate poorly with neuropsychological test performance. Comprehensive neuropsychological testing can identify MS patients with more circumscribed cognitive deficits (see Table 12-1).[122]

Not all patients with MS require formal neuropsychological testing. Clearly, a suitable examination is needed. Four alternative screening examinations for use with MS patients have been developed. Based on preliminary studies, each appears to have considerably greater sensitivity for detecting cognitive impairments

in MS than does the MMSE, while retaining adequate specificity. The Neuropsychological Screening Battery, the Quick Mental Status, the Brief Cognitive Battery, and the Screening Examination for Cognitive Impairment in MS have been the most widely used screening exams.[133,134,155] Evaluation of the usefulness of these instruments is now underway.[131]

Treatment of Cognitive Deficits

Despite the prevalence of MS-related cognitive impairment and its potentially devastating impact on everyday function, no effective treatment is available. A pilot study of intravenous physostigmine demonstrated significant benefit in three out of four MS patients.[156] Cognitive rehabilitation techniques have shown promise in closed head injury, but their generalizability to MS is unclear.[157] Other methods to treat cognitive dysfunction are exploratory at this point.[122]

Depression

Affective disorders are common in MS. When structured interview techniques are used to establish psychiatric diagnosis, the prevalence of major depression among MS clinic patients is estimated to be 14 percent, and the lifetime prevalence to be 47 to 54 percent.[158] The prevalence of bipolar affective disorders also is elevated in MS. Current and lifetime prevalence estimates of bipolar illness among MS clinic attenders are 0 to 2 percent and 13 to 16 percent, respectively.[122]

The median prevalence estimate for clinical depression by practitioners is 30 percent, an estimate nearly twice the actual prevalence of major depression in MS. In a Danish registry survey, suicide risk in MS was conservatively estimated to be almost twice that of age-matched, healthy controls. Risk for suicide is greatest for men under the age of 30 and for the first 5 years after MS diagnosis.[122]

Depression can not be predicted on the basis of traditional disease parameters, such as disease duration or physical disability, as assessed by the EDSS.[158–160] The severity of major depressive episodes increased significantly during exacerbation, especially during ACTH or steroid treatment.[124]

Recent studies have failed to find a relationship between depression and magnetic resonance imaging lesion load.[122] There is empirical evidence of an association between specific psychiatric manifestations, such as flattened affect, thought disorder, and delusions and MS plaque burden in the temporal parietal and frontal lobes and the periventricular region.[122]

Even patients who appear euphoric may be depressed. Therefore, depresssion must be identified by carefully probing of specific vegetative and behavioral symptoms.[30] When more objective validated testing is needed, the Beck Depression Inventory and the Hamilton or Jung depression scales are useful. Objective scales should be used that are complementary in their behavioral and vegetative weighting.

Up to 40 percent, of MS patients with affective or other diagnosable psychobehavioral disorders do not receive treatment.[161] Psychosocial intervention has long been recognized as an important component of comprehensive care in MS.[123] In recent years, studies have demonstrated the efficacy of group therapy, stress management, and cognitively based behavior therapy in MS.[10,122,162] Patients who are less severely depressed benefited from a brief course of cognitive behavioral therapy alone, when compared to controls.[161] In older, more severely physically impaired subjects, longer insight-oriented group psychotherapy significantly reduced self-reported depression when compared to a general discussion group or no treatment.[122,163] Cognitively based behavioral therapy showed long-term benefit of cognitive compensatory training on depression.[164]

PARKINSON'S DISEASE REHABILITATION

Parkinson's disease (PD) is by far the most common movement disorder in this country, affecting 1 percent of individuals age 65 years and over.[165] Many of the symptoms and signs of PD can be seen in other neurodegenerative disorders, as well as in anoxic encephalopathy, multiple lacunar infarcts, drug effects, and the normal aging process (Table 12-4).[166] The benefits of rehabilitation for PD and related disorders are considered.

Parkinson's disease is characterized pathologically by degeneration of pigmented and other brain stem nuclei, particularly the substantia nigra, in association with the formation of eosinophilic neuronal inclusions called Lewy Bodies.[167,168] The primary biochemical defect in PD is the loss of striatal dopamine resulting from the degeneration of dopamine-producing cells in the substant nigra, with the associated hyperactivity of cholinergic neurons in the caudate nuclei contributing to the symptoms.[169] The most prominent hypotheses regarding the etiology of PD are the theories of accelerated aging,

Table 12-4
Clinical features of Parkinson's Disease

Symptoms and Signs
  Rigidity
  Bradykinesia (slowness of movement)
  Resting-postural tremor
  Hypokinesia (small amplitude movement)
  Loss of postural reflexes
  Loss of preparatory and associated movements ("en bloc" movements, decreased arm swing, decreased blinking)
  Akathisia (inability to sit still, relieved by walking about)
  Dementia
  Autonomic dysfunction (orthostatic hypotension, slowed GI motility, urinary retention, impotence)
  Hypokinetic dysarthria
  Festinating gait
  Masked faces (stare with decreased blinking)
  Dystonia
  Flexed posture
  Dysphagia
  Sudden "freezing" of motor activity

Common Presenting Complaints
  Stiffness, aching muscular pain, slowed movements
  Trouble getting out of a chair
  Trouble rolling over in bed
  Falling, tripping over objects on floor
  Tremor, "shaking"
  Depression
  Memory loss
  Stooped posture
  Rapid or whispering speech
  Change in handwriting
  Slowness in activities, dressing, grooming
  Trouble walking
  Slow to respond to questions and requests
  Drooling, trouble controlling saliva

toxin exposure, genetic predisposition, and oxidative stress. The oxidative mechanism theory has received the most support to date, but it is likely that a combination of all four processes contributes to the development of PD.[170]

Although PD can present an array of clinical symptoms and signs (Table 12-4), the cardinal features of the diseases are: (1) resting/postural tremor; (2) bradykinesia; (3) rigidity; and (4) postural instability. In the early stages of PD, rigidity, often described as "stiffness" or "achiness," may be mistaken as a symptom of arthritis. Masked facies and bradykinesia can lead to the most common early misdiagnosis, that of depression. The onset and progression of the disease is slow and insidious. The initial ramifications of PD are protean. Symptoms and signs may begin unilaterally, but eventually spread to involve the other limbs and trunk. Lack of arm swing when walking and changes in handwriting (micrographia) often are early signs.

Although tremor can become disabling, it usually does not impair function as much as bradykinesia and rigidity, which eventually lead to problems in all areas of mobility and activities of daily living (ADL). When ambulating, patients have difficulty in changing directions or moving around objects, and may "freeze," unable to start again. Parkinson's disease patients have great difficulty in carrying out simultaneous but unrelated motor acts, such as talking or taking notes while walking, or throwing or reaching while walking.

Impairment of speech is one of the most frustrating disabilities for patients with PD. Speech becomes rapid, monotonous, and low volume (hypokinetic dysarthria). Speech and handwriting are thus affected by the same phenomenon that causes festinating gait.

Since the basal ganglia play an important role in motor planning and programming, PD patients have difficulty initiating an activity, such as walking or reaching for objects. Normal associated or preparatory movements, such as arm swing during walking, and before rising from a chair.

As PD progresses, autonomic symptoms, including impaired enteric motility, urinary retention and incontinence, and orthostatic hypotension are reported. Dysphagia and postural instability increase the burden of disability. Dementia often is a late feature and ultimately appears in about one-third of the patients. Depression can affect as many as 50 percent of the patients, may be difficult to distinguish from psychomotor retardation. Gradual progression of the PD symptom complex is the general rule.

Before the advent of levodopa therapy, 25 percent of patients with symptom duration of less than 5 years were severely disabled, and 75 percent of survivors with symptom duration of 10 to 15 years were totally disabled. The introduction of levodopa, deprenyl, and novel medication management strategies have prolonged independence. A review of the comprehensive pharmacotherapeutic approach to PD is beyond the scope of this text.

Rehabilitation Approach to PD

Many experts in the treatment of PD recommend rehabilitative services as an adjunct to medical therapy to prevent complications and maintain or assist with function.[171–173] Most patients with PD report that they "feel" or function better with a program of regular exercise. It is not clear whether this results from a general sense of well-being or general conditioning that occurs with exercise. Actual improvement in function, or remediation of specific neurologic deficits of PD has never been demonstrated.

A number of investigators have attempted to assess the efficacy of nonpharmacologic therapy for patients with PD.[174–176] Parkinson's disease patients benefit from exercise programs that focus on improving range-of-motion (ROM), endurance, balance, and gait.[177–181] The efficacy of more functionally oriented programs has not been as thoroughly assessed, although the provision of equipment and instruction in adaptive techniques provided by occupational therapists in the home has been shown to be helpful.[182] Small numbers of subjects, the lack of controls, as well as changes in medication have weakened the scientific rigor of most studies to date.

Comella et al. recently conducted a prospective, randomized, single-blind crossover study of the effects of a 4-week outpatient physical rehabilitation program on mentation, activities of daily living, and motor function as measured by the Unified Parkinson's Disease Rating Scale (UPDRS).[35,181] Sixteen moderate to moderately severe PD patients were seen for 1 hour, three times per week by physical and occupational therapists for 4 weeks. The program consisted of repetitive exercises directed at improving range of motion, balance, fine motor dexterity, gait, and endurance. The intensity of the program was increased as endurance improved. The control group received no intervention. Two 4-week study periods were separated by 6 months. Medication changes were not allowed during the control or therapy phases, but adjustments were permitted during the 6-month interval between study periods as well as during the follow-up period.

Following the physical rehabilitation program there was a significant improvement in activities of daily living and motor function (bradykinesia and rigidity), but no improvement in tremor, timed finger tapping, mentation, or mood. Despite instructions to the subjects to continue the exercise program at home at the completion of the rehabilitation phase, all resumed a more sedentary lifestyle, and at 6-month follow-up the UPDRS scores returned to baseline. Continued exercise might be needed to maintain function, but incorporating such a program into a patient's lifestyle without continuation of an organized program appears unlikely.

Although speech and swallowing disorders commonly are a source of disability in PD, speech therapy is under-utilized.[183,184] Families often complain that speech is improved as long as the patient is receiving therapy, but as soon as the therapy ends, speech reverts to the previous pattern. This clinical experience is supported by the work of Sarno, who noted in a study of 300 PD patients that speech improved only during treatment.[185] Allan also reported rapid deterioration in speech following cessation of formal therapy.[186] Intensive speech therapy (group and individual therapy lasting 3½ to 4 hours per day of 2 weeks duration), produced a positive effect on speech in PD, with some benefits lasting up to 3 months.[187] Therapy should focus on voice and respiratory control, loudness, pitch variation, and control of the rate of speech.

Scott and Caird demonstrated that speech therapy consisting of intonational and prosodic exercises can produce improvements in speech that last up to 3 months.[188,189] The treatment program consists of daily 1-hour sessions carried out in the patient's home over 2 to 3 weeks. The types of motor deficits in PD resulting in both physical and speech impairment, benefit from a program that provides regular and continuing intervention.

Another speech disorder common in PD is palilalia. Palilalia is characterized by the repetition of a word or phrase with increasing rapidity and decreasing intelligibility. The use of pacing boards has been helpful in decreasing palilalia.[178]

Studies addressing the benefits of inpatient rehabilitation in PD are few. Stern et al. studied 47 PD patients admitted to a rehabilitation center who received a course of intensive multidisciplinary rehabilitation in conjunction with the start of levodopa therapy.[190] They noted good to excellent improvements in mobility in 66 percent, with no improvement in 17 percent. A few patients not showing improvement in mobility did show improvement in activities of daily living. When levodopa is initiated in PD outpatients without any concomitant rehabilitation, 60 percent improved and 18 percent worsened or showed no change.

As part of a pilot study to develop appropriate measures to assess the impact of rehabilitation on patients with PD, Cedarbaum et al. looked at the changes in numerous tasks and activities following inpatient rehabilitation.[176] Forty-five patients were studied in an unblinded, open fashion with medication adjustments allowed. No significant change in levodopa dosage occurred. Rehabilitation consisted of an average of 4 hours of therapy a day, 5 days a week. No changes were noted in any of the timed tasks. Statistically significant improvements were noted in ambulation, transfers, dressing, and personal hygiene.

Exercise and Muscle Physiology in PD

Exercise tolerance must be carefully considered in the patient with PD. There is now evidence to indicate that there are some differences in muscle physiology and response to exercise in patients with PD. It is not clear whether this is an effect related to disuse, altered central innervation, or a direct pathologic involvement of muscle. Landin looked at muscle metabolism and physiologic response to exercise in six patients with PD and five healthy controls.[191] Exercise efficiency was reduced in PD subjects, as was muscle adenosine triphosphate (ATP). Reduced efficiency in coupling between respiration and ATP generation by muscles is postulated, a possible result of an altered metabolic state of muscle caused by aberrant innervation. This finding also is consistent with recent reports of alterations of mitochondrial respiration in brain tissue, platelets, and muscle tissue in patients with PD, suggesting a systemic abnormality in mitochondrial function.[191–193]

Reduced mechanical efficiency in leg muscles in PD patients results in twice the work demand of exercise as normal controls.[194] Physical inactivity and deconditioning in subjects with PD may be as important as the altered metabolic state of muscle. However, Gersten et al. demonstrated that levodopa therapy reduced the externally measured work of walking in 46 subjects in varying stages of PD.[195] When clinically appropriate, optimization of levodopa therapy is important to consider prior to embarking on an exercise program, since levodopa produces physiologic changes that impact on the patient's ability to perform and benefit from an exercise program.

Psychological and Social Aspects of PD

Because of the predominance of motor symptoms in PD, psychologic and cognitive impairments and their impact on disability often are overlooked. Although severe dementia can occur late in the disease, most patients with PD perform less well on a wide range of cognitive tests than age- and education-matched controls, even early in the course.[196–199] Adaptation to change in daily routine or environment can be difficult and lead to undue anxiety. Sleep disturbances are common, and particularly difficulty falling asleep. In some patients, levodopa causes a stimulant effect, preventing sleep. Early in the disease, levodopa should be avoided late in the day if possible. If there are no obvious cognitive impairments, diphenhydramine can be used to induce sleep, and may reduce tremor. Trazedone is sedating and can be used as an acceptable alternative. Sleep problems can be accentuated by vivid dreams and hallucinations that occur as a side-effect of dopaminergic medications. Fatigue and an increased tendency to daytime napping also contribute to what eventually can become dysfunctional circadian sleep–wake cycle.

As noted earlier, depression is common in PD. It may be related to a deficit in serotonergic neurotransmission, or to the diminution of cortical levels of norepinephrine and dopamine.[200,201] Depression is difficult to treat in patients with declining mental function, because of the anticholinergic side-effects of the tricyclic (noradrenergic/dopaminergic) antidepressants. A serotonergic agent may be the logical first choice in these patients. If that is ineffective, a tricyclic with low anticholinergic side-effects, such as desipramine or nortriptyline might be worth a try.

Social dysfunction also is quite common, with lack of socialization owing to anxiety related to bodily symptoms as the most common. Patients with akinesia-rigidity tend to experience more emotional stress than those with tremor-predominant PD. In one study, group counseling activities involving both patients and care-givers were helpful in reducing stress in 74 percent of patients.[202]

Driving is a complex cognitive-perceptual-motor task. Maintaining the ability to drive also is important to independence. When motor and/or cognitive function become impaired, the physician should suggest a more detailed driving assessment. In many communities, driver screening is offered as part of a driver's training program for persons with disabilities.

Specific Therapy Approaches

Gait, Station, and Posture The typical patient with moderate PD assumes a flexed posture, has difficulty initiating gait, and ambulates with short shuffling steps at an increasing rate. Base of support usually is narrow. Once walking begins, the patient has great difficulty changing directions, stepping over or moving around objects, or stopping (the festinating gait). Prior to beginning ambulation, the patient with PD does not make the normal preparatory movements of trunk and extremities. During gait, associated movements such as arm swing, trunk rotation, and pelvic motion are reduced or absent. Postural reactions are impaired, so that the PD patient is unable to correct for mild perturbations in the center of gravity (e.g., being brushed by another person or taking a slight misstep), and can topple over at times as if the patient were a statue. "Freezing" can also occur and precipitate a fall. Although helpful in alleviating rigidity and bradykinesia, pharmacologic therapy for PD usually has little or no impact on postural instability. Later in the disease, as fluctuations in response to levodopa occur (the so-called "on-off" effect), performance may be extremely variable and unpredictable.

Useful approaches to these problems include exercises emphasizing trunk extension and lateral and rotational trunk mobility, weight shifting and balance training, and instruction in falling safely and getting up off the floor. Widening stance provides a better base of support. Conscious strategies to initiate gait and maintain cadence often are quite helpful and include mental rehearsal, counting or signing out loud or to oneself, and marching to rhythm. The process can be begun with external cues such as a metronome or music that are gradually withdrawn. Exaggeration of arm swing and leg excursion are also helpful.

Balance activities can be made a part of other functional activities such as washing, grooming, and household activities. A cane can help but also can interfere with function if not properly used. A rolling walker works better than a standard pickupwalker, since patients who need a walker usually cannot incorporate lifting a walker into their gait pattern. Care should be taken to set the walker at a higher height than usual, so as not to further promote flexion posture. Inability to stop once started can be a problem with rolling walkers, and hand brakes on the walker or supervision often are required.

A visit to the patient's home by a physical or occupational therapist can result in environmental safety measures such as the removal of throw rugs, rearrangement of furniture, and the installation of railings grab bars, and other adaptive equipment. Effective home management strategies specific to the patient's home situation can be developed and taught to patients and caregivers.

In the newly diagnosed patient, the opportunity to prevent loss of range of motion and flexed posture is never more important. More vigorous exercise that improves coordination, balance, and general fitness is helpful. Walking, bicycling, dancing, low-impact aerobics, and other group exercise programs will not only improve function, but also provide the opportunity for socialization.

Tremor, Bradykinesia, Hypokinesia, and Rigidity
Although tremor does not usually cause the same degree of impairment as other aspects of PD, it can severely limit function. The tremor is typically a resting-postural tremor that often improves (or at least does not become worse) during movement. Anticholinergic medications can be tried, and may be helpful if tolerated. As the tremor becomes worse with anxiety or stress, relaxation techniques often are helpful. The use of distal weights are not beneficial in the management of tremor.

Bradykinesia (slowness of movement), hypo-kinesia (smallness of movement), and rigidity affecting flexor muscles more than extensors are the key direct neurologic impairments underlying the disability caused by PD. Range of motion and stretching on a daily basis are important in preserving flexibility. Initiation of movement, larger excursions during movement, and co-ordination should be addressed as a part of functional activities. There is increasing evidence that exercise is most effective when it is task-specific.[203] Task-specific exercise might be especially important for the patient with PD in light of the impairments in motor planning and programing characteristic of the disease. Helpful strategies and techniques include measures such as rocking to and fro in the chair before arising and other preparatory motions to provide momentum. A raised chair, toilet seat, and armrests also make rising easier.

One of the most difficult problems is the PD patient's inability to use automatic response during willed functional movement. Repetition improves these responses and the resulting functional movements.[203] Rigidity can result in musculoskeletal pain that often responds to heat, massage, stretching, and range of motion exercises.

Autonomic Dysfunction   Orthostatic hypotension, of all autonomic symptoms, is the most common symptom of end stage PD. Rising slowly from supine and pausing in the sitting position before standing, elevating the head of the bed, and use of pressure garments are conservative approaches that are helpful. Mineralcorticoids also can be beneficial.

Slowed gastric and intestinal motility lead to early satiety, vomiting, poor absorption of medication, and constipation. Useful strategies include frequent small meals, increased fiber intake, bulking agents, stool softeners, suppositories, and timed voiding. Metaclo-pramide facilitates gastric emptying, but should be avoided because of its tendency to cause Parkinsonian side-effects. Cisapride, another such agency, might be a better choice.

Urinary incontinence, difficulty voiding, retention, and infection also can occur. Recurrent urinary infections frequently indicate neurogenic bladder dysfunction, although other causes such as prostatic hypertrophy also are common in this age group. An appropriate investigation typically includes post-void residual, cystoscopy, assessment of renal function, and a cystometrogram-sphincter electromyography (CMG/EMG). These studies guide technical and pharmacologic interventions. An indwelling catheter should only be used as a last resort, usually in the care of a severely disabled patient.

Impotence also can occur as a result of autonomic dysfunction and/or psychological factors. Appropriate assessment and treatment should be considered, as much as any other aspect of disability related to PD.

Sympathetic pain and reflex sympathetic dystrophy can be seen in PD. Pain is often alleviated by levodopa. If it is not, tricyclic antidepressants often are helpful and can decrease tremor. In later stages, the anticholinergic effects on cognition are less well tolerated. The effectiveness of serotonergic reuptake inhibitor antidepressants in alleviating neurogenic pain is unclear.

Cardiopulmonary Function   Flexed posture leads to kyphosis and reduced lung capacity. Rigidity can result in a "restrictive" pulmonary disease pattern, further complicating respiratory function. Endurance often decreases as a result of a sedentary lifestyle. A focus on breathing exercises, proper posture, and trunk extension early in PD is helpful to prevent these musculoskeletal complications that contribute to the high incidence of pulmonary complications. Cardiopulmonary conditioning should also be a component of the early treatment program. Later in the course, breathing and extension exercises should be continued, with the addition of coughing, incentive spirometry, and respiratory therapy techniques. Instruction in energy conservation techniques and pacing can preserve the ability to continue a productive lifestyle.

Management of declining cognitive function becomes an issue in many cases. Although PD has its peak incidence in the sixth decade, the disease begins in some patients in their 40s or 50s. At this point, most will be either employed or responsible for management of the home. Deficiencies in cognitive function very early in the disease may not be apparent on a social level, but may cause problems at work (particularly in highly technical, skilled, or professional occupations). Full neuropsychological assessment is prudent in such cases. In other cases, more limited testing to assess for safety to continue independent living or driving is adequate. Making the family aware of safety issues and providing both the family and patient with compensatory strategies is essential.

A psychologist, psychiatrist, or experienced social worker can all provide helpful input regarding the patient's emotional state. Pharmacologic intervention for depression must be considered for functionally disabling depression. Counseling for both patient and family may be helpful in developing coping skills. Awareness of and encouragement to use community resources and support groups is essential.

ADLs and Adaptive Equipment   As the primary purpose of rehabilitation is to improve or maintain function, a thorough functional assessment is key to the development of an integrated program for the patient with PD. The physical and occupational therapist should work closely together in both the assessment and development of the program. Although ideally the approach is to maintain or improve impairments, to the degree that this becomes impossible, instruction in compensatory techniques and the use of various devices allows the patient to remain functional for a prolonged period. A home visit will help not only in assessing the need for home modification, but also allows the therapists to see how the patient functions in the home.

As in patients with other chronic disabling conditions, patients with PD quickly lose ground when periods of illness restrict their activity or put them at bed rest. Care should be taken to provide range of motion, stretching, proper positioning, breathing exercises, and whatever mobility the patient can tolerate in these situations.

REFERENCES

1. Adams RD, Victor M: *Principles of Neurology,* 6th ed. New York: McGraw-Hill, 1997.
2. Cobble ND, et al, in Delisa JA, Gans B: *Rehabilitation Medicine: Principles and Practice,* 2 ed. Philadelphia: JB Lippincott, 1993.
3. Kocsis JD, Waxman SG: Demyelination: Causes and mechanisms of clinical abnormalilty and functional recovery, in Vinken PJ, Bruyn GW, Klawans HL, Koetsier JC (eds): *Hand-book of Clinical Neurology,* vol. 47. *Demyelinating Diseases.* Amsterdam: Elsevier, 1985, pp. 29–47.
4. Rasminsky M: Pathophysiology of demyelination. *Ann NY Acad Sci* 1984; 436:68–85.
5. McDonald WI, Silberberg DH (eds): *Multiple Sclerosis.* London: Butterworths, 1986, pp. 112–113.
6. Dean G, Kurtzke JF: On the risk of multiple sclerosis according to age at immigration to South Africa. *Br Med J* 1971; 3:725.
7. Kraft GH, Freal JE, Coryell JK, et al: Multiple sclerosis: Early prognostic guidelines. *Arch Phys Med Rehab* 1981; 62:54–58
8. Burks JS, Thompson DS: Multiple sclerosis, in Earnest M (ed): *Therapeutic Emergencies.* New York: Churchill-Livingstone.
9. Percy AK, Bobrega FY, Okazaki H, et al: MS in Rochester, Minn.: A 60 year reappraisal. *Arch Neuro* 1971; 25:105–111.
10. LaRocca NG: *J Neurol Rehab* 1992; 6:3.
11. Weinshenke BG, Ebers GC: The natural history of multiple sclerosis. *Can J Neurol Sci* 1987; 14:255–261.
12. Sadovnick AD, Ebers GC, Wilson RW, Paty DW: Life expectancy in patients attending multiple sclerosis clinics. *Neurology* 1992; 42:991–994.
13. Gay D, Esiri M: Blood-brain barrier damage in acute multiple sclerosis plaques: An immunocytological study. *Brain* 1991; 114:557–572.
14. Adams CW, Poston RN, Buk SJ: Pathology, histochemistry and immunocytochemistry of lesions in acute multiple sclerosis. *J Neurol Sci* 1989; 92:291–306.
15. Paty DW, et al: *J Neurol Rehab* 1993; 7:3/4.
16. Isaac C, Li DK Genton M, et al: Multiple sclerosis: A serial study using MRI in relapsing patients. *Neurology* 1988; 38(10):1511–1515.
17. Willoughby EW, Grochowski E, Li DK, Oger J, Kastrukoff LF, Paty DW: Serial magnetic resonance scanning in multiple sclerosis: A second prospective study in relapsing patients. *Ann Neurol* 1989; 25(1):43–49.
18. Multiple Sclerosis: A National Survey. NIH publication no. 84-2479. Bethesda, MD: United States Depaartment of Health and Human Services, Public Health Service, National Institutes of Health, 1984.
19. McFarland HF, Dhib-Jalbut S: Multiple sclerosis: Possible immumological mechanisms. *Clin Immunol Immunopathol* 1989; 50:96–105.
20. Poser CM: The diagnostic process in multiple sclerosis, in Power CM, Paty DW, Scheinberg L, et al (eds): *The Diagnosis of Multiple Sclerosis.* New York: Thieme-Stratton, 1984, pp. 3–13.
21. Scott TF: Diseases that mimic multiple sclerosis. *Postgrad Med* 1991; 89:187–191.
22. McAlpine D: Multiple sclerosis: A review. *Br Med J* 1973; 2:292–295.
23. Izquerdo G, Gauw J, Lyon-Cain O, et al: Value of multiple sclerosis diagnostic criteria: 70 autopsy confirmed cases. *Arch Neurol* 1985; 42:848–850.
24. McFarllin DE, McFarland HF: Multiple sclerosis. *N Engl J Med* 1982; 307:1183–1188, 1246–1251.

25. McDonald WE, Silberberg DH: The diagnosis of multiple sclerosis, in McDonald WI, Silberberg DH (eds): *Multiple Sclerosis*. London: Butterworths, 1986, pp. 1–10.

26. Paty DW, Oger JJ, Kastrukoff LF, et al: MRI in the diagnosis of MS: A prospective study with comparison of clinical evaluation, evoked potentials, oligoclonal banding, and CT. *Neurology* 1988; 38:180–185.

27. Jacobs L, Kinkel WR, Polachini I, Kinkel RP: Correlations of nuclear magnetic resonance imaging, computerized tomography, and clinical profiles in multiple sclerosis. *Neurology* 1986; 36:27–34.

28. Ormerod IE, Miller DH, McDonald WI: The role of NMR imaging in the assessment of multiple sclerosis and isolated neurological lesions: A quantitative study. *Brain* 1987; 110:1579–1616.

29. Valk J, De Slegte RG, Creqee FC, Hazenberg GJ, et al: Contrast enhanced magnetic resonance imaging of the brain using gadolinium-DTPA. *Acta Radiol* 1987; 28:659–665.

30. Burkes JS: *J Neurorehab* 1992; 6:3.

31. Miller DM: MD. *J Neurorehab* 1994; 8:3.

32. Granger C, Cotter A, Hamilton B, Fiedler R, Hens M: Functional assessment scales: A study of persons with multiple sclerosis. *Arch Phys Med Rehab* 1990; 71:870–875.

33. Verdier-Taillefer MH, Zuber M, Lyon-Caen O, Clanet M, Gout O, Louis C, Alperovitch A: Observer disagreement in rating neurologic impairment in multiple sclerosis: Facts and consequences. *Eur Neurol* 1991; 31:117–119.

34. Kurtzke J: The disability status scale for multiple sclerosis: Apologia pro DSS. *Neurology* 1989; 39:291–302.

35. Goodkin DE, Cookfair D, Wende K, Bourdette D, Pullicino P, Scherokman B, Whitham R: Multiple Sclerosis Collaborative Research Group. Inter- and intrarater scoring agreement using grades 1.0 to 3.5 of the Kurtzke Expanded Disability Status Scale (EDSS). *Neurology* 1992; 42:859–863.

36. Cooperman L, et al: *J Neurorehab* 1994; 8:3.

37. Goodman TL, Hicks RW: Comparison of disability status and exercise performance in patients with multiple sclerosis. *Med Sci Sports Exercise* 1993; 25(suppl):S44.

38. Cohen RA, Kessler HR, Fischer M: The extended disability status scale (EDSS) as a predictor of impairments of functional activities of daily living in multiple sclerosis. *J Neurol Sci* 1993; 115:132–135.

39. Halper J, et al: What do we know about MS care? *J Neurorehab* 1994; 8:3.

40. Syndulko, et al: *J Neurorehab* 1993; 7:3/4.

41. Slater RJ: Scoring techniques and problems in the evaluation of change in patients. *Arch Neurol* 1983; 40:675–677.

42. Willoughby EW, Paty DW: Scales for rating impairment in multiple sclerosis: A critique. *Neurology* 1988; 38:1793–1798.

43. Kurtzke JF: Rating neurologic impairment in multiple sclerosis: An expanded disability status sclae (EDSS). *Neurology* 1983; 33:1444–1452.

44. Noseworthy JH, Vandervoort MK, et al: Group CCMS: Interrater variability with the expanded disability status scale (EDSS) and functional systems (FS) in a multiple sclerosis clinical trial. *Neurology* 1990; 40:971–975.

45. Mickey MR, Ellison GW, Myers LW: An illness severity score for multiple sclerosis. *Neurology* 1984; 34:1343–1347.

46. Sipe JC, Knobler RL, et al: A neurologic rating scale (NRS) for use in multiple sclerosis. *Neurology* 1984; 34:1368–1372.

47. Feigenson JS, Scheinberg L, Catalano M, Polkow L, Mantegazza PM, Feigenson WD, LaRocca NF: The cost effectiveness of multiple sclerosis rehabilitation: A model. *Neurology* 1981; 31(10):1316–1322.

48. Reding MJ, LaRocca NG, Madonna M: Acute hospital care versus rehabilitation hospitallization for management of nonemergent complications in multiple sclerosis. *J Neurol Rehab* 1987; (1):13–17.

49. Francabandera FL, et al: Multiple sclerosis rehabilitation: Inpatient vs. outpatient. *Rehab Nurs* 1988; 13(5):251–253.

50. Haber A, Larocca NG: Minimal record of disability for multile sclerosis. New York: National Multiple Sclerosis Society, 1985.

51. Carey RG, et al: Who makes the most progress in inpatient rehabilitation? An analysis of functional gain. *Arch Phys Med Rehab* 1988; 69:337–343.

52. Greenspun B, Stimeman M, Agri R: Multiple sclerosis and rehabilitation outcome. *Arch Phys Med Rehab* 1987; 68:434–437.

53. Gehlsen G, Beekman K, Assmann N, Winant D, Seidle M, Carter A: Gait characteristics in multiple sclerosis: Progressive changes and effects of exercise on parameters. *Arch Phys Med Rehab* 1986; 67:536–539.

54. Cobble N: *J Neurorehab* 1992; 6:3.

55. Halper J: The functional model in multiple sclerosis. *Rehab Nurs* 1990; 15:77–85

56. Kraft GH, Alquist AD, de Lateur BJ: Unpublished data/personal communication: Effect of resistive exercise on strength in patients with multiple sclerosis.

57. Armstrong LE, Winant DM, et al: Using isokinetic dynamometry to test ambulatory patients with multiple sclerosis. *Phys Ther* 1983; 63:1274–1279.

58. Chen W-Y, Pierson FM, Burnett CN: Force-time measurements of knee muscle functions of subjects with multiple sclerosis. *Phys Ther* 1987; 67:934–940.

59. Kraft GH, Alquist AD, De Lateur BJ: Effect of resistive exercise on physical function in multiple sclerosis, unpublished data.

60. Draft GH: Movement disorders, in Basmajian JV, Kirby L (eds): *Medical Rehabilitation*. Baltimore: Williams & Wilkins, 1984, pp. 19–33.

61. Chan A, Theriot K: *J Neurorehab* 1994; 8:3.

62. Shumway-Cook A, Horak FB: Assessing the influence of sensory interaction on balance. *Phys Ther* 1986; 66:1548–1550.

63. Lewis C: Balance, gait test proves simple yet useful. *PT Bull* 1993; 10:9, 40.

64. Tinetti ME: Performance-oriented assessment of mobility problems in elderly patients. *J Am Geriatr Soc* 1986; 34:119–126.

65. Pratt CA, Horak FB, Herndon RM: Differential effects of somatosensory and motor system deficits on postural dyscontrol in multiple sclerosis patients, in Woolloacott M, Horak F (eds): Posture and Gait: Mechanisms. Eugene, OR: University of Oregon Books, 1992, pp. 118–121.

66. Shepard NT, Telian SA, Smith-Wheelock M: Habituation and balance retraining therapy: A retrospective review. *Neurol Clin* 1990; 8:459–475.

67. Shumway-Cook A, Horak FB: Rehabilitation strategies for patients with vestibular deficits. *Neurol Clin* 1990; 8:441–457.

68. Freal JE, Kraft GH, Coryell JK: Symptomatic fatigue in multiple sclerosis. *Arch Phys Med Rehab* 1984; 65:135–138.

69. Krupp L, Alvarez L, LaRocca N, Scheinberg L: Fatigue in multiple sclerosis. *Arch Neurol* 1988; 45:435–437.

70. Enoka R, Stuart D: Neurobiology of muscle fatigue. *J Appl Physiol* 1992; 72:1631–1648.

71. MacLaren D, et al: A review of metabolic and physiological factors in fatigue, in: Pandolf K (ed): *Exercise and Sport Sciences Reviews*. Baltimore: Williams & Wilkins, 1989, pp. 29–66.

72. Spencer M, et al: Functional response to acute exercise in multiple sclerosis. *Med Sci Sports Exercise* 1993; 25(suppl):S44.

73. Ponichtera-Muncare JA: Exercise in multiple sclerosis. *Med Sci Sports Exercise* 1993; 25(4):451–465.

74. Cohen R, Fisher M: Amantadine treatment of fatigue associated with multiple sclerosis. *Arch Neurol* 1989; 46:676–680.

75. Rosenberg G, Appenzeller O: Amantadine, fatigue, and multiple sclerosis. *Arch Neurol* 1988; 45:1104–1106.

76. Murray TJ: Amantadine therapy for fatigue in multiple sclerosis. *Can J Neurol Sci* 1985; 12:251–254.

77. Weinstein BG, Penman M, Bass B, Ebers GC, Rice GPA: A double-blind, randomized, crossover trial of pemonline in fatigue associated with multiple sclerosis. *Neurology* 1992; 42:1468–1471.

78. Krupp L, LaRocca N, Nuir-Nash J, Steinberg A: The fatigue severity scale: Application to patients with multiple sclerosis and systemic lupus erythematosus. *Arch Neurol* 1989; 46:1121–1123.

79. Brar SP, Smith MB, Nelson LM, Franklin GM, Cobble ND: Evaluation of treatment protocols on minimal to moderate spasticity in multiple sclerosis. *Arch Phys Med Rehab* 1991; 72(3):186–189.

80. Katz RT, Rovai GP, Brait C, Rymer WZ: Objective quantification of spastic hypertonia: Correlation with clinical findings. *Arch Phys Med Rehab* 1992; 73(4):339–347.

81. Bohannon RW, Smith MB: Interrater reliability on a modified Ashworth scale of muscle spasticity. *Phys Ther* 1987; 67:206–207.

82. Robinson CJ, Kett NA, Bolam JM: Spasticity in spinal cord injured patients: Short term effects of surface electrical stimulation. *Arch Phys Med Rehab* 1988; 69(8): 598–604.

83. Bajd T, Gregoric M, Vodovnik L, Benko H: Electrical stimulation in treating spasticity resulting from spinal cord injury. *Arch Phys Med Rehab* 1985; 66(8):515–517.

84. Bajd T, Bowman RG: Testing and modeling of spasticity. *J Biomed Eng* 1982; 4:90–99.

85. Bajd T, Vodovnki L: Pendulum testing of spasticity. *J Biomed Eng* 1984; 6:9–16.

86. Boczko M, Mumenthaler M: Modified pendulousness test to assess tonus of thigh muscles in spasticity. *Neurology* 1958; 8:846–851.

87. Wartenberg R: Pendulouness of the legs as a diagnostic test. *Neurology* 1951; 1:18–24.

88. Vodovnik L, Bowman BR, Hufford P: Effects of electrical stimulation on spinal spasticity. *Med Biol Eng Comput* 1987; 25:439–442.

89. Haber A, LaRocca N (eds): *Minimal Record of Disability for Multiple Sclerosis*. New York: National Multiple Sclerosis Society, 1985.

90. Carey JR: Manual stretch: Effect on finger movement control and force control in stroke subjects with spastic extrinsic finger flexor muscles. *Arch Phys Med Rehab* 1990; 71(11):888–894.

91. Robichaud JA, Agostinucci J, Vander Linden DWV: Effect of air splint application on soleus muscle motoneuron reflex excitability in nondisabled subjects and subjects with cerebrovascular accidents. *Phys Ther* 1992; 72(3):176–184.

92. Tremblay F, Malouin F, Richards CL, Dumas F: Effects of prolonged muscle stretch on reflex and voluntary muscle activations in children with spastic cerebral palsy. *Scand J Rehab Med* 1990; 22(4):171–180.

93. Scherling E, Johnson H: A tone reducing wrist hand orthosis. *Am Occ Ther* 1989; 43(9):609–611.

94. Schapiro RT: *Symptom Management in Multiple Sclerosis*. New York: Demos, 1987, p. 12.

95. Schapiro RT: *Multiple Sclerosis: A Rehabilitation Approach to Management*. New York: Demos, 1991, p. 20.

96. Brar SP, Smith MB, Nelson LM, Franklin GM, Cobble ND: Evaluation of treatment protocols on minimal to moderate spasticity in multiple sclerosis. *Arch Phys Med Rehab* 1991; 72(3):186–189.

97. Cruickshank DA, O'Neill DL: Upper extremity inhibitive cast in a boy with spastic quadriplegia. *Am J Occ Ther* 1990; 44(6):552–555.

98. Yasukawa A: Upper extremity casting: Adjunct treatment for a child with cerebral palsy hemiplegia. *Am J Occ Ther* 1990; 44(9):840–846.

99. Smelt HR: Effect of an inhibitive weight bearing mitt on tone reduction and functional performance in a child with cerebral palsy. *Phys Occ Ther Pediatr* 1989; 9(2):53–80.

100. Langlois S, MacKinnon JR, Pederson L: Hand splints and cerebral spasticity: A review of the literature. *Can J Occup Ther* 1989; 56(3):113–119.

101. Lanflois S, Pederson L, MacKinnon JR: The effects of splinting on the spastic hemiplegic hand. *Can J Occup Ther* 1991; 58(1):17–25.

102. Phillips WE, Audet M: Use of serial casting in the management of knee joint contractures in an adolescent with cerebral palsy. *Phys Ther* 1990; 70(8):521–523.

103. Smith LH, Harris SR: Upper extremity inhibitive casting for a child with cerebral palsy. *Phys Occup Ther Pediatr* 1985; 5(1):71–79.

104. Carlson SJ: A neurophysiological analysis of inhibitive casting: Therapeutic intervention in cerebral palsy. *Phys Occup Ther Pediatr* 1984; 4(4):31–42.

105. Mills VM: Electromyographic results of inhibitory splinting. *Phys Ther* 1984; 64(2):190–193.

106. Booth BJ, Doyle M, Montgomery J: Serial casting for the management of spasticity in the head injured adult. *Phys Ther* 1983; 63(12):1960–1966.

107. McPherson JJ, Kreimeyer D, Alderks M: A comparison of dorsal and volar resting hand splints in the reduction of hepertonus. *Am J Occup Ther* 1982; 36(10):664–670.

108. King TI: Plaster splinting as a means of reducing elbow flexor spasticity: A case study. *Am J Occup Ther* 1982; 36(10):671–673.

109. Nash J, Neilson PD, O'Daiyer NJ: Reducing spasticity to control muscle contracture of children with cerebral palsy. *Dev Med Child Neurol* 1989; 31(4):471–480.

110. Wissel J, Ebersbach G, Gutjahr L, Dahlke F: Treating chronic hemparesis with modified biofeedback. *Arch Phys Med Rehab* 1989; 70(8):612–617.

111. Penn RD: Electrostimulation for spasticity. *Neurosurgery* 1988; 22(2):440–441.

112. Dimitrijevic MR, Sherwood AM: Spasticity: Medical and surgical management. *Neurology* 1980; 30:19–27.

113. Fredriksen TA, Bergmann S, Hesselberg JP, Stolt-Nielsen A, Ringkjob R, Sjaastad O: Electrical stimulation in multiple sclerosis: Comparison of transcutaneous electrical stimulation and epidural spinal cord stimulation. *Appl Neurophysiol* 1986; 49:4–24.

114. Walker JB: Modulation of spasticity. *Science* 1982; 216:203–204.

115. Namey M, et al: *J Neurorehab* 1994; 8:3.

116. Betts CD, Jones SJ, Fowler CG, Fowler CJ: Erectile dysfunction in multiple sclerosis: Associated neurological and neurophysiological deficits, and treatment of the condition. *Brain* 1994; 117:1303–1310.

117. Hirsch H, Smith RL, et al: Use of intracavernous injection of prostaglandin E1 for neuropathic erectile dysfunction. *Paraplegia* 1994; 32:661–664.

118. Heller MD, Okeren O, Aloni R, Davidoff G: An open trial of vacuum penile tumescence: Constriction therapy for neurological impotence. *Paraplegia* 1992; 30:550–553.

119. Larocca NG, et al: Assessment of outcomes in multiple sclerosis. *Neurorehabilitation* 1993; 7:3/4.

120. Rao SM, Leo GJ, Bernardin L, Unverzagt F: Cognitive dysfunction in multiple sclerosis. I. Frequency, patterns, and prediction. *Neurology* 1991; 41:685–691.

121. Heaton RK, Nelson LM, Thompson DS, Burks JS, Franklin GM: Neuropsychological findings in relapsing–remitting and chronic–progressive multiple sclerosis. *J Consult Clin Psychol* 1985; 53:103–110.

122. Fischer J, et al: *J Neurorehab* 1994; 8(3).

123. Rao SM, Leo GJ, Haughton VM, St. Aubin-Faubert P, Bernardin L: Correlation of magnetic resonance imaging with neuropsychological testing in multiple sclerosis. *Neurology* 1989; 39:161–166.

124. Franklin GM, Nelson LM, Filley CM, Heaton RK: Cognitive loss in multiple sclerosis: Case reports and a review of the literature. *Arch Neurol* 1989; 46:162–167.

125. Jennekens-Schinkel A, Sanders EACM: Decline of cognition in multiple sclerosis: dissociable deficits. *J Neurol Neurosurg Psychiatr* 1986; 49:1354–1360.

126. Beatty WW, Goodkin DE, Monson N, Beatty PA: Cognitive disturbances in patients with relapsing remitting multiple sclerosis. *Arch Neurol* 1989; 46:1113–1119.

127. Van den Burg W, Van Zommeren AH, Minderhoud J, Prange AJAM, Beuher NSA: Cognitive impairment in patients with multiple sclerosis and mild physical disability. *Arch Neurol* 1987; 44:722–736.

128. Lyon-Caen O, Jouvent R, Hauser S, et al: Cognitive functioning in recent-onset demyelinating disease. *Arch Neurol* 1986; 43:1138–1141.

129. Peyser JM, Rao SM, LaRocca NG, Kaplan E: Guidelines for neuropsychological research in multiple sclerosis. *Arch Neurol* 1990; 47:94–97.

130. Peyser JM, Edwards KR, Poser CM, Filskov SB: Cognitive function in patients with multiple sclerosis. *Arch Neurol* 1980; 37:577–579.

131. Beatty WW, et al: *J Neurorehab* 1993; 7:3–4.

132. Beatty WW, Goodkin DE: Screening for cognitive impairment in multiple sclerosis: An evaluation of the Mini-Mental State examination. *Arch Neurol* 1990; 47:297–301.

133. Franklin GM, Heaton RK, Nelson LM, Filley CM, Seibert C: Correlation of neuropsychological and MRI findings in chronic/progressive multiple sclerosis. *Neurology* 1988; 38:1826–1829.

134. Rao SM, Leo GJ, Bernardin L, Unverzagt F: Cognitive dysfunction in multiple sclerosis. I. Frenquency, patterns, and prediction. *Neurology* 1991; 41:685–691.

135. Rao SM: Neurosphchology of multiple sclerosis: A critical review. *J Clin Exp Neuropsychol* 1986; 8:503–542.

136. Cummings JL, Benson DF: Subcortical dementia: A review of an emerging concept. *Arch Neurol* 1984; 41:874–879.

137. Canter AH: Direct and indirect measures of psychological deficit in multiple sclerosis. *J Gen Psychol* 1951; 44:3–50.

138. Ron MA, Callanan MM, Warrington EK: Cognitive abnormalities in multiple sclerosis: A psychometric and MRI study. *Psychol Med* 1991; 21:59–68.

139. Litvan I, Grafman J, Vendrell P, Martinez JM: Slowed

information processing in multiple sclerosis. *Arch Neurol* 1988; 45:281–285.

140. Jennekens-Schinkel A, van der Velde EA, Sanders EA, Lanser JB: Memory and learning in outpatients with quiescent multiple sclerosis. *J Neurol Sci* 1990; 95:311–325.

141. Beatty WW, Goodkin DE, Monson N, Beatty PA: Cognitive disturbances in patients with relapsing remitting multiple sclerosis. *Arch Neurol* 1989; 46:1113–1119.

142. Litvan I, Grafman J, Vendrell P, Martinez JM: Slowed information processing in multiple sclerosis. *Arch Neurol* 1988; 45:281–285.

143. Beatty WW, Goodkin DE, Monson N, Beatty PA, Hertsgaard D: Anterograde and retrograde amnesia in patients with chronic progressive multiple sclerosis. *Arch Neurol* 1988; 45:611–619.

144. Grant I, McDonald WI, Trimble MR, Smith E, Reed R: Deficient learning and memory in early and middle phases of multiple sclerosis. *J Neurol Neurosurg Psychiatr* 1984; 47:250–255.

145. Rao SM, Hammeke TA, McQuillen MP, Kharti BO, Lloyd D: Memory disturbance in chronic progressive multiple sclerosis. *Arch Neurol* 1984; 41:625–631.

146. Beatty WW, Monson N, Goodkin DE: Access to semantic memory in Parkinson's disease and multiple sclerosis. *J Geriatr Psychiatry Neurol* 1989; 2:153–162.

147. Caine ED, Bamford KA, Schiffer RB, Shoulson I, Levy S: A controlled neuropsychological comparison of Huntington's disease and multiple sclerosis. *Arch Neurol* 1986; 43:249–254.

148. Fischer JS: Using the Wechsler Memory Scale–Revised to detect and characterize memory deficits in multiple sclerosis. *Clin Neuropsychol* 1988; 2:149–172.

149. Huber SJ, Paulson GW, Shuttleworth EC, et al: Magnetic resonance imaging correlates of dementia in multiple sclerosis. *Arch Neurol* 1987; 44:732–736.

150. Peyser JM, Edwards KR, Poser CM, Filskov SB: Cognitive function in patients with multiple sclerosis. *Arch Neurol* 1980; 37:577–579.

151. Lyon-Caen O, Jouvent R, Hauser S, et al: Cognitive function in recent-onset demyelinating diseases. *Arch Neurol* 1986; 43:1138–1141.

152. Brooks DJ, Leenders KL, Head G, Marshall J, Legg NJ, Jones T: Studies on regional cerebral oxygen utilisation and cognitive function in multiple sclerosis. *J Neurol Neurosurg Psychiatr* 1984; 47:1182–1191.

153. Newton MR, Barrett G, Callanan MM, Towell AD: Cognitive event-related potentials in multiple sclerosis. *Brain* 1989; 112:1637–1660.

154. Sorensen P, Herndon R, et al: *J. Neurorehab* 1994; 8:3.

155. Mahler ME, Davis RJ, Benson DF: Screening multiple sclerosis patients for cognitive impairments, in Jenson K, Knudsen L, Stenager E, Grant I (eds): *Mental Disorders and Cognitive Deficits in Multiple Sclerosis.* London: Libbey, 1989.

156. Leo GJ, Rao SM: Effects of intravenous physostigmine and lecithin on memory loss in multiple sclerosis: Report of a pilot study. *J Neurorehab* 1988; 2:123–129.

157. Prigatano GP, Fordyce DJ, Zeiner HK, Roueche JR, Pepping M, Wood BC: *Neuropsychological Rehabilitation after Brain Injury.* Baltimore: Johns Hopkins, 1986.

158. Joffe RT, Lippert GP, Gray TA, Sawa G, Horvath Z: Mood disorder and multiple sclerosis. *Arch Neurol* 1987; 44:376–378.

159. Foley FW, Traugott U, LaRocca NG, et al: A prospective study of depression and immune dysregulation in multiple sclerosis. *Arch Neurol* 1992; 49:238–244.

160. Schiffer RB, Wineman NM: Antidepressant pharmacotherapy of depression associated with multiple sclerosis. *Am J Psychiatr* 1990; 147:1493–1497.

161. Schiffer RB, Babigian HM: Behavioral disorders in multiple sclerosis, temporal lobe epilepsy, and amyotrophic lateral sclerosis: An epidemiologic study. *Arch Neurol* 1984; 41:1067–1069.

162. Crawford J, McIvor GP: Stress management for multiple sclerosis patients. *Psychol Rep* 1987; 61:423–429.

163. Crawford JD, McIvor GP: Group psychotherapy: Benefits in multiple sclerosis. *Arch Phys Med Rehab* 1985; 66:810–813.

164. Jonsson A, Korfitzen EM, Heltberg A, Ravnborg MH, Byskov-Ottosen E: Effects of neuropsychological treatment in patients with multiple sclerosis. *Acta Neurol Scand* 1993; 88:394–400.

165. Broe CA, Akhter AJ, Andrews CR, et al: Neurological disorders in the elderly at home. *J Neurol Neurosurg Psychiatr* 1976; 39:362–366.

166. ManKovskij N, Karaban I, Mialovickaig: Aging and its relation to Parkinsonism. *Neurology* 1993; 43:2(suppl 1):29.

167. Bethlem J, Den Hartog Jager WA: The incidence and characteristics of Lewy bodies in idiopathic paralysis agitans (Parkinson's disease). *J Neurol Neurosurg Psychiatr* 1960; 23:74–80.

168. Fearnley JM, Lees AJ: Ageing and Parkinson's disease: Substantia nigra regional selectivity. *Brain* 1991; 114:2283–2301.

169. Atadzhanov M, Rakhimdhanov A: "Dopamine deficiency and cholinergic models of the parkinsonia syndrome." *Neurology* 1993; 43:2(suppl 1)S126–129.

170. Jankovic J: "Theories on the etiology and pathogenesis of Parkinson's Disease." *Neurology* 1993; 43:2(suppl 1), S121–123.

171. Stern MB: "Parkinson's disease," in Johnson RT, Griffin (eds): *Current Therapy in Neurologic Disease,* 4th ed. St. Louis: Mosby-Yearbook, 1993, pp. 242–246.

172. Homberg V: "Motor training in the therapy of Parkinson's disease." *Neurology* 1993; 43:12(suppl 6)S45–S46.

173. McDowell FH, Cedarbaum JM: "The extrapyramidal system and disorders of movement," in Joynt R (ed): *Clinical Neurology* rev ed. Philadelphia: JB Lippincott, 1991, ch. 38.

174. Caird FI: Non-drug therapy of Parkinson's disease. *Scott Med J* 1986; 31:129–132.

175. Weiner WJ, Singer C: Parkinson's Disease and nonpharmacologic treatment programs. *J Am Ger Soc* 1989; 37:359–363.

176. Cedarbaum JM, Troy L, Silvestri Metal: Rehabilitation programs in the management of patients with Parkinson's Disease. *J Neurol Rehab* 1992; 6:7–19.

177. Hurwitz A: The benefits of a home exercise regimen for ambulatory patients with Parkinson's disease. *J Neurosci Nurs* 1989; 21:180–184.

178. Mitchel PH, Mertz MA, Catanzaro M-L: Group exercise: A nursing therapy in Parkinson's disease. *Rehab Nurs* 1987; 12:242–245.

179. Franklin S, Cohout LJ, Stern GM, et al: Physical therapy, in Rose F, Capildeo R (eds): *Research Progress in Parkinson's Disease*. London: Pitman Medical, 1981, pp. 397–400.

180. Palmer SS, Mortimer JA, Webster DD, et al: Exercise therapy for Parkinson's disease. *Arch Phys Med Rehab* 1986; 67:741–745.

181. Comella CL, Stebbins GT, Brown-Toms N, et al: Physical therapy and Parkinson's Disease: A controlled clinical trial. *Neurology* 1994; 44:376–378.

182. Beattie A, Caird FI: The occupational therapist and the patient with Parkinson's disease. *Br Med J* 1980; 1:1354–1356.

183. Critchley EMR: Speech disorders of Parkinsonism: A review. *J Neurol Neurosurg Psychiatr* 1984; 47:751–758.

184. Mutch WJ, et al: Parkinson's disease: Disability, review, and management (Medical Practice). *Br Med J* 1986; 293:675–677.

185. Sarno MT: Speech impairment in Parkinson's disease. *Arch Phys Med Rehab* 1968; 49:269.

186. Allan CM: Treatment of nonfluent speech resulting from neurological disease: Treatment of dysarthria. *Br J Disord Commun* 1970; 5:3–5.

187. Robertson S, Thomson F: A study of the efficacy and long term effects of intensive treatment. *Br J Disord Commun* 1984; 19:213–224.

188. Scott S, Caird FI: Speech therapy for Parkinson's disease. *Neurol Neurosurg Psychiatr* 1983; 46:140–144.

189. Scott S, Caird FI: The response of the apparent receptive speech disorder of Parkinson's disease to speech therapy. *J Neurol Neurosurg Psychiatr* 1984; 47:302–304.

190. Stern PH, McDowell FH, Miller JM, et al: Levodopa and physical therapy in treatment of patients with Parkinson's disease. *Arch Phys Med Rehab* 1970; 51:273–277.

191. Lanadin S, Hagenfeldt L, Saltin B, et al: Muscle metabolism during exercise in patients with Parkinson's disease. *Clin Sci Mol Med* 1974; 47:493–506.

192. Parker WD, Boyson SJ, Parks JK: Abnormalities of the electron transport chain in idiopathic Parkinson's disease. *Ann Neurol* 1989; 26:719–723.

193. Bindhoff LA, Birch-Machlin M, Cartlidge NEF, et al: Mitochondrial dysfunction in Parkinson's disease. *Lancet* 1989; 2:49.

194. Saltin B, Landin S: Work capacity, muscle strength and SDH activity in both legs of hemiparetic patients and patients with Parkinson's disease. *Scand J Clin Lab Invest* 1975; 35:531–538.

195. Gersten JW, Marshall C, Dillon T, et al: External work of walking and functional capacity in Parkinsonian patients treated with L-dopa. *Arch Phys Med Rehab* 1972; 53:547–553.

196. Cedarbaum JM, McDowell FH: Sixteen-year follow up of 100 patients begun on Levodopa in 1968: Emerging problems. *Adv Neurol* 1986; 45:469.

197. Mortimer JA, Pirozzolo FJ, Hansch EC, et al: Relationship of motor symptoms to intellectual deficits in Parkinson's disease. *Neurology* 1982; 32:133.

198. Oyebode LR, Barker WA, Blessed G, et al: Cognitive functioning in Parkinson's disease in relation to prevalence of dementia and psychiatric diagnosis. *Br J Psychiatr* 1986; 149:720.

199. Levin BE, Labre MM, Weiner WJ: Cognitive impairments associated with early Parkinson's disease. *Neurology* 1989; 39:557.

200. Mayeux R, Stern Y, Cote L, et al: Altered serotonin metabolism in depressed patients with Parkinson's disease. *Neurology* 1984; 34:642.

201. Scatton B, Javoy-Agid F, Fouquier L, et al: Reduction of cortical dopamine, noradrenaline, serotonin and their metabolites in Parkinson's disease. *Brain Res* 1983; 275:321.

202. Ellgring H, Seiler S, Perleth B, et al: Psychosocial Aspects of Parkinson's disease. *Neurology* 1993; 43:(suppl 6)S41–S44.

203. Gentile AM: Skill acquisition: Action, movement, and neuromotor processes, in Carr JH, Shepart RB (eds): *Movement Science for Physical Therapy in Rehabilitation*. Gaithersburg, MD: Aspen Publishers, 1987, pp. 1–30.

Chapter 13

REHABILITATION MANAGEMENT IN PERIPHERAL NEUROPATHIES

Karen Andrews
Guillermo Suarez
John Michael

Advances in medical rehabilitation have brought significant improvements in the quality of life of patients with peripheral neuropathy of any cause. The clinical manifestations of diabetes mellitus are protean, and offer a useful paradigm for management of symptoms and loss of function in diseases affecting the peripheral nervous system. Diabetic neuropathy is probably the most common form of neuropathy in North America. Comprehensive reviews of the peripheral nervous system, peripheral neuropathies, and specifically diabetic neuropathies have been presented elsewhere and are beyond the scope of this chapter.[1–4]

CLASSIFICATION OF DIABETIC NEUROPATHY

Diabetics are subject to the following clinically distinct neuropathic syndromes: (1) distal sensory motor polyneuropathy; (2) mononeuritis and multiple mononeuropathies including cranial neuropathies; (3) asymmetric proximal motor neuropathy (diabetic amyotrophy); (4) thoracic radiculopathy; (5) acute painful diabetic neuropathy; and (6) small-fiber neuropathy (distal small-fiber neuropathy and diabetic autonomic neuropathy).[4]

Distal Sensory Motor Polyneuropathy

The symptoms and signs of peripheral neuropathy depend on the nerves affected, class and level of axons affected, severity of the underlying pathologic process, age at onset, rate, course, degree of regeneration or sprouting, ectopic impulse generation, and other factors.[5] The symptoms and signs follow a symmetric, length-dependent pattern with the most distal portions of the extremities affected earliest (dying back phenomenon). The sensory system is generally affected first in diabetic neuropathy. Small fiber modalities are especially susceptible, with loss of pain, temperature, and touch before proprioception.[6] The toes are affected first, followed, as the disease progresses, by numbness of the ankles, calves, fingertips, knees, and forearms. This leads to the classic stocking–glove distribution of sensory loss. In severe cases, the shorter intercostal nerves are also involved in a length-dependent manner giving a "teardrop" configuration of sensory loss on the anterior torso.[7] Patients with a distal sensory polyneuropathy may be asymptomatic for years. Symptoms are generally manifested as "numbness, " "tingling," or a "burning" mainly at the toes and feet.[8] Dyck and colleagues found degrees of symptomatic polyneuropathy in 15 percent of patients with insulin-dependent diabetes mellitus and 13 percent of patients with non-insulin-dependent diabetes mellitus.[8] Significant polyneuropathy tends to be associated with diabetic retinopathy, nephropathy, and other end-organ disease. Motor involvement is less apparent and is usually restricted to intrinsic foot and hand muscles until late in the course of the disease. Selective motor polyneuropathy or isolated sensory ataxia are rare in diabetes. Distal symmetrical polyneuropathy is the most common peripheral nerve disorder in patients with diabetes mellitus.[9] Foot pathology is a common cause of morbidity in patients with diabetes. Disease processes range from soft tissue edema, cellulitis, abscess, and skin ulceration, to septic arthritis, osteomyelitis, and neuropathic osteoarthropathy. When there is a history of autonomic and peripheral neuropathy, clinical findings can include decreased perspiration, dry skin, dependent rubor, impaired sensation, and denervation of foot intrinsic muscles with associated claw-foot deformity. Weakness of the peroneal muscles may be compensated during walking by use of the long extensor muscles, especially the extensor hallucis longus muscle to dorsiflex the foot. The subsequent abnormal great toe extension stresses the tip of the toe as it repeatedly strikes the shoe.[10] Charcot changes may be present, including medial tarsal subluxation, pronation, forefoot valgus, increased width, and decreased length that results in abnormal pressure distribution and increased risk for ulceration. Ulcers typically are located at the metatarsal heads, the pulp or tip of a rigid great toe, the heel or midfoot (in the area of collapsed navicula or cuboid bone). Severe motor involvement can result in a "foot drop," with increased pressure distribution at the lateral foot and decreased toe clearance during swing phase.

Mononeuritis and Multiple Mononeuropathies

Although diabetic polyneuropathy has a nonspecific clinical pattern that is indistinguishable from other polyneuropathies, acute mononeuropathies and the proximal motor neuropathy (discussed later) are clinically distinctive and highly associated with coexisting diabetes. Acute cranial mononeuropathies usually occur in middle-aged and older adults. Third-nerve palsy (with sparing of the pupillomotor function) is the most common diabetic cranial mononeuropathy. The abducens, trochlear, and facial nerves are affected in decreasing frequency.[4] Diabetic mononeuropathies appear suddenly and usually have a limited course with spontaneous resolution after weeks or months. It may be difficult to be certain that individual mononeuropathies are due to diabetes, unless other causes of focal neuropathy, such as sarcoidosis, necrotizing vasculitis and leprosy are ruled out. The median, ulnar, lateral femoral cutaneous, and peroneal nerves are most commonly affected. Peripheral nerves may be affected individually or, occasionally, in combination producing a mononeuropathy multiplex. Mononeuropathy multiplex secondary to diabetes is uncommon in relation to the incidence and prevalence of diabetes itself. When present, a superimposed necrotizing vasculitis should be considered.

Proximal Motor Neuropathy

Diabetic proximal motor neuropathy (diabetic amyotrophy or diabetic femoral neuropathy) characteristically occurs in Type II diabetics over the age of 50 with or without evidence of end organ damage either within or outside the nervous system. Onset may be abrupt, over days, or subacute, over weeks. Pain is almost always present, described as deep, aching, and sometimes burning in quality. Although both legs are usually affected, asymmetric weakness and wasting of hip flexors, quadriceps, and hip adductors is common. Other muscle groups, including hamstrings, glutei, and gastrocnemius, are less frequently affected. The quadriceps reflex is reduced or absent on the affected side. Sensory loss other than that seen in an associated subclinical distal sensory motor polyneuropathy is unusual. Functionally, these patients note difficulty with mobility (transfers and ambulation). In general, patients with restricted lumbar plexopathy recover in 3 to 18 months, whereas those with a more diffuse radiculoplexopathy have a poor prognosis.[4] The differential diagnosis should include compression lesions of the lumbosacral roots (predominantly neoplastic or infectious), inflammatory, and autoimmune disorders.

Thoracic Radiculopathy

Thoracic radiculopathy or diabetic truncal neuropathy often begins with pain and dysesthesias in the abdomen, chest, or both. The pain may have a radicular distribution and is usually worse at night. Weakness of the abdominal musculature and a variable pattern of sensory loss also has been reported.[12]

Acute Painful Neuropathy

Painful diabetic sensory neuropathy is a distal sensory neuropathy with severe pain and hyperpathia with little objective evidence of sensory loss. It usually occurs in recently diagnosed insulin-requiring diabetic patients. The onset of painful neuropathic symptoms following vigorous insulin treatment has led to the term "insulin neuritis."[13] In the majority of patients, symptoms subside in 6 to 10 months. When painful symptoms are clearly related to sudden metabolic changes, such as rapid glycemic control, pain remission is more likely.[14] Glycemic control should be maintained as an overall goal of patient management, but symptoms may improve more rapidly if diabetic control is temporarily eased.[4]

Small-Fiber Neuropathy

Small-fiber neuropathy in diabetes and other degenerative disorders of the nervous system is associated with prominent autonomic dysfunction and sensory symptoms. Orthostatic hypotension (postural dizziness, light-headedness, syncope), gastrointestinal symptoms (nocturnal diarrhea, gastroparesis, abdominal bloating), and sexual dysfunction are common. Erythema, mottling, cyanosis, and swelling result from different mechanisms of sympathetic dysfunction (see the following). Painful symptoms often regress after several months, but dysautonomia may persist.

PATHOGENESIS

Polyneuropathy

The pathogenesis of diabetic neuropathy is not known. Many hypotheses, supported by experimental and clinical studies, have been suggested.[15–19] These hypotheses have focused on metabolic, microvascular, and recently, immunologic abnormalities and their interaction. The most important pathologic change in diabetic polyneuropathy is loss of myelinated and unmyelinated nerve axons. Variations in clinical manifestations, severity, and frequency implicate coexisting independent genetic and or environmental variables that may modulate the sensitivity or response to glucose-induced tissue injury. Dyck and associates meticulously demonstrated that the nerves of patients with untreated diabetes and symptoms of neuropathy already showed an increased frequency of segmental demyelination and remyelination, but no increase in axonal degeneration.[15] Nerves of untreated diabetics with symptomatic neuropathy had a mixture of abnormal fibers with segmental demyelination and remyelination, and fibers undergoing axonal degeneration. Nerves of treated diabetics with long-standing symptomatic neuropathy showed mostly axonal degeneration. They propose that an axonal influence initially causes segmental demyelination, then axonal degeneration. The severity of fiber loss and atrophy correlate with the degree of functional impairment in patients with diabetic polyneuropathy.

The Neuropathic Foot

The loss of pain and proprioceptive sensation appears to be of major importance to the pathogenesis of diabetic neuropathic ulcers and osteoarthropathy. Whether neuropathic ulcers can occur with an isolated neuropathic process or only in association with arterial insufficiency remains controversial. Studies by Brand suggest that neuropathic ulcers result from repetitive trauma.[20] Brand studied the histology of rat paws after repetitive stress and determined that an increase in temperature always occurred with repetitive stress. If the temperature increase was followed immediately by a gradual return to normal, this change was thought to be due to simple reactive hyperemia. If temperature increase continued for 10 or more minutes, biopsy showed edema and collection of inflammatory cells. When the repetitions continued at a force equal to walking seven miles per day at a fast pace on hard ground, epithelial hypertrophy with marked inflammation and necrosis of deeper tissues was noted at day three. Ulceration occurred at day 10. When the same experiment was performed with 20 percent fewer daily repetitions and breaks on weekends, hypertrophy occurred without significant breakdown. It can be inferred from this study that in patients with normal sensation, inflammation makes feet tender, and the tender spot is spared further stress until inflammation subsides. With a neuropathic foot, pain is no longer present to provide this feedback.[21] Pecoraro and associates studied 80 consecutive diabetics requiring lower limb amputation and found that an episode of minor trauma preceded the amputation in 69 of 80 patients.[22]

High plantar foot pressures in diabetic patients recently have been found to be strongly predictive of subsequent plantar ulceration, especially in the presence of neuropathy.[23] Patients with rheumatoid arthritis have been compared to diabetic patients with similar foot abnormalities. In the patients with rheumatoid arthritis who have preserved nociception and no evidence of neuropathy, high pressures did not lead to ulceration.[24]

The development of neuropathic joint disease begins with the loss of deep sensation and proprioception. This predisposes the joint to recurrent injury and malalignment. The radiographic manifestations of neuropathic joint disease, heralded by osteopenia, then follow. As the disease progresses, there is loss of articular cartilage, osteophytosis, development of joint effusions, fragmentation of subchondral bone, sclerosis, intra-articular osseous debris, and joint disorganization with subluxation or frank dislocation.[25] In diabetics, the most common location for neuropathic joint disease is the foot, with the midfoot (Lisfranc's joint) being the most common (70 percent), followed by the forefoot (15 percent), and hind foot (15 percent).[26] Pathologically the capsule is thickened. The synovial membrane is indurated and contains osseous and cartilaginous debris. As the joint effusions enlarge, debris may dissect along tissue planes and become far removed from the joint. In long-standing neuropathic osteoarthropathy, the resulting sclerosis, osteophytosis, and fragmentation is dramatic and has been described as "osteoarthritis with a vengeance."[27]

MANAGEMENT

The management program should be individualized to address specific symptoms that appear during the course of the patient's life. The interdisciplinary team approach is important to maximize resources to help the patient maintain or regain function and strive for maximum independence in mobility, activities of daily living, and community re-entry.

Patient and Family Education

Therapeutic success is most likely to occur with an educated patient and family. It is important to discuss in detail diabetes, its complications, and the diffuse and progressive nature of diabetic neuropathy.

A study of the recurrence of neuropathic ulcerations revealed that nearly half were solely attributable to failure to comply with prescribed treatment.[28] In spite of extensive foot ulceration, patients who lack pain sensation often ignore a non-weight-bearing recommendation. Patients should be instructed in proper skin management. They should inspect their feet every day for warmth, swelling, or redness. If erythema or warmth is present in the evening, the foot should be checked again the next morning. If it is still warm, it should be rested by walking less, wearing a different shoe, and taking short steps until the hot spot resolves.[20] If an ulcer develops, the patient should off-weight the foot and seek medical attention. Shoes must fit properly, be comfortable when purchased, gradually broken in, and changed daily to avoid breakdown caused by prolonged pressure.[21] Barefoot walking is forbidden. Decreased protective sensation also increases the risk for thermal injury. Water temperatures of 60–65.6°C (140–150°F) cause full thickness epidermal burns within 2 to 5 seconds. It is recommended that household water temperatures be lowered in the homes of those with diabetic neuropathy to 48.9°C (120°F) to decrease the risk of scalding.[29]

Protective Footwear

Patients with neuropathy should pay careful attention to the selection of footwear. Shoes must fit appropriately when purchased. There is a tendency to select shoes that are too small because they "feel right," especially when small-fiber-mediated nociception is lost, but large-fiber-mediated light touch is preserved. If shoes are too tight, skin breakdown will occur before the shoe is broken in. Footwear for the insensitive foot should generally accommodate, rather than attempt to correct, skeletal deformities. Shoes with an adequate toe box are recommended, to avoid dorsal or mediolateral pressure. A leather upper is recommended to allow heat dissipation and to conform to the foot's shape without causing friction or compression.[30] Extra-depth shoes or shoes with a removable insole are recommended to allow room for an appropriate shoe inlay. A rocker bottom sole can help dissipate the forces of ambulation (Figure 13-1).[20] Silicone-inpregnated socks also may be helpful for shock attenuation and pressure distribution.

Orthoses

Orthoses are used to prevent or correct contractures or to stabilize joints in order to improve function. The force of an orthosis is generally exerted against the body at three points. An orthosis is designed to distribute the force at each point over as large an area as possible to avoid excess pressure. To minimize the forces exerted at the ends of the orthosis, they are designed with as long a lever arm as possible. These principles are extremely important in patients with peripheral neuropathy and anesthetic skin.

Lower Extremity   Accommodative inlays are the most common orthoses used for management of neuropathic foot. Shock-attenuating shoe inserts can serve not only to cushion the stress of ambulation, but also aid in more even pressure distribution on the plantar surface of the foot. If areas of high pressure are noted, as demonstrated by erythema or callous formation, a moderate-density foam insert may be custom-fabricated. Brodsky and associates evaluated the compression, shear-compression, and force distribution of commonly used neoprene, urethane, and polyethylene foams and provide guidelines for the selection of materials for shoe inserts.[31]

Orthotic devices are also used to compensate for paresis or paralysis of the dorsiflexors, subtalar instability, plantar flexor weakness, or knee instability. To compensate for weak dorsiflexors, a dorsi-assist ankle foot orthosis (AFO) is commonly used. This can be fabricated from double metal uprights with spring dorsi-assist, or custom-molded from polypropylene with trim

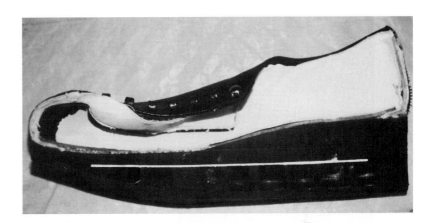

Figure 13-1
Cutaway of shoe modified by placement of steel shank with rocker-bottom sole. This allows forward progression without significant ankle-foot movement, to dissipate forces generated in ambulation.

lines posterior to the malleoli (Figure 13-2). With greater weakness and associated ankle instability, moderate trim lines or trim lines anterior to the malleoli (solid ankle) may be necessary. (Figure 13-3).

With severe weakness of the quadriceps muscle,

Figure 13-2
Custom-molded plastic ankle-foot-orthosis (AFO) with narrow trimline posteriorly, commonly used to provide a dynamic dorsiflexion assist.

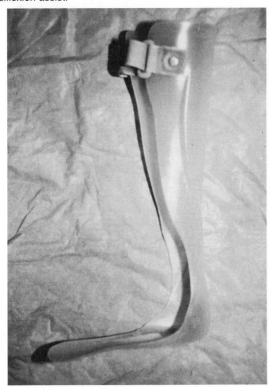

as in diabetic proximal motor neuropathy, especially when hip or knee flexion contractures also are present, a knee-ankle-foot orthosis (KAFO) may be required. This brace provides knee stability and prevents knee buckling during stance phase. When a knee flexion contracture is present, a pretibial shell is commonly recommended. When the quadriceps is weak and the gluteus maximus muscles are strong, knee hyperextension is often evident. Over a period of time, genu recurvatum may develop, leading to pain when it reaches 20–30 degrees. Bracing should be considered to prevent more than 5 degrees of recurvatum while promoting more efficient and safer ambulation (Figure 13-4).

Total contact casting has been shown to be beneficial for the treatment of neuropathic ulcers.[28,32] The total contact cast redistributes weight-bearing forces, decreases edema, protects the wound and surrounding

Figure 13-3
AFO for more involved individual features "solid ankle" trimlines anterior to the malleoli for more powerful control of ankle varus/valgus. This example also includes integral heal-to-sole buildup to accommodate fixed equinus and leg-length discrepancy.

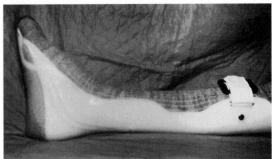

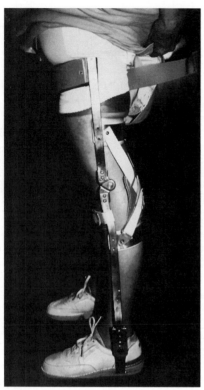

Figure 13-4

This lightweight aluminum knee-ankle-foot-orthosis (KAFO) uses free-motion offset knee joints and ground reaction forces to stabilize the knee in mild recurvatum. By eliminating marked genu recurvatum, this device allows ambulation with knee flexion in swing phase yet prevents further damage to the posterior capsule and cruciate ligaments.

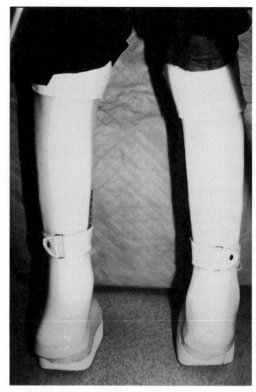

Figure 13-5

Bilateral custom-molded bivalved AFO's that include custom accommodative foam inlays and rocker-bottom crepe soles, are sometimes used in lieu of a total-contact cast when maximum immobilization is required.

tissues, decreases shear forces, localizes infection, protects the foot from outside contamination, and provides immobilization of the wound and Charcot joint.[32] In previous research, casting allowed healing of chronic neuropathic ulcerations in an average of 33–38 days.[32,34] The use of a custom total contact bi-valved polypropylene AFO with custom foot bed has also been described (Figure 13-5).[21,35] These may be especially useful if patients are unable to return for cast changes, wound access is needed, or if a concomitant neuropathic arthropathy is present that requires prolonged immobilization (at least 6 months). Hindfoot Charcot lesions need absolute nonweight-bearing (utilizing the total-contact AFO and crutches for short distances or a wheelchair for community mobility) during the resorptive phase to avoid development of gross deformity.[36]

A double upright patella tendon bearing (PTB) orthosis with double adjustable ankle joints attached to an extra depth shoe with accommodative inlay, steel shank, and rocker sole has been described for use after resolution of the active stage of a neuropathic arthropathy (Figure 13-6).[37] This orthosis is designed to transfer the floor reaction forces to the tibia and proximal musculature to reduce plantar stresses during ambulation. The PTB orthosis should be worn for 1 year, or until radiographs clearly demonstrate resolution of the osteopenia and reconstitution of normal-density bone.[36,37]

Upper Extremity   The ideal upper-extremity orthosis should be lightweight, easy to don and doff, allow optimal sensory input, and maximize function of the hand and forearm. With paralysis of the interossei and lumbricales, a bar across the dorsum of the proximal phalanges facilitates extension of the interphalangeal joints of the

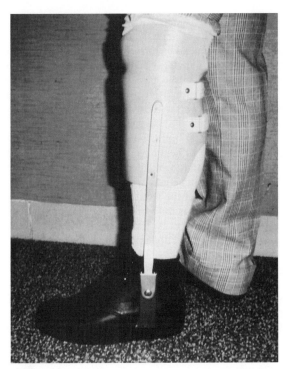

Figure 13-6
One type of AFO designed to partially unload the ankle and protect the foot from the forces of ambulation. This version uses a laminated, total-contact proximal segment connected to an extra-depth shoe via double-adjustable ankle joints. For maximum protection, the joints must limit dorsiflexion to neutral, although plantarflexion is usually permitted. A steel shank and rocker sole, as well as a custom-molded accommodative inlay, protect the fragile foot from excess forces.

fingers by the long extensors. When the long extensors are paralyzed, a support under the volar aspect of the proximal phalanges enables the interphalangeal joints to be extended by the interossei and lumbricales. A static hand orthosis (universal cuff) consists of a flat palmar pocket into which common utensils can be inserted. A C-bar, thumb post, or metacarpal phalangeal (MCP) stop can also be added to the static hand orthosis. Opponens orthoses assist with residual motor power by positioning the thumb in opposition to the other fingers.

Splints for the wrists usually compensate for weakness of the wrist extensors. The wrist is supported in about 25 degrees of extension with respect to the forearm and the thumb continues in the line of the volar plane of the forearm. When the fingers are slightly flexed, the tips of the index and middle fingers lie against

the tip of the thumb. Wrist-control orthoses assist the individual with a weak grasp by preventing flexion of the wrist, thereby creating tension in the finger flexor tendons.

Modalities

Therapeutic heat and cold are not frequently recommended for symptomatic management of peripheral neuropathies and must be used with caution. The most common use of thermal modalities is for pain relief or muscle spasm. A tepid whirlpool bath at about 38°C may be useful in the management of dysesthetic pain. Infrared radiation also may give relief.[38] Radiant heat is probably the safest form of superficial heat in patients with decreased sensation because the skin can be observed during therapy. Deeper heating modalities, such as ultrasound or short wave diathermy, should be avoided. A trial of cryotherapy in conjunction with other therapies may be beneficial to determine its effectiveness. Transcutaneous electrical nerve stimulation (TENS) and direct electrical nerve stimulation (DENS) have been shown to be beneficial for the management of chronic peripheral nerve pain.[39,40] In theory, both procedures activate large fibers, thereby "closing the gate" to the small-fiber neural transmission associated with the production of pain.[41] A central mechanism of action for electrical stimulation is supported by the observation that TENS produces an increase in cerebrospinal fluid endorphins that is blocked by Naloxone.[42] A technique referred to as "acupuncture-like," TENS with low-frequency stimuli (less than 10 per second) of fairly strong intensity has an effect in some cases in which high-frequency stimulation (about 100 per second) is ineffective. For the more invasive DENS, careful patient selection is necessary.[40] Pain must be localized to one peripheral nerve, without a major feature of sympathetically mediated pain.

Exercise

Exercises to regain or preserve the range of motion of joints should be carried out at least twice daily. The disability associated with muscular weakness may be greatly aggravated by contractures. As a conditioning program is initiated, the use of a tilt table and compressive wraps can be beneficial for the management of orthostatic hypotension. Several factors appear to be important in evaluating the possible beneficial or deleterious effects of exercise training. The first is the severity of weakness on initiation of exercise, and the second is the rate of progression of weakness.[43] Overwork weakness has been reported to occur in humans with peripheral nerve lesions.[44] Exercise is useful to those with peripheral neuropathy to counter the negative effects of disuse syndrome.[45] Because of the high incidence of silent cardiovascular disease, caution needs to be used when prescribing exercise intensity, and proper warm up and cool down must be advised. Those with insensate feet or Charcot deformities should have a nonweight-bearing or low-impact exercise program. In these patients, foot inspection needs to be performed after every workout session in addition to their daily routine. Strengthening should be submaximal (avoiding fatigue during exercise).

The first 2 weeks of training should lead to enhanced synchronization and recruitment of motor units.[46] The more efficient use of muscles provided by strengthening and exercises will have early functional and performance implications. Various types of strengthening techniques include isometric, isotonic, isokinetic, and isodynamic. Performing exercises when possible in a closed kinetic chain allows contraction of both agonists and antagonists while joints move in a functional manner. For example, performing squats develops strength for transfer activities. Exercise can prevent or lessen the effects of disuse syndrome, and improve flexibility, strength, aerobic capacity, bone mineral content, and feelings of self-esteem.

Durable Medical Equipment

Gait aids (cane, crutches, walkers) and wheelchairs are beneficial for joint protection and energy conservation. They also broaden the base of support to increase stability for patients with peripheral neuropathy. Although the use of canes, walkers, and crutches are beneficial for off-weighting a neuropathic lower extremity, the potential consequences of upper extremity weight bearing must be considered. Transfer of weight bearing forces to the arms can lead to musculoskeletal injury to the shoulders, degenerative arthritis, carpal tunnel syndrome, and ulnar neuropathy of the wrist.[47]

Medications

The use of medications is reserved for the management of chronic neuropathic pain. Chronic nerve pain is a pathologic state that may require different treatments and outcome expectations. Realistic treatment goals must be established and clearly articulated.

Tricyclic antidepressants, especially the methyl-ated forms (imipramine, amitriptyline, and doxepin) have been shown in animal studies to produce analgesia.[41] Desipramine and amitriptyline have recently been shown to effectively treat neuropathic pain in diabetic humans in a randomized, placebo-controlled trial.[48] Fluoxetine has been reported to be effective in diabetic neuropathic pain only in those with concomitant depression.[48] Amitriptyline alone has been shown to relieve neuropathic pain in both diabetics with normal and depressed moods.[49] Others have advocated the safety and effectiveness of nonsteroidal anti-inflammatory drugs.[50] The mechanisms of action are not well defined, but may involve blockade of the pain–anxiety–depression–pain sequence by increasing cortical inhibition of sensory input, stimulation of central nervous system endorphines, blockade of dopaminergic receptors, or reuptake of brain serotonin.[51] Mexiletine has also recently been shown to offer some benefit in pain management.[52]

Anticonvulsants such as carbamazepine and phenytoin have been used for neuropathic pain because of their potential ability to stabilize neuronal membranes. Both peripheral and central mechanisms are probably involved. Although phenytoin and carbamazepine have proven efficacy in many neuropathic pain syndromes,[53,54] valproic acid and clonazepam may also be effective in certain instances.[55]

Capsaicin is an alkaloid that has been shown to decrease substance P in skin and to reduce chemically induced pain. Local burning may preclude the use in some patients. Initial reports on the efficacy of capsaicin in treating neuropathic pain were encouraging. Diabetics with painful neuropathy studied in an eight-week randomized double-blind vehicle-controlled multicenter study suggest that topical 0.075 percent capsaicin may reduce pain in patients with painful diabetic neuropathy, with subsequent improvement in daily activities, the ability to work and sleep, and enhanced quality of life.[56] However, other studies have shown no evidence of efficacy of capsaicin in chronic painful neuropathy.[57]

REFERENCES

1. Dyck PJ, Thomas PK, Griffin JW, Low PA, Poduslo JF (eds): *Peripheral Neuropathy*. Philadelphia: W.B. Saunders, 1993.
2. Donofrio PD, Albers JW: AAEM Minimonograph 34: Polyneuropathy. Classification by Nerve Conduction Studies and Electromyography. *Muscle Nerve* 1990; 13:889–903.

3. Dyck PJ, Thomas PK, Asbury AK, Winegrad AL, Porte DJ (eds): *Diabetic Neuropathy*. Philadelphia: W.B. Saunders, 1987.

4. Suarez GA, Low PA: Peripheral Nervous System Complications of Diabetes Mellitus and Hypoglycemia, in Vinken PJ, Bruyn GW, Klawans HL (eds): *Handbook of Clinical Neurology*. Amsterdam: Elsevier, in press.

5. Dyck PJ: Detection, Characterization, and Staging of Polyneuropathy: Assessed in Diabetics. *Muscle Nerve* 1988; 11:21–32.

6. LeQuesne PM, Fowler CJ, Parkhouse N: Peripheral Neuropathy Profile in Various Groups of Diabetics. *J Neurol Neurosurg Psychiatr* 1990; 53:558–563.

7. Waxman SG, Sabin TD: Diabetic Truncal Polyneuropathy. *Arch Neurol* 1981; 38:46.

8. Dyck PJ, Kratz KM, Karnes JL, et al: The prevalence by staged severity of various types of diabetic neuropathy, retinopathy, and nephropathy in a population-based cohort: The Rochester Diabetic Neuropathy Study. *Neurology* 1993; 43:817–824.

9. Tuck RR, Schmelzer JD, Low PA: Endoneurial blood flow and oxygen tension in the sciatic nerves of rats with experimental diabetic neuropathy. *Brain* 1984; 107:935–950.

10. Larsen K, Holstein P: Abnormal extension of the big toe as a cause of ulceration in diabetic feet. *Prosthet Orthot Int* 1987; 11:31–32.

11. Ball NA, Stempien LM, Pasupuleti DV, et al: Radial nerve palsy: A complication of walker usage. *Arch Phys Med Rehab* 1989; 70:236–238.

12. Stewart JD: Diabetic truncal neuropathy: Topography of the sensory deficit. *Ann Neurol* 1989; 25:233–238.

13. Ellenberg M: Diabetic neuropathy precipitating after institution of diabetic control. *Am J Med Sci* 1958; 236:466–471.

14. Young RJ, Ewing DJ, Clarke BF: Chronic and remitting painful diabetic polyneuropathy: Correlations with clinical features and subsequent changes in neurophysiology. *Diabetes Care* 1988; 11:34–40.

15. Dyck PJ, Sherman WR, Hallcher LM, et al: Human diabetic endoneurial sorbitol, fructose, and myo-inositol related to sural nerve morphometry. *Ann Neurol* 1980; 8:590–596.

16. Greene DA, Lattimer SA: Sodium- and energy-dependent uptake of myo-inositol by rabbit peripheral nerve competitive inhibition by glucose and lack of an insulin effect. *J Clin Invest* 1982; 70:1009–1018.

17. Kihara M, Zollman PJ, Smithson IL, et al: Hypoxic effect of exogenous insulin on normal and diabetic peripheral nerve. *Am J Physiol* 1994; 266:E980–E985.

18. Low PA: Recent advances in the pathogenesis of diabetic neuropathy. *Muscle Nerve* 1987; 10:121–128.

19. Said G, Slama G, Selva J: Progressive centripetal degeneration of axons in small fibre diabetic polyneuropathy. *Brain* 1983; 106:791–807.

20. Brand PW Project Director: The Cycle of Repetitive Stress on Insensitive Feet (project booklet). SRS grant RC 75 MP0. Carville, Louisiana, United States Public Health Service Hospital, 1975.

21. Andrews KL, Rooke TW, Helm PA: Rehabilitation in vascular diseases, in Braddom (ed): *Textbook of Physical Medicine and Rehabilitation*. Philadelphia: W.B. Saunders, 1996.

22. Pecoraro RE, Reiber GE, Burgess EM: Pathways to diabetic limb amputation: Basis for prevention. *Diabetes Care* 1990; 13(5):513–521.

23. Veves A, Murray HJ, Young MJ, Boulton AJM: The risk of foot ulceration in diabetic patients with high foot pressure: A prospective study. *Diabetologia* 1992; 35:660–663.

24. Masson EA, Hay EM, Stockley I, Veves A, Betts RP, Boulton AJM: Abnormal foot pressure alone may not cause ulceration. *Diabet Med* 1989; 6:426–428.

25. Resnick D: Neuroarthropathy, in Resnick D (ed): *Bone and Joint Imaging*. Philadelphia: W.B. Saunders, 1989, pp. 946–956.

26. Harrelson JM: The diabetic foot: Charcot arthropathy. *Instr Course Lect* 1993; 42:141–146.

27. Wenger DE: Radiographic Evaluation of Diabetic Foot: Differentiation of Osteomyelitis and Neuropathic Osteoarthropathy. Presented at *The Lower Extremity Amputee: A Multidisciplinary Approach* Course, September 1994.

28. Helm PA, Walker SC, Pullium GF: Recurrence of neuropathic ulceration following healing in a total contact cast. *Arch Phys Med Rehab* 1991; 72(12):967–970.

29. Katcher ML, Shapiro MM: Lower extremity burns related to sensory loss in diabetes mellitus. *J Fam Pract* 1987; 24(2):149–151.

30. Weber GA, Cardile MA: Diabetic neuropathies. *Clin Podiatr Med Surg* 1990; 7:1–36.

31. Brodsky JW, Kourosh S, Stills M, Mooney V: Objective evaluation of insert material for diabetic and athletic footwear. *Foot Ankle* 1988; 9(3):111–116.

32. Helm PA, Walker SC, Pullium MG: Total contact casting in diabetic patients with neuropathic foot ulcerations. *Arch Phys Med Rehab* 1984; 65:691–693.

33. Coleman WC, Brand PW, Birke JA: The total contact cast: A therapy for plantar ulceration on insensitive feet. *J Am Podiatr Med Assoc* 1984; 74:548–552.

34. Walker SC, Helm PA, Pullium G: Total contact casting and chronic diabetic neuropathic foot ulcerations: Healing rates by wound location. *Arch Phys Med Rehab* 1987; 68:217–221.

35. Morgan JM, Biehl WC III, Wagner FW Jr: Management of neuropathic arthropathy with the Charcot restraint orthotic walker. *Clin Orthop* 1993; 296:58–63.

36. Harrelson JM: Management of the diabetic foot. *Orthop Clin No Am* 1989; 20(4):605–619.

37. Michael JW, Isbell MA, Harrelson JM: Orthotic management of diabetic neuropathic arthropathy. *J Prosthet Orthop* 1991; 4:45–55.

38. Stillwell GK: Rehabilitative procedures, in Dyck PJ (ed): *Peripheral Neuropathy*, 2nd ed. Philadelphia: W.B. Saunders, 1987.

39. Stillwell GK (ed): *Therapeutic Electricity and Ultraviolet Radiation*, 3rd ed. Baltimore: Williams & Wilkins, 1983, pp. 109–123.

40. Strege DW, Cooney WP, Wood MB, Johnson SJ, Metcalf BJ: Chronic peripheral nerve pain treated with direct electrical nerve stimulation. *J Hand Surg* 1994; 19(6):931–939.

41. Yiannikas C, Shahani BT: Painful sequelae of injuries to peripheral nerves. *Am J Phys Med* 1984; 63(2):53–83.

42. Woolf CJ, Barrett GD, Mitchel D: Naloxone reversible peripheral electroanalgesia in intact and spinal rats. *Eur J Pharmacol* 1977; 45:311–314.

43. Fowler WM Jr: Management of musculoskeletal complications in neuromuscular diseases: Weakness and the role of exercise. *Phys Med Rehab* 1988; 2(4):489–507.

44. Hikok RJ: Physical therapy as related to peripheral nerve lesions. *Phys Ther Rev* 1961; 41:113–117.

45. Graham C, Laskow-McCarthey P: Exercise options for persons with diabetic complications. *Diabetes Educ* 16(3):212–220.

46. Milner-Brown HS, Stein RB, Yemm R: The orderly recruitment of human motor units during voluntary isometric contractions. *J Physiol* (London) 1973;230:359–370.

47. Werner R, Waring W, Davidoff G: Risk factors for median mononeuropathy of the wrist in postpoliomyelitis patients. *Arch Phys Med Rehab* 1989; 70(6):464–467.

48. Max MB, et al: Effects of desipramine, amitriptyline, and fluoxetine on pain in diabetic neuropathy. *NEJM* 1992; 326:1250–1256.

49. Mood MB, et al: Amitriptyline relieves diabetic neuropathy pain in patients with normal or depressed mood. *Neurology* 1987; 37:589–596.

50. Cohen RL, Harris S: Efficiency and safety of nonsteroidal anti-inflammatory drugs in the therapy of diabetic neuropathy. *Arch Intern Med* 1987; 147:1442–1444.

51. Malseed RT, Goldstein FJ: Enhancement of morphine analgesia by tricyclic antidepressants. *Neuropharmacology* 1979; 18:827–829.

52. Dejgard A, et al: Mexiletine for treatment of chronic painful diabetic neuropathy. *Lancet* 1988; 1:9–11.

53. Ellenburg M: Treatment of diabetic neuropathy with diphenylhydration. *NYS J Med* 1968; 68:2653.

54. Bader JL, et al: Carbamazepine for myeloid neuropathy. *NEJM* 1977; 296:596.

55. Dean BZ, Williams FH, King JC, Goddard MJ: Pain rehabilitation: Therapeutic options in pain management. *Arch Phys Med Rehab* 1994; 75:S21–S30.

56. Capsaicin Study Group: Effect of treatment with capsaicin on daily activities of patients with painful diabetic neuropathy. *Diabetes Care* 1992; 15(2):159–165.

57. Low PA, Opter-Gehrking TL, Dyck PJ, Litchy WJ, O'Brien PC: Double-blinded, placebo-controlled study of the application of Capsaicin cream in chronic distal painful polyneuropathy. *Pain* 1995; 62(2):163–168.

Chapter 14

CHRONIC PAIN

Jonathan L. Costa
F. Todd Wetzel

The importance of pain in the spectrum of human experience is emphasized by the monumental amount of medical literature devoted to the subject.[1-6] What we perceive as pain can be generated by virtually any visceral, neuromuscular, or musculoskeletal structure in the body. Pain impulses are shaped and modulated, in turn, in the central nervous system, and coupled closely to our emotional and behavioral states. There are infinite permutations of how pain is perceived and expressed.[1-7]

Nearly all chronic pain begins as acute pain. Any pain lasting more than 6 months is considered chronic pain. Pain of this duration, regardless of cause, appears to lead to multiple physiologic adaptations at the level of the brain, spinal cord, and peripheral nerves.[8,9] In addition, behavioral adaptations are protean and universally accepted (Table 14-1).

Treatment approaches for chronic pain originating outside the central nervous system will be considered first.[2-5] Peripheral sources of chronic pain include musculoskeletal pain originating from tendons and their sheaths, vertebral bodies, ligaments, facet joints, myofascial nodules, and the muscle body itself.[10-11] Neuromuscular pain generators include the more diffuse type driven by irritation of small fibers ("protopathic") and the more localized, sharp pain associated with excessive activity of large fibers ("epicritic").[2] Epicritic pain generators may be induced by inflammation of the nerve itself, apart from mechanical compression or deformity by a space-occupying lesion.[12]

Once pain has evolved to the point of being chronic (persistence for more than 6 months), a special set of requirements dictates the approach to management. First, all diagnostic efforts must have been exhausted in an attempt to find a specific etiology of the pain. Symptom-oriented pain management does not require absolute knowledge of cause. However, all reasonable efforts must be undertaken to identify metabolic or structural pain generators that are reversible.

Second, in the acute phase of pain, all reasonable therapeutic options must be tried. Under most circumstances, efforts are diagnosis-specific. When all reasonable diagnostic and therapeutic options have been exhausted without adequate success, the patient should be considered for a psychobehavioral approach to treatment that encourages adaptation and function.

Any person involved in chronic pain management needs to be aware of a number of precepts. First, chronic pain serves a purpose. In evolution, pain impulses signal internal or external threat. Pain signals get our attention rapidly. If they persist, pain signals easily can expand to occupy a large portion of our attentional focus. Pharmacologic interventions target primary pain generators and their shape, modulation, and magnifications as signals are processed through the central nervous system.

Multidisciplinary management of psychobehavioral dysfunction nearly always is essential to a successful treatment program.

Habituation and attachment to pain is the rule. Pain addiction is no less powerful than drug addiction. The physician should expect a high degree of ambivalence about being weaned from chronic pain behaviors. Most chronic pain patients resist any intervention that alters the dynamic of their relationship with pain. Most chronic pain patients view treatment personnel as a threat, since pain serves a psychologic purpose. Even the most carefully reasoned treatment options may be subject to sabotage, either actively or by passive–aggressive behavior. Firm and clear limits must be set.

The primary outcome variable in monitoring treatment progress should never be self-reporting of pain alone. It is essential that other barometers of progress are used. These include changes in pain behaviors, such as symptom magnification or refusal to perform certain activities, quality of movement, and functional capabilities in recreational, home, and work settings.[1-3] The ultimate objective measure of pain relief is function.

Other components of any program to treat

Table 14-1
Behavioral adaptations to chronic pain

Symptom magnification

Depression

Anger and hostility

Decreased libido

Social isolation

Loss of vocation/avocation

Litigation/disability compensation

Polymedication abuse/dependence

chronic pain include positive reinforcers for "healthy" behavior (exercise, leisure activity, household and work functioning). These must be coupled skillfully to identification and minimization of circumstances in each patient's life that act as reinforcers for maladaptive behavior (secondary emotional gain from a significant other, or financial gain from the workplace). The most important precept of all is acceptance and recognition of a significant failure rate among even the best interdisciplinary pain programs. In about 30 percent of cases, symptoms prove intractable and the patients continue with their previous lifestyles.[2,3,6] No guidelines or practice parameters have been published to date that assist in the identification of patients who will respond favorably. Most physical therapy-based programs geared towards treating chronic pain patients use a three-pronged approach: drug minimization, behavior modification, and physical reconditioning.[3,5,6] Objectives must be realistic and achievable. The patient must be disengaged gradually from the medical-care system and reintegrated into the family and community. Pain-treatment strategies are empowering, and can be used to improve function and quality of life. Nevertheless, chronic pain as a symptom may never be eliminated fully.

A multidisciplinary pain program requires an organized approach and structure to reduce drug dependency.[3,5,6] An experienced pain psychologist is essential. Biofeedback, relaxation, and guided-imagery techniques for pain control and management can be effective. A psychologist is crucial to analyzing family and team dynamics, dependency needs, anger, and other emotional issues that often act as pain modulators.

Physical therapy programs are directed at symptom management, conditioning, endurance, joint mobility, and function. Interventions are *not* curative. Even those who complete a program successfully may need continuing support and therapeutic contact in order to maintain gains in pain management. Given the precarious psychodynamics of the chronic pain patient, program dependency is common. Gradual weaning from the program support system must be engineered, with emphasis on self-help skills and self-control of suffering.

The physician's approach to pharmacologic intervention must be strategically aligned with the three major thrusts of the treatment program.

Reduction of Medication Dependency

Most chronic pain patients are highly dependent on drugs to control pain.[6] There is widespread belief that nociceptive pain is responsive to opioids, whereas neuropathic pain is not.[13] Long-term use of narcotics and tranquilizers rarely is beneficial.[3] Addiction and habituation are common. From the psychobehavioral standpoint, medication overuse feeds into the chronic-pain patient's feelings of lack of control and unwillingness to take responsibility for symptom control. Long-term use of analgesics and sedatives is never curative and may perpetuate suffering and behavioral dysfunction.

The recommendation for chronic pain management is to judiciously taper such medications.[3,5,6] Medication withdrawal should be done under close medical and nursing supervision. On an outpatient basis, a generally safe recommendation for medication withdrawal is to reduce the daily dose by about 10 to 20 percent after each period of five elimination half-lives.[14]

Treatment of Contributing Inflammatory Processes

Anti-inflammatory pharmacotherapy should begin only when there is evidence to suggest that inflammation is a significant contributor to the patient's chronic pain. Oral pulse steroids, given over 1 week, may reduce acute inflammatory components of chronic pain, but rarely are effective over the long term. Topical preparations with local anti-inflammatory activity, such as capsaicin, may be effective on chronic pain from peripheral polyneuropathy or focal neuralgia, such as post-herpetic neuralgia.[15–18]

Treatment of Muscle Spasm and Myofascial Pain

Many patients with pain in the cervical, thoracic, or lumbar regions complain of concomitant muscle spasms in the paraspinal musculature. Thoracic and cervical sprains, scoliosis, or vertebral malalignments also can produce paraspinal muscle spasms. Establishment of a vicious cycle of pain–spasm–pain can be extremely uncomfortable and functionally disabling. Under these circumstances, pharmacological spasmolytics should be considered as adjuvant therapy in the management of chronic pain.

Physical modalities have been tried for centuries in the management of chronic pain. They include dry and moist heat, cryotherapy, vibration, acupuncture, and transcutaneous electrical stimulation (TENS). There has been little to suggest any beneficial aspects to these treatments beyond the expected large placebo effect well-known in the treatment of chronic pain.[19] Acupuncture relief of chronic pain may be endorphin-mediated.[20] There is no substantial body of medical evidence to support the effectiveness of vibration therapy or TENS units, and credible information exists that they are not helpful at all.[21]

SURGICAL APPROACHES

The results of surgical intervention for chronic benign pain syndromes generally are quite poor. This is not surprising given the therapeutic goal: treatment of a persistent pain syndrome without an apparently reversible anatomic cause. The results of one of the earliest interventions, cordotomy, suggested that ablative maneuvers are more efficacious in patients with neoplastic pain.[22] This also is not unexpected, given the time-dependent properties of the principle of neuroplasticity.

The surgical approach to chronic pain syndromes has involved two concepts, interruption of afferent nociceptive pathways (deafferentation), and enhancement of presynaptic inhibition (modulation). The final object of both of these approaches is to diminish nociceptive input. Theoretically, stimulation or interruption could occur at one or several levels of the pain pathway.

In general, the results of surgical intervention are better in cases of pain mediated by nerve-root injury. Unfortunately, many chronic benign pain syndromes really have little to do with cord or root damage. The individual motion segment is itself richly enervated and thus is capable of generating postinjury pain in the absence of frank neural compression (the type-A pain of O'Brien).[23] Of the interventional procedures reviewed, only one, facet rhizotomy, may be appropriate for axial pain syndromes, although spinal cord stimulation is showing increasing promise in this area. Therefore, it is of paramount importance that the patient undergo a detailed evaluation prior to consideration of any of these procedures, ruling out reversible causes of axial and extremity pain. Following such an evaluation, only a very small percentage of chronic patients will be surgical candidates at all. As Shealy has noted, only 5 percent of patients referred for consideration of spinal cord stimulation are implanted.[24]

A review of ablative and modulatory therapies germane to chronic benign pain syndromes follows. The role of all of these therapies is extremely limited. Certainly, the most effective way to deal with chronic benign cervical pain is to avoid creating such a syndrome by judicious initial treatment and rigid surgical indications. In the lumbar spine, Wynn Parry has noted a general belief among specialists that surgery has been overprescribed. By inference, these same concerns must be raised about all aspects of spinal surgery.[25]

ABLATIVE MODALITIES

Cordotomy

Ablation of the anterolateral quadrants to interrupt pain and temperature pathways first was described by Spiller and Martin, and by Förster (Figure 14-1).[22,26] Cordotomy has been a mainstay in the ablative armamentarium for control of pain. Its uses in cases of neoplastic pain have been studied extensively, and the results of cordotomy can be of major benefit in preserving quality of life for these patients.[27–30] Cordotomy also has been employed in nonneoplastic syndromes, such as gastric crises, phantom limb pain, and spondylosis.[31–33] Probst reported results of microsurgical, cervicothoaracic cordotomy in 20 patients with persistent benign radicular

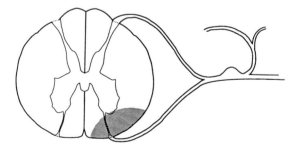

Figure 14-1

Cordotomy (Spiller and Martin, 1912; Förster, 1913). The shaded area represents the surgical lesion created. From Wetzel.[119]

pain caused by epidural fibrosis. All had been previously operated on for lumbar disc herniation. Judging clinical success by greater than 50 percent pain relief, 66 percent were graded as successful at 66 months postoperatively.[33] In a series of 13 patients with 3-year follow-up, Cowrie and Hitchcock report a 23 percent success rate, as measured by curtailment of analgesic medication.[27] White and Sweet note a 33 percent success rate at follow-up greater than 1 year. Lahuerta et al. reviewed 146 patients who underwent 181 percutaneous cervical cordotomies.[34] Only six patients in their group had benign pain syndromes. These include phantom limb, causalgia, postthoracotomy pain, postherpetic neuralgia, and lumbar arachnoiditis. The results of pain relief they reported were variable, but did seem to correlate with the extent of the lesion created. The authors felt that $\frac{1}{5}$ of the cord must be destroyed in order to produce satisfactory pain relief.

Cordotomy can be performed either by an open laminotomy or percutaneously. The selection of technique, in general, is left to the expertise of the surgeon; several authors, however, have recommended the percutaneous technique for cases of neoplastic pain, with open cordotomy in cases of benign pain.[32] Postoperative deficit in pinprick has been shown to correlate with the amount of pain relief.[35]

A persistent problem of cordotomy, however, is the nature and frequency of complications. Reported complications have include ipsilateral weakness, GI dysfunction, fecal incontinence, and impotence. The impact of these complications in a patient with a normal life expectancy obviously is quite significant. Complication rates have ranged from 70 to 93 percent, with higher rates seen in bilateral procedures.[27–29,31,36–41] Additionally, dysesthesias and hypotension may result. The descending vasoconstrictor pathway, terminating in the intermediolateral column of the grey matter, may be divided extensively during the second portion of a bilateral procedure. Typically this produces orthostatic hypotension; however, many authors report that this symptom seldom persists.[31,37,39,41] In the series of Deimeth et al., the orthostatic hypotension persisted in only one patient for 5 years.[31] Horner's syndrome has been reported in 100 percent of patients, ipsilateral leg weakness in 69 percent.[34] Additional complications include transient radicular pain. In general, the utility of cordotomy in chronic benign pain syndromes is quite limited. Aside from the high complication rate, Lipton has observed that the utility of neurodestructive techniques, such as cordotomy, currently are being reevaluated in light of newer techniques of pain control, such as epidural implantation.[42]

DORSAL ROOT ENTRY ZONE (DREZ)

Coagulation of the substantial gelatinosa and structures close to the posterior horn originally was described by Nashold and Ostdahl in a group of patients who had developed pain following avulsion of the brachial plexus (Figure 14-2).[43] The procedure involved creation of radio frequency heat lesions 3 millimeters apart along the line of posterolateral fissure at the site of the rootlet avulsion. Lesions were extended for several centimeters to the first normal rootlets, cranial and caudally to the injuries, so that in total, 10 to 20 lesions were made.

A 60 percent success rate as defined by greater than 50 percent pain relief was reported for DREZ lesioning of brachial plexus injuries by Thomas and Sheehy.[44] A 54 percent success rate was reported by others calling attention to a higher rate of success in plexus avulsion; up to an 82 percent success rate has been reported in cases such as these.[45,46] Neurogenic pain as a result of spinal-cord injury has been treated successfully in approximately 50 percent of patients with the DREZ lesion.[45,47] Higher success rates are noted in distal pain, and lower success rates in diffuse pain syndromes and postherpetic neuralgia. Overall, DREZ lesioning of small series of benign pain syndromes or arachnoiditis have yielded results inferior even to the 25 percent success rates reported for postherpetic lesions.[47,48]

The DREZ lesion may be created by a radio frequency heat probe or argon laser.[43,47–49] Use of intraoperative evoked potential monitoring is recommended. Lunsford and Bennett have reported an increase in P1 latency to be associated with irreversible postoperative sensory motor dysfunction.[50] Overall, the complication rate of the procedure is variable. Young reported ipsilat-

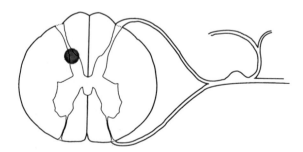

Figure 14-2
Dorsal root entry zone (DREZ): Coagulation of Substantia Gelantinosa. The shaded area represents the surgical lesion created. From Wetzel.[119]

eral leg weakness, and loss of proprioception in 52.3 percent of patients who had undergone radio frequency lesioning; this complication rate dropped to 15 percent in cases performed with the argon laser.[51]

At the present time any recommendations regarding use of the DREZ in chronic benign pain syndromes must be made with extreme caution because of limited experience with this technique and a significant rate of complication.

RHIZOTOMY

Rhizotomy was first described by Abbe in 1896.[52] The sensory rhizotomy had been nearly abandoned by 1925 because of a relatively high failure rate, and subsequent interest in cordotomy.[52,53] Rhizotomy may be performed either by opening the subarachnoid space or by an extradural approach (Figures 14-3 and 14-4). In general, rhizotomy for benign pain syndromes is of the intradural variety. This is owing to anatomic considerations; the cervical root exits the cord directly via the adjacent foramen. In the lumbar spine, when appropriate, extradural rhizotomy is the rule, owing to the arrangement of the cauda equina.

Rhizotomy has been investigated most widely for treatment of neoplastic pain in the head and neck. Specifically, rhizotomy has been shown to be useful in tumors of lung apex and brachial plexus.[54] A variety of benign pain syndromes also have been treated with rhizotomy. Success rates of 60 to 71 percent in the treatment of occipital neuralgia have been noted in multiple series.[41,55,56] In cases of post-traumatic neuralgia, sectioning of the first, second, and third dorsal roots may result in permanent pain relief.[57] The use of rhizotomy in postherpetic neuralgia is less successful, with reported

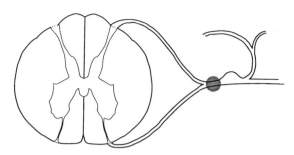

Figure 14-4
Extradural rhizotomy: Lumbosacral. The shaded area represents the surgical lesion created. From Wetzel.[119]

rate of success less than 30 percent.[55] Limb spasticity in patients with cerebral palsy also has been improved by intradural rhizotomy.[58]

In the case of chronic radiculitis, rhizotomy theoretically would yield the desired result; sectioning of the involved root should diminish pain that is peripheral and circumscribed, as the afferent territory of adjacent nerves presumably delineates pain for that region.[54] However, the long-term results of selective sensory rhizotomy or complete rhizotomy fail to support this theoretical benefit. Results may be compromised by imprecise delineation of afferent territory, intersegmental denervation hypersensitivity, intersegmental anastomoses, and ventral afferents.[43,46,59,60–65] Jain has reported benefit in cases of localized intradural scarring; in the lumbar spine, dorsal rhizotomy for the "battered root" syndrome has a very poor success rate.[66,67] Extradural sensory rhizotomy in the treatment of chronic lumbar radiculopathy has been reported to produce pain relief in only 30 percent of patients at an average follow-up of 12.1 months.[68] Hence, rhizotomy to treat chronic benign cervical pain syndromes must be recommended with extreme reluctance.

Seemingly, the most reliable indication for rhizotomy is pain caused by deafferentation itself. Tasker et al. retrospectively reviewed a large series of patients.[69] Patients were divided into two groups: spontaneous and hyperpathic pain. The pain of hyperpathia, produced by normally nonnoxious stimuli, was ameliorated by intravenous sodium thiopental, but not by morphine. Usually it was relieved by proximal local anesthetic blockade. Hyperpathia, which occurred in incompletely deafferentiated areas, was relieved partially by surgical completion of the deafferentation; namely, by completing the rhizotomy. However, the authors did note that pain may persist at the periphery of the sensory loss.

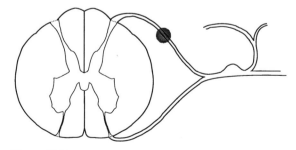

Figure 14-3
Intradural rhizotomy: Cervical, Thoracic. The shaded area represents the surgical lesion created. From Wetzel.[119]

Ganglionectomy

Smith[76] advocated sectioning of the dorsal root ganglion, in addition to rhizotomy, in an effort the improve pain relief (Figure 14-5). Theoretically, afferent fibers convey nociceptive influences from the ganglion to the sympathetic chain and re-enter the cord cranially or caudally to the deafferentiated zone. The anatomical success of dorsal rhizotomy would be confounded further by the presence of afferent fibers in the ventral root. These would permit continued transmission of nociceptive impulses and others signaling pain, such as neuromas or injured roots or nerves.[70–72] Thus it would seem logical that surgical ganglionectomy would overcome these limitations by ablating cell bodies of ventral and dorsal root afferents.[65]

Reported results of ganglionectomy for benign pain syndromes, however, have been disappointing. Sweet and Poletti reported poor results from a small series.[73] Taub, as cited by Sweet and Poletti, reported the results of ganglionectomy for the treatment of intractable sciatica. In his 55 patients, there were no anatomic lesions responsible for the production of sciatica; 56 percent were relieved of their apparent radicular pain at a follow-up of 4.8 years. Similarly discouraging results have been reported by others.[74–76] Recently, North et al. published a long-term follow-up of 13 patients who underwent ganglionectomy for intractable pain on the basis of failed back surgery.[77] Patients were followed at a mean of 5.5 years after dorsal root ganglionectomy. Treatment success, as defined by 50 percent pain relief and patient satisfaction, was recorded in two patients 2 years after surgery, and in no patients at 5.55 years. Thus, at this time, neither ganglionectomy nor rhizotomy can be recommended for chronic benign pain syndromes with any degree of conviction.

FACET RHIZOTOMY

Facet rhizotomy involves interruption of the medial branch of the posterior primary ramus, which supplies the facet joint capsule (Figure 14-6). The medial branch courses through a notch at the base of the transverse process and is covered by a ligament at the anterior–inferior border of the joint. Each posterior primary ramus may supply two facets, with each facet thus receiving innervation from at least two levels.[78,79]

The clinical characteristics of the facet syndrome in the lumbar spine have been well described by Mooney and Robertson.[78] Studies in asymptomatic and symptomatic volunteers have aided in delineation of the cervical facet syndrome.[80,81] The clinical characteristics of "facet pain" differ from conventional anterior or posterior "mechanical" pain. The pain generally is nondermatomal. Some tenderness may be noted, and as a rule, neurological examination is negative. Locally, the key diagnostic maneuver to establish the facet as the primary nociceptor is pharmacologic blockade of the median branch of the posterior primary ramus. This involves percutaneous insertion of a needle into the periarticular region or into the joint itself. The primacy of this maneuver has been emphasized by Slujter.[82]

Rees generally is credited with performing the fast facet rhizotomies. These were done percutaneously, with a knife, and pain relief was obtained in 998 of 1,000 patients.[83] Shealy subsequently reported an unacceptably high incidence of hematoma and adopted a radio frequency probe. He reported a 90 percent success rate in previously operated patients.[84] Schaerer reported results of radio frequency facet rhizotomy in chronic neck and back pain.[85] Using a clinical grading scale of pain intensity, functional limitation, and medication usage, the author reported a 50 percent success rate in a series

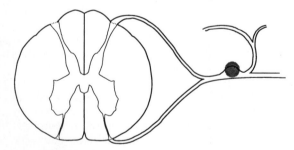

Figure 14-5
Ganglionectomy: Augmentation of thoracic rhizotomy (Smith, 1970). The shaded area represents the surgical lesion created. From Wetzel.[119]

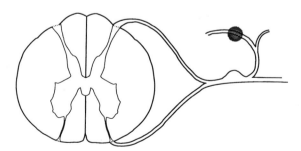

Figure 14-6
Facet rhizotomy (Shealy, 1975). The shaded area represents the surgical lesion created. From Wetzel.[119]

of 50 patients with chronic benign cervical pain syndromes. His average follow-up was 15.4 months. Oudenhoven reported an 83 percent rate of good-to-excellent pain relief in a population of 279 patients suffering from chronic back and extremity pain.[86] Average follow-up was 26 months. He noted a higher success rate in the presence of degenerative changes also. Overall, reported complication rates were very low, and related predominantly to postprocedure spasm, or local wound problems.

Technical guidance is provided by the report of Bogduk et al.[87] The authors investigated the size of experimental lesions made with a radio-frequency probe in egg white and fresh meat. They found that lesions do not extend distal to the tip of the electrode, and that the tissue destruction takes the shape of an oblate spheroid for maximum effective radius of 2 mm. Hence, precise positioning of the probe under fluoroscopic guidance is essential.

After a review of literature, one is tempted to recommend facet rhizotomy following the appropriate diagnostic evaluation. With the exception of the series of Schaerer, however, it is important to recall that there are no studies of long-term efficacy.[85] Certainly it is prudent, however, to consider this procedure prior to the heroic measure of an open arthrodesis for so-called posterior biomechanical column pain.

MODULATORY IMPLANTS

Epidural Implants

Selective nerve-root blockade or epidural blockade has been used successfully in many intraoperative and postoperative situations.[88–91] Implanted epidural narcotic reservoirs have been used in the treatment of intractable spinal and limb pain in a variety of neoplastic conditions as well.[92–98] Downing et al. reported on 23 patients with cancer pain refractory to other methods of pain control. Excellent response rates to implanted reservoirs were noted, with minimal complications.[95] Sjorgren et al. reported on 48 cancer patients receiving long-term treatment with an epidural opioid catheter. The overall effect was satisfactory. Twenty-nine patients were stabilized on epidural opioid treatment, and of these 21 were judged to be clinical successes. Somewhat ominously, however, a tendency toward better relief of nonneurogenic pain was noted.[99] The largest series reported to date is that of Liew and Hui. In their 252 patients, good to excellent pain relief was obtained in 85 percent. For patients who survived more than 3 months, the daily morphine requirement increased progressively from 3.5 to 19.5 mg per day. The authors noted that drug tolerance developed, but not drug addiction.[100]

The use of implantable epidural narcotic reservoirs in patients with chronic benign pain syndromes is less well studied. Several encouraging reports have appeared in the literature, however. In 1985, Auld et al. reported the results of intraspinal narcotic analgesia in 43 patients with chronic benign pain syndromes. Thirty-two of the 43 had continuous delivery systems, and 65 percent reported good to excellent relief of pain in follow-up longer than 2 years. The authors noted neither serious side effects nor evidence of addiction.[101] In an attempt to eliminate the bulkier continuous infusion system, Auld et al. investigated the effects of intraspinal narcotic analgesic on 20 patients using a smaller system consisting of an epidural catheter and subcutaneous reservoir. After an appropriate epidural trial the catheters were inserted. Acceptable pain relief was obtained in 14. The authors believed that the results of this system were comparable with those obtained by using a continuous delivery system and speculated that bolus injections saturated pain receptors as completely as continuous perfusion.[102] Interest in the long-term administration of opioids has continued.[103]

It appears that the implantation of an indwelling epidural narcotic reservoir is a promising new technique that should be considered in the management of chronic pain; however, several notes of caution must be sounded. As previously noted, neuroplasticity in the setting of chronic benign pain does tend to diminish the results of ablative therapies over time. Conceivably, this also may apply to pharmacotherapy. Not all types of pain seem to respond to opioid therapy in the same manner. In general, nociceptive pain, such as somatic, visceral, aching, diffuse, or nonradiating pain, will be more effectively controlled than neuropathic (burning, stinging) pain. However, neuropathic pain may respond with increasing dose.[70] Additionally, the observations of Liew and Hui, noting progressively increasing narcotic requirements in neoplastic patients, must be viewed with some alarm.[39] Keeping these cautions in mind, the following recommendation can be made. An appropriate patient is one who is chronically disabled, not a surgical candidate, not appropriate for behavioral operant therapy, and psychologically sound. After a careful discussion of the potential risks and benefits, a trial of epidural blockade or temporary indwelling intradural therapy may be recommended. If this provides relief, consideration can be given to an epidural narcotic implant.

Table 14-2
Spinal cord stimulation clinical series

Authors	Study design	Study group	Etiology of pain	Follow-up	Results
Clark K: Electrical stimulation of the nervous system for control of pain: University of Texas Southwestern Medical School experience. *Surg Neurol* 1975; 4:164–166.	Retrospective Review	13	Mixed: benign and malignant	Maximum 2 years	53.8% "Good" pain relief
Hoppenstein R: Electrical stimulation of the ventral and dorsal columns of the spinal cord for relief of chronic intractable pain: Preliminary report. *Surg Neurol* 1975; 4:187–194.	Retrospective Review	27 (three underwent ventral implants as well)	"Definite physiopathologic cause of pain"	?	16.2% Complete pain relief 29.6% "Good" pain relief
Hunt WE, Goodman JH, Bingham WG: Stimulation of the dorsal spinal cord for treatment of intractable pain: A preliminary report. *Surg Neurol* 1975; 4:153–156.	Retrospective Review	13	Mixed: benign and malignant	9–51 months	30.7% Excellent or partial benefit
Neilson KD, Adams JE, Hosobuchi Y: Experience with dorsal column stimulation for relief of chronic intractable pain: 1968–1973. *Surg Neurol* 1975; 4:148–152.	Retrospective Review	130	Mixed: mostly low back pain	1–4 years	42.6% "Excellent or good"
Pineda A: Dorsal column stimulation and its prospects. *Surg Neurol* 1975; 4:157–163.	Retrospective Review	76	Not specified	Up to 20 months	25.3% "Excellent" 19% "Satisfactory" relief of pain
Shelden CH, Paul F, Jacques DB, Pudenz RH: Electrical stimulation of the nervous system. *Surg Neurol* 1975; 4:127–132.	Retrospective Review	27	Mixed: neoplasm failed back, diabetic	Not specified	57% "Excellent or good"
Shealy CN: Dorsal column stimulation: Optimization of application. *Surg Neurol* 1975; 4:142–145.	Retrospective Review	80	Not specified	Minimum follow-up 7 months	46% "Excellent or fair" pain relief
Urban BJ, Nashold BS: Percutaneous epidural stimulation of the spinal cord for relief of pain: Long-term results. *J Neurosurg* 1978; 48:323–328.	Retrospective Review	20 (2-week trial)	Mixed: benign and neoplastic	Up to 2 years	6/7 Implanted, "successful"
Young RF: Evaluation of dorsal column stimulating in the treatment of chronic pain. *Neurosurgery* 1978; 3(3):373–379.	Retrospective Review	51	Mixed: degenerative, postoperative, MS, neoplasm, vascular	12–67 months (*m* = 38 months)	8% Pain relief, initially 0% After 4 years
Richardson RR, Siqueira EB, Cerullo LJ: Spinal epidural neurostimulation for treatment of acute and chronic intractable pain: Initial and long-term results. *Neurosurgery* 1979; 5(3):344–348.	Retrospective Review	36	Mixed: neoplasm, diabetic, arachnoiditis	1–3 years	56% Greater than 50% pain relief at 1 year

Reference	Study type	N	Condition	Duration	Results
Leclercq TA, Russo E: La stimulation epidurale dans le traitement des douleurs chroniques. Neurochirurgie 1981; 27:125–128.	Retrospective Review	20	"Failed disc" syndrome	Not specified	50% "Good" results
LeRoy PL: Stimulation of the spinal neuraxis by biocompatible electrical current in the human. Appl Neurophysiol 1981; 44:187–193.	Retrospective Review	49	All chronic benign pain	1–63 months (m = 30.7 months)	50% "Good to excellent" pain relief
Long DM, Erickson D, Campbell J, North R: Electrical stimulation of the spinal cord and peripheral nerves for pain control: A 10-year experience. Appl Neurophysiol 1981; 44:207–217.	Retrospective Review	99	Mixed: radiation neuritis, postsurgical, trauma	7–10 years	"No benefit," 50% of patients originally implanted would "now be rejected"
Blume H, Richardson R, Rojas C: Epidural nerve stimulation of the lower spinal cord and cauda equina for the relief of intractable pain in failed low back surgery. Appl Neurophysiol 1982; 45:456–460	Retrospective Review	28	Failed low back surgery	Not specified	70% "Good" and "fair"
Siegfried J, Lazorthes Y: Long-term follow-up for dorsal cord stimulation for chronic pain syndrome after multiple lumbar operations. Appl Neurophysiol 1982; 45:201–204.	Retrospective Review	89	Mixed: trauma, deformity, failed surgery	3 months to 8 years	74% "Good" or "improved" after 4 years
De la Porte C, Siegfried J: Lumbosacral spinal fibrosis (spinal arachnoiditis): Its diagnosis and treatment by spinal cord stimulation. Spine 1983; 8(6):593–603.	Retrospective Review	94	Arachnoiditis	4 years	60% Subjective improvement
Waisbrod H, Gerbershagen HU: Spinal cord stimulating in patients with a battered root syndrome. Arch Orthop Traumatic Surg 1985; 104:62–64.	Retrospective Review	16	"Battered root"	6–30 months (m = 16 months)	75% Pain free
Kumar K, Wyant GM, Ekong CEU: Epidural spinal cord stimulation for relief of chronic pain. Pain Clin 1986; 1(2):91–99.	Retrospective Review	60	"Varied benign organic etiology"	6 months to 5 years	48% Returned to full-time employment, an additional 13% had greater than 50% relief
Vogel HP, Heppner B, Humbs N, Schramm J, Wagner C: Long-term effects of spinal cord stimulation in chronic pain syndromes. J Neurol 1986; 233:16–18.	Retrospective Review	50	Mixed: benign, phantom, vascular, herpetic	1–5 years	16% "benefit" lasting 3 or more years
Koeze TH, Williams AC de C, Reiman S: Spinal cord stimulation and the relief of chronic pain. J Neurol Neurosurg Psychiatr 1987; 50:1424–1429.	Retrospective Review	20	Mixed: trauma, phantom pain, post-herpetic, arachnoiditis	13.5–42.5 months (m = 28 months)	50% or greater pain relief

Table 14-2

Spinal cord stimulation clinical series (Continued)

Authors	Study design	Study group	Etiology of pain	Follow-up	Results
Mittal B, Thomas DGT, Walton P, Calder I: Dorsal column stimulation (DCS) in chronic pain: report of 31 cases. *Ann Roy Col Surg Eng* 1987; 69:104–109.	Retrospective Review	35	All chronic benign pain	3 months to 8 years	60% "Good to fair pain relief"
Wester K: Dorsal column stimulation in pain treatment. *Acta Neurol Scand* 1987; 75:151–155.	Retrospective Review	35	Mixed: arachnoiditis, phantom pain, MS	4–60 months ($m = 15$ months)	43.5% used stimulation, reported the effect as "weak"
Meglio M, Cioni B, Rossi GF: Spinal cord stimulation in management of chronic pain: A nine-year experience. *J Neurosurg* 1989; 70:519–512.	Retrospective Review	109	Mixed: trauma, herpetic, vascular, neoplasm, failed surgery	2 years	Vascular: 85% success Low back pain: 68% success Paraplegia: 50% success Deafferentation: 33% success Post herpetic: 60% success Neoplasm: 27% success
Meilman PW, Leibrock LG, Leong FTL: Outcome of implanted spinal cord stimulation in the treatment of chronic pain: Arachnoiditis versus single nerve root injury and mononeuropathy. *Clin J Pain* 1989; 5:189–193.	Retrospective Review	20	Mixed	Short-term outcome, 1 month	71.4% "Excellent or good" root injury 23.1% "Excellent or good" Arachnoiditis
Devulder J, De Colvenaer L, Rolly G, Caemaert J, Calliauw L, Martens F: Spinal cord stimulation in chronic pain therapy. *Clin Pain* 1990; 6:51–56.	Retrospective Review	45	Mixed: failed back predominant	Up to 5 years	77% "Very good" pain relief
Devulder J, Vermeulen H, De Colvenaer L, Rolly G, Calliauw L, Caemaert J: Spinal cord stimulation in chronic pain: evaluation of results, complications, and technical considerations in sixty-nine patients. *Clin J Pain* 1991; 7:21–28.	Retrospective Review	69	Mixed: main indication, failed back surgery	Up to 8 years	55% Pain free with SCS or SCS plus non-narcotic drugs
Kumar K, Nath R, Wyant GM: Treatment of chronic pain by epidural spinal cord stimulation: A 10-year experience. *J Neurosurg* 1991; 75:402–407.	Retrospective Review	121	Mixed: most failed back surgery	6 months to 10 years ($m = 40$ months)	40% Pain control by SCS alone An additional 12% pain control with SCS and medication

Reference	Study Type	N	Diagnosis	Follow-up	Results
North RB, Ewend MG, Lawton MT, Kidd DH, Piantadosi S: Failed back surgery syndrome: 5-year follow-up after spinal cord stimulator implantation. *Neurosurgery* 1991; 28(5):692–699.	Retrospective Review Consecutive Series	50	Failed back surgery syndrome	m = 2.2 years and 5.0 years	2.2 years: 53% greater than 50% pain relief 5.0 years: 47% greater than 50% pain relief
North RB, Ewend MG, Lawton MT, Piantadosi S: Spinal cord stimulation for chronic, intractable pain: Superiority of "multi-channel" devices. *Pain* 1991; 44:119–130.	Retrospective Review	62	Mixed: failed surgery, spinal cord injuries, peripheral pathology	.36–4.21 years (m = 2.14 years)	53%, 50% or greater pain relief, satisfied with treatment
Simpson BA: Spinal cord stimulation in 60 cases of intractable pain. *J Neurol Neurosurg Psychol* 1991; 54(3):196–199.	Retrospective Review	60	Mixed: trauma, failed surgery, paresis	2–9 years (m = 29 months)	23.3% "Modest benefit" 46.7% "Significant benefit"
Spiegelmann R, Friedman W: Spinal cord stimulation: A contemporary series. *Neurosurgery* 1991; 28(1):65–71.	Retrospective Review	43	Mixed: RSD, MS, failed surgery	3–33 months (m = 13 months)	63% Pain relief
Tasker RR, Gervasio TC, DeCarvahlo TC, Dolan EJ: Intractable pain of spinal cord origin: Clinical features and implications for surgery. *J Neurosurg* 1992; 77:373–378.	Retrospective Review	35	Mixed: traumatic, iatrogenic, inflammatory, vascular	Cases 1961–1989, specific follow-up not provided	Good result = 50% or more reduction Fair result = 25–50% or more reduction for at least 1 year 27% "Good" for steady pain 20% "Fair" for steady pain
De La Porte C, Van de Kelft E: Spinal cord stimulation in failed back surgery syndrome. *Pain* 1993; 52:55–61.	Retrospective Review	64	Failed back surgery syndrome	1–7 years (m = 4 years)	55% Greater than 50% pain relief
LeDoux MS, Langford KH: Spinal cord stimulation for the failed back syndrome. *Spine* 1993; 18(2):191–194.	Retrospective Review	26	Failed back syndrome	1 month to 5 years	76% "good" at 1 year (n = 21) 74% "good" at 2 years (n = 19) 37.5% "good" at 5 years (n = 8)
North RB, Kidd DH, Zahurak M, James CS, Long DM: Spinal cord stimulation for chronic intractable pain: Experience over two decades. *Neurosurgery* 1993; 32(3):384–395.	Retrospective Review Conservative Case	205	Mixed: failed back, spinal cord injury, peripheral	2–20 years (m = 7.1 years)	52%, 50% or greater pain relief

SPINAL CORD STIMULATION

The Gate Control Therapy revolutionized thinking regarding chronic pain syndromes.[104] According to this model, stimulation of low-threshold primary afferent fibers could result in the central suppression of nociceptive influences. This idea was applied to the treatment of peripheral nerve pain with encouraging results.[72,105] Shealy et al. suggested stimulation of the dorsal columns of the spinal cord to control chronic intractable lower extremity pain; in effect, "closing the gate" at the level of the substantia gelatinosa.[24,106] This idea had the tremendous advantage in that it would allow pain control over a wide region of the body.

Spinal column stimulation has been studied widely.[24,106–108] Initially, electrodes were applied directly to the dorsal columns in a subdural location. Problems were reported with fibrosis, as well as cerebrospinal fluid leakage. Subsequently, Burton recommended an endodural approach that provided comparable results, although initial clinical effect was delayed because of the more rostral location of the stimulator.[109] Thereafter, epidural stimulation has been employed; for this reason it is suggested that the term "dorsal column stimulation" be abandoned in favor of "spinal cord stimulation," as more pathways than the dorsal columns are being stimulated. Larson et al. also have demonstrated that ventral placement can be effective.[110] This is hardly surprising in view of the demonstrated existence of ventral afferents.[65,111] Based on this neurophysiologic information, active pathways are difficult to determine. Additionally, whether or not electrical stimulation activates specific axons inhibiting central transmission or blocks transmissions in nociceptive fibers is unknown.

Indications for spinal cord stimulators include neoplastic and benign pain syndromes. In the latter, spinal cord stimulators have been employed to treat brachial plexus injuries, spinal-cord injuries, and post-amputation pain. The results of a European study group, compiled by Kranick and Thoden, are illustrative.[112] In 1726 patients reviewed shortly after spinal-cord stimulator implantation, greater than 50 percent pain relief was obtained in 38 percent. At long-term follow-up of 468 patients, only 22.5 percent continued to experience this level of relief. Results compiled from a review of the literature, focusing on benign pain syndromes, are shown in Table 14-2. Overall, with technical experience and the use of multichannel programmable devices, results have improved. In Table 14-2, as noted, pain-relief rates ranging from 0 to 85 percent have been obtained. All these studies, however, suffer from the same flaws:

retrospective study design, variable definitions of criteria for success, and outcome comparisons independent of pain etiology.

As the techniques and selection criteria have improved, an overall trend in the literature is apparent, with increased maintenance of pain relief over time. Selection criteria have come to include appropriate psychological screening, and a percutaneous trial ranging from 2 days to 2 months in length. Regarding efficacy in benign pain syndromes, the work of North et al. appears to be illustrative.[29,85] Successful outcomes, as defined by 50 percent or greater pain relief and patient satisfaction, has been realized in 50 to 53 percent of patients for follow-up as long as 20 years.[77] Pain relief rates of up to 60 percent have been reported in arachnoiditis.[113] It should be borne in mind also that most of these implants are for pain syndromes involving the lumber spine and lower extremities; the reported series concerning chronic benign cervical pain syndromes per se are rare. However, by careful consideration, a reasonable degree of extrapolation from these results certainly is merited. In general, results of spinal-cord stimulation are superior in anatomically limited, as opposed to diffuse, pain syndromes; Meilman et al. noted increased efficacy in patients suffering from single-root injury or mononeuropathy as opposed to arachnoiditis; Waisbrod and Gerbershargen also reported that 75 percent of patients who underwent spinal-cord stimulation for a unilateral "battered" lumbar-root syndrome were pain-free after a mean follow-up of 16 months.[114] Patient selection is, as in all cases, of paramount importance. Shealy developed a series of guidelines that include the following: emotional stability, evidence of depression only on the Minnesota Multiphasic Personality Inventory, acceptable medication usage, cooperation with a rehabilitation program, and response to a trial of TENS.[24] Contraindications include: cordotomy, deep brain implant, or previous DREZ lesioning. As noted by Long et al., the majority of failures of spinal-cord simulators may be explained, at least in part, because of psychological overlay.[115] A percutaneous trial is recommended in order to aid in patient selection. In the series of Nielson et al., 96 of 221 had a negative response to a percutaneous trial.[116] Regardless of this, 28 nonresponders were implanted, and one benefited.

Single or multiple leads may be placed percutaneously, or via open laminotomy. In the percutaneous technique, the electrode should be inserted several levels cranial to the site of the puncture; whereas in the open technique, it is inserted at the site of the laminotomy. Quadripolar leads are available for percutaneous or open insertion; an octrode (eight-lead array) is also available. North et al. have commented on the results obtained with multichannel devices.[117] Fifty of the 62 patients suffered from the failed-back syndrome, and in the group, 52 percent reported greater than 50 percent pain relief, at a mean of follow-up of 2.14 years. In general, for upper extremity pain, the lead should be placed between C2 and C4. For chest-wall distal pain syndromes, lead placement between T2 and T7 is recommended.[107] To cover low-back and lower-extremity pain, typically stimulation from T9 to T11 is required.[107]

Complications with spinal-cord stimulation are predominantly technical. Representative rates are found in the report of North et al.[117] The authors reported an 11 percent rate of subcutaneous infection. The predominant complication, however, was lead migration or breakage. Simple bipolar leads required electrode revision in 23 percent; the revision rate in patients with multichannel devices was 16 percent. Fatigue fracture of electrode leads was observed in 13 percent of patients. Migration rates of up to 69 percent have been reported in patients implanted via the percutaneous technique.[118] However, larger, multichannel arrays may be more easily and securely placed at the desired physiological midline with a percutaneous approach. Patients also have reported transient alloynia or paraplegia, although these are rare.

Kranick and Thoden recommended the following guidelines to achieve optimal results.[112] These include the use of multiple electrodes, open placement, cranial positioning of electrodes, absence of secondary gain, and a localized pain syndrome. Although the usage of spinal-cord stimulation in chronic benign pain syndromes must be recommended with caution, this is a promising alternative in patients who meet the selection criteria and in whom other avenues of therapy have proven unrewarding.

CONCLUSION

Overall, the results of intervention, both operative and nonoperative, for chronic pain syndromes are mildly encouraging at best. A central problem in attempting to determine the effectiveness of various treatment approaches based on a literature review is the variety in study design, quality, evaluation standards, and follow-up. Clearly these difficulties only can be resolved by well-controlled prospective studies in the future; these studies may prove difficult for financial and ethical reasons. Additionally, the financial impact of these inter-

ventions needs to be measured quite closely. With the cost of a chronic multidisciplinary pain program measure for measure comparable to the cost of implanted spinal-cord stimulators, future outcome studies directed at both clinical efficacy *and* cost-effectiveness are of paramount importance.

REFERENCES

1. King JC, Kelleher WJ: The chronic pain syndrome: The inpatient interdisciplinary rehabilitative behavioral modification approach. *Phys Med Rehabil: State Art Rev* 1991; 5(1):165–166.
2. Goddard MJ, Dean BZ, King JC: Pain rehabilitation. 1. Basic science, acute pain, and neuropathic pain. *Arch Phys Med Rehabil* 1994; 75(5S):S4–S58.
3. King JC, Goddard MJ: Pain rehabilitation. 2. Chronic pain syndrome and myofascial syndrome. *Arch Phys Med Rehabil* 1994; 75(5S):S9–S14.
4. Williams FH, Maly BJ: Pain rehabilitation. 3. Cancer pain, pelvic pain, and age-related considerations. *Arch Phys Med Rehabil* 1994; 75(5S):S15–S20.
5. Dean BZ, Williams FH, King JC, Goddard MJ: Pain rehabilitation. 4. Therapeutic options in pain management. *Arch Phys Med Rehabil* 1994; 75(5S):S21–S30.
6. Grabois M: Chronic pain evaluation and treatment, in Goodgold J (ed): *Rehabilitation Medicine*. St. Louis: C.V. Mosby, 1988.
7. Graceley RH, McGrath P, Dubnor R: Ratio scales of sensory and affective verbal pain descriptors. *Pain* 1978; 5:5–18.
8. Schieber MH: Physiological bases for functional recovery. *J Neuro Rehabil* 1995; 9:65–71.
9. Stein C: The control of pain in peripheral tissue by opioids. *New Engl J Med* 1995; 332(25):1685–1690.
10. Powney JA, Myers SJ, Gonzales EG, Lieberman JS (eds): *The Physiological Basis of Rehabilitation Medicine*. Boston: Butterworth-Heinemann, 1994, p. 398.
11. Berry CB, Toritani T, Tolson H: Electrical activity and soreness in muscles after exercise. *Am J Phys Med Rehabil* 1990; 69(2):60–66.
12. Ellenberg MR, Honet JC, Treanor WJ: Cervical radiculopathy. *Arch Phys Med Rehabil* 1994; 75:342–352.
13. Jadad AR, et al: Morphine responsiveness of chronic pain: Double-blind randomized crossover study with patient-controlled analgesia. *Lancet* 1992; 339:1367–1371.
14. Rowland M, Tozer TN: *Clinical Pharmacokinetics: Concepts and Applications*. Philadelphia: Lea & Febiger, 1989, pp. 19–31, 33–40.
15. The Capsaicin Study Group: Treatment of painful diabetic neuropathy with topical capsaicin, a double-blind, vehicle controlled study. *Arch Int Med* 1991; 151:2225–2229.
16. Morgenlander JC, et al: Capsaicin for the treatment of

pain in Guillain-Barre syndrome. *Ann Neurol*, 1990; 28:199.

17. Ross DR, Varipapa RJ: Treatment of painful diabetic neuropathy with topical capsaicin. *New Engl J Med* 1989; 321:474–475.

18. Peter C: Post-herpetic neuralgia and topical capsaicin. *Pain* 1988; 33:333–340.

19. Fields HL, et al: Biology of placebo analgesia. *Am J Med* 1981; 70:745–746.

20. Kiser RS, et al: Acupuncture relief of chronic pain syndrome correlates with increased *met*-enkephalin concentration. *Lancet* 1983; 2:1394–1396.

21. Deyo RA, et al: A controlled trial of transcutaneous electrical nerve stimulation and exercise for chronic low back pain. *New Engl J Med* 1990; 143:936–939.

22. Spiller WG, Martin E: The treatment of persistent pain of organic origin in the lower part of the body by division of the anterolateral column of the spinal cord. *JAMA* 1912; 58:1489–1490.

23. O'Brien JP: Mechanisms of spinal pain, in Wall PD, Melzack R (eds): *Textbook of Pain*. New York: Churchill-Livingston, 1989, pp. 240–251.

24. Shealy CN, Mortimer JT, Hagfor NR: Dorsal column electroanalgesia. *J Neurosurg* 1970; 320:560–564.

25. Wynn Parry CB: The failed back, in Wall PD, Melzack R (eds): *Textbook of Pain*. New York: Churchill-Livingston, 1989, pp. 341–354.

26. Förster O: Vorderseitenstrangdurchschneidung im rückenmark zur beseitgung von schmerzen. Berliner Klinische Wochenschrift 1913; 50:1499.

27. Cowie RA, Hitchcock ER: The late results of anterolateral cordotomy for pain relief. *Acta Neurochirugica* 1982; 64:39–50.

28. O'Connell JE: Anterolateral cordotomy for intractable pain in carcinoma of the rectum. *Proc Roy Soc Med* 1969; 62:1223–1225.

29. Raskind R: Analytical review of open cordotomy. *Int Surg* 1969; 51:226–231.

30. Schartz HG: High cervical tractotomy: Technique and results. *Clin Neurosurg* 1960; 8:282–293.

31. Diemath HE, Heppner F, Walker AE: Anterolateral chordotomy for relief of pain. *Postgrad Med* 1961; 29: 485–495.

32. White, JC, Sweet WH: Pain and the neurosurgeon: A 40-year experience. Springfield MA: Charles C Thomas, 1969.

33. Probst C: Microsurgical cordotomy in 20 patients with epi-intradural fibrosis following operation for lumbar disc herniation. *Acta Neurochirurgica (Wien)* 1990; 107: 30–36.

34. Lahuerta J, Bowsher D, Lipton S, Buxton PH: The treatment of chronic thoracic segmental pain by radiofrequency percutaneous partial rhizotomy. *J Neurosurg* 1994; 80(6):986–992.

35. Lahuerta J, Bosher D, Campbell J, Lipton S: Clinical and instrumental evaluation of sensory function before and

after percutaneous anterolateral cordotomy at cervical level in man. *Pain* 1990; 42:233–230.

36. Frankel SA, Prokop JD: The value of cordotomy for the relief of pain. *New Engl J Med* 1961; 264:971–974.

37. French LA: High cervical tractotomy: Techniques and result. *Clin Neurosurg* 1974; 21:239–245.

38. Grant FC, Wood FA: Experiences with cordotomy. *Clin Neurosurg* 1958; 5:38–65.

39. Mansuy L, Sindou M, Fisher G, Brunon J: Spinothalamic cordotomy in cancerous pain. Results of a series of 124 patients operated on by a direct posterior approach. *Neurochirurgie* (Paris) 1976; 22:432–444.

40. Porter RW, Hohmann GW, Bors E, French JD: Cordotomy for pain following cauda equina injury. *Arch Surg* 1966; 92:765–770.

41. Wilkins RH: *Neurosurgical Classics*. New York: Johnson Reprint Corp., 1968, pp. 504–515.

42. Lipton S: Percutaneous Cordotomy. Wall PD, Melzack R (eds): *Textbook of Pain*, 2nd ed. New York: Churchill-Livingston, 1989, pp. 832–839.

43. Nashold BS Jr., Ostdahl RH: Dorsal root entry zone lesions for pain relief. *J Neurosurg* 1979; 51:59–69.

44. Thomas DET, Sheehy J: Dorsal root entry zone coagulation (Nashold's Procedure) in brachial plexus avulsion. *J Neurol Neurosurg Psychiatr* 1982; 45:949.

45. Friedman Ah, Bullitt E: Dorsal root entry zone lesions in the treatment of pain following brachial plexus avulsion, spinal cord injury, and herpes zoster. *Appl Neurophysiol* 1988; 51:164–169.

46. Friedman AH, Nashold BR, Bronee PR: Dorsal root entry zone lesions for the treatment of brachial plexus avulsion injuries: A follow-up study. *Neurosurgery* 1988; 22: 369–377.

47. Powers SK, Adams JE, Edwards MSB, Broggam JE, Hosbuchi Y: Pain relief from dorsal root entry zone lesion made with argon and carbon dioxide microsurgical lasers. *J Neurosurg* 1984; 61:841–847.

48. Powers SK, Barbaro NM, Levy RM: Pain control with laser produced dorsal root entry zone lesions. *Appl Neurophysiol* 1988; 51:243–254.

49. Cosman ER, Nashold BS, Ovelma-Leu JH: Theoretical aspect of radiofrequency lesions in the dorsal root entry zone. *Neurosurgery* 1984; 15:945–950.

50. Lunsford LD, Bennett MH: Evoked potential monitoring during dorsal root entry zone surgery. Patients with chronic pain. *Stereotact Funct Neurosurg* 1989; 53: 233–246.

51. Young RF: Clinical experience with radiofrequency and laser DREZ lesions. *J Neurosurg* 72:715–720.

52. Abbe R: Intradural section of the spinal nerves for neuralgia. *Boston Med Surg J* 1896; 135:329–335.

53. Willner C, Law PA: Pharmacologic approaches to neuropathic pain in Dyck PJ, Thomas PK (ed): *Peripheral Neuropathy*, 3rd ed. Philadelphia: W.B. Saunders, 1993.

54. Dubuisson D: Root surgery, in Wall PD, Melzack R (eds):

Textbook of Pain, 2nd ed. New York: Churchill-Livingston, 1989, pp. 784–794.

55. Onofrio B, Campa H: Evaluation of rhizotomy. *J Neurosurg* 1972; 36:751–755.

56. Scoville WB: Extradural spinal sensory rhizotomy. *J Neurosurg* 1966; 25:94–95.

57. Hunter CR, Mayfield FH: Role of upper cervical roots in the production of pain in the head. *Am J Surg* 1949; 78:743–751.

58. Peacock WJ, Arena LJ: Selective posterior rhizotomy of the relief of spasticity in cerebral palsy. *So Afr Med J* 1982; 62:119–124.

59. Dykes RW, Terzis JK: Spinal nerve distributions in the upper limb: The organization of the dermatome and afferent myotome. *Phil Trans Roy Soc London* [Bio] 1981; 293:509–554.

60. Förster O: The deramatones in man. *Brain* 1933; 56:1–39.

61. Head H: On disturbances of sensation with especial reference to the pain of nerve disease. *Brain* 1893; 16:1–133.

62. Sherrintgon CS: Experiments in the examination of the peripheral distribution of the fibers of the posterior roots of some spinal nerves. *Phil Trans Roy Soc London* [Bio] 1898; 190:45–186.

63. Davis L, Pollock LJ: The peripheral pathway for painful sensation. *Arch Neurol Psychol* 1930; 24:883–898.

64. Pallie W: The intersegmental anastomoses of posterior spinal rootlets and their significance. *J Neurosurg* 1959; 16:188–195.

65. Coggeshall RE, Appplebaum ML, Frazen M, Stubbs TB, Sykes MT: Unmyelinated axons in human ventral roots, a possible explanation for the failure of dorsal rhizotomy to relieve pain. *Brain* 1975; 98:157–166.

66. Jain KK: Nerve root scarring and arachnoiditis as a complication of lumbar intervertebral disc surgery: Surgical treatment. *Neurochirurgia (Stuttgart)* 1974; 17:185–192.

67. Bertrand G: The battered root problem. *Orthopaed Clin No Am* 1975; 6:305–310.

68. Bernard TN, Broussard TS, Dwyer AP, LaRocca SH: Extradural sensory rhizotomy in the management of chronic lumbar spondylosis with radiculopathy. *Orthopaed Trans* 1987; 11:23.

69. Tasker RR, Organ LW, Hawrylyshyn P: Deafferentation and casalgia, in Bonica JJ (ed): *Pain* New York: Raven Press, 1980, pp. 305–329.

70. Portenoy RK, Foley KM, Intarrisi C: The nature of opioid responsiveness and its implications for neuropathic pain: New hypothesis derived from studies of opioid infusions. *Pain* 1990; 43:273–286.

71. Wall PD, Devor M: Sensory afferent impulses originate from dorsal root ganglia as well as from the periphery in normal and injured rats. *Pain* 1983; 17:321–339.

72. Wall PD, Gutrick M: Ongoing activity in peripheral nerves: the physiology and pharmacology of impulses originating from neuroma. *Exp Neurol* 1974; 43:580–593.

73. Sweet WH, Poletti CE: Operations in the brain stem and spinal canal with an appendix on open cordotomy, in Wall PD, Melzack R (eds): *Textbook of Pain,* 2nd ed. New York: Churchill-Livingston, 1989, pp. 812–817.

74. Nash TP: Percutaneous radiofrequency lesioning of dorsal root ganglion for intractable pain. *Pain* 1986; 24:67–73.

75. Osgood CP, Dujovny M, Faille R, Abassy M: Microsurgical ganglionectomy for chronic pain syndromes. Technical note. *J Neurosurg* 1976; 45:113–115.

76. Smith FP: Transpinal ganglionectomy for relief of intercostal pain. *J Neurosurg* 1970; 32:574–577.

77. North RB, Kidd DH, Zahurak M, James CS, Long DM: Spinal cord stimulation for chronic intractable pain: experience over two decades. *Neurosurgery* 1993; 32(3): 384–395.

78. Mooney V, Robertson J: The facet syndrome. *Clin Orthop Rel Res* 1976; 115:149–156.

79. Pedersen HE, Blunck CFJ, Gardener E: Anatomy of lumbosacral posterior rami and meningeal branches of spinal nerves. *J Bone Joint Surg* 1956; 38:377.

80. April CN, Dwyer A, Boduk N: Cervical zygapophyseal joint pain patterns 2: A clinical evaluation. *Spine* 1990; 15(6):458–461.

81. Dwyer A, April CN, Cogduk N: Cervical zygapophyseal joint pain patterns 1: a study in normal volunteers. *Spine* 1990; 15(6):453–457.

82. Sluijter ME: Percutaneous facet denervation and partial posterior rhizotomy. *Acta Anaetheologica Belgica* 1981; 1:63–79.

83. Rees WS: Multiple bilateral subcutaneous rhizolysis of segmental nerves in the treatment of the intervertebral disc syndrome. *Ann Gen Pract* 1971; 16:126.

84. Shealy CN: Percutaneous radiofrequency denervation of spinal facets. Treatment for chronic back pain and sciatica. *J Neurosurg* 1975; 43:448.

85. Schaerer JP: Radiofrequency facet rhizotomy in the treatment of chronic neck and low back pain. *Int Surg* 1978; 63(6):53–59.

86. Oudenhoven RC: The role of laminectomy, facet rhizotomy, and epidural steroids. *Spine* 1979; 4:145–147.

87. Boduk N, MacIntosh J, Marsiana A: Technical limitations to the efficacy of radiofrequency neurotomy for spinal pain. *Neurosurgery* 1987; 20:529–535.

88. Husson JL, Meadeb J, Eudier F, Masse A: Treatment of chronic pain of the musculoskeletal system by epidural stimulation. *J de Chirurgie* (Paris) 1988; 125:522–524.

89. Meglio M, Cioni B, Prezioso A, Talamonti G: Spinal cord stimulation in the treatment of post-therapeutic pain. *Acta Neurochirurgica Suppl. (Wein)* 1989; 46:65–66.

90. Wester K: Dorsal column stimulation in pain treatment. *Acta Neurologica Scandinavica Scandinavia.* 1987; 75: 151–155.

91. Young RF: Evaluation of dorsal column stimulating in the treatment of chronic pain. *Neurosurgery* 1978; 3(3):373–379.

92. Coombs DW, Saunders RL, Gaynor M, Pegean MG: Epidural narcotic infusion reservoir: Implantation and efficacy. *Anesthesiology* 1982; 56:469.

93. Coombs DW, Saunders RL, Pagean MG: Continuous intraspinal narcotic analgesia: Technical aspect of an implantable infusion system. *Reg Anesth* 1982; 7:110.

94. Cosendy BA, Dupaquier G, Buchser E, Chapuis G: Epidural administration of morphine by a completely implantable device. *Helv Chirurgica Acta* 1986; 56:125.

95. Downing JE, Busch EH, Stedman PM: Epidural morphine delivered by a percutaneous epidural catheter for outpatient treatment of cancer pain. *Anesth Anal* 1988; 67:1159.

96. Greenberg HS, Taren J, Ensminger W, Doan K: Benefit from and tolerance to continuous intrathecal infusion of morphine for intractable cancer pain. *J Neurosurg* 1982; 57(3):360–364.

97. Onofrio B, Yaksh T, Arnold D: Continuous low dose intrathecal morphine administration in treatment of chronic pain of malignant origin. *Mayo Clin Proc* 1981; 45–516.

98. St. Marie B: Administration of the intraspinal analgesia in the home care setting. *J Intra Nurs* 1989; 12:164.

99. Sjorgen P, Banning AM, Henriksen H: High dose epidural opioid treatment of malignant pain. *Ugeskrift Laeger* 1989; 151:25–28.

100. Liew E, Hui Y: A preliminary study of long term epidural morphine for cancer pain via a subcutaneously implanted reservoir. *Ma Tsui Hsuech Tsa Chi* 1989; 27:5–12.

101. Auld AW, Maki-Jodela A, Murdoch DW: Intraspinal narcotic analgesia in the treatment of chronic pain. *Spine* 1985; 10:778–781.

102. Auld AW, Murdoch DW, O'Laughlin KA: Intraspinal narcotic analgesic pain management in the failed laminectomy syndrome. *Spine* 1987; 12:953–955.

103. Krames E: Intrathecal infusion therapy for intractable pain: patient management guidelines. *J Pain Sympt Mgmt* 1993; 8:36.

104. Melzack R, Wall PD: Pain mechanism: A new theory. *Science* 1965; 150:971–1070,1965.

105. Sweet WH, Wipsic JG: Treatment of chronic pain by stimulation of fibers of primary afferent nerves. *Trans Am Neurol Assoc* 1968; 93:103–107.

106. Shealy CN, Mortimer JT, Resturek JB: Electrical inhibition of pain by stimulation of the dorsal column. Preliminary clinical report. *Anesth Anal* (Cleveland) 1967; 46:489–491.

107. Nashold BS Jr: Dorsal column stimulation for the control of pain: A three year follow-up. *Surg Neurol* 1975; 4:146–149.

108. Nashold BS Jr., Friedman H: Dorsal column stimulation for control of pain. A three year follow-up: A preliminary report on 30 patients. *J Neurosurg* 1972; 36:590.

109. Burton C: Dorsal column stimulation: optimization of application. *Surg Neurol* 1975; 4:171–179.

110. Larson SJ, Suances A Jr., Cusick JR, Meyer GA, Swiontek T: A comparison between anterior and posterior spinal implant systems. *Surg Neurol* 1975; 4:180–186.

111. Coggeshall RE: Afferent fibers in the ventral root. *Neurosurgery* 1979; 4(5):443–448.

112. Krainick JU, Thoden U: Spinal cord stimulation, in Wall PD, Melzack R (eds): *Textbook of Pain*, 2nd ed. New York: Churchill-Livingstone, 1989, p. 924.

113. De la Porte C, Siegfried J: Lumbosacral spinal fibrosis (spinal arachnoiditis): Its diagnosis and treatment by spinal cord stimulation. *Spine* 1983; (6):593–603.

114. Wisbrod H, Gerbershagen HU: Spinal cord stimulating in patients with a battered root syndrome. *Arch Orthop Traum Surg* 1985; 104:62–64.

115. Long DM, Erickson P, Campbell J, North R: Electrical stimulation of the spinal cord and peripheral nerve for pain control: Ten year's experience. *Appl Neurophysiol* 1981; 44:202–217.

117. North RB, Ewend MG, Lawton MT, Piantadosi S: Spinal cord stimulation for chronic, intractable pain: superiority of "multi-channel" devices. *Pain* 1991; 44:119–130.

118. Racz GB, McCarron RF, Talboys P: Percutaneous dorsal column stimulation for chronic pain control. *Spine* 1989; 14:1–4.

119. Wetzel FT: Chronic benign cervical pain syndromes: Surgical considerations. *Spine* 1992; 17(105):S367–S374.

Chapter 15

EVALUATION AND MANAGEMENT OF BRACHIAL PLEXUS INJURY

Michael Y. Lee
Maureen Nelson
Christine E. Lee

A team approach with the surgeon, neurologist, neuroradiologist, and physiatrist along with the appropriate therapists is optimal in the treatment of brachial plexus injury. After the initial evaluation and treatment, rehabilitation should be instituted as soon as possible. In many instances, brachial plexus injury is discovered during the process of evaluating major brain, spinal, or orthopedic trauma. These injuries in patients may mask or delay the diagnosis of brachial plexus injury. Knowlege of the anatomy of the brachial plexus and signs and symptoms of brachial plexus injury, along with the clinical intuition, will assist in the early diagnosis of injury to the brachial plexus.

ANATOMY

There are several components of the brachial plexus—roots, trunks, divisions, cords, and peripheral nerves. The brachial plexus lies primarily in the lower part of the neck, between the clavicle and the first rib, extending into the axilla. The ventral branches of the C5–C8 and T1 unite to form the brachial plexus, with occasional and highly variable contributions from the ventral branches of C4 or T2. The anterior rami of C5 and C6 nerve roots exit their neural foramina and pass between the anterior and middle scalene muscles. At the lateral border of the anterior scalene muscle, they unite to form the upper trunk of the brachial plexus. The C7 nerve root emerges to form the middle trunk. The lower trunk is formed by the C8 and T1 nerve roots posterior to the anterior scalene muscle.

As the trunks course inferolaterally in the supra-clavicular fossa, each splits into an anterior and a posterior division. The anterior division is composed of the upper and middle trunks to form the lateral cord and the anterior division of the lower trunk is continued as the medial cord. The posterior cord is formed by the posterior division of all three trunks. The cords of the brachial plexus are formed as the divisions pass between the clavicle and the first rib to enter the axilla. Each cord is named for its relationship with the axillary artery. The musculocutaneous, median, and ulnar nerves are formed from the cords in the axilla distal to the inferior border of the pectoralis muscle.[1]

The plexus is divided into two fundamental parts, an anterior (flexor) and a posterior (extensor) portion corresponding to the division of the musculature of the limb. The medial and lateral cords supply the muscles of the pectoral region and all muscles arising on the flexor surface of arm, forearm, and hand. The posterior cord supplies most of the muscles of the shoulder proper and all muscles associated with the extensor surface of the limb. In addition to the branches from the three cords, other important nerves arise proximally or toward the origin of the plexus. The suprascapular nerve and the tiny nerve to the subclavius arise from the upper trunk; and the long thoracic nerve to the serratus anterior arises from the anterior branches of C5, 6, and 7.

ETIOLOGY OF BRACHIAL PLEXUS INJURY

Brachial plexus lesions can occur from diverse causes. Lesions have been identified anywhere from the nerve roots to the peripheral nerves. The most common cause

225

is trauma. Tractional brachial plexus injury following motorcycle accidents occurs in over 80 percent of cases, particularly young adults aged 18–20 years.[2] Traumatic brachial plexus lesions in adults can be differentiated into supraclavicular lesions at root level (75% of cases) and infra- and retroclavicular lesions of the secondary trunks and terminal branches (25% of cases).[3] The mechanisms of injury can be differentiated into direct blunt trauma to the region of the clavicle, often combined with subclavian artery and bone trauma; caudal traction of the shoulder, often combined with hyperflexion of the neck to the contralateral side; and hyperextension of the arm. Nerve-root damage varies from rupture to avulsion. The proportion of total avulsion lesions appears to be rising. The compulsory wearing of crash helmets has meant that many patients now survive more severe lesions with multiple injuries.

Brachial plexopathy in the newborn is also common. The cause for neonatal brachial plexopathy is a matter of debate. How often brachial plexus injury discovered on the neonate is a result of prebirth injury (intrauterine) as opposed to tractional forces experienced during the birth process is not known.[4,5] Neonatal brachial plexus injury has been found after cesarean section.[5a] Brachial plexus lesions are also caused by penetrating injuries, direct compression of the plexus by fascial bands, adjacent skeletal anomalies such as cervical rib, or tumors.[6] A neoplasm may be involved as a direct extension of disease from structures adjacent to the brachial plexus, as well as primary tumors of neural origin or radiation injury. Patients with neoplastic invasion tend to have pain and Horner's syndrome. Prolonged anesthesia with a patient in an unusual posture, and in difficult cases of median sternotomy, cardiac surgery, or radiological procedures may be associated with brachial plexus injury.[7–10] The number of patients who sustain and are treated for open wounds of the brachial plexus is relatively small, and reports are sparse.

In addition, nontraumatic brachial plexopathy can occur as an idiopathic process.[11,12] Some of the rare but well-described associations with the brachial plexus injury include antiallergy injection, Ehlers-Danlos syndrome, systemic lupus erythematosis, familial pressure-sensitive neuropathy, and delayed effects of radiotherapy to the axillary region.[13–18]

EVALUATION OF BRACHIAL PLEXOPATHY

Since the anatomical relationships between the brachial plexus, the components of the neck, thorax, and axilla,

as well as major vessels and pleura involve intimate proximity, it is critical to rule out any acute and serious injury to the vessels, pleura, or intrathoracic contents that can be life-threatening. The focus of the evaluation of brachial plexus injury is to detect the exact nature of the injury, the location of the lesion (including pre- or postganglionic), and completeness of injury.

Clinical Examination

General inspection should note the position of the limb, joints, and presence of any wounds or bone deformities. Any swelling or ecchymosis, trophic changes, sympathetic dysfunction, or changes from vascular insufficiency should be noted. It is essential to assess the passive range of motion of the cervical spine and all joints of the shoulder girdle and upper extremity to detect any instability, pain, or contractures. Joint range of motion can be recorded with a goniometer. Motor examination should be complete, with the strength of each muscle evaluated and recorded.

Sensory examination of the patient with brachial plexus injury should include touch, pain, vibration, and proprioception. The presence of Horner's syndrome should be noted. Because of the intimate relationship of the brachial plexus to the subclavian artery, the vascular status of the peripheral circulation and pulses should be documented.

When the patient has a completely paralyzed arm, clues and clinical signs often indicate whether the lesion is pre- or postganglionic. Tinel's sign is a useful diagnostic maneuver in which the distal tingling is produced by percussing the injured plexus in the neck. A strongly positive Tinel's sign over one or more of the nerve roots in the neck is highly suggestive of a ruptured root.[19] For preganglionic lesions, the presence of characteristically severe burning pain with paroxysmal shoots, Horner's syndrome, and strongly positive Tinel's sign are useful. The Horner's syndrome may disappear after weeks or months. Thus, its absence does not necessarily indicate that the lesion is not preganglionic. Another unfavorable prognostic factor is sensory impairment over the thoracic outlet and the side of the neck, indicating severe disruption of the cervical nerve roots as well as the brachial plexus, and is highly associated with root avulsion. Paralysis of the rhomboids and serratus anterior indicates a preganglionic lesion of at least C5. The presence of vascular injury in the neck and fracture of the neck of the scapula is usually associated with a preganglionic brachial plexus lesion.[19] In contrast, brachial plexus palsy owing to shoulder dislocation has a 90 percent chance of complete recovery.[3] Similarly, incomplete palsy can be regarded as a good prognostic sign.

Clinical Neurophysiological Evaluation

Electrodiagnostic studies are extremely helpful in the clinical evaluation of the extent and severity of a brachial plexus injury. The techniques should include electromyography of limb and shoulder girdle muscles, electromyography of paravertebral muscles, motor and sensory nerve conduction studies, and somatosensory evoked potentials.

Electromyography

The standard needle electromyographic examination in suspected brachial plexus injury involves sampling of selected muscles, at the minimum of two or more muscles supplied by each nerve root. In normal lower motor neuron function, no muscle activity is recorded after insertion of the electromyography needle in the completely relaxed muscle. In the presence of a lower motor neuron lesion involving the nerve root or brachial plexus, spontaneous single muscle fiber discharges (fibrillations and positive sharp waves) can be recorded after electrode insertion 2 to 3 weeks after injury.[20] Unfortunately, signs of muscle denervation are not specific to the level of injury to the lower motor neuron. It occurs after the lower motor neuron has been injured at any level from the root to the distal plexus. Partial damage of the lower motor neuron can show some activation of motor unit action potentials of muscles tested under voluntary contraction. The size, shape, and recruitment pattern of the motor unit action potentials should be carefully studied whenever possible, since the findings changes and the presence of motor unit actions would be essential in determining the level of the injury, status of reinnervation, and prognosis. The detection of spontaneous single muscle fiber discharges in the paraspinal muscles may indicate preganglionic involvement.[20]

Nerve Conduction Studies   Motor and sensory nerve conduction studies of the limb with suspected brachial plexus injury also provide valuable information. Motor nerve conduction studies show distal electrical continuity of peripheral motor neuron to involved muscles. Measurement of the distal latency and the amplitude of compound muscle action potential, and calculation of the conduction velocity are routine components of motor nerve conduction studies. Sensory nerve conduction studies provide information on continuity of sensory neurons distal to the dorsal root ganglion. The presence of sensory nerve action potential in the peripheral nerves of a limb suspected of brachial plexus lesion indicates a lesion proximal to dorsal root ganglion (preganglionic lesion). The absence or significant reduction of the amplitude of sensory nerve action potential is noted in the peripheral nerve with a lesion distal to dorsal root ganglion (post-ganglionic lesion) because of degeneration of the sensory nerve fibers.[20] The absence of a sensory nerve action potential in the presence of anesthesia does not necessarily imply a postganglionic injury, and can indicate both pre- and postganglionic lesion.

Somatosensory Evoked Potentials   Somatosensory evoked potential studies may be useful in the diagnosis of brachial plexus injury when used in conjunction with electromyography and nerve conduction studies.[21] Somatosensory evoked potentials are used to study the afferent pathways including peripheral nerve, plexus, root, and central nervous system by recording responses at selected sites with electrical and mechanical stimuli. The changes in the parameters including onset and peak latencies and peak-to-peak amplitude of somatosensory evoked potentials may be used to detect lesions. Selective stimulation of the digital nerves may be utilized to elicit somatosensory evoked potentials that delineate lesions involving root, plexus, or thoracic outlet.[22] In the evaluation of patients with a brachial plexus lesion, the absence of a somatosensory evoked potential in the presence of a sensory nerve action potential is evidence of a preganglionic sensory root injury. However, the somatosensory evoked potential studies have limited value in the presence of postganglionic lesion.[20]

Transcranial Magnetic Stimulation   Magnetic stimulation has been used in recent years to study and measure central nervous system motor conduction and assess the function of central motor pathways. Magnetic stimulation excites neurons and dendrites presynaptically in order to elicit a motor-evoked potential. The amplitude and latency of the motor-evoked potentials are measured and compared. In very limited studies, motor-evoked potentials have been shown to be useful in brachial plexopathies to document axonal continuity through the injured plexus early in the course of the disease process.[23] More studies are needed to assess the future use of motor-evoked potentials in the evaluation of brachial plexus injury.

Radiographic Imaging Studies Plain radiographs of the cervical spine and shoulder girdle can be helpful to rule out any injury to the cervical spine and cord in traumatic cases. If there is no clinical recuperation with repeated clinical examination within 2 to 4 weeks, computed tomography of the cervical spine with myelography or magnetic resonance imaging (MRI) can be used to obtain more detailed anatomical information. These studies precisely determine the existence of specific lesions, especially root avulsion, and pseudomeningocele. The appearance of the meningocele sheaths and rootlets can also be visualized in great detail. Nonvisualization of a normal nerve root is considered a sign of nerve root avulsion, since normal nerve roots are seen in the neural foramen.[24] Pseudomeningoceles are seen best in coronal and axial planes on MRI as cerebrospinal fluid high-intensity masses.

Recently, MRI has become the preferred imaging modality for the evaluation of suspected brachial plexus pathology. MRI has multiplanar capability, lacks "shoulder artifact" unlike computed tomography, and reliably differentiates vascular from nonvascular structures.[25] MRI is the modality of choice for evaluating suspected neoplasm involving the brachial plexus, and can be used to diagnose nerve root avulsion, neuromas, tumor, and radiation fibrosis.[26,27]

MANAGEMENT

Conservative Management

Seddon's classification of nerve injury into three types—neurapraxia, axonotmesis, and neurotmesis—applies to the brachial plexus.[28] Neurapraxia occurs in brachial plexus injury as a result of moderate stretch. Motor fibers are more affected than sensory, and usually, spontaneous recovery is expected within 6 weeks of injury. Axonotmesis, which results from a greater degree of stretch, involves interruption of axonal continuity, leading to total loss of distal axonal function. Since the neural microtubules are intact and capable of functioning as a conduit for axoplasmic flow in the regenerating axons, spontaneous recovery is possible.

Neurotmesis, the most severe degree of nerve injury, results from complete disruption of all elements of the nerve. Spontaneous recovery is not expected. Preganglionic (or supraganglionic) neurotmesis injury involves avulsion of the root from the spinal cord, whereas postganglionic (or infraganglionic) involves distal rupture of the nerves beyond the dorsal root ganglion. The degree of paralysis may be complete or incomplete, depending on the extent and location of injury. In patients with severe or total paralysis of the upper extremity, effort must be made to prevent further traction of the neurovascular structures that could lead to further injury, and prevent contractures and edema.

Supraclavicular plexus injury is usually caused by traction on the plexus. Damage to the plexus, however, often reaches below the level of clavicle.[29] Involvement of individual neural elements varies from trivial and reversible to catastrophic and irreparable injury. The type of injury to the plexus and its roots is determined both by the magnitude and duration of applied force along the neural pathway. Roots may be avulsed wholly or partially, and differential avulsion of the sensory and motor components can occur. The prognosis for spontaneous recovery of traction injuries depends on the mode and extent of injuries. Patients with ipsilateral Horner's syndrome associated with brachial plexus injury and persistence of severe pain have a poor prognosis.[30]

In contrast, the infraclavicular portion of the plexus is more commonly injured by fractures and dislocations in the region of the shoulder joint. The prognosis for neurological recovery with this mechanism of injury is usually considerably more favorable because of the limited excursion of the fractured or dislocated humerus, as well as the more distal level at which the nerve injury occurs. Since the traction on nerves is usually exerted laterally at a point relatively far removed from an anatomical point of anchorage, the normal elasticity of the nerve roots protects them from more severe damage.[29]

Although the prognosis for mild to moderate neurological injury generally is good, functional recovery may be prevented by a number of factors, including joint stiffness, contractures, edema, atrophy, and pain. Prevention of these complications may enhance functional as well as neurological recovery in the patient with brachial plexus injury. Gentle range of motion exercises, both passive and active-assistive, should be done on a regular basis to prevent or correct mild contractures. This should be done initially by an experienced therapist. Thereafter, the patient and/or care provider can be taught to perform a self range of motion exercise program. Strengthening of the weak muscles should be done by active use of the hand and the upper extremity, and by specific exercises to strengthen specific muscles. Edema of the paralytic limb should be prevented or treated by passive positioning of the arm or hand, elastic garments, massage, active and passive range of motion exercises, a compression pump, continuous passive movement devices, and an orthosis. Further, patients should be instructed to become more independent with one-handedness. For example, if the dominant hand is affected, the patient is taught to write with the other hand, a skill that can be attained within 6 weeks of training in most cases. Adaptive equipment and appliances can be offered to help the patient become more functional with one hand. For those with incomplete loss of muscle strength, the most important consideration is to preserve and/or enhance function, if at all possible.

Orthotic devices are used to provide immobilization, improve alignment, and augment function in the involved extremity. The optimum brace should be comfortable, functional, easy to use, and cosmetically appealing in order to improve patient acceptance. A team approach of physician, therapist, orthotist, patient, and family is required for thorough evaluation and understanding, training, and continued use to achieve maximum benefit.

The airplane shoulder splint, which maintains shoulder abduction at 90 degrees and does not permit glenohumoral motion, has been previously used to manage upper brachial plexus injury in order to keep the arm abducted and externally rotated. It is no longer recommended for this purpose, since it may contribute to high-riding shoulder-girdle movements.[31]

The use of orthotics in complete brachial plexus injury is controversial. Perry and Robinson have described their experience and success of a flail-arm splint in persons with brachial plexus injury.[19,32] They developed the "Redhead roe-hamptom" flail-arm splint, an artificial arm that fits over the patient's own arm to provide some needed and missing upper-extremity function. This device consists of a shoulder support, an elbow locking device, and a forearm trough over the wrist that custom-made or standard appliances can be fitted into. A shoulder harness is provided on the contralateral side to operate opening and closing of the appliance. Through the rehabilitation processes, the patient is encouraged to choose and practice the use of various appliances relevant to his or her lifestyle, including job, hobbies, or recreation. Depending on the extent and location of the brachial plexus injury, modification of the orthosis could be utilized to assist function, improve alignment, and/or prevent contracture formation. As a part of the rehabilitation

program, vocational assessment must begin at the earliest possible stage.

Pain

The avulsion of roots of the brachial plexus is associated with severe pain in the anesthetic limb, characteristically a burning or crushing pain, usually in the hand, occasionally in the forearm, and rarely in the shoulder. In addition to this severe, constant pain, paroxysmal shooting pain through the arm from the shoulder to the hand is reported. Unfortunately, there appears to be no predictable pattern to these paroxysms, and this causes a distressing problem with which patients must cope. Typically, pain is aggravated by cold, wet weather, anxiety or stress, and during an illness. The more severe the lesion, the higher the incidence of severe pain. Although severe pain is not associated with any particular cause of brachial plexus injury, avulsion of C8 and T1 is more likely to lead to pain than avulsion of the upper trunks. Avulsion of C5 and C6 gives burning pain in the thumb and index finger, whereas avulsion of C7, C8, and T1 causes burning pain in the forearm and hand. In some patients, pain relief is accomplished by moving or flexing the fingers, or hitting, massaging, or manipulating the root of the neck or shoulders.[19]

Severe pain can begin at the time of injury or develop days to months later, although it usually appears within 3 months of the injury and rarely after years of injury. In Parry's study of 409 subjects with brachial plexus injury, 51 percent of patients had pain resolved within 3 years, 29 percent had pain longer than 3 years that was tolerable, and 19 percent had severe pain for years that was seriously disruptive.[19] The natural history of pain derived from brachial plexus injury appears to be that the majority of patients will lose their pain within 3 years, and the majority of the remainder will be able to cope with it to live a reasonably normal life.[19]

In the management of pain, it is important to assess the nature of the injury, the interval since onset, as well as the quality, nature, and degree of pain. The longer the patient suffers pain, the more certain that it will become permanent. Pain is not considered nociceptive in origin, but more probably a result of deafferentation. Complete explanation of the cause of pain by the rehabilitation physician is important. Intensive rehabilitation to modify the pain is vital, and may include transcutaneous nerve stimulation, intensive physical exercise, and distraction by meaningful activities, such as work or recreation. As a rule, postganglionic lesions are not associated with pain, although causalgia from partial lesions or regeneration of nerves can occur.

The technique of application of transcutaneous nerve stimulation is important for successful pain control after brachial plexus injury. It is helpful to apply the stimulator in a variety of parameters and different positions over two to three weeks. Careful record keeping is important. For the standard electrode positions, after a total lesion, the electrode should be placed over the back of the neck or the front of the thoracic outlet, stimulating C3 and C4, with another electrode stimulating T2 at the inner side of the upper arm. Thus, nociceptive transmission is blocked by maximum stimulation of the normal nerve roots above and below the site of the lesion. The standard modality is the continuous low-frequency current. which blocks nociceptive transmission from the spinal level to the higher centers. The burst mode activates the reticular formation.

Melzack and Wall showed that the effect of transcutaneous nerve stimulation is cumulative, and that longer usage improves the effectiveness of treatment.[33] Frampton, in describing the technique of electrode application, has advocated continuous stimulation for a minimum of 8 hours a day, for at least a week, before considering the possibility of treatment failure.[34] If stimulation is effective in controlling pain, it should be continued for at least 3 weeks and then diminished only gradually. There are few contraindications for the use of transcutaneous nerve stimulation. It should not be used concomitantly with a pacemaker, or in patients with known arrhythmias. The application over anesthetic skin is useless and should be avoided.

A pharmacological approach to the pain of brachial plexus injury has been used with inconsistent results. Nonsteroidal antiinflammatory agents, acetaminophen, narcotics, antidepressants, and anticonvulsant agents have been used in pain management with varying results.

Invasive procedures should be avoided in the initial stages, since significant nerve regeneration can occur that leads to the abatement of pain and improved motor function. The assessment of nerve regeneration by electrophysiologic criteria can be particularly useful in guiding therapy. Amputation as well as sympathectomy were performed to relieve severe, intractable pain in the first half of the twentieth century. Because the neurologic lesion is proximal to the dorsal root ganglion and the pain is of a deafferentation type, success was limited. Currently these approaches are generally not used. Neurolytic blockade does not appear to have either a diagnostic or a therapeutic role.

However, surgical repair of the brachial plexus can reduce pain as well as restore limb function.[35] When repair is not feasible, dorsal root entry zone (DREZ) lesions can be very effective in pain relief.[35a] Other ablative procedures such as myelotomy and cordotomy do not appear to be useful.

Surgical Management

There has been a dramatic change in the management and potential for recovery after brachial plexus injury, especially after traction lesions.[19,29] Previously, surgery was rarely undertaken. The prevailing belief was that nerve-root avulsion was uncommon, and exploration was pointless, because the probability of finding a surgically reparable lesion was remote. Recently, surgical exploration of traction injuries of the brachial plexus has been considered as early as possible, in the hope of finding surgically reparable lesions.[2,19] Advances in anesthesia, intensive care, neuroimaging, and electrophysiologic monitoring have allowed more complex surgical procedures to successfully repair root avulsion injuries.

The surgical approach should focus on gaining some active control of shoulder and elbow flexion, restoration of simple grip function, protective sensibility, and a reduction of limb pain.[19,29] A thorough preoperative evaluation should carefully assess the patient's goals and needs, and current stage of limb involvement, including range of motion of the joints and manual muscle testing. The goal in the first stage of surgery is to explore and assess the exact location and the extent of the lesion intraoperatively by performing dissection of the brachial plexus in the supra- and infraclavicular region, and axilla if necessary. Depending on the type of the lesion, microsurgical neurolysis, nerve grafting, or reneurotization may be performed.[2] Neurolysis is considered when the peripheral nerves are in continuity and signs of fibrosis are present. If no spinal-cord injury is present, resection of the injured nerve segment and nerve grafting can be performed. For ruptured nerve roots and trunks, nerve grafting has been beneficial to some. Nerve-grafting donor material can be obtained from sensory nerves, such as the sural, or other sensory fibers in the forearm or clavicular region.

In severe injuries with root avulsion, neurotization may be performed with uninjured nerves of the cervical plexus, cranial nerves, or intercostal nerves. Neurotization requires the transfer of a functional, but less important nerve to the distal, more important denervated nerve. For example, nerve transfers for shoulder abduction may include multiple neurotization or double neurotization, with single neurotization for the suprascapular nerve. For elbow flexion, three intercostal nerves can be transferred to the musculocutaneous nerve and, for more distal functions, to the ipsilateral upper trunk.[36]

Since brachial plexus lesions vary extensively, comparative assessment of the postoperative results is difficult, except in a complete root avulsion. The results of neurolysis vary from complete absence to almost full recovery, which reflects the problem of nerve surgery based on the macroscopic appearance of the nerve intraoperatively.[2] The outcome of neurolysis appears to depend significantly on the level of experience of the surgeon. In cases of nerve grafting, motor recovery varies inversely with distance of the graft from the end organ. In other words, better results are seen in the shoulder and upper arm, whereas motor function of the hand remains weak. The nerve transfer or neurotization results depend in part on the number of nerves transferred, but has been shown to restore basic motor functions of the limb, and sensory recovery to regain protective sensibility.

Tendon transfer can also play an important role in the treatment of brachial plexus injuries, especially in the restoration of motor function in the hand. Since there are insufficient motor nerves available for transfer to restore the extensors of the fingers and wrist, the extensor digitorum tenodesis procedure can be used to restore grip function.[37] Tendon transfers are considered when persistent flaccid paralysis, failed nerve repair, or irreparable nerve cases are encountered.[38] Surgical intervention must be combined with appropriate rehabilitative physical and occupational therapies, before and after surgery, to optimize function.

Amputation

Amputation is done far less often now in patients with severe brachial plexus injury but can be offered as one of the management options in selected patients. Usually, some arm function returns with time. If recovery does not occur, amputation can be considered. In 1961 Yeoman and Seddon reported data on 36 patients in whom they compared function after amputation-arthrodesis, limb reconstruction, and no operative treatment.[39] Amputation of the arm with shoulder fusion provided a better result than either reconstruction or nonsurgical management. Patients with severe limb pain are considered poor candidates for surgery, as are those more than 2 years after injury. Ransford and Hughes studied

patients with brachial plexus injuries who had been fitted with a prosthesis following shoulder arthrodesis and found that very few were regular users.[40] Clumsiness of the prosthesis, discomfort from skin contact, and the relative ease with which patients became one-handed were the most frequently cited reasons.

Indications for amputation include patients who find the flail arm becomes a significant hindrance to function, work, or other activities; recurrent infection of the involved arm because of poor hygiene and repeated trauma; other complications including nonunion of long bones, severe posttraumatic joint derangements, and vascular or soft-tissue deficits superimposed upon severe brachial plexus injury.[29] Pain relief, by itself, is not an indication for amputation.

Successful amputation and shoulder arthrodesis requires skillful prosthesis fitting and management. Good patient selection and thorough education on postop management of the residual limb and prosthesis enhances the likelihood of success.

BIRTH BRACHIAL PLEXUS PALSY

Approximately 1 to 2 per 1000 babies are born with a brachial plexus palsy.[41] This number has not changed dramatically, even with improvements in obstetrical techniques. Most have significant recovery on their own, but both the percentage of children recovering and the degree of recovery are quite variable.[41–44] The approach to treatment of infants with brachial plexus palsy is different than that for older children and adults with brachial plexus palsy. Etiology, diagnosis, and treatment options for infants with brachial plexus palsy are discussed.

Risk factors for birth brachial plexus palsy include a multiparous mother, large baby, and shoulder dystocia.[41–44] Most infants with shoulder dystocia do not have brachial plexus injury.[45] Fracture of the clavicle or humerus may occur, and x-rays should be obtained if there is clinical suspicion of a fracture. The etiology most commonly described is traction during the birth process, but reports of intrauterine causes, such as a bicornuate uterus or uterine malpositioning, have become increasingly prevalent.[46]

By far the most common level of involvement is C5–6 (Erb's palsy). The classic waiter's tip posture of an adducted, internally rotated shoulder, extended elbow, and flexed wrist with a pronated forearm is typical. The degree of involvement of C7 along with C5–6 is variable.

Less frequently, the entire plexus is injured. In this case, the entire limb is flaccid. Klumpke's palsy, involving nerve roots C8–T1, is very rare.[47] There is credible, emerging medical opinion that Klumpke's palsy is actually a manifestation of a spinal cord injury, and not the result of injury to the plexus during birth when C8–T1 root involvement is seen on isolation in the newborn, especially if the injury is bilateral.[48] More frequently, infants present for evaluation with only C8–T1 involved, but a careful history reveals entire plexus involvement initially, with subsequent improvement of the upper plexus components. The clinical picture is of intact shoulder and elbow, with wrist and fingers extended, and possibly Horner's syndrome (ptosis, miosis, and anhydrosis).

The phrenic nerve may be involved in upper or total plexus injuries. This can lead to respiratory difficulties in neonates and babies under 1 year, although in older babies, children, and adults, the ineffectiveness of one phrenic nerve does not generally prove problematic.[49]

Evaluation of infants with birth brachial plexus palsy requires some variation in approach, owing to the inability to follow commands or to specify sensation. Physical examination includes visual inspection for differences in size of the upper extremities, color of the hands, or presence of atrophy. Limb palpation may reveal a temperature difference between the hands or a lack of muscle tone in the involved extremity. Fractures of the clavicle or humerus should be ruled out, if necessary by x-ray. Reflexes are absent or decreased at involved levels. Sensation is tested for detection of pin prick in all dermatomes, and a positive response is indicated by facial grimace or by withdrawal, or attempted withdrawal, of the arm. The Moro reflex indicates the ability to abduct the shoulder and to flex the elbows, and is useful in the evaluation of the neonate with suspected brachial plexus injury.

Initial evaluation in some centers includes magnetic resonance imaging or computed tomography of the cervical spine, if spontaneous resolution of motor symptoms is delayed. These studies can determine the presence of avulsions that cannot resolve without surgery. There are conflicting reports on the usefulness of either test. Most studies that advocate neuroimaging involve older children or adults. The small size of the neonate or infant may make these studies less useful in young babies.[50,51] In infants and young children, these tests require conscious sedation or, occasionally, general anesthesia, with the attendant risks, due to the require-

ment of immobility during the examination. Therefore, many large centers have abandoned routine radiographic investigation of young children and neonates with suspected brachial plexus palsy.

Electrodiagnostic evaluation may be quite useful in infants, especially the newborn. Motor and sensory nerve conduction studies and electromyography are regularly performed. Nerve conduction studies provide important information about proximal nerve segment conduction by use of the late waves, particularly the F waves and H reflexes. This electrodiagnostic information can be helpful in determining electrical continuity of the plexus to the spinal cord. Absence of proximal segment conduction may suggest the need for surgical intervention. Motor nerve conduction studies show distal electrical continuity to muscles at involved spinal segments. Sensory nerve conduction studies provide information on continuity distal to the dorsal root ganglion. Paraspinal muscle needle examination provides information on the status of the posterior primary rami. Fibrillations are evidence of a preganglionic lesion, but owing to the overlap of myotomes this is not generally useful. Positive sharp waves and fibrillations are infrequently noted beyond the first few months. Since electrodiagnostic signal abnormalities frequently require a minimum of 10 to 14 days, and often 2 to 3 weeks, from the time of injury to develop, neonates with brachial plexus palsy discovered at birth should have electrodiagnostic examination in the first week of life to establish the nature and onset of injury, as well as prognosis.

Occupational or physical therapy is begun in the first days of life. Parents are instructed in positioning and range of motion of the limb. Proper positioning should begin immediately. The goal of positioning is to minimize contractures and to protect the arm, especially early on, or if the arm is flaccid. Range of motion exercises prevent contractures. The most common problem areas are with contractures of the shoulder in internal rotation, the forearm in pronation, and the wrist in flexion in infants with upper plexus involvement. In infants with lower plexus or posterior cord involvement, an elbow flexion contracture can be seen. Care must be taken in performing range of motion exercises, as overly vigorous stretching can cause subluxation or dislocation of the radial head in supination, or of the humeral head with excessive external rotation.

Splinting should be done to prevent, correct, or minimize contractures. Orthoses are used most frequently at the wrist for positioning or to improve grasp in infants with wrist drop. Splints are also used for protection of the fingers, since frequently infants try to chew on the digits. As strength returns, air splints are occasionally used for a few minutes at a time on the uninvolved arm in order to establish a forced-use paradigm that promotes arm strengthening and improvement in functional skills.

When the limb is completely nonfunctional, an infant may not recognize it as a useful body part. From a developmental stand point, this can be problematic, as the child learns to do activities one-handed. Even if perfect clinical recovery ensues, the palsied limb may not be used. On the other hand, when infants are actively encouraged to look at the arm and to play with it, more function of the arm can be anticipated. A skilled therapist should provide visual, auditory, and tactile stimulation aimed at maximizing development and function of the arm.

Electrical stimulation is not generally used in infants, but is sometimes used as children age. Therapeutic electrical stimulation to the muscle can be provided, but tolerance is variable. There are no large studies that demonstrate the effectiveness of therapeutic electrical stimulation in brachial plexus palsy.

Secondary neuromuscular complications of brachial plexus palsy in infants should be monitored and prevented, where possible. Muscle atrophy generally develops in involved muscles if there is no recovery for extended periods of time. Joint contractures are common, particularly in shoulder adduction and internal rotation, elbow flexion (if biceps function is preserved, but triceps is not), elbow extension (in the opposite case), forearm pronation, wrist flexion, and ulnar deviation at the wrist. Insensate fingers can lead to ulcerations from trauma, including self-inflicted bites. These are seen particularly when the infant is teething, and when sensation appears to be returning. Limb length and circumference discrepancy may develop, presenting some difficulties in clothing the child and general cosmesis. Pain is not a common sequela of birth brachial plexus palsy except, occasionally, in the first few weeks. Similarly, reflex sympathetic dystrophy has not been described after brachial plexus injury discovered at birth. Glenohumeral subluxation is seen occasionally after neonatal bracheal plexus palsy, and can be treated with positioning slings.

If a child with brachial plexus palsy at birth does not show improvement of muscle strength by 3 to 6 months, surgical intervention should be considered, particularly when the deltoid and biceps are severely involved.[42,52] Surgery was initially performed to restore function after brachial plexus injury in the late 1800s, but the morbidity and mortality of this approach was

considerable. Microsurgical advances in the 1970s have improved outcomes.[5] An incision is made along the sternocleidomastoid, over Erb's point, and above the middle third of the clavicle, thus exposing the brachial plexus and the phrenic nerve. A surgical field of the diameter of a tennis ball is optimal. The plexus may reveal neuromas (scar formation) partial or complete physical nerve disruption (rupture); rarely, it may appear visually normal. Avulsions are not typically visualized, as they occur proximal to the operative field. Electrical stimulation can then be performed directly on individual nerve roots, trunks, and branches to evaluate the integrity of the proximal and distal portions of the plexus, using somatosensory evoked potentials and nerve conduction studies.

The anatomical integrity of the plexus at the operative site, together with the electrodiagnostic data, determines the recommended surgical procedure. If scarring and adhesions in the injured plexus can be lysed, and the electrical function is intact, no further operative intervention is indicated. If there is loss of electrical conduction through a neuroma, excision of the mass is performed, followed by placement of nerve grafts. The root selected for grafting to the distal plexus must be intact by somatosensory evoked-potentials criteria. A single nerve root may provide grafts to more than one distal trunk, cord, or nerve. The donor graft nerve is most commonly taken from the sural nerve, although the greater auricular nerve can be used for short segments on occasion.

If there is sufficient nerve length, direct attachment of the proximal and distal nerve portions, without intervening donor nerve tissue, is preferred. If somatosensory evoked potentials, nerve conduction studies, and surgical findings preclude grafting, other surgical options are considered. Intercostal or pectoral nerves can be grafted to the musculocutaneous or axillary nerves in the axilla or proximal arm. Tendon transfers have been successfully used to stabilize or improve movement and function at the wrist. Muscle transfers may be done to improve function of the limb at the elbow or shoulder. The procedures require intensive therapy and good, active cooperation of the child, and therefore are generally deferred until later childhood. Surgical repair of brachial plexus injury does not provide immediate results. Recovery is expected in 4 to 12 months and may continue for up to 2 years postoperatively. Occupational and physical therapy must be continued throughout the recovery process. The arm is generally immobilized for several weeks after a graft, and moved as tolerated after neurolysis.

REFERENCES

1. Hollinshead WH, Jenkins DB: *Functional Anatomy of the Limbs and Back*. Philadelphia: WB Saunders, 1981.
2. Berger A, Becker M: Brachial plexus surgery: our concept of the last twelve years. *Microsurgery* 1994; 15:760–767.
3. Alnot JY: Traumatic brachial plexus lesions in the adult. *Hand Clin* 1995; 11:623–631.
4. Levine MG, Holryode J, Woods JR Jr, et al: Birth trauma: incidence and predisposing factors. *Obstet Gynecol* 1986; 68:784–788.
5. Michlow BJ, Clarke HM, Curtis CG, et al: The natural history of obstetrical brachial plexus palsy. *Plastic Reconstruct Surg* 1994; 93:675–680.
5a. Jennett R, Tarby T, Kreinick CJ: Brachial plexus palsy: An old problem revisited. *Am J Obstet Gynecol* 1992; 166:673–677.
6. Vrettos BC, Rochkind S, Boome RS: Low velocity gun shot wounds of the brachial plexus. *J Hand Surg* 1995; 20B:212–214.
7. Po BT, Hansen HR: Iatrogenic brachial plexus injury: A survey of the literature and of pertinent cases. *Anesth Analog* 1969; 48:915.
8. Graham JG, Pye IF, McQueen INF: Brachial plexus injury after median sternotomy. *J Neurol Neurosurg Psychiatry* 1981; 44:621–625.
9. Lederman RJ, Breuer AC, Hanson MR, et al: Peripheral nervous system complications of coronary artery bypass graft surgery. *Ann Neurol* 1982; 12:297–301.
10. Lyon BB, Hansen BA, Mygind T: Peripheral nerve injury as a complication of axillary arteriography. *Acta Neurol Scand* 1975; 51:29–36.
11. Beghi E, Kurland LT, Mulder DW, et al: Brachial plexus neuropathy in the population of Rochester, Minnesota, 1970–1981. *Ann Neurol* 1985; 18:320–323.
12. Spillane JD: Localized neuritis of the shoulder girdle: A report of 46 cases in the MEF. *Lancet* 1943; 2:532–535.
13. Wolpow ER: Brachial plexus neuropathy: Association with desensitizing antiallergy injections. *JAMA* 1975; 234:620–621.
14. Kayed K, Kass B: Acute multiple brachial neuropathy and Ehlers-Danlos syndrome. *Neurology* 1979; 29:1620–1621.
15. Bloch SL, Jarrett MP, Swerdlow M, et al: Brachial plexus neuropathy as the initial presentation of systemic lupus erythematosus. *Neurology* 1979; 29:1633–1732.
16. Bosch EP, Chul HC, Martin MA, et al: Brachial plexus involvement in familial pressure-sensitive neuropathy: Electrophysiological and morphological findings. *Ann Neurol* 1980; 8:620–624.
17. Lederman RJ, Wilbourn AJ: Brachial plexopathy: Recurrent cancer or radiation? *Neurology* 1984; 34:1331–1335.
18. Thomas JE, Colby MY, Jr: Radiation-induced or metastatic brachial plexopathy? A diagnostic dilemma. *JAMA* 1972; 222:1392–1395.
19. Parry CBW: Thoughts on the rehabilitation of patients with brachial plexus lesions. *Hand Clin* 1995; 11:657–675.
20. Kimura J: *Electrodiagnosis in Disease of Nerve and Muscle: Principles and Practice,* 2nd ed. Philadelphia: FA Davis, 1989.
21. Jones S: Investigation of brachial plexus traction lesions by peripheral and spinal somatosensory evoked potentials. *J Neurol Neurosurg Psychiatry* 1979; 42:107–116.
22. Synek VM: Somatosensory evoked potials after stimulation of digital nerves in upper limb: Normative data. *Electroencephalogr Clin Neurophysiol* 1986; 65:460–463.
23. Eisen AA, Shytybel W: *Clinical Experience with Transcranial Magnetic Stimulation.* AAEM Minimonograph #35, Rochester, Minnesota, AAEM, 1990.
24. Reede DL: Magnetic resonance imaging of the brachial plexus. *MRI Clin N Am* 1993; 1:185–193.
25. Panasci DJ, Holliday RA, Shpizner B: Advanced imaging techniques of the brachial plexus. *Hand Clin* 1995; 11:545–553.
26. Bilbey JH, Lamond RG, Mattrey RF: MR imaging of disorders of the brachial plexus. *J Magn Reson Imag* 1994; 4:13–18.
27. Castagno AA, Shuman WP: MR imaging in clinically suspected brachial plexus tumor. *AJR* 1987; 149:1219–1222.
28. Seddon HJ: Three types of nerve injury. *Brain* 1943; 66:237.
29. Leffert RD: *Brachial Plexus Injuries.* London: Churchill Livingstone, 1985.
30. Barnes R: Traction injuries of the brachial plexus in adults. *J Bone Joint Surg* 1949; 31B:10.
31. Johnson EW, Alexander MA, Koenig WC: Infantile Erb's palsy (Smellie's palsy). *Arch Phys Med Rehabil* 1977; 58:175.
32. Robinson C: Brachial plexus lesions. Functional splintage. *Br J Occup Ther* 1986; 49:311–334.
33. Melzack R, Wall PD: *The Challenge of Pain.* London: Penguin, Harmondsworth, 1983.
34. Frampton V: Transcutaneous nerve stimulation and chronic pain. In Wells, Frampton, Bowsher (eds): *Pain Management by Physiotherapy,* Butterworth Heinemann, 1994.
35. Narakas AO: The effects on pain of reconstructive neurosurgery in 160 patients with traction and/or crush injury to the brachial plexus, in Siegfried, Zimmerman M (eds): *Phantom and Stump Pain.* New York, Springer-Verlag, 1981, pp. 126–147.
35a. Thomas DG, Kitchen ND: Long-term follow-up of dorsal root entry zone lesions in brachial plexus avulsion. *J Neurol Neurosurg Psych* 1994; 57(6):737–738.
36. Chuang DC: Neurotization procedures for brachial plexus injuries. *Hand Clin* 1995; 11:633–645.
37. Ochiai N, Nagano A, Yamamoto S: Tenodesis of extensor digitorum in treatment of brachial plexus injuries involving C5, 6, 7 and 8 nerve roots. *J Hand Surg* 1995; 20B:671–674.
38. Dunnet WJ, Housden PL, Birch R: Flexor to extensor tendon transfers in the hand. *J Hand Surg* 1995; 20B:26–28.

39. Yeoman PM, Seddon J: Brachial plexus injuries. Treatment of the flail arm. *J Bone Joint Surg* 1961; 43B:493–500.

40. Ransford AO, Hughes PF: Complete brachial plexus lesions. *J Bone Joint Surg* 1977; 59B:417–422.

41. Greenwald AG, Schute PC, Shively JL: Brachial plexus birth palsy: A 10 year report on the incidence and prognosis. *J Pediatr Orthop* 1984; 4:689–692.

42. Meyer RD: Treatment of adult and obstetrical brachial plexus injuries. *Orthopedics* 1986; 9:899–903.

43. Brown KLB: Review of obstetrical palsies: Non-operative treatment. *Clin Plas Surg* 1984; 11:181–187.

44. Eng GD, Koch G, Smokvina MD: Brachial plexus palsy in neonates and children. *Arch Phys Med Rehabil* 1978; 59:458–464.

45. Baskett TF, Allen AC: Perinatal implications of shoulder dystocia. *Obstet Gynecol* 1995; 86:14–17.

46. Koenigsberger MR: Brachial plexus palsy at birth: Intrauterine or due to delivery trauma? *Ann Neurol* 1980; 8:228.

47. al-Qattan MM, Clarke HM, Curtis CG: Klumpke's birth palsy. Does it really exist? *J Hand Surg* (British) 1995; 20:19–23.

48. Eng GD, Binder H, Getson P, O'Donnell R: Obstetrical brachial plexus palsy: Outcome with convservative management. *Muscle Nerve* 1996; 19:884–891.

49. Clarke HM, Curtis CG: An approach to obstetrical brachial plexus injuries. *Hand Clin* 1995; 11:563–581.

50. Hashimoto T, Mitomo M, Hikabuki N, et al: Nerve root avulsion of birth palsy: Comparison of myelography with CT myelography and somatosensory evoked potential. *Radiology* 1991; 178:841–845.

51. Zidek KA, Nelson MR, Laurent JP, et al: The efficacy of computerized tomography/ myelography and magnetic resonance imaging in the evaluation of birth brachial plexus injuries. *Arch Phys Med Rehabil* 1996; 77:929–930.

52. Gilbert A, Razaboni R, Amar-Khodja S: Indications and results of brachial plexus surgery in obstetrical palsy. *Ortho Clin N Am* 1988; 19:91–105.

Chapter 16

REHABILITATION OF RADICULOPATHY

Michelle S. Gittler
David J. Weiss

In this chapter the anatomy, biomechanics, pathophysiology, clinical presentations, differential diagnosis, evaluation, and treatment for radiculopathy are reviewed. The earliest record of root compression can be found in Edward Smith's Surgical Papyrus, an Egyptian manuscript that dates back to between 2500 and 4500 B.C. Its report focused on a patient with back and leg pain that worsened on leg elevation. Despite the fact that root compression has been a source of human suffering for thousands of years, it was not until this century that radiculopathies were recognized as a distinct clinical entity. In 1934, Mixter and Barr[1] established a link between disorders of the lumbar intervertebral disc and root compressions. In 1943, Semmes and Murphy outlined cervical disc disorders and radiculopathies as causes of neck and upper-extremity pain.[2] Influential articles by Verbiest (1949), concerning the narrowing of the lumbar canal, and Brain (1952) on cervical spondylosis, soon followed.[3,4] Finally, in the 1950s, thoracic root compressions were recognized. The delay in appreciation of thoracic radiculopathies stems from their infrequent incidence and the coexistence of spinal-cord compressions.[5]

ANATOMY

The spinal column consists of 33 bony vertebrae (seven cervical, 12 thoracic, five lumbar, five sacral, four coccygeal), 23 fibrocartilaginous discs, and multiple ligaments and muscles. All of the vertebrae and discs have the same basic structure and function with some variations in different regions.[6] Each vertebra can be thought of as a functional unit that is made up of an anterior body that is the main weight-bearing structure of the spinal column, and a posterior spinal arch that protects the neural elements of the spine (Figure 16-1).[7] The vertebral body is a rounded bony structure with flattened superior and inferior surfaces that are covered by hyaline cartilage (or end plates). Unique to the cervical spine are the uncovertebral joints or joints of Luschka, which are osseous elevations (exostoses) on the posterior lateral aspects of the vertebral bodies (Figure 16-2). These elevations form pseudojoints that protect the contents of the spinal canal from intervertebral disc protrusion but also can compromise the spinal cord and/or the spinal roots if they hypertrophy in conjunction with degenerative joint disease.

Two pedicles jutting out in a posterolateral direction from the vertebral body along with two laminae form the neural arch or posterior portion of the functional unit. The junction of the superior and inferior pedicles creates an intervertebral foramen that is the pathway for the spinal nerves to exit the neural arch. The posterior portion also gives rise to two transverse processes and a central spinous process that serve as attachment sites for ligaments and paraspinal musculature. The arch supports superior and inferior zygopaphyseal (facet) joints that start at the junction of the pedicle and lamina. These facet joints articulate to guide movement of the spinal column.

In flexion, the adjacent pedicles and lamina separate and the intervertebral foramen, through which spinal nerves travel, enlarges. With extension, these foram-

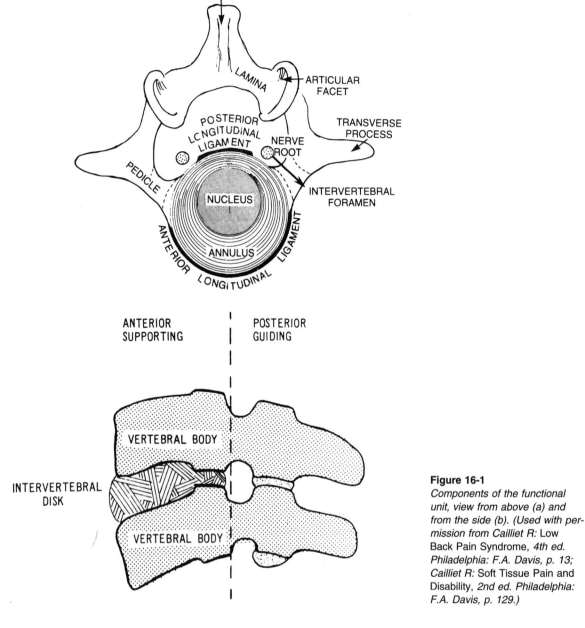

Figure 16-1
Components of the functional unit, view from above (a) and from the side (b). (Used with permission from Cailliet R: Low Back Pain Syndrome, 4th ed. Philadelphia: F.A. Davis, p. 13; Cailliet R: Soft Tissue Pain and Disability, 2nd ed. Philadelphia: F.A. Davis, p. 129.)

ina become smaller. In lateral flexion, or side bending, the intervertebral foramina on the side of flexion narrow with the opposite foramina enlarging.

The cervical spine is the most mobile part of the spinal column.[8] The atlas and axis (C_1 and C_2) are unique structures that allow for flexion, extension, and rotation of the cervical spine. The C_1–C_2 articulation and the occipitoatlantal articulation generate the most motion in the cervical spine. Fifty percent of cervical spine flexion and extension occurs at the occipitoatlantal joint and 50 percent of cervical axial rotation takes place at the atlantoaxial joint. Next to

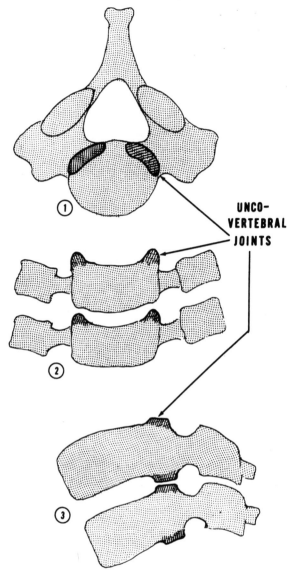

Figure 16-2

Uncovertebral joints. Superior view (1) depicts the posterolateral placement of the uncovertebral joints. Also shown are anteroposterior (2) and lateral (3) views. (Used with permission from Cailliet R: Soft Tissue Pain and Disability, 2nd ed. Philadelphia: F.A. Davis, p. 128.)

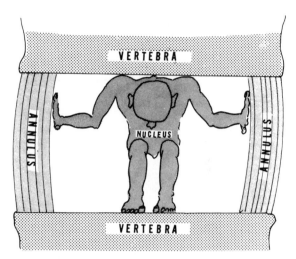

Figure 16-3

Function of the nucleus pulposus (schematic) (Used with permission from Cailliet R: Low Back Pain Syndrome, 4th ed. Philadelphia: F.A. Davis, p. 9.)

spinous processes all limit thoracic movement to only slight lateral flexion and some rotation, with flexion and extension essentially being eliminated.[10,11]

Large vertebrae and intervertebral discs characterize the lumbar spine. Flexion and extension, along with lateral bending, all are undertaken easily in this part of the spinal column. Lumbar facet orientation, or actual locking of adjacent facets, results in severe limitation of rotation. The greatest amount of motion is in the L_{4-5}, $L_5–S_1$ region; disc herniation and facet degeneration commonly are found in this area of the lumbar spine.

From the $C_2–C_3$ intervertebral space through the $L_5–S_1$ space there are 23 discs located between each vertebral body. These fibrocartilaginous intervertebral discs function to both separate the adjacent vertebrae and act as shock absorbers for the spinal column. Each disc is made up of an outer annulus fibrosis and an inner nucleus pulposus. Ten to twenty obliquely oriented circumferential collagenous lamellar sheets form the flexible, yet resilient, outer annulus fibrosis. Within is contained the gel-like mucopolysaccharide nucleus pulposus (Figure 16-1). This nucleus reacts to outside pressure by reconforming and transmitting the force equally and in all directions to the outer annular fibers (Figure 16-3).[10]

In flexion, the anterior aspect of the disc is compressed while the posterior portion is elongated. The exact opposite occurs with spine extension; the posterior

these two joints, the greatest mobility is seen at $C_5–C_6$, $C_4–C_5$, and $C_6–C_7$.[8,9]

The thoracic portion of the spinal column allows the least amount of motion and is the most stable. Facet orientation, thoracocostal articulations, and overlapping

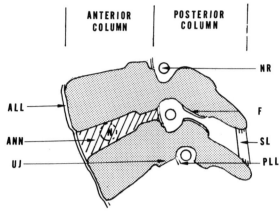

Figure 16-4

The ligaments of the functional unit. ALL = anterior longitudinal ligament, ANN = annulus fibrosis, UJ = uncovertebral joint, NR = nerve root, F = facet, SL = superior ligament, PLL = posterior longitudinal ligament. (Used with permission from Cailliet R: Neck and Arm Pain, 5th ed. Philadelphia: F.A. Davis, p. 5.)

disc is compressed with elongation of the anterior aspect. To help reinforce the outer annular sheets, anterior and posterior longitudinal ligaments blend in with the lamellar fibers. Other ligaments that help support the spinal column include the interspinous ligament, the ligament nuchae, the supraspinous ligament, and the ligamentum flavum (Figure 16-4).[10]

Intervertebral discs are avascular and receive their nutrition through a process of disc compression and dehydration that sets the stage for subsequent diffusion and imbibition of nutrients into the disc substance.[12,13]

All of the previous structures serve to protect the spinal cord and its roots. There are 31 pairs of spinal nerves that arise as dorsal and ventral roots from the spinal cord: eight cervical, 12 thoracic, five lumbar, five sacral, and one coccygeal. The ventral roots originate from the anterior and lateral grey columns of the spinal cord. The axons that form the dorsal root begin in the dorsal root ganglia (DRG) located within the intervertebral foramen (Figure 16-5). These two roots join soon after the DRG, within the intervertebral foramen, to form the spinal nerves. In the foramen, the motor root is closest to the disc and the sensory root is closest to the facet joint. These nerves occupy one third to one half of the intervertebral foramen.[7,14] The sensory root is twice the size of the motor root (Figure 16-6).

After the spinal nerves exit the intervertebral foramen they terminate as anterior and posterior rami. The anterior rami are the larger of the two, and supply the anterolateral aspect of the trunk and the muscles of the limbs. The posterior rami innervate the skin and deep muscles of the back and neck (Figure 16-5).

In the cervical region all the nerves exit their foramina above their corresponding vertebrae. This rule holds true except for the C_8 nerve, which exits below C_7 and above T_1. All thoracic and lumbar nerves exit *below* their same-numbered vertebrae, that is, the L_4 root, for example, exits between the L_4 and L_5 vertebrae. Thus, with a disc herniation at C_5–C_6, the C_6 nerve would be compromised, whereas a herniation at L_4–L_5 likely would jeopardize the L_4 nerve. The spinal cord ends at approximately L_1 as the conus medullaris. Its lower motor-neuron continuation, the cauda equina, descends through the spinal canal. Because of the orientation of the individual nerve roots in the cauda equina, a disc herniation may affect many roots, depending on the direction the disc herniates. For example, an L_4 disc herniation in a posterolateral direction will compress the L_5 root, and a central herniation affects the S_1 root (Figure 16-7).

The area of skin that is supplied by a single root is called a dermatome. Myotomes refer to muscle fibers innervated by single spinal segments. Specific myotomal and dermatomal distributions are expressed in Figure 16-8 and in Tables 16-1 and 16-2.

RADICULOPATHY: PATHOPHYSIOLOGY

Most radiculopathies may be attributed to root compression or nerve root tension resulting from degeneration or prolapse of an intervertebral disc.[15–17] The mechanism for the generation of radicular pain is still unclear. There has been spirited discussion in the literature as to the anatomic correctness of the phrase "nerve root compression secondary to disc herniation" as the etiology for radiculopathy. Rupture of the intervertebral disc or extruded disc herniation, as a cause of lumbar radiculopathy, was first described in 1934 by Mixter and Barr.[1] In 1941 Dandy described "concealed intervertebral discs," discs that are too small to produce compression of any of the nerves in the lumbar canal; these concealed discs produce symptoms by becoming adherent to a nerve root.[16] In 1943 O'Connell described "stretching of an intraspinal nerve in its extradural portion over or around the protruded disc" as producing the clinical syndrome of radiculopathy.[16] Movements

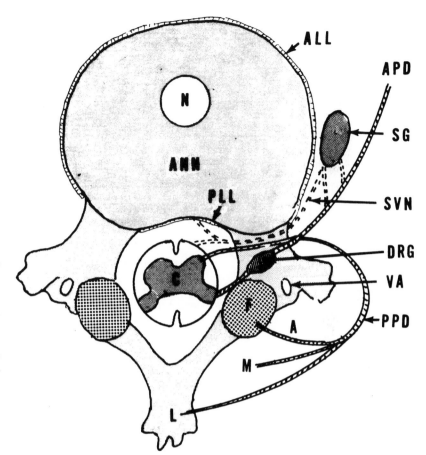

Figure 16-5

Component fibers of a cervical nerve. A view of a functional unit depicts the components of a cervical nerve. C = spinal cord, SG = stellate ganglion, DRG = dorsal root ganglion, APD = anterior primary division, PPD = posterior primary division, A = articular branch of PPD, M = muscular branch of PPD, L = ligamentous branch of PPD, SVN = sinuvertebral nerve; branches to dura and PLL, N = disc nucleus, ANN = disc annulus, ALL = anterior longitudinal ligament, PLL = posterior longitudinal ligament, F = facet, VA = vertebral artery foramen. (Used with permission from Cailliet R: Neck and Arm Pain, 3rd ed. Philadelphia: F.A. Davis, p. 26.)

and positions that increase this tension would thus aggravate radicular pain, whereas rest and postures that minimize the stretch relieve pain. Spinal nerves usually are placed under tension by disc herniation and only rarely compressed.

It is fairly well accepted in the literature that spinal nerves adjacent to a prolapsed disc are inflamed and highly sensitive to the slightest manipulation, whereas uninflamed nerves may be mobilized with very little, if any, discomfort.[17] Slight tension on an inflamed spinal nerve may cause radicular pain. Pain experienced on stimulation of a spinal nerve can be quite variable in quality, depending on the magnitude and duration of the stimulus, but in all cases the presence of inflammation is necessary to evoke a painful sensation.[17,18]

When Mixter and Barr first described the radicular pain of sciatica and related this compression of a spinal root by a herniated lumbar intervertebral disc, it was presumed that the radicular symptoms were second-

ary to prolonged repetitive firing in the injured sensory fibers and this led to perception of pain in the peripheral distribution of these fibers. This concept was challenged on the basis that acute peripheral nerve compression neuropathies are, as a rule, painless.[18,19]

Compression of peripheral nerves or nerve roots may induce numbness and/or weakness (Saturday-night palsy) but typically does not cause pain.[18,19] Experimental investigations in vivo have indicated that numbness is typically a result of ischemia (which may later result in demyelination) and not the mechanical deformation of a nerve fiber. It is apparent that the pathophysiology of compressive nerve lesions should not be oversimplified and expressed only in terms of mechanical injury.[20]

Although no one argues that mechanical factors are involved in nerve-root injury in connection with intervertebral disc herniations, it has been speculated that breakdown products from the degenerating nucleus

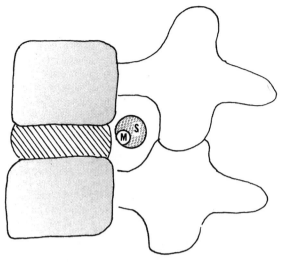

Figure 16-6
Sensorimotor aspect of nerve root. Within the intervertebral foramen, the motor roots are smaller than the sensory and are inferior and posterior near the disk.

pulposus may induce a "chemical radiculitis."[21] Since inflammation is known to occur in sections of nerve roots adjacent to degenerating discs, it would appear that the inciting agent is most likely a chemical product of disc degeneration itself.[22]

Nachemson has found very high hydrogen ion concentrations in some patients who have had extensive adhesion formations around the nerve root.[21] Saal demonstrated extraordinarily high levels of the potentially inflammatory phospholipase A_2 in extracts of human intervertebral discs.[22]

The leakage of proteins or other chemical mediators into the endoneurial space is problematic because there is no lymphatic system in the endoneurial space. Proteins that have leaked into the space will be cleared with great difficulty.[20] When this exudate is invaded by inflammatory cells, there is an inevitable conversion to intraneural fibrosis. It is this intraneural fibrosis that causes an irreversible focus of potential irritation. This occurs because: (1) fibrosis alters the biomechanics of the nerve root; (2) fibrosis interferes with the normal intrinsic vascular supply; and (3) the presence of interneural fibrosis can cause a "choking out" of axons in this area.[17,18,20] Multiple studies have demonstrated that acute compression of dorsal roots and peripheral nerves does not produce sustained repetitive discharge of these nerves. Repetitive firing secondary to acute mechanical injury is of short duration.[18] However, minor

compression of the normal dorsal root ganglion can produce prolonged repetitive firing.[18,19] It would appear that radicular pain associated with a herniated intervertebral disc or other intraspinal masses may be due initially to compression of the dorsal root ganglion.[18,19] The more chronic component of radicular pain then would be attributed to chemical radiculitis.

Pain also may be referred from other structures in the vertebral column, including the richly innervated outer third of the annulus, the periosteum, ligaments, fascia, as well as the facet joints. A thorough clinical exam should distinguish these pain generators from true radicular pain.

INCIDENCE

The incidence of cervical radiculopathies (5–36 percent) is second only to root lesions of the lumbar spine (62–90 percent).[23] Thoracic root lesions are rare and account for less than 2 percent of all radiculopathies.[23] In the cervical region, C_6 and C_7 are recognized as having the highest clinical incidence of injury.[24–27] The L_5 and S_1 roots are by far the most commonly involved in the lumbar sacral region because of abnormalities of the fourth and fifth lumbar discs.[28]

BIOMECHANICS

The biomechanics of radiculopathies surround changes in the functional unit; the anterior portion, consisting of the vertebral body and the disc, and the posterior part, made up of the neural arch that includes the intervertebral foramina and, in the cervical region, the uncovertebral joints. Kirkaldy-Willis and both Scoville and Hanflig eloquently make the argument that there is a continuum of wear and tear or a cascade of degeneration that these structures undergo that predisposes the roots to damage.[25,29,30] Changes in the outer annular fibers, nucleus pulposus, vertebral body, pedicles, laminae, facet joints, or uncovertebral joints lead to situations where an everyday movement or minor trauma (e.g., rotation of the neck or back while changing lanes on the highway) in addition to the major traumas (e.g., severe whiplash injury) will cause the final breakdown and may result in a radiculopathy. Disc and skeletal degeneration by themselves do not necessitate root injury. Factors that determine the changes in these structures include genetics, work-related activities, and trauma. This may explain why

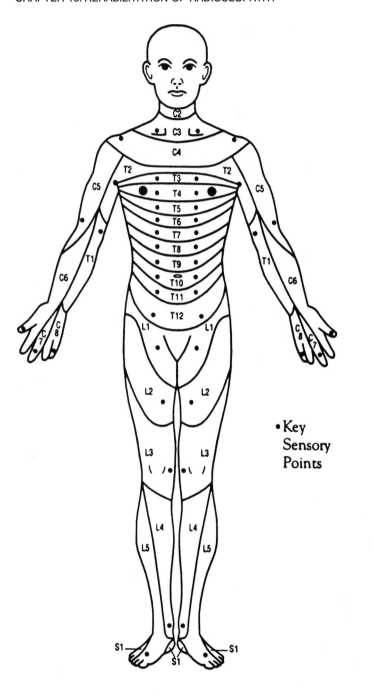

• Key
Sensory
Points

Figure 16-7
Cross section of the cauda equina at L₂–L₃.

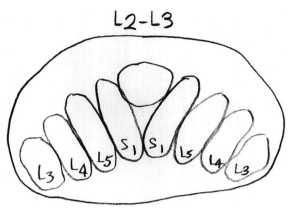

Figure 16-8
Dermatomal map.

all people with radiographic changes do not all have radiculopathies.

By age 20 the disc has reached its maximum development.[10] Therefore, the start of this degenerative cascade can be expected to start some time after age 20. Phase I on this continuum reflects abnormal movements of the different parts of the functional unit.[29] The first manifestations are intervertebral disc annular tears. Facet joint dysfunction also occurs and places increased

stress on the outer layers of the disc. Sudden dynamic overloads can result in the classic discogenic radiculopathy (herniated or extruded disc; see Figure 16-9). These are called "soft" discs and have been shown to cause radiculopathies by direct mechanical compression or through an intense inflammatory process.[31,32] It is now accepted that intervertebral disc protrusion is the most common cause of radiculopathies in patients younger than 40–50 years of age.[33–35] More complex degenerative changes of the bones and supporting structuring are usually responsible in older populations.[33,34,36]

The direction of the herniation determines the neurologic sequela (see Figure 16-10). In the cervical spine, a central herniation may cause a myelopathy, whereas a more posterior–lateral herniation results in a radiculopathy of the nerve root adjacent to the disc herniation (e.g., a C_{5-6} disc herniation will cause a C_6 radiculopathy). The anatomy of the cauda equina makes manifestations of lumbar-disc herniations harder to predict. Far lateral disc herniations cause nerve roots to be damaged at the foramen's exit zone. Thus, the nerve root affected is of the level above the herniation (e.g., an L_{4-5} lateral disc herniation affects the L_4 nerve root). The posterior lateral disc herniation is the most common herniation that results in lumbosacral radiculopathy, and this affects roots below the disc level. Recent anatomic studies of the cauda equina have revealed an organized system where the lower sacral roots (S_{2-5})

Table 16-1
Cervical myotomes

Rhomboids	C_5			Pronator teres	C_6	C_7	
Supraspinatus	C_5	C_6		Flex carpi radialis	C_6	C_7	
Infraspinatus	C_5	C_6		Flex dig sublimis	C_7	C_8	T_1
Deltoid	C_5	C_6		Flex pol. longus	C_8	T_1	
Biceps brachii	C_5	C_6		Pronator quadratus	C_8	T_1	
Serratus ant.	C_5	C_6	C_7	ABD pol. brevis	C_8	T_1	
Brachioradialis	C_5	C_6		Flex carpi ulnaris	C_8	T_1	
Anconeus	C_7	C_8		Flex digit profundus	C_8	T_1	
Triceps	C_7	C_8		Abd dig. minim.	C_8	T_1	
Ext. carpi radialis	C_6	C_7		Add pollicis	C_8	T_1	
Ext. dig. communis	C_7	C_8		First dorsal interos.	C_8	T_1	
Ext. carpi ulnaris	C_6	C_7	C_8				
Ext. pol. brevis	C_7	C_8					
Ext. pol. longus	C_7	C_8					
Ext. indicis	C_7	C_8					

Table 16-2

Lumbar-sacral myotomes

Iliacus	L_2	L_3	L_4	abd hallucis	S_1	S_2	
Thigh adductors	L_2	L_3	L_4	Quad femoris	L_2	L_3	L_4
Glut. medius	L_4	L_5	S_1	Glut maximus	L_5	S_1	S_2
Int. hamstrings	L_4	L_5	S_1	Ext. hamstrings	L_5	S_1	
Tib. anterior	L_4	L_5		Ext. hal. long	L_4	L_5	S_1
Ext. dig. brev.	L_5	S_1		Peronei	L_5	S_1	
Tibialis post.	L_5	S_1		Flex dig. long	L_5	S_1	
Gastrocnemius	L_5	S_1	S_2	Soleus	S_1	S_2	

are located in the most dorsal aspect of the thecal sac.[37] Each preceding lumbosacral root lies in a progressively more anterior lateral location (Figure 16-8). Therefore, the more posterior and central the lumbosacral disc herniation, the more distal the root that is affected. This is the case until a posterior–central herniation causes a cauda equina syndrome, a compressive neuropathy involving multiple lumbar and sacral roots.

In the cervical region, there is a discreet separation of the motor (ventral) and sensory (dorsal) roots.[38,39] This accounts for the isolated compromise of either the ventral or dorsal roots in the cervical spine. As a result, painless motor weakness in a myotomal distribution as well as numbness and/or parasthesias without any motor deficits in a dermatomal pattern may be the only symptoms of a cervical radiculopathy. This is rarely seen in a lumbosacral radiculopathy, where the motor and sensory roots travel closely together from the conus medullaris to their respective intervertebral foramina separated only by a thin piece of arachnoid.[40] Thus, motor and sensory deficits commonly appear together with lumbosacral radiculopathies. In both cervical and lumbosacral radiculopathies, pain can accompany the other symptoms. The exact mechanism behind radicular pain is still unclear.[41] As mentioned previously, the proposed biomechanics include compression of the dorsal root ganglion (DRG) and/or mechanical sensitivities in the chronically injured nerve root.[42]

Phase II in the degenerative cascade refers to excessive motion of the functional unit and, at times, frank instability. This is more common in the middle-aged spine. At this point further disc abnormalities appear including multiple outer annular tears allowing multiple frank nuclear herniations throughout the disc (Figure 16-11). The resulting reduction in disc space

height places more stress on the facet joints increasing facet-joint laxity and dynamically narrowing the intervertebral foramen. Root damage can accompany these changes by direct pressure from dynamic lateral entrapment in the foramen or can be mediated by the inflammatory process.[22,31]

Segmental stabilization of the functional unit is the last phase in this degenerative cascade.[29] Here facet joints become fibrosed, discs are increasingly degenerated and desiccated, allowing the approximation of vertebral end plates and subsequent osteophyte formation. This is the stage of spondylosis, frank osteoarthritis, or degenerative joint disease (DJD) and commonly is referred to as "hard discs."[24,25,29,33,43] At this point the majority of radiculopathies are caused by fixed lateral foraminal stenosis from facet joint osteophytes, vertebral body osteophytes and, in the cervical spine, uncovertebral joint pathology (Figure 16-12).[29]

In the lumbar spine, spinal stenosis has become a catch-all phrase first described by Verbiest[3] as an anatomic variation that leads to specific neurologic symptoms. The definition of spinal stenosis in the context of the preceding biomechanic description is a narrowing of the spine that leads to paroxysmal mechanical compression of the cauda equina and thus transient multilevel neurologic symptoms most commonly manifesting as neurologic caudication or pseudocaudication. Further information on lumbar spinal stenosis can be found elsewhere.[29,36,44]

In this last stage, degenerative spondylolisthesis of the lumbar spine can cause radiculopathy by allowing forward displacement of the upper vertebral body on the lower body, trapping the exiting nerve root.[44] Typically it is the L_5 root that is impinged by an L_{4-5} degenerative spondylolisthesis.[44]

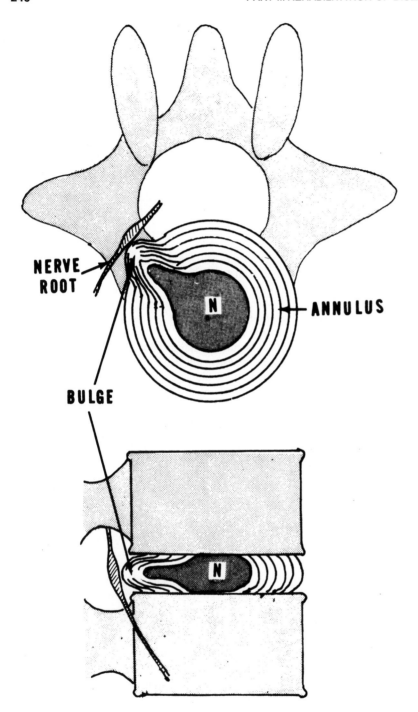

Figure 16-9
Internal extrusion of the nucleus in a posterior lateral direction. (Used with permission from Cailliet R: Neck and Arm Pain, 3rd ed. Philadelphia: F.A. Davis, p. 132.)

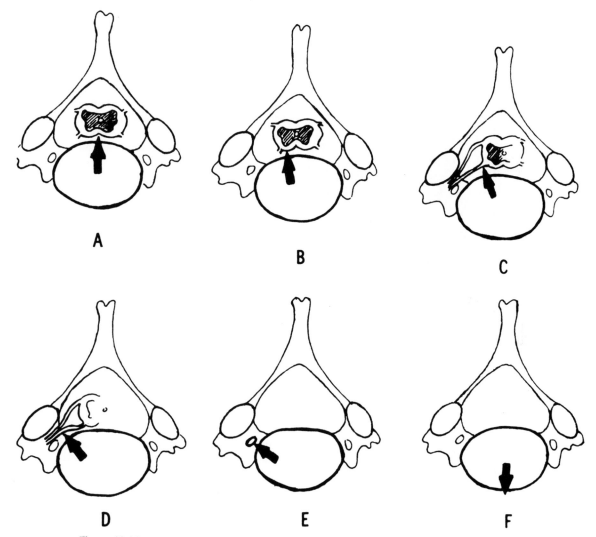

Figure 16-10

Possible results from direction of disc herniation. A = dorsomedial herniation may cause bilateral cord compression. B = paramedical herniation: unilateral cord compression. C = dorsolateral protrusion: unilateral cord and nerve root compression. D = intraforaminal protrusion: radical nerve root compression. E = lateral protrusion: vertebral artery and nerve compression. F = ventral protrusion causes no nerve root, cord, or vertebral artery compression. (Used with permission from Cailliet R: Neck and Arm Pain, 3rd ed. Philadelphia: F.A. Davis, p. 133.)

HISTORY/SYMPTOMS OF CERVICAL RADICULOPATHY

The majority of patients (80–100 percent) will present with symptoms of pain, parasthesia, numbness, and/or weakness that they cannot relate to a precipitating event.[24–26,45–49] The most common sites of pain are: the intrascapular region, the shoulder, the upper arm, the forearm and the occiput.[27,50] Radicular pain can be achy, dull, deep, sharp, burning, or electric in quality, depending on whether the dorsal root or ventral root or both are affected.[30,47] Other well-defined presentations

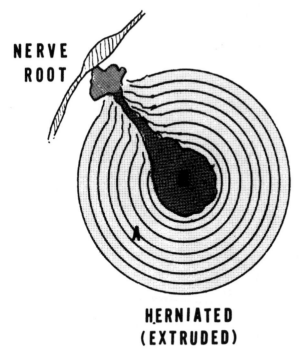

NERVE ROOT

HERNIATED (EXTRUDED)

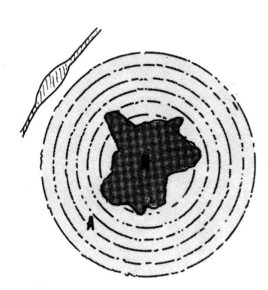

DEGENERATED

of cervical radicular pain include cervical angina, breast pain and regional facial pain. Table 16-3 outlines common pain patterns.[24,26,33,30,46,48,51–53] Further information needed includes: precipitating events, distribution, quality and duration of the pain, sensory or motor changes, nocturnal symptoms, lower-extremity symptoms, and bowel or bladder symptoms. Exacerbating and relieving activities or positions should always be noted. Patients often, for example, describe exacerbation of symptoms with overhead activities and valsalva-producing maneuvers, owing to the elevation of interforaminal pressure on the nerve roots. Lying down may provide relief, whereas neck extension worsens symptoms. Unlike the pain with lumbar radiculopathies, movements of involved upper extremities do not aggravate the symptoms.[41] Neck pain that awakens a person from sleep must be pursued with a high suspicion for malignancy.[54] Lower extremity symptoms and/or bowel or bladder changes suggest cervical myelopathy and require aggressive evaluation.[54]

PHYSICAL EXAM FOR CERVICAL RADICULOPATHY

The physical exam in cervical radiculopathies begins with general observations of the patient. Does the patient assume a protective neck posture? Does the patient avoid certain motions? Is there any muscle atrophy? Atrophy helps to both delineate the specific root involved and date the lesion (acute vs. chronic). Specific muscles that are atrophied with root lesions are identified in Table 16-3.

Neck range of motion both passively and actively can be limited by pain. In radiculopathy this pain is made worse with extension and rotation to the affected side; it improves with lateral bending away from this side.[50]

Loss of motor strength in a myotomal distribution has the highest diagnostic specificity for radiculopathies.[27,51] True weakness must be differentiated from

Figure 16-11
Disc herniation and degeneration. Top. An extruded nucleus in which the nucleus has "herniated" out of the torn annulus fibers. Bottom. Degenerated nucleus with fragmented annular fibers. (Used with permission from Cailliet R: Soft Tissue Pain and Disability Syndrome, *2nd ed. Philadelphia: F.A. Davis, p. 87.)*

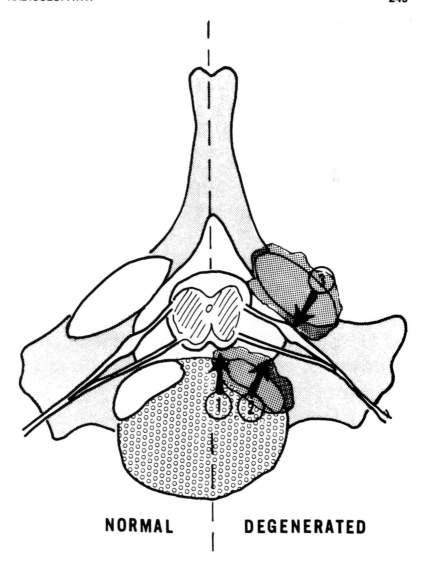

Figure 16-12

Osteoarthritis of the cervical spine. Left side reveals normal facet joint and uncovertebral joint with no encroachment on the nerve root or cord. Right side shows osteophytosis of unco-vertebral joint encroaching into spinal canal (1) and into interver-tebral foramen (2). Degenerative changes of facet joint (3) cause encroachment into foramen. All three osteophytes can cause neu-rologic dificit of cord or nerve root. (Used with permission from Caillet R: Soft Tissue Pain and Disability, *2nd ed. Philadelphia: F.A. Davis, p. 156.)*

NORMAL   **DEGENERATED**

pain-induced weakness. Table 16-3 highlights the specific patterns of muscle weakness in the cervical radiculopathies. The sensory exam of cervical dermatomes can help localize root levels, but owing to overlap and indistinct anatomic borders, this exam should not be relied upon as the primary delineator of affected root levels. Dermatomes from C_6, C_7, and C_8 roots are the most specific because of their discreet finger representations (Figure 16-13). Deep tendon reflexes are a reliable tool in helping to localize a lesion to one of two root levels.[27,51] The most common motor, sensory, and reflex findings with specific cervical radiculopathies are listed

in Figures 16-14 to 16-16. In order to rule out cervical spinal-cord compression, the lower extremities must be carefully examined for weakness, changes in sensation, increase in muscle stretch reflexes, and other upper-motor signs.[55]

There are many provocative tests that can help confirm cervical nerve-root compression within the fo-ramina. The most popular of these tests are Spurling's neck-compression test and L'Hermitte's sign. Spurling's test is performed by having the patient seated with the head extended, rotated, and laterally flexed toward the side of pain. The examiner then applies an axial force

Table 16-3

Specific cervical root level

Root	Referred pain	Paresthesia	Weakness	Reflex
C_5	Shoulder and upper arm	None in digit	Shoulder	Biceps
C_6	Radial aspect forearm	Thumb	Biceps Brachioradialis Wrist extensor	Biceps
C_7	Dorsal aspect forearm	Index and middle fingers	Triceps	Triceps
C_8	Ulnar aspect forearm	Ring and little fingers	Finger intrinsics	Triceps

From Cailliet R: *Neck and Arm Pain,* 3rd ed., Philadelphia: F.A. Davis, p. 142, with permission.

Figure 16-13

Dermatomes of cervical nerve roots C_5 to C_8. (Used with permission from Cailliet R: Neck and Arm Pain, *3rd ed. Philadelphia: F.A. Davis, p. 137.)*

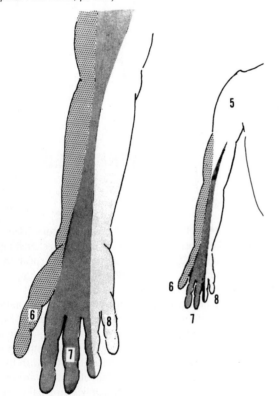

on the head.[34,46] This accentuated neck extension causes posterior disc bulging, while the lateral flexion with rotation narrows the ipsilateral neural foramina.[56] Replication of the pain, sensory changes, and/or motor strength loss is a positive Spurling's test.

L'Hermitte's sign, first described in 1932, requires the patient to be seated with the neck being actively flexed. A positive response is an "electric" sensation down the spine and sometimes down the upper extremities. Cervical cord tumors, spondylosis, and multiple sclerosis are also associated with a positive L'Hermitte's sign. Other provocative tests used include the axial manual traction test and the arm-abduction test. Both of these tests relieve symptoms of a radiculopathy when they are positive. In the axial manual traction test, the examiner physically elongates the cervical spine and thus opens the intervertebral foramina. The arm-abduction test relieves traction on the involved root by abduction overhead arm raising. These four tests can establish the presence or absence of nerve-root compression at the foraminal level, but are poor at localizing specific root levels.[34] After a comprehensive history and physical exam, 75–80 percent of specific root levels of injury can be determined.[57]

DIFFERENTIAL DIAGNOSIS— CERVICAL RADICULOPATHY

Cervical disc herniation resulting in nerve-root compression, tension, and/or inflammation is only one of the etiologies for the clinical presentation of radiculopathy.

Cervical myelopathy owing to degenerative disease of the spine is the second most common cause of the radicular syndrome. Nerve roots may be compressed by osteophytic overgrowth, which usually involves the

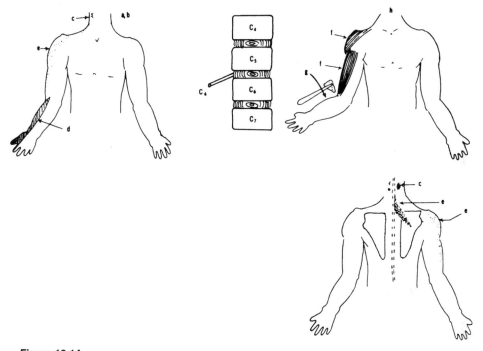

Figure 16-14

Sixth cervical nerve root irritation. a = Neck rigidity. Limited extension and rotation to the right. b = Pain and paresthesia aggravated by coughing and sneezing. c = Tenderness over exit of C_6 nerve root. d = Paresthesia and hypasthesia of thumb and some of index finger (from history and physical examination). e = Subjective pain and tenderness over deltoid and rhomboid muscle areas. f = Weakness of deltoid and biceps muscles. g = Depressed biceps jerk. h = x-ray studies equivocal. (Used with permission from Cailliet R: Neck and Arm Pain, 3rd ed. Philadelphia: F.A. Davis, p. 142.)

lower cervical vertebrae and narrows the spinal canal and intervertebral foramina. It may cause progressive injury of the spinal cord or roots or both. Although there is a characteristic triad of painful stiff neck, brachialgia, and spastic weakness with variable ataxia of the legs, each of these components may occur separately or in variable combinations and sequences. Although ruptured discs occur chiefly at the C_5–C_6 or C_6–C_7 interspace, the formation of osteophytes in transverse bony ridges may extend much higher than this and occur at several levels.[58]

When signs and symptoms of cervical radiculopathy occur with myelopathy, amyotrophic lateral sclerosis (ALS) also should be considered. The clinical presentation of ALS is usually painless, but cramping may occur, mimicking radiculopathy. Electrodiagnostic findings in ALS usually are widespread, involving many segments of the cervical region, and are not consistent with a single root compression. Findings of generalized lower motor-neuron dysfunction with electrodiagnostic evidence of reinnervation (large motor unit potentials) in ALS help differentiate the condition from cervical radiculopathy.

Both primary and metastatic tumors to the cervical region may result in nerve-root compression. Metastatic tumors typically involve more than a single spinal cord or nerve-root segment, whereas primary tumors often are heralded by bilateral findings. Spinal imaging studies, particularly magnetic resonance imaging, are the gold standard for differentiating benign cervical root compression from neoplastic myeloradiculopathy.

Pancoast tumors, or tumors of the apex of the lung, also may simulate cervical herniated discs. However, the pain tends to be acute, and clinical findings are most consistent with involvement of the lower trunk of the brachial plexus, including a Horner's syndrome.

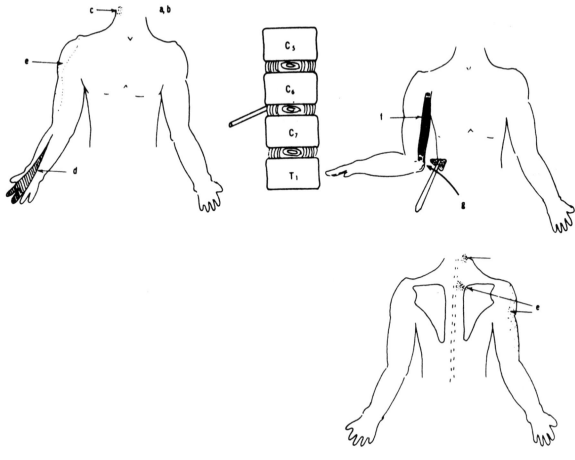

Figure 16-15
Seventh cervical nerve root irritation. a = Neck rigidity. Limited extension and rotation to the involved side. b = Pain and paresthesia aggravated by coughing and sneezing. c = Tenderness over exit of C_7. d = Paresthesia and hypasthesia of index and middle finger. e = Subjective deep pain and tenderness of dorsolateral upper arm and superior medial angle of scapula. f = Weakness of triceps (also possibly biceps). g = Depressed triceps jerk. (Used with permission from Cailliet R: Neck and Arm Pain, 3rd ed. Philadelphia: F.A. Davis, p. 143.)

Additionally, compression of the lower trunk of the brachial plexus by a cervical rib may mimic a radicular syndrome. Again, findings will not be limited to a single root.

Additional disorders to consider in the workup of cervical radiculopathy include Parsonage Turner Syndrome, also known as neurologic amyotrophy, idiopathic brachial plexopathy, and brachial neuritis. This brachial plexus syndrome, presumably of viral origin, may affect any combination of nerves in the upper limb or, even less commonly, a single upper-limb nerve. Although typically it presents with pain, followed by weak-

ness and eventual atrophy, its onset may be difficult to distinguish from cervical radiculopathy, particularly when the upper trunk of the plexus is involved.

Severe median neuropathy at the wrist may contribute to the development of proximal arm as well as neck pain. Carpal-tunnel syndrome is marked by pain, parasthesias, and weakness only in the distribution of the median nerve, in contrast with the multiple-nerve pattern seen in the entrapment of a single cervical root. Of note, carpal-tunnel syndrome may coexist with cervical radiculopathy, as reported in the "double crush" phenomenon.[59]

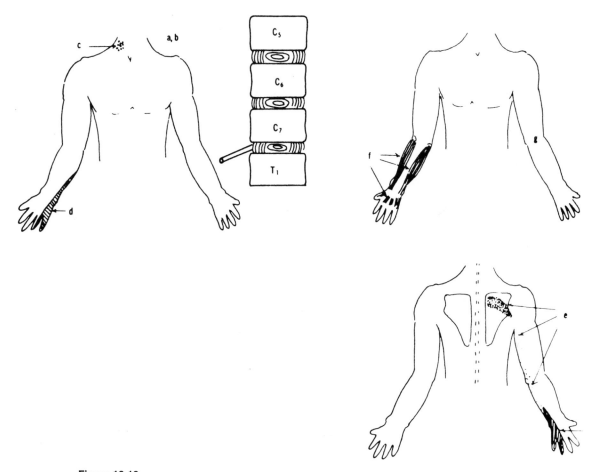

Figure 16-16

Eighth cervical nerve root irritation. a = Neck rigidity. Limited extension and rotation to the involved side. b = Pain and paresthesia aggravated by coughing and sneezing. c = Tenderness over exit of C_8. d = Paresthesia and hypasthesia of inner forearm and little finger. e = Subjective deep pain and tenderness from scapula down inner side of upper arm, inner forearm, to little finger. f = Weakness of hand muscles. g = No reflex changes. (Used with permission from Cailliet R: Neck and Arm Pain, 3rd ed. Philadelphia: F.A. Davis, p. 143.)

Musculoskeletal disorders, such as rotator cuff tears, subacromial bursitis, and bicipital tendinitis, may all result in neck and upper-limb pain. They are differentiated from cervical radiculopathy through the clinical evaluation. If the history, physical exam, and subsequent treatment do not result in acceptable resolution of the problem, electrophysiologic studies and imaging studies should be performed.

Other considerations in a differential diagnosis of cervical radiculopathy include: spinal vascular malformations, myofascial pain syndrome, epidemic neuromyasthenia, and postherpetic neuralgia. The entrapment

mononeuropathies (the most common being crutch paralysis and Saturday-night palsy) usually are differentiated easily from radiculopathy based on single nerve involvement.[60]

RADICULOPATHY—THORACIC

Compressive thoracic root lesions may occur as a result of tumor, disc degeneration, or herniation. The majority of patients who present with a clinical picture consistent with a thoracic radiculopathy are diabetic and typically have one or more lower thoracic roots affected. There are no electrophysiologic studies that can differentiate a compressive from a metabolic root lesion. However, the classic finding in a diabetic thoracic radiculopathy is the presence of paraspinal fibrillation potentials, along with findings typical of diabetic peripheral neuropathy.[61]

If a patient's medical history indicates that metastatic tumor is possible, spinal imaging studies may be necessary.

HISTORY/SYMPTOMS OF THE LUMBOSACRAL RADICULOPATHY

Many of the specific symptoms seen in cervical radiculopathies are also found with lumbosacral radiculopathies. It is the location of these symptoms that is different. Similarities include the fact that the majority of patients lack the ability to recall an antecedent precipitating event (64–76 percent).[28,62] Pain, parasthesias, numbness, and/or weakness are common. Pain in the low back or buttock is a frequent complaint.[63,64] This pain, along with numbness and/or parasthesias, often extends below the knee in dermatomal patterns. Valsalva maneuvers (coughing, sneezing, defecating) may worsen their symptoms by increasing intraforaminal pressure on the roots.[28,62,63] Not infrequently, clearly demonstrable objective weakness is present before the patient becomes aware of it.[28,62] As with cervical radiculopathies, nocturnal pain should spur inquiry about weight loss or other signs or symptoms of malignancy. Finally, saddle numbness with or without sphincter problems signals a true surgical emergency (cauda equina syndrome).

PHYSICAL EXAM FOR THE LUMBOSACRAL RADICULOPATHY

As in cervical radiculopathies, the physical exam in patients with lumbosacral radiculopathies begins by observing the patient. Initial inspection may indicate a functional scoliosis, or listing of the spine away from the side of root pain.[10,28,62,64] A loss of the normal lumbar lordosis, restricted mobility of the spine, and a "corkscrew" phenomenon on straightening up from a lumbar flexed position are common.[64]

On physical exam, spasm of paraspinal muscles and atrophy of specifically affected limb muscles may be observed.[10,62] Hypaesthesia, paresis, and/or reflex changes also are observed.[28,65] Specific patterns of motor, sensory, and reflex deficits serve to localize the lesion (Table 16-4).[10] The sensory changes of L_5 and S_1 dermatomes, located on the foot, are the most specific of the sensory exam.[10,28] The loss of the Achilles reflex is seen in both L_5 and S_1 radiculopathies. Loss of the medial hamstring reflex reflects an L_5 lesion, whereas a decreased lateral hamstring reflex points to an S_1 injury. No lumbosacral radiculopathy physical exam is complete without a full rectal exam. This includes a sensory check of the S_{3-5} dermatomes, an evaluation of rectal tone, and the proper bulbocavernosis reflex to rule out a cauda equina syndrome.

Confirmatory root tension maneuvers for the lumbosacral radiculopathies include the straight leg raise (SLR), the crossed straight leg raise, the Lasègue's maneuver and the femoral stretch test.[10,28,62] A SLR is performed with the patient lying down and the examiner flexing the hip while keeping the knee extended and the foot in a neutral or dorsiflexed position. Pain that extends down the leg to the foot at 30–70° of hip flexion has the highest specificity and points to L_5 and S_1 root injuries.[10,44] A positive crossed SLR, pain extending down the involved leg while performing a SLR on the uninvolved leg, suggests an extruded or sequestered disc fragment at $L_{4,5}$ or L_5S_1 and/or a significant L_4, L_5, or S_1 radiculopathy.[10,44] Lasègue's maneuver is similar to the SLR, but is performed with the patient seated. The hip is flexed with the knee extended; the examiner actively dorsiflexes the foot. A positive test produces radicular pain with each dorsiflexion of the foot. The femoral stretch test is the L_{2-4} equivalent of the SLR. This is done by having the patient lie on the uninvolved side while extending the involved hip. The examiner then actively flexes the involved knee, which stretches the femoral nerve and, if positive, stretches inflamed L_{2-4} nerve roots producing radicular pain.

DIFFERENTIAL DIAGNOSIS—LUMBAR

The differential diagnosis of lumbosacral radiculopathy must encompass all causes of back pain. Low back pain may arise from multiple potential pain generators, including: (1) musculoligamentous injuries; (2) degenerative changes (discs and facets); (3) intervertebral disc herniation; (4) spinal stenosis; (5) anatomic spinal anomolies (spondylolisthesis, scoliosis); (6) underlying systemic disorders; and (7) visceral diseases (aorta, pelvic organs).[66]

Most causes of low back pain emanate from musculoligamentous injury or degenerative changes. Common diagnostic considerations include: myofascial pain,

Table 16-4

Schematic dermatome and myotome level of lumbosacral nerve root impingement

Nerve root	Inter-vertebral space	Subjective pain radiation	Sensory area	Bladder bowel dysfunction[a]	SLR[b]	Ankle jerk[c]	Knee jerk[c]	Motor dysfunction (myotome)[d]
L_3	L_2–L_3	Back to buttocks to posterior thigh to anterior knee region	Hypalgesia in knee region	+/−	Usually −	+	+	Quadriceps weakness
L_4	L_3–L_4	Back to buttocks to posterior thigh to inner calf region	Hypalgesia inner aspect of lower leg	+/−	Usually − Maybe +	+	−	Quadriceps and possible anticus weakness
L_5	L_4–L_5	Back to buttocks to dorsum of foot and big toe	Hypalgesia in dorsum foot and big toe	+/−	+ +	+	+	Weakness of anterior tibialis, big toe extensor, gluteus medius
S_1	L_5–S_1	Back to buttocks to sole of foot and heel	Hypalgesia in heel or lateral foot	+/−	+ + +	−	+	Weakness of gastrocnemius, hamstring, gluteus maximus

From Cailliet R: *Low Back Pain Syndrome,* 4th ed. Philadelphia, F.A. Davis, p. 224, with permission.

[a] Bladder and bowel dysfunction can occur at any level.

[b] Related to extent of nerve root movement at each level.

[c] Ankle jerk is absent only at L_5–S_1; knee jerk at L_3–L_4.

[d] Only the more obvious and functional muscles are listed.

bursitis, osteoarthritis, sacroiliac dysfunction, coccydynia, and piriformis syndrome (sciatic nerve entrapment).

Spinal stenosis, a polyradicular syndrome, usually causes bilateral symptoms that are exacerbated by walking or merely standing, which disappear with sitting or lying down, and are worsened with extension.[67] Activities that depend on spinal flexion, such as bicycle riding, dancing, or pushing a shopping cart often can be performed with ease.

If the history of bilateral leg pain is accompanied by a description of urinary retention or fecal incontinence, cauda equina syndrome must be evaluated emergently. Physical findings of decreased anal sphincter tone and perineal or saddle anesthesia confirm the diagnosis. Cauda equina compression is a true surgical emergency.

Anatomic and structural anomalies of the spine that may cause low back pain include scoliosis and spondylolisthesis. Although frequently asymptomatic, these spinal variants may cause pain when severe or combined with other degenerative changes. Traumatic vertebral fractures and compression fractures from osteoporosis (either primary or secondary) will generate considerable localized pain, typically worsened with any movement, and often with a discrete onset.

Underlying systemic diseases that commonly cause low back pain include: systemic cancer, infections, and ankylosing spondylitis. Back pain owing to malignancy is often present day and night and unrelieved by bed rest.[68] Multiple myeloma and adenocarcinomas of the breast, prostate, and lung account for a large majority of osseous metastases, with the most common sites including the vertebrae, pelvis, and femur.[69] Epidural metastasis, common in breast, prostate or lung cancer, multiple myeloma, melanoma, or renal cell carcinoma generates pain that is usually midline and progresses to neurologic deficits (spinal-cord compression) approximately 7 weeks after the onset.[70]

Spinal infections, chiefly epidural abscesses, are an important cause of low back pain. Sources include the urinary tract, skin infections, and injection sites for intravenous drug use. Dissemination is hematogenous. Tuberculosis may be disseminated, as in the immuno-compromised host, or have a primary vertebral source (Pott's disease). Spine tenderness in response to percussion has a high sensitivity for bacterial infection, but poor specificity.[68,71]

The spondyloarthropathies, or seronegative spondyloarthritides, are characterized by involvement of the sacroiliac joints, peripheral inflammatory arthropathy, and the absence of rheumatoid factor. Ankylosing spondylitis is a disease of insidious onset in persons under 40, associated with morning stiffness lasting at least 3 months and improvement with exercise. X-rays reveal bilateral sacroiliitis. Other disorders with a component of inflammatory spine disease include: Reiter's syndrome (usually sudden onset), psoriatic arthropathy, intestinal arthropathy, juvenile ankylosing spondylitis, and reactive arthropathy (associated with Yersinia infections or other enteric pathogens).[72]

Visceral sources of back pain include diseases of the kidneys, intestinal viscera, and pelvic organs (ovaries, uterus). The aorta (as in dissection) and iliofemoral vasculature may give rise to back and lower extremity pain, respectively. Vascular claudication causes cramping in both lower extremities (typically the calves) after walking a specific distance. The cramping pain is relieved when the individual stops walking. Changing position usually is unnecessary, unlike spinal stenosis.

DIAGNOSTIC STUDIES IN RADICULOPATHY

Imaging Studies—Cervical

Confirmation or further evaluation of a clinical diagnosis may require confirmation by imaging studies. The imaging studies currently utilized in evaluation of the cervical spine include: plain film evaluation, computed tomography (CT) including postmyelogram CT (PMCT), and magnetic resonance imaging (MRI).

While plain film evaluation of the spinal column is frequently the first diagnostic examination ordered in the evaluation of suspected disease, the information obtained from plain films is frequently limited because of a lack of specificity and sensitivity. Anterior/posterior and lateral radiographs provide no information about the presence or location of a disc herniation even if a narrowed disc space is observed.[73] Plain x-rays are helpful in the initial evaluation of chronic degenerative changes of the uncovertebral joints, spondylosis, infection, and possible osseous metastasis. However, abnor-

malities are detected relatively late in the natural history of most of these disorders. By age 60–65, 95 percent of asymptomatic men, and 70 percent of asymptomatic women, have at least one degenerative change on x-ray.[74] There are no criteria for selective use of plain x-rays in cervical pain.

Myelography alone is a reliable way to evaluate the thecal sac and its contents, but it is an invasive procedure with the potential for rare but serious complications, particularly with cervical puncture.[75]

Modern imaging protocols now use both CT and MRI to maximize the information obtained from each of these studies, based on their specificity and sensitivity. CT provides superior information about osseous structures, and MRI is unsurpassed in soft-tissue evaluation.

Because of the very small size of the anatomic components of the cervical spine, imaging with high resolution is required. It is important to delineate the normal neural structures within the spinal canal as well as those in the intervertebral foramina. The cervical spine survey must include the vertebral bodies, intervertebral discs, the spinal cord, as well as the thecal sac and posterior elements. CT provides excellent delineation of the vertebral bodies, laminae, facet joints, spinal canal, and intervertebral foramina. PMCT may be the best means for evaluation of lateral cervical disc herniations and cervical foraminal narrowing.[75] High-resolution CT is able to identify unsuspected fractures in a suspicious vertebra, as well as fractures in adjacent vertebrae.[75]

MRI provides excellent evaluation of the spinal cord and nerve-root anatomy, paraspinal soft tissues, intervertebral canal, and posterior spinal elements. The evaluation of small disc herniations, chrondro-osseous spurs, and hypertrophied or calcified ligaments is difficult. Therefore, to achieve a contrast difference between the posterior margin of the discovertebral joint and the thecal sac, T_1 and T_2 weighted sequences are required. The cervical spine can also be evaluated by oblique sequences through the intervertebral foramina, as well as by multiple-angled sections through individual disc spaces.[73] MRI technology has progressed to the point that it has essentially replaced other imaging studies of the spine. However, there is a significant false-positive rate with MRI. It may demonstrate a major abnormality in the cervical spine in 14 percent of asymptomatic individuals less than 40 years old, and 28 percent of those older than 40.[70] The level most frequently associated with a false positive study is C_{5-6}, followed by C_{6-7}. Degeneration of a disc is seen in 37 percent of asymptomatic individuals.[70] MRI results must be strictly matched with clinical signs and symptoms in order to validate specific imaging signals as pain generators. In the setting of ferromagnetic bioprostheses or claustrophobia, when MRI can not be used, PMCT is the procedure of choice.

IMAGING STUDIES—LUMBAR

Plain radiographs are readily available, and offer a relatively inexpensive evaluation of bony structures. Their primary limitation is poor visualization of soft tissues. Abnormalities of the spinal cord and intervertebral discs cannot be identified until secondary osseous changes have occurred.[76] In acute low back pain, plain x-rays remain controversial.[77-79] Deyo and Diehl have proposed selective use of anteroposterior and lateral views in the acute stage of low back pain according to specified criteria (Table 16-5).[77]

Lumbar spine radiography is the largest source of gonadal irradiation in the United States.[79] A single lumbar spine series results in gonadal radiation doses equivalent to a daily chest x-ray for over 6 years.[80] Many studies of oblique views have demonstrated little diagnostic gain, while doubling the radiation exposure.[81,82] The World Health Organization recommends that oblique views not be routinely obtained, but reserved only for special problems after thorough review of A-P and lateral views.[83] These suggestions will reduce cost and radiation exposure associated with each exam.

Routine radiographs provide no information

Table 16-5

Proposed criteria for use of plain anterior-posterior and lateral radiograms in the evaluation of acute low back pain[a]

Age over 50

Fever

Clinical findings suggestive of ankylosing spondylitis

Suspicion of malignancy

History of significant antecedent trauma

Motor neurologic deficit

Litigation considerations

Steroid use

Drug or alcohol abuse

[a] Deyo RA, Diehl AK: Lumbar spine films in primary care; current use and effects of selective ordering criteria. *J Gen Int Med* 1986; 1:20–25.

about the presence or location of disc herniation, even when a narrowed disc space is observed. CT scanning, myelography, or magnetic resonance imaging are indicated when surgical intervention is being considered or when exam and symptoms suggest a tumor or infectious process. The most important caveat is correlation of the patient's signs and symptoms with the imaging studies. Wiesel demonstrated that over 30 percent of lumbar spine CT scans were abnormal in an asymptomatic population.[84] In those under age 40, a diagnosis of herniated nucleus pulposus was made in 19.5 percent of people. In those over age 40, 50 percent of CT scans were read as abnormal, with the most common diagnoses being canal stenosis and facet degeneration. CT and myelography have similar sensitivity (80–95 percent) and specificity (68–88 percent) in the diagnosis of herniated lumbar discs.[79,85] CT does provide superior visualization of lateral vertebral structure and pathology, such as lateral disc protrusions, lateral recess stenosis, and foraminal stenosis.

In the late 1980s, magnetic resonance imaging was predicted to be the procedure of choice for lumbar spine imaging.[79] In a prospective study of MRI of the lumbar spine in asymptomatic patients, Boden et al. found that 20 percent of patients under age 60 had herniated discs. Fifty-seven percent of asymptomatic patients over age 60 had evidence of a herniated disc or canal stenosis.[86] In another study of MRI of the lumbar spine in people without back pain, Jensen et al. found that only 36 percent of those examined had a normal study.[87] Approximately 50 percent of people had a bulge in at least one intervertebral disc, and 25 percent had at least one disc protrusion.[88] Eight percent of subjects had facet arthropathy. MRI examination of 41 asymptomatic women revealed disc bulge or herniation in 54 percent of those studied.[89]

Bulging discs may be regarded as normal findings, since they are found in over half of asymptomatic adults.[88-90] Terminology may be helpful in determining which lesions are meaningful. Extruded discs (focal, obvious extension of the disc beyond the interspace, with a base narrower than the diameter of the extruding material) appear to be unusual in people without symptoms, and may warrant more concern than discs that merely protrude.[89] A patient's clinical situation must be evaluated carefully in conjunction with the results of MRI studies because bulges and protrusions on MRI in people with radiculopathy may be coincidental.[88]

In older patients, degenerative, bony changes are the most likely source of radiculopathy. CT scans may be reasonable imaging studies in this population. Disc pathology tends to be the etiology for radiculopathy in those younger than 40: MRI is an appropriate study in this age group for evaluation of low back pain.

ELECTRODIAGNOSIS

Comprehensive electrodiagnosis includes nerve conduction studies and electromyography. Electromyography is the most useful qualitative method for evaluating radiculopathies.[87]

Although the most common clinical presentation of radiculopathy is with signs and symptoms of sensory fiber compromise, sensory-nerve action potentials (SNAPS) typically are unaffected. This is because the lesion usually is proximal to the dorsal-root ganglion. It has no effect on the dorsal-root ganglia and its peripheral fibers are intact. If sensory conduction is abnormal in the area of sensory loss, the possibility of a peripheral nerve injury must be considered.[91]

The motor conduction velocities also usually are normal in monoradiculopathies, as most peripheral nerves contain fibers from more than one root. When the root lesion is causing axonal degeneration one may see a decrement in the amplitude of the compound muscle action potential (CMAP) in the motor-nerve conduction study. A very weak muscle will have a good prognosis for recovery if the CMAP remains large ($\geqq 30$ percent of the unaffected side).[91]

F-waves are late responses recorded from a muscle following maximal stimulation of its nerve. The F-wave is obtained from the antidromic pathway in the motor nerve activating the anterior horn cells, then causing an orthodromic impulse back to the muscle being recorded. The F-wave measurement has proved to be disappointing in the evaluation of patients with radiculopathies and other proximal nerve lesions, which are inaccessible to more conventional nerve conduction studies.[92] The studies frequently are normal. When they are abnormal, needle electromyographic abnormalities also are present. Thus, F-wave examination usually does not provide additional useful information.[91]

The H-wave, or H reflex, is a monosynaptic spinal reflex. It is obtained consistently from adults only by recording from the gastrocnemius-soleus muscles while stimulating the tibial nerve. Only S1 fibers are evaluated, so there are limitations to its use. Unfortunately, the H-wave occasionally is normal with proven S1 radiculopathy, owing to incomplete root involvement. An abnormal H-reflex is not synonymous with S1 radiculopathy, as a lesion anywhere along the course of the tibial nerve,

sacral plexus, or spinal cord may yield an abnormality. Finally, H reflexes often are absent in persons over 60, persons with polyneuropathy, or in the setting of previous S1 radiculopathy.

Somatosensory evoked potentials (SEPs) are obtained by electrical stimulation of a mixed motor and sensory nerve, a pure sensory nerve, or the skin innervated by a specific nerve root. SEPs are carried in the posterior columns of the spinal cord. Vibration and position sense usually are normal in radiculopathy. In unilateral cervical radiculopathy studies, a high false-negative rate occurs on the symptomatic side, with many false-positives on the asymptomatic side.[92] Side-to-side latency differences, amplitude or configuration differences are used by some investigators. The usefulness of SEPs in the evaluation of radiculopathy is unclear, and therefore the diagnosis should not be based on SEPs alone.[92,93]

Needle electromyography (EMG) is the oldest electrophysiologic method to evaluate patients with suspected radiculopathy. It is still the single most useful procedure, and has the highest diagnostic yield of any electrophysiologic technique currently available. Needle EMG evaluates only *motor* root fibers that have axonal loss. In the needle EMG, several muscles should be strategically assessed specific limb myotomes. The study is considered positive if abnormalities are present in two or more muscles that receive innervation from the same root, preferably supplied by different peripheral nerves. EMG abnormalities include positive waves and fibrillation potentials (also referred to as fibrillation potentials of the biphasic spike or positive sharp wave form) that indicate denervation (motor-axon loss). Fasciculation potentials and complex repetitive discharges are spontaneous electrical discharges seen in chronic denervation. Nerve root irritation leads to abnormal motor unit potential (MUP) recruitment. Abnormal MUP recruitment results are present from the onset, and are attributed to both myelin and axonal degeneration. Several EMG-determined myotomal charts have been devised (see Figures 16-1 and 16-2). Paraspinal musculature may be normal in an otherwise abnormal EMG. This occurs when the posterior primary rami are uninvolved, or if reinnervation to these muscles has already occurred (late changes).

Seven to ten days after the nerve-root compromise, positive waves and increased insertional activity can be seen in the paraspinal musculature.[93] Fibrillation potentials and positive waves in the extremities typically occur in a root distribution 18–21 days after the onset of neck, back, or extremity pain or painless motor loss.[23,87,91,92] Fibrillation potentials are the most sensitive indicator of motor-axon loss, developing in a proximal–distal gradient. Three to six weeks after the onset of root compromise, sustained positive waves appear in the limb musculature. Spontaneous activity begins to disappear after 3 months in more proximal muscles as reinnervation occurs.

The EMG abnormalities seen with radiculopathy are intimately related to the chronicity of the nerve-root lesion. Fibrillation potentials unaccompanied by abnormalities of the motor unit potential configuration suggest a recent-onset radiculopathy. MUP abnormalities of a chronic nature, such as polyphasia, and small fibrillations (<100 μV) suggest a more remote onset. A combination of small and large fibrillation potentials as well as chronic motor unit potential changes indicate a chronic but actively discharging radiculopathy.

Paraspinal muscle evaluation may be abnormal in patients who have undergone spine surgery. The absence of EMG abnormality in the post-surgical paraspinal musculature may help rule out a new or recurrent lesion.[91]

After acute injury, it may be necessary to obtain a baseline EMG, in order to establish the presence or absence of preexisting injury. For example, in an injured worker, a baseline EMG at the onset of symptoms may demonstrate actively discharging denervation potentials, ruling out the acute incident as the precipitant cause.

In general, EMG evaluation of a suspected radiculopathy will be the most fruitful when performed between 3 and 6 weeks after the onset of symptoms.

C_5–C_6 Radiculopathies Lesions of the C_5 and C_6 roots (the C_4 and C_5 discs) typically are difficult to distinguish one from another. With both of these lesions, abnormalities may be seen in the biceps, brachioradialis, deltoid, and infra- and supraspinatus. If denervation potentials are seen in rhomboids as well, then the C_5 root is the root of involvement. Conversely, if the pronator teres and/or the flexor carpi-radialis is involved, then the compromised root is probably C_6. In many patients, none of these identifying muscles will show abnormalities: Thus, localization to a single root, C_5 versus C_6, remains elusive.

C_7 Radiculopathies Lesions of the C_7 root (C_6 disc) are the most common cervical radiculopathy, accounting for up to 70 percent of all cervical radiculopathies.[23,91] It is far easier to localize these lesions to the root level. Denervation potentials will be found in one or more of the C_7 radial-innervated muscles, such as the triceps and extensor carpi radialis, as well as in the C_7 median innervated muscles, such as the flexor carpi radialis and pronator teres.

C_8–T_1 Radiculopathies As with the C_5–C_6 radiculopathies, lesions of the C_8 and T_1 roots often are grouped together because of their extensive myotomal overlap. Although it is difficult to differentiate one from another by needle exam, most lesions appear to affect the C_8 root (because of involvement of the C_7 disc).

Partial brachial plexopathies may mimic cervical radiculopathies. Needle examination of the extremity may not help with differentiation of a C_5–C_6 radiculopathy from an upper trunk plexopathy, or a C_8–T_1 radiculopathy from a lower trunk plexopathy. Evaluation of the appropriate sensory-nerve action potential, as well as assessment of the cervical paraspinal muscles, will be helpful.

Although most cervical radiculopathies are unilateral lesions, it is advisable to examine at least one muscle in the contralateral limb, preferably of the muscle that had shown abnormalities on the symptomatic side. When evidence of multilevel radiculopathy is found, needle examination of the contralateral limb is mandatory. Findings in multiple root distributions suggest cervical spinal stenosis, an intramedullary lesion, or, perhaps, metastatic root entrapment as a source of symptoms. Further, if bilateral multiple root changes are found, an examination of a lower extremity is important to evaluate the possibility of motor-neuron disease.

L_2, L_3, L_4 Radiculopathies These are difficult to distinguish from one another because of extensive myotomal overlap. Almost all muscles in the L_2–L_4 myotomes are innervated by the femoral (L_2, L_3, L_4) or obturator (L_2, L_3, L_4) nerves. There is no reliable sensory NCS for evaluating these fibers to distinguish plexopathy from radiculopathy. In diabetics, L_2, L_3, or L_4 radiculopathy may be difficult to differentiate from diabetic amyotrophy by electrodiagnostic criteria.

L_5 Radiculopathy Lesions of the L_5 root will result in EMG abnormalities in all peroneal innervated muscles, the medial hamstring, the gluteus medius, tensor fascia lata, tibialis posterior, flexor digitorum, and the paraspinal muscles. Peroneal sensory studies should be normal. This, in addition to the extensive L_5 representation in the lower extremity, will readily separate common peroneal neuropathy from an L_5 radiculopathy.

S_1, S_2 Radiculopathies EMG abnormalities commonly are seen in the gastrocnemius, soleus, intrinsic foot muscles, lateral hamstrings, and the glutei, particularly the gluteus maximus. Unfortunately, many of these muscles also receive some innervation from S_2, and thus, S_1 and S_2 lesions may be difficult to separate. In the S_1 radiculopathy, the H-wave may be abnormal, with a normal sural sensory nerve action potential. Of all the radiculopathies S_1 and S_2 are most often bilateral, because these fibers are located medially in the cauda equina and are thus more vulnerable to midline compression. Whenever an S_1 or S_2 radiculopathy is found, needle examination of the contralateral limb should be performed.

TREATMENT OF RADICULOPATHY

The therapeutic approach to radiculopathy includes anything from relative bed rest and nonsteroidal anti-inflammatory drugs to surgery. Commonly used modalities include traction, heat, cold, active physical therapy, isometric and range-of-motion exercises, and dynamic stabilization. The purpose is to reduce nerve-root inflammation and edema. Patient education in body mechanics and appropriate exercises are essential to avoid recurrence. A clinical-care pathway for evaluation and treatment of nerve-root compression is presented (Figure 16-17).

Activity limitations may range from the avoidance of moderate to heavy activities to a few days of relative bedrest in the case of an acute, severe radiculopathy.

Positioning and postural awareness to avoid further irritation of the involved nerve root must be part of conservative treatment. In cervical radiculopathy, ipsilateral neck flexion (as in using a phone) and neck extension (bifocal wearer at the computer) must be avoided.

Soft collars are frequently prescribed by physicians, but there is no consensus on proper use or effectiveness.[94] Soft foam collars do little to limit cervical motion. Rigid plastic collars are somewhat more effective.[95] In a questionnaire survey on the use of a soft cervical collar for cervical pain, Naylor and Mulley found that 76 percent of users reported pain reduction.[96] There is agreement that collars should only be worn for a limited amount of time.[14,97] The wide part of the collar is placed posteriorly with the narrow part anteriorly to limit neck extension. There is no literature supporting the use of lumbar orthotics in acute radiculopathy.

Nonsteroidal anti-inflammatory drugs usually are the first line of pharmacologic intervention in treating radiculopathy. They provide pain relief and reduce inflammation. A short course of oral steroids in a burst-and-taper method of administration has been tried in acute, severe radiculopathy. However, this is controversial and has not been thoroughly studied.[14] A comparison of dexamethasone and placebo in patients with lumbosacral radicular pain found no benefit from treatment with dexamethasone.[98] Many questions have been raised in subsequent investigations regarding the conclusions of this study, and anecdotal reports continue to discuss the usefulness of oral steroids in the treatment of lumbosacral radiculopathy.[98–102] High-dose, rapidly tapered intramuscular dexamethasone injections also have led to marked pain relief in an uncontrolled study of one hundred patients with radicular pain owing to herniated lumbar intervertebral discs.[100]

Additional adjunctive medications that are useful include low-dose tricyclic antidepressants to decrease pain and improve sleep, and muscle relaxants and spasmolytic agents to break the cycle of patient anxiety and painful spasm. If absolutely necessary, narcotic analgesics can be administered on a short-term basis for acute, particularly intense pain at the onset. They are never to be given on a long-term basis for chronic pain management.

Extensive medical evidence supports the use of epidural steroid and local anesthetic in the treatment of lumbosacral radiculopathy.[102–106] In both lumbar and cervical epidural steroid injections for radiculopathy, improvement in neurologic deficit as well as in pain have been reported.[106,107] Fully 86 percent of patients with clinical sciatica and radiologic evidence of nerve-root entrapment were treated successfully by serial epidural administration or periradicular infiltration of steroid and local anesthetic.[102] Epidural steroids also have been reported to be beneficial in cervical radiculopathy in patients with pain refractory to conservative treatment.[107–109] Over half of those who have no relief of pain from conservative therapy have good to excellent responses after epidural steroid injection.[109]

Those with acute radiculopathy have a better response to epidural steroids than those with chronic symptoms.[110] Significant improvement in pain should be felt 1 to 3 weeks after the procedure, lasting up to 3 months.

Physical modalities are for pain modulation. They include heat, cold, traction, and electrical stimula-

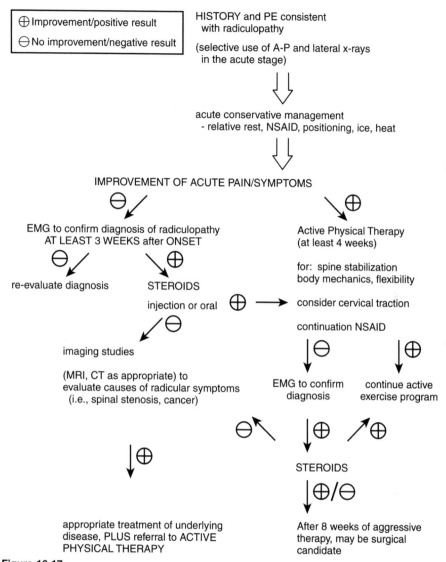

Figure 16-17
Flowchart for rehabilitation of radiculopathy.

tion. Heat decreases muscle spasm and joint stiffness, increases collagen tissue extensibility and blood flow, and is effective in pain relief.[111] There are two forms of therapeutic heat: deep and superficial. Superficial heat penetrates less than 1 cm, generates a slow rise in subcutaneous tissue temperature, and has a short duration of temperature elevation. There are few well-designed studies that evaluate the efficacy of superficial heat. Hot packs can relax muscles and relieve pain.

Deep heat given by therapeutic ultrasound penetrates to a depth of 6 centimeters below the skin surface. Deep heat should be avoided in the acute phase of nerve root irritation. It has the potential for exacerbating the inflammation of an affected nerve, leading to greater pain.

Cold also decreases muscle spasm, and is effective in pain relief. Cold packs may be applied for 15–30 minutes several times per day. The effectiveness of cryotherapy compared to other physical modalities is unknown.

The decision whether to use superficial heat or cold in acute conservative management is primarily based on the patient's perception of efficacy. Both will relieve paraspinal muscle spasm and pain. The patient should be instructed to begin with one modality 15–20 minutes several times daily. A second modality may be tried as well. A single modality or alternate heat and cold can be effective.

Traction

The effects of traction include distraction of vertebral bodies, separation of apophyseal joints, enlargement of the intervertebral foramina, and stretching of muscles and ligaments. Traction can be performed manually by a therapist, or mechanically. Traction is contraindicated in patients with spinal ligamentous instability, spondylytic myelopathy, and in conditions associated with atlantoaxial subluxation (such as Down syndrome and rheumatoid arthritis).

Pain frequently is relieved after cervical traction.[112–114] Although traction can relieve pain at the time it is applied and perhaps for hours afterward, it does not influence the rate of recovery.[113] In order to counterbalance the weight of the head, at least 10 pounds of force must be used. Colachis has found that an angle of 24 degrees of neck flexion with a force of 30 pounds applied for 7 seconds yielded maximum vertebral separation at 25 minutes. The greatest separation posteriorly occurs at the C_6–C_7 level, and anteriorly at the C_4–C_5 level.[115] Instruction in proper techniques for home traction is essential to prevent errors in positioning. The patient should have responded well in the clinic to traction before home traction is suggested.

Lumbar or pelvic traction may be useful to provide symptomatic relief of some types of disc pathology. There are no studies, however, that document the benefits of lumbar traction in lumbosacral radiculopathy. There is minimal experimental or clinical support for the efficacy of pelvic traction, and it may lead to deconditioning and adverse psychological consequences.[116]

Traction generally is *not* accepted as a treatment modality in lumbosacral radiculopathy. A force equal to at least 26 percent of the patient's weight is necessary to overcome the surface resistance of the lower half of the body.[117] Bed traction cannot overcome this resistance, and leads to little or no separation of vertebral elements. Bed traction basically ensures bedrest. Using a split table reduces frictional forces, but 50 pounds

of force must be used to achieve posterior interbody separation. This amount of force may not be tolerated well, and no residual separation has been noted 30 minutes after traction.[118]

Indications for surgical intervention in radiculopathy include disc extrusion, progressive neurologic deficits, and failed conservative management with intractable pain that correlates with a recognizable clinical and radiologic pain generator. There is no consensus on the duration of conservative treatment before surgery is considered.

Surgical intervention in lumbar and cervical radiculopathy frequently involves decompression of the root involved, but is beyond the scope of this text.

OUTCOMES

The major objectives for the treatment of radiculopathies are the reduction or resolution of pain, restoration of sensory or motor loss, return to normal activities of daily living, and prevention of further episodes of radicular symptoms. Treatment sequencing is based on the individual and thus must be guided by the physical exam, the patient's unique circumstances, and the results of current treatments.[14]

There are no studies that directly compare the outcomes of surgery with those of conservative management for cervical radiculopathies. However, retrospective outcome studies on patients treated by medical management, medical management then surgery, and with surgery alone are plentiful. Between 80 and 90 percent of patients with radiculopathies respond well to conservative care.[49,119,120] Analyses of outcome after medical management have not scientifically controlled for specific treatment types to date. Surgical outcomes also have impressive results. Studies that have retrospectively examined outcomes for both surgery after failed conservative management and acute surgical intervention have found good to excellent results in 64 to 90 percent of their patients.[24,25,33,43,45,47,48,121]

Recently there also has been an increasing emphasis on the nonoperative treatment of lumbosacral radiculopathies. The proponents of conservative management can point to success rates of up to 70 to 90 percent.[63–65,122,123] This is, again, comparable to surgical outcomes of good to excellent results in 56 to 90 percent of patients.[124,125] Many studies have directly compared surgical to conservative management within patient populations and found outcomes to be equal.[28,64,126,127] Coexisting spinal stenosis is a major adverse outcome predictor for conservative therapy of lumbosacral radiculopathy.[128]

The best surgical outcomes are seen in patients with symptoms less than 2 months in duration and in discs with frank herniations as opposed to small protrusions.[127] Interestingly, the size of disc herniation or protrusion need not correlate with outcome of either medical or surgical therapy.[65,123,129]

Additional outcome predictors for both surgical and conservative therapy include poor motivation, psychosocial distress, lower education levels, and personality disorders and psychopathology.[124,125,130,131] When medical and surgical therapy fail to relieve pain after 6 months, a diagnosis of chronic pain is established. The diagnosis and treatment of chronic pain are covered elsewhere in this book.

REFERENCES

1. Mixter W, Barr J: Rupture of the intervertebral disc with involvement of the spinal canal. *New Engl J Med* 1934; 211:210–214.
2. Semmes RE, Murphey F: The syndrome of unilateral rupture of the sixth cervical nerve root: A report of four cases with symptoms simulating coronary disease. *JAMA* 1943; 121:1209–1214.
3. Verbiest H: *Neurogenic Intermittent Claudication*. New York: American Elsevier, 1976.
4. Brain WR, Northfield DWC, Wilkinson M: Neurological manifestations of cervical spondylosis. *Brain* 1952; 75:187–225.
5. Wilbourn AJ: Radiculopathies: History and pathophysiology. In Syllabus: AAEE Course D: Radiculopathies. Rochester, MN: American Association of Electromyography and Electrodiagnosis, 1989: 7–10.
6. Netter FH: Musculoskeletal system, Part I, in CIBA Collection Medical Illustrations. Summit NJ, CIBA Geigg Corp. Vol. 5, pp. 9–17.
7. Cailliet R: *Soft Tissue Pain and Disability*. 2nd ed., Philadelphia: F.A. Davis, 1988.
8. Kottke FJ, Mundle MD: Range of mobility of the cervical spine. *Arch Phys Med Rehab* 1959; 40:379–382.
9. Delisa JA: *Rehabilitation Medicine Principles and Practice*, 2nd ed. Philadelphia: J.B. Lippincott, 1993, p. 477.
10. Cailliet R: *Low Back Pain Syndrome*, 4th ed. Philadelphia: F.A. Davis, 1991.
11. Hoppenfeld S: *Physical Examination of the Spine and Extremities*, 1st ed. Norwalk, CT: Appleton Century-Crofts, 1976.
12. Cole AJ, Forral JP, Stratton SA: Cervical Spine Athletic Injuries, in *PM&R Clinics of North America*. Philadelphia: W.B. Saunders, 1994.
13. Bogduk N, Twoney LT: *Clinical Anatomy of the Lumbar Spine*, 2nd ed. New York: Churchill Livingstone, 1991.
14. Ellenberg MR, Honet JC, Trevnor WJ: Cervical radiculopathy. *Arch Phys Med Rehabil* 1994; 75:345–352.
15. Garvey TA, Eismont FJ: Diagnosis and treatment of cervical radiculopathy and myelopathy. *Orthop Rev* 1991; 20:595–603.
16. O'Connell JE: Sciatica and the mechanism of the production of the clinical syndrome in the protrusions of the lumbar intervertebral discs. *Br J Surg* 1942–1943; 30: 315–327.
17. Murphy R: Nerve roots and spinal nerves in degenerative disc disease. *Clin Orthop* 1977; 129:46–60.
18. Rydeuick B, Brown M, Lundburg G: Pathoanatomy and pathophysiology of nerve root compression. *Spine* 1984; 9:7–15.
19. Howe J, Loeser JD, Calvin WH: Mechanosensitivity of dorsal root ganglia and chronically injured axons: a physiologic basis for the radicular pain of nerve root compression. *Pain* 1977; 3:25–41.
20. Lundburg G, Myers R, Powell H: Nerve compression injury and increased endoneurial fluid pressure: A "miniature compartment syndrome." *J Neurol Neurosurg Psychiat* 1983; 46:1119–1124.
21. Nachemson A: A critical look at the treatment for low back pain. *Scand J Rehab Med* 1979; 11:143–147.
22. Saal JS, Franson RC: High levels of inflammatory phospholipase A2 activity in lumbar disc herniations. *Spine* 1990; 15:674–678.
23. Wilburn AJ, Aminoff MJ: AAEM Minimonograph #32: The electrophysiologic examination in patients with radiculopathies. *Am Assoc Electrodiag Med* 1988; 11:1099–1144.
24. Odom GL, Finney W, Woodhall B: Cervical disk lesions. *JAMA* 1958; 166:23–38.
25. Scoville WB, Dohrmann GV, Corkill G: Late results of cervical disc surgery. *J Neurosurg* 1976; 45:203–210.
26. Murphy F, Simmons JCG, Brunson B: Surgical treatment of laterally ruptured cervical discs. *J Neurosurg* 1973; 38:679–683.
27. Yoss RE, Corbin KB, McCarthy CS, Love JG: Significance of symptoms and signs in localization of involved root in cervical disc protrusion. *Neurology* 1957; 7:673–683.
28. Hakelius A: Prognosis in sciatica: A clinical follow up of surgical and non-surgical treatment. *Acta Orthop Scand Supp* 1970; 129:1–70.
29. Kirkaldy-Willis WH: *Managing Low Back Pain*, 1st ed. New York: Churchill Livingstone, 1983.
30. Hanflig SS: Pain in the shoulder girdle, arm and precordium due to foraminal compression of nerve roots. *Arch Surg* 1943; 46:652–663.
31. Saal JS, Saal JJ, Herzog R: The natural history of lumbar intervertebral disk extrusions treated nonoperatively. *Spine* 1990; 15:683–686.

32. Marshall L, Trethewie E, Curtain C: Chemical irritation of nerve root in disc prolapse. *Lancet* 1973; 2:320.

33. Lundsford LD, Bissonette DJ, Jannetta PJ, Sheptak PE, Zorub DS: Anterior surgery for cervical disc disease. Part 1: Treatment of lateral cervical disc herniation in 253 cases. *J Neurosurg* 1980; 53:1–11.

34. Viikari-Juntura E, Porras M, Laasonen EM: Validity of clinical tests in the diagnosis of root compression in cervical disc disease. *Spine* 1989; 14:253–257.

35. Frymoyer JW: Back pain and sciatica. *NEJM* 1988; 318(5):291–300.

36. Garfin SR: A 50-year-old woman with disabling spinal stenosis. *JAMA* 1995; 274(24):1949–1954.

37. Wall EJ, Cohen MS, Mansic JB, et al: Cauda equina anatomy I: Intrathecal nerve root organization. *Spine* 1990; 15(12):1244–1247.

38. Cailliet R: *Functional Anatomy in Neck and Arm Pain*, 3rd ed. Philadelphia: F.A. Davis, 1991.

39. Marzo JM, Simmons EH, Kallen F: Intradural connections between adjacent cervical spinal roots. *Spine* 1987; 12:964–968.

40. Wall EJ, Cohen MS, Abithal JJ, et al: Organization of intrathecal nerve roots at the level at the conus medullaris. *JBJS* 1990; 72(10):1495–1499.

41. Atkinson R, Ghelman B, Tsairis P, Warren RF, Jacobs B, Lavyne M: Sarcoidosis presenting as cervical radiculopathy, a case report and literature review. *Spine* 1982; 7:412–416.

42. Howe JF, Loeser JD, Calvin WH: Mechanosensitivity of dorsal root ganglia and chronically injured axons: A physiological basis for the radicular pain of nerve root compression. *Pain* 1977; 3:25–41.

43. Herkowitz HN, Kurz LT, Overholt DP: Surgical management of cervical soft disc herniation: a comparison between the anterior and posterior approach. *Spine* 1990; 15:1026–1030.

44. McNab I, McCulloch J: *Backache*, 2nd ed. Baltimore: Williams & Wilkins, 1990.

45. Bertalanffy H, Eggert HR: Clinical long-term results of anterior discectomy without fusion for treatment of cervical radiculopathy and myelopathy: A follow-up of 164 cases. *Acta Neurochir* 1988; 90:127–135.

46. Spurling RG, Scoville WB: Lateral rupture of the cervical intervertebral discs: A common cause of shoulder and arm pain. *Surg Gynecol Obstet* 1944; 78:350–358.

47. Yu YL, Woo E, Huang CY: Cervical spondylitic myelopathy and radiculopathy. *Acta Neurol Scand* 1987; 75:367–373.

48. Murphy F, Simmons JCH: Ruptured cervical disc: Experience with 250 cases. *Am Surg* 1966; 32:83–88.

49. Honet JC, Puri K: Cervical radiculitis: treatment and results in 82 patients. *Arch Phys Med Rehabil* 1976; 57:12–16.

50. Braddom RL: *Physical Medicine & Rehabilitation*, 1st ed. Philadelphia: W.B. Saunders, 1996.

51. Henderson CM, Hennessy RG, Shuey HM, Shackelford

EG: Posterior-lateral foraminotomy as an exclusive operative technique for cervical radiculopathy: A review of 846 consecutively operated cases. *Neurosurgery* 1983; 13(5):504–512.

52. Booth RE, Rothman RIE: Cervical angina. *Spine* 1976; 1:28–32.

53. LaBan MM, Mecrschoert JR, Taylor RS: Breast Pain: A Symptom of Cervical Radiculopathy. *Arch Phys Med Rehab* 1979; 60:315–317.

54. Langfitt TW, Elliott FA: Pain in the back and legs caused by cervical spinal cord compression. *JAMA* 1967; 200(5):112–115.

55. Liversedge LA, Hutchinson EC, Lyons JB: Cervical spondylosis simulating motor neuron disease. *Lancet* 1953; 2:652–659.

56. Ehni B, Ehni G, Patterson RH Jr: Extradural spinal cord and nerve root compression from benign lesions of the cervical area, in Youmans JR (ed): *Neurologic Surgery*. Philadelphia: W.B. Saunders, 1990, pp. 2878–2916.

57. Hunt WE, Miller CA: Management of cervical radiculopathy. *Clin Neurosurg* 1986; 33(29):485–502.

58. Adams RD, Victor M (eds): *Principles of Neurology*, 5th ed. New York: McGraw-Hill, 1993, pp. 1100–1103.

59. Upton RM, McConas AJ: The double crush nerve entrapment syndromes. *Lancet* 1973; 2:359.

60. Marianacci AA: A correlation between the operative findings in cervical herniated discs with the electromyograms and opaque myelograms. *Electromyography* 1966; 6:5–29.

61. Langstreth G, Newcomer A: Abdominal pain caused by diabetic radiculopathy. *Ann Int Med* 1977; 86:166–169.

62. Dvorak J, Gavchat MH, Valach L: The outcome of surgery for lumbar disc herniation. I. A 4–17 years' follow-up with emphasis on somatic aspects. *Spine* 1988; 13(12):1418.

63. Johnson EW, Fletcher FE: Lumbosacral radiculopathy. Review of 100 consecutive cases. *Arch Phys Med Rehabil* 1981; 62:321.

64. Weber H: Lumbard disc herniation: A controlled prospective study with ten years of observation. *Spine* 1983; 8(2):131–140.

65. Bush K, Cowen N, Katz DE, Gishen P: The natural history of sciatica associated with disc pathology. *Spine* 1992; 17:1205.

66. Deyo RA, Rainville J: What can the history and physical examination tell us about low back pain? *JAMA* 1992; 268:760–765.

67. Petropoulos B: Lumbar spinal stenosis. *Clin Orthop Rel Res* 1989; 246:70–80.

68. Deyo RA, Diehl AK: Cancer as a cause of back pain: frequency, clinical presentations and diagnostic strategies. *J Gen Int Med* 1988; 3:230–238.

69. U.S. Dept. of Health and Human Services. Clinical Practice Guideline Management of Cancer Pain. 1994; 9:30.

70. Boden SD, Mecowin PR: Abnormal magnetic resonance

Chapter 17

VESTIBULAR DI
AND REHABILIT

Susan J. Herdman

Vestibular rehabilitation techniques provid
to medical and surgical management of p
vestibular disorders. For some disorders, i
mary treatment. Not all vestibular disorde
are effectively treated with these technique
ter will focus on rehabilitation approach
specific vestibular conditions: benign paro
tional vertigo, unilateral vestibular paresis,
disequilibrium. Benign paroxysmal positi
essentially is a biomechanical problem in v
probably fragments of otoconia, move int
semi-circular canals, causing that canal to b
tive to the pull of gravity. The goal of trea
disorder is to provide relief from the vertig
as possible by moving the debris out of the c
eral vestibular paresis is the result of an a
vestibular receptors or neurons. The goal
ment is to improve gaze and postural stabi
disequilibrium may be due to an uncompen
eral or to bilateral vestibular loss. The goal
postural stability and to reduce the perce
balance.

BENIGN PAROXYSMAL
POSITIONAL VERTIGO

Presentation and Pathophysiology

Benign paroxysmal positional vertigo (BPl
terized by periods of vertigo, lasting only
occur when the subject moves his or her h

scans of the cervical spine in asymptomatic subjects. *JBJS* 1990; 72A:1178–1184.

71. Chandrasekar PH: Low back pain and intravenous drug abusers. *Arch Int Med* 1990; 150:1125–1128.

72. Schumacher HR (ed): *Primer on Rheumatic Diseases*, 10th ed. Atlanta: Arthritis Foundation, 1993, pp. 151–168.

73. Herzog R: State of the art imaging of spinal disorders in PM&R *State Art Rev* 1990; 4:221–270.

74. Gore DR, Sepic SB: Roentgenographic Findings of the Cervical Spine in Asymptomatic People. *Spine* 1986; 11(6):521–524.

75. Bates D, Ruggien P: Imaging Modalities for evaluation of the spine. *Radio Clinics N Am* 1991; 29(4):675–690.

76. Deyo RA: Early Diagnostic Evaluation of low back pain. *J Gen Int Med* 1986; 1:331–338.

77. Deyo RA, Diehl AK: Lumbar spine films in primary care; current use and effects of selective ordering criteria. *J Gen Int Med* 1986; 1:20–25.

78. Frymoyer JW: Back pain and sciatica. *NEJM* 1988; 318:291–300.

79. Deyo RA, Bigos SJ: Diagnostic Imaging Procedures for the lumbar spine (editorial). *Ann Int Med* 1989; 111:865–867.

80. Hall FM: Back pain and the radiologist. *Radiology* 1980; 137:861–863.

81. DeLuca SA, Rhea JT: Are routine oblique roentgenograms of the lumbar spine of value? *JBJS* 1981; 63:846.

82. Eisenberg RL, Akin JR: Single, well centered lateral view of lumbosacral spine: is coned view necessary? *Am J Radiol* 1979; 133:711–713.

83. World Health Organization: A rational approach to radiodiagnostic investigations. *WHO Tech Rep Ser* 589. WHO Geneva, 1983; 31.

84. Wiesel SW, Tsourmas N: A study of computer assisted tomography: The incidence of positive CAT scans in an asymptomatic group of patients. *Spine* 1984; 9:549–551.

85. Haughton VM, Eldevik OP: A prospective comparison of computed tomography and myelography in the diagnosis of herniated lumbar disks. *Radiology* 1982; 142:103–110.

86. Boden SD, Davis DO: Abnormal magnetic resonance scans of the lumbar spine in asymptomatic patients. *JBJS* 1990; 72A:403–408.

87. Aminoff MJ: Clinical electromyography, in *Electrodiagnosis in Clinical Neurology,* 2nd ed. New York: Churchill Livingstone, 1986, pp. 231–263.

88. Jensen MC, Brant-Zawadzki MN: Magnetic resonance imaging in people without back pain. *NEJM* 1994; 331:69–73.

89. Weinreb JC, Wolbarsht LB: Prevalence of lumbosacral intervertebral disc abnormalities in MR images in pregnant and asymptomatic nonpregnant women. *Radiology* 1989; 170:125–128.

90. Deyo RD: Magnetic resonance imaging of the lumbar spine: Terrific test or tar baby? (editorial). *NEJM* 1994; 331:115–116.

91. Spindler HA, Felsenthal G: Electrodiagnostic evaluation of acute and chronic radiculopathy, in Electromyography: A Guide for Referring Physicians. *PM&R Clin North Amer* 1990; 1:53–68.

92. Weichers DO: Radiculopathies, STARS. *Clin Electrophysiol* 1989; 3:4, 713–724.

93. Kimura J: Abuse and misuse of evoked potentials as a diagnostic test. *Arch Neurol* 1985; 42:78–80.

94. Teale C, Mulley GP: Support collars: A preliminary survey of their benefits and problems. *Clin Rehabil* 1990; 4:33.

95. Johnson RM, Hart DL: Cervical Orthoses: A study comparing their effectiveness in restricting cervical motion in normal subjects. *JBJS* 1977; 59A:332–339.

96. Naylor JR, Malley GP: Surgical collars: A survey of their prescriptions and use. *Br J Rheumatol* 1991; 30:282.

97. Tan JC, Nordin M: The role of physical therapy in the treatment of cervical disc disease. *Orth Clin North Am* 1992; 23:435–449.

98. Haimovic IC, Beresford HR: Dexamethasone is not superior to placebo for treating lumbosacral radicular pain. *Neurology* 1986; 36:1593–1594.

99. Harris MI, Glass JP: Steroids for lumbar radiculopathy (letter). *Neurology* 1987; 37:1689.

100. Green LN: Steroids for lumbar radiculopathy (letter). *Neurology* 1987; 37:1689–1690.

101. Longstreth WT: Steroids for lumbar radiculopathy (letter). *Neurology* 1987; 37:1690.

102. Bush K, Conan N: The natural history of sciatica associated with disc pathology. *Spine* 1992; 17:1205–1212.

103. Bush K, Hillier S: A controlled study of caudal epidural injections of triamcinolone plus procaine in the management of intractable sciatical. *Spine* 1991; 16:572–573.

104. Dilke TFW, Burry HC: Extradural corticosteroid injection in management of lumbar nerve root compression. *BMJ* 1973; 2:635–637.

105. Ridley MG, Kingsley GH: Out-patient lumbar epidural corticosteroid injection in the management of sciatica. *Br J Rheumatol* 1988; 27:295–299.

106. Bowman SJ, Wedderburn L: Outcome assessment after epidural corticosteroid injection for low back pain and sciatica. *Spine* 1993; 18:1345–1350.

107. Shulman J: Treatment of neck pain with cervical epidural steroid injection. *Reg Anesthesiol* 1986; 11:92–94.

108. Rowlingson JC, Kirschenbaum LP: Epidural analgesic techniques in the management of cervical pain. *Anesthesiol Analg* 1986; 65:938–942.

109. Warfield Ca, Biber MP: Epidural steroid injection as a treatment for cervical radiculitis. *Clin J Pain* 1988; 4:201–204.

110. Benzon HT: Epidural steroid injections for low back pain and lumbosacral radiculopathy. *Pain* 1986; 24:277–295.

111. Lehmann JF (ed): *Therapeutic Heat and Cold*. Philadelphia: Williams & Wilkins, 1990, pp. 417–581.

112. Martin G, Corbin K: An evaluation of conservative treatment for patients with cervical disk syndrome. *Arch Phys Med Rehab* 1954; 35:87–92.

113. British Association of Physical Medicine: Pain and arm: A multicentre trial of the effects of apy. *Br Med J* 1966; 1:253–258.

114. Goldie I, Landquist A: Evaluation of the effec ent forms of physiotherapy in cervical pain. *Scc Med* 1970; 2–3:117–121.

115. Colachis S, Strohm B: Effect of duration of i cervical traction on vertebral separation. *Arci Rehab* 1966; 47:353–359.

116. Cheatle MD, Esterhai JL: Pelvic traction as tr acute back pain: Efficacious, benign or delete 1991; 16;12:1379–1381.

117. Judovich BD: Lumbar traction therapy—eli physical factors that prevent lumbar stre 1955; 159:549.

118. Colachis SC, Strohm BR: Effects of intermitt on separation of lumbar vertebrae. *Arch Phys* 1969; 50:251–258.

119. Rubin D: Cervical radiculitis: Diagnosis anc *Arch Phys Med Rehabil* 1960; 41:580–586.

120. Martin GM, Corbin KB: Evaluation of conser ment for patients with cervical disc syndrome *Med Rehabil* 1954; 35:87–92.

121. Henderson CM, Hennessy RG, Shuey HM, EG: Posterior-lateral foraminotomy as an exc ative technique for cervical radiculopthy: A r consecutively operated cases. *Neurosui* 13(5):504–512.

122. Pearce J, Moll JMH: Conservative treatment history of acute lumbar disc lesions. *J Neurc Psychiatr* 1967; 30:13–17.

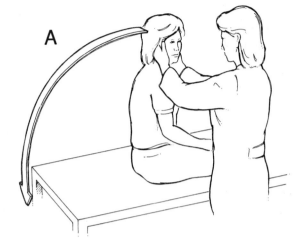

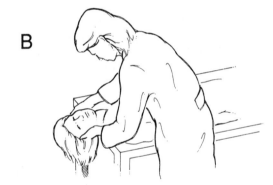

Figure 17-1
Hallpike-Dix maneuver. The patient is moved rapidly from sitting into a supine position with the head turned so that the affected ear is 30 degrees below the horizontal in order to stimulate the posterior canal and produce vertigo and nystagmus in most patients with BPPV. (Reprinted with permission from Herdman SJ (ed): Vestibular Rehabilitation. *Philadelphia, FA Davis, 1994.)*

(Figure 17-2A,B). The resulting excitation of the sensory receptors produces vertigo, nystagmus, and nausea. Although this theory adequately accounts for the latency of onset of the nystagmus and vertigo of BPPV, it does not explain the brief duration of the nystagmus and vertigo. Debris adhering to the cupula would cause the cupula to be deflected for as long as the head remained in the provoking position. Although there might be a gradual decrease in vertigo and nystagmus owing to central adaptation, the vertigo and nystagmus should persist.

A second theory, canalithiasis, was proposed by Hall, Ruby, and McClure, who suggested that the degenerative debris is not adherent to the cupula of the posterior canal but instead is floating freely in the endolymph within the semicircular canal.[5] When the head is moved into the provoking position, the debris slowly moves to the most dependent position within the canal (Figure 17-2C,D). The falling otoconia moves the endolymph, which in turn overcomes the inertia of the cupula, exciting the neurons. The latency of the response is related to the time it takes for the cupula to be deflected by the movement of the endolymph. The increase in vertigo and nystagmus that occurs is related to the relative deflection of the cupula. The decrease in vertigo and nystagmus as the position is maintained is due to cessation of endolymph movement and the return of the cupula to its normal alignment. This theory recently has been supported by the observation of a milky debris within the long arm of the posterior canal in patients with BPPV.[6] The debris clearly moves when the position of the head is altered.

Treatment Approaches

Several approaches have been developed to treat patients with BPPV. Some treatments are based on the idea that debris embedded in the cupula of the posterior canal can be dislodged by repeatedly moving the patient into the position that provokes the vertigo. An alternative treatment attempts to move the debris out of the posterior canal by moving the patient's head through a series of positions.

Brandt-Daroff Habituation Exercises Proposed by Brandt et al., the treatment requires the patient to move into the provoking position repeatedly, several times a day.[7] The patient is first sitting and then rapidly moves into the position that causes the vertigo and nystagmus (Figure 17-3). The severity of the vertigo usually is directly related to how rapidly the patient moves into the provoking position. The patient stays in that position

Table 17-1
Clinical features of benign paroxysmal positional vertigo

Positional vertigo

Latency of onset of symptoms from provocative position

Nystagmus, concomitant with symptoms

Fatiguable symptoms and nystagmus (<60 seconds)

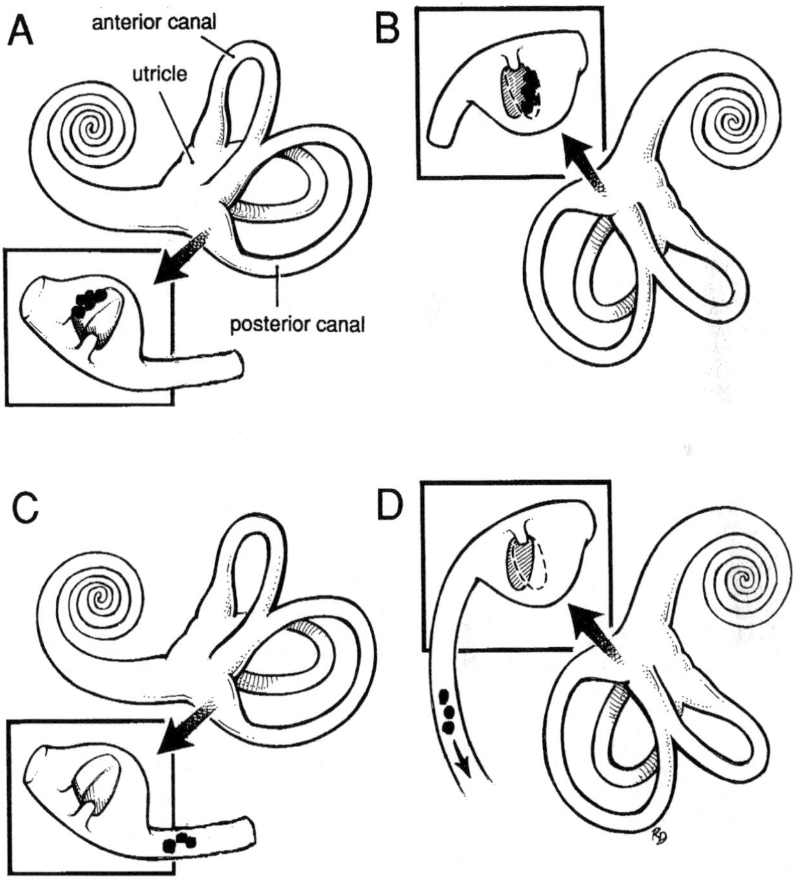

Figure 17-2
When the debris is adhering to the cupula of the posterior canal (A), movement of the patient into the Hallpike-Dix position (B) will result in distortion of the cupula owing to the pull of gravity. Debris floating freely in the long arm of the posterior canal (C) will drift to the most dependent position in the canal (D) when the patient is moved into the Hallpike-Dix position, also resulting in movement of the cupula. (Reprinted with permission from Herdman SJ et al: Single-treatment approaches to benign paroxysmal positional vertigo. Arch Otolaryngol Head Neck Surg 1993; 119:450.)

until the vertigo stops, plus an additional 30 seconds, and then sits up. Moving into the sitting position usually results in vertigo, although this "rebound effect" will be less severe and of a shorter duration. Nystagmus, if it reoccurs, will be in the opposite direction. The patient remains in the upright position for 30 seconds and then moves rapidly into the mirror-image position on the other side, stays there for 30 seconds and then sits up. The patient then repeats the entire maneuver 10 to 20 times. The entire sequence is repeated three times a day until the patient has two consecutive days without vertigo.

Patients must work through the vertigo and the accompanying nausea that may occur while performing these exercises. Usually these complaints disappear quickly when the patient is moved out of the provoking position or as the vertigo decreases. Repeated positional changes may cause a prolonged and generalized disequi-

librium with persistent nausea, however. This may be disturbing enough that the patient stops the exercises. Patients should be warned that this may occur and that it is only a temporary effect. Usually modifying the exercises (reducing the repetitions for a while) or regulating the time during the day when the exercises are performed effectively controls these problems, but medication, such as Phenergan, can be taken half an hour before the exercises are performed.

It is not clear why these exercises result in a decrease in the vertigo and nystagmus. One explanation is that the debris becomes dislodged from the cupula of the posterior canal and moves to a location no longer affecting the cupula during head movement. This would seem to be most likely if the debris were adhering to the utricular side of the cupula. A second possibility is that habituation occurs, reducing the nervous system response to the signal from the posterior canal. Brandt

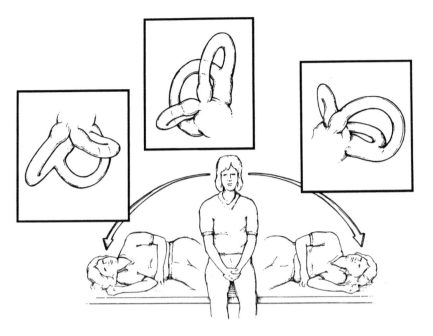

Figure 17-3
Brandt-Daroff habituation exercises. The patient moves quickly from sitting into the side-lying position that produces vertigo and stays in that position until the vertigo stops plus an additional 30 seconds. The patient then sits up again and remains in the upright position for at least 30 seconds. Then the patient moves rapidly into the mirror-image side-lying position, stays there for 30 seconds, and then sits up. The entire maneuver is repeated until the vertigo diminishes. (Modified from Brandt T, Daroff RB: Physical therapy for benign paroxysmal positional vertigo. Arch Otolaryngol 1980; 106:484–485.)

and Daroff argue against habituation as a mechanism for recovery because many patients recover abruptly.[7]

Liberatory Maneuver This treatment also is based on the theory that the debris is adherent to the cupula. In the Liberatory maneuver, as in the Brandt and Daroff habituation exercises, the provoking position must be identified first.[7,8] Once the side of involvement has been identified, the patient is quickly moved into the provoking side-lying position with the head turned into the plain of the posterior canal and is kept in that position for 2 to 3 minutes (Figure 17-4). The patient is then rapidly moved up through the sitting position and down into the opposite side-lying position, with the therapist maintaining the alignment of the neck and head on the body (the face then is angled down toward the bed). Typically, nystagmus and vertigo reappear in this second position. If the patient does not experience vertigo in this second position, the head is abruptly shaken once or twice, using low amplitude movements, presumably freeing the debris. The patient stays in this position for several minutes. The patient then is slowly taken into a seated position. The patient must then keep his head in a vertical (upright) position for 48 hours (including while sleeping) and must avoid the provoking position for 1 week following the treatment. We recommend that the patient be fitted with a soft cervical collar to wear during the first 48-hour period as a reminder to keep the head upright. Unlike the exercises suggested by Brandt and Daroff, the Liberatory maneuver usually requires only a single treatment. Presumably this treatment is effective because the debris is dislodged from the cupula during the maneuver.

Canalith Repositioning Maneuver This treatment approach is based on the theory that the debris is floating in the endolymph in the long arm of the semicircular canal.[9] Hall, Ruby, and McClure hypothesized that with repeated movement of the head into the precipitating position, some of the debris moves out of the posterior canal, thereby reducing the response.[5] This idea was refined by Epley, who described a specific sequence of head positions that would result in movement of the debris out of the posterior canal, through the common crus and into the vestibule.[9] Several modifications of the treatment Epley developed have been used, most involving changes in the timing of the movements.[10,11] First, the patient is moved rapidly into the Hallpike-Dix position that provokes the symptoms and is kept in that position for several minutes (Figure 17-5). The head then is slowly turned to the opposite Hallpike-Dix position, keeping the neck extended during the move-

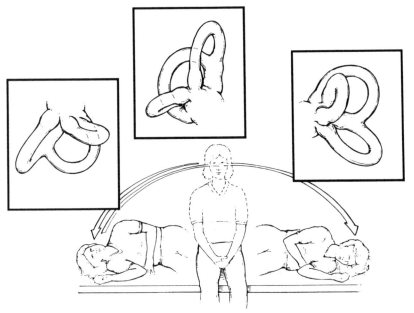

Figure 17-4
Liberatory maneuver. The patient turns his head 45 degrees away from the affected side and then moves quickly into the position that provokes the vertigo, staying in that position for 2 to 3 minutes. He then is turned rapidly to the opposite ear down with the therapist maintaining the alignment of the neck and head on the body. The patient stays in this position for 5 minutes. The patient is then slowly taken into a seated position. He must remain in a vertical position for 48 hours and must avoid the provoking position for 1 week. (Reprinted with permission from Herdman SJ et al: Single-treatment approaches to benign paroxysmal positional vertigo. Arch Otolaryngol Head Neck Surg 1993; 119:450.)

ment. The patient then rolls into the opposite side-lying position with the head turned 45 degrees toward the floor. The patient remains in this position for several minutes and then slowly sits up. As with the "Liberatory maneuver," the patient must then remain in an upright position for 48 hours and avoid bending forward, looking up or down with the head, or lying down. For 5 more days the patient is advised not to lie on the affected side. Epley suggests using vibration over the mastoid during the treatment to facilitate the movement of the debris. The use of vibration is not universally accepted. Concern that more debris could be dislodged from the utricle and float into the posterior canal has been raised by some who advocate against vibration. Treatment results are similar to those of Epley and others who advocate the use of vibration.[9,10,12]

Treatment Efficacy

Studies on the efficacy of these treatments indicate that they facilitate the remission of vertigo in patients with BPPV.[7–10] The results of these studies must be interpreted cautiously, however, because of the high incidence of spontaneous remission that occurs in patients with BPPV. Several authors have reported spontaneous remission in as many as 60 percent of all patients with BPPV within 3 to 4 weeks, although Brandt and Daroff suggest that it may be months before the vertigo disappears, if left untreated.[7,8,13]

Brandt and Daroff studied a series of 67 patients with histories of BPPV of 2 days' to 8 months' duration.[7] None of these patients had evidence of other neurological or neuro-otological disease. Fully 95 percent of subjects had no symptoms after 3 to 14 days of exercises. The only subject who did not respond to treatment had a

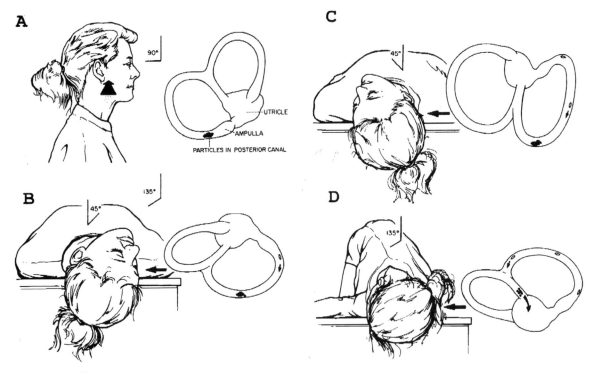

Figure 17-5

Canalith repositioning maneuver. The patient is quickly moved from sitting (A) into the Hallpike-Dix position with the affected ear down (B). The patient is kept in that position for 2 to 3 minutes and then the head slowly is moved through extension until the opposite ear is down (C). The patient stays in that position briefly (until any vertigo stops) and then is rolled onto the shoulder opposite the affected ear so that the head is pointed 45 degrees toward the floor (D). The patient stays in that position for 2 to 3 minutes and then slowly sits up. The patient must then remain with the head in an upright position for 48 hours and must avoid lying on the affected side for 5 days after that. (Reprinted with permission from Parnes LS, Price-Jones RG: Particle repositioning maneuver for benign paroxysmal positional vertigo. Ann Otol Rhinol Laryngol 1993; 102:325.)

perilymph fistula requiring surgical repair. Anecdotally, the time until patients are symptom-free or have at least a moderate reduction in symptoms may be more protracted in patients with a prolonged history of the disorder. The more protracted the course, the more resistant BPPV is to treatment.

The Liberatory maneuver also appears to be an effective treatment. Semont et al. report a "cure" rate of 84 percent after a single treatment and 93 percent after two treatments in a series of 711 patients with BPPV treated with the Liberatory maneuver over an 8-year period.[8] In a different study of 30 patients with posterior canal BPPV, the remission rate after a single treatment using the Liberatory maneuver was 70 per-

cent, with improvement in symptoms in another 20 percent.[10]

Epley and others have reported remission of vertigo in better than 85 percent of subjects treated using the Canalith repositioning maneuver.[9–12] It is clear that it is important with this treatment to move the patient's head to the 45-degree nose-down orientation, in order for the treatment to be effective. In one study, the maneuver was first performed with the patient's head moved only into the opposite Hallpike-Dix orientation (Figure 17-5C) and the effectiveness of the treatment in achieving complete remission of vertigo with a single treatment was only 57 percent.[10] The results after repeated treatments using a complete "roll" (Figure 17-

5D), however, were similar to those reported by Epley and others (92 percent asymptomatic).[9,10] The more complete roll assures that the debris will move from the long arm of the posterior canal into the common crus.

In summary, comparison of studies of the different treatment approaches for BPPV would suggest that there is similar success with all treatments. We can design treatments suited to individual patients, therefore, with the confidence that the final outcome will be similar.

Anterior and Horizontal Canal BPPV

BPPV involving the anterior or horizontal canals has been reported in several studies.[14–16] Infra-red recordings of the eye movements made while patients were moved into the provoking position and when they returned to a sitting position in 161 patients with a diagnosis of benign paroxysmal positional vertigo have been reviewed carefully.[14] Of these patients, 65 percent had nystagmus consistent with posterior semicircular canal involvement (upbeating and torsional), 12 percent had nystagmus consistent with anterior canal involvement (downbeating and torsional), and 2.5 percent had nystagmus consistent with horizontal canal involvement (geotropic horizontal nystagmus suggesting canalithiasis or ageotropic horizontal nystagmus suggesting cupulolithiasis). In 20.5 percent, the particular canal involved could not be determined. Seventy-three percent ($n = 24$) of these later patients had torsional nystagmus, indicating that either the posterior or the anterior canal was involved, but there was no obvious vertical component. In only 5.5 percent of the 161 patients was it impossible to identify any canal component. These patients closed their eyes with the onset of the vertigo, made excessive saccadic eye movements, or blinked rapidly, and the direction of the nystagmus could not be determined. The identification of canal involvement was made by examining the initial nystagmus when the patient was moved into the provoking position in only 79 percent of the patients. In the other patients, the identification of the canal involved was based on the observation of the reversal phase of the nystagmus as the patient remained in that position, or of the nystagmus that occurred when the patient returned to a sitting position.

The identification of the specific canal involved influences which treatment approach will be effective. It has been suggested that the Canalith repositioning maneuver is appropriate for treatment of anterior canal BPPV, but the Liberatory maneuver is unlikely to result in remission of symptoms because of the orientation of the anterior canal during the maneuver.[14] It has been suggested also that a modification of the Canalith repositioning maneuver can be used in the treatment of horizontal canal BPPV.[17] Often it is difficult to determine the affected side in horizontal canal BPPV, because the patient develops nystagmus and vertigo when moved into both the right and the left sidelying positions (Figure 17-6) as the debris in the endolymph of the horizontal canal shifts toward or away from the cupula.[15] The side that results in greater symptomatic complaints usually is considered to be the affected side in horizontal canal BPPV. In treatment, the patient would first be moved into a supine position, with the head turned toward the affected side. The head is then turned away from that side toward the less symptomatic side. The patient is then rolled onto the less symptomatic side, onto the stomach, and then over into the supine position. The patient then sits up.[17] As in treatment for posterior and anterior canal BPPV, the patient is advised not to lie down or bend over for 48 hours. The efficacy of treatment for horizontal canal BPPV has not yet been determined, primarily because this disorder is much less common that either posterior or anterior canal BPPV and because its spontaneous remission rate has not been established.

Postural Disturbances

Patients with BPPV also may complain of disequilibrium and may have abnormal postural responses.[18,19] The basis for this instability is not known. One possibility is that it is related directly to the abnormal signal from the affected canal that results from the presence of debris. Second, it may be related to horizontal canal paresis. Statistically significant abnormal responses to caloric irrigations have been reported to occur in up to 47 percent of patients with BPPV, suggesting that decreased horizontal canal function may contribute to the patient's complaints of instability. Voorhees suggests that the postural instability in some patients may be related to concurrent head injury. Tests of postural stability should be an integral part of the assessment of patients with BPPV who complain of balance problems, in order to develop an appropriate treatment plan.

Treatment Guidelines

A rare complication of the Canalith repositioning maneuver is the conversion of posterior canal BPPV to either anterior or horizontal canal BPPV, presumably because of movement of the free-floating debris from

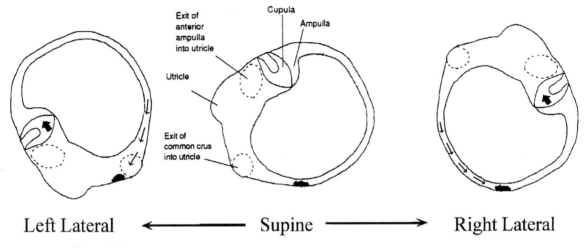

Figure 17-6
Proposed mechanism for horizontal canal BPPV if debris is floating freely in the long arm of the canal. Moving the patient to either the right or the left lateral position will result in movement of the debris within the endolymph of the canal and therefore cause the cupula to move, resulting in nystagmus and vertigo. (Modified from Baloh et al: Horizontal semicircular canal variant of benign positional vertigo. Neurology *1993; 43:2542.)*

one canal into another.[20] In a retrospective study of a consecutive sample of 85 patients diagnosed with posterior canal BPPV and treated with the Canalith repositioning maneuver, 5.8 percent developed anterior canal ($n = 2$) or horizontal canal ($n = 3$) positional vertigo following use of this maneuver. Careful observation of the direction of the nystagmus is necessary for correct identification of which canal is involved in those patients who do not respond to the initial treatment using the Canalith repositioning maneuver. Also it is advisable to observe the direction of the nystagmus during the treatment because if the debris is moving toward the common crus, the nystagmus always should be in the same direction. A change in the direction would indicate that the debris has moved back into the posterior canal or into another canal.

Patients, especially those with long histories of BPPV, may have anxiety about moving into the provoking position. Brandt's exercises may be modified so that the patient has more control over the position change and gradually becomes less fearful of provoking the vertigo and nausea. Also, patients may prefer to perform the exercises on the floor, rather than on the bed, since they know they will not fall. The anxious patient, however, may move out of the provoking position too quickly when attempting to do the exercises on his or her own, or may move too slowly into the position in order to avoid provoking the vertigo.

The impact of anxiety on the patient should not be underestimated. Patients with longstanding BPPV may become so fearful of provoking the vertigo that they tie one arm down at night to keep from rolling over onto the "bad side." Those who are especially anxious or fearful may be treated more easily using either the Liberatory or the Canalith repositioning maneuver, because they will experience the vertigo only one or two times.

Cervical and back pain may preclude the use of the Liberatory or Canalith repositioning maneuvers, or may be aggravated by the repeated positional changes of Brandt's exercises. Older patients may be less tolerant of the Liberatory and Canalith repositioning maneuvers, especially if they move cautiously because of other conditions, such as arthritis. In the Canalith repositioning maneuver, neck extension can be avoided by using a tilted treatment table (achieving the same orientation of the vertical canals during treatment). The positional changes used in Brandt's exercises also can be modified to enable the patient to perform them with ease. Care should be taken, however, in using any of these procedures in patients with osteoporosis or after previous neck injury or surgery.

VESTIBULAR PARESIS AND LOSS

Presentation and Pathophysiology

Vestibular paresis and loss typically disrupt gaze and postural stability, leading to vertigo, disequilibrium, and oscillopsia during head movements. Treatment of these vestibular deficits must address the problems associated with changes in the vestibulo-ocular reflex, postural control, and general physical condition. Results from studies on experimental animals and in human beings with unilateral or bilateral vestibular deficits suggest that a proper program of exercises enhances compensation.[21–26]

Unilateral Vestibular Paresis The underlying causes of unilateral vestibular loss include viruses and other inflammatory processes, vascular events, and trauma. Patients with sudden onset of unilateral vestibular loss usually complain of severe vertigo and nausea that lasts for 12 hours or more and gradually resolves over several days. Vertical diplopia and inability to stand up are common. The imbalance in the tonic or resting firing rate of the vestibular system results in spontaneous nystagmus, a skew deviation, and an asymmetry in postural muscle activity even when the patient is standing quietly. Recovery of the tonic vestibular system occurs spontaneously, within a few days from onset. The persistence of spontaneous nystagmus in the light or of a skew deviation for more than 1 week suggests a central lesion that may be preventing or slowing compensation. Patients with unilateral vestibular dysfunction also have an imbalance in the dynamic vestibular system that results in decreased gain of the vestibular-ocular reflex (VOR) and a gait ataxia.

The disruption of the vestibulo-ocular reflex during the acute stage after unilateral vestibular loss is well documented in both animals and human beings.[27–32] After unilateral neuronitis, labyrinthectomy, or vestibular nerve section, VOR gain is decreased to 30 to 50 percent of normal.[30,32] Halmagyi et al. reported average VOR gain of .25 1 week after unilateral vestibular nerve section at head velocities of approximately 120 deg/sec.[31] Recovery of the dynamic function of the vestibular system does not occur spontaneously. The VOR, and probably the vestibulospinal reflex (VSR), requires a combination of head movement and a visual input to produce an error signal to induce an increase in the gain of the vestibular response. This recovery period can be expected to last 6 weeks or more.

Bilateral Vestibular Loss The most common cause of bilateral vestibular loss (BVL) probably is the use of ototoxic medications, such as certain aminoglycosides and chemotherapeutic drugs. BVL also can occur as the result of spontaneous, sequential unilateral loss, or as a consequence of an autoimmune process. Unless the loss occurs sequentially or is asymmetric, patients with BVL do not complain of vertigo, nor do they have spontaneous nystagmus or a skew deviation. Patients with BVL do manifest a profound oscillopsia and have severe gait ataxia initially. Although some recovery of the vestibular system itself may occur in patients with BVL, functional recovery of gaze and postural stability primarily occurs as the result of other compensatory mechanisms. The recovery period can be prolonged. Changes in postural stability, for example, continue to occur for 2 years after bilateral vestibular loss.

Goals of Rehabilitation

The goals of physical therapy intervention in patients with unilateral vestibular paresis or with bilateral vestibular loss are to improve the patient's functional balance and mobility, general physical condition and activity level, safety during ambulation and other gait-related activities, and to decrease the magnitude of the patient's symptoms. Patients usually are seen on an outpatient basis and are instructed in a home exercise program. In some cases, the initial treatments will occur while the patient is in the hospital. The physical therapist must clarify to the patient the treatment goals and the potential effects of exercise in order to motivate the patient to perform the exercises on a regular basis.

Gaze Stability The functional equivalent of the VOR is the ability to see clearly during head movements. Movement of the head while attempting to fixate on a target has the potential to cause significant retinal slip, and therefore degradation of visual acuity, unless the VOR and other mechanisms can produce an appropriate compensatory eye movement. The compensatory eye movement does not have to perfectly match the head movement because 2 to 4 deg/sec of retinal slip can be tolerated without degradation of visual acuity.[33,34]

The requirements to achieve gaze stability vary with the task the person is performing. When the body is relatively stable, such as while sitting or standing, there is little head movement, and the requirements for gaze stability are minimal. Visually guided eye movements, such as visual tracking, are sufficient to maintain gaze stability.[35–37] During locomotion, however, the velocity and frequency of head movements are above the compensatory ability of visually guided eye movements and are random.[38,39] This "randomness" is a significant factor, because under these conditions, predictive eye movements will not help to stabilize gaze, and some degradation of visual acuity might be expected even in normal subjects.

Mechanisms involved in the recovery of gaze stability following vestibular loss include the recovery of the vestibular system itself, potentiation of the cervico-ocular reflex, improved visual tracking, central preprogramming, changes in saccadic amplitude, and restricting head movements.[40–43] Various studies support the premise that there is considerable variability among patients as to which compensatory mechanisms will be utilized.[40,43,44]

Vestibulo-Ocular Reflex (VOR) Recovery of gaze stability may result in part from recovery of the VOR itself. Allum et al. and Paige report that VOR gain improves with time after unilateral vestibular loss and is within normal limits in 1 to 3 months.[30,32] Other studies suggest an even more prolonged recovery period, lasting up to 3 years.[45] Halmagyi et al., however, found no significant increase in horizontal VOR gain at 1 year post-surgery, presumably because they used rapid, unpredictable head movements.[31] VOR gain recovers partially in some patients with bilateral vestibular loss as well, but only to relatively low velocity head movements.[46] Recovery of vestibular function itself, therefore, may contribute to the recovery of gaze stability, but only with lower velocity, predictable head movements.

Cervico-Ocular Reflex (COR) The COR is a compensatory eye movement generated by inputs from receptors in ligaments and joints in the upper cervical region.[47] These somatosensory inputs go to the contralateral vestibular nuclei, and presumably produce a compensatory eye movement that parallels the VOR. In normal individuals, the presence of the COR is variable and, when present, accounts for, at most, a gain of 0.2 eye velocity over rotation.[41,43,48,49]

The COR does not appear to contribute to the recovery of gaze stability following UVL.[44] In contrast, the COR in patients with bilateral vestibular loss appears to have a higher gain, and to produce significant eye movements across a wider range of frequencies than in normal subjects. For example, the gain of the COR in BVL patients rotated at 0.5 Hz in the dark varies from 0.36 to 1.01, depending on the test conditions.[40] Bronstein et al. found the gain of the COR to be as high as 0.8 in some subjects at low frequencies.[41] Although the gain decreased to approximately 0.24 at 0.3 Hz, it was still greater than that of normal subjects (0.02). Chambers et al. suggest that the COR can function to produce compensatory eye movements for the unpredictable head movements of normal activities.[43] The frequency range of the COR appears to be too low to contribute significantly during activities such as walking, however.

Central Pre-programming The role of central preprogramming of compensatory eye movements to improve gaze stability has been demonstrated in normal and in vestibular-deficient subjects in numerous studies, primarily by comparing the gain of the compensatory eye movements during active and passive head movements.[38,40,41,44,46] Kasai and Zee demonstrated the influence of centrally pre-programmed eye movements in several experiments on patients with bilateral vestibular loss.[40] They showed that when subjects could anticipate the next position of a target that moved between two positions, gaze stability improved.[40]

Saccadic Eye Movements and Visual Tracking Numerous studies have demonstrated that patients with bilateral vestibular deficits alter saccadic eye movements as a part of a compensatory strategy adopted to improve gaze stability. Saccade amplitude may be attenuated during combined eye and head movements, or both slow-phase and saccadic eye movements executed in the same direction during trunk on body rotation.[40,50]

Postural Stability Most patients with vestibular loss complain of postural instability only when they are standing or, especially, walking. The exception would be during the immediate period after onset when the patient may be disoriented because of severe vertigo. Maintaining postural stability during quiet stance is not a difficult task and most patients are able to perform this normally within a few days from onset. Movement of the head, however, will result in a decrease in postural stability. The velocity and frequency of horizontal head movements during walking, for example, range from 20 to 79 deg/sec and from 0.7 to 1.2 Hz, and can cause considerable instability.[51,52] Furthermore, during ambulation these head movements occur in a random and unpredictable manner.

The mechanisms of recovery of postural stability are less well understood than is recovery of gaze stability. This is, at least in part, because it is difficult to assess the contribution of just the vestibulo-spinal system to postural stability. In general, it is believed that recovery is in part due to recovery of the vestibular system itself. The substitution of visual and somatosensory cues for lost vestibular function also is significant, especially in those patients with severe vestibular deficits. A study on the course of recovery of patients with complete bilateral vestibular deficits over a 2-year period has shown that patients switch the sensory cues on which they rely.[53] Initially, patients rely on visual cues as a substitute for the loss of vestibular cues. Over time, they become more reliant on somatosensory cues to maintain balance. In this study, patients were required to maintain balance when facing a moving visual surround. Over a 2-year study period, they recovered the ability to maintain their balance to within normal limits in the testing paradigm, except at high frequencies. The vestibular system functions at higher frequencies than the visual or somatosensory systems. This accounts for why neither visual nor somatosensory cues can substitute completely for loss of vestibular cues.

Treatment Approaches

The use of exercises in the treatment of patients with vertigo owing to peripheral vestibular disorders was introduced by Sir Terence Cawthorne, an otolaryngologist, and by F. S. Cooksey, a physiotherapist, in the 1940s.[54,55] The use of these and similar exercises has continued to be advocated as an important intervention strategy in the rehabilitation of vestibular patients and have been modified as our knowledge about vestibular function has changed.[56-64]

Cawthorne-Cooksey Exercises The Cawthorne-Cooksey exercises were developed for patients with unilateral vestibular deficits and post-concussive disorders.[54,55] These exercises consist of a sequence of progressively more complex movements, including movements of the head, tasks requiring coordination of eye and head movement, total body movements, and balance tasks (Table 17-2). Cawthorne and Cooksey also suggested that patients should be trained to function in "busy" environments, such as grocery stores and malls. These environments are particularly challenging to patients with vestibular disorders because of the rich visual environment and movement. Although no controlled studies have been performed to determine the effectiveness of the Cawthorne-Cooksey exercises, Hecker et al. reported that 84 percent of a group of patients with vestibular disorders showed improved function following a course of rehabilitation using these exercises.[57]

Table 17-2

Cawthorne-Cooksey exercises for patients with vestibular hypofunction

A. In bed
  1. Eye movements—at first slow, then quick
    a. up and down
    b. side to side
    c. focusing on finger moving from 3 feet to 1 foot away from face
  2. Head movements at first slow, then quick; later with eyes closed
    a. bending forward and backward
    b. turning from side to side
B. Sitting (in class)
  1. 2 as above
  2. shoulder shrugging and circling
  3. bending forward and picking up objects from the ground
C. Standing (in class)
  1. as A1 and A2 and B3
  2. changing from sitting to standing position with eyes open and shut
  3. throwing a small ball from hand to hand (above eye level)
  4. throwing ball from hand to hand under knee
  5. changing form sitting to standing and turning round in between
D. Moving about (in class)
  1. circle round center person who will throw a large ball and to whom it will be returned
  2. walk across room with eyes open and then closed
  3. walk up and down slope with eyes open and then closed
  4. walk up and down steps with eyes open and then closed
  5. any game involving stooping and stretching and aiming such as skittles, bowls, or basketball

  Diligence and perseverance are required but the earlier and more regularly the exercise regimen is carried out, the faster and more complete will be the return to normal activity.

Reprinted with permission from Dix MR: The rationale and technique of head exercises in the treatment of vertigo. *Acta Oto-Rhino-Laryngol Belg* 1979; 33:370.

Vestibular Adaptation Exercises Adaptation exercises take into consideration the mechanisms identified to induce changes in gain in the vestibular system.[60,61] Movement of images across the retina (retinal slip) during head movement is one error signal that produces adaptive changes in the vestibular system, although retinal slip alone can also produce significant changes in vestibular gain.[65,66]

Experimentally, several different approaches have been used to induce adaptation of the VOR in normal subjects. These approaches include the use of magnifying or minifying glasses, and forced oscillations inside an optokinetic drum.[65,67,68] These paradigms are used to modify the vestibular system slowly, over a period of days, which would not be appropriate for patients with vestibular disturbances. Several studies have shown, however, that VOR gain changes can occur within minutes.[69–72] Post and Lott have obtained changes in VOR gain in normal subjects with four minutes of active head rotation, while fixating a target moving in a direction opposite to the head motion.[73] Furthermore, Pfaltz has shown that brief periods of unidirectional optokinetic stimulation (30 sec, 10 times daily for 10 days) can produce VOR changes in human beings following unilateral vestibular loss compared to non-treated patients.[74]

Exercises to induce vestibular adaptation in patients with vestibular loss use brief periods of exercises, performed several times daily, to attempt to induce recovery of gaze stability and to improve visual acuity in patients with vestibular deficits. These exercises are designed to produce retinal slip in order to induce vestibular adaptation. They also are performed actively, which may potentiate the cervico-ocular reflex and central pre-programming (Figure 17-7). In each exercise, the "error signal" is the small amount of retinal slip produced during the head movement because of the inadequate VOR. Normal movement occurs over a wide range of velocities and frequencies of head movement. Therefore, patients should perform the head movement exercises at many different velocities and frequencies for optimal effects.[69]

Different head positions can also be used to vary the exercise.[72] Mental effort also may help improve the gain of the system. It is well documented that VOR gain can be increased even in the dark, if the subject simply imagines that he is looking at a stationary target on the wall, while the head is moving.[75,76] Patients should be encouraged to concentrate on the task and not be distracted by conversation and other activities.

Balance and Gait Training Patients with peripheral vestibular deficits most commonly complain of unsteadiness during walking. Complaints of balance problems when sitting or supine are unusual. Patients also have difficulty walking in the dark such as in a movie theater, on uneven surfaces and uphill grades, and through cluttered rooms. Although balance training may begin with static tasks, it is critical to incorporate dynamic balance activities as early as possible. These exercises must be performed as part of a home program. Exercises must also be performed in other environments, such as grocery stores, parks, and malls. A general fitness program can be initiated, with a physician's approval.

Exercises to Foster the Substitution of Alternative Strategies The treatment approach for patients with complete loss of vestibular function involves the use of exercises to enhance the use of visual and somatosensory information to improve postural stability and to develop the use of compensatory strategies in situations where balance is stressed maximally. Additionally, patients often learn to turn on lights at night if they have to get out of bed or to wait, sitting at the edge of the bed, before getting up in the dark, for their eyes to adjust to the darkened room. Lights that come on automatically and emergency lighting in and outside the house in case of a power failure are often recommended. Anticipatory planning for visual environments, such as shopping malls, should be encouraged. For some patients, negotiating a busy environment may require the use of an assistive device, such as a shopping cart or a cane. For others, with bilateral vestibular loss, no assistive devices are needed.

Exercises to improve gaze stability of patients with bilateral vestibular deficits are similar to those used in the treatment of patients with incomplete vestibular lesions. Theoretically, the COR can be potentiated by having the patient perform head movements while maintaining visual fixation on a target (Figure 17-7). The exercise, therefore, is the same as that used to increase VOR gain. This is fortunate, because if there is any remaining vestibular function in these patients, the exercises may increase the gain of the vestibular system as well. Kasai and Zee found that individual patients used different sets of strategies to attempt to maintain gaze stability in the absence of a VOR, including corrective saccades and alterations in pursuit eye movements, as well as enhancement of the COR.[40] Exercises to improve gaze stability, therefore, should not be designed to emphasize any particular strategy. Instead, they should provide situations where patients can develop their own strategies to maintain gaze stability. No mechanism to improve gaze stability will fully compensate for the loss of the VOR. Some patients will continue to have difficulty seeing during rapid head movements.[50]

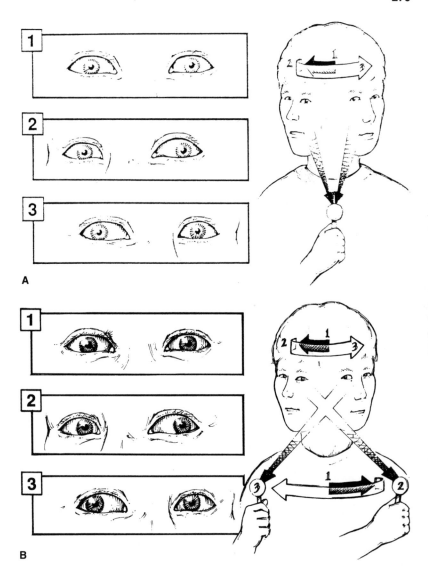

Figure 17-7
Exercises to increase the gain of the vestibular system can include a X1 viewing paradigm (A) and a X2 viewing paradigm (B). In the X1 viewing paradigm, the visual target is stationary and the subject moves his head back and forth while trying to maintain visual fixation on the target. In the X2 viewing paradigm, the target and the head move in opposite directions while the subject again keeps the target in focus. These exercises are performed using a small visual target (foveal stimulus) and a large visual target (full-field stimulus) with the head moving either horizontally or vertically. (Reprinted with permission from Johnson R, Griffin J (eds): Current Therapy in Neurologic Disease, 4th ed. St. Louis, Mosby Year-Book, 1993; p. 12.)

Treatment Efficacy

Exercise Facilitates Recovery   Studies of the effect of unilateral and bilateral vestibular loss in animals support the concept that visuo-motor experience shortens the recovery time of the dynamic vestibular reflexes.[77–79] Mathog and Peppard demonstrated that following unilateral labyrinthectomy, cats given exercises recovered faster than a non-exercised control group.[77] Igarashi et al. found that specific exercises resulted in a more rapid recovery of dynamic postural stability when a control group (non-exercise) was compared with an exercise group after unilateral and bilateral vestibular lesions in squirrel monkeys.[21,78]

Although there is considerable anecdotal evidence that exercises are helpful, only recently have prospective, controlled studies in human beings provided evidence that the use of vestibular rehabilitation techniques is beneficial for patients with unilateral or bilateral vestibular loss.[22–24] These studies have primarily emphasized outcome measures such as changes in postural stability, disability, and subjective complaints as a result of therapeutic interventions.

Horak et al. studied patients with chronic unilateral vestibular hypofunction, inner ear concussive syndrome, and benign paroxysmal positional vertigo.[22] The effects of a 6-week course of customized vestibular exercises, consisting of vestibular habituation, eye–head, balance, and conditioning exercises were compared with the use of vestibular suppressant medications. Although both groups had a decrease in subjective complaints, only the group performing vestibular exercises had improved postural stability. Krebs et al. studied the effectiveness of vestibular exercises on postural stability during ambulation and stair-climbing in patients with chronic bilateral vestibular deficits.[23] Using a placebo-controlled trial, they found that patients performing customized exercises had better stability while walking and stair-climbing, and were able to walk faster than did patients performing isometric and conditioning exercises. During the acute stage after unilateral vestibular loss, the use of vestibular adaptation exercises results in improved postural stability during stance and ambulation and a decrease in disequilibrium when compared with a control group.[24]

Generic versus Customized Exercises

The original exercises proposed by Cawthorne and Cooksey were not customized to the needs of the individual patient. In more recent studies, the exercises usually are customized based on the results of the examination. Recent studies have clearly shown that customized, supervised physical therapy results in more patients achieving complete remission of symptoms (85 percent) compared with generic, unsupervised home-based exercise programs (64 percent).[25,26,79]

Factors in Recovery

Several studies have attempted to identify factors that affect the potential for recovery in patients with vestibular deficits. In general, the results of these studies suggest that patients with stable unilateral vestibular deficits, motion-provoked symptoms, lesser initial disability or with a more recent time of onset have a better recovery.[63,80] Some studies have suggested that patients with head injury tend to have a poorer prognosis, although many do show a decrease in symptoms with treatment.[63,80] Keim et al., however, found little difference in recovery between patients with central and peripheral vestibular deficits using vestibular and balance exercises.[54,55,60,81] These results were based on clinical improvement in standing and walking balance, as well as resumption of activities of daily living. The effect of age on recovery is not clear. Norre reported slower recovery

in patients 60 years and older, but Shepard et al. found that age did not affect the length of the recovery process or the final level of outcome.[63,80,82] Shepard et al. found that therapy takes longer to be effective in mixed central and peripheral lesions, or if the patient were on medications or had increased long-latency responses to sudden perturbations of the support surface.[83,93]

Potential for Recovery

Unilateral Vestibular Paresis   Recovery from unilateral vestibular lesions usually is quite good. Most patients return to normal activities. The rate and final level of recovery will be affected by (1) the presence of other medical problems, particularly those affecting the visual and somatosensory system, central vestibular structures, and the neck; (2) the use of vestibular suppressant medications; and (3) the age of the patient. The adaptive capability of the vestibular system itself is diminished with age, a fact that is compounded by age-related changes in visual and somatosensory inputs.[32]

Assessment of the patient prior to initiation of an exercise program is essential to establishing the goals and treatment. During the initial stage following unilateral vestibular loss, complaints of severe vertigo, nausea, and vomiting are common. Head movement usually aggravates symptoms. The patient usually prefers to lie quietly, often in a darkened room or with eyes closed. At this stage, medications to suppress vegetative responses, and intravenous fluid replacement commonly are administered. Optimum visual inputs (bright room lights, curtains open) should be encouraged during the first days after the acute onset of a vestibular deficit.

After 1 to 3 days, the symptoms of nausea and vertigo should resolve, and spontaneous nystagmus and skew deviation usually decrease as the resting state of the vestibular neurons recovers. Patients can begin exercises as early as *2 or 3 days* after the onset of vestibular loss, using gentle, active head movement. Although early initiation of exercises may increase vertigo or disequilibrium, neither symptom should preclude timely treatment. If vomiting occurs, exercises may be terminated. As patient improvement is noted, usually within a few days to a week or more, the exercise regimens can be expanded.

Recovery of postural stability occurs more gradually. Within 1 to 2 days after the onset of the vestibular deficit, getting out of bed should be encouraged, with necessary assistance. Assistance with ambulation may be required for several days. Most patients can stand with feet together and eyes closed within 4 to 5 days of onset of vestibular loss, albeit with increased sway. Gait may be grossly ataxic for the first week. After that, most are sufficiently steady to walk independently.

During this initial stage of recovery, several different balance and gait exercises are appropriate. Goals include increasing endurance while walking, improving stability while standing with a more narrow base of support (Romberg position) with eyes both open and closed, and beginning to turn the head while walking. Exercises to improve balance in sitting or other positions usually are not necessary. For post-operative patients, bending over must be avoided. Within 2 or 3 days of onset, the VOR adaptation exercises should be performed while standing, as a preparation to walking as well as improving head turning.

Recovery from unilateral vestibular neuronitis, labyrinthitis, or from a surgical procedure such as vestibular nerve section usually takes 6 weeks. However, recovery may take up to 6 months in some patients. Patients with vestibular nerve section, for example, often are back at work within 3 weeks. Recovery from resection of an acoustic neuroma typically takes longer, although most of the recovery usually occurs within the first few weeks. After the first 2 or 3 weeks, persistent complaints of fatigue, instability while turning quickly, and some difficulty walking in the dark are common. Walking on uneven surfaces or when there is a change in light intensity (opening a door to the outside, walking through intermittent shadows, such as tree shadows) may prove difficult. Driving is almost always a matter of concern. Before this can be recommended, clear vision during rapid and abrupt head movements is essential.

Chronic Disequilibrium   Chronic vestibular dysfunction, as a rule, is not associated with persistent vertigo or vomiting. The exception is episodic vestibular disorders such as Meniere's disease. Frequently, head and trunk movements are limited in an attempt to avoid precipitating disequilibrium and nausea. Head movements must be encouraged. The vestibular rehabilitation program may begin with the same adaptation exercises used during the acute stage following unilateral vestibular loss. Starting slowly may be necessary. Some will complain that they feel worse as they stress the vestibular system by performing head movements that they had been avoiding. A clearly articulated explanation in advance is helpful. Improvement within 6 weeks in compliant patients is the rule. The longer vestibular paresis persists, the more the time necessary to see improved function. Once the patient is able to perform the initial

vestibular exercises, it may be necessary to institute more complex movements in order to habituate vestibular responses and to make the patient less fearful of movements that might precipitate vertigo.

Gait exercises can be extremely useful for chronic vestibular dysfunction. A good starting point may be simple static balance exercises with eyes open and closed, on a stable support surface or on foam. A series of exercises that stress balance by gradually decreasing the base of support is helpful. Even if station can not be maintained successfully for the required period of time, practice will improve balance. More difficult balance exercises include walking and turning suddenly, or walking in a circle while gradually decreasing the circumference of the circle, first in one direction and then in another. The practice of walking in different environments, such as on grass, in malls, and at night often is particularly beneficial. Precautions to prevent falls always should be taken.

Bilateral Vestibular Loss   Bilateral peripheral vestibular deficits make it particularly difficult to see clearly during head movements, besides causing balance problems. Disequilibrium becomes particularly evident during standing or walking. When bilateral vestibular paresis develops during the course of a prolonged illness (e.g., following antibiotic therapy) balance problems may not become apparent until the patient tries to get out of bed. Even then, the balance problem often is attributed to weakness.[84] Although many motor systems are critical to postural stability, they cannot compensate completely for the loss of vestibular function. Unlike exercises for unilateral vestibular deficits, therapy must be aimed at fostering the substitution of visual and somatosensory cues for lost vestibular function.

When incomplete bilateral vestibular loss is present, return to activities such as driving at night and some sports often is possible. When severe bilateral vestibular loss is present, driving at night may not be possible because of the gaze instability. Activities such as sports are usually limited because of gaze and postural problems.

Recovery following bilateral vestibular loss is slower than for unilateral paresis and can continue for a 2-year period. Gradually, reliance on visual cues for postural stability decreases and reliance on somatosensory cues increases.[53] Maintenance of vestibular function may require ongoing exercises, at least intermittently.

Recovery can be reversed by medical illness. Upper respiratory infection, fatigue, or treatments such as chemotherapy may make balance worse. A return to vestibular exercises may be necessary in order to regain postural stability.

Treatment Guidelines

A comparison summary of the clinical features of acute and chronic unilateral and bilateral vestibular loss is presented in Table 17-3. Several points concerning the assessment and development of treatment need to be emphasized.

First, it is important to know whether there is any residual vestibular function. Vestibular function should be documented using rotary chair or caloric tests. If remaining vestibular function can be detected on the pathologically involved side(s), vestibular adaptation exercises are recommended to enhance vestibular function (Figure 17-7). If *no* remaining vestibular function can be detected, exercises must be directed at the substitution of visual and somatosensory cues to improve gaze and postural stability. The presence of residual vestibular function can be used to predict recovery.

Second, it is particularly important with bilateral vestibular loss to identify the presence of progressive disorders affecting the visual and somatosensory systems, such as macular degeneration and cataracts. These comorbid degenerative disorders adversely affect bal-

Table 17-3
Vestibular loss

Test	Acute UVL	Chronic UVL	Acute BVL	Chronic BVL
Nystagmus	Spontaneous in light and dark; gaze-evoked follows Alexander's Law; may have head-shaking induced	Spontaneous in dark; head-shaking induced	None	None
Vestibulo-ocular reflex	Abnormal with slow and rapid rotations, often in both directions	Abnormal with rapid head thrusts toward side of lesion	Abnormal with slow and rapid rotations bilaterally	Abnormal with rapid head thrusts bilaterally, sometimes with slow as well
Romberg	Often positive	Negative	Positive	Negative
Tandem Romberg	Cannot perform	Normal with eyes open; cannot perform with eyes closed	Cannot perform	Sometimes can perform with eyes open; not with eyes closed
Single-legged stance	Cannot perform	Normal	Cannot perform	Normal in many patients with eyes open
Altered visual and somatosensory cues	Most have loss of balance when both are altered	Normal	Loss of balance when both are altered	Loss of balance when both are altered
Fukuda's stepping test	Cannot perform	Normal	Cannot perform	Normal with eyes open; cannot perform with eyes closed
Gait	Wide-based, decreased rotation; slow; may need assistance for few days	Normal	Wide-based, decreased rotation, slow; may need assistance	Wide-based, decreased rotation; most do not need assistance
Turn head while walking	Cannot keep balance	Normal or slight unsteadiness	Cannot keep balance	Some can keep balance if walk slowly

ance. Visual field and acuity also affect postural stability and should be assessed. The assessment of vibration, proprioception, and kinesthesia in the lower extremities is essential. Although mild deficits in sensation in the feet may have no effects on postural stability in otherwise normal individuals, in those with vestibular loss, somatosensory deficits may have profound effects on balance and the potential for functional recovery. The detection and awareness of concomitant disorders affecting somatosensory function is important.

Third, many exercises used in the treatment of vestibular disorders increase symptoms initially. This may be disconcerting, and reassurance may be crucial to treatment compliance. Excessive symptom exacerbation during the initiation of treatment often can be avoided by beginning with only a few key exercises. Exercises are attempted two to five times per day based on tolerance. Limiting initial therapy regimens to only a few exercises is especially important when a significant anxiety component is present. This may be critical to successful initiation of the rehabilitation process. Counseling by a psychologist or a psychiatrist may be especially useful as an adjunct to treatment.

SUMMARY

Vestibular rehabilitation appears to be an important adjunct to medical and surgical treatments of vestibular disorders. Three primary types of vestibular problems are amenable to these techniques: benign paroxysmal positional vertigo, unilateral vestibular paresis, and bilateral vestibular loss. New treatments for BPPV have been developed based on the theory of canalithiasis. These treatments result in the remission of vertigo in 85 to 90 percent of all patients with a single treatment. BPPV can occur in any of the semicircular canals and treatment can and should be directed accordingly. Patients with unilateral vestibular deficits can be expected to recover from the vertigo and/or disequilibrium they first experience. The final level of recovery should be to return to all or most activities. Other nervous system disorders can delay or limit the level of recovery. Studies on animals and human beings suggest that exercises facilitate recovery of vestibular system function. Early intervention also seems to be important in optimizing recovery. Restricting movement or visual inputs, and the use of vestibular suppressant medications, may delay and limit recovery. Bilateral vestibular deficits are also amenable to physical therapy, but the prognosis is not as good. After complete bilateral vestibular loss, substi-

tution of other sensory modalities for lost vestibular function may be effective.

REFERENCES

1. Barany R: Diagnose von Krankheitserscheinungen im Bereiche des Otolithenapparatus. *Acta Oto-Laryngol* 1921; 2:434.
2. Dix MR, Hallpike CS: Pathology, symptomatology and diagnosis of certain disorders of the vestibular system. *Proc R Soc Med* 1952; 45:341.
3. Baloh RW, Honrubia V, Jacobson K: Benign positional vertigo: Clinical and oculographic features in 240 cases. *Neurology* 1987; 37:371.
4. Schuknecht HF: Cupulolithiasis. *Arch Otolaryngol* 1969; 90:765.
5. Hall SF, Ruby RRF, McClure JA: The mechanisms of benign paroxysmal vertigo. *J Otolaryngol* 1979; 8:151.
6. Parnes LS, McClure J: Free-floating endolymph particles: A new operative finding during posterior semicircular canal occlusion. *Laryngoscope* 1992; 102:988.
7. Brandt T, Daroff RB: Physical therapy for benign paroxysmal positional vertigo. *Arch Otolaryngol* 1980; 106:484.
8. Semont A, Freyss G, Vitte E: Curing the BPPV with a Liberatory maneuver. *Adv Oto-Rhino-Laryngol* 1988; 42:290.
9. Epley JM: The Canalith repositioning procedure: for treatment of benign paroxysmal positional vertigo. *Otolaryngol Head Neck Surg* 1992; 107:399.
10. Herdman SJ, Tusa RJ, Zee DS, Proctor LP, Mattox DE: Single treatment approaches to benign paroxysmal positional vertigo. *Arch Otolaryngol Head Neck Surg* 1993; 119:450.
11. Parnes LS, Price-Jones RG: Particle repositioning maneuver for benign paroxysmal positional vertigo. *Ann Oto Rhino Laryngol* 1993; 102:325.
12. Li JC: Mastoid oscillation: A critical factor for success in the Canalith repositioning procedure. *Otolaryngol Head Neck Surg* 1995; 112:670.
13. Gyo K: Benign paroxysmal positional vertigo as a complication of postoperative bedrest. *Laryngoscope* 1988; 98:332.
14. Herdman SJ, Tusa RJ, Clendaniel RA: Eye movement signs in vertical canal benign paroxysmal positional vertigo, in Fuchs AF, Brandt T, Buttner U, Zee D (eds): *Contemporary Ocular Motor and Vestibular Research: a Tribute to David A. Robinson.* Stuttgart, Thieme, 1994; pp. 385–387.
15. Baloh RW, Jacobson K, Honrubia V: Horizontal semicircular canal variant of benign positional vertigo. *Neurology* 1993; 43:2542.
16. McClure J: Horizontal canal BPV. *J Otolaryngol* 1985; 14:30.
17. Epley JM: Positional vertigo related to semicircular canalithiasis. *Otolaryngol Head Neck Surg* 1995; 112:154.

18. Black FO, Nashner LM: Postural disturbance in patients with benign paroxysmal positional nystagmus. *Ann Oto Rhino Laryngol* 1984; 93:595.

19. Voorhees RL: The role of dynamic posturography in neurotologic diagnosis. *Laryngoscope* 1989; 99:995.

20. Herdman SJ, Tusa RJ: Complication of the Canalith repositioning maneuver. *Arch Otolaryn Head Neck Surg* 1996; 122:281–286.

21. Igarashi M, Ishikawa K, Ishii M, et al: Physical exercise and balance compensation after total ablation of vestibular organs, in Pompeiano O, Allum JHJ (eds): *Progress in Brain Research*. Elsevier, Amsterdam, 1988; pp. 395–401.

22. Horak FB, Jones-Rycewicz C, Black FO, Shumway-Cook A: Effects of vestibular rehabilitation on dizziness and imbalance. *Otolaryngol Head Neck Surg* 1992; 106:175.

23. Krebs DE, et al: Double-blind, placebo-controlled trial of rehabilitation for bilateral vestibular hypofunction: Preliminary report. *Otolaryngol Head Neck Surg* 1993; 109:735.

24. Herdman SJ, Clendaniel RA, Mattox DE, Holliday MJ, Niparko JK: Vestibular adaptation exercises and recovery: Acute stage after acoustic neuroma resection. *Otolaryngol Head Neck Surg* 1995; 113:77.

25. Shepard NT, Telian SA: Programmatic vestibular rehabilitation. *Otolaryngol-Head Neck Surg* 1995; 112:173.

26. Szturm T, Ireland DJ, Lessing-Turner M: Comparison of different exercise programs in the rehabilitation of patients with chronic peripheral vestibular dysfunction. *J Vest Res* 1994; 4:461.

27. Fetter M, Zee DS: Recovery from unilateral labyrinthectomy in Rhesus monkeys. *J Neurophys* 1988; 59:370.

28. Maoli C, Precht W, Reid S: Short- and long-term modifications of vestibulo-ocular response dynamics following unilateral vestibular nerve lesions in the cat. *Brain Res* 1983; 50:259.

29. Honrubia V, Garland K, Marco J, et al: Vestibulo-ocular reflex changes following peripheral labyrinthine lesions, in Ruben RW (ed): *The Biology of Change in Otolaryngology*. Elsevier, 1986, pp. 155–170.

30. Allum JHJ, Yamane M, Pfaltz CR: Long-term modifications of vertical and horizontal vestibulo-ocular reflex dynamics in man. *Acta Otolarngol (Stockh)* 1988; 105:328.

31. Halmagyi GM, Curthoys IS, Cremer PD, et al: The human horizontal vestibulo-ocular reflex in response to high-acceleration stimulation before and after unilateral vestibular neurectomy. *Exp Brain Res* 1990; 81:479.

32. Paige GD: Nonlinearity and asymmetry in the human vestibulo-ocular reflex. *Acta Otolaryngol (Stockh)* 1989; 108:1.

33. Westheimer G, McKee SP: Visual acuity in the presence of retinal-image motion. *J Optical Soc Am* 1975; 65:847.

34. Demer JL, Goldberg J, Porter FI: Effect of telescopic spectacles on head stability in normal and low vision. *J Vest Res* 1991; 1:109.

35. Leigh RJ, Brandt T: A reevaluation of the vestibuloocular reflex: new ideas of its purpose, properties, neural substrate, and disorders. *Neurology* 1993; 43:1288.

36. Leigh RJ, Sawyer RN, Grant MP, Seidman SH: High-frequency vestibuloocular reflex as a diagnostic tool. *Ann NY Acad Sci* 1992; 656:305.

37. Demer JL: Evaluation of vestibular and visual oculomotor function. *Otolaryngol Head and Neck Surg* 1995; 112:16.

38. Demer JL, Amjadi F: Dynamic visual acuity of normal subjects during vertical optotype and head motion. *Invest Ophthalmol Vis Sci* 1993; 34:1894.

39. Burgio DL, Blakley BW, Myers SF: The high-frequency oscillation test. *J Vestibular Res* 1992; 2:221.

40. Kasai T, Zee DS: Eye-head coordination in labyrinthine-defective human beings. *Brain Res* 1978; 144:123.

41. Bronstein AM, Hood JD: The cervico-ocular reflex in normal subjects and patients with absent vestibular function. *Brain Res* 1986; 373:399.

42. Dichgans J, Bizzi E, Morasso P, Tagliasco V: Mechanisms underlying recovery of eye-head coordination following bilateral labyrinthectomy in monkeys. *Exp Brain Res* 1973; 18:548.

43. Chambers BR, Mai M, Barber HO: Bilateral vestibular loss, oscillopsia, and the cervico-ocular reflex. *Otolaryngol Head Neck Surg* 1985; 93:403.

44. Barnes GR: Head-eye coordination in normals and in patients with vestibular disorders. *Adv Oto-Rhino-Laryngol* 1979; 25:197.

45. Imate Y, Sekitani T: Vestibular compensation in vestibular neuronitis: Long-term follow-up evaluation. *Acta Otolaryngol (Stockh)* 1993; 113:463.

46. Takahashi M, Hoshikawa H, Tsujita N, Akiyama I: Effect of labyrinthine dysfunction upon head oscillation and gaze during stepping and running. *Acta Otolaryngol (Stockh)* 1988; 106:348.

47. Hikosaka O, Maeda M: Cervical effects on abducens motorneurons and their interaction with vestibulo-ocular reflex. *Exp Brain Res* 1973; 18:512.

48. Barlow D, Freedman W: Cervico-ocular reflex in the normal adult. *Acta Otolaryngol* 1980; 89:487.

49. Sawyer RN, Thurston SE, Becker KR, Ackley CV, Seidman SH, Leigh RJ: The cervico-ocular reflex of normal human subjects in response to transient and sinusoidal trunk rotations. *J Vestibular Res* 1994; 4:245.

50. Segal BN, Katsarkas A: Long-term deficits of goal-directed vestibulo-ocular function following total unilateral loss of peripheral vestibular function. *Acta Otolaryngol (Stockh)* 1988; 106:102.

51. Grossman GE, Leigh RJ, Abel LA, Lanska DJ, Thurston SE: Frequency and velocity of rotational head perturbations during locomotion. *Exp Brain Res* 1988; 70:470.

52. Grossman GE, Leigh RJ, Bruce EN, Huebner WP, Lanska DJ: Performance of the human vestibuloocular reflex during locomotion. *J Neurophysiol* 1989; 62:264.

53. Bles W, Vianney de Jong JMB, de Wit G: Compensation for labyrinthine defects examined by use of a tilting room. *Acta Otolaryngol* 1983; 95:576.

54. Cawthorne T: The physiological basis for head exercises. *J Chart Soc Physiother* 1944; 30:106.

55. Cooksey FS: Rehabilitation in vestibular injuries. *Proc R Soc Med* 1946; 39:273.

56. McCabe BF: Labyrinthine exercises in the treatment of diseases characterized by vertigo: Their physiologic basis and methodology. *Laryngoscope* 1970; 80:1429.

57. Hecker HC, Haug CO, Herndon JW: Treatment of the vertiginous patient using Cawthorne's vestibular exercises. *Laryngoscope* 1974; 84:2065.

58. Dix MR: The rationale and technique of head exercises in the treatment of vertigo. *Acta Oto-Rhino-Laryng. Belg.* 1979; 33:370.

59. Norre ME, DeWeerdt W: Treatment of vertigo based on habituation. *J Laryngol Oto* 1980; 94:971.

60. Zee DS: Vertigo: Current therapy in neurological disease. 1985; 8.

61. Herdman SJ: Exercise strategies for vestibular disorders. *Ear, Nose, Throat* 1989; 68:961.

62. Shumway-Cook A, Horak FB: Vestibular rehabilitation: An exercise approach to managing symptoms of vestibular dysfunction. *Semin Hear* 1989; 10:196.

63. Telian SA, Shepard NT, Smith-Wheelock M, Kemink JL: Habituation therapy for chronic vestibular dysfunction: Preliminary results. *Otolaryngol Head Neck Surg* 1990; 103:89.

64. Tokumasa K, Fujino A, Noguchi H: Prolonged dysequilibrium in three cases with vestibular neuronitis: Efficacy of vestibular rehabilitation. *Acta Otolaryngol (Stockh)* 1993; 503:39.

65. Gauthier GM, Robinson DA: Adaptation of the human vestibuloocular reflex to magnifying lenses. *Brain Res* 1975; 92:331.

66. Shelhamer M, Tiliket C, Roberts D, Kramer PD, Zee DS: Short-term vestibulo-ocular reflex adaptation in humans II. Error signals. *Exp Brain Res* 1994; 100:328.

67. Harris LR, Cynader M: Modification of the balance and gain of the vestibulo-ocular reflex in the cat. *Exp Brain Res* 1981; 44:57.

68. Lisberger SG, Miles FA, Optican LM: Frequency-selective adaptation: evidence for channels in the vestibulo-ocular reflex. *J Neuroscience* 1983; 3:1234.

69. Collewijn H, Martins AJ, Steinman RM: Compensatory eye movements during active and passive head movements: fast adaptation to changes in visual magnification. *J Physiol* 1983; 340:259.

70. Jones GM, Guitton D, Berthoz A: Changing pattrens of eye-head coordination during 6 h of optically reversed vision. *Exp Brain Res* 1988; 69:532.

71. Demer JL, Porter FI, Goldberg J, et al: Adaptation to telescopic spectacles: vestibulo-ocular reflex plasticity. *Invest Ophthalmol Vis Sci* 1989; 30:159.

72. Shelhamer M, Robinson DA, Tan HS: Context-specific adaptation of the gain of the vestibulo-ocular reflex in humans. *J Vest Res* 1992; 2:89.

73. Post RB, Lott LA: The relationship between vestibulo-ocular reflex plasticity and changes in apparent concomitant motion. *Vision Res* 1992; 32:89.

74. Pfaltz CR: Vestibular compensation. *Acta Otolaryngol* 1983; 95:402.

75. Baloh RW, Lyerly K, Yee RD, et al: Voluntary control of the human vestibulo-ocular reflex. *Acta Otolaryngol (Stockh.)* 1984; 97:1.

76. Furst EJ, Goldberg J, Jenkins HA: Voluntary modification of the rotatory-induced vestibulo-ocular reflex by fixating imaginary targets. *Acta Otolaryngol (Stockh.)* 1987; 103: 231.

77. Mathog RH, Peppard SB: Exercise and recovery from vestibular injury. *Am J Otolaryngol* 1982; 3:387.

78. Igarashi M, Levy JK, O-Uchi T, et al: Further study of physical exercise and locomotor balance compensation after unilateral labyrinthectomy in squirrel monkeys. *Acta Otolaryngol* 1981; 92:101.

79. Courjon JH, Jeannerod M, Ossuzio I, et al: The role of vision on compensation of vestibulo ocular reflex after hemilabyrinthectomy in the cat. *Exp Brain Res* 1977; 28:235.

80. Shepard NT, Telian SA, Smith-Wheelock M: Habituation and balance retraining therapy. *Neurol Clin* 1990; 5:459.

81. Keim RJ, Cook M, Martini D: Balance rehabilitation therapy. *Laryngoscope* 1992; 102:1302.

82. Norre ME, Beckers A: Vestibular habituation training for positional vertigo in elderly patients. *J Am Ger Soc* 1988; 36:425.

83. Shepard NT, Telian SA, Smith-Wheelock M, Raj A: Vestibular and balance rehabilitation therapy. *Ann Otol Rhinol Laryngol* 1993; 102:198.

84. JC (anonymous): Living without a balance mechanism. *N Engl J Med* 1952; 246:458.

85. Jacobson GP, Newman CW: The development of the dizziness handicap inventory. *Arch Otolaryngol Head Neck Surg* 1990; 116:424.

86. Watanabe T, Hattori Y, Fukuda T: Automated graphical analysis of Fukuda's stepping test, in Igarashi M, Black FO (eds): *Vestibular and Visual Control of Posture and Locomotor Equilibrium* Karger, Basel, 1985; p. 80.

Part III

MANAGEMENT OF CONDITIONS ASSOCIATED WITH CHRONIC NEUROLOGIC DYSFUNCTION

Chapter 18

NEUROGENIC BLADDER AND BOWEL

David A. Gelber

Bladder and bowel dysfunction occur commonly in patients with neurologic disease. Urinary incontinence affects 5 to 15 percent of elderly patients living in the community and over 50 percent of patients in institutions.[1] The prevalence of fecal incontinence is 0.5 to 1.5 percent in the general population and approximately 10 percent in elderly institutionalized patients.[2,3] Management of the complications of neurogenic bowel and bladder is costly. For example, it is estimated that $400 million is spent on adult diapers in the United States each year, whereas a total of $1 to 10 billion is spent annually in caring for patients with urinary incontinence.[2,4–6] Neurogenic bowel and bladder can lead to medical complications including urinary tract infections, development of renal or bladder calculi, and skin excoriation.[7] In addition, urinary and fecal incontinence may be associated with serious psychological and social sequelae. Incontinence often results in social embarrassment and a feeling of lost autonomy. The need to address excessive time to one's bodily functions may be demoralizing to patients. Finally, the presence of bowel or bladder dysfunction is often a major factor in determining whether a patient will be able to be managed at home or require placement in a skilled-care facility.[7]

This chapter will focus on bladder and bowel dysfunction as it relates to patients with neurologic diseases. The anatomy, physiology, and assessment of bowel and bladder function will be reviewed. Management of neurogenic bladder and bowel, particularly with emphasis on the rehabiliation patient, will be discussed in detail.

NEUROGENIC BLADDER

Anatomy and Physiology

Anatomy of the Lower Urinary Tract   The bladder wall consists primarily of the detrusor muscle, which is composed of intertwined smooth-muscle bundles.[8] Distally, the bladder tapers into the bladder neck and urethra.[9] The urethra is composed of inner and outer smooth-muscle layers, which are contiguous with those in the bladder and separated by the prostate gland in males.[10] In the lower urinary tract there are two distinct sphincter mechanisms that facilitate urinary continence. The internal urinary sphincter is formed by the outer smooth-muscle layer of the urethra; this encircles the proximal urethra ventrally and allows for closure of the bladder neck and proximal urethra.[11] More distally lies the external urinary sphincter that, in contrast, is composed of skeletal muscle. There are two separate components to the external sphincter. The first is periurethral striated muscle that surrounds the distal urethra. The second component is a reflection downward from the pelvic-floor musculature (urogenital diaphragm) that surrounds the urethra as a "pelvic sling."[11,12] Voluntary contraction of the external sphincter results in constriction of the urethra and thus helps prevent leakage of urine at inappropriate times.

Neural Control of Micturition Bladder emptying is facilitated by activation of the parasympathetic nervous system. Parasympathetic neurons originate in the pelvic nucleus, located in the interomediolateral cell column of the sacral spinal cord at levels S2–S4.[13] Motor neurons course through the ventral nerve roots and pelvic nerves and synapse in ganglia located in and adjacent to the bladder wall. Most of the postganglionic parasympathetic fibers terminate in the detrusor muscle. Parasympathetic afferent nerve fibers, responsible for the sensation of bladder filling, return via the pelvic nerves to the sacral spinal cord, thus completing a reflex loop.[14] Activation of the parasympathetic nerves results in contraction of the bladder wall.

The sympathetic nervous system acts in reciprocal fashion, with activation resulting in storage of urine. Sympathetic neurons originate in the interomediolateral cell column of the thoracolumbar spinal cord, at levels T11–L2, course through the ventral roots, and synapse in the prevertebral ganglia.[14] Postganglionic sympathetic axons travel with the hypogastric nerves and terminate in the bladder wall, bladder neck, and urethra.[15] Activation of the sympathetic nerves result in relaxation of the bladder wall, mediated by beta-adrenergic receptors, and contraction of the internal sphincter, mediated by alpha-adrenergic receptors.[16]

The somatic nervous system also plays a major role in urine storage through its innervation of the external urinary sphincter. The motor neurons innervating the external sphincter arise in the pudendal nucleus, located in the ventral horn of the sacral spinal cord at levels S2–S4.[15,17] Efferent motor nerves course along the wall of the pelvis in the pudendal nerve and innervate the pelvic-floor musculature and periurethral striated muscle. Activation of the somatic nerves result in contraction of the pelvic-floor muscles and external sphincter resulting in constriction of the distal urethra. In contrast to parasympathetic and sympathetic function, the somatic nervous system, and therefore external sphincter function, is under conscious, voluntary control.

During micturition, the parasympathetic system is activated while the sympathetic and somatic systems are inhibited. This results in contraction of the bladder wall and relaxation of the bladder neck and proximal urethra (internal sphincter) and external sphincter. This is mediated primarily through the caudal spinal cord reflex loops described. Spinal cord intersegmental

reflexes also are thought to modulate this system.[14] In addition to the cholinergic parasympathetic pathways and adrenergic sympathetic pathways described, other neurotransmitters, including vasoactive intestinal peptide (VIP), *leu*-enkephalin, neuropeptide Y, substance P, somatostatin, calcitonin gene-related peptide (CGRP), ATP, and histamine may be involved as neuromodulators of the neuromicturition pathways.[18–25]

Bladder and sphincter activity is coordinated so that when the bladder contracts, the internal and external urinary sphincters relax in a coordinated fashion. The bladder and sphincter neuronal centers in the caudal spinal cord are believed to be coordinated by descending neural pathways that arise in a pontine micturition center located in the region of the reticular formation rostral to the locus ceruleus.[26–29] Efferent fibers descend from the pontine micturition center through the reticulospinal tracts and terminate on the pelvic and pudendal nuclei in the sacral spinal cord. Afferent proprioceptive input from stretch receptors in the bladder wall and sphincters ascend in the spinal cord in the posterior columns and terminate in the pontine micturition center, completing another reflex loop.[15] Ascending sensory pathways also terminate in the cerebral sensory cortex allowing for conscious awareness of bladder filling and the urge to void.

In addition to afferent input from the caudal spinal cord, the pontine micturition center receives facilatory and inhibitory input from various cortical and subcortical structures that allows for voluntary control of micturition (Figure 18-1). In animal studies, the red nucleus, midbrain tegmentum, ventrolateral nucleus of the thalamus, substantia nigra, subthalamus, pallidum, supermedial frontal lobe, anterior cingulate gyrus, genu of the corpus callosum, and the fastigial nucleus of the cerebellum have been shown to inhibit micturition.[15,30,31] Conversely, the medulla, mesencephalon, rostral hypothalamus, and septum have been shown to facilitate micturition via connections to the pontine micturition center.[32] However, in humans, these pathways have not been definitively identified.

In summary, as the bladder fills, there is conscious awareness of the urgency to void. This is mediated by stretch receptors located in the bladder wall that project via sensory afferent nerves to the sacral spinal cord and then on to the sensory cortex of the brain by the posterior column pathway. If it is not a socially appropriate time to void, micturition can be consciously inhibited via descending cortical inhibitory influences on the pontine micturition center. Inhibition of the pontine micturition

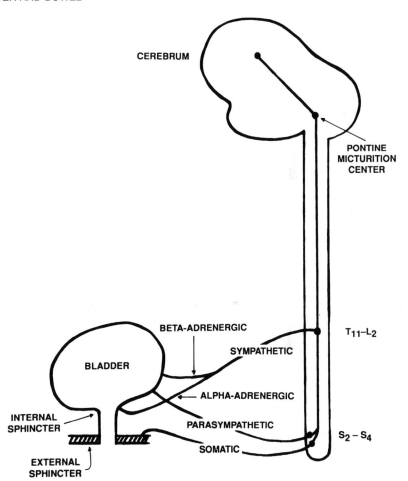

Figure 18-1

Innervation of the lower urinary tract. The pontine micturition center coordinates bladder and sphincter activity through descending pathways to the caudal spinal cord. Its activity is modulated by cortical and subcortical influences that allow for conscious control of micturition. Parasympathetic innervation to the bladder wall originates in the sacral spinal cord (S2–S4). Sympathetic innervation to the bladder wall (beta-adrenergic) and internal sphincter (alpha-adrenergic) arises in the thoracolumbar cord (T11–Tl2). Somatic innervation to the external sphincter originates in the sacral cord (S2–S4).

center, in turn, results in decreased parasympathetic activity, and an increase in sympathetic and somatic outflow from the caudal spinal cord. This leads to relaxation of the bladder wall and contraction of the bladder neck, proximal urethra, and external sphincter, which act in concert to maintain urinary continence.

Once it is an appropriate time to void, cortical inhibition over the pontine micturition center is consciously removed, resulting in activation of the parasympathetic pathways and inhibition of the sympathetic and somatic micturition pathways. This causes vigorous contraction of the bladder wall with coordinated relaxation of the urinary sphincters, resulting in bladder emptying. External sphincter activity ceases at the onset of bladder contraction and remains silent throughout the duration of the contraction.

Urologic Evaluation

Urologic assessment should include a history and physical examination. One should inquire about a past history of childhood eneuresis, renal or bladder stones, urinary tract infections, previous urologic surgery, sexual dysfunction, and neurologic disease. A detailed history of current urologic symptoms, including incontinence, urinary hesitancy or retention, frequency, urgency, and nocturia, as well as a thorough neurologic review of symptoms also should be obtained. Physical examination includes a genitourinary and neurologic examination. In addition to the routine assessment of cognitive, sensory, and motor function, there are several cutaneous reflexes that indirectly test the integrity of the sacral micturition pathways. The bulbocavernosus reflex, elicited by squeezing the glans penis or clitoris, results in reflex contraction of the external anal sphincter. The anal wink, elicited by stimulation of the perianal skin, also results in reflex contraction of the anal sphincter. Both of these cutaneous reflexes are mediated by spinal cord segments S2–S4 and are lost with lesions affecting the sacral spinal cord or sacral nerve roots at these levels.[33]

Laboratory evaluation on all patients should at least include urinalysis and measurement of blood urea nitrogen and creatinine. If there is a suspicion of renal dysfunction, an intravenous pyelogram, renal genitourinary ultrasound, abdominal CAT scan, or measurement of creatinine clearance may be indicated. Evaluation should also include measurement of postvoid residual urine volumes (PVR). PVR can be measured by intermittent straight catheterization or ultrasound after voluntary voiding.[34–37] A PVR of greater than 50 mL is considered abnormal and is indicative of an impairment in bladder emptying.[38] One should be cautious in interpreting PVR measurements in patients with severe language or cognitive impairments. These patients often are unable to understand the instructions for the procedure, or fail to notify staff on a timely basis after voiding, leading to falsely elevated PVR in these individuals.[39]

The most definitive diagnostic procedure for evaluation of micturition physiology is a urodynamic study.[40] An optimal study should at least include a cystometrogram (CMG) and external sphincter electromyogram (EMG). The procedure involves passing a catheter into the bladder and filling it with either fluid (usually isotonic saline) or gas (carbon dioxide). Pressures are measured by transducers located in the bladder and urethra.[38,40] The cystometrogram graphs bladder pressure versus volume in response to bladder filling and emptying. The bladder volume at which the patient first senses filling is noted. In normal individuals this is approximately 25 percent of bladder capacity, or 125 to 200 mL.[41] Bladder capacity, defined as the volume at which the patient expresses the urge or desire to void, or when strong uninhibited detrusor contractions are noted on the CMG, also is recorded.[42] A normal bladder capacity is 400 to 500 mL. Once filling is complete, patients are asked to voluntarily void. During voiding intravesical pressures normally reach 40 to 80 cm H_2O, and bladder emptying should be complete.[41]

If needed, additional information can be obtained during the urodynamic study. For example, at the conclusion of the study, as the catheter is being withdrawn, pressure measurements along various points of the urethra can be obtained to give a "urethral pressure pro-

file."[38,42] This may provide additional information about the function of the internal and external urinary sphincters. Bladder emptying into a uroflowmeter allows for measurement of urine flow rate. Urine flow rate may be slowed by bladder outlet obstruction or a poorly contracting bladder.[36]

External urethral sphincter EMG provides direct measurement of sphincter activity. It is generally performed concurrently with the cystometrogram and allows for the assessment of the coordination of bladder and urethral sphincter function.[40] In normal individuals external sphincter activity ceases at the onset of a bladder contraction and remains silent throughout the duration of the contraction.[43] Direct needle electromyography of the periurethral striated muscle is the preferred method. However, the electrodes may be difficult to place, especially in young children.[43] Alternative techniques include the use of perineal surface electrodes or needle electrodes placed into the pelvic-floor muscles. Because there is a strong correlation between the electrical activity of the external urethral sphincter and the external anal sphincter, urinary sphincter activity may be studied indirectly by needle EMG of the external anal sphincter or by use of an anal plug electrode.[44]

Classification of Bladder Dysfunction

Numerous classification schemes of bladder dysfunction have been developed.[45–53] Unfortunately, this has created confusion in the literature because of the different terminology used in each. To help standardize this terminology, the International Continence Society developed a system that classifies both detrusor and urethral (sphincter) function as normal, overactive, or underactive, on the basis of urodynamic studies.[54] Detrusor function is considered "normal" if there is no significant rise in bladder pressure during filling, if there are no involuntary bladder contractions during filling, and if normal voiding can be voluntarily initiated, sustained, and suppressed. Detrusor function is considered "overactive" if there are involuntary bladder contractions during filling that cannot be suppressed voluntarily. If there is no apparent neurological cause for the bladder overactivity this is termed an "unstable detrusor." If there is a neurological lesion felt to be responsible for the bladder overactivity this is termed "detrusor hyperreflexia." It is recommended that the use of the terms "hypertonic bladder," "upper motor neuron bladder," "reflex," "spastic," and "uninhibited bladder"—all of which have been used in the literature to describe an overactive bladder—be avoided.[54]

Conversely, the bladder is defined as "underactive" if there are no bladder contractions during filling, and if a poorly sustained contraction or no contraction occurs during attempts to voluntarily void. If there is neurologic disease to explain the bladder dysfunction, this is termed "detrusor areflexia." It is likewise recommended that the use of the terms "atonic," "hypotonic," "autonomic," and "flaccid bladder" be abandoned.[54]

Internal and external urethral sphincter activity also is defined as normal, overactive, or incompetent. Urethral closure is considered "normal" if there is positive urethral closure pressure during bladder filling and a decrease in urethral pressure during voiding to allow for unobstructed urine outflow. Sphincter activity is defined as "overactive" if the urethra fails to relax or if it contracts involuntarily during a bladder contraction. The latter also is referred to as "detrusor–sphincter dyssynergia." The urethral sphincters are defined as underactive or "incompetent" if there is diminished urethral closure pressure or a decrease in external sphincter EMG activity during bladder filling.[54]

Lesion Localization

Cerebral Lesions Urinary incontinence is common in patients with diseases of the brain, including stroke, neoplasm, normal pressure hydrocephalus, multiple sclerosis, cerebral palsy, and Parkinson disease. Lesions that directly affect the neuromicturition pathways between the cerebrum and pontine micturition center result in detrusor hyperreflexia with normal urethral sphincter activity (Table 18-1).[55–58] Abnormal perception of bladder fullness and inability to consciously inhibit micturition leads to urgency incontinence.[59] Urodynamic studies demonstrate uninhibited bladder contractions greater than 15 cm H_2O that occur during bladder filling.[28] Bladder capacity may be significantly reduced. Because the urethral sphincters do relax appropriately during a detrusor contraction, bladder emptying usually is complete.

Urinary incontinence occurs in 37 to 60 percent of stroke patients and persists in up to half of these patients after 1 year.[55,58,60–62] Of these incontinent patients, bladder hyperreflexia is seen in 37 to 82 percent, and has been correlated, in several series, with lesions of the frontoparietal cortex, basal ganglia, internal capsule, and putamen.[55,56,63–66]

Urinary incontinence after stroke may also develop as a result of specific focal neurologic deficits.[58] This subgroup of patients is typically aphasic or demented and unable to communicate the need to void (situational incontinence). Urodynamic studies typically are normal.

Urinary incontinence is common with Parkinson disease. The incidence of bladder hyperreflexia is 50 to 93 percent of patients with urologic symptoms.[57,67–71] This is consistent with the presumption that the basal ganglia are involved in the modulation of micturition. As is expected with suprapontine lesions, urethral sphincter activity is coordinated in most cases. However, in a small percentage of patients (7–18 percent), sphincter pseudodyssynergia occurs.[28,71] In contrast to true sphincter dyssynergia, in which involuntary sphincter contraction occurs during bladder contraction, pseudodyssynergia is defined as a voluntary contraction of the perineal muscles that occurs during an uninhibited bladder contraction in order to prevent leaking. External sphincter bradykinesia also has been described, defined as the slowed relaxation of the external sphincter during bladder contraction, in 11 percent of those with Parkinson disease.[71] However, this finding has not been confirmed in a subsequent study.[57]

Neurogenic bladder also is common in multiple sclerosis, with 78 to 94 percent of those affected experiencing urologic symptoms at some point in the course of their disease.[72–74] Bladder hyperreflexia with normal sphincter activity is the most common urodynamic pattern, occurring in 52 to 78 percent of symptomatic patients.[75]

Suprasacral Spinal-Cord Lesions Lesions located between the pontine micturition center and caudal spinal cord, most commonly associated with traumatic spi-

Table 18-1
Urodynamic study pattern based on lesion localization

Lesion localization	Urodynamic study pattern
Rostral to pons	Detrusor hyperreflexia with coordinated sphincters
Between pons and sacral spinal cord	Detrusor hyperreflexia with sphincter dyssynergia
Sacral spinal cord	Detrusor and sphincter areflexia
	Detrusor areflexia with normal sphincter function
	Sphincter areflexia with normal detrusor function
Sacral nerve root or peripheral nerves	Detrusor and sphincter areflexia

nal-cord injuries, spinal-cord tumors, multiple sclerosis, and transverse myelitis, result in an overactive bladder with uncoordinated sphincters (detrusor hyperreflexia with urinary sphincter dyssynergia) (Table 18-1).[76–78] During voiding the bladder contracts against a closed sphincter, leading to urinary retention. Because extremely high intravesical pressures (often in excess of 100 cm H_2O) are generated, if left untreated renal damage (hydronephrosis) can develop. Urodynamic studies usually reveal a reduced bladder capacity, with vigorous bladder contractions occurring at low bladder volumes. EMG of the external urinary sphincter shows sphincter contraction occurring simultaneously with bladder contractions.[76] The internal urinary sphincter also may be dyssynergic, particularly with lesions affecting the cervical or upper thoracic spinal cord.

Eighty-nine percent of patients with complete suprasacral spinal-cord injuries eventually develop a hyperreflexic bladder with sphincter dyssynergia.[28] However, initially, during the period of spinal shock, bladder and urinary sphincters are completely areflexic. Although the sphincters usually regain function within days of the injury, detrusor activity generally does not return until 6 to 12 weeks post-injury.[79] Incomplete suprasacral traumatic spinal-cord injuries also can lead to development of bladder hyperreflexia, although the incidence of sphincter dyssynergia is lower (44 percent).[28]

Sphincter dyssynergia is common in suprasacral meningomyelocele and can be complicated by development of intrarenal reflux, renal scarring, and recurrent urinary-tract infections.[80] Sphincter dyssynergia occurs in approximately 30 percent of patients with multiple sclerosis, because of the development of spinal-cord plaques.[73]

Lesions of Sacral Spinal Cord, Sacral Nerve Roots, and Peripheral Nerves   Lesions affecting the peripheral nerves, cauda equina, or conus medullaris, most commonly associated with peripheral neuropathies, myelomeningocele, sacral spinal-cord tumors, trauma, or spinal stenosis, typically result in an underactive bladder with an areflexic external sphincter (Table 18-1).[80–86] Urodynamic studies show diminished sensory awareness of bladder filling, an increase in bladder capacity, and absent or nonsustained bladder contractions.[41] Occasionally, conus medullaris lesions are associated with normal sphincter function if the pudendal nucleus is spared. Conversely, sacral-cord lesions that spare the pelvic nucleus may result in an areflexic sphincter with normal detrusor function.[76]

Neurogenic bladder is present in 27 to 85 percent of diabetes mellitus owing to development of somatic and autonomic neuropathy.[87] The initial symptom usually is diminished sensation of bladder filling. As the disease progresses the bladder becomes hyporeflexic with ineffectual contractions, resulting in urinary retention.[88] This, in turn, predisposes the diabetic to the development of urinary-tract infections, bladder or renal stones, and injury to the upper urinary tract. As the bladder fills beyond its capacity, urine leaks out, resulting in overflow incontinence. This may be exacerbated by an underactive external urinary sphincter.[76]

Detrusor areflexia is present in 33 percent of multiple sclerosis patients, whereas sphincter areflexia occurs in 15 percent.[72] Bladder and urinary sphincter areflexia also is seen in the spinal-shock phase following acute suprasacral spinal-cord injuries, as described.

Treatment

Methods commonly used for treatment of the neurogenic bladder include nonpharmacologic interventions, such as timed voiding programs, biofeedback, medications, and surgical procedures (Tables 18-2 and 18-3). Treatment should be individualized, with the benefits of treatment carefully considered. Most important, therapeutic decisions should be based on the knowledge of abnormal voiding physiology, as demonstrated by urodynamic study.[39,58] Treatment strategies should be based on neurologic lesion localization, in addition to the results of urodynamic evaluation.

Cerebral Lesions   Focal or diffuse cerebral lesions may lead to urinary incontinence, despite normal urodynamic studies. Typically, aphasia or dementia leads to situational incontinence, with inability to communicate the need to void.[58] Nonpharmacologic treatment, such as implementation of a timed voiding program, often results in improvement in incontinent episodes in these individuals.[58] A typical program involves offering the patient a urinal or bedpan, or placing him or her on the commode on a regularly scheduled basis. In incontinent male patients, use of a condom catheter also is an option.

Detrusor hyperreflexia with coordinated sphincters is the urodynamic pattern most often associated with suprapontine lesions, and results clinically in urgency incontinence. Treatment is geared toward diminishing reflex bladder activity.[76]

Urinary-tract infection itself may cause bladder hyperreflexia.[89] Therefore, a urinalysis should be obtained on all incontinent patients, and if infection is

Table 18-2
Treatment of detrusor dysfunction

Detrusor hyperreflexia	*Detrusor hyporeflexia*
Nonpharmacologic interventions	Nonpharmacologic interventions
Scheduled voiding program	Fluid restriction
Biofeedback	Credé or Valsalva technique
External collection device	Intermittent catheterization
Electrical nerve stimulation	Indwelling catheter
	Electrical nerve stimulation
Medications	Medications
Anticholinergics	Cholinergics
Antispasmodics	Naloxone
Alpha-adrenergic blockers	
Verapamil (intravesical)	
Capsaicin (intravesical)	
Surgical procedures	Surgical procedures
Sacral rhizotomy	Urinary diversion
Presacral neurectomy	Vesicostomy
Cystolysis	
Augmentation cystoplasty	

found, antibiotic therapy instituted promptly. When bladder hyperreflexia and infrequent incontinent episodes are present, or anticholinergic medications contraindicated, implementation of a scheduled voiding program may be beneficial.[90–96] Biofeedback may also be an option in selected patients.[97]

If these measures are ineffective, pharmacologic intervention may be necessary. The hallmark of treatment has been the use of anticholinergic medications, such as propantheline, which act by blockade of muscarinic receptors located in and about the bladder wall.[98] However, anticholinergic side effects often limit their use. These include dry mouth, blurred vision, tachycardia, constipation, orthostasis, and impotence.[99] Oxybutynin has both anticholinergic and antispasmodic activity, and has been shown to be as effective as propan-

Table 18-3
Treatment of urinary sphincter dysfunction

Overactive external sphincter	Areflexic external sphincter
Medications	Nonpharmacologic interventions
Baclofen	External collection device
Diazepam	Indwelling catheter
Dantrolene	
Botulinum toxin injections	
Surgical procedures	Surgical procedures
External sphincterotomy	Artificial sphincter placement
Pudendal neurectomy	Bladder-neck reconstruction
Sacral rhizotomy	Fascial-sling bladder suspension
Overactive internal sphincter	Areflexic internal sphincter
Medications	Medications
Alpha-adrenergic blockers	Alpha-adrenergic agonists
Methyldopa	Beta-adrenergic blockers
Clonidine	Conjugated estrogens

theline in the treatment of bladder hyperreflexia.[100] Oxybutynin has fewer side effects and may be preferable, especially in the elderly population.[101] Oxybutynin also may be administered intravesically in patients who are unable to tolerate the oral preparation.[102,103] Imipramine, dicyclomine, and flavoxate, with both anticholinergic and antispasmodic properties, are useful alternatives in the treatment of bladder hyperreflexia, although flavoxate has been shown to be somewhat less effective than the other drugs noted.[76,104–106]

Other medications may be effective in selected cases. Alpha-adrenergic blockers, such as phenoxybenzamine, phentolamine, prazosin, and terazosin, have their major site of action on alpha-adrenergic receptors located in the bladder neck, resulting in relaxation of the internal sphincter. In normal individuals, alpha blockers have little direct effect on the bladder wall. However, these medications have been shown to diminish detrusor hyperreflexia and improve bladder compliance with overactive bladders.[107–110] Alpha-adrenergic blockers are probably most useful in combination with anticholinergic medications. Intravesical administration of verapamil and capsaicin also have been shown to diminish bladder hyperreflexia.[111,112]

In cases of refractory bladder hyperreflexia, surgical neurologic ablation procedures may be considered. In general, these procedures diminish reflex bladder activity by selectively lesioning the peripheral neural reflex arc connecting the caudal spinal cord and bladder. However, these procedures are often limited by loss of other functions subserved by sacral segments. For example, a sacral rhizotomy at levels S2–S4 abolishes detrusor hyperreflexia, but causes loss of reflex erections, loss of vaginal lubrication, and impaired anal sphincter activity.[113,114] An alternative procedure involves selective lesioning of the S2–S4 dorsal nerve roots in combination with placement of an electrical stimulator on the ventral nerve roots.[114,115] This allows for adequate urine storage with electrically triggered bladder emptying at socially appropriate times. A nerve plexus–presacral neurectomy, which sections the sympathetic chain and divides the presacral nerve, interrupts the sensory limb of the sacral micturition reflex arc and diminishes bladder hyperreflexia.[116] Cystolysis, or selective denervation of the bladder, also abolishes reflex bladder activity. Although this is a more complicated procedure, it has the advantage of sparing urinary sphincter function.[117]

Electrical stimulation may be helpful in refractory cases of detrusor hyperreflexia. Various methods are effective, including stimulation of the pelvic floor, dorsal penile nerve, pelvic nerves, and pudendal nerves.[118–121] Stimulation increases the afferent signals to the spinal cord, which, in turn, by reflex inhibition, inhibits bladder contractions.

When detrusor hyperreflexia and a small noncompliant bladder are present, it may be difficult to achieve adequate urine storage, even with the interventions described. Augmentation cystoplasty may be necessary.[122,123] This procedure involves enlarging the bladder with an interposed piece of colon or small bowel.

Both medical and surgical treatment of bladder hyperreflexia often causes a conversion of the bladder to an areflexic state, resulting in urinary retention. Therefore the PVR must be followed closely after treatment is initiated.[99] Fortunately, a hyporeflexic bladder generally is more easily managed, especially with an intermittent catheterization program (described in the following).[124]

Suprasacral Spinal-Cord Lesions   Detrusor hyperreflexia with urinary sphincter dyssynergia is associated with lesions located between the pons and caudal spinal cord. Either the external or internal urinary sphincter (or both) may be dyssynergic, depending on the spinal-cord level involved. A dyssynergic pattern can cause serious clinical sequelae. Because the bladder is contracting against a closed sphincter, bladder emptying is incomplete and high intravesical pressures are generated that can lead to upper urinary-tract injury. Overall, treatment is geared toward elimination of sphincter and bladder overactivity, and facilitating complete bladder emptying.

Alpha-adrenergic blockers are most useful in the treatment of internal sphincter dyssynergia. These drugs act to relax the bladder neck and proximal urethra. Phenoxybenzamine is effective but is limited by side effects, including orthostatic hypotension, diarrhea, tachycardia, and retrograde ejaculation.[109] Prazosin and terazosin, selective alpha$_1$ blockers, are alternatives.[107–110] Methyldopa also has been shown to improve bladder emptying by acting centrally to diminish sympathetic outflow.[125] Clonidine, an alpha$_2$ agonist, also has been shown to be effective, and probably acts, as well, through inhibition of central sympathetic activity.[126,127]

Several medications can be used to treat external sphincter overactivity. Baclofen, administered orally or intrathecally, has been shown to directly inhibit both bladder and external-sphincter contractions through its inhibition of polysynaptic spinal-cord reflexes.[128–130] Diazepam may be used as adjunctive therapy, although its use is limited by sedative side effects and habituation.[76]

Dantrolene sodium reduces external-sphincter activity by a direct inhibitory effect on skeletal-muscle contraction.[131,132] However, because the major side effect is generalized weakness, this medication probably is best used in the bedridden quadriplegic patient.

Botulinum toxin also has been studied in the treatment of external sphincter hyperreflexia.[133] Injection of toxin directly into the sphincter results in a significant drop in urethral pressure and postvoid residual urine volumes. The drawbacks of this procedure are that several injections usually are required and the beneficial effect is relatively short-lived (average of 50 days).

If urinary retention persists, other treatment options include an intermittent catheterization program or placement of an indwelling catheter.[134] Unfortunately, most quadriplegic patients do not have the manual dexterity to catheterize themselves and use of chronic indwelling catheters increases the risk of urinary-tract infection, bladder-stone formation, urethral stricture, and squamous-cell carcinoma.[76]

If pharmacotherapy fails, surgical options for the treatment of sphincter dyssynergia should be considered. Transurethral external sphincterotomy is commonly used in male patients.[113] The major drawbacks of this procedure are that it is irreversible and often results in overflow incontinence by rendering the sphincter incompetent. As a result, many patients subsequently require condom/catheter drainage or a urinary-diversion procedure.[135] Pudendal neurectomy and sacral rhizotomy are other options, but may result in loss of reflex erections and reflex bowel activity, as described earlier.[136] A recent series reported favorable outcomes following placement of an intraurethral sphincter stent prosthesis.[137]

Despite management of the sphincter dyssynergia, urinary incontinence often persists because of concurrent bladder hyperreflexia. Management options for this component are described in the preceding section. Often a combination of treatments, such as anticholinergic medications plus alpha-adrenergic blockers or anticholinergic medications plus external sphincterotomy, are needed.

Lesions of Sacral Spinal Cord, Sacral Nerve Roots, and Peripheral Nerves Detrusor areflexia with sphincter areflexia is the urodynamic pattern most commonly associated with severe peripheral neuropathies or lesions of the conus medullaris or cauda equina.[113] This pattern also is seen during the acute spinal-shock phase following suprasacral spinal-cord injuries.[138] Clin-

ically, urinary retention with overflow incontinence is the rule.

Treatment is geared toward preventing overfilling of the bladder and facilitating complete bladder emptying. Fluid restriction (1800–2400 mL/day) is recommended as an initial step. An intermittent catheterization program is often necessary and should be performed with frequency to keep bladder volumes below 500 mL.[76,79] Symptomatic urinary-tract infections should be treated promptly. There is little evidence to support the use of prophylactic antibiotics or the treatment of asymptomatic urinary-tract infections.[139] An intermittent straight catheterization program is preferred over use of an indwelling catheter or urinary-diversion procedure.

Bladder emptying often can be enhanced by the Credé or Valsalva techniques, which allow for passive voiding by increasing intravesical pressure.[140] The major drawback to these procedures is that they can cause ureteral reflux owing to the high retrograde pressures required to open the bladder neck.

Medications may be used to improve detrusor contractility and bladder emptying. The cholinergic medications, such as benthanechol chloride, are most commonly used.[141,142] Unfortunately, these medications are effective in facilitating bladder-wall contractions only if the detrusor is capable of generating low-amplitude contractions. They are not effective in the completely areflexic bladder.[141,143] Furthermore, use of these drugs is limited by side effects, including vomiting, diarrhea, bradyarrythmias, sweating, and bronchospasm. Finally, the use of cholinergic medications is contraindicated if there is evidence of bladder-outlet obstruction, such as in males with prostatic disease, in order to avoid development of a pseudodyssynergic state.[76] Naloxone has been shown to improve detrusor contractility in select patients with incomplete spinal-cord injuries. It is thought to act by potentiating spinal-cord reflexes through inhibition of enkephalins.[144]

Electrical stimulation also has been shown to improve detrusor contractility and bladder emptying. Stimulation of the sacral ventral nerve roots causes bladder wall contractions and improves bladder emptying, but side effects, including penile erection, pelvic pain, and piloerection, are intolerable for some.[145] Stimulation of the pelvic nerves also facilitates detrusor contractions, but may cause pain, and may increase internal sphincter activity and outflow resistance.[119]

Significant sphincter areflexia may lead to persistent leakage of urine. Condom catheter drainage can be considered in men. If the internal sphincter is incompetent, medications may be effective in increasing tone in the bladder neck and proximal urethra. Alpha-adrenergic medications, including ephedrine, pseudoephedrine, and phenylpropanolamine, have been shown to be effective in this regard.[76] Side effects of these medications include hypertension, anxiety, and insomnia. Beta-adrenergic blockers may be effective in increasing internal sphincter tone, probably by unmasking alpha-adrenergic receptors located in the bladder neck. Conjugated estrogens also improve sphincter function, although the mechanism of action is unknown.[76] For external sphincter incompetence, surgical interventions, including placement of an artificial urinary sphincter, bladder neck reconstruction, or fascial sling bladder-neck suspension can be considered.[113]

NEUROGENIC BOWEL

Anatomy and Physiology

Anatomy of the Lower Gastrointestinal Tract   The colon is primarily responsible for absorption of water and electrolytes from liquid chyme, formation of semisolid feces, and storage of fecal material until an appropriate time for defecation. The colon ends distally at the rectum, a tube composed of smooth muscle approximately 5 inches in length, which is contiguous with the sigmoid colon superiorly and the anal canal inferiorly. The anal canal is approximately $1\frac{1}{2}$ inches in length and ends distally in the external opening, the anus. Inferiorly, the rectal smooth muscle fibers are thickened and form the internal anal sphincter.[146-148] The external anal sphincter, composed of striated muscle, envelops the distal rectum and anal canal. Its deepest portion is contiguous with the puborectalis muscle, which forms a muscular sling around the rectum.[2]

Neural Control of Defecation   Similar to the lower urinary tract, the distal bowel and anal sphincters are innervated by autonomic and somatic nerves. Parasympathetic innervation to the stomach, duodenum, small bowel, and proximal two thirds of the colon is from the vagus nerve. The distal colon and rectum are innervated by the pelvic nerves, originating in the interomediolateral cell column of the sacral spinal cord at levels S2–S4.[149,150] Sympathetic innervation to the gastrointestinal tract originates in the interomediolateral cell column of the thoracolumbar cord. Segments T4–T12 supply the stomach, duodenum, small bowel, and right colon

through the superior mesenteric plexus, whereas segments L1–L3 supply the left colon and rectum through the inferior mesenteric plexus.[149] Both parasympathetic and sympathetic activity are under involuntary control. Defecation is facilitated by action of the parasympathetic nervous system, which increases gastrointestinal motility and relaxes the internal anal sphincter. The sympathetic system acts in opposite fashion, to decrease peristalsis and increase activity of the internal anal sphincter.

In contrast, the external anal sphincter is innervated by the somatic nervous system and is under voluntary control. Contraction of the external sphincter helps maintain fecal continence.[2] Efferent somatic fibers arise in the ventral horns of the sacral cord, levels S2–S4, and are carried by the pudendal nerves.[2,148,151] The pudendal nerves also contain somatic sensory afferent fibers that transmit information from stretch receptors in the anal canal and external sphincter back to the spinal cord to complete a reflex loop (Figure 18-2).

Movement of stool is facilitated by two major types of motor activity in the colon. Segmental contractions, called haustrations, allow for slow propulsion of stool. This activity predominates in the cecum and ascending colon. Mass action contractions, which predominate in the transverse colon and sigmoid, propel fecal material in bulk toward the rectum to allow for expulsion of stool. These mass movements are facilitated by several means. Distension of the stomach and duodenum by food induces reflex contractions in the rectum. These gastrocolic and duodenocolic reflexes occur during the first hour after meals and are strongest after breakfast.[152] Distension of the rectum by stool or by chemical or mechanical irritation (e.g., suppository, enema, digital stimulation) induces mass contractions of the distal colon and rectum.[153] These reflex contractions are facilitated by an increase in parasympathetic activity, which is mediated through the sacral spinal-cord reflex arc, described previously.

In the normal continent state, both the internal and external anal sphincters are tonically active. The internal sphincter accounts for 50 to 85 percent of the resting anal tone.[2,147] As stool fills its distal end, the rectum contracts and stretch receptors in the anal wall are activated, sending afferent information back to the caudal spinal cord centers. In response, the internal anal sphincter relaxes and the external anal sphincter transiently contracts (rectoanal inhibitor reflex). This allows stool to come into contact with the sensory receptors in the anal mucosa.[2] This reflex may be coordinated by a defecation center located in the anterior pons, akin

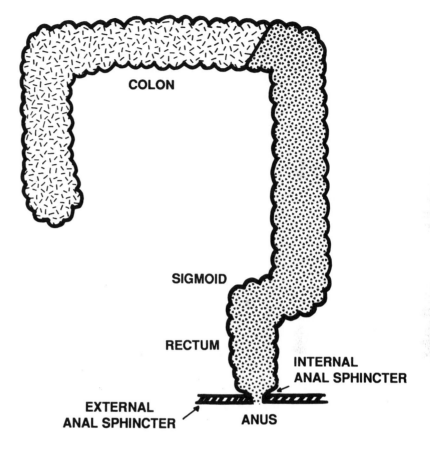

Figure 18-2

Innervation of the lower gastrointestinal tract. The proximal two-thirds of the colon is innervated by the vagus nerve (parasympathetic) and superior mesenteric plexus (sympathetic, segments T4–T12). The distal third of the colon, including the rectum, is innervated by the pelvic nerves (parasympathetic, segments S2–S4) and inferior mesenteric plexus (sympathetic, segments L1–L3). The external anal sphincter is innervated by the pudendal nerve (somatic, segments S2–S4).

to the pontine micturition center, described previously.[154] Anal sensations are relayed through ascending neural pathways to the cerebral cortex, providing the sense of the urge to defecate. If it is not a socially appropriate time to defecate, one can consciously inhibit the urge to defecate. This is mediated by cortical inhibitory influences on the neural defecation pathways.[2] In addition, one can voluntarily contract the external sphincter and puborectalis muscle to help maintain fecal continence.

If it is an appropriate time for defecation, this cortical inhibition is removed, and the parasympathetic system is activated, resulting in colonic mass action. The latter is facilitated by straining (Valsalva maneuver).[153] Simultaneously, there is inhibition of the sympathetic and somatic nervous system pathways, which results in relaxation of the internal and external sphincters, allowing for voluntary expulsion of stool.

Evaluation of Neurogenic Bowel

Clinical evaluation should include a detailed history of bowel habits. One should inquire as to the frequency of bowel movements, consistency of stool, sensation at time of defecation, and the frequency and severity of fecal incontinence.[2] Associated symptoms, such as rectal pain, rectal bleeding, mucous discharge, urinary incontinence, and presence of concurrent disease, such as diabetes mellitus, may provide clues as to the cause of bowel dysfunction. An obstetric history is also important, given the association of fecal incontinence with obstetrical trauma. Physical examination should include inspection of the anus and perianal skin for evidence of perineal soiling, hemorrhoids, anal fissures or tears, and rectal prolapse.[2] A digital rectal examination allows for bedside assessment of the resting and squeeze tone of the anal sphincters, evaluation for sphincter defects, rectoceles, and rectovaginal fistulae. Proctoscopy can rule out additional pathology in the anus and rectum. Detailed neurologic examination also should be performed, including assessment of sacral spinal cord reflexes, discussed previously.

There are several widely available anorectal physiologic tests that are often part of the standard evaluation of fecal incontinence.[155] These include anorectal manometry, pudendal nerve conduction studies, and anal sphincter electromyography (EMG).

Anorectal manometry involves passage of a soft plastic, small diameter, multichannel catheter into the rectum. The rectum can be distended by either water perfusion or balloon catheters and pressures along various segments of the rectum can be measured.[156] Anal manometry allows for determination of resting anal pressure (normal 30–60 mmHg), which primarily reflects internal sphincter tone, squeeze pressure (normal 100–180 mmHg), which measures voluntary contraction of the external sphincter, and the presence or absence of the rectoanal inhibitor reflex, which assesses coordination of the sacral defecation reflex.[2]

Pudendal nerve function can be evaluated electrophysiologically. The nerve is stimulated transrectally and the evoked response of the external sphincter is measured to provide measurement of the pudendal-nerve terminal motor latency (PNTML).[155,159,160] The PNTML is prolonged in patients with pudendal-nerve injuries and polyneuropathies. A prolonged PNTML is a poor prognostic sign with regard to improvement following sphincteroplasty in the treatment of fecal incontinence.[161]

Anal sphincter EMG is useful in the diagnosis of lower motor neuron injuries to the external sphincter.[155,162,163] Typically both sides of the external anal sphincter are studied. Acute injuries to the sacral nerve roots, sacral plexus, or pudendal nerves result in spontaneous electrical activity, including fibrillation potentials and positive sharp waves, suggestive of ongoing denervation. During voluntary contraction of the anal sphincter there may be decreased recruitment of motor units. The presence of polyphasic motor units of increased amplitude and duration suggest a chronic neuropathic process with reinnervation.[155,156]

Other diagnostic studies, including single-fiber EMG, cinedefecography, and anal endosonography, may provide additional diagnostic information in select cases of fecal incontinence.[155] However, details of these studies are beyond the scope of this chapter.

Lesion Localization

Cerebral Lesions   Cerebral lesions, including stroke, dementia, and brain tumors, often lead to fecal incontinence. This may be owing to interruption of the connections between the cerbral cortex and the pontine and spinal defecation centers, or to altered mentation and decreased sensory awareness associated with the neurologic disease itself.[2] Gastrointestinal motility is normal and spinal-cord defecation reflexes are intact. Therefore, stool is delivered to the rectum automatically and there is normal reflexive relaxation of the internal sphincter. However, conscious inhibition of defecation is difficult, and impaired voluntary contraction of the external sphincter in response to rectal distension leads to fecal incontinence.[153]

Suprasacral Spinal-Cord Lesions   Lesions of the cervical, thoracic, and lumbar spinal cord, most commonly caused by traumatic spinal-cord injuries, multiple sclerosis, and transverse myelitis, result in fecal incontinence owing to interruption of the connections between the brain and reflex centers in the caudal spinal cord. Bowel dysfunction is more commonly associated with cervical and upper thoracic spinal-cord injuries, and with complete as opposed to incomplete cord injuries.[150] After acute spinal-cord injury, during spinal shock, there is generally a 3- to 4-day period of paralytic ileus with gastric dilatation, because of diminished gastrointestinal peristalsis.[150] Following this early period, peristalsis in the small bowel and right colon returns, owing to normal vagus nerve activity. However, the parasympathetic innervation to the distal colon, arising from the sacral cord, remains inhibited, resulting in fecal impaction in the transverse colon.[150,164–166] Overflow fecal incontinence also may occur owing to external anal sphincter areflexia.

Complications associated with gastric and small-bowel distension include vomiting and respiratory distress, caused by interference with movement of the diaphragm. Fecal impaction also may precipitate episodes of autonomic dysreflexia, characterized by hypertension, bradycardia, sweating, and headache, especially in patients with cervical or upper thoracic spinal cord lesions.[165]

Following the acute spinal-shock phase, reflex defecation generally becomes possible. This may be induced naturally, by rectal distension with stool, or artificially, by mechanical (digital) stimulation or chemical irritation (suppository or enema) of the rectal mucosa.[153] Because of the interruption of the neural pathways connecting the brain to caudal spinal-cord centers, there is loss of cortical inhibition of defecation. This results in parasympathetic overactivity and mass colonic contractions facilitating expulsion of stool. Patients with spinal-cord injuries also may be unable to contract their external sphincters forcefully, leading to episodes of urgent fecal incontinence.[167]

Fecal incontinence occurs in 39 to 68 percent of patients with multiple sclerosis because of lesions in both the brain and spinal cord.[168–170] Abnormalities of both anorectal sensory and motor function have been described. Resting anal sphincter pressures generally are normal, but rectal sensation can be impaired. Diminished external sphincter contraction occurs in response to rectal distension.[168–170]

Lesions of the Sacral Spinal Cord, Sacral Nerve Roots, and Peripheral Nerves

Lesions of the caudal spinal-cord defecation centers, sacral-nerve roots, and peripheral nerves innervating the colon, rectum, and anal sphincters result in decreased colonic motility and external anal sphincter areflexia.[165] This pattern is seen most commonly in traumatic sacral spinal-cord injuries, myelomeningocele, and polyneuropathy, and results clinically in constipation with overflow fecal incontinence.

Neurogenic bowel is common in diabetes owing to development of both somatic and autonomic neuropathy. Manometric studies demonstrate decreased sensory perception of rectal distension, and decreased anal resting and squeeze pressures, owing to hyporeflexic internal and external sphincters.[147,169,171] The postprandial gastrocolic reflex also is diminished.[172] Chronic constipation, which occurs in 20 to 60 percent of diabetics, may alternate with diarrhea.[173,174] The cause of diarrhea probably is multifactorial. Sympathetic dysfunction, owing to autonomic neuropathy, results in impaired colonic fluid absorption. In addition, bowel bacterial overgrowth, abnormalities of bile acid, and exocrine pancreatic dysfunction, common in diabetic patients, may be factors.

External sphincter areflexia, with overflow fecal incontinence, may result from pudendal nerve injuries sustained during childbirth or pelvic surgery.[157] In addition, many patients with "idiopathic" fecal incontinence actually have pudendal neuropathies, diagnosed by prolonged pudendal-nerve terminal motor latencies on nerve-conduction study testing.[160]

Treatment

The goal of treatment of neurogenic bowel is to achieve regular bowel movements, avoid accidents, and prevent medical complications, such as fecal impaction and diarrhea. Nonpharmacologic measures, medications, and surgical interventions may be considered, depending on the individual and severity of the neurogenic bowel (Table 18-4). Treatment options based on lesion localization and abnormalities of bowel and sphincter function now are reviewed.

Cerebral Lesions Cerebral lesions cause fecal incontinence, most commonly because of diminished ability to inhibit the urge to defecate. Neurologic deficits, such as decreased sensory perception, aphasia, and severe motor deficits, which impact a patient's ability to communicate the urge to defecate or to manage the physical aspects of toileting, also may be contributing factors. For these patients, a habit-training program should be considered. This involves placing the patient on the commode at regularly scheduled times, often following breakfast or supper, to take advantage of the gastrocolic reflex.[175] A reward system also can be initiated. If a habit-training program alone is ineffective, other modalities may be useful to help induce bowel movements at scheduled times. These techniques involve stimulation of the anal mucosa to trigger the spinal defecation reflex, including digital stimulation of the anal wall, use of rectal suppositories (glycerin or bisacodyl), or enemas.[153,166,167] If fecal incontinence persists, adult diapers may be required.

Table 18-4
Treatment strategies for neurogenic bowel

Treatment of constipation	Treatment of anal sphincter incompetence
Valsalva maneuver	Biofeedback
Abdominal massage	Surgical procedures
Bulk cathartics	Anterior sphincteroplasty
Stool softeners	Encirclement procedures
Rectal suppositories	Muscle transposition procedures
Enemas	
Digital stimulation	
Manual disimpaction	

Suprasacral Spinal-Cord Lesions   During the acute spinal-shock period following spinal-cord injury, there is loss of reflex gastrointestinal function, resulting in constipation and overflow fecal incontinence. Paralytic ileus may be present during the first few days and may cause abdominal distension, vomiting, and respiratory distress. Management during this period includes nasogastric suctioning and intravenous hydration, with close monitoring of fluid balance.

Following the acute spinal-shock phase, the ability to defecate reflexively usually returns. Oral feedings are initiated as soon as bowel sounds return. Fluid intake of at least 1,500 to 2,000 mL daily is encouraged, and should be combined with a diet high in fiber. Bulk cathartics, such as psyllium hydrophilic colloid and milk of magnesia, and use of stool softeners, such as docusate sodium, help create a softer, bulkier stool that is more easily passed.[2,165]

The next goal of treatment is to induce bowel movements at regular and socially appropriate times (daily or every other day). To trigger the defecation reflex, digital stimulation or use of rectal suppositories, as described previously, often are used.[2,153,165,166] If fecal impaction develops, manual disimpaction may be necessary. Care must be taken, particularly in patients with cervical or upper thoracic spinal-cord injuries, to prevent precipitation of autonomic dysreflexia.[165] The risk may be lessened by use of lidocaine jelly applied to the anal mucosa prior to disimpaction and by avoiding the use of enemas.[152,176]

Lesions of the Sacral Spinal Cord, Sacral-Nerve Roots, and Peripheral Nerves   Injury to the sacral spinal cord, nerve roots, or pudendal nerves often leads to constipation owing to impairment of the sacral spinal-cord defecation reflexes. It may help to have patients defecate while sitting on the commode, as gravity may assist with stool evacuation. Vigorous straining (Valsalva maneuver) and abdominal massage from right to left also help propel stool toward the rectum. If these methods are ineffective in regulating bowel habits, use of bulking agents, stool softeners, rectal suppositories, and enemas, as described earlier, may be needed.[177–179]

Peripheral neuropathy or sacral spinal-cord lesions often cause diminished sensory perception of rectal distension and weakness of the external anal-sphincter contraction, leading to leakage of stool. Biofeedback has reduced fecal incontinence in myelomeningocele and diabetic neuropathy.[2,178,180–183] In a typical program, the rectum is distended with an inflatable balloon and the patient is asked to voluntarily contract his or her anal sphincter in response to the sensation of rectal distension. The amount of distension is gradually diminished until an effective response can be generated to small distensions. Sphincter exercises to improve strength of contraction may be added. Biofeedback may be most effective when combined with a behavior-modification program.[178]

Diarrhea may be associated with fecal incontinence, especially in diabetic autonomic polyneuropathy. Treatment with loperamide or diphenoxylate with atropine is useful under these circumstances.[2,179]

Persistent fecal incontinence owing to an incompetent external anal sphincter may necessitate surgical repair of the sphincter to prevent fecal incontinence. Various procedures, including anterior sphincteroplasty, encirclement procedures, and muscle transpositions, have been used.[2,161,184,185] If fecal incontinence persists, diversion procedures, such as colostomy or ileostomy, may be needed, under extreme circumstances (nonhealing decubitus ulcer).

SUMMARY

Neurogenic bowel and bladder are commonly associated with diseases affecting either the central or peripheral nervous system and have potential medical and psychosocial consequences. A thorough diagnostic evaluation should be performed to determine the specific abnormal micturition or defecation patterns in order to help design therapy. Although there are a variety of potential treatment options for neurogenic bowel and bladder, management should be individualized and geared toward prevention of long-term complications.

REFERENCES

1. Resnick NM, Yalla SV: Management of urinary incontinence in the elderly. *NEJM* 1985; 13:800–805.
2. Jorge JM, Wexner SD: Etiology and management of fecal incontinence. *Dis Colon Rectum* 1993; 36:77–97.
3. Tobin GW, Brocklehurst JC: Faecal incontinence in residential homes for the elderly: Prevalence, aetiology and management. *Age Ageing* 1986; 15:41–46.
4. Hu T: Impact of urinary incontinence on health-care costs. *JAGS* 1990; 38: 292–295.
5. Ouslander JG, Kane RL, Abrass IB: Urinary incontinence in elderly nursing home patients. *JAMA* 1982; 248:1194–1198.
6. Sier H, Ouslander J, Orzeck S: Urinary incontinence

among geriatric patients in an acute-care hospital. *JAMA* 1987; 257:1767–1771.

7. Whitehead WE, Schuster MM: Behavioral approaches to the treatment of gastrointestinal motility disorders. *Med Clin No Am* 1981; 65:1397–1411.

8. Tanagho EA, Pugh RC: The anatomy and function of the ureterovesical junction. *Br J Urol* 1962; 35:151–165.

9. Tanagho EA, Smith DR: The anatomy and function of the bladder neck. *Br J Urol* 1966; 38:54–71.

10. Hutch JA, Rambo ON, Jr: A new theory of the anatomy of the internal urinary sphincter and the physiology of micturition. III. Anatomy of the urethra. *J Urol* 1967; 97:696–704.

11. Hutch JA: A new theory of the anatomy of the internal urinary sphincter and the physiology of micturition. IV. The urinary sphincter mechanism. *J Urol* 1967; 97:705–712.

12. Koyanagi T: Studies on the sphincteric system located distally in the urethra: The external urethral sphincter revisited. *J Urol* 1980; 124:400–406.

13. Awad SA, Downie JW: The adrenergic component in the proximal urethra. *Urol Int* 1977; 32:192–197.

14. de Groat WC, Booth AM: Physiology of the urinary bladder and urethra. *Ann Intern Med* 1980; 92:312–315.

15. Bradley WE, Timm GW, Scott FB: Innervation of detrusor muscle and urethra. *Urol Clin No Am* 1974; 1:3–27.

16. Awad SA, Bruce AW, Carro-Ciampi G, Downie JW, Lin M: Distribtution of α- and β-adrenoceptors in human urinary bladder. *Br J Pharmacol* 1974; 50:525–529.

17. Rockswold GL, Bradley WE, Chou SN: Innnervation of the external urethral and external anal sphincters in higher primates. *J Comp Neurol* 1980; 193:521–528.

18. Milner P, Crowe R, Burnstock G, Light JK: Neuropeptide Y- and vasoactive intestinal polypeptide-containing nerves in the intrinsic external urethral sphincter in the areflexic bladder compared to detrusor-sphincter dyssynergia in patients with spinal cord injury. *J Urol* 1987; 138:888–892.

19. Alm P, Alumets J, Brodin E, Hakanson R, Nilsson G, Sjoberg NO, Sundler F: Peptidergic (substance P) nerves in the genito-urinary tract. *Neuroscience* 1978; 3:419–425.

20. Burnstock G, Cocks T, Crowe R, Kasakov L: Purinergic innervation of the guinea-pig urinary bladder. *Br J Pharmacol* 1978; 63:125–138.

21. Crowe R, Moss HE, Chapple CR, Light JK, Burnstock G: Patients with lower motor spinal cord lesion: A decrease of vasoactive intestinal polypeptide, calcitonin gene-related peptide and substance P, but not neuropeptide Y and somatostatin-immunoreactive nerves in the detrusor muscle of the bladder. *J Urol* 1991; 145:600–604.

22. Dray A, Metsch R: Opioid receptor subtypes involved in the central inhibition of urinary bladder motility. *Eur J Pharmacol* 1984; 104:47–53.

23. Gu J, Blank MA, Huang WM, Islam KN, McGrego GP, Christofides N, Allen JM, Bloom SR, Polak JM: Peptide-containing nerves in human urinary bladder. *Urology* 1984; 24:353–357.

24. Khanna OP, DeGregorio GJ, Sample RG, McMichael RF: Histamine receptors in urethrovesical smooth muscle. *Urology* 1977; 10:375–381.

25. Gu J, Restorick JM, Blank MA, Huang WM, Polak JM, Bloom SR, Mundy AR: Vasoactive intestinal polypeptide in the normal and unstable bladder. *J Urol* 1983; 55:645–647.

26. Bradley WE, Conway CJ: Bladder representation in the pontine-mesencephalic reticular formation. *Neurology* 1966; 16:237–249.

27. Tang PC: Levels of brain stem and diencephalon controlling micturition reflex. *J Neurophysiol* 1955; 18:583.

28. Siroky MB, Krane RJ: Neurologic aspects of detrusor-sphincter dyssynergia, with reference to the guarding reflex. *J Urol* 1982; 127:953–957.

29. Bhatia NN, Bradley WE: Neuroanatomy and physiology: Innervation of the lower urinary tract, in Raz S (ed): *Female Urology*. Philadelphia: W.B. Saunders, 1983, pp. 13–32.

30. Lewin RJ, Dillard GV, Porter RW: Extrapyramidal inhibition of the urinary bladder. *Brain Res* 1967; 4:301–307.

31. Andrew J, Nathan PW: The cerebral control of micturition. *Proc R Soc Med* 1965; 58:553–555.

32. Carlsson CA: The supraspinal control of the urinary bladder. *Acta Pharmacol Toxicol* 1978; 43:8–12.

33. Bors E, Blinn KA: Bulbocavernosus reflex. *J Urol* 1959; 82:128.

34. Massagli TL, Jaffe KM, Cardenas DD: Ultrasound database. *J Reprod Med* 1990; 35:925–931.

35. Kjeldsen-Kragh J: Measurement of residual urine volume by means of ultrasonic scanning: A comparative study. *Paraplegia* 1988; 26:192–199.

36. Churchill BM, Gilmour RF, Williot P: Urodynamics. *Pediatr Clin No Am* 1987; 34:1133–1157.

37. Revord JP, Opitz JL, Murtaugh P, Harrison J: Determining residual urine volumes using a portable ultrasonographic device. *Arch Phys Med Rehab* 1993; 74:457–462.

38. Norton C: Urodynamic and medical investigations of urinary incontinence. *Geriatr Nurs Home Care* May 1987; 11–14.

39. Gelber DA, Jozefczyk PB, Good DC, Laven LJ, Verhulst SJ: Urinary retention following acute stroke. *J Neuro Rehab* 1994; 8:69–74.

40. Bump RC: The urodynamic laboratory. *Urogynecology* 1989; 16:795–816.

41. Saxton HM: Urodynamics: The appropriate modality for the investigation of frequency, urgency, incontinence, and voiding difficulties. *Radiology* 1990; 175:307–316.

42. Diokno AC: Diagnostic categories of incontinence and the role of urodynamic testing. *JAGS* 1990; 38:300–305.

43. McGuire E: Electromyographic evaluation of sphincter function and dysfunction. *Urol Clin No Am* 1979; 6:121–124.

44. Lose G, Andersen JT: A disposable anal plug electrode for pelvic floor/anal sphincter electromyography. *J Urol* 1987; 137:249–252.

45. Krane RJ, Siroky MB: Classification of neuro-urologic disorders, in Krane RJ, Siroky MB (eds): *Clinical Neurourology*. Boston: Little, Brown & Co., 1979, pp. 143–158.

46. Krane RJ, Siroky MB: Classification of voiding dysfunction: value of classification systems, in Barrett DM, Wein AJ (eds): *Controversies in Neuro-Urology*. New York: Churchill Livingstone, 1984, pp. 233–238.

47. Barrett DM, Wein AJ: Classification of voiding dysfunction: a simple approach, in Barrett DM, Wein AJ (eds): *Controversies in Neuro-Urology*. New York: Churchill Livingstone, 1984, pp. 239–250.

48. Staskin DR: Classification of voiding dysfunction, in Krane RJ, Siroky MB (eds): *Clinical Neuro-Urology*, 2nd ed. Boston: Little, Brown & Co., 1991, pp. 411–424.

49. Bors E, Comarr AE: *Neurologic Urology*. Baltimore: University Park Press, 1971.

50. Bradley WE: Physiology of the urinary bladder, in Walsh P, et al (eds): *Campbell's Urology*. Philadelphia: W.B. Saunders, 1986, pp. 129–185.

51. Hald T, Bradley WE: *The Urinary Bladder*. Baltimore: Williams & Wilkins, 1982.

52. Wein AJ: Classification of neurogenic voiding dysfunction. *J Urol* 1981; 125:605.

53. Lapides J: (1967) Cystometry. *JAMA* 1967; 201:618.

54. Bates CP, Bradley WE, Glen ES, Melchior H, Rowan D, Sterling AM, Sundin T, Thomas D, Torrens M, Turner-Warwick R, Ziner NR, Hald T: Fourth report on the standardisation of terminology of lower urinary tract function. *J Urol* 1981; 53:333–335.

55. Khan Z, Starer P, Yang WC, Bhola A: Analysis of voiding disorders in patients with cerebrovascular accidents. *Urology* 1990; 35:265–270.

56. Reding MJ, Winter SW, Hochrein SA, Simon HB, Thompson MM: Urinary incontinence after unilateral hemispheric stroke: A neurologic-epidemiologic perspective. *J Neurol Rehab* 1987; 1:25–30.

57. Decter RM, Bauer SB, Khoshbin S, Dyro FM, Krarup C, Colodny AH, Retik AB: Urodynamic assessment of children with cerebral palsy. *J Urol* 1987; 138:1110–1112.

58. Gelber DA, Good DC, Laven LJ, Verhulst SJ: Causes of urinary incontinence after acute hemispheric stroke. *Stroke* 1993; 24:378–382.

59. Geirsson G, Fall M, Linström S: Subtypes of overactive bladder in old age. *Age Ageing* 1993; 22:125–131.

60. Borrie MJ, Campbell AJ, Caradoc-Davies TH, Spears GF: Urinary incontinence after stroke: A prospective study. *Age Ageing* 1986; 15:177–181.

61. Brocklehurst JC, Andrews K, Richards B, Laycock PJ: Incidence and correlates of incontinence in stroke patients. *J Am Geriatr Soc* 1985; 33:540.

62. Gelber D, Jozefczyk P, Good D: Measures that predict improvement in post-stroke urinary incontinence. *J Neuro Rehab* 1994; 8:86.

63. Khan Z, Hertanu J, Yang WC, Melma A, Leite E: Predictive correlation of urodynamic dysfunction and brain injury after cerebrovascular accident. *J Urol* 1981; 126:86–88.

64. Linsenmeyer TA, Zorowitz RD: Urodynamic findings in patients with urinary incontinence after cerebrovascular accident. *Neurol Rehab* 1992; 2:23–26.

65. Feder M, Heller L, Tadmor R, Snir D, Solzi P, Ring H: Urinary incontinence after stroke: Association with cystometric profile and computerized tomography findings. *Eur Neurol* 1987; 27:101–105.

66. Fall M, Ohlsson BL, Carlsson CA: The neurogenic overactive bladder: Classification based on urodynamics. *Br J Urol* 1989; 64:368–373.

67. Berger Y, Blaivas JG, DeLaRocha ER, Salinas JM: Urodynamic findings in Parkinson's disease. *J Urol* 1987; 138:836–838.

68. Andersen JT, Hebjorn S, Frimodt-Moller C, Walter S, Worm-Petersen J: Disturbances of micturition in Parkinson's disease. *Acta Neurol Scand* 1976; 53:161–170.

69. Andersen JT, Bradley WE: Cystometric, sphincter and electromyelographic abnormalities in Parkinson's disease. *J Urol* 1976; 116:75–78.

70. Greenberg M, Gordon HL, McCutchen JJ: Neurogenic bladder in Parkinson's disease. *So Med J* 1972; 65:446–448.

71. Pavlakis AJ, Siroky MB, Goldstein I, Krane RJ: Neurologic findings in Parkinson's disease. *J Urol* 1983; 129:80–83.

72. Andersen JT, Bradley WE: Abnormalities of detrusor and sphincter function in multiple sclerosis. *Br J Urol* 1976; 48:193–198.

73. Miller H, Simpson CA, Yeates WK: Bladder dysfunction in multiple sclerosis. *Br Med J* 1965; 1:1265–1269.

74. Bradley WE, Logothetis JL, Timm GW: Cystometric and sphincter abnormalities in multiple sclerosis. *Neurology* 1973; 23:1131–1139.

75. Betts CD, D'Mellow MT, Fowler CJ: Urinary symptoms and the neurological features of bladder dysfunction in multiple sclerosis. *J Neurol Neurosurg Psychiatr* 1993; 56:245–250.

76. Gelber DA: Bladder dysfunction, in Good DC, Couch JR (eds): *Handbook of Neurorehabilitation*. New York: Marcel Dekker, 1994, pp. 373–402.

77. Weinstein MS, Cardenas DD, O'Shaughnessy EJ, Catanzaro ML: Carbon dioxide cystometry and postural changes in patients with multiple sclerosis. *Arch Phys Med Rehab* 1988; 69:923–927.

78. Wyndaele JJ: Urethral sphincter dyssynergia in spinal cord injury patients. *Paraplegia* 1987; 25:10–15.

79. O'Donnell WF: Urological management in the patient with acute spinal cord injury. *Crit Care Clin* 1987; 3:599–617.

80. Van Gool JD, De Jong TP, Van Wijk AA: Urodynamics in children with myelomeningocele: early assessment of obstruction and incontinence. *Acta Urol Belg* 1989; 57:497–501.

81. Frimodt-Moller C: Diabetic cystopathy I: A clinical study of the frequency of bladder dysfunction in diabetics. *Dan Med Bull* 1976; 23:267–278.

82. Kirby RS: Studies of the neurogenic bladder. *Ann R Coll Surg Engl* 1988; 70:285–289.

83. Smith AY, Woodside JR: Urodynamic evaluation of patients with spinal stenosis. *Urology* 1988; 32:474–477.

84. Snape J, Duffin HM, Castleden CM: Urodynamic findings in sacrococcygeal chordoma. *Br J Urol* 1987; 59:50–52.

85. Gelber DA, Pfeifer MA: Management of diabetic neuropathy, in Marshall SM, Home PD (eds): *The Diabetes Annual,* vol. 8. Amsterdam: Elsevier, 1994, pp. 349–363.

86. Greene DA, Gelber DA, Pfeifer M, Carroll PB: Diabetic neuropathy, in Becker KL (ed): *Principles of Endocrinology & Metabolism*, 2nd ed. Philadelphia: J. B. Lippincott, 1995, pp. 1270–1280.

87. Kaplan SA: Bladder dysfunction, in Lebovitz HE (ed): *Therapy for Diabetes Mellitus and Related Disorders.* Alexandria, VA: American Diabetes Association, 1991, pp. 288–292.

88. Buck AC, Reed PI, Siddiq YQ, Chisholm GD, Fraser TR: Bladder dysfunction and neuropathy in diabetes. *Diabetologia* 1976; 12:251.

89. Schoenberg HW, Gutrich JM: Management of vesical dysfunction in multiple sclerosis. *Urology* 1980; 16:444–447.

90. Pengelly AW, Booth CM: A prospective trial of bladder training as treatment for detrusor instability. *Br J Urol* 1980; 52:463–466.

91. Greengold BA, Ouslander JG: Bladder retraining for elderly patients with post-indwelling catheterization. *J Gerentol Nurs* 1986; 12:31–35.

92. Frewen WK: The management of urgency and frequency of micturition. *Br J Urol* 1980; 52:367–369.

93. Frewen WK: A reassessment of bladder training in detrusor dysfunction in the female. *Br J Urol* 1982; 54:372–373.

94. Long ML: Incontinence: The way you react to your clients' incontinence influences their attitudes about the problem. *J Gerentol Nurs* 1985; 11:30–41.

95. Holmes DM, Stone AR, Bary PR, Richards CJ, Stephenson TP: Bladder retraining, 3 years on. *Br J Urol* 1983; 55:660–664.

96. Hadley EC: Bladder training and related therapies for urinary incontinence in older people. *JAMA* 1986; 3:372–379.

97. Cardozo LD, Abrams PD, Stanton SL, Feneley RC: Idiopathic bladder instability treated by biofeedback. *Br J Urol* 1978; 50:521–523.

98. Benson GS, Wein AJ, Raezer DM, Corriere JN: Adrenergic and cholinergic stimulation and blockade of the human bladder base. *J Urol* 1976; 116:174–175.

99. Fowler CJ, van Kerrebroeck P, Nordenbo A, Van Poppel H: Treatment of lower urinary tract dysfunction in patients with multiple sclerosis. *J Neurol Neurosurg Psychiatr* 1992; 55:986–989.

100. Moisey CU, Stephenson TP, Brendler CB: The urodynamic and subjective results of treatment of detrusor instability with oxybutynin chloride. *J Urol* 1980; 52:472–475.

101. Ouslander JG, Blaustein J, Connor A, Orzeck S, Yong CL: Pharmacokinetics and clinical effects of oxybutynin in geriatric patients. *J Urol* 1988; 140:47–50.

102. Brendler CB, Radebaugh LC, Mohler JL: Topical oxybutynin chloride for relaxation of dysfunctional bladders. *J Urol* 1988; 141:1350–1352.

103. Greenfield SP, Fera M: The use of intravesical oxybutynin chloride in children with neurogenic bladder. *J Urol* 1991; 146:532–534.

104. Thompson IM, Lauvetz R: Oxybutynin in bladder spasm, neurogenic bladder, and enuresis. *Urology* 1976; 8:452–454.

105. Fischer CP, Diokno A, Lapides J: The anticholinergic effects of dicyclomine hydrochloride in uninhibited neurogenic bladder dysfunction. *J Urol* 1978; 120:328–329.

106. Finkbeiner AE, Welch LT, Bissada NK: Uropharmacology: IX. Direct-acting smooth muscle stimulants and depressants. *Urology* 1978; 12:231–235.

107. Jensen D, Jr: Uninhibited neurogenic bladder treated with prazosin. *Scand J Urol Nephrol* 1981; 15:229–233.

108. Petersen T, Husted SE, Sidenius P: Prazosin treatment of neurological patients with detrusor hyperreflexia and bladder emptying disability. *Scand J Urol Nephrol* 1989; 23:189–194.

109. Scott MB, Morrow JW: Phenoxybenzamine in neurogenic bladder dysfunction after spinal cord injury. II. Autonomic dysreflexia. *J Urol* 1978; 119:483–484.

110. Swierzewski SJ, Gormley EA, Belville WD, Sweetser PM, Wan J, McGuire EJ: The effect of terazosin on bladder function in the spinal cord injured patient. *J Urol* 1994; 151:951–954.

111. Mattiasson A, Ekstrom B, Andersson KE: Effects of intravesical instillation of verapamil in patients with detrusor hyperactivity. *J Urol* 1989; 141:174–177.

112. Fowler CJ, Beck RO, Gerrard S, Betts CD, Fowler CG: Intravesical capsaicin for treatment of detrusor hyperreflexia. *J Neurol Neurosurg Psychiatr* 1994; 57:169–173.

113. Madersbacher H: The various types of neurogenic bladder dysfunction: an update of current therapeutic concepts. *Paraplegia* 1990; 28:217–229.

114. MacDonagh RP, Forster MC, Thomas DG: Urinary continence in spinal injury patients following complete sacral posterior rhizotomy. *J Urol* 1990; 66:618–622.

115. Koldewijn EL, Van Kerrebroeck PE, Rosier PF, Wijkstra H, Debruyne FM: Bladder compliance after posterior sacral root rhizotomies and anterior sacral root stimulation. *J Urol* 1994; 151:955–960.

116. Leach GE, Goldman D, Raz S: Surgical treatment of detrusor hyperreflexia, in Raz S (ed): *Female Urology*. Philadelphia: W.B. Saunders, 1983, pp. 326–334.

117. Freiha FS, Stamey TA: Cystolysis: A procedure for the selective denervation of the bladder. *J Urol* 1980; 123:360–363.

118. Ohlsson BL, Fall M, Frankenberg-Sommar S: Effects of external and direct pudendal nerve maximal electrical stimulation in the treatment of the uninhibited overactive bladder. *Br J Urol* 1989; 64:374–380.

119. Tanagho EA, Schmidt RA: Electrical stimulation in the clinical management of the neurogenic bladder. *J Urol* 1988; 140:1331–1339.

120. Ishigooka M, Hashimoto T, Izumiya K, Katoh T, Yaguchi H, Nakada T, Handa Y, Hoshimiya N: Electrical pelvic floor stimulation in the mangement of urinary incontinence due to neuropathic overactive bladder. *Frontiers Med Biol Engng* 1993; 5:1–10.

121. Wheeler JS, Walter JS, Sibley P: Management of incontinent SCI patients with penile stimulation: Preliminary results. *J Am Paraplegia Soc* 1994; 17:55–59.

122. Sidi AA, Reinberg Y, Gonzalez R: Comparison of artifical sphincter implantation and bladder neck reconstruction in patients with neurogenic urinary incontinence. *J Urol* 1987; 138:1120–1122.

123. Kass EJ, Koff SA: Bladder augmentation in the pediatric neuropathic bladder. *J Urol* 1983; 129:552–555.

124. Bennett CJ, Young MN, Adkins RH, Diaz F: Comparison of bladder management complication outcomes in female spinal cord injury patients. *J Urol* 1995; 153:1458–1460.

125. Raz S, Kaufman JJ, Ellison GW, Mayers LW: Methyldopa in treatment of neurogenic bladder disorders. *Urology* 1977; 9:188–190.

126. Nordling J, Meyhoff HH, Christensen NJ: Effects of clonidine (Catapresan) on urethral pressure. *Invest Radiol* 1979; 16:289–291.

127. Herman RM, Weinberg MC: Clonidine inhibits vesicosphincter reflexes in patients with chronic spinal lesions. *Arch Phys Med Rehab* 1991; 72:539–545.

128. Leyson JFJ, Martin BF, Sporer A: Baclofen in the treatment of detrusor-sphincter dyssynergia in spinal cord injury patients. *J Urol* 1980; 124:82–84.

129. Kiesswetter H, Schober W: Lioresal in the treatment of neurogenic bladder dysfunction. *Urol Int* 1975; 30:63–71.

130. Nanninga JB, Frost F, Penn R: Effect of intrathecal baclofen on bladder and sphincter function. *J Urol* 1989; 142:101–105.

131. Hackler RH, Broecker BH, Klein FA, Brady SM: A clinical experience with dantrolene sodium for external urinary sphincter hypertonicity in spinal cord injured patients. *J Urol* 1980; 124:78–81.

132. Murdock MM, Sax D, Krane RJ: Use of dantrolene sodium in external sphincter spasm. *Urology* 1976; 8:133–137.

133. Dykstra DD, Sidi AA, Scott AB, Pagel JM, Goldish GD: Effects of botulinum A toxin on detrusor-sphincter dyssynergia in spinal cord injury patients. *J Urol* 1988; 139:919–922.

134. Geraniotis E, Koff SA, Enrile B: The prophylactic use of clean intermittent catherization in the treatment of infants and young children with myelomeningocele and neurogenic bladder dysfunction. *J Urol* 1988; 139:85–86.

135. Vapnek JM, Couillard DR, Stone AR: Is sphincterotomy the best management of the spinal cord injured bladder? *J Urol* 1994; 151:961–964.

136. Stark G: Pudendal neurectomy in management of neurogenic bladder in myelomeningocele. *Arch Dis Child* 1969; 44:698.

137. Chancellor MB, Rivas DA, Linsenmeyer T, Abdill CA, Ackman CFD, Appell RA, Bennett J, Binard J, Boone TB, Chetner MP, Defalco A, Foote J, Gajewski J, Green B, Juma S, MacMillan R, Mayo M, Roehrborn CG, Stone A, Thorndyke WC, Vazquez A: Multicenter trial in North America of UroLume urinary sphincter prosthesis. *J Urol* 1994; 152:924–930.

138. Yasuda K, Yamanishi T, Murayama N, Sakakibara R, Shimaza J: Lower urinary tract dysfunction in the anterior spinal artery syndrome. *J Urol* 1993; 150:1182–1184.

139. Mohler JL, Cowen DL, Flanigan RC: Suppression and treatment of urinary tract infection in patients with an intermittently catheterized neurogenic bladder. *J Urol* 1987; 138:336–340.

140. Resnick NM, Yalla SV: Management of urinary incontinence in the elderly. *NEJM* 1985; 313:800–805.

141. Diokno AC, Koppenhoefer R: Bethanechol chloride in neurogenic bladder dysfunction. *Urology* 1976; 8:455–458.

142. Lapides J: Urecholine regimen for rehabilitating the atonic bladder. *J Urol* 1964; 91:658–659.

143. Light JK, Scott FB: Bethanechol chloride and the traumatic cord bladder. *J Urol* 1982; 128:85–87.

144. Vaidyanathan S, Rao MS, Chary KS, Sharma PL, Das N: Enhancement of detrusor reflex activity by naloxone in patients with chronic neurogenic bladder dysfunction. Preliminary report. *J Urol* 1981; 126:500–502.

145. Grimes JH, Nashold BS, Anderson EE: Clinical application of electronic bladder stimulation in paraplegics. *J Urol* 1975; 113:338–340.

146. Beersiek F, Parks AG, Swash M: Pathogenesis of anorectal incontinence. *J Neurol Soc* 1979; 42:111–127.

147. Sun WM, Read NW, Donnelly TC: Impaired internal anal sphincter in a subgroup of patients with idiopathic fecal incontinence. *Gastroenterology* 1989; 97:130–134.

148. Frenckner B: Function of the anal sphincters in spinal man. *Gut* 1975; 16:638–644.

149. Devroede G, Lamarche J: Functional importance of extrinsic parasympathetic innervation to the distal colon and rectum in man. *Gastroenterology* 1974; 66:273–280.

150. Gore RM, Mintzer RA, Calenoff L: Gastrointestinal complications of spinal cord injury. *Spine* 1981; 6:538–544.

151. Snooks SJ, Barnes PRH, Swash M: Damage to the innervation of the voluntary anal and periurethral sphincter musculature in incontinence: an electrophysiological study. *J Neurol Neurosurg Psychiatr* 1984; 47:1269–1273.

152. Opitz JL, Thorsteinsson G, Schutt AH, Barrett DM, Olson PK: Neurogenic bowel and bladder, in DeLisa JA (ed): *Rehabilitation Medicine*. Philadelphia: J.B. Lippincott, 1988, pp. 492–518.

153. Munchiando JF, Kendall K: Comparison of the effectiveness of two bowel programs for CVA patients. *Rehab Nurs* 1993; 18:168–172.

154. Weber J, Denis P, Mihout B, Muller JM, Blanquart F, Galmiche JP, Simon P, Pasquis P: Effect of brain-stem lesion on colonic and anorectal motility: study of three patients. *Dig Dis Sci* 1985; 30:419–425.

155. Jorge JM, Wexner SD: A practical guide to basic anorectal physiology investigations. *Contemp Surg* 1993; 43:214–224.

156. Wexner SD, Marchetti F, Salanga VD, Corredor C, Jagelman DG: Neurophysiologic assessment of the anal sphincters. *Dis Colon Rect* 1991; 34:606–612.

157. Cheong DM, Vaccaro CA, Salanga VD, Wexner SD, Phillips RC, Hanson MR: Electrodiagnostic evaluation of fecal incontinence. *Muscle Nerve* 1995; 18:612–619.

158. Kiff ES, Swash M: Slowed conduction in the pudendal nerves in idiopathic (neurogenic) fecal incontinence. *Br J Surg* 1984; 71:615–616.

159. Swash M, Snooks SJ: Motor nerve conduction studies of the pelvic floor innervation, in Henry MM, Swash M (eds): *Coloproctology and the Pelvic Floor*, 2nd ed. Oxford: Butterworth-Heinemann, 1992, pp. 196–206.

160. Vernava AM, Longo WE, Daniel GL: Pudendal neuropathy and the importance of EMG evaluation of fecal incontinence. *Dis Colon Rect* 1993; 36:23–27.

161. Wexner SD, Marchetti F, Jagelman DG: The role of sphincteroplasty for fecal incontinence: A prospective physiologic and functional review. *Dis Colon Rect* 1991; 34:22–30.

162. Bartolo DC, Jarratt JA, Read NW: The use of conventional electromyography to assess external sphincter neuropathy in man. *J Neurol Neurosurg Psychiatr* 1983; 46:1115–1118.

163. Felt-Bersma RJ, Strijers RL, Janssen JJ, Visser SL, Meuwissen SG: The external anal sphincter: relationship between anal manometry and anal electromyography and its clinical relevance. *Dis Colon Rect* 1989; 32:112–116.

164. Glick ME, Meshkinpour H, Haldeman S, Hoehler F, Downey N, Bradley WE: Colonic dysfunction in patients with thoracic spinal cord injury. *Gastroenterology* 1984; 86:287–294.

165. Comarr AE: Bowel regulation for patients with spinal cord injury. *JAMA* 1958; 167:18–21.

166. Dunn KL, Galka ML: A comparison of the effectiveness of Therevac SB and bisacodyl suppositories in SCI patients' bowel programs. *Rehab Nurs* 1994; 19:334–338.

167. Stiens SA: Reduction in bowel program duration with polyethylene glycol based bisacodyl suppositories. *Arch Phys Med Rehab* 1995; 76:674–677.

168. Sorensen M, Lorentzen M, Petersen J, Christiansen J: Anorectal dysfunction in patients with urologic disturbance due to multiple sclerosis. *Dis Colon Rect* 1991; 34:136–139.

169. Caruana BJ, Wald A, Hinds JP, Eidelman BH: Anorectal sensory and motor function in neurogenic fecal incontinence. *Gastroenterology* 1991; 100:465–470.

170. Jameson JS, Rogers J, Chia YW, Misiewicz JJ, Henry MM, Swash M: Pelvic floor function in multiple sclerosis. *Gut* 1994; 35:388–390.

171. Schiller LR, Santa Ana CA, Schmulen AC, Hendler RS, Harford WV, Fordtran JS: Pathogenesis of fecal incontinence in diabetes mellitus: evidence for internal-anal-sphincter dysfunction. *N Engl J Med* 1982; 307:1666–1671.

172. DePonti F, Fealey RD, Malagelada JR: Gastrointestinal syndromes due to diabetes mellitus, in Dyck PJ, Thomas PK, Asbury AK, Winegrad AI, Porte D (eds): *Diabetic Neuropathy*. Philadelphia: W.B. Saunders, 1987, pp. 155–161.

173. Feldman M, Schiller L: Disorders of gastrointestinal motility associated with diabetes mellitus. *Ann Intern Med* 1983; 98:378–384.

174. Goyal RK, Spiro HM: Gastrointestinal manifestations of diabetes mellitus. *Med Clin No Am* 1971; 55:1031–1044.

175. Whitehead WE, Schuster MM: Behavioral approaches to the treatment of gastrointestinal motility disorders. *Med Clin No Am* 1981; 65:1397–1411.

176. Liptak GS, Revell GM: Management of bowel dysfunction in children with spinal cord disease or injury by means of the enema continence catheter. *J Pediatr* 1992; 120:190–194.

177. Sullivan-Bolyai S, Swanson M, Shurtleff DB: Toilet training the child with neurogenic impairment of bowel and bladder function. *Issues Comp Pediatr Nurs* 1984; 7:33–43.

178. Whitehead WE, Parker L, Bosmajian L, Morrill-Corbin D, Middaugh S, Garwood M, Cataldo MF, Freeman J: Treatment of fecal incontinence in children with spina bifida: Comparison of biofeedback and behavior modification. *Arch Phys Med Rehab* 1986; 67:218–224.

179. Cohen M, Rosen L, Khubchandani I, Sheets J, Stasik J, Riether R: Rationale for medical or surgical therapy in anal incontinence. *Dis Colon Rect* 1986; 29:120–122.

180. MacLeod JH: Management of anal incontinence by biofeedback. *Gastroenterology* 1987; 93:291–294.

181. Wald A: Use of biofeedback in treatment of fecal incontinence in patients with meningomyelocele. *Pediatrics* 1981; 68:45–49.

182. Wald A: Biofeedback for neurogenic fecal incontinence: Rectal sensation is a determinant of outcome. *J Pediatr Gastroenterol Nutr* 1983; 2:302–306.

183. Wald A, Tunuguntla AK: Anorectal sensorimotor dysfunction in fecal incontinence and diabetes mellitus: Modification with biofeedback therapy. *N Engl J Med* 1984; 310:1282–1287.

184. Orrom WJ, Miller R, Cornes H, Duthie G, Mortensen NJ, Bartolo DC: Comparison of anterior sphincteroplasty and postanal repair in the treatment of idiopathic fecal incontinence. *Dis Colon Rectum* 1991; 34:305–310.

185. Corman ML: Follow-up evaluation of gracilis muscle transposition for fecal incontinence. *Dis Colon Rect* 1980; 23:552–555.

Chapter 19

CONTRACTURE AND LIMB DEFORMITIES

Kathleen R. Bell
Krista Vandenborne

DEFINITIONS AND FUNCTIONAL EFFECTS OF CONTRACTURES

Joint contractures and congenital or acquired limb deformities are a common problem encountered in the rehabilitation of neurologic and musculoskeletal disorders. A joint contracture is best defined as a fixed loss of mobility at a joint that may originate with any of the components of the joint, including the soft tissue, tendons, bony articulation, or intra-articular ligaments. Joint contractures should not be confused with the abnormal limb posturing or spasticity associated with disorders of tone, although posturing and contracture often coexist. Posturing or "functional joint contractures" seen with severe spasticity or muscle imbalance across a joint must be treated along with the "fixed" contracture, if improved limb function is to result.

The importance of limb contractures and deformities lies in their devastating effects on health maintenance, function, and emotional or social state. For persons with severe cognitive and physical impairment, the presence of contractures in the upper and lower limbs greatly complicates nursing care, by interfering with hygiene and positioning in bed and wheelchair. For those confined to a bed or wheelchair, the presence of contractures can predispose to the formation of pressure ulcers over bony prominences. Insufficient attention to range of motion in the cognitively impaired can compound the effects of the primary illness or injury, limiting functional mobility and the ability to perform activities of daily living.

Significant loss of joint mobility often can mean the difference between independent and dependent mobility. For instance, most unilateral trans-tibial amputees can be functional community ambulators with an appropriate prosthesis. However, the presence of hip and knee flexion contractures can complicate or prevent the successful fit of a prosthesis, resulting in increased use of assistive devices or dependence on wheelchair use. Even if a prosthesis can be fitted, standing or walking with knee flexion contractures causes increased expenditure of energy because of increased demands on knee extensor muscles.[1]

Head, neck, and trunk contractures may interfere with the ability to communicate effectively and lessen opportunities for socialization for the disabled person. Self-awareness of distorted body image can adversely affect motivation for successful reintegration. This may be a particular issue with the adolescent population during development. There is also evidence that temporomandibular joint contracture can restrict normal oral–motor function in children with severe spastic quadriplegia.[2]

Contractures and limb deformities are often given low priority during medical treatment of the patient with neurologic or musculoskeletal disorders. Bax and Brown observed that the effectiveness of interventions that prevent deformity may be difficult to demonstrate, but that the presence of a contracture with resulting decreased independence and increased medical costs is readily apparent.[3] The surgical and hospitalization costs for correcting functionally significant joint contractures in patients with brain injuries has been estimated to exceed 20,000 dollars per surgical procedure.[4]

Although in most instances contractures are detrimental to function and health maintenance, there are a few situations in which relatively mild contractures may enhance function by stabilizing an otherwise weak limb.[5] For example, a minor degree of contracture of the long finger flexors in a patient with spinal cord injury and quadriplegia may facilitate passive pinch. For an ambulatory patient with weak plantar flexors, a mild ankle contracture may be useful during push-off, minimizing the need for bracing.[6] The importance of careful, individualized functional analysis of contractures is essential to planning treatment. A careful consideration of the expense and risks of treatment must always take into account the possibility that therapeutic intervention may lead to an irreversible decline in function.

PREVALENCE

Limited data are available on the prevalence of joint contracture in most diagnostic categories. Of those admitted to a spinal-cord rehabilitation unit, Yarkony et al. have reported that 15 percent had functionally significant contractures.[7] After traumatic brain injury (TBI), 84 percent of those sent for acute medical rehabilitation have contractures of greater than 15 percent of joint range of motion.[8] Contractures after brain trauma most frequently occur in the hips (81 percent), shoulders (76 percent), and ankles (76 percent).[8]

The geriatric population is particularly at risk for the development of contractures. Studies have shown elderly people to have less compliant soft tissue than younger people.[9] Although healthy elderly persons living in the community have a low prevalence of joint contracture, the prevalence among those with dementia or living in nursing facilities is greater.[10] More than three-quarters of elderly patients followed at a dementia research center who were unable to walk had multi-limb contractures (defined as a loss of 50 percent of normal range of motion [ROM] at the joint). On the other hand, only 11 percent of ambulatory patients have been reported to have contractures.[11] Institutionalized elderly persons with dementia are much more likely to have contactures interfering with function than those living in the community.[11,12]

Contractures are commonly associated with pediatric neurological disorders. In children with myelomeningocele, for instance, the average range of hip contracture for children with thoracic level lesions is 11–21 degrees, for upper lumbar levels 10–32, for lower lumbar levels 6–27.[13] Although no figures are readily available for children with cerebral palsy, 75 percent of adults with spastic quadriplegia from cerebral palsy have sig-

nificant joint contractures, particularly those who are nonambulatory.[14]

PATHOLOGY AND PATHOPHYSIOLOGY OF CONTRACTURES

There is general agreement that the development of fixed contractures is mainly related to biomechanical and biochemical changes in intra-articular and peri-articular structures, although early stages of stiffness often are linked to ultrastructural changes in skeletal muscle.[15,16]

Prolonged joint immobilization, whether the consequence of orthopedic treatment, bed rest, or joint pain, invariably leads to joint contractures as well as other musculoskeletal changes and is the single most frequent cause of fixed contractures. The normal mechanical stresses experienced during routine motor activities are essential for the maintenance of many cellular metabolic activities. Reduction of such stresses by inactivity or immobilization results in large structural changes, causing joint stiffness. Morphological description of the intra-articular, peri-articular, and myopathic changes related to fixed joint contractures is now being studied.

Anatomical Changes in the Synovial Joint

The effect of immobilization on synovial joints has been studied in both humans and animals, using different models, including plaster casts, internal splints, neurectomy, and compression devices.[17–20] Irrespective of the method of immobilization or whether weight-bearing was permitted, alterations in the synovial joint are strikingly similar, even among species.

The first gross alteration in the immobilized joint is the progressive infiltration of fibrofatty connective tissue into the joint space.[17,19,21–23] This fibrofatty connective tissue is composed of mature fat cells and wisps of fibrous connective tissue and blood vessels, and is lined with several layers of synovial cells.[21] During prolonged immobilization, hyperplastic fibrofatty connective tissue progressively covers intra-articular soft tissue structures (e.g., ligaments) and non-articulating cartilage surfaces. With the passage of time, adhesions also develop between the exposed tissue surfaces, eventually causing complete obliteration of the joint cavity. (Figure 19-1). In humans, fibrofatty tissue typically envelops the cruciate ligaments and fills the intercondylar notch.

In a more advanced stage, the lack of activity also

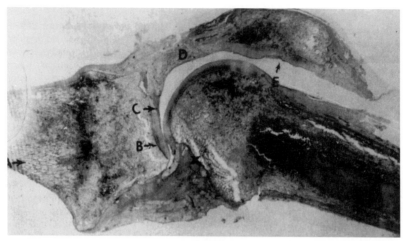

Figure 19-1

Photograph of post mortem dissected knee joint of patient with advanced knee flexion contracture. Fibrofatty tissue from the infrapatellar fat pad (D) has covered the distal pole of the patella and has become welded to the articular surface of the tibia (C). Fibrofatty tissue of the suprapatellar pouch has covered the proximal pole of the patella and has completely enveloped the posterior cruciate ligament (x). (Reprinted from J Bone and Joint Surg, 54-A, Enneking WF and Horowitz M, The intra-articular effects of immobilization on the human knee, 973–985, Copyright [1972].)

affects the articular cartilage and subchondral bone.[18–22] Pathological changes affecting articular cartilage can be separated into those in noncontact areas and those in contact areas.

Structural changes in noncontact areas have been attributed to the proliferation of the fibrofatty connective tissue.[22] Initially, adhesions are formed between the proliferating fibrofatty connective tissue and cartilage. With time, fibrofatty connective tissue blends imperceptibly with the superficial layers of cartilage and assumes a fibrous appearance. Continued immobilization leads to gradual atrophy of the cartilage and further replacement by fibrofatty tissue.

In contact areas, mild to severe changes of articular cartilage develop, depending on the duration and position of immobilization and, most importantly, on the degree of compression.[17,18,24] At the onset, articular cartilage becomes fibrillated and cartilage ulcerations are observed.[18,19,21,24] As time evolves, articular cartilage is replaced by a more mature fibrous tissue, which may extend into the depths of cartilage down to subchondral bone.[19,21,22] Concomitant tissue repair processes lead to hyperemia and fibrovascular proliferation in the subjacent marrow spaces. In advanced cases, penetration into the deep strata of cartilage with destruction of the subchondral plate has been demonstrated.[21] Gradually, hyaline cartilage is replaced by primitive mesenchymal tissue and undergoes enchondral ossification. With further progression, mature fibrous tissue replaces articular cartilage, causing joint ankylosis (Figure 19-2).[21]

Pressure necrosis of articular cartilage is not produced by simple mechanical destruction, but may be caused by nutritional depletion.[17] Since articular cartilage is avascular, chondrocytes receive most of their nourishment by diffusion of nutritional factors from synovial fluid, and to a lesser extent from subchondral blood vessels. Continuous compression of cartilage not only prevents the synovial fluid from reaching the surface under pressure, but it also prevents diffusion of the nutrient fluids through the intercellular substance of cartilage.[17,20]

Biochemical Changes in the Periarticular Fibrous Connective Tissue

The most recognized feature of a joint contracture is progressive contracture of the capsule and pericapsular structures. The mechanism by which the periarticular connective tissue loses its flexibility subsequent to the inhibition of motion has been the subject of considerable interest. The decreased flexibility of connective tissue has been associated with biochemical changes in all

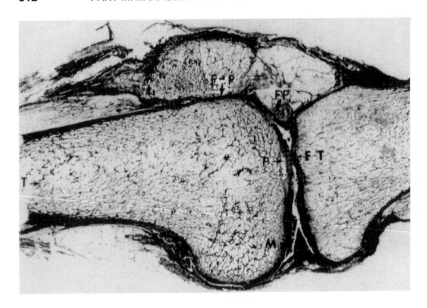

Figure 19-2
Photograph of post mortem dissected knee joint of patient with clinically fused knee. The articular cartilage of the patella, femoral condyle, and tibia has been replaced by mature fibrous connective tissue. Only small islands of articular cartilage remain. The femoral condyle and patella and the femoral condyle and tibia are fused together by mature fibrous connective tissue. The joint cavity is completely obliterated. (Reprinted from J Bone Joint Surg, 54-A, Enneking WF and Horowitz M, The intra-articular effects of immobilization on the human knee, 973–985, Copyright [1972].)

three of its major constituents: extracellular water, collagen, and glycosaminoglycan.[22,25–29]

The periarticlar connective tissue in tendons, ligaments, and capsules consists mostly of organic collagen.[30] With the exception of a small amount of elastine in some connective tissues, collagen is the only tensile resistant protein in these tissues. Collagen fibers are laid down in a very specific pattern, which determines the mechanical properties of the connective tissue (e.g., the relatively linear pattern of the collateral ligaments). The other major constituents of periarticular connective tissue are water and proteoglycan. Together they allow collagen fibers to glide independently of each other. Hyaluronic acid, an important proteoglycan bound to water, is considered the principal fibrous connective tissue lubricant.[31] The interstitial fluid serves as a spacer between individual collagen fibers.[22,25–27]

Stress deprivation affects all three constituents of connective tissue. Akeson has shown that the water content of connective tissue decreases as much as six percent with immobilization.[27] In the same study, the total amount of glycosaminoglycans was reduced by 20 percent, and hyaluronic acid by 40 percent. This large decline in water and hyaluronic acid content decreases the spacing and lubrication efficiency of the matrix, causing fibril–fibril friction, as well as adhesions or cross-linkings between adjacent collagen fibrils.[22,25–29]

Amiel et al. demonstrated, in association with a decrease in extracellular water and proteoglycan, an

increase in both collagen synthesis and degradation, leading to a net increase in the amount of immature collagen.[28,29,32] However, when new immature fibrils are laid down without mechanical input, they are dispersed randomly, bridging or cross-linking existing fibers with divergent tracking patterns (Figures 19-3A and 19-3B).[26] This increase in the intrafiber and interfiber cross-links interferes incrementally with the functional gliding of the individual collagen fibers.

Structural Changes in Skeletal Muscle

The adverse clinical effects of immobilization on skeletal muscle include muscle atrophy, rigidity, weakness, and a shift in fiber type composition from slow twitch to fast twitch. The most obvious adaptation to immobilization clinically is a decrease in muscle mass and strength. Magnetic resonance imaging studies have demonstrated up to a 30 percent decrease in the muscle cross-sectional area following 6 weeks of immobilization.[33] This decrease in muscle mass is associated with an even greater decline in muscular strength. Several authors have reported a 50 percent loss in muscular strength after only 6 weeks of immobilization.[34,35]

Morphological changes in intramuscular connective tissue are not well recognized, but just as important.[36–40] In rat calf muscles, immobilization has been shown to alter the architecture and increase the total volume of intramuscular connective tissue.[37] Increase

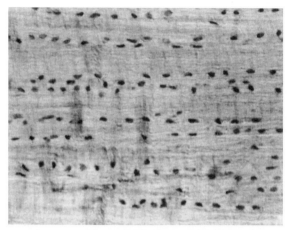

A

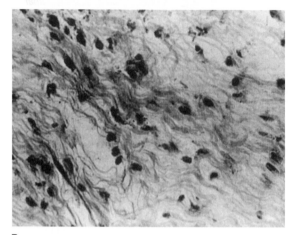

B

Figure 19-3

A. Anterior cruciate ligaments from nonimmobilized and B. 9-weeks immobilized rabbit knee. Note that the pattern of cellular alignment is distorted in the immobilized periarticular connective tissue. (Reprinted from Biorheology, *17, Akeson WH, Amiel D, and Woo SL-Y, Immobility effects on synovial joints. The pathomechanics of joint contracture, 95–110, Copyright [1980], with kind permission from Elsevier Science Ltd, The Boulevard, Langford Lane, Kidlington 0X5 1GB, UK)*

in connective tissue volume is a function of the duration of immobilization. As shown in Figure 19-4A, only a few delicate collagen fibers are present in the healthy muscle, whereas 1 week of immobilization produces a dense network of collagen fibers throughout the muscle. By 3 weeks of immobilization, each muscle

fiber is surrounded by a thick connective tissue layer, isolating muscle cells from each other and their surrounding capillaries (Figure 19-4B). Based on quantitative analysis, Josza et al. demonstrated that during 3 weeks of immobilization in the lengthened position, the proportion of connective tissue in rat calf muscles increased from 2.8 percent in the soleus and 3.1 percent in the gastrocnemius to 54 percent and 30 percent, respectively.[37] Similar changes were observed following immobilization in the shortened position and following tenotomy of the achilles tendon. The increase in connective tissue involved both endomysial and perimysial collagen.

Associated with changes in intramuscular connective tissue, changes in muscle length following immobilization also have been described.[39,41] Cat soleus muscles immobilized in the lengthened position have 20 percent more sarcomeres in series, whereas those immobilized in a shortened position had 40 percent fewer sarcomeres compared to normal muscles. Shortened muscle shows a significant decrease in extensibility.

Finally, Kannus has demonstrated that immobilization causes degenerative changes in the myotendinous junction.[42] These changes are characterized by a decrease in the contact area between the muscle cells and tendon collagen fibers, a reduction in the glycosaminoglycan and proteoglycan content, and an increase in the less mature type III collagen at the myotendinous junction.

Functional Contractures and Their Neurological Origin

Unlike fixed contractures, functional contractures (or posturing) are the result of an imbalance in the muscle tone of agonist and antagonist muscle groups across a joint, usually produced by an upper motor neuron lesion. A major function of the upper motor neurons and their descending pathways (corticospinal, corticobulbar, reticulospinal, vestibulospinal, and rubrospinal) is to provide descending inhibitory influences that regulate lower motor neuron activity.[43] Following upper motor neuron lesions, inhibitory control is lost and spasticity develops.[43–45]

What forces a joint into a fixed position or posture is the combination of muscle weakness and excessive muscle contraction owing to spasticity and/or rigidity.[45] Functional (reducible) contractures are often difficult to distinguish from fixed contractures without using temporary anesthesia or motor nerve blocks to diminish the spastic response.[43] If the spastic limb is allowed to

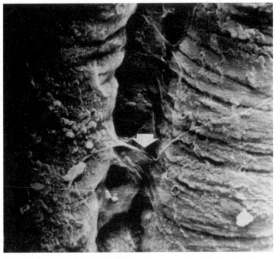 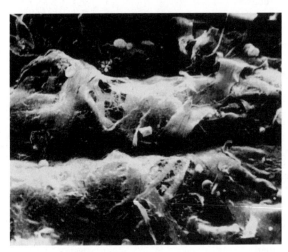

A   B

Figure 19-4

A. Electron micrograph of normal rat muscle tissue, with few collagen fibers connecting the myocytes.
B. Electron micrograph of soleus muscle, 3 weeks after tenotomy. Note the dense network of
connective tissue isolating the muscle cells. (Reprinted from J Bone Joint Surg, 72-B, Josza L,
Kannus P, Thoring J, Reffy A, Jarvinen M, and Kvist M, The effect of tenotomy and immobilisation
on intramuscular connective tissue: A morphometric and microscopic study in rat calf muscles,
293–297, Copyright [1990].)

remain fixed in an imbalanced posture without mobilization, collagen tissue changes eventually will occur and fixed contractures will develop.

Effect of Aging and Other Developmental Considerations

Structural changes in connective tissue with normal aging predispose the elderly to the development of joint contractures. Cross-linking stabilizes collagen fibers, and provides them with the tensile strength and viscoelasticity necessary to stabilize joints.[30] The degree of cross-linking, number and density of fibers, and their orientation and diameter, are the major determinants of function. Aging has been shown to affect both the nature and organization of collagen fibers, altering their function. Using stress–strain measurements, Heikkinen and others demonstrated an increase in stiffness of rat skin with age.[52–56] Reduced collagen fiber elasticity is caused by an increase in the number of intramolecular and intermolecular cross-links.[57–59] Changes in the con-

centration and composition of proteoglycans also may play a major role.[30]

Concomitant with the changes in collagen, the elderly also experience changes in both the quality and quantity of skeletal muscle. Between the ages of 50 and 80, muscular strength decreases approximately 40 percent, with the largest change occurring after the age of 70.[60] Muscle strength is well maintained up to the age of 50, and then declines by 15 percent between the sixth and seventh decade of life, and by 30 percent during the following decades.[61–65] These age-related reductions in muscle strength are a direct result of and proportionate to decreases in muscle mass.[60,66–69] Young et al., using ultrasound, showed a 25–30 percent reduction in the muscle cross-sectional area of elderly men and women compared to younger controls.[67,70] Computed tomography and magnetic resonance imaging studies show similar age-related reductions in muscle cross-sectional area, along with large increases in fat and connective tissue.[60,71,72] Non-muscle tissue in the quadriceps and hamstrings of elderly subjects has been demonstrated to increase 59 percent and 127 percent, respectively, when compared to younger persons.[71] Even in the absence of any specific disease, large increases in collagen stiffness and disproportionate contributions of fat and connective tissue to muscle morphology, combined with muscle atrophy, set the stage for contracture formation in the geriatric patient.

Contractures in Children At the opposite end of the spectrum are children. Neurological disorders are most commonly the cause of contractures in children. Because of skeletal immaturity, muscle imbalance across a joint often is more deforming in the young compared to adults.[73,74] Elbow flexion and pronation, as well as hip flexion and adduction contractures, are common in cerebral palsy, regardless of a heterogeneous picture of rigidity, spasticity, dystonia, and weakness.[75,76] In addition to directly influencing the formation of contracture through muscle weakness, intrinsic muscle disease in children results in delayed muscle growth, encouraging further weakness and imbalance as children age.[77] Daily stretching of muscle for as little as 30 minutes has been shown to significantly augment weight and cross-sectional area of normal and dystrophic muscle.[78]

Acquired Contractures

Bed rest and immobilization have been used for decades in the management of trauma and acute illness. As early as the time of Hippocrates (400 B.C.), immobilization of some type was used to cure the injured or diseased limb.[79] The concept of immobilization as a therapeutic procedure became especially popular in the late nineteenth century, popularized chiefly by the great British orthopedic pioneers, Hugh Owen Thomas and Sir Robert Jones, for various joint disorders.[79,80] Others, including Lewis Sayre, strongly opposed long-term immobilization, pointing to the adverse effects of inactivity.[81] Today, it is clear that prolonged immobilization has many adverse effects, and that a careful balance between rest and motion is essential to uncomplicated recovery.

The single most important factor in contracture formation is lack of joint movement. Immobilization of a person in a flexed bed or wheelchair for prolonged periods without frequent movement of the joints through the entire range of motion may result in contracture without any underlying disease.[82] The presence of certain disease processes or neurological syndromes may accelerate the formation of contractures.

Systemic Diseases and Contractures Some systemic diseases, such as diabetes mellitus, appear to predispose to limited joint mobility. In diabetics, collagen abnormalities have been demonstrated, with aberrant cross-linkages and glycosylation of collagen fibers resulting in limited joint motion, particularly in the small joints of the hands (Figure 19-5).[83,84] Dupuytren's contracture also is commonly seen in type I and type II diabetics. Both limited joint motion and Dupuytren's contractures occur in about 20–35 percent of all diabetic patients.[83,85,86] Although hand abnormalities are the most prevalent, contracture at other joints may also occur.

Degenerative muscle disorders, such as muscular dystrophy, characterized by muscle-fiber destruction and the progressive replacement of muscle cells with fat and fibrous tissue, can result in contractures.[93–96] The plantar flexion contracture typically seen in muscular dystrophy is caused by weakness in the tibialis anterior and peronei muscles, which oppose plantar flexion, and the proliferation of connective tissue in the gastrocnemius muscle, which shortens the muscle. Pathological changes observed in inflammatory myopathies include muscle fiber degeneration and necrosis, with prominent perivascular, perimysial, and endomysial inflammatory infiltration. In chronic polymyositis, degenerated muscle fibers are replaced by fat and fibrous tissue, leading to contracture formation.[97]

Contractures commonly are seen in stroke, brain injury, spinal-cord injury, multiple sclerosis, Parkinson's disease, and other degenerative or traumatic diseases

Figure 19-5

The hands of a 57-year-old diabetic male demonstrating both limited joint mobility of the interphalangeal joints of the fingers and Dupuytren's contracture.

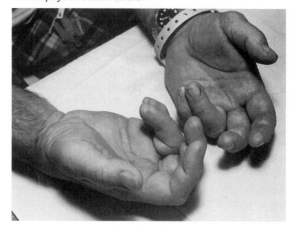

of the nervous system as a result of imbalances of muscle tone and strength that occur across immobilized joints. Poliomyelitis, still commonly reported in underdeveloped countries, stems from the viral-induced loss of anterior horn cells. This results in isolated muscle weakness and primary strength imbalance across joints with no constriction of tone. Common contracture deformities after polio include flexion–abduction deformity at the hip, knee flexion, and pes valgus contractures.[98,99] Movement disorders, such as athetosis or ataxia, generally are not associated with fixed contractures.[100]

Other Associated Conditions   Trauma may be associated with the development of joint contracture, stemming from ligamentous or muscle damage, especially in the hand. Ischemia owing to partial muscle rupture or compartment syndrome also can result in muscle fibrosis, with subsequent shortening.[101] Sufficient muscle damage can occur during intramuscular injections to result in significant muscle shortening.[102]

Heterotopic ossification (HO), resulting from local muscle trauma or nervous system injury, also can lead to joint contracture, caused by the deposition of bone rather than collagen changes. HO has been attributed to both immobilization and overaggressive ranging of a neurologically impaired limb.[103] Extraskeletal bone develops from disordered differentiation of pluripotential mesenchymal cells into osteoblastic cells located in muscle or fascial planes, leading to mechanical obstruction of joint motion.[104]

Congenital Limb Deformities

Congenital limb deformities have numerous causes, including genetic, muscle and nerve disorders, perinatal central nervous system insults, and peripheral nerve injuries. Generalized involvement, as in osteogenesis imperfecta, or segmental effects, as in clubfoot, have been well described. In osteogenesis imperfecta, contractures are part of the defining characteristics of the disease. Virtually 100 percent of those affected have hip contractures.[105]

Congenital clubfoot, a complex deformity with elements of varus, equinus, adductus, and cavus, is a common abnormality seen in children with neurologic disorders. It is most commonly treated with early manipulation and casting of the foot, continuing application of corrective Denis Browne splints and footwear until age seven or eight, and in some cases, surgery.[108]

MANAGEMENT

Prevention

Prevention is the cornerstone of managing contractures. Positioning is the first level of prevention. When bedrest is required, the flexed hip and knee position should be avoided: Sandbags, splints, or foam wedges can be used to prevent excessive limb rotation. Adequate seating support will maintain normal trunk-to-limb position and prevent joint contracture as well. Daily range-of-motion exercises must be performed with or without an assistant. Splinting in functional positions may be necessary when consciousness is impaired and spontaneous change of position is impossible.

Physical Examination

Careful physical examination remains the most important evaluation tool in contracture management. In addition to examining the joint in question, it is important to examine the adjacent joints and the surrounding muscles. Accurate measurements of ROM may require analgesic, medication and/or the use of superficial heat. ROM tests that rely heavily on the identification of anatomic landmarks may be less accurate in the pediatric population where anatomic development may be influenced by spasticity or paresis.[109] There is no clear indication that radiographic techniques add much information to the careful physical examination in determining ROM, except when suspicion of ectopic bone formation, joint dislocation, ankylosis, or other bone deformity exists.[110] However, in the child with spasticity, radiographic examination of the hips and spine often is necessary in the overall development of a management plan that may involve surgery.

Muscle testing and evaluation of spasticity or weakness is essential to determining proper treatment methods for contractures. Recurrence of contracture after treatment often is owing to persistence of the underlying problem of muscle imbalance across a joint in a spastic limb. In addition to "static" muscle testing, observation in a more functional setting are helpful. The spontaneous use of a limb prior to treatment is often an excellent guide to predicting outcome. For instance, the persistence of primitive head–limb reflexes (such as in cerebral palsy), may prevent functional use of a hand even if contractures are reduced successfully.[111]

Sensory testing also contributes to overall assessment. Surgical procedures, particularly in the upper limb and hand, are much more likely to result in improved function in a limb with some preserved two-point discrimination and stereognosis. Certain types of splints (e.g., dynamic splints) may be relatively contraindicated in an insensate limb.

Cognitive and behavioral abilities are also factors in therapeutic assessment. Intricate tendon transfer procedures are unlikely to produce desired results if cognitive function is significantly depressed. Agitation or involuntary limb movements necessitate the use of soft splints, medications, or blocks rather than solid casts, in order to protect against injury.

The physical examination can be augmented by the use of temporary blocks or general anesthesia. Voluntary muscle activity and joint motion often are masked by the presence of spasticity. Temporary nerve blocks allow separation of the effects of spasticity from the effects of muscle or tendon contracture. General anesthesia may be required to obtain a reliable joint examination when severe spasticity is present.

For complex problems of contracture involving limb deformity and spasticity, dynamic electromyography and gait analysis assist in analyzing individual muscle contribution to abnormalities of function, allowing for better selection of muscles and tendons to be treated.[112–115] Studies of torque production, elasticity, and viscosity of the ankle joint also can distinguish between the contribution of spasticity and passive mechanical properties.[116–118]

Timing and Duration of Intervention

Generally, in acquired contractures, the earlier intervention is performed, the better the outcome. In contractures associated with spasticity, the timing for intervention is more problematic, especially if the neurological status fluctuates. Use of neurolytic blocks only after the neurological status has stabilized, perhaps as long as 12 months after stroke or traumatic brain injury, has been suggested by some.[119] Early intervention in the treatment of spasticity in acquired brain injury may result in altered neural pathways, diminishing the likelihood of spasticity and contracture development.[120] A phenol block performed within the first few months following traumatic brain injury may result in preserved joint ROM and avoid the necessity of later surgery. The established risks of increasing motor paresis and temporary dysesthesia should be considered.[121,122]

Considerable controversy exists regarding the timing of surgical intervention in contracture management. For children with Duchenne muscular dystrophy, there is debate whether early surgical intervention in the correction of ankle plantar flexion and hip and knee flexion contractures prolongs the ability to walk and stand. Proponents of early intervention report rapid postoperative rehabilitation and decreased need for orthoses.[123–126] In cerebral palsy, surgery is deferred until after motor development is complete, but before the adolescent growth spurt occurs.[114]

Types of Intervention

As is always the case with joint contracture, positioning is the basis for all other types of treatment. Prone positioning in bed or on a mat is an excellent way to treat shoulder, hip, and knee contractures; wedges and pillows can be used for comfort for those with significant range-of-motion limitations. Standing unsupported or supported in standing tables and other apparati permits good stretch not only for the Achilles tendon but also for the pelvis, hips, and knees, but may not correct existing contractures.[127]

Independent of the modality used, it is important to clearly identify the goal of treatment. This is especially true for surgical procedures. The goal may be as simple as improving the ease of passively positioning in a wheelchair or as complex as improving the quality of ambulation. The goals likely will dictate very different conservative and surgical treatments.

Physical Modalities The most commonly applied physical modality for the treatment of contracture is range-of-motion exercises, both passive and active. Sustained stretching by the patient or therapist is essential for increasing joint flexibility. Prolonged, low-load stretching is the most effective intervention for permanently elongating collagen tissue.[128,129] In addition to elongating collagen, experimental animal models support the contention that stretch is necessary for muscle growth at the musculotendinous junction and for maintenance of the number of sarcomeres in muscle.[77,130] This is a particularly compelling idea when applied to the child with spasticity and contracture. Tendon lengthening by itself may not result in improved function, only increased ROM (a situation sometimes encountered after tendon-lengthening surgery). Muscle lengthening, however, improves the function of the muscle, allowing more effective force generation along an increased range of lengths.[131,132]

The crucial question in stretching is how long is long enough? It appears that at least 6 hours of stretch to a muscle must be applied over a 24-hour period in order to gain a significant degree of stretch. Experimental evidence indicates that the longer the stretch is applied, the better the result.[133,134] However, stretching should be done with care, especially in pediatric and geriatric patients, or following prolonged immobilization or lack of weight-bearing, in order to avoid possible limb fracture.[135] Static positioning devices can help in maintaining desired positions of the limbs. In addition to traditional splints, intermittent compression devices and air splints have been successful in partially correcting elbow and knee contractures.[136]

The ability to increase range of motion can be improved with the use of a variety of heating modalities. Heating connective tissue at about 45°C enhances elongation and decreases tissue damage associated with stretching.[128,137] For small joints that are not endowed with a great deal of subcutaneous tissue, paraffin dips are very well tolerated and often can be performed independently by the patient and family. Ultrasound application is necessary for deeper joints or areas with thick tendon attachments. Performing sustained stretches or range-of-motion exercises may be better tolerated when performed in warm water, especially when multiple joint contractures are present.

Techniques such as joint mobilization or capsular distraction and deep friction massage may be helpful in mobilizing soft-tissue contractures. Another method of applying stretch to soft tissues, static progressive stretch, recently has been described.[138] A device is used to generate incremental increases in stretch intermittently over a 30-minute period, allowing some "relaxation" of the stretched tissue to a new resting length before initiating the next stretch.[138] This approach permits better patient control of stretching, preventing soft-tissue injuries from overstretching.

Although the literature dealing with the use of intra-articular corticosteroid injections to treat stiff or contracted joints is sparse, some published and verbal reports support the limited use of such treatment to improve range of motion and decrease stiffness.[139]

As with any rehabilitation program, encouraging functional activities that emphasize use of the joint in question will help maintain gains in range of motion and preserve anatomic alignment. Swimming and cycling, for example, can be adapted to many functional levels and encourage active limb use.

Serial Casting and Dynamic Orthotics   The application of a cast about the involved joint is a safe, low-cost method of delivering a low-load prolonged stress or stretch to a joint contracture (Figure 19-6). In fact, serial casting appears to be a superior method to others in

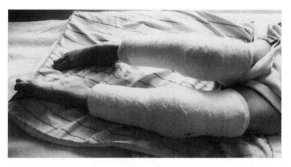

Figure 19-6
Serial casts applied to correct long-standing knee flexion contractures in a 65-year-old women with spastic quadriparesis due to a cerebral cyst and hydrocephalus. In this case, flexion contractures were interfering with the ability to position the patient adequately in a wheelchair. (Photograph courtesy of Stephanie Gephardt.)

reducing contractures.[120,140] Serial casts, as well as other methods of stretch, lengthen the muscle or tendon or both. In addition, serial casting may impact on the modulation of reflex activity of a spastic limb, and diminish spasticity through physiological mechanisms that are not entirely clear.[141–143]

In order for a serial cast to be effective, it must remain in place for a substantial period of time, usually 5–10 days. Although the ideal duration for casting has not been established, the longer the cast is worn, the greater the increase in ROM. The increased length of time may induce more basic alterations in connective tissue and muscle physiology.[134] Vigilant monitoring of the condition of skin beneath the cast is important for prevention of pressure ulcers, and can be facilitated by cast bivalving (Figure 19-7).

Figure 19-7
After maximal correction of a joint contracture is obtained with serial casting, the casts may be converted into removeable splints and used to maintain the limb in the corrected position. (Photograph courtesy of Stephanie Gephardt.)

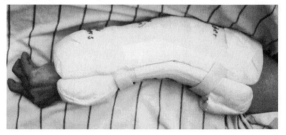

Dynamic splinting is another method of correcting limited joint motion.[144] A splint that allows free movement in the direction of the agonist muscles, but applies a prolonged, low-load stretch in the antagonist direction, is applied to the restricted joint when the limb is not in functional use. This is particularly useful for the small joints of the hand, where relatively small forces are used to produce a stretch.[119] The advantage of this procedure is the preservation of limb function and the ability to remove the splint for hygiene and comfort. Tolerance to the prolonged stretch generated by dynamic splinting is variable. Proper splint application is required to avoid joint damage. Dynamic splinting also can be provided by the continuous passive motion devices typically used after joint surgery.[119]

Control of Spasticity and Heterotopic Ossification

Even though reduction of tone across a joint may occur following reduction of a joint contracture, persistent spasticity or muscle weakness often leads to contracture recurrence.

Peripheral nerve blocks can be used as adjunctive therapy in the treatment of contractures (Figure 19-8).[121] Temporary nerve trunk blocks using lidocaine or bupivicaine allow transient relaxation of spastic muscles and attenuate the discomfort of stretching.[145] Temporary blocks used prior to applying serial casts allow improved position of the limb within the cast and better cast tolerance.[119,121] Phenol nerve blocks are particularly well suited to controlling spasticity and preventing contracture during recovery from traumatic brain and spinal-cord injury.[146] Recently, intramuscular injection of botulinum toxin has been shown to reduce muscle tone and improve active and passive range of motion in non-fixed contractures.[147] The effects of botulinin toxic block are temporary, and injection may need to be repeated every 3–4 months.

Heterotopic bone formation may impede the reduction of joint contractures. Specific non-surgical treatments to inhibit the formation of ectopic bone include the use of diphosphonates that diminish the mineralization of osteoid matrix, nonsteroidal anti-inflammatory agents that interfere with the synthesis of prostaglandin E_2, and low-dose radiation to prevent cell proliferation and bone growth.[104] Maintenance of joint ROM once bone formation has started is essential. Once heterotopic bone formation is mature, surgery can be performed for contracture reduction. Nonsteroidal anti-inflammatory agents for 3 months or low-dose radiation postoperatively have been shown to prevent reformation of osteoid matrix.[148]

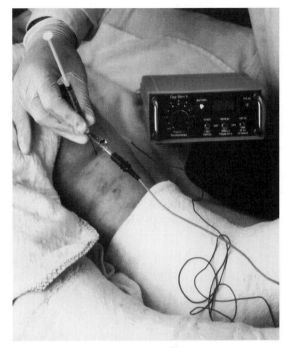

Figure 19-8
Anesthetic or phenol nerve or motor branch blocks can be performed at the bedside or in the clinic as an adjunct to serial casting or stretching in the patient with spasticity.

Corrective Surgery   Generally, surgical intervention should be deferred until at least 18 months after initial central nervous system injury to permit neurological stabilization.[13,149,150]

Improvement in ROM that occurs immediately after surgical release of contractures will almost always decrease to some extent over the first few months.[148] It is not clear what factors cause recurrence of contractures after surgical correction. Age, preoperative ability, and postoperative immobilization are not correlated with the recurrence of knee contractures after distal hamstring release in patients with cerebral palsy.[151]

Tendon transfer surgery of the upper or lower limb has achieved increasing popularity in the long-term management of joint contracture. The muscle tendon being transferred will continue to fire in the same pathophysiologic sequence established preoperatively. Dynamic electromyography is very useful in identifying the sequence and duration of muscle firing. Even if a muscle fires continuously, it is possible to use that muscle to provide countervailing balance against another hyperactive antagonist muscle.[111]

A number of reports on the use of the Ilizarov technique of bone and soft tissue external distraction to correct foot deformities and limb contractures are available now.[152,153] This treatment typically requires the use of a bone distraction apparatus for months and places high demands on the cooperation and vigilance of both patient and caregivers. The most common complication is pin-site infection. External distraction for knee contracture deformity may lead to posterior subluxation requiring surgical correction. Outcome results and healing time are comparable to conventional osteotomies.[152,153] Postoperative splinting, cast immobilization, and continuous passive motion devices may be required. Postoperative care will depend on the type of surgical procedure used, patient tolerance, and ability to cooperate.

MANAGEMENT OF SPECIFIC JOINTS

Shoulder

Shoulder movement depends to a large degree on the elasticity of soft tissue, including the capsule, rotator cuff, and supporting ligaments. In addition to the shoulder muscles and cartilaginous structures, the movement of scapular muscles (subscapularis, latissimus dorsi, and trapezius) also is essential for normal ROM. Inflammation, injury, spasticity, or weakness of any of these elements may result in contracture. However, almost half of the total shoulder ROM can be lost before function is severely affected, since contributions from scapulothoracic motion can accommodate for losses of glenohumeral function and vice versa. Physical examination of the shoulder reveals characteristics that identify the location of muscle or collagen tissue shortening. For instance, because of the diagonal orientation of the fibers of the shoulder capsule, external rotation of the shoulder is first and most severely affected in capsulitis. When muscles bridging the scapula and the humerus are shortened in children with poorly developed trunk control, winging of the scapula occurs when the arm is ranged in flexion or abduction.

Frozen shoulder or capsulitis can be associated with stroke or other neurological disease, diabetes mellitus, thyroid disease, isolated trauma, chronic repetitive tendinous injury, and degenerative joint disease. In some instances, a cause or associated condition is not established. Idiopathic capsulitis generally resolves after 1–2 years and can usually be treated conservatively.[119]

In neurological disease, limitations of the shoulder may be owing primarily to contracture of the subscapularis and pectoralis major muscles, resulting in adduction and internal rotation of the limb. Mild degrees of shoulder contracture respond to the use of ultrasound and stretching. In stretching the shoulder in abduction or flexion, application of sliding and compression force within the glenoid fossa will help avoid inducing subluxation of the humeral head. Treatment of pectoralis major muscle spasticity with phenol or botulinum toxin injections may be used as an adjunct to ROM therapy. Release or lengthening of both the subscapularis and pectoralis major muscles in extreme cases may be necessary. Postoperative stretching of the shoulder capsule is important for optimal results.[111]

Elbow and Forearm   Elbow and forearm contractures are a frequent complication of major trauma. The elbow joint consists of two joints with the accompanying ligaments and capsules. The ulnohumeral joint subserves flexion and extension, whereas the radioulnar joint controls pronation and supination. Structurally, most of the muscle mass crosses the elbow joint anteriorly, creating force production imbalance. Contracture at the elbow adversely affects the function and ROM of the adjacent shoulder and wrist joints.[148]

The use of light wrist weights for stretch, after the application of hot packs while maintaining position in dynamic and/or static extension splints has been recommended.[148] Stretch deformation also has been obtained with the use of static progressive stretch devices controlled by the patient.[138] In addition, dynamic splinting and serial casting have been shown to provide long-term improvement in joint function.[140,144] Intermittent compression garments have been successful in resolving elbow contractures of traumatic origin and have the advantage of simplicity.[154]

Surgery is not recommended for elbow contractures with less than 30 percent loss of ROM. Particular care must be taken during these procedures to avoid damaging the median or ulnar nerves. Surgical correction may be limited in chronic contracture because of the risk of overstretching the median and posterior interossesous nerves and brachial artery. Procedures used to resolve a "simple" elbow contracture include open or arthroscopic capsulectomy, biceps tendon lengthening, brachialis myotomy, and release of the anterior fibers of the collateral ligaments. In the spastic limb, functional use of the elbow can be improved by brachioradialis myotomy, with z-lengthening of the biceps tendon and fractional lengthening of the brachialis.[115,155,156] Complication rates as high as 17 percent may be seen following surgery for elbow contractures.[155]

Wrist and Hand The presence of multiple joints and an intricate system of ligaments and tendons makes therapeutic decision making for treatment of hand contractures complex. In Dupuytren's disease, damage to the collateral ligaments and volar plate can result in continued ROM limitations even after fascial release is performed.[158] The hand joints are particularly well suited to treatment with dynamic splinting and joint distraction, as small joints respond favorably to low force applications. Surgical release procedures with postoperative dynamic splinting is effective for hand contractures.[159]

Complex surgical procedures are most successful if the patient has sufficient cognitive ability to cooperate with intensive postoperative rehabilitation. Other favorable determinants for operative success include retained sensation and functional limb use.[115] Improvement in tenodesis of the spastic hand may be a limited but worthwhile objective of surgery.[159] Simple procedures, such as tenotomy of the deep and superficial tendons at the wrist, may facilitate hygiene or improve positioning.[160]

Typically, the weak hand and wrist will assume a flexed position with or without spasticity present. With spastic paresis of the limb, a thumb-in-palm deformity may be present. In certain syndromes, such as arthrogryposis multiplex, a "windblown hand" deformity comprised of contracted web space, flexion contracture, subluxation of the metacarpophalangeal joint, and very weak thenar muscles exists.[161]

Muscle tendon transfers are also used to treat forearm pronation and wrist flexion deformities. The Green transfer, which involves the transfer of the flexor carpi ulnaris to the extensor carpi radialis brevis or extensor carpi radialis longus, in combination with pronator releases if necessary, has resulted in functional use of the limb as an assist, while improving cosmetic appearance.[162,163] Prior to tendon transfer surgery, a combination of dynamic electromyography and peripheral nerve blocks help determine the level of motor control present.

Hip Hip flexion contractures in conjunction with knee flexion contractures are a common consequence of positioning in adjustable hospital beds and wheelchairs. When muscle tone is elevated in the spastic limb, adductor tightness may be present. Because of the proximity of the hip joint to the trunk, there is no orthosis or splint that can control hip positioning in the spastic

patient. Positioning, therefore, is particularly important in the prevention of hip flexion contracture. The prone position is highly effective in maintaining full hip ROM. In addition, control of the position of the hip can be facilitated by controlling the knee. Immobilizing the knee in an extension position will prevent extreme flexion of the hip. Conversely, mobilizing the knee by passive range of motion will concomitantly mobilize the hip.

In analyzing a hip contracture, the function of the rectus femoris, hamstrings, and tensor fascia lata is crucial. Each one controls function at the hip and knee. The Thomas test or prone hip extension are the most reliable methods to measure hip ROM, and are easy to perform.[109] To perform the Thomas test correctly in spastic limbs, the examiner must keep the hip adducted. Examination of the hip in abduction may mask the appearance of contracture.[163]

Stretch applied to the hip is most effective when preceded with pre-stretch heating by ultrasound followed by prolonged prone positioning. Care should be taken not to be overzealous with passive stretching, especially after prolonged immobilization, where demineralized osteoporotic bone is susceptible to pathologic fracture.

Shortening of the iliopsoas muscle is a common cause of hip flexion contracture. In the mature hip flexion contracture, surgery (z-lengthening of the psoas major tendon) may be the only effective means of increasing range of motion.[114,150] However, the risk of decreasing ambulatory function by increasing hip flexor weakness should always be considered.[150]

When adductor contractures require surgery, adductor myotomy alone is preferable to myotomy combined with obturator neurectomy, especially for those who ambulate.[150] Soft-tissue releases are effective in enhancing range of motion at the hips and knees in arthritis or spastic lower extremity paresis.[164]

In spastic children, the presence of elevated muscle tone and progressive shortening of the hip flexors and adductors can lead to hip deformities, subluxation, and eventual dislocation. Hip dislocation is associated with pain and progressive pelvic deformity, causing positioning difficulties even in the nonambulatory child. Surgical intervention to prevent progressive subluxation and dislocation in children at risk should be performed before skeletal deformities progress, usually before age five.[150,165]

In nonambulatory children with established hip dislocations, the indications for surgical repair are controversial. If the dislocation is not painful or interfering with positioning, waiting may be appropriate. As the children grow and develop, pain may increase and pose significant functional limitations. Established hip dislocations can be surgically addressed using soft-tissue releases, open reduction and osteotomies, resection arthroplasties, and arthrodesis and arthroplasty.[106] Surgical outcome can be adversely affected by severe pelvic obliquity or heterotopic bone formation.[166]

Knee   The knee is a complex joint because of its intra-articular arrangement of ligaments, menisci, collateral ligaments, and the joint capsule. The knee joint is crossed by several two-joint muscles, including the rectus femoris, hamstrings, and gastrocnemius.

The knee functions in a closed-kinetic chain. It reciprocally is affected by the position of the hip and ankle. Knee flexion posture can be caused by changes at the knee joint, or in response to hip or ankle position. The biomechanical pathophysiology of knee function is the major determinant of therapeutic decision making in the treatment of knee contractures. In the child with cerebral palsy and crouch gait, for instance, the knee flexion during gait may be owing to tight hamstrings, hip flexion contracture, or overly lengthened Achilles tendon.

Examination of the knee joint should isolate knee ROM and measure changes in ROM with changes in hip and ankle position. Gait analysis often yields important information on whether shortening of the hamstrings is promoting pelvic stabilization.[167] The use of a gait laboratory, anesthetic peripheral nerve blocks, and videotaping all promote more pathophysiologically specific therapeutic decision making. Simple remediation of hip flexion deformity may be all that is required to correct knee-flexion deformity.

The ability to compensate for knee flexion contractures appears to be limited. Flexion beyond 20 degrees has been shown to severely impair ambulation. Increased energy requirements related to augmented quadriceps and other muscle activity have been offered as one explanation.[168–170] In neurologically-induced knee weakness, hyperextension of the knee maintains stability in stance.[169] Knee-flexion contractures prevent this compensatory technique and decrease gait stability. Limited knee ROM also has been shown to affect balance, further stressing adjacent joints and muscles used for compensation.[1]

Rehabilitative techniques used to treat knee contractures include serial casting and dynamic splints. Forceful stretching of the knee may result in damage to the soft tissue structures or long bone fractures when osteopenia is present. Adjustable external bone fixators (such as the Ilizarov or Orthofix devices) provide a sustained stretch by promoting serial positioning. Complications, such as pin-site infection, should always be considered.[164]

Surgical soft-tissue releases include distal hamstring tenotomy or lengthening, posterior capsulotomy and deep tissue dissection, or proximal hamstring tenotomy.[172] Overly aggressive correction may result in sciatic nerve injury. Distal hamstring lengthening may also result in overcompensation by the rectus femoris muscle, leading to a "stiff-legged" gait. Addition of transfer of the distal rectus femoris tendon posteriorly has improved knee extension in stance and knee flexion in the swing phase.[114] However, how often the actual degree of functional ambulation is affected by loss of knee flexion in the presence of rectus spasticity and who will benefit from muscle transfer remains unclear.[173]

Knee extension contractures are uncommon and are generally associated with trauma, infection, or heterotopic ossification. Traumatic knee extension contractures respond better to surgical intervention than do those caused by infection.[175]

Ankle and Foot   Ankle plantar flexion contractures may involve isolated gastrocnemius, soleus, or combined shortening of both plantar flexor muscles. Lengthening of the Achilles tendon to improve ankle range of motion can cause impaired push-off during gait. Computer simulations suggest that correcting gastrocnemius and soleus contractures independently by lengthening the aponeurosis of each muscle or correcting the Achilles tendon length for the soleus contracture and lengthening the gastrocnemius aponeurosis may result in preserved strength.[176]

Deep posterior compartment syndrome of the leg can result in severe scarring of the posterior tibialis, flexor digitorum longus, and flexor hallucis longus muscles, resulting in equinovarus positioning of the foot. Excision of the offending muscle and tendon may be necessary for treatment, along with soft tissue releases.[177] The Ilizarov method of external graduated traction has been used successfully in the reduction of ankle contractures.[178]

Calcaneus deformities can be treated by resection or tenotomy of the anterior tibial tendon, sometimes in conjunction with tenodesis to the tibia. Another technique used for correction of a calcaneus deformity of the foot (commonly seen with myelomeningocele) is posterior transfer of the anterior tibialis muscle through the interosseous membrane to the calcaneus. Optimum results are seen in all age groups in more distal lesion levels (L5–S1).[179]

Spasticity in foot muscles often leads to equinus, varus, equinovarus, or toe-flexion deformities. Release of the long-toe flexors and interphalangeal joint arthrodesis can improve foot stability, in conjunction with aggressive treatment of spasticity.[180] When equino-varus deformity is recurrent, a triple arthrodesis or joint fusion may be necessary.

REFERENCES

1. Potter P, Kirby R, MacLeod D: The effects of simulated knee-flexion contractures on standing balance. *Am J Phys Med Rehab* 1990; 69:144.

2. Pelegano J, Nowysz S, Goepferd S: Temporomandibular joint contracture in spastic quadriplegia: effect on oral-motor skills. *Dev Med Child Neurol* 1994; 36:487.

3. Bax MCO, Brown JK: Contractures and their therapy. *Dev Med Child Neurol* 1985; 27:423.

4. Kaplan M, Yablon S, Ivanhoe C, et al: Surgical correction of contracture: The costs of failed joint management in acquired brain injury. *Arch Phys Med Rehab* 1995; 76:1082.

5. Willig T, Bach J, Rouffet M, et al: Correlation of flexion contractures with upper extremity function and pain for spinal muscular atrophy and congenital myopathy patients. *Am J Phys Med Rehab* 1995; 74:33.

6. Perry J, Mulroy S, Renwick S: The relationship of lower extremity strength and gait parameters in patients with post-polio syndrome. *Arch Phys Med Rehab* 1993; 74:165.

7. Yarkony GM, Bass LM, Keenan V, et al: Contractures complicating spinal cord injury: incidence and comparison between spinal cord centre and general hospital acute care. *Paraplegia* 1985; 23:265.

8. Yarkony GM, Sahgal V: Contractures: a major complication of craniocerebral trauma. *Clin Orthop* 1987; 219:93.

9. Vandervoort A, Chesworth B, Cunningham D, et al.: An outcome measure to quantify passive stiffness of the ankle. *Can J Pub Health* 1992; 83:S19.

10. Bergstrom G, Aniansson A, Bjelle A, Grimby G, Lundgren-Lindquist B, Svanbory A: Functional consequences of joint impairment at age 79. *Scand J Rehabil Med* 1985; 17:183.

11. Mollinger LA, Steffen TM: Knee flexion contractures in institutionalized elderly: prevalence, severity, stability and related variables. *Phys Ther* 1993; 73:437.

12. Souren LEM, Franssen EH, Reisberg B: Contractures and loss of function in patients with Alzheimer's disease. *J Am Ger Soc* 1995; 43:650.

13. Broughton N, Menelaus M, Cole W, et al: The natural history of hip deformity in myelomeningocele. *J Bone Joint Surg (British)* 1993; 75:760.

14. Turk M, Weber R, Pavin M, et al: Musculoskeletal problems among adults with cerebral palsy: Findings among persons who reside at a developmental center (Abs). *Arch Phys Med Rehab* 1995; 76:1055.

15. Finsterbush A, Friedman B: Early changes in immobilized rabbits knee joints: A light and electron microscopic study. *Clin Orthop* 1973; 92:305.

16. Stuart C, Shangraw R, Prince M, et al: Bed-rest induced resistance occurs primarily in muscle. *Metabolism* 1988; 37:802.

17. Salter R, Field P: The effects of continuous compression on living articular cartilage. *J Bone Joint Surg Am* 1960; 42A:31.

18. Thaxter T, Mann R, Anderson C: Degeneration of immobilized knee joints in rats. *J Bone Joint Surg* 1965; 47A:567.

19. Evans E, Burke G, Eggers W, et al: Experimental immobilization and remobilization of rat knee joints. *J Bone Joint Surg Am* 1960; 42A:737.

20. Hall M: Cartilage changes after experental immobilization of the knee joint of the young rat. *J Bone Joint Surg Am* 1963; 45A:36.

21. Enneking W, Horowitz M: The intra-articular effects of immobilization on the human knee. *J Bone Joint Surg Am* 1972; 42A:973.

22. Akeson W, Amiel D, Woo S-Y: Immobility effects on synovial joints: the pathomechanics of joint contracture. *Biorheology* 1980; 17:95.

23. Baker W, Thomas T, Kirkaldy-Willis W: Changes in the cartilage of the posterior intervertebral joints after anterior fusion. *J Bone Joint Surg* 1969; 4:737.

24. Trias A: Effect of persistent pressure on the articular cartilage. *J Bone Joint Surg* 1961; 43B:376.

25. Akeson W: An experimental study of joint stiffness. *J Bone Joint Surg Am* 1961; 43A:1022.

26. Akeson W, Amiel D, Mechanic G, et al: Collagen cross-linking alterations in joint contractures: Changes in the reducible cross-links in periarticular connective tissue collagen after 9 weeks of immobilization. *Conn Tiss Res* 1977; 5:15.

27. Akeson W, Woo S-Y, Amiel R, et al: The connective tissue response to immobility: Biochemical changes in periarticular connective tissue of the immobilized rabbit knee. *Clin Orthop Rel Res* 1973; 93:356.

28. Amiel D, Akeson W, Harwood R, et al.: Effect of immobilization on the types of collagen synthesized in periarticular connective tissue. *Conn Tiss Res* 1980; 8:27.

29. Amiel D, Woo S-Y, Harwood F, et al: The effect of immobilization on collagen turnover in connective tissue: A biochemical-biomechanical correlation. *Acta Orthop Scand* 1982; 53:325.

30. Nimni M: Collagen: Structure, function, and metabolism in normal and fibrotic tissue. *Semin Arth Rheum* 1983; 13:1.

31. Swann D, Radin E, Nazimiec M, et al: Role of hyaluronic acid in joint lubrication. *Ann Rheum Dis* 1974; 33:318.

32. Klein L, Dawson M, Heiple K: Turnover of collagen in the adult rat after degeneration. *J Bone Joint Surg Am* 1977; 59A:1065.

33. Hather B, Adams G, Tesh P, et al: Skeletal muscle responses to lower limb suspensions in humans. *J Appl Physiol* 1992; 72:1493.

34. Macdougall J, Elder G, Sale D, et al: Effects of strength training and immobilization on human muscle fibres. *Eur J Appl Physiol* 1980; 43:24.

35. Veldhuizen J, Verstappen F, Vroemen J, et al: Functional and morphological adaptations following four weeks of knee immobilization. *Int J Sports Med* 1993; 14:283.

36. Jozsa L, Thoring M, Jarvinen P, Letho M, Kivist M: Quantitative alterations in intramuscular connective tissue following immobilization: an experimental study in the rat calf muscles. *Exp Mol Pathol* 1988; 49:267.

37. Jozsa L, Kannus P, Thoring J, et al: The effect of tenotomy and immobilisation on intramuscular connective tissue. *J Bone Joint Surg Br* 1990; 72B:293.

38. Salonen V, Lehto M, Kalimo H, Penttinen R, Aro H: Changes in intramuscular collagen and fibronectin in denervation atrophy. *Muscle Nerve* 1985; 8:125.

39. Tabary JC, Tabary C, Tardieu C, Tardieu G, Goldspink G: Physiological and structural changes in the cat's soleus muscle due to immobilization at different lengths by plaster casts. *J Physiol* 1972; 224:231.

40. Williams PE, Goldspink G: Connective tissue changes in immobilized muscle. *J Anat* 1984; 138:343.

41. Herbert RD, Balnave RJ: The effect of position of immobilisation on resting length, resting stiffness, and weight of the soleus muscle of the rabbit. *J Orthop Res* 1993; 11:358.

42. Kannus P, Jozsa L, Kvist M, et al: The effect of immobilization on myotendinous junction: An ultrastructural, histochemical and immunohistochemical study. *Acta Physiol Scand* 1992; 144:387.

43. Perry J: Determinants of muscle function in the spastic lower extremity. *Clin Orthop Rel Res* 1993; 288:10.

44. Botte M, Nickel V, Akeson W: Spasticity and contracture: Physiologic aspects of formation. *Clin Orthop Rel Res* 1988; 233:7.

45. Young R, Wiegner A: Spasticity. *Clin Orthop Rel Res* 1987; 219:50.

46. Landau W: Spasticity: What is it? What is it not? in Feldman R, Young R, Koella W (eds): *Spasticity-Disordered Motor Control*, Chicago, Yearbook Medical Publishers, 1980.

47. Crone C, Hultborn H: Spinal pathophysiology of spasticity, in Pederson E, Clausen J, Dades L. (eds): *Actual Problems in Multiple Sclerosis Research*. Copenhagen: FADL's Forlag, 1983, p. 87.

48. Delwaide P: Human monosynaptic reflexes and presynaptic inhibition: An intrepretation of spastic hyper-reflexia, in Desmedt J (ed): *New Developments in Electromyogra-phy and Clinical Neurophysiology*. Basel: Karger, 1973, p. 508.

49. Pierrot-Deseilligny E, Mazieres L: Spinal mechanisms underlying spasticity, in Delwaide P, Young R (eds): *Clinical Neurophysiology in Spasticity*. Amsterdam: Elsevier, 1985, p. 63.

50. Lance J: Symposium Synopsis, in Feldman R, Young R, Koella W (eds): *Spasticity-Disordered Motor Control*. Chicago: Yearbook Medical Publishers, 1980, p. 485.

51. Gilman S, Newman S: *Manter and Gatz's Essentials of Clinical Neuroanatomy and Neurophysiology*. Philadelphia: F.A. Davis, 1987.

52. Heikkinen E: Transformations of rat skin collagen: with special reference to the aging process. *Acta Physiol Scand (Suppl)* 1968; 317:5.

53. Heikkinen E, Kulonen E: Age factor in the maturation of collagen. Intramolecular linkages in mildly denatured collagen. *Experientia* 1964; 20:310.

54. Rasmussen D, Wakim K, Windelmann R: Effect of aging on human dermis: Studies of thermal shrinkage and tension, in Montagna W (ed): *Advances in Biology of Skin*, New York: Pergamon Press, 1965, p. 151.

55. Rigby B: Increase with time in the thermal stability of rat tail tendon stored in 0.9% NaCl. *Biochem Biophys Acta* 1967; 140:548.

56. Verzar F: Aging of the collagen fiber, in Hall D, Jackson D (eds): *International Review of Connective Tissue Research*. New York: Academic Press, 1964, p. 244.

57. Smith E, Serfass R: *Exercise and Aging: The Scientific Basis*. Hillside, NJ: Enslow, 1981.

58. Butzow J, Eichhorn G: Physical chemical studies on the age changes in rat tail tendon collagen. *Biochem Biophys Acta* 1968; 145:208.

59. Heikkinen E, Mikkonen L, Kulonen E: Age factor in the maturation of collagen. Cross-links in heat-denatured collagen in tail tendon and skin of rat. *Exp Gerontol* 1964; 1:31.

60. Rice C, Cunningham D, Paterson D, et al: Strength in an elderly population. *Arch Phys Med Rehab* 1989; 70:391.

61. Dakofod V, Nneskiold-Samsoe B, Munter J, et al: Muscle strength and functional capacity in 78–81 year old men and women. *Eur J Appl Physiol* 1984; 52:310.

62. Harries U, Bassey E: Torque-velocity relationships for the knee extensors in women in the 3rd and 7th decades. *Eur J Appl Physiol* 1990; 60:187.

63. Larsson L: Morphological and functional characteristics of the ageing skeletal muscle in man. *Acta Physiol Scand Suppl* 1978; 457:1.

64. Murray M, Duthie E, Gambert S, et al: Age-related differences in knee muscle strength in normal women. *J Gerontol* 1985; 40:275.

65. Vandervoort A, Hayes K Belanger A: Strength and endurance of skeletal muscle in the elderly. *Physiother Can* 1986; 38:167.

66. Larsson L, Grimby G, Karlsson J: Muscle strength and

speed of movement in relation to age and muscle morphology. *J Appl Physiol* 1979; 46:451.

67. Young A, Stokes M, Crowe M: The size and strength of the quadriceps muscle of old and young women. *Eur J Clin Invest* 1984; 14:282.

68. Bruce S, Newton D, Woledge R: Effect of age on voluntary force and cross-sectional area of human adductor pollicis muscle. *Q J Exp Physiol* 1989; 74:359.

69. Frontera W, Hughes V, Evans W: A cross-sectional study of upper and lower extremity muscle strength in 45–78 year old men and women. *J Appl Physiol* 1991; 71:644.

70. Young A, Stokes M, Crowe M: Size and strength of the quadriceps of muscles of old and young men. *Clin Physiol* 1985; 5:145.

71. Overend T, Cunningham D, Patterson D, et al: Thigh composition in young and elderly men determined by computed tomography. *Clin Physiol* 1992; 12:629.

72. Conley K, Cress M, Jubrias S, et al: From muscle properties to human performance, using magnetic resonance. *J Gerontol Ser A* 1995; 50A:35.

73. Binder H, Eng G: Rehabilitation management of children with spastic diplegic cerebral palsy. *Arch Phys Med Rehab* 1989; 70:481.

74. Berman B: Selective posterior rhizotomy: Does it do any good? *Neurosurg State Art Rev* 1989; 4:431.

75. Winters TJ, Gage J, Hicks R: Gait patterns in spastic hemiplegia in children and young adults. *J Bone Joint Surg* 1987; 69A:437.

76. Halpern D: Rehabilitation of children with brain damage, in Kottke F, Stillwell G, Lehmann J (eds): *Krusen's Handbook of Physical Medicine and Rehabilitation*, 4th ed. Philadelphia: W.B. Saunders, 1990, 746.

77. Ziv I, Blackburn N, Rang M, et al: Muscle growth in normal and spastic mice. *Dev Med Child Neurol* 1984; 26:94.

78. Frankeny J, Holly R, Ashmore C: Effects of graded duration of stretch on normal and dystrophic skeletal muscle. *Muscle Nerve* 1983; 6:269.

79. Bick E: *Source Book of Orthopaedics*. Baltimore: Williams & Wilkins, 1948.

80. Thomas H: *Diseases of the Hip, Knee and Ankle Joints with Their Deformities, Treated by a New and Efficient Method*. London: Lewis, 1878.

81. Sayre L: *Orthopedic Surgery and the Diseases of the Joints*. New York: D'Appleton and Co, 1876.

82. Wright J, Menelaus M, Broughton N, et al: Natural history of knee contractures in meylomeningocele. *J Pediatr Orthop* 1991; 11:725.

83. Campbell RR, Hawkins SJ, Maddison PJ, et al: Limited joint mobility in diabetes mellitus. *Ann Rheumatol* 1985; 44:93.

84. Renard E, Jacques D, Chammas M, et al: Increased prevalence of soft tissue hand lesions in type 1 and type 2 diabetes mellitus: various entities and associated significance. *Diabete Metab (Paris)* 1994; 20:513.

85. Gamstedt A, Holm-Glad J, Ohlson C-G, et al: Hand ab-normalities are strongly associated with the duration of diabetes mellitus. *J Int Med* 1993; 234:189.

86. Chammas M, Bousquet P, Renard E, et al: Dupuytren's disease, carpal tunnel syndrome, trigger finger, and diabetes mellitus. *J Hand Surg* 1995; 20A:109.

87. Convery F, Conaty J, Nickel V: Flexion deformities of the knee in rheumatoid arthritis. *Clin Ortho* 1971; 74:90.

88. Banwell B: Exercise and mobility in arthritis. *Nurs Clin No Am* 1984; 19:605.

89. Fam A, Schumacher HJ, Clayburne G, et al: Effect of joint motion on experimental calcium pyrophosphate dihydrate crystal induced arthritis. *J Rheumatol* 1990; 17:644.

90. Van Lent P, Wilms F, Van Den Berg W: Interaction of polymorphonuclear leucocytes with patellar cartilage of immobilized arthritic joints: a scanning electron microscopic study. *Ann Rheum Dis* 1989; 48:832.

91. Van Lent P, Van Den Bersselaar L, Van De Putte L, et al: Immobilization aggravates cartilage damage during antigen-induced arthritis in mice. *Am J Pathol* 1990; 136:1407.

92. Buckley S, Skinner S, James P, et al: Focal scleroderma in children: an orthopaedic perspective. *J Pediatr Orthop* 1993; 13:784.

93. Demichele S, Brown R: Connective tissue metabolism in muscular dystrophy. Levels of collagen and mucopolysaccharides in embryonic chickens with genetic muscular dystrophy. *Comp Biochem Physiol* 1984; 79B:203.

94. Spencer H, Morgulis S, Wilder V: A micromethod for the deterinatin of gelatin and a study of the collagen content of muscle from normal and dystrophic rabbits. *J Biol Chem* 1937; 120:257.

95. Thomson E, Yasin R, Van Beers G, et al: Myogenic defects in human muscular dystrophy. *Nature* 1977; 268:241.

96. Dubowitz V: *Muscle Disorders in Childhood*. London: Saunders, 1978.

97. Jones D, Round J: *Skeletal Muscle in Health and Disease: A Textbook of Muscle Physiology*. Manchester: Manchester University Press, 1990.

98. Sharma JC: Residual poliomyelitis of lower limb: pattern and deformities. *Ind J Pediatr* 1991; 58:233.

99. Watts HG: Management of common Third World orthopaedic problems: paralytic poliomyelitis, tuberculosis of bones and joints, Hansen's disease (leprosy), and chronic osteomyelitis. *Instruct Course Lect* 1992; 41:471.

100. Molnar G: Cerebral palsy, in Molnar G (ed): *Pediatric Rehabilitation*, Baltimore: Williams & Wilkins, 1985, p. 446.

101. Matsusue Y, Yamamuro T, Ohta H, et al: Fibrotic contracture of the gastrocnemius muscle. A case report. *J Bone Joint Surg Am* 1994; 76:739.

102. Napiontek M, Ruszkowski K: Paralytic drop foot and gluteal fibrosis after intramuscular injections. *J Bone Joint Surg Br* 1993; 75:83.

103. Daud O, Sett P, Burr R, et al: The relationship of heterotopic ossification to passive movements in paraplegic patients. *Dis Rehab* 1993; 15:114.

104. Hastings H, Graham T: The classification and treatment of heterotopic ossification about the elbow and forearm. *Hand Clin* 1994; 10:417.

105. Binder H, Conway A, Gerber L: Rehabilitation approaches to children with osteogenesis imperfecta: A ten-year experience. *Arch Phys Med Rehab* 1993; 74:386.

106. Gamble J, Rinsky L, Bleck E: Established hip dislocations in children with cerebral palsy. *Clin Orthop* 1990; 253:90.

107. Delgado-Baeza E, Albinana-Cilveli J, Miralles-Flores C: Why does the pelvic deformity occur in experimental dislocation of the growing hip? *J Pediatr Orthop* 1992; 12:376.

108. Ponseti I: Treatment of congenital club foot. *J Bone Joint Surg Am* 1992; 74A:448.

109. Bartlett M, Wold L, Shurtleff D, et al: Hip flexion contractures: a comparison of measurement methods. *Arch Phys Med Rehab* 1985; 66:620.

110. Bar-On E, Malkin C, Eilert R, et al: Hip flexion contracture in cerebral palsy. The association between clinical and radiologic measurement methods. *Clin Orthop* 1992; 281:97.

111. Skoff H, Woodbury D: Management of the upper extremity in cerebral palsy. *J Bone Joint Surg Am* 1985; 67A:500.

112. Perry J, Hoffer M, Antonelli D, et al: Electromyography before and after surgery for hip deformity in children with cerebral palsy. A comparison of clinical and electromyographic findings. *J Bone Joint Surg Am* 1976; 58:201.

113. Perry J, Hoffer M: Preoperative and postoperative dynamic electromyography as an aid in planning tendon transfers in children with cerebral palsy. *J Bone Joint Surg Am* 1977; 59:531.

114. Nene A, Evans G, Patrick J: Simultaneous multiple operations for spastic diplegia. Outcome and functional assessment of walking in 18 patients. *J Bone Joint Surg Br* 1993; 75:488.

115. Kozin S, Keenan M: Using dynamic electromyography to guide surgical treatment of the spastic upper extremity in the brain-injured patient. *Clin Orthop* 1993; 288:109.

116. Hillstrom H, Perlberg G, Siegler S, et al: Objective identification of ankle equinus deformity and resulting contracture. *J Am Pod Med Assoc* 1991; 81:519.

117. Price R: Mechanical spasticity evaluation techniques. *Crit Rev Phys Rehab Med* 1990; 2:65.

118. Lehmann F, Price R, deLateur B, et al: Spasticity: Quantitative measurements as a basis for assessing effectiveness of therapeutic intervention. *Arch Phys Med Rehab* 1989; 70:6.

119. Bell K: Contractures: Prevention and management. *Crit Rev Phys Rehabil Med* 1990; 1:231.

120. Hill J: The effects of casting on upper extremity motor disorders after brain injury. *Am J Occup Ther* 1994; 48:219.

121. Bell K: The use of neurolytic blocks for the management of spasticity. *Phys Med Rehab Clin No Am* 1995; 6:885.

122. Glenn M: Nerve blocks, in Glenn M, Whyte J (eds): *The Practical Management of Spasticity in Children and Adults*, Philadelphia: Lea & Febiger, 1990, p. 227.

123. Forst R, Forst J: Importance of lower limb surgery in Duchenne muscular dystrophy. *Arch Orthop Trauma Surg* 1995; 114:106.

124. Shapiro F, Specht L: Current concepts review. The diagnosis and orthopaedic treatment of inherited muscular diseases of childhood. *J Bone Joint Surg Am* 1993; 77A:439.

125. Bach J, McKeon J: Orthopedic surgery and rehabilitation for the prolongation of brace-free ambulation of patients with Duchenne muscular dystrophy. *Am J Phys Med Rehab* 1991; 70:323.

126. Bonnet L, Burgot D, Bonnard C, et al: Surgery of the lower limbs in Duchenne muscular dystrophy. *French J Orthop Surg* 1993; 5:160.

127. Kunkel C, Scremin A, Eisenberg B, et al: Effect of "standing" on spasticity, contracture, and osteoporosis in paralyzed males. *Arch Phys Med Rehab* 1993; 74:73.

128. Warren C, Lehmann J, Koblanski J: Heat and stretch procedures: an evaluation using rat tail tendon. *Arch Phys Med Rehab* 1976; 57:122.

129. Kottke F, Pauley D, Ptak R: The rationale for prolonged stretching for correction of shortening of connective tissue. *Arch Phys Med Rehab* 1965; 47:345.

130. Holly R, Barnett J, Ashmore C, et al: Stretch-induced growth in chicken wing muscles: a new model of stretch hypertrophy. *Am J Phys* 1980; 238:C62.

131. Tardieu G, Tardieu C, Colbeau-Justin P, et al: Effects of muscle length on an increased stretch reflex in children with cerebral palsy. *J Neurol Neurosurg Psychiat* 1982; 45:348.

132. Tardieu C, Tabary J, Tabary C, et al: Comparison of the sarcomere number adaptation in young and adult animals. Influence of tendon adaptation. *J de Physiol* 1977; 73:1045.

133. Tardieu C, Lespargot A, Tabary C, et al: For how long must the soleus muscle be stretched each day to prevent contracture? *Dev Med Child Neurol* 1988; 30:3.

134. Flowers K, LaStayo P: Effect of total end range time on improving passive range of motion. *J Hand Ther* 1994; 7:150.

135. Simonian P, Staheli L: Periarticular fractures after manipulation for knee contractures in children. *J Pediatr Orthop* 1995; 15:288.

136. Yates P, Cornwell J, Scott G, et al: Treatment of haemophilic flexion deformities using the Flowtron intermittent compression system. *Br J Haematol* 1992; 82:384.

137. Lehmann J, Masock A, Warren C, et al: Effect of therapeutic temperatures on tendon extensibility. *Arch Phys Med Rehab* 1970; 51:481.

138. Bonutti P, Windau J, Ables B, et al: Static progressive stretch to reestablish elbow range of motion. *Clinical Orthop* 1994; 303:128.

139. Namba R, Kabo J, Dorey F, et al: Intra-articular corticosteroid reduces joint stiffness after an experimental periarticular fracture. *J Hand Surg* 1992; 16:1148.

140. Zander C, Healy N: Elbow flexion contractures treated

with serial casts and conservative therapy. *J Hand Surg* 1992; 17:694.

141. Anderson J: Efficacy of soft splints in reducing severe knee-flexion contractures. *Develop Med Child Neurol* 1988; 30:502.

142. MacKay-Lyons M: Low-load prolonged stretch in treatment of elbow flexion contractures secondary to head trauma: A case report. *Phys Ther* 1989; 69:296.

143. Phillips W, Audet M: Use of serial casting in the management of knee joint contractures in an adolescent with cerebral palsy. *Phys Ther* 1990; 70:521.

144. Shewring D, Beaudet M, Carvell J: Reversed dynamic slings: results of use in the treatment of post-traumatic flexion contractures of the elbow. *Injury* 1991; 22:400.

145. O'Laughlin T, Klima R, Kenney D: Rehabilitation of eosinophilic fasciitis. A case report. *Am J Phys Med Rehab* 1994; 73:286.

146. Botte M, Abrams R, Bodine-Fowler S: Treatment of acquired muscle spasticity using phenol peripheral nerve blocks. *Orthopedics* 1995; 18:151.

147. Calderon-Gonzalez R, Calderon-Sepulveda R, Rincon-Reyes M: Botulinum toxin A in management of cerebral palsy. *Pediatr Neurol* 1994; 10:284.

148. Weiss A, Sachar K: Soft tissue contractures about the elbow. *Hand Clin* 1994; 10:439.

149. Keenan M: Surgical decision making for residual limb deformities following traumatic brain injury. *Orthop Rev* 1988; 17:1185.

150. Bleck E: Management of the lower extremities in children who have cerebral palsy. *J Bone Joint Surg Am* 1990; 72:140.

151. Dhawlikar S, Root L, Mann R: Distal lengthening of the hamstrings in patients who have cerebral palsy. Long-term retrospective analysis. *J Bone Joint Surgery Am* 1992; 74:1385.

152. Atar D, Grant A, Lehman W: New approach to limb deformities in neuromuscular patients. *Bull Hosp Joint Dis Orthop Inst* 1990; 50:99.

153. Stanitski D: Treatment of deformity secondary to metabolic bone disease with the Ilizarov technique. *Clin Orthop Rel Res* 1994; 301:38.

154. Karachalios T, Maxwell-Armstrong C, Atkins R: Treatment of post-traumatic fixed flexion deformity of the elbow using an intermittent compression garment. *Injury* 1994; 25:313.

155. Jones G, Savoie F: Arthroscopic capsular release of flexion contractures. *Arthroscopy* 1993; 9:277.

156. Nowicki K, Shall L: Arthroscopic release of a posttraumatic flexion contracture in the elbow: A case report and review of the literature. *Arthroscopy* 1992; 8:544.

157. Andrew J: Contracture of the proximal interphalangeal joint in Dupuytren's disease. *J Hand Surg Br* 1991; 16:446.

158. Rives K, Gelberman R, Smith B, et al: Severe contractures of the proximal interphalangeal joint in Dupuytren's disease: Results of a prospective trial of operative correction and dynamic extension splinting. *J Hand Surg* 1992; 17:1153.

159. Treanor W, Moberg E, Buncke H: The hyperflexed seemingly useless tetraplegic hand: a method of surgical amelioration. *Paraplegia* 1992; 30:457.

160. Needoff M, Moulton A: Surgical treatment of fixed flexion contractures in the hands of institutionalised patients. *J Hand Surg Br* 1991; 16:449.

161. McCarroll HJ, Manske P: The windblown hand: correction of the complex clasped thumb deformity. *Hand Clin* 1992; 8:147.

162. Beach W, Strecker W, Coe J, et al: Use of the Green transfer in treatment of patients with spastic cerebral palsy: 17 year experience. *J Ped Orthop* 1991; 11:731.

163. Green N: The orthopaedic care of children with muscular dystrophy. *Instr Course Lect* 1987; 36:267.

164. Moreno-Alvarez M, Espada G, Maldonado-Cocco J, et al: Longterm followup of hip and knee soft tissue release in juvenile chronic arthritis. *J Rheumatol* 1992; 19:1608.

165. Kalen V, Bleck E: Prevention of spastic paralytic dislocation of the hip. *Dev Med Child Neur* 1985; 27:17.

166. Perlmutter M, Synder M, Miller F, et al: Proximal femoral resection for older children with spastic hip disease. *Dev Med Child Neurol* 1993; 35:525.

167. Hoffinger S, Rab G, Abou Ghaida H: Hamstrings in cerebral palsy crouch gait. *J Pediatr Orthop* 1993; 13:722.

168. Cerny K, Perry J, Walker J: Adaptations during the stance phase of gait for simulated flexion contractures at the knee. *Orthopedics* 1994; 17:501.

169. Hsu AT, Perry J, Gronley JK, Hislop HJ: Quadriceps force and myoelectric activity during flexed knee stance. *Clin Orthop* 1993; 288:254.

170. Potter P, Kirby R: Relationship between electromyographic activity of the vastus lateralis while standing and the extent of bilateral simulated knee-flexion contractures. *Am J Phys Med Rehab* 1991; 70:301.

171. Herzenberg J, Davis JDP, et al: Mechanical distraction for treatment of severe knee flexion contractures. *Clin Orthop* 1994; 301:80.

172. Atar D, Zilberberg L, Votemberg M, et al: Effect of distal hamstring release on cerebral palsy patients. *Bull Hosp Jt Dis* 1993; 53:34.

173. Damron T, Breed A, Cook T: Diminished knee flexion after hamstring surgery in cerebral palsy patients: Prevalence and severity. *J Pediatr Orthop* 1993; 13:188.

174. Firestone T, Krackow K, Davis JD IV, et al: The management of fixed flexion contractures during total knee arthroplasty. *Clin Orthop Rel Res* 1992; 284:221.

175. Falkiewisz C, Fengler F, Hein W: The surgical treatment of knee joint extensor muscle contractures. *Beitrage Zur Orthopadie Und Traumatologie* 1990; 37:225.

176. Delp S, Statler K, Carroll N: Preserving plantar flexion strength after surgical treatment for contracture of the triceps surae: a computer simulation study. *J Orthop Res* 1995; 13:96.

177. Manoli A, Smith D, Hansen SJ: Scarred muscle excision for the treatment of established ischemic contracture of the lower extremity. *Clin Orthop* 1993; 292:309.

178. Calhoun J, Evans E, Herndon D: Techniques for the management of burn contractures with the Ilizarov Fixator. *Clin Orthop* 1992; 280:117.

179. Georgiadis G, Aronson D: Posterior transfer of the anterior tibial tendon in children who have a myelomeningocele. *J Bone Joint Surgery Am* 1990; 72A:392.

180. Harkless L, Bembo G: Stroke and its manifestations in the foot. A case report. *Clin Podiatr Med Surg* 1994; 11:635.

Chapter 20

HYPERTONIA: DIAGNOSIS AND MANAGEMENT

Robert R. Young

Hypertonia ranges in magnitude from so severe that no movement is possible at the joint, to so slight that clinicians debate whether or not it is present. When limbs have been paralyzed for years, the ankle, for example, may become fused in plantar flexion. It cannot be flexed or extended, but the resistance to passive movement may reflect contracture of fibrous tissue at the joint rather than muscle contraction. In these situations it is not possible to stretch the muscles crossing the ankle. An orthopedic operative approach to these joint contractures occasionally is necessary as it also is to provide relief of joint immobilization secondary to heterotopic ossification. However, the remainder of this chapter will deal with hypertonia of skeletal muscle consequent to excessive activity of spinal motor neurons. For further discussion of joint contractures, see Chapter 19.

Spasticity, the most common cause of hypertonia, has been defined as a velocity-dependent increase in tonic stretch reflexes (muscle tone) following damage to the upper motor neuron.[1] This definition is more restricted than the one usually employed by clinicians; they use the term spasticity to include other positive symptoms (exaggerated tendon jerks, a Babinski response, other increased cutaneous reflexes, dystonic postures, contractures) and negative symptoms such as paresis, lack of dexterity, and fatigability.[2] To emphasize fundamental differences between the positive and negative symptoms and signs, the term spastic paresis has been used to describe or characterize the whole complex syndrome.[3] Within it, there are different subtypes, including those seen with lesions of the spinal cord (spinal spasticity with particularly hyperactive triple flexion reflexes and tonically flexed limbs) and those following supraspinal lesions (hemiplegic spasticity in which stretch reflexes are prominently exaggerated, lower limbs extended, and upper limbs flexed).

Although, by definition, muscles are always hypertonic if spasticity is present, only in a subgroup of spastic patients is muscle tone dramatically increased so that abnormal postures are seen as a result. The paraplegic or hemiplegic varieties of this spastic dystonia—tight flexion at all joints in the upper limb with strong flexion or, more commonly, extension at hip, knee, and ankle—present much more of a rehabilitative problem than simple increased stretch reflexes.[4] Certain treatments outlined in the following are used primarily to reduce spastic dystonia, not to treat spasticity or spastic paresis in general. Spastic dystonia has a characteristic temporal profile. With rare exceptions, muscle tone is normal or reduced immediately after an acute lesion of the motor system. A Babinski response is present immediately and the bulbo-cavernosus reflex returns within a few hours, but tonic and phasic stretch reflexes do not reappear or become hyperactive for at least several days. They then continue to increase for weeks, unless the concomitant paresis lessens, at which time hypertonia may also lessen, although not always. When the limb remains densely paretic or plegic, hypertonia becomes maximal and permanent by 6 months. In some patients, especially those with spinal cord lesions, after 10 or 20 years, tendon reflexes and muscle tone decrease, but the latter usually is not significant because by then joint contractures keep the limb in the posture originally determined by muscle hypertonia.

Rigidity is seen in pure form in patients with Parkinson's disease and less often in those with rarer conditions that also do not produce visible lesions on CT or MRI. It is defined as increased muscle tone that is length- rather than velocity-sensitive, is present at rest, is seen without a Babinski response, and is not accompanied by increased tendon jerks. Although present in both extensor and flexor muscles throughout the range of movement (and even before stretching begins), it tends to be stronger in flexor muscles and is easiest to feel during slow stretch.[5]

Although these simple definitions clearly differentiate spasticity from rigidity, that differentiation often may be difficult in practice. If one restricts the examination simply to muscle tone without regard to the etiology of the condition, the nature of the plantar response, and so on, rigid muscle groups appear in limbs of paraplegic and hemiplegic patients, often in the same limb in which the antagonist muscles are spastic. Mixed forms of hypertonia exist and a practical approach should be taken to guide therapy. Diagnostic and therapeutic categories based on etiology and location of CNS lesions are preferable to those based simply on whether the hypertonia is velocity- or length-sensitive.

SHOULD THE HYPERTONIA BE TREATED?

Not all the symptoms and signs listed in the preceding can be treated, and others that can be treated should not be. Hyperactive tendon jerks, as manifest by clonus, sometimes are troublesome for patients. Patients never complain of a Babinski response. On the other hand, increased muscle tone and the resultant abnormal flexor or extensor postures may make it difficult for a patient to dress, transfer, bathe, receive toilet care, ride in a wheelchair, and so on. If so, treatment should be considered. Flexor spasms are uncomfortable or sometimes painful, inconvenient, potentially damaging to patients or their surroundings, and cause frequent awakenings at night. They can and should be treated.

However, heightened flexor reflexes may be used to get a patient onto a bedpan or to help with dressing and ambulation. Patients, using their exaggerated cutaneous reflexes to help with activities of daily living (ADL), may complain if treatments reduce those reflexes. Similarly, extensor hypertonia in the leg can serve as a built-in crutch, so treating that hypertonia will produce buckling of the leg when it is used to bear weight during transfers or ambulation; that will produce an unhappy patient. Fingers with spastic dystonia in flexion may be useful for carrying things. These are examples of situations where alleviating spastic dystonia or spastic hyperreflexia, although possible, is counterproductive. Theoretically at least, spasticity may help reduce muscular atrophy, reduce osteoporosis, and improve venous return. If it is not producing disabilities in that particular patient's life, why treat spasticity?

A more frequent source of patient and physician disappointment with therapy for hypertonia is emphasized by the term spastic paresis. Although therapies exist that reduce positive symptoms such as flexor spasms and spastic dystonia, almost nothing can be done to overcome the negative paretic symptoms caused by lesion-induced disconnections within the central motor system. Treating the spasticity thus usually does nothing for the paresis. Patients or physicians who expect treatments for spastic paresis to alleviate the paresis will almost always be disappointed when only the spasticity or spastic dystonia responds.

Rarely, especially in patients with nonspastic hypertonia, alleviation of the dystonia will unmask some useful voluntary function that had been submerged by the continuous muscle activity. This is particularly true with Parkinson's disease and idiopathic torsion dystonia. But when spastic dystonia is alleviated, little if any voluntary function usually is found to exist in the normotonic limb. Theoretically, in a spastic paretic limb where some voluntary contraction remains (e.g., in triceps surae), normal or increased reciprocal inhibition may make the antagonist muscle (tibialis anterior) appear weaker than it would if the excessive discharge of gastrosoleus motoneurons could be reduced. Frequent improvement in strength of dorsiflexion consequent to reduction of spasticity in plantar flexors remains to be demonstrated.

If treatments for hypertonia are to be considered effective, appropriate therapeutic goals must be agreed on beforehand. If the patient expects therapy for spastic paresis to result in his getting out of the wheelchair or using his hand to write, he will almost certainly be disappointed. If painful spasms are a significant problem, treatment can reduce or eliminate them, and patients are grateful for such relief even if they must remain in the wheelchair. Children with spastic equinus ankle deformities who walk on their toes ambulate much better and more securely when they can get their feet flat on the floor. That happens when spastic dystonia in the triceps surae muscles is eliminated medically or, if that is not satisfactory, surgically.[6] Care must be taken not to discredit therapies because they fail to make the paralyzed muscles function again.[7] If therapeutic goals are set based on the patient's significant but treatable dysfunctions and the correct therapy is chosen, the outcome should be satisfactory.

Finally, one reasonable goal is to return spasticity, which has flared up after being stable for years, back to its chronic level. For example, a urinary tract infection, a poorly functioning catheter, fecal impaction, pressure sores, ingrown toenails, tight clothing, renal stones, an entrapment neuropathy, or any situation that would be painful if the person could feel it, will increase spasticity or, in a patient with minimal deficits, cause it to become evident. Appropriate treatment to alleviate these exacerbating factors will result in spasticity receding to its former level.

PHYSICAL THERAPIES

A very effective but often overlooked physical therapy for hypertonia involves muscle stretching. Judging by the results of immobilizing a neurologically normal limb (e.g., in a cast) or of experiments of a similar nature, everyday activities put joints through full ranges of motion and, by stretching muscles that cross that joint, keep them at their normal lengths. Disuse of muscles owing to spastic paresis or bradykinesia (with failure to stretch their antagonists) and development of the flexor or extensor postures consequent to spastic dystonia or rigidity, as noted previously, both result in spastic or bradykinetic muscles becoming shorter and stiffer than normal. To prevent or reverse this sort of hypertonia, frequent passive stretching of muscles (putting joints through full ranges of motion at least several times a day) should begin as soon as possible after the diagnosis is made of a stroke, Parkinson's disease, and so on. Joint contractures are much easier to prevent than treat. Once such a deformity occurs, it is uncomfortable, increases spasticity, and interferes with many activities of daily living.

Proper positioning, when the patient is in bed or in a chair, helps prevent abnormal dysfunctional postures. But if, despite this, contractures do develop, as often is the case, the limbs and trunk should at least be in a natural position. Braces, splints, or casts cannot prevent the development of spastic dystonia, Parkinsonian flexed postures, or other dystonic postures (including torticollis). At best, bracing can retard the development of these abnormal postures or result in a slightly less extreme posture. At worst, serial casting, for example, can help minimize an extreme posture that has developed already. On the other hand, braces provide useful compensation for weak muscles. When weak foot dorsiflexion produces a steppage gait or the patient's toes catch on the floor or door-sill during the swing through phase of gait, a light ankle-foot orthosis normalizes the gait, for which the patient is grateful. A cock-up splint at the wrist can increase prehension function there, but only if the wrist and finger flexors are not very hypertonic. For a more thorough discussion of these topics, see Chapter 26.

Cooling limbs or reducing body temperature alters mechanical properties of muscle and increases its stiffness as well as that of connective tissue around joints. Patients with hypertonia complain of becoming even stiffer when they are cold. On the other hand, local cooling with ice, which can easily and cheaply be used at home, or ethyl chloride spray, also slows or blocks nerve conduction, particularly in cutaneous afferents as well as in muscle efferents if deep cooling is obtained, and, in the latter circumstance, may also reduce muscle spindle discharge. All of this reduces spinal reflexes and hence muscle tone and spasms. These effects appear to outlast the actual lowering of temperature, but cooling is not particularly useful as a chronic therapy for muscle hypertonia.

Heating a limb also alters mechanical properties of muscle and periarticular tissues, making them more compliant and less stiff, thus reducing hypertonia. Heat, as with hot packs or infrared radiation, is also somehow soothing and relieves muscle spasms, even when the heat is superficial and does not appear to affect muscles or joints directly. The latter deep tissues can be warmed by microwave or short-wave diathermy or by using ultrasound. Heating, providing tissues are not burned, is inexpensive and readily available. It is comforting but must be repeated frequently.

Electrotherapy has a long history but at present is used most often as transcutaneous electrical nerve stimulation (TENS) to relieve acute pain following various surgical procedures and as functional electrical stimulation (FES) to activate muscles that are paralyzed but not denervated. TENS is less effective for chronic pain or for muscle hypertonia worsened by pain, but in some patients is associated with generalized relaxation and modest reduction in muscle tone that lasts for 45 minutes after the stimulation is finished.[8] FES is used to stimulate contraction of muscles in the upper or lower extremity whose spinal motoneurons are intact and connected to the muscle but disconnected from higher CNS centers for voluntary control. The aim is to produce grasping (extension followed by flexion of the fingers), for example, or stance/transfer and gait.[9] However, some of these patients are also found to have reduced spastic dystonia, not only during stimulation but for a few hours afterwards. Nonfunctional, simple electrical stimulation of muscles antagonistic to those that are hypertonic may produce similar long-lived relaxation of the latter. Whether this is caused by increased reciprocal inhibition of the agonist is unknown. In other patients, stimulation of the hypertonic muscle itself is followed by its relaxation. Dorsal column stimulators will be discussed in the following.

PHARMACOTHERAPIES

After attention to noxious inputs to the cord and stretching or positioning the affected limbs, medical treatment or management of spasticity usually involves the use of oral (or, occasionally, intravenous or intramuscular) medications. Selective applications of baclofen to the caudal cord, of botulinum toxin to the motor endplate zones of hypertonic muscles, or of alcohol/phenol to peripheral nerves are discussed elsewhere in this chapter.

Baclofen, in its commercially available racemic form, is a GABA-B (gamma amino butyric acid, receptor type B) agonist. The L-form is probably the active principle and the D-form may antagonize the response to L-baclofen.[10] Baclofen reduces the release of excitatory neurotransmitters and has been the most useful of the anti-spastic agents available in the United States. Like all of these agents—except dantrolene, botulinum toxin and alcohol/phenol—oral baclofen alleviates hypertonia and spasms in patients with lesions of the spinal cord and is not effective when lesions are rostral to the cord. Side effects, such as drowsiness, leg weakness, dizziness, mental changes, or upset stomach, are infrequent, providing doses are increased slowly from 5 mg twice a day to 120 mg per day or more in divided doses. In some patients, several hundred mg per day are needed and tolerated. Adverse events affecting liver function or other organ systems are rare.[11]

Tizanidine, which has been used for more than 10 years around the world but only recently became available in this country, is an alpha-2 noradrenergic agonist that also may act on imidazoline receptors, for which agmatine (decarboxylated arginine) is the endogenous central nervous system ligand. Tizanidine, like baclofen, is recommended for spasms and hypertonia owing to spinal cord lesions. Side effects, such as dry mouth, sedation, or fatigue, are not common if the dose is slowly increased, using 2-mg and then 4-mg tablets, to 8 mg three times a day; maximum doses are 12 mg three times a day. Serious systemic adverse events are rare. Despite its structural similarity to clonidine, tizanidine almost never produces symptomatic hypotension. It also seems to produce less muscle weakness than baclofen.[12] Tizanidine is not available for intrathecal injection.

Clonidine, also an alpha-2 noradrenergic agonist, is approved by the FDA for treatment of hypertension. In doses of 0.05 to 0.2 mg three or four times a day, it also relieves spastic dystonia in the legs of patients with spinal lesions, but now that tizanidine is available, may be used less often.[13]

Dantrolene blocks release of calcium from sarcoplasmic reticulum in muscle and thus prevents contraction when a muscle action potential is generated ("excitation contraction uncoupling"). In a dose-related manner, it weakens all muscles, including hypertonic ones. Although sometimes this may be helpful in the care of completely paralyzed patients leading a bed–chair existence, it is rarely useful for less severely affected patients, particularly those with supraspinal lesions in whom hypertonic and normotonic muscles would be weakened.

Doses can be increased over 1 month from 25 mg per day to as much as 400 mg per day. Side effects in addition to generalized weakness include sedation, diarrhea, and nausea. Serious adverse events include hepatotoxicity, especially in older patients, those receiving more than 200 mg per day, and those who have received dantrolene previously. Liver function tests must be monitored throughout treatment.[11] Few spastic patients receive long-term dantrolene therapy but it is life-saving for emergency treatment of anesthesia-induced malignant hyperthermia. Also it may be useful as acute therapy for sudden, severe increases in spasticity, as when intrathecal therapy fails and there is sudden withdrawal from baclofen.

Diazepam and other benzodiazepines (such as alprazolam, clonazepam, and tetrazepam) increase the affinity of GABA for GABA-A receptors and thus increase GABA-mediated presynaptic inhibition as well as inhibition of descending facilitatory pathways. They are most effective in decreasing spasms and spastic dystonia in patients with disorders of the spinal cord but may help certain patients with cerebral lesions too. Side effects are relatively frequent and include drowsiness, sedation, depression, irritability, loss of coordination, and increased fatigue. Therapy begins with 2 mg once or twice a day and increases slowing to as much as 15 mg four times a day. These large doses often are very well tolerated if increases are gradual. Adverse events affecting liver, renal function, or other bodily systems are uncommon.[11]

Many other pharmacologic agents have been used systemically to treat muscle hypertonia, but studies of most of them have shown little or no benefit versus placebo. Many reports are anecdotal, and none is widely used. They include alpha-adrenergic blockers (thymoxamine), beta-blockers (propranolol), carisoprodol, cyclobenzaprine, cyproheptadine, oral glycine (an inhibitory neurotransmitter), its precursor threonine, ivermectin, memantine, mexiletine, phenothiazines, phenytoin, piracetam, progabide (another GABA agonist), and tetrahydrocannabinol.[14–16] The FDA recently has approved a stronger warning about hepatotoxicity caused by chlorzoxazone, a centrally acting muscle relaxant. Hepatitis and extensive necrosis leading to death from hepatic failure have been reported and are unpredictable. Its antispastic actions are questionable, therefore its use for that indication is not recommended. Further studies and more useful drugs clearly are necessary.

Several pharmacologic agents have been injected locally with relief of excess muscle activity. Intramuscular and perineural injections, sometimes done using an open operative technique or ultrasound or CT for localization, of 50 percent ethanol or 2 to 10 percent phenol damage motor and sensory nerves, block conduction of all impulses for a few months and produce local fibrosis. This makes further injections more difficult, and sometimes produces painful dysesthesias. The "prolonged local anesthesia" permits more natural positioning of the arms or legs.

Botulinum toxin, serotype A (Btx), injected intramuscularly, diffuses to end plate zones where it is quickly and avidly bound presynaptically, preventing release of acetylcholine from motor axon terminals. This results in chemical denervation of that muscle that lasts several months. Because the toxin also can diffuse to neighboring muscles, they may be weakened as well. Btx does not affect sensory nerves and is not damaging to tissues. Injections of Btx are effective in weakening a few crucial muscles in any one spastic patient and have been proven safe, without serious or systemic side effects. This weakness may not improve function but can help with comfort by reduction in pain owing to muscle contraction or spasms and improve nursing care, hygiene, and positioning of limbs. It also can help prevent the foot from pistoning out of an ankle-foot orthosis so the brace can be more useful. In children with an equinus deformity caused by cerebral palsy, Btx injections into triceps surae permit the foot to be dorsiflexed at the ankle so the heel and plantar surface of the foot can be placed flat on the floor, improving balance and gait.[17] Repeated injections, every 6 months or less often, avoid the need for heel-cord lengthening operations until the child is fully grown. The formulation of Btx available in the United States (Botox, Allergan) is not identical in strength to that manufactured in Great Britain (Dysport, Porton). The maximum recommended dose of the former is 400 units or less *in toto* in a 70-kg adult, divided among several hypertonic muscles. Beneficial results in patients with spasticity and rigidity have been reported.[18]

SURGICAL THERAPIES

Since spastic dystonia and Parkinsonian rigidity are both clinical manifestations of tonic stretch reflexes, damage to the stretch reflex arc will eliminate the hypertonia. Such damage may involve afferent fibers in peripheral nerve or dorsal roots, efferent fibers in peripheral nerve or ventral roots, or the cord itself. Dorsal or ventral rhizotomies were employed in the first half of this century but produced complete anesthesia of large parts of the limb or complete flaccidity, neither of which is ideal.

Neurectomies produce similar permanent effects but, since they involve damage to muscle nerves, there is less superficial anesthesia and fewer muscles are involved. An interesting and useful accompaniment to such neurectomies (e.g., an obturator neurectomy) is reduction in spastic dystonia in other parts of the limb than those innervated by the nerve that has been damaged. This may imply that with upper motor neuron lesions, hyperactive lower motor neurons and their interneurons are activated in a generalized, mass-action fashion by peripheral inputs coming from regions of the limb other than that which they innervate.

Removal of the hyperactive distal spinal cord (cordectomy) will eliminate hypertonia in muscles innervated by that portion of the cord but, even when restricted to patients with a profound rostral cord lesion, produces a flaccid, anesthetic state and eliminates any useful reflex function of the bladder, bowels, and blood pressure. It is no longer done. Spinothalamic cordotomy will disconnect pain afferents from their intracranial targets but will not disconnect them from caudal spinal circuits and thus will not reduce the nociceptive enhancement of spastic hyperreflexia.

On the other hand, dorsal root entry zone lesions (DREZtomy), a particularly precise form of myelotomy, can do just that and have been employed successfully in the treatment of spastic hypertonia, usually in the lower limbs.[19] In addition, selective dorsal rhizotomies are undertaken in an attempt to transect just those nociceptive and muscle afferents responsible for the hypertonia, sparing cutaneous and other afferents.[20] They often are successful, even though techniques for identifying the offensive afferents are questionable. It seems that the number of afferent fibers cut may be the determining factor in success of the procedure rather than the type of afferents transected.[21]

Scattered reports describe success in alleviating spastic hypertonia by stereotactic lesions in ventrolateral thalamus, the anterior pulvinar, and dentate nucleus of the cerebellum, but others report no success with these procedures. Unfortunately the literature does not make clear exactly which sort of hypertonia was being treated and these procedures are no longer popular. On the other hand, ventrolateral or ventrointermediolateral thalamotomy or ventroposterolateral pallidotomy clearly reduce or eliminate the hypertonic rigidity seen with Parkinson's disease.[22,23]

As noted herein, baclofen is a very effective oral therapy for spasticity caused by spinal lesions. However, in some patients with particularly severe spinal spasticity, it is not possible, with oral therapy, to reach optimally effective concentrations of baclofen in the cord without producing systemic side effects. In such patients, single intrathecal test injections (using a lumbar puncture needle and, on successive days, increasing from 50 to 75 to 100 μg of commercially available racemic D-L-baclofen) will permit patient and physician to evaluate its efficacy as well as any adverse events, such as loss of extensor tone of the legs. Intrathecal baclofen is useful primarily to treat spasms as well as more tonic aspects of spastic hypertonia in the lower extremities. Significant concentrations around the rostral cord and medulla, as would be necessary to treat hypertonic arms, may compromise respiration. There are, however, suggestions that intrathecal baclofen used to treat spastic lower extremities can also reduce tone and increase function in the upper limbs and in muscles of speech in children with cerebral palsy. If test doses of intrathecal baclofen produce satisfactory relief of spasms and/or spastic hypertonia and so on, a subcutaneous pump can be implanted to effect chronic infusions of baclofen intrathecally.[24]

Although intrathecal baclofen is recommended for patients with disorders of the spinal cord (caused by trauma, multiple sclerosis, compression, or infarction) whose spastic dystonia and painful spasms cause significant disability and interfere with care, there also have been reports of success with patients with spastic cerebral palsy, head injury, and stiff-man syndrome. One report of a single patient with spastic diplegic cerebral palsy treated with intrathecal L-baclofen is promising.[25] Intrathecal morphine, useful for chronic pain, also temporarily alleviates symptoms and signs of spasticity.

Barolat, Myklebust, and Wenninger described beneficial effects of electrical stimulation of the spinal cord (known, perhaps inaccurately, as dorsal column stimulation) for the relief of pain in patients with spasms and spastic dystonia owing to spinal lesions.[26] This technique is used to treat intractable pain but, since pain afferents also produce or enhance spasms and spastic dystonia, especially in patients with spinal lesions, it also may relieve symptoms of spasticity in carefully selected patients.

SUMMARY

Each individual patient with muscle hypertonia must be carefully evaluated clinically to answer such questions as: What type of hypertonia is this and is it amenable to therapy? Does it seriously affect the patient's quality of life or performance? Should it be treated, and if so, how? Which, among the least invasive therapies, should be used initially? How will the treatment be monitored? Under what circumstances will the therapy be deemed satisfactory; that is, what goals are appropriate? What outcomes will be unsatisfactory and will require institution of other therapies?

As a general rule, reasonable therapeutic goals include relief of pain owing to tonic contraction of muscle or muscle spasms (which also cause frequent awakenings at night) and restoration of more normal limb position (which aids hygiene, simplifies dressing, improves transfers and sitting, and permits the use of braces). Restoration of function requires regeneration of damaged CNS tissue and reestablishment of appropriate connections, neither of which is a therapeutic possibility at this time. Improvement in function, such as in activities of daily living, may follow treatment for muscle hypertonia, but more often does not. However, it must be emphasized that the various therapies outlined herein, even if they do not restore the ability to walk or use the hand, are valuable. Spasticity, rigidity, and dystonia can be painful, unpleasant, and handicapping; when they are, they should be treated.

REFERENCES

1. Lance JW: Symposium synopsis, in Feldman RG, Young RR, Koella WP (eds): *Spasticity: Disordered Motor Control.* Chicago: Yearbook Medical, 1980, pp. 485–494.
2. Young RR: Spastic paresis, in Young RR, Woolsey RM (eds): *Diagnosis and Management of Disorders of the Spinal Cord.* Philadelphia: W.B. Saunders, 1955, pp. 363–376.
3. Young RR: Treatment of spastic paresis. *New Engl J Med* 1989; 320:1553–1555.
4. Young RR: Spasticity: a review. *Neurology* 1994; 44(suppl 9):S12–S20.

5. Marsden CD: Motor dysfunction and movement disorders, in Asbury AK, McKhann GM, McDonald WI (eds): *Diseases of the Nervous System*. Philadelphia: W.B. Saunders, 1992, pp. 311–312.

6. Koman LA, Mooney III JF, Smith B, et al: Management of cerebral palsy with botulinum-A toxin: preliminary investigation. *J Pediatr Orthop* 1993; 13:489–495.

7. Young RR: Special correspondence reply. *Neurology* 1995; 45:2296.

8. Potisk KP, Gregoric M, Vodovnik L: Effects of transcutaneous electrical nerve stimulation (TENS) on spasticity in patients with hemiplegia. *Scand J Rehab Med* 1995; 27:169–174.

9. Scott TRD, Peckham PH: Functional electrical stimulation and its application in the management of spinal cord injury, in Young RR, Woolsey RM (eds): *Diagnosis and Management of Disorders of the Spinal Cord*. Philadelphia: W.B. Saunders, 1995, pp. 377–396.

10. Fromm GH, Shibuya T, Nakata M, et al: Effects of D-baclofen and L-baclofen on the trigeminal nucleus. *Neuropharmacology* 1990; 29:249–254.

11. Young RR, Delwaide PJ: Spasticity. *New Engl J Med* 1981; 304:28–33, 96–99.

12. Young RR (ed): Role of tizanidine in the treatment of spasticity. *Neurology* 1994; 44(suppl 9):S1–S80.

13. Donovan W, Carter R, Rossi C, et al: Clonidine effect on spasticity: a clinical trial. *Arch Phys Med Rehabil* 1988; 69:193–194.

14. Costa JL, Diazgranados JA: Ivermectin for spasticity in spinal-cord injury. *Lancet* 1994; 343:739.

15. Bauer HJ, Hanefeld FA: *Multiple Sclerosis*. Philadelphia: W.B. Saunders, 1993.

16. Jimi T, Wakayama Y: Mexiletine for treatment of spasticity due to neurological disorders. *Muscle & Nerve* 1993; 16:885.

17. Cosgrove AP, Corry IS, Graham HK: Botulinum toxin in the management of the lower limb in cerebral palsy. *Dev Med Child Neurol* 1994; 36:3886–3896.

18. Grazko MA, Polo KB, Jabbari B: Botulinum toxin A for spasticity, muscle spasms, and rigidity. *Neurology* 1995; 45:712–717.

19. Sindou M: Microsurgical DREZ-tomy for the treatment of pain and spasticity, in Young RR, Delwaide PJ (eds): *Principles and Practice of Restorative Neurology*. Oxford: Butterworth/Heinemann, 1992, pp. 144–151.

20. Kasdon DL, Lathi ES: A prospective study of radiofrequency rhizotomy in the treatment of post-traumatic spasticity. *Neurosurgery* 1984; 15:526–529.

21. Logigian EL, Wolinsky JS, Soriano SG, Madsen JR, Scott RM: H reflex studies in cerebral palsy patients undergoing partial dorsal rhizotomy. *Muscle & Nerve* 1994; 17:539–549.

22. Struppler A: Stereoencephalotomy and control of skeletal muscle tone. *Stereotact Func Neurosurg* 1989; 52:205.

23. Laitinen LV, Hariz MI: Movement disorders, in Youmans JR (ed): *Neurological Surgery*. Philadelphia: W.B. Saunders, 1996, pp. 3575–3609.

24. Coffey RJ, Cahill D, Steers W, et al: Intrathecal baclofen for intractable spasticity of spinal origin: results of a long-term multicenter study. *J Neurosurg* 1993; 78:226–232.

25. Albright AL, Barry MJ, Hoffmann P: Intrathecal L-baclofen for cerebral spasticity: case report. *Neurology* 1995; 45:2110–2111.

26. Barolat G, Myklebust JB, Wenninger W: Effects of spinal cord stimulation on spasticity and spasms secondary to myelopathy. *Appl Neurophys* 1988; 51:29–44.

Chapter 21

PRESSURE ULCERS

Gary M. Yarkony
Mark J. Goddard

Pressure ulcers are a common consequence of immobility for neurologically compromised patients. Skin ulcerations caused by pressure and shear are frequently referred to as decubitus ulcers, bed sores, ischemic ulcers, and pressure sores. Pressure ulcer is the most appropriate term to denote the principal etiologic factor that results in the sloughing of necrotic tissue, causing an ulceration. A pressure ulcer is defined as any lesion caused by unrelieved pressure resulting in damage of underlying tissue.[1] Although prolonged pressure is certainly the essential pathophysiologic event predisposing tissues to breakdown, a complex array of factors contributes to their development. These include biomechanical, biochemical, neurophysiologic, and nutritional forces that impact the tissue environment.

Reports of the incidence and prevalence of pressure ulcers vary and are related to the facility and underlying medical condition and age of the persons involved. A recent survey of persons in acute care hospitals revealed a prevalence of 9.2 percent, with the sacrum, heel, and ischium being the most common sites.[2] A survey of a single acute care hospital showed a prevalence of 4.7 percent.[3] Nursing homes in one study had a prevalence at the time of admission of 17.4 percent.[4] Incidence during a 1-year period of pressure ulcer development in the nursing home study ranged from 9.5 percent at year one to 21.6 percent by year two. Previous estimates of pressure ulcer prevalence in acute care hospitals ranged from 3 to 14 percent among hospitalized patients between 15 and 25 percent on admission to skilled nursing facilities.[1] The most common sites of development are the sacrum, ischium, trochanter, and about the ankles and heels.[5] Tremendous efforts to curtail expanding health care costs should bring prevention and early detection of pressure ulcers to the forefront of diligent rehabilitation care. Pressure ulcer prevalence in acute care hospitals is noted to range from 3 to 14 percent, and they are more common in extended care facilities, occurring in from 15 to 25 percent of nursing home residents.

Several populations have been identified that are particularly at risk: spinal cord injured patients, elderly with femoral fractures, and those in a critical care setting. The treatment of pressure ulcers in the United States has a signficiant economic impact.[3] The total national cost of presure ulcer treatment exceeds $1.33 billion.[1] Recent research into growth and metabolic factors and new technologies for pressure relief offer new hope for pressure sore prevention and treatment in the population at risk.

RECOGNITION

The most important first step in managing pressure ulcers is recognizing those individuals at risk and providing preventive measures. Several scales have been developed to categorize risk assessment. The Norton and Braden scales have been the most extensively studied.[6] The Norton scale has been used mainly for elderly patients in hospital settings, whereas the Braden scale has been used mainly in medical-surgical units, intensive care units, and extended care facilities. Examples of those two scales are provided (Tables 21-1 and 21-2). Incorporation of these assessment scales enables the health care team to recognize the high-risk patient. Individuals with prolonged immobility, incontinence, impaired nutritional status, and altered level of consciousness are at increased risk for pressure ulcer formation.

PERSONS AT RISK

Any person who is immobilized or has an immobilized body part in a cast is at risk for pressure ulcer development.[7] Hospitalized patients who are bedridden or chair-bound are at increased risk of developing pressure ulcers if they have hypoalbuminemia, fecal incontinence, and fractures.[3] Malnourished or vitamin-deficient patients are at increased risk of pressure develop-

Table 21-1
Norton Scale

Physical condition		*Mental condition*		*Activity*		*Mobility*		*Incontinent*	
Good	4	Alert	4	Ambulant	4	Full	4	Not	4
Fair	3	Apathetic	3	Walk/help	3	Slightly limited	3	Occasional	3
Poor	2	Confused	2	Chairbound	2	Very limited	2	Usually/urine	2
Very bad	1	Stupor	1	Bed	1	Immobile	1	Doubly	1

Name   Date

ment.[4,5] Elderly persons, particularly those in hospitals or nursing homes, are at risk. Norton and Braden[6] have developed scales that assess physical and mental activity, continence, sensation, and other factors to identify persons at risk.[6] The elderly may be at particular risk of pressure ulcer development for several reasons. Ischemia may be induced more easily in elderly persons than younger persons and they may develop more shear while sitting.[10,29] Mean pressure and the calculated total pressure per bed occupation hour (referred to as impulse pressure in the study) on the sacrums of elderly persons are increased in elderly as compared to younger subjects who are in bed.[11] Aging skin, with its associated physical, structural, physiological, and immunological changes, may have a major impact on pressure ulcer development.[12,13] Aged skin has a diminished barrier function, increased susceptibility to shearing forces, and a decreased vascularity and barrier function. Body build may impact on an individual's susceptibility to pressure ulcer development. Thinner persons may develop higher pressures over bony prominence than average weight or obese patients.[14,15]

Psychosocial adjustment affects a person's ability to follow through on prescribed skin care regimens. Depressed persons and those prone to self-neglect may develop pressure ulcers owing to lack of follow-through on self-care needs.[16,17] Poor home care, poor advice from caregivers, and inadequate care in general by persons not familiar with skin care principles in paralyzed persons may contribute to pressure ulcer development.[18] Persons with spinal cord injury are a group well known to be at high risk for pressure ulcer development.[19] A spinal cord injured person's risk may be enhanced immediately after injury by prolonged immobilization on spine boards, and the risk is inversely related to systolic blood pressure.[20]

PRESSURE ULCER DESCRIPTION

Adequate description of a pressure ulcer is essential to allow communication between staff and to assess wounds for research purposes. Generally an ulcer is given a grade or stage based on erythema of the skin or depth of the ulcer (Table 21-1).[21–23] The most commonly used system is that developed by Shea, which includes four grades. In addition, the Shea classification uses the description "closed pressure sore" to record the presence of large cavities accessible through a small sinus of the skin surface. A scale developed by Yarkony and Kirk has been compared to the Shea classification in a study that indicated a higher interrater reliability for the Yarkony-Kirk scale.[21] This scale includes a distinct classification of a red area and a healed area to allow for recognition of sites of future breakdown (Table 21-3). It also describes the depth of a wound by the tissue observed at the base of the wound. This scale also had improved utility in spite of having more grades. The National Pressure Ulcer Advisory Panel has developed a scale that they described as combining several of the most commonly used staging systems. It was developed as a step toward developing a universally accepted classification but has not been verified and accepted as a standard.[23] A classification has also been developed by the International Association for Enterostomal Therapy.[24] No study exists comparing the use of

Table 21-2
The Braden Scale

Patient's Name: _____   Evaluator's Name: _____   Date of Assessment _____

	1	2	3	4	
Sensory Perception Ability to respond meaningfully to pressure related discomfort	1. Completely limited: Unresponsive (does not moan, flinch, or graph) to painful stimuli, owing to diminished level of consciousness or education, or limited ability to feel pain over most of body surface.	2. Very limited: Responds only to painful stimuli. Cannot communicate discomfort except by moaning or restlessness, has a sensory impairment that limits the ability to feel pain or discomfort over ½ of body.	3. Slightly limited: Responds to verbal commands but cannot always communicate discomfort or need to be turned, has some sensory impairment that limits ability to feel pain or discomfort in one or two extremities.	4. No impairment: Responds to verbal commands. Has no sensory deficits that would limit ability to feel or voice pain or discomfort.	
Moisture Degree to which skin is exposed to moisture	1. Constantly moist: Skin is moist almost constantly by perspiration, urine, etc. Dampness is detected every time patient is moved or turned.	2. Model: Skin is often but not always moist. Linen must be changed at least once a shift.	3. Occasionally moist: Skin is occasionally moist, requiring an extra linen change approximately once a day.	4. Rarely moist: Skin is usually dry; linen requires changing only at routine intervals.	
Activity Degree of physical activity	1. Bedfast	2. Chairfast: Ability to walk severely limited or nonexistent. Cannot bear own weight and/or must be assisted into chair or wheelchair.	3. Walks occasionally: Walks occasionally during day but for very short distances, with or without assistance. Spends majority of each shift in bed or chair.	4. Walks frequently: Walks outside the room at least twice a day and inside room at least once every 2 hours during waking hours.	
Mobility Ability to change and control body position	1. Completely immobile: Does not make even slight changes in body or extremity position without assistance.	2. Very limited: Makes occasional slight changes in body or extremity position, but is unable to make frequent or significant changes independently.	3. Slightly limited: Makes frequent but slight changes in body or extremity position independently.	4. No limitations: Makes major and frequent changes in position without assistance.	
Nutrition Usual food intake pattern	1. Very poor: Never eats a complete meal. Rarely eats more than 1/3 of any food offered. Eats two servings or less of protein (meat or daily products) per day. Takes fluids poorly. Does not take a liquid diet supplement, or is NPO[a] and/or maintained on clear liquids of IV[b] for more than 5 days.	2. Probably inadequate: Rarely eats a complete meal and generally eats only about ½ of any food offered. Protein intakes includes only three servings of meat or daily products per day. Occasionally will take a dietary supplement or receives less than optimum amount of liquid diet or tube feeding.	3. Adequate: Eats over half of most meals. Eats a total of four servings of protein (meat, dairy products) each day. Occasionally will refuse a meal, but will usually take a supplement if offered, or is on a tube feeding or TPN[c] regimment, which probably meets most nutritional needs.	4. Excellent: Eats most of every meal. Never refuses a meal. Usually eats a total of four or more servings of meat and dairy products. Occasionally eats between meals. Does not require supplementation.	
Friction and shear	1. Problem: Requires moderate or maximum assistance in moving. Complete lifting without sliding against sheets is impossible. Frequently slides down in bed or chair, requiring frequent repositioning with maximum assistance. Spasticity, contractures, or agitation leads to almost constant friction.	2. Potential problem: Moves feebly or requires minimum assistance. During a move skin probably slides to some extent against sheets, chair restraints, or other devices. Maintains relatively good position in chair or bed most of the time, but occasionally slides down.	3. No apparent problem: Moves in bed and chair independently and has sufficient muscle strength to lift up completely during move. Maintains good position in bed or chair at all times.		

Total Score: _____

---

[a] NPO: Nothing by mouth.
[b] IV: Intravenously.
[c] TPN: Total parenteral nutrition.

339

Table 21-3
Clinical practice guidelines

Stage I
Nonblanchable edema of intact skin; the heralding lesion of skin ulceration. Note: Reactive hyperemia normally can be expected to be present for one-half to three-fourths as long as the pressure occluded blood flow to the area (Lewis and Grant, 1925). This should not be confused with a Stage I pressure ulcer.

Stage II
Partial thickness skin loss involving epidermis and/or dermis. The ulcer is superficial and presents clinically as an abrasion, blister, or shallow crater.

Stage III
Full thickness skin loss involving damage or necrosis of subcutaneous tissue that may extend down to, but not through, underlying fascia. The ulcer presents clinically as a deep crater with or without undermining of adjacent tissue.

Stage IV
Full thickness skin loss with extensive destruction, tissue necrosis, or damage to muscle, bone, or supporting structures (for example, tendon or joint capsule). Note: Undermining and sinus tracts may also be associated with Stage IV pressure ulcers.

these numerous systems to each other and their utility in the evaluation and treatment of pressure ulcers. This is an area in which future research is needed. Wounds covered with necrotic tissue or eschar should be debrided to determine the grade of the wound.

Other systems include the use of color to describe wounds.[25,26] This is not specific to any type of wound. Yellow wounds indicate soft necrotic tissue, black indicates adherent necrotic tissue, and red indicates a wound ready to heal with granulation tissue. Assessment of pressure ulcers requires a description of the wound and surrounding tissue, assignment of a grade, and measurement of its size.

Numerous techniques have been described to measure the size and depth of a pressure ulcer. Generally the ulcer is measured and its maximum dimensions and depth are indicated. It is then diagrammed, traced, or photographed.[27] Acetate tracing, the Kundin device, (a six-pronged measuring device), and photography with digital analysis were recently compared. Acetate tracings can provide the most accurate description of wound area, but require manual or computer planimetry once the tracings are completed.[28] The photographic method required special equipment and an image analysis sys-

tem. The Kundin measuring device underestimated areas consistently.[29] Other more complex techniques not generally applicable in the clinical setting included dental impression materials, and analyzing photographs with a computer taken over a polyester grid.[30-32] Sinography may be used with clinical assessment of a tunneling ulcer is not adequate. A radiopaque dye is instilled into the wound and plain x-ray allows a determination of the depth and extent of the lesion. These are the wounds that Shea describes as closed.[33-35]

Bates-Jensen et al. have developed a Pressure Sore Status Tool as a means of clinically describing a pressure ulcer.[36] It described the location, shape, and 13 items, including size, depth, edges, undermining necrotic tissue, exudate, surrounding skin, and evidence of healing. They proposed future research areas to study use of this tool. This tool's complexity and associated need for training make the use of this technique in all care settings questionable.

ETIOLOGY

Although numerous factors are involved in formation of a pressure ulcer it is clear that pressure over bony prominences is the key etiologic factory. Trumble described the relationship between pressure intensity and duration in 1930.[37] Kosiak's classic studies were the first to define the relationship between pressure and time.[38-40] He described a parabolic relationship between pressure and time, indicating that higher pressures require a shorter time period to cause ulceration than lower pressures. This relationship was determined using dogs, which is not as relevant an animal model to humans as pigs, whose skin more closely resembles human skin.

Daniel's studies in pigs showed a curve similar to the one described by Kosiak.[41] The curve for paraplegic animals was similar in shape but the orders for time and magnitude were reduced. This was attributed to impaired mobility and sensation, incontinence leading to skin maceration, and atrophy of soft tissues leading to increased interface pressure at bony prominences. Pressure that exceeds the mean blood pressure on the back can lead to cessation of skin blood flow.[42] Pressure is more concentrated in the area of the muscle and fat adjacent to the bone.[43] In contrast to Kosiak, Daniel determined that these tissues are more susceptible to pressure and may show signs of damage prior to evidence of damage to the skin.[44,45] Tissue that is atrophied, scarred, or secondarily infected has an increased susceptibility to pressure.[41,46] Skin can be damaged by intermittent pressures in excess of mean capillary pressures that results in endothelial damage and platelet thrombosis.[47] Moderate stresses, although within physiological limits, can result in damage to the skin if repeated frequently.[48]

Shearing force is the second key factor in the development of "presshear ulcers." The word *presshear* indicates the two major factors in the development of skin ulceration owing to pressure and shear. This is proposed as a more accurate term than pressure ulcers to describe these lesions.[49] Shear is an applied force that causes an opposite parallel sliding motion in the planes of an object.[50] It has been described as "more disastrous than the more vertical pressure" as it cuts off large areas of vascular supply. An example of a situation in which shearing forces occur is on the sacrum when the head of the bed is elevated for an immobilized person who is supine.[51] Shear can significantly decrease the amount of pressure needed to occlude blood flow.[52,53] Elderly persons tend to develop higher shearing forces while sitting, further predisposing them to pressure ulcers. Friction applies mechanical forces to the epidermis resulting in increased susceptibility to ulceration.[54]

Moisture secondary to incontinence or perspiration can result in skin maceration and predispose patients to pressure ulceration.[43] Anaerobic waste products that accumulate owing to occlusion of lymphatic vessels have been hypothesized to contribute to tissue necrosis and can theoretically be mediated by emotional stress.[55,56] It has been suggested in small, poorly controlled study groups that smoking cigarettes, which contain nicotine, a peripheral vasoconstrictive agent, increases the risk of pressure ulceration.[57]

Although pressure and shear are still considered the major causes of pressure ulcers, the summary above indicates a multifactorial problem. These many aspects must be considered in the treatment plan for those persons considered to be at risk.

PATHOPHYSIOLOGY

The skin is the body's largest organ and contains the most extensive vascular supply. Its functions include regulation of body temperature, protecting against environmental factors such as infection and ultraviolet radiation, and mediation of sensory modalities (pain, pressure, temperature).[58] Understanding the anatomic and physiologic properties of skin leads to a clear sense of how pressure ulcers develop.

The epidermis consists of three layers of keratinocytes that differentiate through their life cycle.[59] The basal layer of germinative (mitotically active) cells in the stratum germinativum give rise to differentiating (metabolically active) cells in the stratum spinosum that finally differentiate into cornified (nonviable) cells in the stratum corneum. Transit time from the basal layer to the stratum corneum is approximately 14 days, whereas the final shedding phase in the corneum is 14 days. Injury to the skin, therefore, may take at least 28 days for recovery.

Two other epidermal cells, the melanocytes and the Langerhans cell, also play important roles.[60] Melanocytes protect the skin against solar radiation. Langerhans cells are intimately involved with the skin's immune response.

Other epidermal structures contribute to skin function. Sebaceous glands aid in maintaining skin surface lipid sufficient to protect against water loss. Apocrine glands are vestigial nonsecretory glands in humans until after puberty, and account for body odor. Eccrine glands are responsible for thermal regulation. In the febrile debilitated patient, however, this process may lead to maceration and eventually fungal supra-infection, especially in the infra-mammary and perineal areas. Hair functions include heat conservation, tactile probing, and physical protection of the skin.

The dermal layer anatomically consists of a rich supply of vasculature, connective tissue, and nerve receptors. Blood flow is constricted following adrenergic stimulation, as well as the vasopressor action of angiotensin. Vasodilatation occurs through effects from histamine, alcohol, prostaglandins, and heat.

Collagen accounts for 70 to 80 percent of the dry weight of human skin and structurally limits deformation. Collagen is formed by crosslinking of molecules and is remodeled depending on pressure forces. Elastic tissues provide skin turgor or tone.

Finally, afferent transmission of sensory input occurs at the dermal level. Thick myelinated $A\beta$ fibers conduct touch and vibration quickly, whereas the $A\delta$ fibers conduct pain, temperature, and itching at slower rates. Intermediate myelinated $A\mu$ fibers transmit light touch and pressure.

As the name implies, pressure is certainly one of the most significant biomechanical factors leading to pressure ulceration. None of the biomechanical factors described in this section work in isolation in the clinical setting. Nevertheless, there has been increasing evidence demonstrating the role of these variables for development of pressure ulcers in high-risk patients.

Kosiak was one of the first to demonstrate the relationship between pressure and time in a classic article in 1961 using dog models. Even at very high pressures of 400 to 500 mm Hg, skin ulceration did not occur if relieved before 2 hours.[44] Dinsdale reinforced this concept, demonstrating that when applied pressure exceeds capillary closing pressure (i.e., 35 mm Hg) for at least 2 hours ischemia occurs.[45] During activity, high pressures can be generated at focal tissue points. The flexible walls of blood and lymph vessels collapse when these pressures exceed the capillary closing pressure, resulting in ischemic deprivation of oxygen and nutrients, tissue acidosis, increased capillary permeability, and even vascular thrombosis.[46] Through the work of Rogers and others, the threshold for pressure in humans has been established to be 60 mm Hg for 1 hour before tissue ischemia occurs.

Daniel et al. evaluated pressure effects in paraplegic animal models noting that less time and pressure were needed to develop skin ulceration.[41] Impaired mobility and sensation, incontinence, and soft tissue atrophy all contributed to heightened tissue pressure adjacent to bony prominences. In fact, Daniel established that the tissues closer to the bone were more susceptible to pressure effects than the skin.[47]

Early in the investigation of pressure ulcers, Reichel noted the importance of shearing as a contributing factor. He found that shear can decrease by 50 percent the amount of pressure needed to cause a pressure ulcer.[51] The significance of shear as a contributing factor is emphasized by Yarkony, who coined the term "presshear ulcers" as a better description of these lesions.[52] The most common scenario for this occurs in the bed-bound patient. If the hip line is not at the middle crease of the bed, the sacrum can shear downward when the head of the bed is elevated.

Brand has demonstrated the significance of repetitive application of even low pressure to the development of soft tissue breakdown.[48] Necrosis could be induced when repetitive critical loads were applied to the foot pads of rats over a 3-week period. However, he also found that the soft tissue could hypertrophy and withstand greater loads than expected if rest intervals followed by restressing was implemented.[53]

Another significant biomechanical factor predisposing to tissue breakdown is moisture. Even as early as 1852, Brown-Sequard recognized that soiling and moisture increased the effects of pressure sores.[54] The incidence of pressure ulcers increases in nursing home populations with urinary and fecal incontinence.[61] Allman investigated variables affecting pressure ulcer development in bedridden hospitalized patients and found fecal incontinence was one the most significant factors

($p < 001$).[3,55] The impact of incontinence is multifactorial. Moist skin can be macerated and exposed to chemical irritation (with urinary incontinence) and even bacterial contamination (with fecal incontinence).[61,62] Finally, adherence of linens and clothing to moist skin increases the likelihood of further shearing. Rises in temperature can produce marked effects on tissues by increasing the metabolic demands of the cells.

Multiple medical factors have been associated with higher risk for pressure ulcer development. Immobility, with all its accompanying sequelae, is one of the most important risk factors. Nutrition is a crucial consideration particularly after multiple trauma.[63] Because of a negative nitrogen balance, patients may require 3500 to 4000 calories per day with protein content to effect tissue healing and prevent breakdown. Poor nutrition will result in weight loss and depletion of tissue padding, predisposing to breakdown at bony prominences. Low protein states can lead to edema and even anasarca. The skin will become less elastic with compromised vascular transfer. Allman found hypoalbuminemia as the most significant laboratory value in 634 patients who developed pressure ulcers.[3]

Anemia likewise ranks as a major medical risk factor for tissue breakdown.[63] Hemoglobin below 8 to 10 g/dL results in decreased blood oxygen carrying capacity compromising tissue capacity for maintenance and healing. Macrocytic anemia may be secondary to low folate or B$_{12}$ levels. Microcytic indices may be related to iron deficiency anemia. In both cases, supplement is required to correct the anemia.

Although pressure ulcers do not typically require antibiotic therapy, infection can be responsible for nonhealing sores.[64,65] In one study, pressure ulcers have been established as the probable source of bacteremia in approximately 1.7 cases per 10,000 hospital discharges. Yet the mortality in hospitalized persons was greater than 50 percent among patients over the age of 60 with evidence of bacteremia. Organisms most frequently identified include Proteus mirabilia, E. coli, Klebsiella, Pseudomonas (23–45 percent), Staph aureus, Group A Strep, enterococci (19–39 percent), and anaerobics (Bacteroides fragilis, 16–50 percent). Infections should be suspected if there is surrounding erythema, purulent drainage, and a foul odor. All open wounds may be contaminated. Therefore, culture and treatment should be reserved for ulcers with the aforementioned signs of infectious complication. Underlying osteomyelitis should be suspected in any patient with a nonhealing ulcer. A combination of positive plain x-ray, erythrocyte sedimentation rate of 120 mm/hr, or white blood cell count of 15,000 mm, or greater, may be an indication of underlying osteomyelitis. The combination of all three has a positive predictive value of 69 percent.[66] Technetium bone scans often are positive. However, bone biopsy is the most definitive diagnostic procedure as Sugarman demonstrated in 26 percent of his study patients.[71]

Edema, as mentioned previously, is a risk factor associated with low protein states.[9] However, as dependent edema is a common phenomenon in the neurologically compromised patient, it must be considered a separate factor. Edema may decrease cellular transport of oxygen and nutrients placing tissues at risk for injury. The skin at the feet and sacrum, in particular, must be monitored. Appropriate compression garments, leg elevation when seated, and even mild diuretics may be warranted.

Diabetes, in conjunction with fecal incontinence, is a major independent risk factor in nursing homes with higher incidence of pressure ulcers.[68] Tissue integrity in diabetics may be compromised by a multiplicity of etiologies. Tissue ischemia can be secondary to large- and small-vessel disease. Anesthetic areas can be produced by peripheral neuropathy leading to pressure susceptibility. Local blood flow control in the dermal layer via adrenergic modulation may be compromised in the diabetic with autonomic neuropathy. Close blood glucose monitoring and management with appropriate diet, exercise, traditional hypoglycemics, insulin, as well as newer hypoglycemic agents, such as glucophage, may be indicated.

Spasticity is another common medical problem in neurorehabilitation.[57] Increased shearing is a significant factor and, because of predominant synergy patterns, prone lying can be difficult to achieve. The skin overlying the sacrum, trochanters, lateral malleoli, and epicondyle are especially at risk. Pressure ulcers, once developed, can exacerbate spasticity in a vicious cycle. With the exception of spinal cord injury, effectiveness of oral anti-spasticity medications for central nervous system processes can be limited. Other options may include neurolytic blocks (botulinum toxin or phenol), intrathecal baclofen, and surgical options (posterior rhizotomy).

Prolonged spasticity and immobility may eventually lead to contractures. The skin over a contracted joint eventually becomes less plastic. Contractures are classified as arthrogenic, soft tissue, or myogenic.[69] If the periarticular tissues become warm and swollen, heterotopic ossification must be considered in the differential diagnosis. Heterotopic ossification is noted predominantly in traumatic brain injury and spinal cord injury

with "new bone" formation in connective tissue planes.[70] Disodium etidronate may limit the extent of ossification if therapy is started early. Contracture management includes therapeutic stretching, positioning, and possible surgical release or transfer if severe.

Medications such as analgesics, sedatives, and hypnotics may alter sensorium, especially in the elderly who are already very susceptible to the effect of polypharmacy. Medications should be monitored on a weekly basis to determine effective length of treatment. Even "benign" medications such as antiepileptics and H_2 receptor antagonists may interfere with cognitive processing.

Patients with varying degrees of dementia (Alzheimer's and multiinfarct) are very much at risk for pressure ulcer development.[68] Minimental status exams can identify high-risk patients. Endogenous depression should be treated appropriately with antidepressant medications. Seratonin reuptake inhibitors, such as sertraline and paroxetine are less sedating. Functional capacities markers, such as difficulty ambulating, transferring, and feeding have been identified by Brandeis as risk factors for pressure ulcer development in the nursing home setting.[68]

PATHOLOGY

Kosiak, based on a study of dogs, proposed that pressure degeneration occurs equally in tissue at all levels, as opposed to only from bone outward.[39] He later described edema, loss of cross striations and myofibrils, hyalinization, phagocytosis by neutrophils, and macrophages in normal and paraplegic rats. There were no differences in paraplegic and normal rats, but these studies were done less than 24 hours after section of the spinal cord.[40]

Dinsdale described changes in swine due to friction.[71] Friction initially removes the stratum corneum. The superficial cells at the epidermis separate from the basal cells because their bridges are brittle. With pressure and friction, superficial dermis become hyperemic, then eosinophilic, and with increasing pressure hemorrhage and leukocyte infiltration occur in the capillaries of the dermis. The superficial dermis then became necrotic.[71] Friction can be affected by the amount of moisture on the skin.[72] With low rates of sweating, friction increases, but with maximal sweating there is a decrease, compared to dry skin. Daniel's studies in swine showed that initial damage occurs in deep muscle with progression towards the skin.[41] The animal model in swine is more appropriate than Kosiak's dog model. At high pressures of short duration (500 mm Hg 9 hours) or low pressures of long duration (100 mm Hg 10 hours) skin remains intact but deep muscle damage occurs. At high pressures of long duration (800 mm Hg 10 hours) or low pressures of prolonged duration (200 mm Hg 15 hours) damage from muscle to the subcutaneous tissue and lower dermis is seen, but superficial skin and hair growth were intact. With long duration pressure (600 mm Hg 11 hours, 200 mm Hg 16 hours) a visible skin lesion can be found after 1 week and full thickness destruction occurs.[14] With septicemia, bacteria can localize at the sites of pressure application and encourage breakdown at lower pressure.[41] These studies of early muscle damage serve as a basis for turning patients at least every 2 hours to prevent pressure ulcerations.[7,39,40]

Witkowski and Parish have described changes in human skin.[73] A sequence of capillary and venule dilation, followed by edema of the papillary dermis and a perivascular infiltrate has been observed. Platelet aggregation, red blood cell engorgement, and perivascular hemorrhage follows. As vascular changes occur, sweat glands and subcutaneous fat show signs of cell death, with eventual epidermal necrosis. Although biopsies were taken from various sites, there was no correlation with pressure amount and duration, and no indication of shearing. Deep tissues were not studied.[73]

MANAGEMENT

Any management regimens must first begin with close and regular inspection of the skin. Measurement of the dimensions and exact locations of pressure ulcers is crucial. Ulcer staging is always appropriate, as recommended by a consensus panel for the Clinical Practice Guideline outlines (Table 21-3).[23]

PREVENTION

The methods and technologies used to prevent pressure ulcers depend on the setting. In a hospital setting, the basis for prevention is vigilant nursing care.[74] Most persons can be treated with proper bed positioning and turns every 2 hours. Bony prominences should be checked every 2 hours and hyperemia of the skin should resolve in 30 minutes. Turning techniques should avoid shearing the soft tissues. Patients should be alternated between positioning on their backs and sides, and placed prone if medically indicated. Care should be taken to avoid pressure over bony prominences. The prone position has larger low-pressure areas and smaller high-pressure areas.[75] Difficulties develop in the acute care setting when turning is limited or not possible owing to the medical condition, or when a person has pressure ulcers that prohibit various positions. As a result, the development of numerous beds and bed overlays to prevent pressure ulcers has burgeoned over the past decade. A large number of products are now commercially available. There is insufficient literature to make recommendations as to cost effectiveness and appropriate patient characteristics for a specific mattress, and further study is needed in this area. The majority of investigative efforts to date are case reports or uncontrolled studies.

Mattress overlays are designed to reduce pressure during recumbency.[76] They can be static pads or alternating pressure mattresses. The alternating pressure pads will have periods of high and low pressure, and there appears to be a great variability in their effectiveness. Two inch convoluted foam provides no protection for the trochanter. At least 4 inches of foam is needed.[76] Although these pads may reduce pressures below a standard bed, pressure can be raised by spasm, posture (changes), and muscle contractions. Alternating-pressure air mattresses require a constant supply of electricity, are noisy, and are subject to puncture and breakdown.[77] Waterbeds are bulky, make turns and lifting difficult, and make it difficult for the patient to sit up.[77] Skin pressure is high over the shoulder on water beds.[78]

Low air-loss beds (air flotation) support the patient on an air permeable fabric through which air is continuously pumped. They produce consistently less pressures than standard beds or water beds.[79] Pressure in the areas of bony prominences is consistently less than capillary pressures.[79] Pressure on low air loss beds is equivalent to air fluidized beds, when adjusted properly. If not, they can be less effective than static beds.[80]

Air fluidized beds use a process that makes a granule behave like a liquid by forcing warm air through beads covered by a woven polyester sheet.[81,82] Adverse effects include fluid loss, dehydration, dry skin, scaly skin, and epistaxis from the flow of dry air. Confusion and disorientation can occur owing to the sensation of floating. The development of thick pulmonary secretions can occur. Turning and repositioning may be difficult and pressure ulcers can develop. The size and weight of the bed can be problematic, and microspheres can leak. The therapy is expensive and can have a bactericidal effect owing to the sequestration and desiccation of microorganisms by the ceramic beads.[83–85]

One large controlled study done over a 10-day period in an acute care hospital comparing alternating air mattress overlays and water beds with standard mattresses demonstrated a decrease in pressure ulcer development with air or water mattresses. The study was done over a 10-day period in an acute care hospital.[77] Low air loss beds, compared to foam mattresses, led to improvement in the healing of pressure ulcers in a nursing home study.[86] A recent study in an intensive care unit setting demonstrated the clinical utility and cost-effectiveness of low air loss beds in preventing the development of pressure ulcers.[87]

The majority of studies testing the effectiveness of air fluidized beds have been uncontrolled. Allman et al. compared air fluidized beds to standard therapy in a large general hospital population.[81] Pressure ulcer healing improved, although the development of new ulcers was not eliminated. Further study is needed to determine the cost effectiveness of these beds and optimal treatment periods. These beds may be particularly useful in the intensive care unit or for postoperative pressure ulcer patients, although controlled studies in these areas are needed.[68] Rotating beds are used in trauma units for conditions such as acute spinal cord injury. These beds are not practical in rehabilitation or home settings because they interfere with transfers and therapy. They are useful to prevent pressure ulcers in persons who must be immobilized in the supine position.

In the rehabilitation setting minimal air loss and air fluidized beds are generally used for short time periods because they are not practical or are too expensive for home use. The rehabilitation team must determine turning tolerance on a mattress and overlay suitable for home use. Patient and family education for prevention and early intervention at home are the key to preventive measures.

Wheelchair cushions are available in several forms to help prevent pressure ulcers. They are generally gel, foam, air, or water filled. They do not eliminate the need for pressure relief in the wheelchair and do not decrease ischial pressure below capillary pressure.[89] There is a high degree of variability in benefits, and no ideal cushion. Gel cushions will maintain instant skin temperature, but cooling of the cushion after 3 hours is necessary to maintain this effect. Foam cushions increase temperature of the seating surface, whereas water-filled cushions cause a decrease. An air-filled cushion with multiple cells causes an increase in humidity and temperature of the seating surface as well, but this increase is less than that resulting from foam cushions.[90,91] Air-filled cushions require the user to monitor air pressure, which can be a problem in the noncompliant patient. Foam cushions have a life span of 6 months.[92] Contoured foam cushions will reduce pressure and improve posture and balance when compared to standard foam, gel, and multiple cell air-filled cushions in studies involving less than 10 patients.[93,94]

Pressure relief should be encouraged to prevent ulceration. Numerous devices have been developed to measure their frequency and encourage follow-through.[75,95] Many spinal cord injured persons can sit for prolonged periods and not develop pressure ulcers, although this is not universal.

Numerous supports have been designed to reduce or totally eliminate pressure on the heel while in bed. The most effective of these devices are the ones designed to elevate the heel from the bed completely to eliminate pressure.[96] Doughnut-shaped devices decrease blood flow to the area in the center and should not be used. Electrical stimulation is currently being studied as a means to prevent pressure ulcers. Electrical stimulation of the gluteus maximus muscles increases local blood flow and produces a change in the contour of these muscles. The utility and cost effectiveness of this technique requires further study.[97,98]

MEDICAL MANAGEMENT

Identifying patients at risk and reducing the intrinsic and extrinsic factors predisposing to pressure ulcer development is crucial. Indirect treatment includes comprehensive medical management. Malnutrition is common in acute medical and extended care settings. Nutritional support (including tube feedings) should maintain patients in a positive nitrogen balance—typically 30 to 35 calories/kg/day and 1.25 to 1.50 grams of protein/kg/day.[99] Total parenteral nutrition should be considered if the gastrointestinal tract is not functional.[100]

Wound healing occurs in a continuum that has been described by three stages.[101] The inflammatory phase lasts up to 3 days. A fibrin clot is formed as platelets aggregate to prevent bleeding. Platelets release substances to cause further platelet aggregation: factors chemotactic for leukocytes, proteolytic enzymes that initiate couplement activation, and growth factors. Thrombocytopenia may diminish the rate of wound healing. Leukocytes remove foreign material and macrophages remove bacteria and debris. Macrophages are essential cells and release angiogenic substances and stimulate fibroblasts. Fibroblasts appear at 48 to 72 hours and their growth is enhanced by low oxygen and high lactate levels. They synthesize collagen elastin and proteoglycans. The proliferation phase occurs next until the wound is healed. Granulation tissue develops and contracts. Collagen synthesis and angiogenesis occurs as new epithelium with its silver appearance, covers the wound. A maturation process occurs after the wound is healed. This phase continues for years as the scar is observed to shrink and thin out from reorganization. Fading of the scar is secondary to regression of capillaries.

Assuring adequate nutrition should be a routine part of medical management of any patient irrespective of his or her risk for pressure ulcers. When a pressure ulcer develops, nutritional status must be reassessed. Mulholland et al. were the first to demonstrate diminished plasma protein levels in persons with pressure ulcers.[8] Malnutrition may occur in hospitalized patients in general, medical, and surgical wards.[102] Nursing home patients with pressure ulcers may have low cholesterol, albumin, and zinc levels and be anemic in spite of a high protein calorie diet administrated via feeding tubes.[63] A study using serum albumin, total lymphocyte count, and somatic protein as markers in nursing home patients determined that those with pressure sores were more severely malnourished.[68] Inadequate protein intake correlates with potential for ulcer healing.[81]

Maintaining adequate protein, calorie, and fluid intake to prevent negative nitrogen balance and dehydration is essential.[103,104] Water is needed in excess of 1.6 L/day, and 1.5 to 2 g of protein are needed per kilogram of body weight.[103] The major source of calories should be from carbohydrates.[103] Protein balance can be assessed by serum albumin and transferrin levels, but nitrogen balance studies may be helpful. Zinc and its impact on pressure ulcers has been the subject of numerous studies.[105] Zinc is required for protein synthesis and repair.[106] Zinc levels, if elevated (>400 mg/dL), can interfere with macrophage function and should only be supplemented in persons who are zinc deficient.[103,107,108] Iron should only be supplemented in iron-deficient individuals. Vitamin C is required for collagen synthesis and is needed in levels above the basic requirement. It has been the subject of several studies.[109,110] In a double-blind placebo-controlled study on 20 patients with pressure ulcers, vitamin C supplementation of 1 g per day in divided doses has been shown to improve the rate of pressure ulcer healing. Excess ascorbic acid is metabolized to oxalic acid and may increase kidney stone risk.[63] This risk has not been studied in pressure ulcer patients. Persons with pressure ulcers should receive the basic requirements of all vitamins and trace elements and appropriate treatment should be given when anemia is present.

TREATMENT OF THE ULCER

There is no definitive study on the most effective way to treat pressure ulcers. This treatment algorithm is based on the results of both animal and human studies. Very few investigations systematically compare one treatment with a standard nontoxic control. Clinically, an individual patient may respond better to a dressing that is supposed to result in slower healing. A common example is when a patient is switched from wet-to-dry dressings to an occlusive dressing as the wound improves. Healing may stop until the saline dressing is reapplied. The generally accepted principles of pressure ulcer management are described. Further study is needed to determine the ideal moist-wound healing environment as products proliferate without adequate study.

The first step in treatment of a pressure ulcer after removing pressure, is the elimination of necrotic tissue. Debridement may be surgical, mechanical osmotic, chemical enzymatic, or autolytic.[112,113] Necrotic tissue is a barrier to wound contraction and epithelialization, and a nidus for infection. Surgical debridement is the most efficient method of debridement and generally is done with a scalpel. A newer method of surgical debridement is vaporization with a carbon dioxide laser. The laser can debride bone, as well as soft tissue. Wet-to-dry dressing can remove small amounts of necrotic tissue and is a useful technique to remove residual necrotic tissue after a partial surgical debridement. These dressings will remove healthy tissue as well, and should be discontinued when the wound is clean. Hydrotherapy is especially labor intensive and is generally not necessary.

Autolytic debridement under an occlusive dressing can occur, but this technique is slow and it is more efficient to debride a wound before using an occlusive dressing. Enzymatic debridement agents contain either fibrinolysin-deoxyribonuclease trypsin, papain, collagenase, or sutilians. These materials require several treatments and are more expensive than simple debridement or wet-to-dry dressing changes.

It is not possible to review the risks and benefits of all dressings, positions, salves, and liniments that have been proposed to treat pressure ulcers. Adherence to basic principles of wound care is essential, and some commonly used toxic substances should be avoided. Research in pressure ulcer treatment includes numerous controlled studies and those discussing potentially useful dressings, in comparison with "control" dressings containing toxic substances.[113,114] When a new device for pressure ulcers is used, observational effects on the part of staff are important to consider. In a recent study, a placebo device that supposedly emitted electromagnetic waves was judged to be effective by hospital staff.[115] However, when the study began, staff awareness increased, calling into question the benefits of the treatment.

A great deal of interest in the contribution of a moist environment to wound healing began with Winters' study in domestic pigs.[111] A moist-wound environment resulted in enhanced epithelialization that stimulated growth of underlying connective tissues.[116] Hinman and Maibach confirmed these benefits in humans, and described how eschar in an air-exposed wound inhibits migration of epithelium.[117] Knighton studied the hypoxic wound environment under occlusive dressings, and concluded that local wound hypoxia encourages angiogenesis and capillary growth.[118] Comparisons of hydrocolloid dressings, wet-to-dry dressing, polyurethane film, and air exposure by Alvarez et al. in an animal model confirmed improved wound healing in a moist environment and described damage to the new epithelium when removing the polyurethane films and gauze.[119]

Concern about infection under occlusive dressings have been raised by several authors. Infection rates are low with occlusive dressings, and they may pose a protective barrier to invasion by bacteria. They should not be applied to grossly infected wounds. The comparative value of one occlusive dressing over another has been reviewed by Falanga.[120] Premature removal can cause epithelial damage, and granulating wounds that are covered with an occlusive dressing that do not epithelialize should be changed to a nonadherent dressing. Occlusive dressings should not be placed over a severe dermatitis surrounding a wound. Hydrocolloid dressings may have a modest cost benefit in treating pressure ulcers when compared to saline-soaked gauze, but may not be as effective as gauze in lesions that expose muscle.[121,122] Calcium alginate dressings, a polysaccharide from brown seaweed, have recently been introduced in the United States.[123,124] They are devised to handle wounds with large amounts of exudate, but scientific documentation of their benefit is lacking. Most studies on occlusive dressings and other moist dressing do not uniformly control for the nutritional and metabolic status of cohort study groups.

Careful consideration must be given to the application of topical agents to pressure ulcers. Povidone-iodine, a topical antiseptic, contains iodine that can be absorbed through the skin and mucosal surfaces, resulting in increased serum iodine concentrations.[125–127] Iodine absorption can result in metabolic acidosis, hypernatremia, hyperosomolarity, and renal failure, as well as hypothryoidism and hyperthyroidism. Povidone-iodine (1 percent) is also toxic to fibroblasts, as is 3 percent hydrogen peroxide, 0.5 percent sodium hypochlorite, and 0.25 percent acetic acid.[128] These substances are not recommended.

Topical antibiotics, such as bacitracin, silver sufladizine, and combination of neomycin, bacitracin, and polymyxin B may enhance epidermal healing.[111,120,128] This effect may not be explained by antimicrobial activity alone.[129] Although the clinical uses of topical antibiotics have not been well established, our clinical experience suggests that they are especially beneficial when used with a nonadherent gauze on superficial ulcerations. This is particularly helpful on superficial open areas that cannot hold an occlusive dressing or are unresponsive to one.

Electrical stimulation to promote wound healing has been the subject of numerous studies over the years that have recently been reviewed.[130–135] Many of these studies have insufficient sample size or have been poorly controlled. The clinical use of electrical stimulation techniques has not been established, and further study is needed.

GROWTH FACTORS

Growth factors are naturally occurring proteins secreted by platelets and macrophages that are believed to direct the migration of cells into wounds and orchestrate the process of repair.[101,136] Epidermal growth factor increases mitosis in epidermal cell cultures and granulation tissue, and may enhance epithelialization. It increases glycosaminoglycan synthesis in dermal fibroblast cultures and it increases glycolysis, fibronectin, and nucleic acid synthesis. In animal studies, recombinant epidermal growth factor has been shown to enhance wound epithelialization of partial thickness wounds.[138,139]

Both acidic and basic forms of fibroblast growth factor (FGF) have been demonstrated. FGF stimulates endothelial cell growth and blood vessel growth in vivo.[27,138] Transforming growth factor beta (TGFB1) is released from platelets and has a direct effect on collagen synthesis, and accelerating maturation.[138,139]

TGFB1 inhibits the differentiation of fibroblasts in myofibroblasts, most likely by reducing the need for wound contraction as increased cellular matrix is synthesized.

Platelet derived growth factor (PDGF) is chemotactic for fibroblasts, smooth muscle cells, neutrophils, and mononuclear cells.[138,140] It induces an inflammatory response and a provisional matrix synthesis in wounds that exceeds that generated by the normal healing process. The differentiation of fibroblasts is affected in the same manner as TGFB1, described earlier. Platelet-derived growth factor derived from recombinant DNA is currently being studied in humans. Autologous-platelet-derived wound-healing factors are also being used in nonhealing wounds.[141–143] This is prepared by using platelet-rich plasma, extracting the platelets, and suspending them in a buffer solution that is activated with thrombin and made into a salve. Robson reported that persons treated with high doses of recombinant platelet-derived growth factor BB showed improved healing in pressure ulcer response of 100 mg/mL doses.[144] Lower doses tested were not effective. This study is inconclusive, because of the small sample size and statistical significance of $p = 0.12$.[136] Studies by Knighton and Atril using platelet extracts may contain a more natural combination of factors needed to stimulate wound healing, as opposed to a single growth factor.[141–143] In these studies, the types of patients and the content of the extracts were uncontrolled and the sample size was small. The content of the growth factors in each extract was not known. Further studies using defined preparations in large, well-controlled studies are needed. Although platelet-derived growth factor and its preparations are the most extensively studied, it is too early to recommend their usage.

Growth factors or extracts of autologous human platelets may play a major role in the treatment of pressure ulcers in the future. Further study is needed to determine the indications, cost effectiveness, and type of ulcers that will benefit optimally from growth factors and how they should be incorporated in overall patient management.

Vitamins should be supplemented in deficient states. Microcytic anemia may be an indication of an iron-deficient state. Zinc is an integral element for protein synthesis and can be supplemented in the deficient individual. Vitamin C is necessary for collagen synthesis and supplementation of 1 g/d has been shown to improve the rate of pressure ulcer healing.[105]

Initial direct care of a pressure ulcer involves debridement of devitalized tissues. Sharp debridement can be accomplished with scalpel or scissor, and should be executed until good granulation is demarcated. Extensive Stage IV lesions should be debrided in the operating room, where the need for a bone biopsy is assured.

Mechanical debridement can be accomplished by wet-to-dry dressing, hydrotherapy, wound irrigations, and dextranomers. Normal saline is typically used for wet-to-dry applications. However, care must be taken to moisten the edges of the ulcer bed so that new granulation tissue is not removed.

Enzymatic debridement agents contain either fibrinolysin-deoxyribonuclease trypsin, papain, collagenase or sutilains. Autolytic debridement involves the use of synthetic (usually occlusive) dressings to cover the wound. These dressings buffer the wound from incontinence, and allow necrotic tissues to self-digest from inherent wound enzymes.[111] One exception to the rule of debridement is heel ulcers with a dry eschar. These do not require debridement unless edema, erythema, fluctuance, or drainage are present.

Antiseptic agents such as povidone-iodine, hydrogen peroxide, sodium hypochlorite (Dakin's solution), and acetic acid are not recommended owing to cytotoxicity. Topical antibiotics (bacitracin, silver sulfadiazine) may be useful in conjunction with nonadherent gauze for superficial ulceration. Wound cleaning can also be accomplished by hydroponic ulcer irrigation, between 4 to 15 pounds per square inch (psi).[145]

Other adjunctive therapies have been studied, including: hyperbaric oxygen, infrared, ultraviolet, low energy laser irradiation, ultrasound, various topical agents (sugar, vitamins, hormones) and systemic drugs (vasodilators, hemorrheologis, serotonin inhibitors, fibrinolytic agents).

COMPLICATIONS

Pressure ulcers may become infected, lead to local abscess formation, and cause septicemia or osteomyelitis. Infection of an ulcer is recognized by extensive surrounding inflammation and induration, purulent drainage, and fever.[146] A foul odor generally is associated with the presence of anaerobes.[147] Swab cultures do not always concur with the results of deep tissue culture, and deep tissue cultures vary depending on the site of the lesion.[147] A technique known as irrigation-aspiration has been shown to have a 97.6 percent concordance for aerobes and a 91.8 percent concordance for anaerobes when compared with biopsy.[148] As pressure ulcers heal and granulation tissue appears, the bacterial counts drop. Common organisms include aerobic organisms

(Staphylococcus aureus, Streptococcus, Pseudomonas, Proteus) and anaerobic organisms (Clostridia, Bacteroides). Although there has been some debate in the past on treatment of pressure ulcers with antibiotics, their use is generally limited to systemic infection and lesions with surrounding cellulitis.[7,64,146,147,149] Foul-smelling necrotic tissue can be removed with debridement, wound cleansing, and saline wet-to-dry dressing. Topical or oral metronidazole may be beneficial in treating infected ulcers not responsive to local care.[150,151]

Soft tissue and pelvic abscesses can develop owing to pressure ulcers. A soft tissue abscess may present with spontaneous rupture or may be diagnosed by aspiration. Computerized tomography and ultrasound are valuable in identifying these abscesses.[152,153]

Osteomyelitis in bone beneath a pressure ulcer can impair healing of an ulcer, result in repeated breakdown, impair healing of surgically repaired wounds, and result in spread of infection. Many methods have been proposed to diagnose osteomyelitis.[154,155] Nuclear medicine scans are often positive, owing to local, nonspecific bone disease and soft tissue infection and plain x-rays alone do not always correlate directly with osteomyelitis.[67,155] Bone biopsy is still the definitive diagnostic procedure of choice for osteomyelitis. A positive plain x-ray, a white cell count of 15,000 mm³ or an erythrocyte sedimentation rate of 120 mm/h or greater is presumptive evidence of osteomyelitis. A recent study indicates that plain x-ray can identify osteomyelitis with greater accuracy than computerized tomography.[66]

Bacteremia is a potentially life-threatening complication of pressure ulcers, but fortunately is rare. Mortality in one series has been reported at over 50 percent.[64] Surgical debridement of the ulcer along with appropriate antibiotics is essential.[65,156]

"Marjolins ulcer," a malignant degeneration of a chronic pressure ulcer present for more than 20 years, is a rare (<0.5 percent) complication.[157–161] Clinical signs include pain, increasing discharge, foul odor, and bleeding and verrucous hyperplasia.[162–166] Biopsy remains the definitive diagnostic method.[167,168] Metastasis to inguinal nodes is common.

Stage II, III, and IV ulcers are invariably colonized with bacteria, but usually are not clinically infected. Appropriate cleansing and debridement will generally prevent bacterial colonization from proceeding to clinically significant infection.

Topical antibiotics can be utilized for a 2-week trial for clean ulcers that are not healing or continue to produce an exudate. Antibiotics, such as silver sulfadiazine or triple antibiotics, are most effective against Gram-negative, Gram-positive, and anaerobic organisms.[169]

Appropriate systemic antibiotic therapy is required for patients with soft tissue infection (fluid obtained by needle aspiration with bacterial levels exceeding 10 organisms per gram of tissue), bacteremia, sepsis (tachycardia, hypotension, deterioration in mental status), advancing cellulitis, or osteomyelitis.

SURGICAL TREATMENT

Davis is credited with the first report of a skin flap in treatment of a pressure ulcer.[170] He undercut and shifted flaps of skin and subcutaneous tissue. A large series of repairs reported by Conway and Griffith in 1956 described several principles of surgical treatment.[171] They included excision of the ulcer surrounding scar tissue, underlying bursas, and removal of underlying bone. Surgical management included careful hemostasis and a muscle flap to fill in deep holes and provided a well-vascularized bed for healing. Split thickness skin grafts and advancement or rotation flaps have been extremely successful in those who are conscientious about personal care. Large flaps with skin and fat have been used, avoiding large scars over the site of the ulcer. Myocutaneous flaps are now the primary means of surgical management.[171]

Muscle is metabolically more active than skin and more sensitive to pressure. Its effectiveness as a cover for pressure ulcers has been called into question. Anatomical dissections reveal that myocutaneous flaps are being placed over bony prominences not normally covered by muscle. The muscle in these flaps will atrophy.[45,46] New flaps are being studied that rotate innervated, vascularized tissue, allowing for skin afferentiation, and hopefully reduce recurrence.[173–175] These flaps may require multiple surgical stages. Further study is needed to determine the indications for and effectiveness of these innervated flaps.

One recent series indicates that 69 percent of patients experience ulcer recurrence as early as 9.3 months after surgical repair.[172] Clearly, myocutaneous flaps are not a definitive cure for pressure ulcers. Repair of a pressure ulcer should be accompanied by an educational program in the rehabilitation setting to teach methods to prevent occurrence and to reassess equipment and attendant care needs. Specific surgical techniques have been described and illustrated by Agris and Spira.[5] Pressure sores not responding to medical management and not amenable to surgical repair have resulted in amputation of the lower extremities. This generally occurs with multiple ulcerations and severe osteomyelitis.[176] Although in the past this has been considered a surgical technique to aid rehabilitation, it is now used as a last resort when standard medical and surgical repair are not possible.[177]

Stage III and IV ulcers will usually require surgical intervention. Skin grafting (usually split thickness) can be utilized for superficial full thickness ulcers that are small and relatively clean, as well for massive ulceration. Skin flaps that incorporate a cutaneous vascular supply can be useful for Stage IV ulcers.

Musculocutaneous flaps incorporate the adjacent skin with its perforating vessels, as well as the muscle and fascia. Customary flaps include the tensor fascia lata, posterior hamstring, and gluteal muscle. Free flaps are donor sites distant from the wound and are reserved for very large ulcers. The latissimus dorsi flap typically is used for these procedures.

Prophylactic ischiectomy is not recommended.[178] This procedure often results in perineal ulcers and urethral fistulas. Postoperatively, patients are generally managed in air-fluidized beds.

CONCLUSION

The physical and psychosocial costs of pressure ulcers is astronomical. As the aging U.S. population increases, more individuals will be at risk to develop debilitating conditions placing them at risk for pressure ulcer development. Comprehensive education and management strategies must be implemented in any health care facility. Excellent algorithms for predictions, prevention, nutritional assessment, management, and infection control and have been outlined in the 1994 Clinical Practice Guidelines.

REFERENCES

1. National Pressure Ulcer Advisory Panel: Pressure ulcers: Incidence Economic Risk Assessment. Consensus Development Conference Statement. National Pressure Ulcer Advisory Panel. Rockville, MD. 1989; 5–6.
2. Meechan M: Multisite Pressure Ulcer Prevalence Survey. Decubitus 1990; 3:14–17.
3. Allman RM, Larade CA, Noel LB, et al: Pressure sores among hospitalized patients. *Ann Int Med* 1986; 105:337–342.
4. Brandeis AH, Morris JN, Nash DJ, Lipsitz VA: The epidemiology and natural history of pressure ulcers in elderly nursing home residents. *JAMA* 1990; 264:2905–2909.
5. Agris, J, Spiro M: Pressure ulcers; prevention and treatment. CIBA Clinical Symposia 32(S) 1979, CIBA Pharmaceutical Company.
6. Agency for Health Care Policy and Research: Pressure ulcers in adults prediction and prevention. Agency for Health Care Policy and Research Publication No. 92-0047. US Department of Health and Human Services. 1992; 13–17.
7. Allman RM: Pressure ulcers among the elderly. *N Engl J Med* 1989; 320:850–853.
8. Mulholland JH, Tui C, Wright AM, Vinci V, Shartroff B: Protein metabolism and bed sores. *Ann Surg* 1943; 118:1015–1023.
9. Pinchcofsky-Devis GD, Kaminski MU Jr: Correlation of pressure sores and nutritional status. *J Am Geriatr Soc* 1986; 34:435–440.
10. Bennett L, Kavner D, Lee BY, Trainer FS, Lewis JM: Skin blood flow in seated geriatric patients. *Arch Phys Med Rehabil* 1981; 52:392–398.
11. Clark M, Rowland LB: Comparison of contact pressures measured at the sacrum of young and elderly subjects. *J Biomed Eng* 1989; 11:197–199.
12. Yarkony GM: Aging skin, pressure ulcerations, and spinal cord injury, in Whiteneck GG (ed): *Aging with Spinal Cord Injury.* New York: Demos, 1993, pp. 39–52.
13. Kligman AM, Grove GL, Balin AK: Aging of human skin, in Finch CE, Schneider EL (eds): *Handbook of the Biology of Aging.* New York: Van Nostrand Reinhold, 1985.
14. Garber SL, Krouskop TA: Body build and its relationship to pressure distribution in the seated wheelchair patient. *Arch Phys Med Rehabil* 1982; 63:17–20.
15. Garber SL, Campion LJ, Krouskop TA: Trochanteric pressure in spinal cord injury. *Arch Phys Med Rehabil* 1982; 63:549–552.
16. Anderson TP, Andberg MM: Psychosocial factors associated with pressure sores. *Arch Phys Med Rehabil* 1979; 60:341–346.
17. Gordon WA, Harasymiw S, Bellile S, Lehman L, Sherman B: The relationship between pressure sores and psychosocial adjustment in persons with spinal cord injury. *Rehabil Psych* 1982; 27:185–191.
18. Thiyagorajan C, Silver JR: Aetiology of pressure sores in patients with spinal cord injury. *Br Med J* 1984; 289:1487–1490.
19. Yarkony, GM, Heinemann, AW: Pressure ulcers, in Stover SL, Delisa JA, Whiteneck GG: *Rounds. Spinal Cord Injury Clinical Outcomes from the Model Systems.* Gaithersburg, MD: Aspen Publishers, 1995, pp. 100–119.
20. Mawson AR, Biundo PR Jr, Neville P, et al: Risk factors for early occurring pressure ulcers following spinal cord injury. *Am J Phys Med Rehabil* 1988; 67:123–127.
21. Yarkony GM, Kirk PM, Carlson C, et al: Classification of pressure ulcers. *Arch Dermatol* 1990; 126:1218–1219.

22. Shea JD: Pressure sores: Classification and management. *Clin Orthop* 1975; 112:89–100.

23. National Pressure Ulcer Advisory Panel: Pressure ulcers: incidence, economics, risk assessment. Consensus Development Conference Statement. West Dundee, IL: S-N Publications Inc, 1989.

24. Mash N: Standards of Care dermal wounds: pressure sores. Irving, CA: International Association of Enterostomal Therapy, 1987.

25. Cuzzell JZ: The New RYB Color Code. *Am J Nurs* 1988; 88:1342–1346.

26. Moriorty MB: How color can clarify wound care. *RN* 1951; 51:49–54.

27. Dealy C: Measuring a wound. *Nursing* 1991; 4:29.

28. Thomas AC, Wysocki AB: The healing wound: A comparison of three clinical useful methods of measurement. *Decubitus* 1990; 3:18–25.

29. Kundin JI: A new way to size up a wound. *Am J Nurs* 1989; 89:206–207.

30. Covington JS, Griffin JW, Mendiw RK, et al: Measurement of pressure ulcer volume using dental impression materials: Suggestion from the field. *Phys Ther* 1989; 69:690–694.

31. Resch CS, Kerner E, Robson MC, et al: Pressure sore volume measurement: A technique to document and record wound healing. *J Am Geriatr Soc* 1988; 36:444–446.

32. Anthony D, Barnes E: Measuring pressure sore accurately. *Nursing Times* 1984; 80:33–35.

33. Putnam T, Calenoff L, Betts HB, Rosen JS: Sinography in management of decubitus ulcers. *Arch Phys Med Rehabil* 1978; 59:243–246.

34. Borgstrom PS, Ekberg O, Lasson A: Radiography of pressure ulcers. *Acta Radiologica* 1988; 29:581–584.

35. Hooker EZ, Sibley P, Nemchausky B, Lopez E: A method for quantifying the area of closed pressure sores by sinography and disitometry. *J Neurosci Nurs* 1988; 20:118–127.

36. Bates-Jensen BM, Uredevoe DL, Brecht ML: Validity and reliability of the pressure sore status tool. *Decubitus* 1992; 5:20–28.

37. Trumble HC: The skin tolerance for pressure and pressure sores. *Med J Aust* 1930; 2:724–726.

38. Kosiak M, Kubicek WG, Olson M, Danz JN, Kottke FJ: Evaluation of pressure as factor in production of ischial ulcer. *Arch Phys Med Rehabil* 1958; 39:623–629.

39. Kosiak M: Etiology and pathology of ischemic ulcer. *Arch Phys Med Rehabil* 1959; 42:62–68.

40. Kosiak M: Etiology of decubitus ulcers. *Arch Phys Med Rehabil* 1961; 42:19–29.

41. Daniel RK, Wheatley D, Priest D: Pressure sores and paraplegics: An experimental model. *Ann Plast Surg* 1985; 15:41–49.

42. Larsen B, Holstein P, Lassen NA: On the pathogenesis of bedsores. *Scand J Plast Reconstr Surg* 1979; 13:347–350.

43. Rueler JB, Cooney TG: The pressure sore: pathophysiology and principles of management. *Ann Intern Med* 1981; 94:661–666.

44. Daniel RK, Priest DL, Wheatley DC: Etiologic factors in pressure sores an experimental model. *Arch Phys Med Rehabil* 1981; 62:492–498.

45. Nola GT, Vistnes LM: Differential response of skin and muscle in the experimental production of pressure sores. *Plast Reconstr Surg* 1980; 66:728–733.

46. Daniel RK, Farbusoff B: Muscle coverage of pressure points: The role of myocutaneous flaps. *Ann Plast Surg* 1982; 8:446–452.

47. Barton AA: The pathogenesis of skin wounds due to pressure, in Kenedi RM, Couden JM, Scales JT (eds): *Bedsore Biomechanics*. Baltimore: University Park, 1916, pp. 55–62.

48. Brand PW: Pressure sores the problem, in Kenedi RM, Couden JM, Scales JT (eds): *Bedsore Biomechanics*. Baltimore: University Park, 1916, pp. 19–23.

49. Yarkony GM: Pressure ulcers: A review. *Arch Phys Med Rehabil* 1994; 75:908–917.

50. *Dorland's Illustrated Medical Dictionary*, 27th ed. Philadelphia: WB Saunders, 1988, p. 1514.

51. Reichel SM: Shearing force as a factor in decubitus ulcer in paraplegics. *JAMA* 1958; 166:762–763.

52. Bennett L, Kavner D, Lee BY, Trainer FA: Shear vs pressure as causative factors in skin blood flow occlusion. *Arch Phys Med Rehabil* 1979; 60:309–314.

53. Realer JB, Cooney TG: The pressure sore: Pathophysiology and principles of management. *Ann Intern Med* 1985; 15:41–49.

54. Dinsdale SM: Decubitus ulcers role of pressure and friction in causation. *Arch Phys Med Rehabil* 1974; 55:147–152.

55. Krouskop TA, Reddy NP, Spencer WA, Secor JW: Mechanisms of decubitus ulcer formation: a hypotheses. *Med Hypoth* 1978; 4:37–39.

56. Krouskop TA: A syntheses of the factors that contribute to pressure sore formation. *Med Hypoth* 1983; 11:255–267.

57. Lamid S, El Ghatit AZ: Smoking, spasticity and pressure sores in spinal cord injured patients. *Am J Phys Med* 1983; 62:300–306.

58. Kligman AM, Grove, GL, Balin AK: Aging of human skin, in Finch CE, Schenider EL (eds): *Handbook of the Biology of Aging*. New York: Van Nostrand Reinhold, 1985.

59. Geneser F: *Textbook of Histology*. Philadelphia: Lea & Febiger, 1987.

60. Cormack DH: *Ham's Histology*. Philadelphia: JB Lippincott, 1987.

61. Keller PA, Sinkovic SP, Miles SJ: Skin dryness: A major factor in reducing incontinence dermatitis. *Ostomy Wound Manage* 1990 Sep–Oct:30:60–64.

62. Shipes E, Stanley I: Effects of a liquid copolymer skin barrier for preventing skin problems. *Ostomy Manage* 1981 Spring 4:19–23.

63. Bruslow RA, Hallfrish J, Goldberg AP: Malnutrition in tube feed nursing home patients with pressure sores. *J Parent Enteral Nutr* 1991; 15:663–668.

64. Bryan CS, Dew CE, Reynolds KL: Bacteremia associated with decubitus ulcers. *Arch Int Med* 1983; 143:2093–2095.

65. Galpin JE, Chow AW, Bayer AS, Guze LB: Sepsis associated with decubitus ulcers. *Am J Med* 1976; 61:346–350.

66. Lewis VL Jr, Bailey MH, Pulawski G, et al: The diagnosis of osteomyelitis in patients with pressure sores. *Plast Reconstr Surg* 1988; 81:229–232.

67. Sugarman B: Osteomyelitis in spinal cord injury. *Arch Phys Med Rehabil* 1984; 65:132–134.

68. Brandeis GH, et al: A longitudinal study of risk factors associated with the formation of pressure ulcers in nursing homes. *JAGS* 1994; 42:388–393.

69. Bell KR, Halar EM: Contractures: Prevention and management. *Crit Rev Phys Med Rehabil* 1990; 1:231–246.

70. Hassard G: Heterotopic bone formation about the hip and unilateral decubitus ulcers in spinal cord injury. *Arch Phys Med Rehabil* 1975; 56:355–358.

71. Dinsdale SM: Decubitus ulcers in swine: Light and electron microscopy study of pathogenesis. *Arch Phys Med Rehabil* 1973; 54:51–56.

72. Sulzberger MB, Cortese TA Jr, Fishman L, Wiley HS: Studies on blisters produced by friction I. results of linear rubbing and twisting techniques. *J Invest Dermatol* 1966; 47:456–465.

73. Witkowski JA, Parish LC: Histopathology of the decubitus ulcer. *J Am Acad Dermatol* 1982; 6:1014–1021.

74. Rehabilitation Institute of Chicago: *Division of Nursing: Rehabilitation Nursing Procedures Manual*. Rockville, MD: Aspen, 1990, pp. 179–203.

75. Lindan O, Greenway RM, Piozza JM: Pressure distribution on the surface of the human body: I. evaluation in lying and sitting positions using a "bed of springs and nails." *Arch Phys Med Rehabil* 1965; 46:378–385.

76. Krouskop TA, Williams R, Krubs M, Herszkowicz I, Garber S: Effectiveness of mattress overlays in reducing interface pressures during recumbency. *J Rehabil Res Dev* 1985; 22:7–10.

77. Andersen KE, Jensen O, Kuarning SA, Bach E: Decubitus prophylaxis: A prospective trial on the efficiency of alternating-pressure air mattresses and water mattresses. *Acta Dermatovener* 1982; 63:227–270.

78. Redfern SJ, Jeneid PA, Gillingham ME, Lunn HF: Local pressures with ten types of patient support systems. *Lancet* 1973; 2:277–280.

79. Dean LS, Krall S, Wharton GW: A comparison study of the pressure relief characteristics of two air floatation beds. San Francisco: American Spinal Injury Association Abstracts, 1986, p. 274.

80. Krouskop TA: The role of mattresses and beds in preventing pressure sores, in Lee BY, Ostrande LE, Cochran GVB, Shaw WW (eds): *The Spinal Cord Injured Patients: Comprehensive Management*. Philadelphia: WB Saunders, 1991, pp. 244–250.

81. Allman RM, Walker JM, Hart MK, et al: Air-fluidized beds or conventional therapy for pressure sores: A randomized trial. *Ann Int Med* 1987; 107:641–648.

82. Thomson CW, Ryan DW, Dunkin LJ, Smith M, Marshall M: Fluidized-bead bed on the intensive therapy unit. *Lancet* 1980; 1:568–570.

83. Nimit K: Public health service assessment guidelines for home air-fluidized bed therapy. Washington, DC: US Government Printing Office, 1989.

84. Sharbaugh RJ, Hargest TS: Bactericidal effect of the air-fluidized bed. *Am J Surg* 1971; 37:583–586.

85. Sharbaugh RJ, Hargest TS, Wright FA: Further studies on the bactericidal effect of the air fluidized bed. *Am J Surg* 1973; 39:253–256.

86. Ferrell BA, Osterwell D, Christenson P: A randomized trial of low-air-loss beds for treatment of pressure ulcers. *JAMA* 1993; 269:494–497.

87. Inman KJ, Sibbald WJ, Rutledge FS, Clark BJ: Clinical utility and cost-effectiveness of an air suspension bed in the prevention of pressure ulcers. *JAMA* 1993; 269:1139–1143.

88. Dolezai R, Cohen M, Schultz RC: The use of clinitorn therapy unit in the immediate postoperative care of pressure ulcers. *Ann Plastic Surg* 1985; 14:33–36.

89. Souther SG, Carr SD, Vistnes LM: Wheelchair cushions to reduce pressure under bony prominences. *Arch Phys Med Rehabil* 1974; 55:460–464.

90. Seymour RJ, Lacefield WE: Wheelchair cushion effect on pressure and skin temperature. *Arch Phys Med Rehabil* 1985; 66:103–108.

91. Stewart SFC, Palmieri V, Cochran GVB: Wheelchair cushion effect on skin temperature heat flex, and relative humidity. *Arch Phys Med Rehabil* 1980; 61:229–233.

92. Ferguson-Pell M, Cochran GVB, Palmieri V, Branski JB: Development of a modular wheelchair cushion for spinal cord injured persons. *J Rehabil Res Dev* 1986; 23:63–76.

93. Sprigle SH, Faisant JE, Chung KC: Clinical evaluation of custom-contoured cushions for the spinal cord injured. *Arch Phys Med Rehabil* 1990; 71:655–658.

94. Sprigle S, Chung KC, Brubaker CE: Reduction of sitting pressures with custom contoured cushions. *J Rehabil Res Dev* 1990; 27:135–140.

95. Patterson RP, Fisher SV: Sitting pressure-time patterns in patients with quadriplegia. *Arch Phys Med Rehabil* 1986; 67:812–814.

96. Pinzur MS, Schumacher D, Reddy N, Osterman H, Havey R, Patwordin A: Preventing heel ulcers: A comparison of prophylactic body support systems. *Arch Phys Med Rehabil* 1991; 72:508–510.

97. Levine SP, Kett RL, Gross MD, Wilson BA, Cederna PS, Juni JE: Blood flow in the gluteus maximus of seated individuals during electrical muscle stimulation. *Arch Phys Med Rehabil* 1990; 71:682–686.

98. Levine SP, Kett RL, Cederna PS, Brooks SV: Electrical muscle stimulation for pressure sore prevention: Tissue shape variation. *Arch Phys Med Rehabil* 1990; 71:210–215.

99. Chernott, R, Milton K, Lipshitz D: The effect of a very

high protein liquid formula on decubitus ulcer healing in long-term fed institutionalized patients (abstract). *J Am Diet Assoc* 1990; 90(9):A 1–30.

100. Kaminski MU Jr: Enteral hyperalimentation. *Surg Gynecol Obstet* 197; 143:12–16.

101. Rudolph R, Shannon ML: The normal healing process, in Eaglstein WH (ed): *New Directions in Wound Healing.* Princeton: ER Squibb & Sons, 1990.

102. Bristian BR, Blackburn GL, Vitale J, Cochran D, Naylor J: Prevalence of malnutrition in general medical patients. *JAMA* 1976; 235:1567–1570.

103. Silane M, Oot-giromini B: Systemic and other factors that affect wound healing, in Eaglstein WH (ed): *New Directions in Wound Healing.* Princeton: ER Squibb & Sons, 1990.

104. Constantian MB, Jackson HS: Biology and care of the pressure ulcer wound, in Constantian M (ed): *Pressure Ulcers: Principles and Techniques of Management.* Boston: Little, Brown. 1980, pp. 69–100.

105. Breslow R: Nutritional status and dietary intake of patients with pressure ulcers review of research literature 1943–1989. *Decubitus* 1991; 4:16–21.

106. Hallbook J, Lanner E: Serum-zinc and healing of venous leg ulcers. *Lancet* 1972; 2:780–782.

107. Williams CM, Lines CM, McKay EC: Iron and zinc status in multiple sclerosis patients with pressure sores. *Eur J Clin Nutr* 1988; 42:321–328.

108. Norris JR, Reynolds RE: The effect of oral zinc sulfate on decubitus ulcers. *JAGS* 1971; 19:793–797.

109. Hunter T, Rajai KT: The role of ascorbic acid in the pathogenesis and treatment of pressure sores. *Paraplegia* 1971; 8:211–216.

110. Taylor TV, Rimmer S, Day B, et al: Ascorbic acid supplementation in treatment of pressure sores. *Lancet* 1974; 11:544–546.

111. Witkowski JA, Parish LC: Debridement of cutaneous ulcers: medical and surgical aspects. *Clin Dermatol* 1992; 9:585–591.

112. Baxter CR, Rodeheaver GT: Interventions: hemostasis, cleansing, topical, antibiotics, debridement and closure, in Eaglstein WH (ed): *New Directions in Wound Healing.* Princeton: ER Squibb & Sons, 1990, pp. 71–82.

113. Yarkony GM, Kramer E, King R, et al: Pressure sore management: Efficacy of a moisture reactive occlusive dressing. *Arch Phys Med Rehabil* 1984; 65:597–600.

114. Gorse GT, Messner RL: Improved pressure sore healing with hyrocolloid dressings. *Arch Dermatol* 1987; 123:766–771.

115. Fernie GR, Dornan J: The problems of clinical trials with new systems for preventing or healing decubiti, in Kenedi RM, Couden JM, Scales JT (eds): *Bedsore Biomechanics.* Baltimore: University Park, 1916, pp. 315–320.

116. Winter GD: Formation of scab and rate of epithelialization of superficial wounds in skin of young domestic pig. *Nature* 1962; 193:293–294.

117. Hinman CD, Maibach H: Effect of air exposure and occlusion on experimental human skin wounds. *Nature* 1963; 200:377–378.

118. Knighton DR, Silver IA, Hunt TK: Regulation of wound-healing angiogenesis-effect of oxygen gradients and inspired oxygen concentration. *Surgery* 1981; 90:262–270.

119. Alvarez OM, Mertz PM, Eaglstein WH: Effect of occlusive dressings on collagen synthesis and re-epithelialization in superficial wounds. *J Surg Res* 1983; 35:142–148.

120. Falanga V: Occlusive wound dressings: Why when which? *Arch Dermatol* 1988; 124:872–877.

121. Xakellis GC, Chrischilles EA: Hydrocolloid vs. saline-gauze dressings in treating pressure ulcers: A cost-effectiveness analysis. *Arch Phys Med Rehabil* 1992; 73:463–439.

122. Seburn MD: Pressure ulcer management in home health care: Efficacy and cost effectiveness of moisture vapor permeable dressing. *Arch Phys Med Rehabil* 1986; 67:726–729.

123. Fower E, Papen JC: Evaluation of an alginate dressing for pressure ulcers. *Decubitus* 1991; 4:(3):47–52.

124. Chapius A, Dollfus P: The use of calcium alginate dressings in the management of decubitus ulcers in patients with spinal cord lesions. *Paraplegia* 1990; 28:269–271.

125. Dela Cruz F, Brown DH, Leikin JB, et al: Iodine absorption after topical administration. *W J Med* 1987; 146:43–45.

126. Shetty KR, Duthie EH Jr: Thyrotoxicosis induced by topical iodine application. *Arch Int Med* 1990; 150:2400–2401.

127. Aronott GR, Friedman SJ, Doedeus DJ, Lavelle KJ: Increased serum iodide concentration from iodine absorption through wounds treated topically with povidone-iodine. *Am J Med Sci* 1980; 279:173–176.

128. Lineaweaver W, Howard R, Soucy D, et al: Topical antimicrobial toxicity. *Arch Surg* 1985; 120:267–270.

129. Geronemus RG, Mertz PM, Eaglstein WH: Wound healing: The effects of topical antimicrobial agents. *Arch Dermatol* 1979; 115:1311–1314.

130. Kloth LC, Feedar JA: Acceleration of wound healing with high voltage, monophasic, pulsed current. *Phys Ther* 1988; 68:503–508.

131. Wolcott LE, Wheeler PC, Hardwicke HM, Rowley BA: Accelerated healing of skin ulcers by electrotherapy: Preliminary clinical results. *So Med J* 1969; 62:795–801.

132. Carley PJ, Wainapel SF: Electrotherapy for acceleration of wound healing, low intensity direct current. *Arch Phys Med Rehabil* 1985; 66:443–446.

133. Alvarez OM, Mertz PM, Smerbeck RV, Eaglstein WH: The healing of superficial skin wounds is stimulated by external electrical current. *J Invest Dermatol* 1983; 81:144–148.

134. Akers TK, Gabrielson AL: The effect of high voltage galvanic stimulation on the rate of healing of decubitus ulcers. *Biomed Sci Instrum* 1984; 20:99–100.

135. Yarkony GM, Roth EJ, Cybulski GR, Jaeger RJ: Neuromuscular stimulation in spinal cord injury II: Prevention

of secondary complications. *Arch Phys Med Rehabil* 1992; 73:195–200.

136. Hotta SS, Holohan TV: Procurren: A platelet-derived wound healing formula. Health Technology Review No. 2. Agency for Health Care Policy and Research, Department of Health and Human Services. 1992; Aug. AHCOR Pub No. 92-0065.

137. Mertz PM, Davis SC, Arakawa Y, Cohen A: Pulsed rh EGF treatment increased epithelialization of partial thickness wounds [abstract]. *J Invest Dermatol* 1988; 90:558.

138. Falanga V, Zitelli JA, Eaglstein WH: Wound healing. *J Am Acad J Dermatol* 1988; 191:559–563.

139. Pierce GF, Vande Berg T, Rudolph R, Torpley T, Mustoe TA: Platelet-derived growth factor and transforming growth factor Beta selectively modulate glycosaminoglycans, collagen and myofibroglasts in excisional wounds. *Am J Pathol* 1991; 138:629–646.

140. Pierce GF, Brown D, Mustoe TA: Quantitative analysis of inflammatory cell influx, procollagen type I synthesis and collagen cross linking in incisional wounds; influence of PDGF-BB and TGF B therapy. *J Lab Clin Med* 1991; 117:373–382.

141. Knighton DR, Ciresi KF. Fiegel VD, et al: Classification and treatment of chronic nonhealing wounds: Successful treatment with autologous platelet-derived wound healing factors (PDWHF). *Ann Surg* 1986; 204:322–330.

142. Knighton DR, Ciresi KF, Fiegel VD, et al: Stimulation of repair in chronic, nonhealing, cutaneous ulcers using platelet-derived wound healing formula. *Surg Gynecol Obstet* 1990; 170:56–60.

143. Atri SC, Misra J, Bisht D, Misra K: Use of homologous platelet factors in achieving total healing of recalcitrant skin ulcers. *Surgery* 1990; 108:508–512.

144. Robson MC, Phillips LG, Thomason A, Robson LE, Pierce GF: Platelet-derived growth factor BB for the treatment of chronic pressure ulcers. *Lancet* 1992; 339:23–25.

145. Rodeheaver GT, Pettry D, Thacker JG, Edgerton MT, Edlich RF: Wound cleaning by high pressure irrigation. *Surg Gynecol Obstet* 1975; 141:357–362.

146. Sugarman B: Infection and pressure sores. *Arch Phys Med Rehabil* 1985; 66:177–179.

147. Sapico FL, Ginunas VJ, Thornhill-Joyner M, et al: Quantitative microbiology of pressure sores in different stages of healing. *Diag Microbiol Infect Dis* 1986; 5:31–38.

148. Ehrenkranz NJ, Alfonso B, Nerenberg D: Irrigation-aspiration for culturing draining decubitus ulcers: Correlation of bacteriological findings with a clinical inflammatory scoring index. *J Clin Microbiol* 1990; 28:2389–2393.

149. Daltrey DC, Rhodes B, Chattwood JG: Investigation into microbial flora of healing and non-healing decubitus ulcers. *J Clin Pathol* 1981; 34:701–705.

150. Baker PG, Haig G: Metronidazole in the treatment of chronic pressure sores and ulcers. *Practitioner* 1981; 225:561–573.

151. Gomulin IH, Brandt JL: Topical metronidazole therapy

for pressure ulcers of geriatric patients. *J Am Geriatr Soc* 1983; 31:710–712.

152. Firooznia H, Rafii M, Golimbu C, et al: Computerized tomography of pressure sores, pelvic abscess, and osteomyelitis in patients with spinal cord injury. *Arch Phys Med Rehabil* 1982; 63:545–548.

153. Firooznia H, Rafaii M, Golimbu C, Sokolow J: Computerized tomography in diagnosis of pelvic abscess in spinal-cord-injured patients. *Comput Radiol* 1983; 7:335–341.

154. Sugarman B: Pressure sores and underlying bone infection. *Arch Int Med* 1987; 147:553–555.

155. Thornhill-Joynes M, Gonzales F, Stewart CA, et al: Osteomyelitis associated with pressure ulcers. *Arch Phys Med Rehabil* 1986; 67:314–318.

156. Rissing JP, Crowder JG, Dunfee T, White A: Bacteroides bacteremia from decubitus ulcers. *So Med J* 1974; 67:1179–1182.

157. Berkwits L, Yarkony GM, Lewis V: Marjolin's ulcer complicating a pressure ulcer: case report and literature review. *Arch Phys Med Rehabil* 1986; 67:831–833.

158. Dumurgier C, Pujol G, Chevalley J, et al: Pressure sore carcinoma: A late but fulminant complication of pressure sores in spinal cord injury patients case report. *Paraplegia* 1991; 29:390–395.

159. Treves N, Pack GT: Development of cancer in burn scars: Analysis and report of thirty-four cases. *Surg Gynecol Obstet* 1930; 51:749–782.

160. Schlosser RJ, Kanar EA, Harkins HN: Surgical significance of Marjolin's ulcer with report of three cases. *Surgery* 1956; 39:645–653.

161. Giblin T, Pickrell K, Pitts W, Armstrong D: Malignant degeneration in burn scars: Marjolin's ulcer. *Ann Surg* 1965; 162:291–297.

162. Bereston ES, Ney C: Squamous cell carcinoma arising in chronic osteomyelitic sinus tract with metastasis. *Arch Surg* 1941; 43:257–268.

163. Dunn JE Jr, Levin EA, Linden G, Harzfeld L: Skin cancer as cause of death. *Cal Med* 1965; 102:361–363.

164. Fitzgerald RH, Brewer NS, Dahlin DC: Squamous-cell carcinoma complicating chronic osteomyelitis. *J Bone Joint Surg (Am)* 1976; 58:1146–1148.

165. Johnson LL, Kempson RK: Epidermoid carcinoma in chronic osteomyelitis: Diagnostic problems and management: Report of ten cases. *J Bone Surg (Am)* 1965; 47:133–145.

166. McNally AK, Dockerty MB: Carcinoma developing in chronic draining cutaneous sinuses and draining cutaneous sinuses and fistulas. *Surg Gynecol Obstet* 1949; 88:87–96.

167. Taylor GW, Nathanson IT, Shaw DT: Epidermoid carcinoma of extremities with reference to lymph node involvement. *Ann Surg* 1941; 113:268–275.

168. Glass RL, Spratt JS Jr, Perez-Mesa C: Fate of inadequately excised epidermoid carcinoma of skin. *Surg Gynecol Obstet* 1966; 122:245–248.

169. Kucahn JO, Robson MC, Hegers JP, Ko F: Comparison

of silver sulfadizine, povidine iodine, and physiodesic saline in the treatment of chronic pressure ulcers. *J Am Geriatr Soc* 1981; 29:232–235.

170. Davis JS: The operative treatment of scars following bedsores. *Surgery* 1938; 3:1–7.

171. Conway H, Griffith BH: Plastic surgery for closure of decubitus ulcers in patients. *Am J Surg* 1956; 91:946–975.

172. Disa JJ, Carlton JM, Goldburg NH: Efficacy of operative care in pressure sore patients. *Plast Surg* 1992; 89:272–278.

173. Spear SI, Kroll SS, Little JW III: Bilateral upper-quadrant (intercostal) flaps the value of protective sensation in preventing pressure sore recurrence. *Plast Reconstr Surg* 1987; 80:734–736.

174. Daniel RK, Terzis JK, Cunningham DM: Sensory skin flaps for coverage of pressure sores in paraplegic patients: A preliminary report. *Plast Reconstr Surg* 1976; 58:317–328.

175. Dibbell DG: Use of a long island flap to bring sensation to the sacral area in young paraplegics. *Plast Reconstr Surg* 1974; 54:220–223.

176. Lawton RL, DePinto V: Bilateral hip disarticulation in paraplegics with decubitus ulcers. *Arch Surg* 1987; 122:1040–1043.

177. Chase RA, White WL: Bilateral amputation and rehabilitation of paraplegics. *Plast Reconstr Surg* 1959; 24:445–455.

178. Hackler RH, Zampiers TA: Urethal complications following ischiecomy in spinal cord injury patients: A urethal pressure study. *J Urol* 1987; 137:253–255.

Chapter 22

CEREBELLAR TREMOR AND ATAXIA

Charles R. Smith

Few in the field of rehabilitation would argue that the patient with cerebellar impairment presents a particularly challenging problem. Cerebellar symptoms can be a significant source of disability. Unfortunately, rehabilitation strategies are often limited. All too frequently, attempts at rehabilitation are unsuccessful despite genuine and concerted efforts. Although a variety of drugs have been alleged to improve cerebellar tremor, which is a cause of severe disability, responses often are unpredictable, and many therapeutic claims are unconfirmed by others. Because of these difficulties, some rehabilitation specialists avoid patients with cerebellar symptoms, adopting a pessimistic attitude. They believe that such patients are refractory to treatment, and many are denied access to rehabilitation.

In this chapter, the rehabilitation approach for the patient with cerebellar symptoms is considered, focusing primarily on cerebellar tremor and ataxia. Brief discussions of relevant cerebellar anatomy and physiology will be followed by a description of cerebellar symptoms and the pathophysiology of cerebellar tremor. The rehabilitative strategies for the patient with cerebellar symptoms will follow, including medical management, physical and occupational therapy, and recent advances in assistive technology.

NEUROANATOMY

The cerebellum is divided into three functional subdivisions. The vestibulocerebellum, which includes the flocculonodular lobe, has reciprocal connections with the vestibular complex of the pons. It is primarily concerned with coordination of eye movements and truncal stability. The cerebellar hemispheres, which contain the other two functional subdivisions, can be conceptualized as containing three sagittally arranged zones on each side: a midline zone (or vermis), an intermediate zone, and a lateral zone.[1] The second functional subdivision, also called the spinocerebellum, includes the midline and intermediate zones. The inputs to the spinocerebellum, as its name suggests, come from the spinal cord. Clinically, the midline zone is primarily associated with disorders of stance, gait, truncal stability, and head posture. Lesions of the intermediate zone, especially on the left, can cause disturbances of speech.[2]

The third functional subdivision, the cerebrocerebellum, is represented by the lateral zone. The cerebrocerebellum plays a special role in planning and initiation of movement.[3] Dysfunction of the lateral zone or its connections may cause several movement disorders: the latency to make volitional movements is increased, normally smooth movements become irregular causing incoordination, and rhythmic oscillations may be induced by goal-directed movement or with maintenance of antigravity postures.

The cerebellar cortex is composed of three layers: the outermost molecular layer, containing the stellate and basket cells; the granular layer, which is innermost and primarily populated by densely packed granule cells; and the Purkinje cells, a monolayer of large, flask-shaped neurons between the molecular and the granular layers. The cells of the molecular and granular layers make synaptic connections with the dendrites of the Purkinje cells.

The primary inputs to the cerebellum include the mossy fibers and the climbing fibers. The mossy fibers emanate from the spinocerebellar tracts and many brain stem nuclei, including the pontine and trigeminal nuclei, vestibular complex, and reticular formation. Fibers from the pontine nuclei relay information from the cerebral cortex, permitting the cerebral cortex to modulate lateral zone activity. The mossy fibers terminate in the granular layer of the cerebellar cortex. Climbing fibers originate in the inferior olivary complex and send their terminals to the molecular layer of the cerebellar cortex, where they synapse on dendrites of the Purkinje cells. Both mossy and climbing fibers send collaterals to the deep cerebellar nuclei.

The paired, deep cerebellar nuclei constitute the cells of origin for the primary outflow tracts from the cerebellum. The largest and most lateral of these, the dentate nuclei, receive their inputs from the Purkinje cells (except those afferents from the vermis), the inferior olives, and other brain stem nuclei. The axons of the dentate cells make up a large part of the dentatorubrothalamic tract, the principal pathway through which the cerebrocerebellum influences the motor and premotor cortex of the frontal lobes.

The fastigial nuclei, the most medially placed, receive afferents from the spinal cord and some brain stem nuclei and send efferents to the vestibular complex and reticular formation. The emboliform and globose nuclei, which together lie between the fastigial and dentate nuclei (hence the collective term *interposed nuclei*), receive their afferents from the inferior olivary complex and the red nucleus and send their projections primarily to the red nucleus. Purkinje cells in the vermis project to the fastigial nuclei and, from the intermediate zones, to the globose and emboliform nuclei to influence ongoing execution of limb movement.

SYMPTOMS OF CEREBELLAR DYSFUNCTION

If the cerebellar hemispheres are affected, patients complain of clumsiness or abnormal movements of the upper limb on the side of the lesion. With subtle lesions, patients may first notice problems requiring fine motor control, such as writing, or fastening buttons and earrings. With more-extensive involvement, difficulties will be noticed when reaching for objects. Lesions of the dentate nucleus or its projections, including the superior cerebellar peduncle, can lead to even-more-severe dif-

ficulties because of tremor that may make many activities of daily living difficult or even impossible.

The most frequently recognized complaint associated with cerebellar lesions is gait imbalance. Typically, patients describe their gait as drunken. They may also use the imprecise term "dizzy." Falling is common, especially when attempting to turn. When the lesion is lateralized to one cerebellar hemisphere, patients tend to fall ipsilateral to the involved side. If the lesion is in the cerebellar outflow tract after its decussation in the inferior midbrain, the gait abnormality will be appreciated on the side opposite the lesion and may be conjoined with hemiparesis if the adjacent cerebral peduncle or posterior limb of the internal capsule also is involved. With more-severe impairment, patients may be unable to stand or sit without support.

Speech and swallowing also are frequently affected by cerebellar disease. Patients report that their speech is slurred, which may be severe enough to interfere significantly with communication. When swallowing problems are added, patients describe choking or coughing after swallowing. For many, liquids may be the source of the greatest difficulty.

SIGNS OF CEREBELLAR DISEASE

The cardinal signs of cerebellar dysfunction include reduced muscle tone, incoordination of voluntary movement, and impairment of truncal stability and gait. Involvement of the upper limbs is commonly observed with more laterally placed cerebellar hemisphere lesions and their connections. The classic clinical abnormalities are hypotonia, ataxia, and incoordination. The terms *dysmetria, dyssynergia,* and *dysdiadokokinesia* are often used interchangeably with *ataxia*. All refer essentially to the same phenomenon; that is, abnormalities in range, rate, and force of voluntary movement.[4]

Hypotonia is frequently most obvious in acute cerebellar hemispheric lesions and is appreciated less often in more chronic lesions. Several bedside tests can determine if subtle hypotonia is present. For example, when the upper limbs are extended with the hands in the prone position, there may be "spooning" of the hand on the side of the lesion, characterized by slight flexion of the wrist and extension of the metacarpalphalangeal joints. There may be a subtle limpness of the affected hand, especially noticeable when the hand is shaken and compared to the normal side. When the outstretched upper limbs are tapped, there is a wider excursion of displacement on the affected side, indicating inadequate fixation because of reduced tone at the shoulder. Hypotonia may contribute to disability, but its impact usually is difficult to separate from that of other coincidental cerebellar impairments.

Patients with cerebellar disease cannot quickly or accurately change from one voluntary motor activity to another, especially if the new activity is diametrically opposite to the first. The inability to smoothly execute rapid, alternating movements is called dysdiadoko-kinesia. In the upper limbs, it is commonly tested at the bedside by asking the patient to rapidly tap, regularly alternating between supination and pronation, one hand on the other. The unpredictable decomposition of rate, force, and rhythm is readily apparent. Rapid tapping of the one heel on the opposite knee demonstrates the same phenomenon in the lower limbs.

Cerebellar tremor associated with goal-directed motor activities, such as reaching for an object, is termed *intention (kinetic or action) tremor*. Typical cerebellar intention tremor is 3 to 5 Hz and is coarse and somewhat irregular. It worsens as the limb approaches the target. It can be adequately demonstrated by asking the patient to perform the finger-to-nose test in the upper limbs or the heel-knee-shin test in the lower limbs. It is important to have the patient fully extend their limb when doing the finger-to-nose test, as the tremor is most pronounced when the limb is in this position. Intention tremor can be a source of severe disability.

Postural tremor, so called because it is most reliably induced by maintaining the limb in an antigravity posture, often occurs coincidentally with intention tremor and both may cumulatively increase disability. A third type of tremor, titubation, involves the trunk, including the head, and occurs at rest. Associated with it may be tremor of speech. Titubation is more rhythmic, whereas intention and postural tremor are not true sinusoidal oscillations but are somewhat irregular. Resting tremor can occur with cerebellar disease but is uncommon. It is quite different from the resting tremor seen in Parkinson's disease, a condition in which resting tremor is regularly associated.

Dysmetria, referred to as serial dysmetria by Sabra and Hallett, presents as a low-frequency, irregular tremorlike movement.[5] Typically, patients with dysmetria, like those with intention tremor, will overshoot or undershoot their target. Because the frequency of the tremor is low, however, compensatory adjustments seem more successful. Frequently, dysmetria by itself is less a source of impairment than kinetic or postural tremor, but there are frequent exceptions. As for intention tremor, dysmetria can be readily evaluated on the finger-to-nose test in the upper limbs or the heel-knee-shin test in the lower limbs.

Cerebellar gait disturbances, referred to as gait ataxia, result from postural instability and incoordination of lower limb movements. Patients typically lurch from side to side and, to lower the center of gravity, walk with their feet spaced widely apart. Performing a tandem gait is frequently impossible for all but the most minimally impaired. Even those with mild impairment walk apprehensively and often will do so only with another's support or a gait aid. When the disturbance of function is more severe, standing with the feet close together will cause the patient to sway and fall, whether or not the eyes are open. Truncal instability independent of visual cues helps to distinguish sensory ataxia resulting from dorsal column disease or peripheral neuropathy (rombergism).

When gait ataxia is the primary cerebellar problem, the lesion usually is traced to the midline region of the cerebellum (anterior superior vermis). However, more laterally placed bilateral lesions can also be responsible. Coincident cerebellar signs in the upper limbs will indicate that the lesion is more extensive.

Other common signs of cerebellar dysfunction include ipsilateral head tilt, slurred or scanning speech, and a variety of ocular motility problems, including nystagmus, ocular dysmetria, and opsoclonus. Weakness is not a feature of cerebellar disease, although patients may use this term to describe their symptoms. Deep tendon reflexes may be pendular in cerebellar disease, but not as frequently as medical textbooks might suggest.

PATHOPHYSIOLOGY OF CEREBELLAR TREMOR

Tremor may be defined as a more or less rhythmic oscillation of a body part around a fixed point. Although the exact pathology responsible for intention tremor is unknown, the cerebellar outflow pathways, including the dentate nucleus and the superior cerebellar peduncle, are frequently implicated.[6]

Studies in laboratory animals have provided considerable insight into the mechanisms of cerebellar tremor. Gilman, Carr, and Hollenberg performed cerebellar ablations in macaque monkeys and observed ipsilateral 4 to 5 Hz tremor with goal-directed movements in the upper extremities that worsened as the hand approached its target.[7] The tremor was not abolished by dorsal rhizotomy, indicating that the movement disorder was not modulated by stretch-reflex pathways.

Vilis and Hore, however, showed that stretch-reflex oscillation may play a role in the genesis of cerebellar tremor.[8] They demonstrated that the frequency of cerebellar tremor induced by reversible cooling of the deep cerebellar nuclei of awake and unanesthetized monkeys using implantable electrodes could be increased by the addition of spring loads to the limbs or decreased by inertial limb loads. This is strong supportive evidence that specific cerebellar lesions may alter the function of somatosensory reflex pathways.

Cerebellar intention tremor may result from an inability to make appropriate correctional movements following a movement error. These inappropriate corrections lead to further errors, resulting in a series of oscillations collectively observed as intention tremor. Specifically, intention tremor results from the absence of phase-advanced information necessary for the limb to stop on target.[9] The absence of this information allows the limb to pass by the target until stretching of the antagonist muscles initiates movement termination.

As cerebellar intention tremor is associated with precise voluntary movement, long-loop reflexes and higher motor control centers also may play a contributory role. With the execution of a voluntary movement, the dentate and interposed nuclei of the cerebellum and the lateral zones of the cerebellar hemispheres (cerebrocerebellum) receive efferent information from the frontal and parietal lobes by way of the nuclei of the basis pontis, pontine reticular formation, and the inferior olives.[10] Normally, impulses from the cerebellum precede, and thereby regulate, those from the motor cortex regarding the initiation and termination of voluntary movement.[11] Since the cerebellum also receives somatosensory feedback through the spinocerebellar pathways, providing an ongoing analysis of the dynamics and kinematics of motor activity, the cerebellum is poised for the optimization of movement based on internal desires, prior experience, and external constraints. With the cerebellum, the nervous system is capable of using sensory feedback to anticipate deviations from the desired movement and is thereby capable of formulating an effective response to external and internal disturbances. Cerebellar dysfunction disrupts this control process and compromises voluntary control of intentional movements.

As a number of segmental and transcortical neural loops are under the influence of cerebellar modulation, oscillation in one or more of these loops could be responsible for cerebellar tremor. Lesions of the deep cerebellar nuclei or their outflow pathways, but not the cerebellar cortex alone, have been shown to be sufficient to produce intention tremor. Other pathophysiologic mechanisms almost certainly exist. These different mechanisms conceivably could be distinguished by their unique characteristics or "fingerprints" on quantitative motor testing.

Serial dysmetria, another cerebellar movement disorder, may create the appearance of an irregular tremor and is due to successive inaccurate movements during goal-directed behavior.[5] This also results from an inability to make appropriate correctional movements following a movement error. Attempts to correct prior mistakes lead to further errors, which collectively are observed as an irregular, slow tremor. It is distinguished from intention tremor in that serial dysmetria is of low frequency and not rhythmic, and therefore not a tremor in the strict sense.

There have been very few analyses of cerebellar movement disorders in human subjects. Rondot and Bathien evaluated patients with several cerebellar disorders and observed an increase in reaction time and a delay in the contraction of the antagonist muscles during goal-directed motor behavior.[12] In their review of 11 multiple sclerosis (MS) patients, Sabra and Hallett distinguished two groups of patients presenting with cerebellar tremor and three distinct types of tremor: serial dysmetria, intention tremor, and postural tremor.[5] They used electromyography (EMG) to measure tremor frequency and averaged EMG burst-duration in agonist and antagonist muscles to categorize each tremor type. The first group did not have postural tremor but did have a low amplitude intention tremor ranging from 5 to 8 Hz. Serial dysmetria, however, appeared to be the major functional problem for these patients. The second patient group had large amplitude postural tremor that persisted and worsened with intention. They labeled this combination of postural tremor and intention tremor "action tremor," which ranged from 2.5 to 4 Hz. Serial dysmetria was also a considerable problem for these patients.

REHABILITATION OF CEREBELLAR SYMPTOMS

In the most general terms, the rehabilitation specialist confronts three general categories of functional impairment in patients with cerebellar disease: upper limb incoordination; truncal instability affecting sitting, standing, and gait; and speech and swallowing disorders. Upper limb cerebellar tremor, either postural, intention, or both, can be a source of severe disability. The most

tions provide unsatisfactory relief of the symptoms. Occupational therapists are particularly focused in teaching compensatory skills for upper limb impairments. For example, the occupational therapist can instruct the patient to use the unaffected upper limb to assist the involved extremity when feeding, grooming, and dressing. The occupational therapist also can try the myriad equipment adaptations that can compensate for upper limb incoordination. These tools include: modified eating utensils, for example, weighted cutlery, rocker knives, covered drinking cups, nonskid placemats, and various feeding devices; grooming aids such as electric toothbrushes, electric razors, and modified hair brushes; dressing aids including the liberal use of Velcro® fasteners, and weighted button hooks. There are many other gadgets and compensatory adaptations, both in the home and workplace, that a clever and resourceful occupational therapist can devise to maximize independence and self-esteem.

Intention tremor has sometimes been improved by the application of lead-containing Velcro® wrist or ankle weights.[29,30] The weights, typically between 240 and 720 grams in the upper limb applications, may function, at least in part, by increasing proprioceptive awareness during limb activities. They may also assist in dampening other unwanted movements interfering with desired task completion. Greatest benefit is observed in those with moderate tremor, whereas function is frequently worsened in patients with mild or very severe tremor. Further, these attempts often result in fatigue, especially in patients who are also weak. Although always worth trying, wrist weights are rarely effective enough for most patients to persist in using them, and those with the most severe intention tremor are not helped at all.

Assistive Technology   Other mechanical methods of restoring independence have become increasingly pursued in recent years, and have been reviewed recently by Michaelis.[31] Robotic devices, such as page turners that respond to the push of a button, are quite acceptable but, at mealtime, many patients prefer to be fed by another person rather than a machine. Most of these feeding instruments also are prohibitively expensive. Another approach, esthetically more acceptable to a broader range of patients, is the elimination of relatively high frequency oscillations, such as intention tremor, by mechanical methods. For example, viscous damping can successfully reduce the impact of unwanted movements while permitting the desired activity. These techniques function essentially as shock absorbers. Such viscous

dampers are now commercially available to assist with feeding (e.g., Neater Eater) or operating a computer (e.g., MouseTRAP).[31] There is evidence to suggest that viscous damping may not only reduce the amplitude of oscillation resulting from intention tremor, but that the feedback effects may actually decrease the severity of the tremor force.[31] Other experimental devices use computer-controlled systems, such as computer-controlled magnetic particle brakes.[32]

Truncal Ataxia

Midline cerebellar dysfunction results in defective control of posture and gait instability. Truncal adjustments necessary for the execution of limb movements are impaired and contribute to limb incoordination. Normal postural control requires the coordinated contraction of the muscles of the head and trunk to ensure stability of the body against gravitational forces. Otherwise, balance will be compromised, and the patient will topple over while seated or fall while standing. As for the limbs, the cerebellum receives information regarding the position of the trunk muscles through joint receptors, muscle spindles, and cutaneous afferents, so that moment-to-moment adjustments can be made to maintain stability.

Physical Therapy   There are no pharmacologic treatments to alleviate gait ataxia. When it appears that gait has become hazardous or inefficient, the patient should be referred for physical therapy. The physical therapist focuses on developing truncal stability before teaching functional gait. Training of neck control is followed, in order of development, by training of independent trunk balance and motion, training of the upper extremities for protective extension and support to balance the trunk, hip balance and motion, knee balance and motion, and free standing.[27]

Safety is the primary initial objective. Gait training for patients with ataxia impaired enough to compromise safety begins with learning balance control and how to recover from sudden loss of balance. Only after the patient has mastered truncal stability, weight shifting, and recovery should functional gait be attempted. If gait is attempted before these skills have been mastered, injury may result, and progress may be hampered.

To improve postural stability, the physical therapist will utilize a variety of different weight-bearing antigravity postures, depending on the degree of impairment. These include lying prone with the elbows supporting the upper trunk, sitting, standing on all fours, kneeling, and standing upright on two feet and then

Table 22-1
Frenkel's exercises

Exercises while supine

The patient lies on a bed or plinth with a smooth surface along which the heels may slide easily. A caster shoe rolling on a large board positioned under the lower extremities may be used to make the activities easier by reducing friction. The various motions to be practiced may be indicated by lines painted on the board. The head should be supported so that the patient can see the legs and feet.

1. Flex the hip and knee of one extremity, sliding the heel along in contact with the bed. Return to the original position. Repeat with the opposite extremity.
2. Flex as in exercise 1. Then abduct the flexed hip. Return to the flexed position and then to the original position.
3. Flex the hip and knee only halfway and then return to the extended position. Add abduction and adduction.
4. Flex one limb at the hip and knee, stopping at any point in flexion or extension on command.
5. Flex both lower extremities simultaneously and equally; add abduction, adduction, and extension.
6. Flex both lower extremities simultaneously to the halfway position; add abduction and adduction to the half-flexed position. Extend. Stop in the pattern on command.
7. Flex one extremity at the hip and knee with the heel held 2 in above the bed. Return to the original position.
8. Flex as in exercise 7. Bring the heel to rest on the opposite patella. Successively add patterns so that the heel is touched to the middle of the shin, to the ankle, to the toes of the opposite foot, to the bed on either side of the knee, and to the bed on either side of the leg.
9. Flex as in exercise 7 and then touch the heel successively to the patella, shin, ankle, and toes. Reverse the pattern.
10. Flex as in exercise 7 and then on command touch the heel to the point indicated by the therapist.
11. Flex the hip and knee with the heel 2 in above the bed. Place the heel on the opposite patella and slowly slide it down the crest of the tibia to the ankle. Reverse.
12. Use the pattern in exercise 11, but slide the heel down the crest of the opposite tibia, over the ankle and foot to the toes. If the heel is to reach the toes, the opposite knee must be flexed slightly during this exercise. Stop in the pattern of command.

Table 22-1
Frenkel's exercises (Continued)

Exercises while supine

13. With malleoli and knees in apposition, flex both lower extremities simultaneously with the heels 2 in above the bed. Return to the original position. Stop in the pattern on command.
14. Perform reciprocal flexion and extension of the lower extremities with the heels touching the bed.
15. Perform reciprocal flexion and extension of the lower extremities with the heels 2 in above the bed.
16. Perform bilateral simultaneous flexion, abduction, adduction, and extension with the heels 2 in above the bed.
17. Place the heel precisely where the therapist indicates with the finger on the bed or the opposite extremity.
18. Follow with the toe the movement of the therapist's finger in any combination of lower extremity motion.

Exercises while sitting

1. Practice maintaining correct sitting posture for two minutes in an armchair with the back supported and the feet flat on the floor. Repeat in a chair without arms. Repeat without back support.
2. Mark time to the counting of the therapist by raising only the heel from the floor. Progress to alternatively lifting the entire foot and replacing it precisely in a marked position on the floor.
3. Make two cross marks on the floor with chalk. Alternately glide the foot over the marked cross; forward, backward, left and right.
4. Practice rising from and sitting on a chair to the therapist's counted cadence: (a) Flex the knees and draw the feet under the front edge of the seat. (b) Bend the trunk forward over the thighs. (c) Rise by extending the knees and hips and then straightening the trunk. (d) Bend the trunk forward slightly. (e) Flex the hips and knees to sit. (f) Straighten the trunk and sit back in the chair.

Exercises while standing

1. Walking sideways. Balance is easier during sidewards walking because the patient does not have to pivot over the toes or heels, which decreases the base of support. The exercise is performed to a counted cadence: (a) Shift the weight to the left foot. (b) Place the right foot 12 in to the right. Shift the weight to the right foot. (d) Bring the left foot over to the right foot. The size of the step taken to the right or left may be varied.

Table 22-1
Frenkel's exercises (Continued)

Exercises while standing

---

2. Walk forward between two parallel lines 14 inches apart, placing the right foot just inside the right line and the left foot just inside the left line. Emphasize correct placement. Rest after 10 steps.

3. Walk forward, placing each foot on a footprint traced on the floor. Footprints should be parallel and 2 inches lateral to the midline. Practice with quarter steps, half steps, three-quarter steps, and full steps.

4. Turning. (a) Raise the right toe and rotate the right foot outward, pivoting on the heel. (b) Raise the left heel and pivot the left leg inward on the toes. Bring the left foot up beside the right.

---

one foot. Specific exercise techniques are taught that facilitate stability by including truncal muscles and joints as well as muscles and joints of the limbs. As improvement occurs, dynamic postural responses can be challenged by incorporating controlled mobility activities such as weight shifting, moving in and out of postures, or movement transitions. The patient can practice such activities as supine-to-sit, sit-to-stand, or scooting on a mat. Distal extremity movements can be superimposed on proximal stability to further challenge control.

Once the necessary balance skills have been mastered through practice, functional gait training should start. If balance control has not been attained before walking is initiated, gait is lurching, hazardous, and fatiguing. Therefore, the ability to maintain balance should be the primary focus during the initial period of gait training.

The first gait exercise is standing on both feet with balance provided by the upper limbs. The patient then learns to shift weight from one foot to the other and establish balance while bearing full weight on one lower limb. The upper limbs are used only to maintain balance. This is followed by walking with a walker and, if possible, crutches, with one or two canes, and, finally, without gait aids.

The individual components of gait are practiced in a protected environment until mastered. When needed, selective external stabilization, such as the use of parallel bars, is provided to maintain safety and to permit the patient to focus on learning the component of gait being practiced. Practice should continue until each component has been mastered and becomes automatic.

Patients frequently become frustrated with the slowness of their progress. Many complain that they are not proceeding at a fast enough pace and become impatient. The therapist must be constantly alert to the frustration experienced by the patient and provide ongoing encouragement. Otherwise, the patient will not learn the components of gait in their proper sequence and, worse yet, may learn mistakes that will be more difficult to undo once they have become fixed.

Gait Aids   The therapist will also need to determine what adaptations are needed to ensure safe and efficient gait. For many, a simple cane or a quad cane may be all that is necessary. However, for others, a walker will be required. Many patients with mild to moderate ataxia will walk quite well with a rolling walker such as the Nova®. Those who have significant tremor or more severe degrees of truncal instability will have more difficulty using any type of gait aid and may require a wheelchair. Patients with significant ataxia rarely do well with forearm crutches, and for most this is not a safe option.

Frenkel's Exercises   Frenkel's exercises (Table 22-1) have been suggested for the treatment of ataxia. This series of exercises of increasing difficulty, from simple movements with gravity eliminated to more complicated patterns, improves lower extremity proprioceptive control. The exercises are done in each of four positions: lying, sitting, standing, walking. By careful concentration and by slow repetition, some degree of coordination may be restored by the utilization of other senses. If proprioceptive impairment is severe, visual cues are substituted.

These exercises are physiologically sound insofar as they use total patterns, righting reflexes, and stabilization mechanisms while stressing prime movements. Some of Frenkel's exercises also stress normal daily activities. However, their greatest value is in compensating for loss of proprioception by enhancing visual cues. Success is thus limited when dysfunction arises from cerebellar lesions.[34]

REFERENCES

1. Jansen J, Brodal A: *Aspects of Cerebellar Anatomy.* Oslo: Gruntd Tanum, 1954.
2. Amarenco P, Chevrie-Muller C, Roullet E, et al: Paravermal infarct and isolated cerebellar dysarthria. *Ann Neurol* 1991; 30:211–213.

3. Allen GI, Tsukahara N: Cerebrocerebellar communication systems. *Physiol Rev* 1974; 54:957–1006.

4. Holmes G: The cerebellum of man. *Brain* 1939; 62:1–30.

5. Sabra AF, Hallett M: Action tremor with alternating activities in antagonist muscles. *Neurology* (Cleveland) 1984; 34:151–156.

6. Fahn S: Cerebellar tremor: Clinical aspects, in Findley LJ, Capildeo R (eds): *Movement Disorders: Tremor.* London: Macmillan, 1984, pp. 355–363.

7. Gilman S, Carr D, Hollenberg J: Kinematic effects of deafferentation and cerebellar ablation. *Brain* 1976; 99:311–330.

8. Vilis T, Hore J: Effects of changes in mechanical state of limb on cerebellar intention tremor. *J Neurophysiol* 1977; 40:1214–1224.

9. Vilis T, Hore J: Central neural mechanisms contributing to cerebellar tremor produced by limb perturbations. *J Neurophysiol* 1980; 43:279–291.

10. Ghez C: The cerebellum, in Kandel ER, Schwartz JH, Jessell TM (eds): *Principles of Neural Science*, 3rd ed. New York: Elsevier, 1991, pp. 626–646.

11. Meyer-Lohmann J, Hore J, Brooks VB: Cerebellar participation in generation of prompt arm movements. *J Neurophysiol* 1977; 40:1038–1050.

12. Rondot P, Bathien N: Motor control in cerebellar tremor, in Findley LJ, Capildeo R (eds): *Movement Disorders: Tremor.* London: Macmillan, 1984, pp. 365–376.

13. Wade DT: *Measurement in Neurological Rehabilitation.* Oxford: Oxford Medical Publications, 1992.

14. Hauser SL, Dawson DM, Lehrich JR, et al: Intensive immunosuppression in progressive multiple sclerosis: A randomized, three-arm study of high-dose intravenous cyclophosphamide, plasma exchange, and ACTH. *N Engl J Med* 1983; 308:173–180.

15. Collen FM, Wade DT, Bradshaw CM: Mobility afer stroke: Reliabilty of measures of impairment and disability. *Int Dis Stud* 1990; 12:6–9.

16. Mathiowetz V, Weber K, Kashman N, et al: Adult norms for the nine-hole peg test of finger dexterity. *Occup Ther J Res* 1985; 5:24–37.

17. Kurtzke JF: Rating neurological impairment in multiple sclerosis: An Expanded Disability Status Scale (EDSS). *Neurology* 1983; 33:1444–1452.

18. Sabra AF, Hallett M, Sudarski L, et al: Treatment of action tremor in multiple sclerosis with isoniazid. *Neurology* 1982; 32:912–913.

19. Hallett M, Lindsay JW, Dov Adelstein B, et al: Double-blind trial of isoniazid for severe postural tremor in patients with multiple sclerosis. *Neurology* 1984; 34(suppl I):128.

20. Duquette P, Pleines J, du Souich P: Isoniazid for tremor in multiple sclerosis: A controlled study. *Neurology* 1985; 35:1772–1775.

21. Jancovic J: The clinical spectrum and treatment of tremors. *Neuroview* 1986; 2:1–6.

22. Trelles L, Trelles JO, Castro C, et al: Successful treatment of two cases of intention tremor with clonazepam. *Ann Neurol* 1984; 16:621.

23. Jancovic J, Schwartz K: Botulin toxin treatment of tremors. *Neurology* 1991; 41:1185–1188.

24. Cooper IS: Neurosurgical treatment of the dyskinesias. *Clin Neurosurg* 1977; 24:367–390.

25. Richardson RR: Rehabilitative neurosurgery: Posttraumatic syndromes. *Stereotac Funct Neurosurg* 1989; 53:105–112.

26. Brice J, McLelland DL: Suppression of cerebellar ataxia by contingent electrical stimulation in the basal ganglia. *Lancet* 1980; 1:1221–1222.

27. Kottke FJ: Therapeutic exercise to develop neuromuscular coordination, in Kottke FJ, Lehmann JF (eds): *Krusen's Handbook of Physical Medicine and Rehabilitation,* 4th ed. Philadelphia: WB Saunders, 1990, pp. 452–479.

28. Brooks VB, Thach WT: Cerebellar control of posture and movement, in Brooks VB (ed): *Handbook of Physiology, Section 1: The Nervous System,* vol. II. *Motor Control,* Part 2. Bethesda, MD: American Physiological Society, 1981, pp. 877–946.

29. Chase RA, Cullen JK, Sullivan SA, et al: Modification of intention tremor in man. *Nature* (London) 1965; 206:485–487.

30. Haver RL, Cooper R, Morgan MH: An investigation into the value of treating intention tremor by weighting the affected limb. *Brain* 1972; 95:579–590.

31. Michaelis J: Mechanical methods of controlling ataxia. *Balliere's Clin Neurol* 1993; 2:121–139.

32. Rosen MJ, Arnold AS, Baiges IJ, et al: Design of a controlled energy-dissipation orthosis (CEDO) for functional suppression of intention tremors. *J Rehab Res* 1995; 32:1–16.

33. Frankel HS: *The Treatment of Tabetic Ataxia* (Freyberger L, trans). Philadelphia: Blakiston's, 1902.

34. Cailliet R: Exercise in multiple sclerosis, in Basmajian IV (ed): *Therapeutic Exercise.* Baltimore: Williams & Wilkins, 1984, pp. 407–420.

Chapter 23

FATIGUE AND REHABILITATION OF NEUROLOGIC DISORDERS

Jack H. Petajan

THE PERCEPTION OF FATIGUE

In association with most illnesses that bring people to the doctor, fatigue is a common complaint. The observation that there is a specific disease and then a separate state of being "sick" is very likely dependent, to a considerable extent, upon the fatigue that accompanies stimulation of the immune system by infection or injury. Anyone who has experienced dysfunction in any system of the body soon becomes aware of how specific dysfunction soon generalizes to impair nearly every activity of daily living. This generalization sometimes makes it very difficult to discover the specific function that is at fault. This fact alone has major implications for methods of therapy and rehabilitation. It is not enough to focus on correction of a specific dysfunction alone. The impact of the dysfunction on daily life and mechanisms of adaptation must be examined.

An example of how a specific illness might impact the patient is congestive heart failure (CHF), a common source of fatigue. This, of course, is a non-neurological disorder, but the patient may complain of muscle weakness, moderate chest discomfort or tightness, shortness of breath, orthopnea, cough, ankle edema, awareness of heartbeat, sweating, and increased lassitude. Involvement of a number of systems are suggested in these complaints. The chief complaint may be any one of these. If the complaint is that of muscle weakness, then attention may be drawn to the neuromuscular system. If the complaint is lassitude and trouble sleeping, a depressive component may be present. The physical examination will yield important clues to the diagnosis: swollen ankles, venous congestion, rales at the lung bases, and perhaps some evidence of cardiac pathology. Application of the appropriate medical therapy may relieve many of the symptoms that are associated with these complaints. The meaning of the diagnosis to the patient ("My heart is failing. When will this end?") all add up to loss, the consequence of which is depression. There is adjustment of daily activities to accommodate the limits imposed by heart disease. The physician supporting the patient in his or her effort to cope with disability often finds him- or herself in the position of a cognitive therapist providing information, encouragement, and specific philosophical viewpoints that may be helpful in the process of adjustment.

It cannot be emphasized enough that the context within which the illness occurs must be considered carefully. The religious and philosophical beliefs of the patient must be considered as well as historical evidence for prior depression and anxiety disorders requiring medical or psychiatric intervention. It has been demonstrated that individuals with a prior history of such disorders experience more fatigue, less ability to cope, and prolonged recovery following viral infection, as well as enhanced skin reaction to experimental antigens.[1-5] Since the complaint of "fatigue" arises from diverse sources and multiple systems are involved, a detailed history and physical examination will be required to uncover what may be multiple sources for the complaint.

FACTORS CONTRIBUTING TO THE SYMPTOM OF FATIGUE

Psychological Factors

Disorders associated with long-term depression and/or anxiety may predispose to the complaint of fatigue. So-

367

matization, commonly associated with the disorder "borderline personality" and a history of physical or sexual abuse, may result in a long-standing history of fatigue. Interpersonal isolation, and a history of protracted stress, often associated with an extremely rich past medical history, may be obtained. Association with individuals who have been chronically ill or caring for those who are chronically ill may result in a syndrome of identification with the sick patient, resulting in chronic fatigue. There has been insufficient emphasis on the role of modeling "sick" behavior in childhood. Somatization and complaints of fatigue can be multigenerational. This is often detected when obtaining the history in the presence of other family members. Pediatricians are aware of the strong parental influence on reporting symptoms of pain and fatigue by the child.

The sports medicine and exercise literature contain references to the importance of psychological preparation for exercise and the influence of such preparation on training.[6] Maximal effort is influenced by suggestion and group identification. Chronic pain and disability can influence rest and produce mental distractions that diminish the ability to cope with normal daily activities. Measures of the impact of illness such as the Sickness Impact Profile can help to quantify the role of chronic illness on such daily activities as mobility and social interaction.[7]

The perception of illness is extremely important in the production of the symptom of fatigue. The perception of the seriousness of illness has a great impact on the degree of fatigue and disability that results from a particular deficit. It is important to ask a patient to elaborate on his own perception of the cause of his fatigue and the perception of his illness if it has been diagnosed. Cognitive therapy can be applied that can help the patient define some symptoms as more benign than others and less threatening. Fear of isolation and abandonment, pain, and progressing disability, may be the primary contributors to the symptom of fatigue. Along with rehabilitation directed toward a specific disability, psychological counseling and support of the patient and his or her family will be extremely important. Compliance with any rehabilitation program or medical regimen can be improved greatly by attachment to a supportive group.[8–10]

Immune Factors

Fatigue commonly is associated with a wide variety of infections, both acute and chronic. Indeed, a state of fatigue may persist for months following some acute infections. Studies have demonstrated that the administration of specific cytokines can induce the symptom of fatigue.[11] Cytokines such as IL-1 and interferons alpha, beta, and gamma that permit communication between T-cells also may interact directly with the central nervous system to modify behavior and induce the symptom of fatigue.[12] Fatigue in AIDS patients is probably present as a consequence of CNS involvement since no evidence of muscle involvement is usually found.[13] The role of neurokines (cytokines that react with the CNS) in producing fatigue in acquired infections is unknown. There is increasing awareness of the role cytokines may play in producing the symptoms of "sickness" and fatigue that accompany infection. In some illnesses, such as multiple sclerosis, specific cytokines such as interleukin-beta, soluble interleukin 2 receptors, and interleukin 6 have been identified that may be associated with the severe fatigue experienced by 80–90 percent of these patients.[14] Interleukin (IL-1) can interact directly with the diencephalon and can produce fatigue, malaise, muscle pain, and cognitive deficits when administered to patients. Tumor necrosis factor and IL-1 induce slow-wave sleep. These cytokines have been studied extensively in chronic fatigue syndrome (CFS).[11,12,15–21]

Neuroendocrine Factors

Deficiencies of specific hormones, such as cortisol and thyroid hormone, may lead to profound fatigue. Indeed, fatigue and lassitude may be the presenting complaint in these disorders. Too rapid withdrawal of steroid therapy or steroid–induced hypoadrenalism, may result in severe fatigue. Dysautonomia may accompany neuroendocrine disorder, the chief complaint of which is orthostasis. Dysautonomia produces very profound fatigue, which may respond to replacement therapy. Abnormalities of the hypothalamic pituitary adrenal axis have been reported in the chronic fatigue syndrome.[22]

SYSTEMIC ROLE IN FATIGUE

Neuromuscular Systems

The classical disorders that conform best with the physiological definition of fatigue are myasthenia gravis (MG) and the myasthenic syndromes. Decrements in muscle force with repetitive or sustained muscle contraction are found in these disorders. It is common to be able to demonstrate muscle weakness in these patients and to detect the decrement in muscle force on clinical examination applying various maneuvers of muscle testing. The key feature of these disorders is that the muscle weakness and fatigue may be highly focal, mimicking isolated neuropathic or muscular disorders. The muscle weakness is painless and unassociated with paresthesia. A complaint of episodic muscle weakness that cannot be demonstrated on physical examination should raise the concern that MG or myasthenic syndrome is not the correct diagnosis. That MG may be a focal disease, despite the elevation of antibody against the nicotinic acetylcholine receptor, indicates that the antigenicity of the receptor is a mosaic with varying degrees of susceptibility throughout the body.

Motoneuron disease and polyneuropathies, which can affect the level of innervation of skeletal muscle, will produce a shortened exercise tolerance along with weakness. The patient usually complains of significant muscle weakness rather than fatigue but finds that he or she cannot sustain muscle activity for a normal period of time. Repetitive nerve stimulation often reveals a decrement in CMAP amplitude not unlike myasthenia gravis.[23] Severe muscle weakness that reduces the baseline level of force results in a premature loss of function. This effect is relatively more significant than the increased rate of fatigue.[24] The same can be said for a variety of myopathies, including the muscular dystrophies, which can also result in a reduced level of baseline muscle force. A variety of metabolic myopathies produce a decreased exercise tolerance, depending on the specific enzyme abnormality present. For example, myophosphorolase B deficiency diminishes the tolerance to sustained isometric muscle contraction.[25] The patient may be asymptomatic until middle age, when some unaccustomed activity, such as lifting furniture, may result in signs and symptoms of rhabdomyolysis and myoglobinuria. Following this experience the patient may experience other episodes of muscle contracture in association with isometric exercise that limits his or her physical performance. Adenylate deaminase deficiency, another common disorder, may produce muscle aching with exercise that limits exercise performance.[26] Mitochondrial myopathies may limit endurance exercise in a patient, produce small muscles, and yet not impact significantly on activities of daily living. Reduced endurance for physical activity associated with muscle cramps and myoglobinuria characterizes patients with carnitine palmitoyl-transferase deficiency inherited as a recessive trait. Muscle or systemic carnitine deficiency

produces a similar syndrome. In these disorders fatty acid transport into muscle mitochondria is impaired.

The postpolio syndrome or symptoms resulting from the late effects of poliomyelitis include muscle aching and increased fatigue, which usually make their onset in middle age or later.[27] Most patients have adapted to significant muscle weakness by maintaining relatively high levels of physical activity. One view of the decreased exercise tolerance is that during normal aging motor neurons are lost, placing a greater burden on those that remain. The results of studies conflict in supporting this point of view. Occasionally, one will find a patient with normal strength and little or no evidence for chronic neurogenic atrophy who complains of excessive fatigue, with a background of having had poliomyelitis producing paralysis. Encephalitis resulting from poliomyelitis may play a role in the genesis of fatigue. Brain-stem lesions in these patients, especially in the reticular formation, may be of significance.[28]

Muscle-membrane disorders, such as periodic paralysis producing myotonia, are associated with altered exercise tolerance and inability to achieve maximal effort. The physical and electrodiagnostic findings are most helpful in understanding these conditions, which can now be diagnosed by molecular techniques.[29]

Central Nervous System

The CNS disorders that have been studied the most with respect to fatigue are those that affect mobility. Parkinson's disease commonly is associated with reports of fatigue, but there have been few studies to document changes in motor performance over time or that have assessed exercise tolerance.[30] Improved aerobic conditioning in patients with Parkinson's disease may diminish the symptom of fatigue. Other extrapyramidal disorders, especially those that produce ongoing involuntary movements, also are commonly associated with a complaint of fatigue. Not only is there increased muscle activity during the day but an inability to rest.

Fifty to 90 percent of patients with multiple sclerosis complain of severe fatigue that often has a diurnal pattern; in most patients fatigue worsens with increased environmental temperature.[31–34] Cooling techniques, medications, and improvement in aerobic fitness can be important in diminishing the symptom of fatigue. Spinal-cord disease and spinal trauma will produce physical disability, and because the mobility depends to a considerable extent on upper extremity function, excessive

Table 23-1

Sample measures of fatigue

Rand Index of Vitality	*Score*
1. During the past 2 weeks, how much energy, pep, or vitality have you had or felt?	
___ (a) Very full of energy, lots of pep	(6)
___ (b) Fairly energetic most of the time	(5)
___ (c) My energy level varies quite a bit	(4)
___ (d) Generally low in energy, pep	(3)
___ (e) Very low in energy or pep most of the time	(2)
___ (f) No energy or pep at all, I feel drained, sapped	(1)
2. During the past 2 weeks, have you felt tired, worn out, used up, or exhausted?	
___ (a) All of the time	(1)
___ (b) Most of the time	(2)
___ (c) A good bit of the time	(3)
___ (d) Some of the time	(4)
___ (e) A little of the time	(5)
___ (f) None of the time	(6)
3. During the past 2 weeks, have you felt active and vigorous, or dull and sluggish?	
___ (a) Very active, vigorous every day	(6)
___ (b) Mostly active, vigorous; never dull, sluggish	(5)
___ (c) Fairly active, vigorous; seldom dull, sluggish	(4)
___ (d) Fairly dull, sluggish; seldom active, vigorous	(3)
___ (e) Mostly dull, sluggish; never really active, vigorous	(2)
___ (f) Very dull, sluggish every day	(1)
4. During the past 2 weeks, have you been waking up feeling fresh and rested?	
___ (a) All of the time	(6)
___ (b) Most of the time	(5)
___ (c) A good bit of the time	(4)
___ (d) Some of the time	(3)
___ (e) A little of the time	(2)
___ (f) None of the time	(1)

Fatigue Scale of Chalder

(Instructions): For each statement, reply as either: "same as usual"= 0; "worse"= 1; or "much worse"= 2.

Physical Fatigue
1. I get tired easily.
2. I need to rest more.
3. I feel sleepy or drowsy.
4. I can no longer start anything.
5. I am always lacking in energy.
6. I have less strength in my muscles.
7. I feel weak.
8. I can start things without difficulty, but get weak as I go on

Mental Fatigue
1. I have problems concentrating
2. I have problems thinking clearly
3. I make more slips of the tongue, or have problems finding the correct word
4. I have problems with eyestrain
5. I have problems with memory

fatigue may result. Rehabilitative techniques to improve upper-extremity function can be helpful in diminishing fatigue. Most head trauma patients complain of fatigue, but there is no relationship to the period of unconsciousness following the head trauma.[35] Fatigue is associated with decreased attentiveness, reduced mental capacity, depression, sleepiness, and lassitude. These symptoms gradually may decrease during the year following the head trauma and can be ameliorated to a considerable extent by stimulation and physical exercise. Other

Table 23-1
Sample measures of fatigue (Continued)

Fatigue Severity Scale (FSS)

Patients are instructed to choose a number from 1 to 7 that indicates their degree of agreement with each statement where 1, indicates strongly disagree and 7, strongly agree.

Statement:

1. My motivation is lower when I am fatigued.
2. Exercise brings on my fatigue.
3. I am easily fatigued.
4. Fatigue interferes with my physical functioning.
5. Fatigue causes frequent problems for me.
6. My fatigue prevents sustained physical functioning.
7. Fatigue interferes with carrying out certain duties and responsibilities.
8. Fatigue is among my three most disabling symptoms.
9. Fatigue interferes with my work, family, or social life.

Fatigue questionnaire

Questions	Completely disagree						Completely agree

(*Instructions*): Below are a series of statements regarding your fatigue. By fatigue we mean a sense of tiredness, lack of energy, or total body giveout. Please read each statement and choose a number from 1 to 7, where 1 indicates you completely disagree with the statement and 7 indicates you completely agree. Please answer these questions as they apply to the past 2 weeks. Circle the appropriate number on the answer sheet.

Questions	1	2	3	4	5	6	7
1. I feel drowsy when I am fatigued.	1	2	3	4	5	6	7
2. When I am fatigued, I lose my patience.	1	2	3	4	5	6	7
3. My motivation is lower when I am fatigued.	1	2	3	4	5	6	7
4. When I am fatigued, I have difficulty concentrating.	1	2	3	4	5	6	7
5. Exercise brings on my fatigue.	1	2	3	4	5	6	7
6. Heat brings on my fatigue.	1	2	3	4	5	6	7
7. Long periods of inactivity bring on my fatigue.	1	2	4	5	6	7	
8. Stress brings on my fatigue.	1	2	3	4	5	6	7
9. Depression brings on my fatigue.	1	2	3	4	5	6	7
10. Work brings on my fatigue.	1	2	3	4	5	6	7
11. My fatigue is worse in the afternoon.	1	2	3	4	5	6	7
12. My fatigue is worse in the morning.	1	2	3	4	5	6	7
13. Performance of routine daily activities increases my fatigue.	1	2	3	4	5	6	7
14. Resting lessens my fatigue.	1	2	3	4	5	6	7
15. Sleeping lessens my fatigue.	1	2	3	4	5	6	7
16. Cool temperatures lessen my fatigue.	1	2	3	4	5	6	7
17. Positive experiences lessen my fatigue.	1	2	3	4	5	6	7
18. I am easily fatigued.	1	2	3	4	5	6	7

Table 23-1
Sample measures of fatigue (Continued)

Questions	Completely disagree						Completely agree

Below are a series of statements regarding your fatigue. By fatigue we mean a sense of tiredness, lack of energy, or total body giveout. Please read each statement and choose a number from 1 to 7, where 1 indicates you completely disagree with the statement and 7 indicates you completely agree. Please answer these questions as they apply to the past 2 weeks. Circle the appropriate number on the answer sheet.

19. Fatigue interferes with my physical functioning.	1	2	3	4	5	6	7
20. Fatigue causes frequent problems for me.	1	2	3	4	5	6	7
21. My fatigue prevents sustained physical functioning.	1	2	3	4	5	6	7
22. Fatigue interferes with carrying out certain duties and responsibilities.	1	2	3	4	5	6	7
23. Fatigue predated other symptoms of multiple sclerosis.	1	2	3	4	5	6	7
24. Fatigue is my most disabling symptom.	1	2	3	4	5	6	7
25. Fatigue is among my 3 most disabling symptoms.	1	2	3	4	5	6	7
26. Fatigue interferes with my work, family, or social life.	1	2	3	4	5	6	7
27. Fatigue makes other symptoms worse.	1	2	3	4	5	6	7
28. I experience prolonged fatigue after exercise	1	2	3	4	5	6	7

diseases that are associated with chronic pain and chronic motor and sensory disability customarily are associated with fatigue. Patients with painful peripheral neuropathy not only are unable to rest but also frequently take medications that induce fatigue and sleepiness. Epilepsy may be associated with increased somnolence and fatigue.[36] Often it is difficult to sort out the consequences of the primary disorder from medication side effects.

Immune System and Other Factors

Acute infection and the post-infectious states commonly are associated with severe fatigue. Several disorders, such as Epstein-Barr virus infection, CMV infection, and HIV infection are associated commonly with fatigue and long-standing alteration of the immune system.[37] Rheumatologic disorders such as rheumatoid arthritis, system lupus erythematosus, and Lyme disease commonly are associated with chronic fatigue.[38–41] Sleep disorders are a common cause of fatigue and daytime

somnolence.[43–46] Correction of these disorders or the cause of sleep loss may ameliorate fatigue. Age itself is not a cause of increased fatigue within the limits of normal function.[47] Workplace or occupationally induced fatigue may result from loss of sleep or interruption of circadian rhythms.[48–50] The chronic fatigue syndrome may result from immune abnormalities associated with fatigue.[17] There are conflicting reports of immune abnormalities.

ASSESSMENT AND MEASUREMENT OF FATIGUE

The physiological definition of fatigue is the decrement in muscle force that occurs with repetitive or sustained muscle contraction. Such determinations usually are made under controlled conditions of muscle activation and muscle-force recording. In neuromuscular diseases, such as MG, characterized by significant decrements in muscle force with repetitive or sustained stimulation,

Table 23-1
Sample measures of fatigue (Continued)

Fatigue impact scale	
Questions	*Responses*

(Instructions): The fatigue impact scale asks subjects to rate how much of a problem fatigue has caused them during the past month, including the day of testing, in reference to the statements listed below. The subject is asked to put the appropriate response: 0 = no problem; 1 = small problem; 2 = moderate problem; 3 = big problem; 4 = extreme problem.

1. I feel less alert. ___
2. I feel that I am more isolated from social contact. ___
3. I have to reduce my workload or responsibilities. ___
4. I am more moody. ___
5. I have difficulty paying attention for a long period. ___
6. I feel like I cannot think clearly. ___
7. I work less effectively (this applies to work inside or outside the home). ___
8. I have to rely more on others to help me or do things for me. ___
9. I have difficulty planning activities ahead of time. ___
10. I am more clumsy and uncoordinated. ___
11. I find that I am more forgetful. ___
12. I am more irritable and more easily angered. ___
13. I have to be careful about pacing my physical activities. ___
14. I am less motivated to do anything that requires physical effort. ___
15. I am less motivated to engage in social activities. ___
16. My ability to travel outside my home is limited. ___
17. I have trouble maintaining physical effort for long periods. ___
18. I find it difficult to make decisions. ___
19. I have few social contacts outside of my own home. ___
20. Normal day-to-day events are stressful for me. ___
21. I am less motivated to do anything that requires thinking. ___
22. I avoid situations that are stressful for me. ___
23. My muscles feel much weaker than they should. ___
24. My physical discomfort is increased. ___
25. I have difficulty dealing with anything new. ___
26. I am less able to finish tasks that require thinking. ___
27. I feel unable to meet the demands that people place on me. ___
28. I am less able to provide financial support for myself and my family. ___
29. I engage in less sexual activity. ___
30. I find it difficult to organize my thoughts when I am doing things at home or at work. ___
31. I am less able to complete tasks that require physical effort. ___
32. I worry about how I look to other people. ___
33. I am less able to deal with emotional issues. ___
34. I feel slowed down in my thinking. ___
35. I find it hard to concentrate. ___
36. I have difficulty participating fully in family activities. ___
37. I have to limit my physical activities. ___
38. I require more frequent or longer periods of rest. ___
39. I am not able to provide as much emotional support to my family as I should. ___
40. Minor difficulties seem like major difficulties. ___

the description of the pathological state conforms nicely with conditions pertaining in the physiology laboratory. However, a wide variety of pathological states exist in which the complaint of fatigue is present and there is no documentation of declining muscle force with continued activity. Performance of common daily functions may decline with time or a feeling of lassitude may be present in the absence of any sign of muscle weakness or objective measure of fatigue. If the patient reports loss of function below his customary level of performance, the disease process will determine the anatomical site and nature of the dysfunction. Although a specific pathophysiological mechanism responsible for fatigue or decline in performance may not be known, it has been presumed possible in most instances to characterize fatigue simply by asking questions referable to specific symptoms. The problem with this approach is that the subjective experience of fatigue can be suggested by the questions themselves. Thinking about the answer to the question "Do you feel tired most of the time?" may elicit a positive response from anyone. The Fatigue Severity Scale (FSS) is such a scale.[51] This scale has good reproducibility but is relatively insensitive and unlikely to detect changes in the level of fatiguability in response to some intervention. The FSS contains nine items that are rated from 1 to 7 with respect to the impact of a specific activity on the symptom of fatigue. Visual analog scales of fatigue severity suffer from the same problem.[33,34,52] They may be answered impulsively and do not allow for the description of the quantitative aspects of fatigue.

Another approach that more fully describes the effect fatigue has on various aspects of life is to question the subject about specific activities of daily living. Components of the Sickness Impact Profile (SIP) and the Fatigue Impact Scale utilize this approach.[7,31] The SIP detected improvement in mobility, increased energy level, and reduced depression in a group of ambulatory multiple sclerosis patients participating in a 15-week aerobic exercise program.[53] The Fatigue Impact Scale differentiated fatigue experienced by MS patients from that experienced by a group of hypertensive patients. It contains 40 statements and is completed using a 1 to 4 rating scale.

The Medical Outcome Survey subset items on fatigue measure mental and psychological states as well as general health.[54] It includes a four-item question designed to evaluate energy level (the Rand Index of Vitality). It does not obtain information concerning the impact of fatigue on activities of daily living and does not evaluate factors that modify fatigue.

Simple self-administered assessments of function can be carried out by patients themselves. An ambulation test consisting of a timed 25-foot walk and steps counted can be administered at different times of the day or weekly to assess the course of an illness such as multiple sclerosis as well as its diurnal pattern of fatigue. A description of some of these scales is presented in Table 23-1.

EVALUATION OF THE PATIENT WITH FATIGUE

The patient may present with fatigue as the primary complaint. Such disorders as hypothyroidism, hypoadrenalism, multiple sclerosis, occult infection, or occult neoplasm may be present. A careful assessment of medication is essential, since fatigue is a common side-effect of such drugs as tricyclic antidepressants, beta blockers, benzodiazepines, and anticonvulsants. A change in dose may be sufficient to relieve the symptoms of fatigue. Patients presenting with fatigue as the primary symptom should have a thyroid function test, serum chemistries, complete blood count, antinuclear antibody panel, erythrocyte sedimentation rate, and urinalysis. In 50 percent of patients presenting in a primary-care center, this group of tests yielded a positive diagnosis.[55] Treatable causes of fatigue, such as hypothyroidism, anemia, renal disease, diabetes mellitus, occult inflammation, neoplasm, autoimmune diseases, and infections were detected.

Fatigue presenting within the context of another illness will require special attention to the impact of that illness on the fatigue symptom. For example, occult infection worsens fatigue in multiple sclerosis patients and may presage an exacerbation. Chronic pain, present in painful peripheral neuropathy, may prevent sleep and rest. Psychological stress, superimposed on disability caused by neurological disease, may suddenly enhance fatigue. The severity of chronic pain and its impact on daily life may be grossly underreported, since it is a daily companion. Rheumatoid arthritis, cancer, eosinophilic myalgic syndrome, chronic low-back pain, chronic headache, and neuropathic pain all fit into this category.[38]

The presence of sleep disorder should be assessed. The patient him- or herself may be a poor reporter of this problem. Long driving trips for a patient with sleep apnea require a constant battle with daytime sleepiness. Complaints of fatigue and weakness may resolve with a correction of sleep apnea. Obesity, snoring, nocturnal awakenings, narcolepsy, and daytime sleeping must be noted.[56–60]

Depressed patients commonly report fatigue and abnormal sleep patterns. Depression accompanies many illnesses that in turn produce fatigue. The loss of function produced by neurological disease, especially cognitive deficits, may induce severe reactive depression or worsen preexisting endogenous depression.[61] It is important to note losses occurring in the recent past, to assess the familial, social, situational, and occupational support system, and to ask the patient directly about self-esteem and the presence of morbid thinking.

The Beck Depression Inventory and the Center for Epidemiological Studies Depression Scale (CES-D) are simple tests that can be administered in the clinic.[62,63] Those with medical and neurological illnesses are expected to have somewhat higher scores. For the CES-D, a threshold scale of 16 indicates depression, but for those with coexisting illness the threshold is elevated to 25, at which point a psychiatric referral usually is indicated.

Neurological disorders that affect cognition, such as multiple sclerosis, may present with severe fatigue, even when little objective neurological deficit is present. Neuropsychological testing (WAIS-R) can be helpful in sorting out those patients in whom fatigue is related to a severe inability to adapt to changes in the environment owing to cognitive deficits.[61]

TREATMENT

The initial step in treatment is to acknowledge that fatigue exists. The possible mechanism of fatigue must be discussed and the patient and his or her family must be educated concerning factors that may play a role in worsening fatigue. For example, the fatigue present in many neurological diseases is exacerbated by heat. The most common of such disorders is multiple sclerosis.[33] On exposure to heat or vigorous exercise neurological disability may worsen or develop anew. Various techniques, including a cool bath in the afternoon, swimming, and air conditioning, can assist in promoting optimum function. When a physical or neurological deficit is present, relatives and associates must understand that fatigue by itself can produce disability. In myasthenia gravis, weakness may be considered functional, because at times it is minimal or absent.

In some disorders, improving aerobic fitness and muscle strength can improve exercise tolerance and reduce fatigue. A balance between an appropriate exercise program and rest must be achieved. The influence of rest on fatigue in pathological states has not been studied adequately. Many factors must be considered, such as regulation of blood pressure and heart rate, electrolyte balance, and recovery of muscle function following exercise. Patients frequently report that even 10 minutes of recumbent rest in the afternoon restores strength and improves endurance. The quality of sleep also is important. Fatigue is a common complaint in sleep-deprived individuals. When illness compromises the quality of sleep, then fatigue results from multiple factors derived from the illness itself as well as from lack of rest.

MEDICATIONS APPLIED TO THE TREATMENT OF FATIGUE

The first and oldest medications applied to fatigue management are the central nervous system stimulants. These include caffeine, a mild stimulant with a wide dose range, and pemoline 18.75–112.5 mg daily, which can produce irritability in some and palpitations as adverse side-effects. Pemoline has been used for treating the fatigue associated with multiple sclerosis.[64] In a double-blind study, 46 percent improved versus 19.5 percent utilizing a placebo.[64] There were 25 percent with side effects. Methylphenidate (Ritalin), 2.5–20 mg daily, also produces side effects such as insomnia, headache, and restlessness. The primary adverse effects of the central nervous system stimulants is their adverse effect on the quality of rest. Brief periods of sleep have been shown to be as effective as stimulants in restoring function in sleep-deprived normal subjects.

Amantadine hydrochloride, 100 mg b.i.d., has been demonstrated to help with the diurnal fatigue commonly associated with multiple sclerosis.[34,64–66] Higher levels of beta endorphin and betalipoprotein, and lower levels of pyruvate and lactate were found in patients whose fatigue responded to treatment. Although dopaminergic activity has been found, its mechanism of action is unknown. In one study, cognitive function also was found to improve. Some patients complained of excessive sleepiness, decreased cognition, and fatigue, with these symptoms responding in varying degrees. Others have not been able to duplicate these findings.[67] How Amantadine affects these symptoms, especially cognitive function, is unclear. Increased irritability, sleeplessness, and uncomfortable psychological effects may be adverse side effects. Livido reticularis may be severe in some, and is particularly disturbing to women.

Other drugs, such as selegiline, a monoamine oxidase B inhibitor, has been purported to relieve fatigue in multiple sclerosis. A strong placebo effect in treating fatigue is clearly recognized. Anecdotal reports of benefits must be verified by controlled trials. Four aminopyridine, a K$^+$ channel blocker, has been reported to increase muscle strength and reduce fatigue in multiple sclerosis patients.[68]

Depression and anxiety play a strong part in producing and amplifying the symptoms of fatigue. Common experience verifies that recovering from fatigue resulting from pleasant activities seems to occur more rapidly than from fatigue resulting from a painful experience. It is essential to identify depression as an accompanying problem in many neurological illnesses and to recognize that most patients will not admit outright to queries about depression. Only when a list of daily activities relinquished, relationships constricted or severed, and thoughts darkened by morbidity is elicited can some perception of the severity of depression be established. Societal and cultural influences may interfere with the diagnosis of depression. Using an abbreviated pencil-and-paper assessment of mood, such as the Beck Depression Inventory, the Profile of Mood States, or a guided interview prior to or during a clinic visit, has been found to be very useful.[62,69]

Antidepressant drugs that do not sedate may be of most help for patients with significant depression without agitation or anxiety. These agents include desipramine, sertaline, and fluoxitine. When agitation and sleeplessness accompany depression, a tricyclic antidepressant taken before bedtime may be more useful. These also help to reduce troublesome nocturnal flexor/extensor spasms, and may augment spasmolytic agents such as lioresal.

Anxiety often accompanies depression and fatigue. Anxiolytic drugs such as the benzodiazepines often sedate and may worsen fatigue, and in some individuals may worsen depression. It is essential to begin with small doses, usually given at night, or at times of high anxiety, and to recognize the importance of drug interaction. Referral to a psychotherapist is essential for such patients. The State Trait Anxiety Inventory can be used to assess the level of anxiety.[70]

Sleep disorders often are associated with fatigue. A sleep history must be obtained, and if necessary, data obtained on the patient's sleep pattern. It is not unusual to find very poor sleep hygiene. Simple modifications in the sleep ritual may greatly enhance the quality of sleep. It is helpful not to engage in physical exercise late in the day, use the bedroom for such activities as television, or attempt to use alcohol for sedation.

Individual relaxation technique must be encouraged. A simple technique may be as simple as having a patient recall a place or experience that produced joy and a sense of safety. He or she is told to close the eyes and elaborate this image in the imagination. This should be practiced daily. The relaxation technique itself involves moving into the image step by step in the imagination. With each step the state of relaxation deepens. The depth of self-hypnosis and relaxation deepens with practice. To develop proficiency in meditation techniques of different types requires discipline and practice.

FATIGUE IN SPECIFIC DISORDERS

Multiple Sclerosis

Clinical Pathophysiology The critical lesion of multiple sclerosis is demyelination that occurs secondary to a T-cell–mediated autoimmune response to myelin antigens. There is focal perivascular demyelination and infiltration with inflammatory cells.[71] Several theories have been posed to explain the autoimmune attack on myelin, including molecular mimicry between the viral antigen and various components of myelin-based protein, elaboration of new antigens, and occult viral infection with predilection for oligodendrocyte.[71–73] A genetic factor predisposing to autoimmunity possibly related to reduced expression of HLA class I antigens may be present along with activation of an autoimmune process by infection.[74] Exacerbation commonly follows infection, whereas a polyclonal hyperimmune state decreases susceptibility to infection. There is latitudinal-dependent and age-associated residence influence on the incidence of multiple sclerosis.[71]

MRI reveals areas of inflammation and edema associated with demyelination distributed predominantly in subcortical white matter, often with a periventricular distribution. Lesions may be present in the cerebrum, brain stem, cerebellum, and spinal cord.

Demyelination is associated with remyelination as well as axonal loss. The functional consequence of this is slowed or blocked impulse conduction within the central nervous system. Delay of somatosensory-evoked potentials and motor-evoked responses are common, even when no apparent abnormality is present. IgG is increased in proportion to albumin in the cerebrospinal fluid and there is decreased variation in the molecular weight and charge of these proteins leading to the phenomenon of oligoclonal banding on electrophoresis.[71] During an acute attack and early in the course of the disease oligoclonal banding may not be present despite elevated IgG. This phenomenon usually becomes apparent later. Lymphocytic pleocytosis in the CSF is present during acute exacerbations. Comparison of serum IgG with CSF IgG reveals synthesis within the central nervous system and decreased blood-brain barrier.[71] MRIs taken weekly or monthly reveal lesions that come and go with only a moderate correlation with the clinical status.

Impaired impulse conduction in the central nervous system is sensitive to slight alterations in body temperature that increase sodium conductance, so that there is less net flow of transmembrane current over time. The depolarization/repolarization process takes place more rapidly, so that there is less current available for depolarization at the next node of Ranvier essential for saltatory conduction. The demyelination process begins paranodally and widens the node where sodium channels are concentrated. As a consequence current density is reduced and it may be insufficient to cause membrane depolarization, leading to conduction block.

The remyelination process creates more nodes of Ranvier, results in fewer myelin lamellae, and may leave wide gaps of unmyelinated axon. Thus, conduction is slowed or blocked. Recent studies support the view that astrocytic processes may play a role in repair of nodal membrane and may be capable of inserting sodium channels.[75] Conduction properties of demyelinated and remyelinated axons may make them susceptible to activity or exercise-induced conduction block. This may play a role along with elevated temperature in reducing exercise tolerance and producing fatigue.

Muscle Strength and Endurance A variety of neurological syndromes may be produced by multiple sclerosis. A common presentation is spastic paraparesis. Force generation in limbs with spastic paraparesis is abnormal. Maximal force is achieved more slowly than normal and fatigue develops more rapidly. Central fatigue is increased and there is a delay in recovery of pH and phosphocreatine to control levels as determined by magnetic-resonance spectroscopy when exercise is produced by repetitive peroneal motor-nerve stimulation activating tibialis anterior.[76] The abnormality may result from an altered pattern of innervation on the inadequately activated tibialis anterior. No direct relationship appears to exist between the excessive systemic fatigue experienced by the multiple sclerosis patient and the degree of muscle involvement.

Performance A diurnal pattern of fatigue affects 50–90 percent of MS patients with some acquiring new neurological deficits later in the day, such as fluctuations in walking ability between morning and afternoon. Fatigue is associated with physical and not mental activity.[77] This relationship is not seen in patients with systemic lupus erythematosus, Lyme disease, or controls.[77] Many patients (90 percent) experiencing this pattern of involvement usually are very temperature-sensitive.[33] Physical activity may result in a gradual, although temporary, loss of function. Spastic paresis with stiffness also worsens in some patients as a consequence of immobility. A limb maintained in one position undergoes an increase in thixotropy. A patient may be able to walk to the clinic and after sitting quietly for 20–30 minutes may be unable to walk into the examining room. Studies using an isokinetic dynamometer for investigation of the stiffness and knee flexion have revealed that brief periods of rest in the extended position significantly increased nonreflex stiffness.[78]

Motivation Depression affects 50–65 percent of multiple sclerosis patients and cognitive deficit is present in about as many. However, a study of severely fatigued multiple sclerosis patients revealed less than 10 percent to be suffering from major depression.[79] Recommendations for therapy, especially exercise, are unlikely to be complied with unless adequate attention is paid to factors that influence communication and motivation. Attachment to a group and repeated reinforcement of the plan are essential to compliance.

Treatment and Rehabilitation Appropriate rest, including a nap in the afternoon, may be the most logical treatment for excessive fatigue. A cool bath in the afternoon also may reduce fatigue significantly. Filling the tub with tepid water to which cold water then is added is the best method for graduated exposure to cold and avoidance of gross flexor and extensor spasms that may occur as a mass reflex owing to cold exposure. Gentle agitation of the water is essential to facilitate deep tissue cooling. A shower or evaporative cooling is much less effective. Cooling vests utilizing gel pads or circulating coolant also have been found to be effective and may be more convenient.

As mentioned earlier, amantadine hydrochloride, 100 mg twice daily, and pemoline also may reduce the symptom of fatigue.[34,64] Finally, improving exercise tolerance utilizing an aerobic training program can reduce fatigue and alleviate depression.[53] Neurological deficits require that a specific exercise prescription be given the patient.

Treatments of exacerbation with prednisone or methylprednisolone will shorten the duration of exacerbations and reduce fatigue. Long-term immune modulation therapy may be indicated.

Parkinson's Disease

Clinical Pathophysiology   In idiopathic Parkinsonism, dopaminergic cells of the substantia nigra pars compacta (SNPc) are lost or degenerate, resulting in both decreased excitation and inhibition that is GABAergic onto striatal neurons (STR) that in turn project to the globus pallidus externa (GPe), where input is inhibitory, and to the globus pallidus interna (GPi), where input is excitatory (inhibition is "external" and excitation is

"internal"). Loss of SNPc neurons results in greater inhibition of GPi and diminished excitation of GPe. GPe neurons also are GABAergic and inhibit SNPc neurons. SNPc neurons are in turn excitatory to GPi. GPi neurons also are GABAergic and inhibit neurons of nucleus ventralis lateralis (VL) that provide excitatory input to the supplementary motor area (SMA) and motor cortex (MC). An excitatory feedback from SMA and MC onto STR GPe and STR GPi also is present (see Figure 23-1).[79]

Current models of Parkinsonism predict increased activity in GPi, increased inhibition of VL, and loss of activation or drive to MC. This is believed to be the basis for bradykinesia and akinesia. Two pathways, a direct and indirect pathway, involving the basal ganglia (BG) VL-MC circuit, result in increased GPi activity. The direct pathway results in less inhibition of GPi and the indirect pathway—GPe to subthalamic nucleus

Figure 23-1

Schematic representation of the BG-VL-MC circuits. Arrows represent the predicted changes in neuronal activity consequent to destruction of the Snpc. Asterisk indicates supplemental connection from SMA and motor cortex. (Modified from Montgomery.[79])

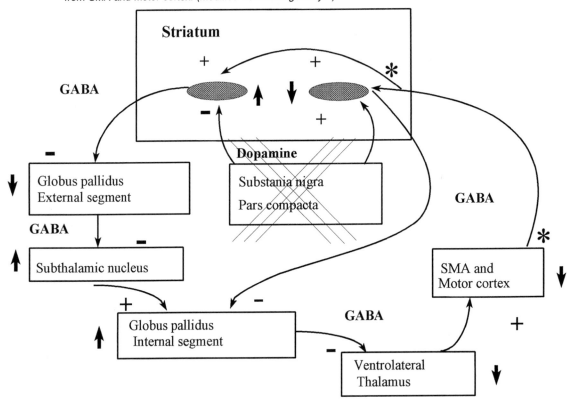

(STN)—results in loss of inhibitory activity to GPi. This results in increased STN activity and excitation of GPi, which in turn imposes more inhibition on VL-MC, resulting in bradykinesia.

The neurotoxin 1-methyl-4-phenyl-1,2,3,6-tetra-hydropyridine (or MPTP) produces a hypokinetic rigid syndrome similar to Parkinson's disease.[80–82] This syndrome has been produced in nonhuman primates given this drug. Increased activity in GPi and STN has been found. STR neurons increase firing rate following 6-hydroxypyridine lesions of SNPc in rats and MPTP in nonhuman primates. These data suggest that the indirect pathway is most important in Parkinsonism.[80–82]

The model predicts that lesions of GPi or STN should reduce symptoms of Parkinsonism, especially bradykinesia. Lesions of GPi and STN improve symptoms in MPTP-treated nonhuman primates and PD patients. Bradykinesia may result from impaired motor planning, increased antagonistic muscle activity, or altered recruitment of motor units, especially their firing rate. Failure to modulate the output of a postural motor generator, especially its ability to produce fine adjustments in motor-unit firing rate, may constitute the functional lesion of Parkinsonism.

Not all investigators support the proposed model, since lesions of the GPi produced by carbon monoxide can produce Parkinsonism. Selective cooling of the GPi will slow arm movements. Modification of the model by including in it a "motor generator" with a functional capacity for frequency modulation of output might help explain such inconsistencies. In other words, loss of frequency modulation would include failure to activate the BG-VL-MC circuit from 0 or any given "idling level" of activity. The model does not help in understanding tremor. However, interposition of the "motor generator" that idles at tremor frequency and results in cyclic activation of the VL-ML circuit might explain tremor. Microelectrode recordings from VLGP1 and STN have determined that such activity exists in MPTP-treated nonhuman primates.[83] Spontaneous rhythmic activity in neuronal networks occurs at multiple locations in the central nervous system, such as the respiratory center in the medulla, the vestibulocerebellar system, and oculomotor systems. Corticomotor neurons themselves have rhythmic discharges. Cholinergic interneurons of the striatum (STR) may play a part in this rhythmic modulation. The sleep–wake cycle also represents an oscillation of the nervous system but with a very long time constant. The phenomenon of fatigue or loss of performance over time is crucially dependent on the adjusted activities of such oscillating systems.

Muscle Power and Endurance Parkinson's disease produces immobility, usually in elderly persons. Loss of muscle mass, decreased compliance of the chest with restricted breathing, and malnutrition were severe problems prior to the advent of L-dopa therapy. Still, Parkinson's disease is progressive and loss of muscle strength and endurance is consistently observed in patients followed in the clinic. Aerobic exercise programs may be helpful in increasing tolerance for activities of daily living.

Studies of motor control have suggested delayed time for movement despite near-normal onset times of agonist EMG activity. Reaction time, defined as EMG activity and movement, are prolonged in MPTP-treated nonhuman primates. Abnormal movement latency may be explained by the presence of tonic activity in antagonistic muscles. Prolonged EMG latency may relate to impairment of motor-unit frequency modulation. In MPTP-treated nonhuman primates abnormal patterns of frequency modulation of neurons have been found in the putamen.[79]

Performance Scales for assessment of activities of daily living (Parkinson's disease severity scale of Hohn and Yahr) have been utilized to evaluate the response to medication and the diurnal pattern of change in performance affected by bradykinesia, rigidity, and tremor.[84] Dramatic changes in response to L-dopa medication are seen in which the patient may progress from being immobilized in a chair or bed to being fully ambulatory and capable of all aspects of self-care. In other patients, changes in performance may be more subtle and time of day may be as important as medication dose.

Fatigue Parkinson's disease patients commonly experience fatigue. Over half of patients surveyed report fatigue among their most severe symptoms and one-third the most disabling symptom.[30,84] Although depression correlates with fatigue, patients who are not depressed also experience fatigue. Only a low positive correlation between fatigue and Parkinson's disease severity using the Parkinson's disease severity scale has been found.[30] A diurnal pattern of fatigue has not been found, nor does there seem to be a relationship to motor activity in treated patients.[30]

The effect of sleep on fatigue in Parkinson's disease has been investigated. Parkinson's disease patients and age-control subjects do not differ in the degree of sleep disturbance.[30] Although Parkinson's disease patients with excessive daytime sleepiness reported disturbed sleep and worsening of symptoms, no relationship has been found between fatigue, abnormal sleep patterns, diurnal fluctuation, and symptoms or medication.[30]

There have been no quantitative performance measures of fatigue and Parkinson's disease in relation to performance of motor activities or time of day.

Treatment and Rehabilitation The accepted treatment of Parkinson's disease is the replacement of L-dopa or improvement in dopaminergic synaptic transmission by such medications as pergolide. Anticholinergic medication, possibly suppressing the effect of putamenal cholinergic interneurons, also benefit symptoms. Amantadine, an antiviral drug, also has dopaminergic activity and may amplify the effect of L-dopa as well as reduce the symptom of fatigue. Selegiline, a monamine oxidase B inhibitor, reduces the required dose of L-dopa and slows the progression of Parkinson's disease.[85] Protein intake also influences the required dose of L-dopa by influencing the availability of dopamine.

Maintenance of the range of motion, strength, and aerobic fitness in a fashion coordinated with the benefits of medication is essential for the successful management of Parkinson's disease. Some patients report a reduced requirement for medication and less fatigue associated with improved fitness. Further studies to document this relationship must be done.

Stroke

Clinical Pathophysiology The size of the infarct is a function of the caliber of vessel occluded and the extent of collateral circulation. In most stroke patients, cerebrovascular disease does not confine itself to a single vessel. Thus, the watershed area surrounding the area of primary infarction producing neuronal death is highly variable. Since the MCA distributes blood to the area about the Sylvian fissure and central sulcus and deep structures of the internal capsule containing cortical afferent and efferent axons, basal ganglia, and thalamus, the face, tongue, and upper extremity function is most severely impaired. Watershed areas shared with the anterior cerebral artery account for variation in the degree of lower-extremity involvement.[94]

Surrounding the volume of brain containing irreversibly damaged neurons (area of primary injury) a penumbra of edematous and hypoxic brain tissue exists. About this region, a breakdown of the blood-brain barrier occurs, resulting in edema, cellular diapedesis, sometimes hemorrhage, and at the margins, vasodilatation causing increased blood flow. Changes in the size of the penumbra affect the functional outcome. Neurons within this region are not necrotic but owing to an abnormal extracellular environment, abnormal ionic concentration of calcium, sodium, potassium, and decreased pH, these neurons become inexcitable. In addition, many neurons lose both axonic and dendritic connections, which changes the function of neural networks.

It is the goal of medical therapy to (1) prevent extension of the zone infarcted; (2) reduce the zone of edema and arrested circulation; (3) prevent neuronal death; and (4) facilitate activation of viable neurons capable of assuming function or reorganizing networks with establishment of new connections.

Muscle Strength The pattern of muscle weakness in the hemiplegic patient is the familiar flexed and plegic upper extremity and the extended circumducted and paretic lower extremity. The greater involvement of the upper extremity suggests that it will recover more slowly but its relative improvement is quite similar to that of the lower extremity.[95] Motor recovery for brief, short contractions follows a stereotypic pattern. Flaccid paralysis, the period of diaschisis first described by Von Manakow, is followed by flexor synergy and then spasticity. Flexor activity spreads across joints from proximal to distal muscles. Finally, volitional movements and extension become possible as spasticity diminishes. Minimal spontaneous recovery 2 months poststroke was found in 441 patients with the majority having poor recovery and prolonged flaccidity.[90] Recovery may arrest at the stage of synergistic movements. Other variables affect outcome. These include age, general medical condition, cognitive deficits, and psychosocial support, important for day-to-day stimulation. Nondominant cerebral involvement, hemisensory neglect, and homonymous hemianopsia greatly impair performance of activities of daily living.

Endurance Improvement in motor function is measured by improvement in strength as well as in the period of time an activity can be sustained. The ability to ambulate 150 feet determined by the time and number of steps required assess the speed and efficiency of gait.[96] The patient's complaint is that of weakness. Immobility and its effect on cardiovascular fitness results in decreased endurance for physical activity of all kinds. The primary impact is on useful performance of activities of daily living.

Performance   Performance of activities of daily living depends on many factors. Motor deficits may in fact contribute only a small amount to limiting the functional outcome. Added deficits such as homonymous hemianopsia, hemisensory loss, cognitive impairment, and additional medical problems, especially cardiopulmonary disease, greatly limit outcome in comparison to the effects of hemiparesis alone.

Measures of Motor Function and Performance   Muscle strength can be measured using hand dynamometers or techniques such as the Tuft's Quantitative Neurological Examination or isokinetic dynamometers.[97] It is apparent that force generation in patients with central nervous system disorders is abnormal. Peak forces are not achieved as rapidly as normal and there is more variability. Therefore, maximal voluntary contraction alone does not fully describe motor deficit.

Comprehensive assessment of extremity motor function is accomplished with such instruments as the Fugl-Meyer Motor Assessment Scale, and the Rivermead Motor Assessment Score.[98,99] Activities of daily living are assessed by such instruments as the Barthel Index, a functional independence measure, and Katz Activities of Daily Living Scale.[100,101]

Fatigue   Recovery following stroke is dependent to a considerable extent on the level of arousal. Frequent stimulation through passive and active body movements and social interaction contribute to enhanced arousal. Mortality from stroke is related to the level of consciousness and its duration. There are no measures of strength or endurance or changes in performance over time as a function of the period of unconsciousness or level of consciousness. One would predict that all factors increasing, the level of consciousness and arousal would impact favorably on such measures of fatigue. This view is compatible with the observed effect of amphetamine on stroke recovery and the deleterious effect of sedation and GABAergic drugs.

Treatment and Rehabilitation   Once cerebral thrombosis has occurred it is important to ascertain the underlying cause and prevent progression. Therapy to control hypertension and anticoagulation may be applied. Agitation with hyperventilation may be treated by sedation or anxiolytic medications such as diazepam. Experiments on the rat following a cortical ablation clearly demonstrated that sedation, use of GABAergic drugs and betaadrenergic blockade can increase neurologic deficit and delay recovery.[102,103] Deficit is reduced by amphetamine and the effects can be abolished by haloperidol. Haloperidol can cause defects to reappear in animals that are recovered.[104–106]

Cortical activation and stimulation of adrenergic mechanisms appear to enhance recovery. Psychomotor stimulation would seem to play a similar role. Reduction in the period of diaschisis, "unmasking" of connections such as those provided by the supplementary motor area that can facilitate movement, especially complex movements, and activation of adrenergic arousal mechanisms can be achieved by appropriate medications and physical stimulation. Measurements of fatigue and decrements in performance are very likely to respond favorably to the same measures. A variety of approaches to physical therapy have claimed effectiveness in improving stroke recovery. However, there are no control studies to verify such claims. Spontaneous recovery, possibly influenced by various modalities of stimulation, may be the common factor facilitating recovery.

Head Injury

Muscle Strength and Endurance   Motor deficits are a function of the site of injury. As with the stroke patient the motor deficit is among a number of factors that contribute to disability and fatigue. Depression and anxiety have been found positively associated with the complaint of fatigue 9 months after brain injury. Tests of muscle fatigue did not reveal significant differences from controls.[107]

The level of arousal as well as cognitive deficits, sensory loss, and visual deficits play a major role in determining the level of disability. A period of immobility lasting weeks or longer results in decreased muscle mass, lower blood volume, and deconditioning. Early stimulation and ambulation can help to reduce these adverse consequences.

Performance   ADLs are significantly limited less as a consequence of motor deficits than of the lack of ability to organize behavior and to respond appropriately to situational stimuli. Inappropriate behavior, emotional lability, and impaired memory contribute more to disrupted performance than motor deficit. Tolerance for social stimuli and impulse control are poor and demonstrate major fluctuations in fatiguability. These clinical observations are not substantiated by quantitative testing of performance over time. Fatigue, irritability, anxiety, and headaches not soley related to the injury were found to vary as a function of the severity of injury and time out from the injury.[108]

Fatigue   In response to a survey of head-injury patients at 1 and 12 months after the injury and discharge from the rehabilitation service, fatigue was a common complaint.[108] The relationship between the symptom of fatigue and the location of the cerebral lesion, duration of coma or amnesia, or the Glasgow outcome scores have not been determined. The history of drug abuse and the risk of fatigue also must be determined. Sedatives, anxiolytic drugs, and anticonvulsant drugs can be expected to lessen fatigue when discontinued. Using cortical evoked responses, the P3 has been found to be delayed in recovered head-injury patients. The results suggested that patients could be classified into two groups: those that underprocess information and those that overprocess information (needless processing of irrelevent information), resulting in fatigue.[109]

Treatment and Rehabilitation   The acute treatment of the head-injured patient requires management of the intracerebral hemorrhage and edema, maintaining a clear airway, supporting ventilation when necessary, prevention of aspiration pneumonia, adequate alimentation, and fluid balance. In most patients there are multiple injuries, such as limb fractures, that complicate management. Surgery may be required for ruptured spleen, perforated viscera, and severe chest trauma. Fracture of the cervical spine accompanied by cervical trauma may be present and not recognized in the patient with severe head injury.

In the subacute recovery phase, usually occurring in the first 6 weeks, passive movement of extremities and social stimulation are applied. Contact with others, especially family members, helps to reduce agitation and facilitate the reorganization of behavior. As mentioned in the preceding, sessions of social interactions may be followed by hours of sleep. Gradually, tolerance for physical and social activity improves. In the long term, measured in years, special consideration must be given to cognitive deficits and impulse control. Depending on the age of the patient, improvement can be detected years after the injury has occurred.[108]

Postpolio Syndrome (PPS)

Clinical Pathophysiology   In a patient 50 years or older with a history of poliomyelitis and symptoms of increased weakness and fatigue developing about 30 years after the acute infection, postpolio syndrome is present.[27] The postpolio syndrome occurs in 25–40 percent of survivors.[27] Residual weakness is present in the majority of patients. A history of additional involvement of other limbs and bulbar involvement can be elicited. Some patients report full recovery and no impairment of motor function, even for sports. The primary complaint is increased weakness, especially of the most severely involved limbs. Progression is continuous and present for many months. Muscle pain with activity is not uncommon. Cold intolerance and extreme fatigue also are reported.[110–112] In response to progressive weakness, some patients increase the intensity of their exercise programs, including muscle strengthening exercises. This may accelerate weakness and cause more pain. The crucial historical data should include benchmarks for loss of activities of daily living; a cane, walker, and then a wheelchair may be required in succession over a period of many months. Bulbar function may worsen. Depression commonly results from these losses, which recall the terrors of the initial illness.

Electromyographic studies can be used to ascertain the extent of neurogenic atrophy with reinnervation. It is common to find that involvement is much more extensive than that recalled by the patient. Motor-unit action potentials are polyphasic, prolonged in duration, increased in amplitude, and fire rapidly with minimal effort. Rarely, little evidence for prior denervation is found. In these cases, other causes for increased weakness, fatigue, and muscle weakness should be sought.

The simplest explanation for loss of strength and decreased performance recognized in late middle age in the postpolio patient is that the process has not occurred suddenly but gradually over time, with a subtle adjustment of physical activities to compensate for motor deficits. The loss of specific benchmarks, such as the need for a cane or inability to climb stairs, brings the patient to the clinic. The most likely basis for slowly progressive weakness is the well-recognized loss of motoneurons occurring with age that becomes relatively more significant as the numbers of motor units decrease and the capacity for reinnervation declines.

Electrophysiological studies supporting this impression include declining CMAP, decreasing recruitment of motor units and increased firing rates of motor units at moderate effort. It is not unusual to discover one to two large single motor units firing at rates greater than 60 cycles per second and the patient unable to recruit additional motor units. Studies that have investigated motor-unit firing rate at varying percentages of maximal voluntary contraction may not disclose this phenomenon, since maximum voluntary contraction is so dramatically reduced.[113] Kinesiologic studies of gait have recorded nearly 100 percent recruitment of motor units during normal pacing, whereas in normal subjects less than 25 percent of motor units were recruited.[114] Biopsy of these atrophic muscles, especially leg muscles of ambulatory patients, often reveals evidence for necrosis and associated inflammation. Overuse of muscle fibers driven at excessively high rates leads to abnormal increases in intracellular calcium, triggering a cascade of autolytic processes.[115]

PPS may represent an interesting phenomenon of reactivated viral infection. Dalakis has proposed five different mechanisms for PPS.[27] The first is *attrition*. Motoneurons responding to the process of denervation by axonal branching become "overstressed." The process of denervation and reinnervation is ongoing throughout the life of the patient, as evidenced by abnormal jitter and histochemical changes. These "overstressed" neurons die prematurely. The second is *normal aging*. The normal loss of motoneurons is expected to be much more significant when the total number is decreased. However, normal aging does not impact motoneuron numbers until age sixty and PPS can occur prior to this age. Further, the patients selected for study were under age 60. The third is *immune dysregulation:* inflammation in the spinal cord in stable patients not succumbing to the effects of poliomyelitis; endomypseal inflammation consisting of CD8+ and CD4+ lymphocytes surrounding healthy muscle fiber expressing MHC-1 class antigens, inconsistently abnormal peripheral blood subsets, high GM, antibodies (IgM not IgG); and high interleukin 2, IL2 receptors, and oligoclonal bands in the CSF. The fourth is possible association with HLA-DQ17 haplotype, suggesting genetic susceptibility. The fifth is response to persistent polio RNA and viral mutants. The presence of polio-specific IgG, intrathecal synthesis of polio-specific IgM present in oligoclonal bands in 21 of 36 patients, high serum IgM polio virus–specific antibodies, and early positive results using PCR-amplifying polio viral RNA in CSF of 4/37 and serum of 7/37 patients all support a role for persistent viral infection.[116–119] Dalakis proposes that "change in biological properties of the virus could result in restrained RNA synthesis that allows for persistence without replication." Further mutation of the virus may induce immunologic response that may include upregulation of self-antigen, resulting in an inflammatory response.

Extensive involvement in the CNS by polio virus previously described by Bodian to include neurons in spinal cord, cerebral cortex, cerebellum, and brain stem is compatible with MRI findings of hypodense areas in the brain stem of a high percentage of patients with fatigue and PPS. Not only degeneration of motoneurons, but also brain-stem reticular neurons responsible for arousal may play a significant role in the fatigue process.[120]

In a small number of patients no history of muscle involvement was obtained, but there was EMG evidence for prior denervation. Some patients may have experienced delayed onset of weakness despite an absent history of weakness during a polio epidemic in which they were immersed. The siblings of these patients were hospitalized with the disease. None of these 12 patients were restudied for reinfection.[121]

Studies of muscle fatigue in PPS patients have not revealed increased slopes of the fatigue curve, but rather weakness resulting in earlier loss of force below critical levels. Fiber-type predominance may be seen in reinnervated muscles, which may account for altered fatigue. A predominance of fast fatigue, Type II fibers may lead to a more rapid loss of muscle force during maximal voluntary contraction, and vice versa. The degree of involvement, evidence for reinnervation, fiber-type predominance, as well as inflammation and myopathic change would seem to be crucial to understanding abnormal fatigue. The ongoing process of denervation and reinnervation results in diminished neuromuscular transmission, as evidenced by increased jitter throughout the course of the illness.[122,123]

Fatigue Fatigue, either related to specific muscle functions or systemic, was found to be a symptom in 47–89 percent of post-polio patients.[124,125] Physical exercise was found to worsen fatigue in 48 percent, whereas in normal subjects controlled exercise lessened fatigue. The degree of fatigue was not age-related. Post-polio patients reported some depression but depression did not affect the progression of fatigue. Systemic symptoms such as less energy, inability to concentrate, and heaviness in the limbs were more common in depressed patients.[124,125]

Postpolio patients manifest little evidence for psychopathology in comparison to patients with other chronic illnesses and fatigue utilizing the MMPI and the Beck Depression Inventory.[126]

Treatment and Rehabilitation Understanding the mechanism of fatigue and reassuring the patient that rapid progression of weakness is unlikely to occur can relieve many of the associated depressive symptoms and lead to appropriate modification of behavior designed to protect muscles from further injury and to conserve energy. Rating of perceived exertion is the same in symptomatic, asymptomatic, and control subjects.[112,127] This means that appropriate pacing of physical activity in the symptomatic patient can be achieved and this will help to prevent local muscle fatigue as well as overuse. Short periods of rest have been found to be very helpful.[128]

Medical treatment of depression, prescribed exercise, relaxation techniques such as meditation, and family education are essential to delaying the consequences of increased weakness. Medical treatment, such as pyridostigmine HCL, may be tried to improve neuromuscular transmission. Bulbar symptoms are more likely to respond. More specific treatments may be developed as viral and autoimmune mechanisms become identified.

Chronic Fatigue Syndrome

Clinical Physiology The patient with the Chronic Fatigue Syndrome (CFS) usually is a middle-aged woman who has experienced severe fatigue for a number of months (women are three times more likely than men to have this syndrome, and the prevalence is 37.1(F), 7.6(M) per 100,000).[129,130] The onset of fatigue may be associated with a flu-like illness or upper-respiratory infection, or other signs of infection that may include fever. In some cases, a recurrence of symptoms of infection such as a sore throat, muscle aches, "swollen glands," or symptoms of gastroenteritis may be reported. A fatigue history documenting a significant withdrawal from daily activities and reduced performance of these activities is common. Work outside the house often is discontinued. Help in performance of household tasks and an afternoon rest usually are required. Little or no primary or secondary gain arise from these changes. Interpersonal relationships frequently are disturbed, even at the cost of substantial income. Despite these changes, a history of specific disability cannot be obtained. There is no history of developing muscle weakness or loss of any specific function. Difficulty in thinking and concentration may be elicited. Changes in sleep habits also occur. These symptoms of malaise, low energy, and loss of interest in all activities eventually create or are associated with significant depression. However, many patients deny depression as a primary complaint. It is customary for a patient to have seen a number of physicians. All routine laboratory studies described previously for the evaluation of a fatigue patient are normal.

Physical findings are unremarkable. The presence of any neurological signs suggesting multiple sclerosis, polyneuropathy, myopathy, or a connective-tissue disorder require further laboratory investigation such as cerebrospinal fluid examination, electromyography, or muscle biopsy.

There is little understanding of this syndrome. Since its earliest report in the 1700's and through subsequent designations as the myalgic encephalomyelitis syndrome and the immune dysfunction syndrome, CSF has remained an extremely mysterious illness.[131] At one time, Epstein-Barr virus infection was believed to account for fatigue occurring in epidemic proportions, but this has been disproven.[132–134]

Center for Disease Control criteria for the diagnosis have been established, but these are so restrictive that modifications have been suggested that include post-infectious fatigue, somatiform disorders, nonpsychotic depression, and panic disorders (Table 23-2).[135,136] Revised criteria are shown in Table 23-3.[137] Virtually all of the findings are historical and difficult to document. Patients with CFS often have other organic conditions that produce systemic fatigue as a

Table 23-2
CDC case definition of CFS

Clinically evaluated, unexplained persistent or relapsing chronic fatigue that is of new or definite onset (has not been life-long) is not the result of ongoing exertion, is not substantially alleviated by rest, and results in substantial reduction of educational, occupational, social, or personal activities; and concurrence of 4 or more of the following symptoms (all of which have persisted or recurred during 6 or more consecutive months of illness). Symptom Criteria— beginning at or after onset of fatigue and persisting or recurring for more than 6 months

1. Self-reported impairment in short-term memory or concentration severe enough to substantially reduce activities of daily living
2. Sore throat
3. Tender cervical or axillary lymph nodes
4. Muscle pain
5. Multijoint pain without swelling or redness
6. Headaches of a new type, pattern, or severity
7. Unrefreshing sleep
8. Postexertional malaise lasting more than 24 hours

Source: Krupp LB, LaRocca NC, Muir-Nash J, et al: The fatigue severity scale applied to patients with multiple sclerosis and systemic lupus erythematosus. *Arch Neurol* 1989; 46:1121–1123.

Table 23-3
Recommended modifications of CFS case definition

Exclusions
  Psychiatric disorders
    Psychoses
      Psychotic depression
      Bipolar disorder
      Schizophrenia
    Substance abuse
  Postinfectious fatigue
    Documented infection
    Etiologic agent is known to produce chronic active
      infection
    Clinical picture compatible with ongoing active
      infection
      Chronic hepatitis B or C with active liver disease
      Infection with human immunodeficiency virus
        (HIV-I)
      Lyme disease (inadequately treated)
      Tuberculosis (TB)

Inclusions (in patients who otherwise meet CDC case
    definition)
  Fibromyalgia
  Postinfectious fatigue
    Lyme disease with persistent fatigue after appropriate
      antibiotic therapy
    Brucellosis with persistent fatigue after appropriate
      antibiotic therapy
    Acute infectious mononucleosis (documented) followed
      by chronic debilitating fatigue
    Acute cytomegalovirus infection
    Acute toxoplasmosis (adequately treated)
  Nonpsychotic depression
  Somatoform disorders
  Generalized anxiety disorder/panic disorder

prominent symptom. About 60 percent of patients with CFS have an organic or psychological disorder as the basis for their fatigue. The majority of CFS patients have psychiatric disease, whereas 20–45 percent have organic disease.[39,138–142]

Comparison of CFS patients with multiple sclerosis or postpolio patients with comparable degrees of fatigue reveals that CFS patients have more depression.[143,144] Response to an experimental psychological stressor has been shown to be significantly greater in CFS patients compared to those with muscular dystrophy or neurosis.[145] CFS patients have more depressive symptoms and less cognitive impairment than their counterparts experiencing fatigue with multiple sclerosis.[146]

Systemic Evaluation of CFS

The cardiopulmonary response to exercise is normal, but maximal levels of work appropriate for age are often not achieved.[147,148] Tests of muscle strength and endurance, as well as muscle histomorphometry, also are normal.[149,150] Jitter studies utilizing single fibers are normal.[151]

Although the course of CFS is protean, there is evidence for chronic infection that includes a febrile onset in some patients, recurrent low-grade fever, sore throat, adenopathy, and epidemic occurrences. Specific viruses and bacteria that have been excluded as causative agents include Epstein-Barr virus, cytomegalovirus, herpes simplex viruses 1, 2, and 6, and mycoplasma.[134,152–157] Elevated antibody titers to some, but not all viruses indicate that the immune response is not simply polyclonal.[157] Recurrent signs of infection suggest reactivation of latent infection. This is supported by data on markers of infection in CFS patients in comparison to controls.

A number of immune factors are altered in CFS. These include decreased NK lymphocytes and increased NK adhesion molecules.[17] Total lymphocyte count (CD3) is unchanged but CD8 (suppressor/cytotoxic)/ CD56 (NK) ratio is increased.[158] Interleukin-2 and IgG are increased, whereas IgA and IgE are decreased.[159] IgG is increased and the cytokine TGF beta also is elevated, as is leukocytic enzyme 2′,5′-oligoadenylate synthetase, leading to increased RNase levels and reduced cell metabolism.[17] TNF alpha and beta have been found elevated.[160] The overall picture is one of immune system activation with symptoms suggesting chronic infection.[161]

The clinical analysis can be difficult, because all patients are most likely not experiencing the same illness. Endogenous depression can cause some of these changes, and patient groups that have been studied differ significantly in severity of illness and completeness of evaluation. In general, the severity of CFS does not bear any relation to the degree of immunologic abnormality.[158] Physical exercise did not affect the level of cytokines: interferon gamma and alpha, interleukin-1 and beta, or tumor necrosis factor. With exercise, symptoms of fatigue, depression, and confusion have been shown to improve.[162]

The possibility that endocrinopathy is the cause of CFS has been investigated. Basal glucocorticoid levels are reduced, 24-hour urinary free cortisol is below normal, and adrenocorticotropin hormone (ACTH) is elevated.[163] Adrenocortical sensitivity to ACTH is increased, but response to bovine corticotropin-releasing hormone (CRH) is diminished.[163] This has been interpreted as resulting from central adrenergic insufficiency, possibly related to a deficiency of CRH or other factors relating to central dysautonomia.

By history and testing instruments, the majority of CFS patients have psychiatric diagnoses, most commonly depression. Depression is three times more common in CFS patients than in those with other illnesses. Twenty-four to 50 percent of CFS patients have a prior psychiatric diagnosis. It is well known that severe depression and situational stress can adversely affect the immune system, predisposing to infection in association with CFS.[138,140–142,164–167]

Sleep complaints have been reported in 33–81 percent of CSF patients.[56,59] Alpha-delta sleep has been correlated with chronic fatigue without depression.[56,59,168,169]

Studies of autonomic function in patients meeting the strict CDC criteria for CFS may provide a basis for linking together the symptom of fatigue, immune abnormality, endocrinopathy, and exercise data. Neurologically mediated hypotension was diagnosed by tilt table and response to isoproterenol in 22 of 23 patients with CFS versus 4 of 14 controls. Seventy percent of CFS patients and no controls had an abnormal response to stage 1 of the tilt, 45 minutes at 70 degree tilt. Nine patients reported complete or nearly complete resolution of symptoms after therapy using fludrocortisone, beta-adrenergic blocking agents, or disopyramide, to treat neurologically mediated hypotension.[170]

Patients with dysautonomia complain of profound fatigue. The most common finding on examination is orthostatic hypotension. During routine physical examination, slowly developing orthostatic hypotension may go unnoticed. The restoration of normal blood pressure through the use of fludrocortisone is helpful in these patients. Central dysautonomia may cause severe fatigue and be a component of CFS, as well as other conditions such as multiple sclerosis.[171–172]

Treatment and Rehabilitation The recognition that CFS is the result of several factors guides treatment. Psychological issues must be addressed, especially depression. Chronic pain must be managed effectively. If a sleep disorder is present, it must be treated. Encouragement and introduction of a graduated exercise program is helpful. The presence of fatigue can begin a cycle of morbidity in which reduced physical activity progressively reduces exercise tolerance. Exercise can even accelerate recovery from an illness that improves spontaneously.[8,173,174]

A number of medical therapies, such as acyclovir, have been tried without success.[52,175–177] Mild improvement has been reported following gamma globulin treatment in two of four studies. Ampligen, a synthetic ribonucleic acid that has both antiviral properties and immune modulating properties decreases CFS symptoms following 24 weeks of treatment.[178] These results support the concept that CFS results from an immune response not unlike that present in chronic infection. These results require confirmation.

Since CFS, depression, and fibromyalgia syndrome share many common affective features, including dysphoria and depression, antidepressants have been tried. CFS appears to respond favorably with smaller doses of antidepressant medication than those required for depression.[179]

Myasthenic Syndrome, Motoneuron Disease, Channelopathies

Clinical Pathophysiology The patient with a neuromuscular disorder complains of weakness and fatigue, and usually can differentiate between the two. For example, the patient with myasthenia gravis (MG) demonstrates the classical picture of what has been called "pathological fatigue." Continued or repetitive use of a muscle results in a decrement in force that leads to disability. Repetitive chewing produces such weakness of the masseter that the mouth cannot be closed. Reading causes diplopia. Even the effort to keep the eyes open produces ptosis. In most instances, substantial recovery occurs with rest. It is this pattern of weakness induced by exercise then recovery with rest that characterizes MG. A diurnal pattern of weakness often is present with symptoms more evident in the afternoon. The Lambert-Eaton syndrome also produces weakness with activity but strength may transiently increase when exercise is begun from a condition of complete rest.

Motor neuron disease leads to a progressive loss of strength that results in disability measured month by month. Loss of spinal (lower) motoneurons, as well as spasticity from loss of cortical motoneurons is common. Fatigue, manifested by hourly or diurnal variations in strength may be noticeable. Similarly, patients with dystrophy or other diseases that produce muscle-fiber loss complain of more weakness than fatigue.

The myotonic disorders are influenced by muscle activity so that the patient may observe changes in stiffness that may increase with rest, activity, or ambient temperature. A warm-up helps most patients to reduce stiffness. Under certain circumstances, including exposure to cold, stiffness may increase, and it may be possible to measure the actual induction of myotonia.

The physical examination for most disorders reveals a particular pattern of involvement that can be helpful in diagnosis. For example, in MG, involvement often is highly focal, with early involvement of ocular and bulbar muscles common. Weakness may develop only in isolated muscles. Weakness in proximal muscles is characteristic of many dystrophic disorders. In myotonic muscular dystrophy, there is distal muscle wasting, a "myopathic facies," and often ptosis. Frontal balding, cataracts, cardiac conduction defects and smooth-muscle disorders fill out the spectrum of involvement. MG is the only condition in which significant disability occurs as the result of muscle activity over time and recovery occurs with rest. Such changes do not occur in myopathies where weakness is the chief complaint.

Muscle Strength and Endurance In MG neuromuscular transmission is impaired, as a result of autoimmune injury to post-junctional acetylcholine receptors.[180,181] The amount of acetylcholine that is released with each action potential decreases steadily with each impulse, so that by the fourth or fifth impulse a nadir is reached. If the number of receptors is reduced, then the amount of acetylcholine secretion may be insufficient to activate individual muscle fibers. The safety factor for neuromuscular transmission is exceeded, and conduction failure results.[181]

In motoneuron disease, weakness predominates, but as the illness progresses, physical activity may result in increased weakness. The impression of increased fatiguability may result from the more rapid loss of function, whereas the rate of fatigue development is normal. The weak muscle starts its fatigue curve at a lower point. However, repetitive motor-nerve stimulation in amyotrophic lateral sclerosis (ALS) patients may reveal a decrement in amplitude similar to that seen in myasthenia gravis.[23] This may result from impaired neuromuscular transmission present as a result of motor axons dying back and nascent neuromuscular junctions occurring with reinnervation. In some cases fatigue and muscle strength may improve with the judicious use of anticholinesterase medications. Studies of fatigue in selected muscle groups with mild-to-moderate weakness have revealed increased rates of fatigue development.[182] Decreased work capacity and oxygen consumption have been demonstrated using cycle ergometry.[183] Higher

rates of inorganic phosphate to creatine phosphate as well as lower intracellular pH in comparison to controls have been found.[184,185] Mechanisms of fatigue in ALS require further investigation. In the postpolio syndrome, rates of fatigue development also are increased, but no difference in muscle phosphagen metabolism in comparison to controls has been found.[186,187]

In some channelopathies, such as paramyotonia, muscle contraction may increase stiffness and worsen disability. In other myotonic disorders, such as myotonia congenita, a warm-up may reduce stiffness and limit fatigue.[29] In metabolic myopathies fatigue results from failure to utilize energy sources for muscle contraction. The first disorder of this type was identified by McCardle in 1951 as a defect in muscle glycogen utilization.[188] Ischemic exercise resulted in painful contracture. Myophosphorylase deficiency was subsequently identified.[189] Unaccustomed isometric muscle contractions may lead to contracture and severely limit exercise performance. Ischemic exercise test reveals normal elevation of ammonia but no elevation of lactate. Patients with this disorder may exercise normally with little consequence. When exercise exertion is increased, painful contracture may develop. Serum creatine phosphokinase and myoglobin levels may be elevated, leading to myoglobinuria. Despite such changes nuclear magnetic resonance spectroscopy does not reveal reduction in levels of adenosine triphosphate (ATP).[190] Phosphofructokinase deficiency and other glycolytic enzyme deficiencies may mimic this disorder in many respects.[191,192]

Myoadenylate deaminase deficiency results in failure to elevate ammonia during ischemic exercise.[193] Exercise intolerance is common, experienced as aching muscles characteristic of overuse. Complaints may be minimized, or passed off as a normal response to exertion. This is the most common metabolic myopathy.

Fatty-acid transport into muscle mitochondria may be limited by deficient muscle or systemic carnitine and carnitine palmitoyltransferase deficiency inherited as an autosomal recessive trait.[194] Endurance exercise relying on fatty acids for fuel is limited, and myoglobinuria is common. A variety of abnormalities of the cytochrome complex exist. In Luft's disease ATP synthesis is diverted to heat production. Cytochrome b deficiency also has been identified as a cause of limited endurance.[195,196]

In general, the neuromuscular disorders are characterized by muscle weakness that leads to disability that is relatively constant throughout the day. Myasthenia gravis and the Eaton-Lambert syndrome are exceptions. A great many factors may alter the rate of fatigue development in neuromuscular disorders. Denervating disorders associated with reinnervation may result in significant alteration in the population of different types of motor units. Fast-fatigue motor units may replace those that are fatigue-resistant. The size of motor units is grossly affected with enlargement, followed by reduction in size as disease progresses. Individual fibers may become hypertrophic. Twitch characteristics and fatigue properties are affected by fiber size. Normal fibers are juxtaposed with reinnervated and denervated fibers. The distribution of fibers within the motor unit is abnormal, characterized by fiber-typed grouping and group atrophy. The normal intermingling of fibers from different motor units is abnormal. During exercise, inactive muscle fibers adjacent to active fibers act like sponges that absorb the extracellular byproducts of exercise. Sodium and potassium pumping by these fibers is capable of limiting the increase in extracellular potassium that accumulates around active fibers. An excess of extracellular potassium diminishes sarcolemmal membrane excitability and slows conduction speed of the muscle-fiber action potential. This, in turn, slows contraction rate and attenuates other contractile properties of muscle, thereby contributing to great fatigue.[197]

Disuse resulting from immobilization or altered patterns of innervation present in spastic paresis result in increased fatigability in response to tetanic nerve stimulation.[198,199]

Defects can exist at any step in the neuromuscular activation process, causing fatigue as the primary net result.

Involvement of Other Systems in Neuromuscular Diseases

Many neuromuscular disorders are associated with involvement of other organs and systems that may contribute to the symptom of fatigue. Cardiac involvement in Emery-Dreyfuss, Duchenne muscular dystrophy, Becker's muscular dystrophy, and polymyositis may lead to cardiogenic fatigue. It is essential to identify fatigue as a symptom separate and distinct from weakness and to be aware that it may have multiple and nonmuscular causes.

Treatment and Rehabilitation

The presence of muscle weakness supports the development of the "morbidity cycle." Failure to perform even the simplest activities of daily living may result in withdrawal, depression, and unwillingness to engage in activities that can be easily accomplished. Even MG patients, under successful treatment, may benefit from exercise to improve endurance and strength. Similarly, patients with Duchenne muscular dystrophy may improve strength and delay progression of weakness, through the application of selective exercises.

Fatigue in the Elderly

Clinical Pathophysiology   Unless confronted by specific symptoms or disability, the elderly patient may come into the clinic only for routine examination. Aging is associated with decreased muscle mass, increased localized pain from such processes as osteoarthritis, and decreased cardiopulmonary function. A gradual and subtle adjustment of physical activity occurs that allows performance of daily activities within a zone of comfort. It is not uncommon for a spouse to be unaware of the gradual and insidious development of congestive heart failure in his or her partner owing to the subtle adjustment of activity over time that must occur if symptoms are to be avoided. This in part explains why elderly persons do not complain of fatigue unless significant illness or depression is present. In studies of the relationship between fatigue and depression in the older patient, age was not associated with the severity of fatigue.[42,200]

The pathophysiology of aging depends to some extent on the loss of neurons in the central nervous system that occurs decade by decade. Estimates of the number of motor units decline steadily after the age of 50 to 60. Muscle-fiber minimum diameter becomes smaller. There is no evidence for reinnervation phenomena, such as fiber-type grouping. Fiber-type distribution remains the same, but Type II atrophy may be present if physical activity has been limited by such factors as joint pain.

Muscle Strength and Endurance   Studies of the twitch torque produced by tibialis anterior muscle have revealed no significant difference between young and elderly subjects, but twitch potentiation is significantly greater in the young. Contraction time, time to peak torque, and one-half relaxation times also are slowed in the elderly.[201] Training does not change contraction characteristics in the elderly but response to potentiation is significantly increased.[202] Thus, twitch potentiation is the single most important feature of muscle contraction influenced by both age and training. Torque decline in tibialis anterior muscle in response to repetitive stimulation at 20 Hz is more rapid in elderly than young subjects but at 30 and 40 Hz no significant difference is found. M wave amplitude and area are lower for elderly subjects but the rate of decline during repetitive stimulation is not different from that of young subjects. Thus, neuromuscular transmission is not demonstrated to be less adequate in older subjects.[201,202]

Significant improvement in aerobic fitness measures of well-being (Profile of Mood States) and cortical evoked responses have been demonstrated to occur as a result of an exercise training program for elderly subjects.[203]

Motivation Since depression has been highly correlated with symptoms of fatigue as well as decreased passive short-term memory in elderly subjects, situational factors such as retirement, loss of a spouse, separation from family members, and concomitant illness must be addressed. Attachment to groups with similar goals and objectives and participation in exercise and recreational programs are important to health maintenance and the overall quality of life for elderly persons.

Fatigue in Patients with Epilepsy

Clinical Pathophysiology At a tertiary care center, most patients with epilepsy are those with difficult-to-control mixed seizure disorders. These patients have a wide variety of etiologies for their seizures and may have associated neurological deficits. Most are on a variety of medications and experience disorders of mood, attention, and cognition. Fatigue occurs in nearly 44 percent of epileptics by Fatigue Severity Scale criteria. Fatigue was correlated with depression in this group ($R = 0.56$, $P < 0.001$). Depression in turn was correlated with seizure frequency and was independent of the type of anticonvulsant used.[36]

Motivation Depression related to seizure frequency and possibly anticonvulsant side-effect plays a significant role in the production of fatigue in epileptics on multiple antiepileptic drugs. Altering the mode of delivery of carbamazepine from conventional to controlled release forms results in a 34 percent (44/131) reduction in side-effects and medication tolerance.[212]

Treatment and Rehabilitation Combination antiepileptic drug therapy can contribute to symptoms of fatigue and depression. Simplifying the medical regimen when appropriate, institution of monotherapy when possible, use of controlled formulas, and treatment of depression can help diminish the symptom of fatigue.

Postoperative Fatigue (POF)

Clinical Pathophysiology Following major abdominal surgery, fatigue and pain are a common experience. Current practice is to mobilize patients as quickly as possible and to begin ambulation within hours of recovery from anesthesia. The peak level of fatigue in 38 patients occurred after one week and returned to preoperative levels at one month.[213] Three months later the level of fatigue was less than at preoperative levels.[213] In women undergoing hysterectomy fatigue was substantially reduced at 6 months.[214] POF is correlated most closely with preoperative levels of fatigue and also correlates with age, presence of cancer, and the degree of pain.[215]

Studies of POF have not found a primary muscular or nutritional cause for its presence. However, muscle protein synthesis has been found to be decreased for up to 13 days after abdominal surgery.[216] Studies of adductor pollicis brevis muscle using repetitive stimulation of ulnar nerve revealed no effect of surgery, but grip strength fell after operation and returned to normal after 3 months.[213] Perceived effort increased after surgery and returned to normal in 3 months. Total body nitrogen fell in the first 2 weeks after surgery, and normalized by 3 months. Experimental evidence indicates that fatigue following surgery is not accompanied by any muscular defect, but rather results from increased central fatigue.[217]

Factors considered responsible for POF are decreased phosphocreatine in muscles, proton accumulation in muscle, depletion of muscle glycogen stores, hypoglycemia, and an increase in the ratio of free tryptophan/branch chain amino acids. Supplying branch chain amino acids may reduce fatigue. Supplemental glutamine counteracted a decline in postoperative muscle protein synthesis as long as it was given, but had no effect on the perceived level of fatigue.[218,219]

Reduction in stress during surgery is a function of the operative procedure and its duration, type of anesthesia, and method of postoperative pain relief. The role of these factors in the development of POF has been studied. POF is reduced significantly following laparoscopy in comparison to orthodox laparotomy.[220–222] Epidural anesthesia produced equivalent degrees of POF in comparison to general anesthesia.[223] POF was enhanced using patient-controlled analgesia in comparison to administration of morphine given on demand.[224] POF correlates with the degree of surgical trauma, but not with the duration of anesthesia and surgery or the perioperative nutritional status, age, or sex.[225] Postoperative complications manifested as deterioration in nutritional status, loss of muscle strength, and cardiovascular response to exercise are highly correlated with POF.[225] POF has been found higher in coronary-artery bypass patients with higher levels of perioperative catacholamines.[226] Most investigations of the role of psychological factors in POF have deemphasized their relative importance, but 30-day POF has been correlated with concurrent levels of depression and anxiety.[225]

Treatment and Rehabilitation   POF can be reduced through reduction in surgical stress. The most dramatic example of reduced surgical trauma is laparoscopic surgery compared to orthodox laparatomy. Minimizing tissue destruction intraoperatively is more important than the duration of surgery or type of anesthesia in prevention of POF.

Restoration of normal nutrition and physical activity postoperatively is also important. Patient-controlled analgesia may improve patient comfort, at the expense of greater POF.[22]

The key to reduced POF is to reduce the magnitude of surgical trauma, and to maximize nutritional and physical activity as soon as possible.

Infectious and Postinfectious Fatigue

Clinical Pathophysiology   Fatigue is a universal feature of major systemic infections. Viral infections known to be associated with severe fatigue include hepatitis, influenza, and EBV. Bacterial infections, such as Lyme disease and brucella also cause severe fatigue. Major systemic infectious illness may be followed by months of chronic fatigue. Out of 166 patients seen in an infectious-disease clinic, 83 percent of chronic-fatigue cases began with an acute illness, usually an upper-respiratory infection.[37] Stress during the acute illness was perceived as responsible for chronic fatigue.[2] Attempts to identify specific viruses commonly associated with chronic fatigue have produced variable results. In 35 patients with postinfectious fatigue, recurrent persistent HHV-6 infection was found in 73 percent, and EBV infection in 34 percent; 7 percent had evidence for infection by both viruses.[227] Consistent identification of EBV infection in chronic fatigue has never been established.[229] Dual infection with EBV and adenovirus type 2 was found in four patients experiencing severe chronic fatigue.[230] The difficulty in establishing such relationships stem from the high prevalence of antibody against common

viruses in the general population. Large population-based studies of chronic-fatigue patients compared to control groups have not demonstrated consistent patterns of viral infections.

Human immunodeficiency virus (HIV) infection is associated with fatigue, muscle wasting, and myalgia.[13] No alteration in muscle metabolism or azothiaprine-related mitochondrial disorders were found.[13] Fatigue in HIV infection may result from the direct influence of the virus on the central nervous system. CD4 receptors are present on neurons within the CNS. Viral involvement of these neurons may explain acquired immunodeficiency syndrome (AIDS) dementia as well as fatigue.

In some patients treated for Lyme disease, fatigue persisted despite disappearance of all acute infectious symptoms. In these patients, serum IgM was elevated in comparison to controls.[41] CSF abnormalities were present and the clinical picture often resembled multiple sclerosis. Persistent fatigue, depression, and cognitive deficit is associated with B. burgdorferi antigen in cerebrospinal fluid.[41] Studies of T-cell subsets in patients with the post-viral fatigue syndrome have indicated a decreased percentage of CD56+ Fc gamma receptor (CD16) + MK cells suggesting a reduced capacity of antibody-dependent cellular cytotoxicity.[231] In 26 patients with elevated EBV titers, serial cultures for this and HHV-6 virus obtained over time were no different from those found in a control population. However, patients with chronic fatigue demonstrated higher in vitro natural killer-cell activity and lower interleukin-2 production than controls. Improvement in fatigue symptoms over time was not associated with any changes in antibody titers to EBV or HHV-6.[232]

Treatment and Rehabilitation   The prognosis for recovery from postviral fatigue syndrome is good. Antiviral therapy has not been found to be effective in reducing fatigue levels. Antibiotic treatment of patients suspected of having Lyme disease on a serological basis alone, without objective signs, has not been found to be cost-effective.[233] Support groups have been helpful for many-patients, but their composition is very heterogeneous and includes patients with somatoform disorders, depression, and other chronic-fatigue syndromes.

Encouragement must be offered to remain active; participation in a comfortable, low- level aerobic exercise program can be beneficial. Improved fitness can reduce the symptoms of fatigue.

Fatigue in the Workplace

Clinical Pathophysiology Work-related fatigue often leads to specific musculoskeletal complaints that may be intimately intertwined with issues of motivation and secondary gain. It is essential to outline daily activities in detail, the physical and cognitive requirements of the job, and the work schedule. Examination of the latter may reveal an adverse impact on sleep cycles.

Workers may suffer from sleep deprivation when working 12-hour shifts that rotate biweekly. Job stress has been documented to be associated with an increased incidence of serious illness among workers, including myocardial infarction.[234]

Ergonomic studies can be used to investigate assumptions about the causes of fatigue and musculoskeletal complaints in the workplace. Changes in the work environment that are often very simple can sometimes be immensely helpful. Early investigations have proven the value of task-specific analysis of occupationally individual fatigue. For example, fatigue in fingers resulting from typing has been analyzed by studying the tremor spectra. Changes in power spectra over time documented the development of fatigue.[235,236] Following a cranking exercise carpenters were found to have more trouble nailing than sawing or screwing.[237] Cardiovascular and muscular criteria of fatigue were found to be the same for carrying.[238] It was found that carrying loads greater than six kilograms for women or ten kilograms for men led to "cardiovascular nonsteady states" and EMG signs of fatigue.[238] Muscle tension and divergent patterns of muscle activation were not found to be responsible for neck and shoulder complaints in women performing repetitive short-cycle industrial tasks.[239] Musculoskeletal complaints in sewing-machine workers were found to be significantly less in the stronger workers.[240]

For centuries, the optimum duration of the work week has been the subject of debate. Evaluation of occupational fatigue across a wide variety of industries reveals little attention to sleep cycles or the advantages of periodic rests. Overtime work (greater than 12 hours) has been reported as a source of power-plant operator error.[242] Fatigue was not recognized sufficiently as a cause of accidents among truck drivers, whose income is based on working extra hours.[243] Rotating 8-hour shifts among firefighters was demonstrated to depress mood and create sleepiness on the job.[244] Erratic schedules were found to impair work performance in ferry pilots, mates, and masters.[245]

Sleep loss leads to sleep debt, which can be made up by sleeping deeply for 2 or 3 days. When sleep/wake patterns (circadian rhythms) are interrupted, hormonal regulation, body temperature, work performance, mood, a variety of vegetative functions, and information processing are all disrupted.[43–50] Older individuals are more severely affected by such changes.[246] Depression and situational family stressors have been found to induce fatigue and impair work performance.[247,248]

Preoccupation with the welfare of children, sick individuals at home, or disturbed marital relations can also disrupt work performance and cause fatigue.

Treatment and Rehabilitation An occupational history must be obtained that includes an adequate description of the work process. The work schedule must be reported. A detailed sleep history is essential. Loss of sleep affects most aspects of psychomotor performance and depresses mood, suggesting a change in schedule may be all that is necessary. Contributing stress factors at work and at home must be discussed and addressed.

SUMMARY

The physiologic definition of fatigue as a decline in muscle force with a repetitive or sustained contraction is operationally useful for some but not all types of neurologically based fatigue. Some neuromuscular disorders such as myasthenia gravis manifest decrements in muscle force that result from a defect in neuromuscular transmission. In chronic fatigue syndrome or postinfectious fatigue, fatigue complaints may be disabling, and even prevent gainful employment, yet no muscle weakness or decrements in muscle force with exercise can be detected. In multiple sclerosis, combinations of both central and peripheral fatigue may be present.

Depression, psychosocial stressors, and chronic pain contribute in varying degrees to the symptom of fatigue. Lack of rest and interrupted sleep contribute strongly to fatigue in a variety of settings, especially in the workplace or in association with chronic pain.

A common feature in several disorders is an alteration of the immune response, sometimes in response to infection, autoimmune state, or psychological stress. The fatigue associated with immune-system activation suggests immune regulation of energy-conservation processes from within the central nervous system

In each disorder described the symptom of fatigue is common, or the most common symptom. The pathophysiologic basis for fatigue in different settings is quite diverse. Mechanisms range from central fatigue that may result from impaired impulse conduction, defective synaptic transmission, or neuronal cell death to muscle membrane disorders and impaired muscle contraction. Finally, the immune system and psychological factors, especially depression, may play a major role in the production of fatigue. As specific mechanisms are understood it is likely that a common thread will emerge that will clarify our concepts of fatigue and improve its treatment.

Acknowledging the presence of fatigue and maintaining activity within its limits can help prevent the "morbidity cycle" in which tolerance for activitiy becomes progressively lower. Appropriate medications, a supportive environment, and an exercise prescription are essential ingredients of the rehabilitative process.

REFERENCES

1. Canter A, Cluff LE, Imboden JB: Hypersensitive reactions to immunization innoculations and antecendent psychological vulnerability. *J Psychosomat Res* 1972; 16:99–101.

2. Cohen S, Tyrrell AJ, Smith AP: Psychological stress and susceptibility to the common cold. *N Engl J Med* 1991; 325:606–612.

3. Cope H, David A, Pelosi A, Mann A: Predictors of chronic "postviral" fatigue. *Lancet* 344:864–868, 1994.

4. Imboden JB, Canter A, Cluff LE: Convalescence from influenza. A study of the psychological and clinical determinants. *Arch Intern Med* 1961; 108:393–399.

5. Imboden JB, Canter A, Cluff LE, Trevor RW: Brucellosis: Psychologic aspects of delayed convalescence. *Arch Int Med* 1959; 103:406–444.

6. Cramer SR, Neiman DL, Lee JW: The effects of moderate exercise training on psychological well-being and mood state in women. *J Psychosom Res* 1991; 35:437–449.

7. Gilson BS, Bergner M, Bobbit RA, et al: The sickness impact profile: Final development and testing, 1975–1978. Seattle Department of Health Services, School of Public Health and Community Medicine, University of Washington, 1979.

8. Butler S, Chalder T, Ron M, Wessely S: Cognitive behaviour therapy in CFS. *J Neurol Neurosurg Psychiatr* 1991; 54:153–158.

9. Friedberg F, Krupp LB: A comparison of cognitive behavioral treatment for chronic fatigue syndrome and primary depression. *Clin Infec Dis* 1994; 18(Suppl):105–110.

10. Lloyd AR, Hickie I, Brockmand A, et al: Immunological and psychological therapy for patients with chronic fatigue syndrome: A double-blind placebo controlled trial. *Amer J Med* 1993; 94(2):197–203.

11. Chao CC, DeLa Hunt M, Hu S, et al: Immunologically mediated fatigue: a murine model. *Clin Immum Immunopathol* 1992; 64:161–165.

12. Chao CC, Janoff EN, Hu S, et al: Altered cytokine release in peripheral blood mononuclear cell cultures from patients with the CFS. *Cytokine* 1991; 3:292–298.

13. Miller RG, Carson PJ, Moussani RS, et al: Fatigue and myalgia in AIDS patients. *Neurology* 1991; 41:1603–1607.

14. Bertolone K, Coyle PK, Krupp LB, et al: Cytokine correlates of fatigue in MS. *Neurology* 1993; 43:A356.

15. Barker E, Fujimura SJ, Fadem MB, et al: Immunologic abnormalities associated with CFS. *Clin Infect Dis* 1994; 18:S136–S141.

16. Gupta S, Vayuvegula BA: Comprehensive immunological analysis in CFS. *Scan J Immunol* 1991; 33:319–327.

17. Klimas NG, Salvato FR, Morgan R, Fletcher MA: Immunologic abnormalities in CFS. *J Clin Microbiol* 1991; 28:1403–1410.

18. Landay AL, Jessup C, Jennette ET, Levy JA: CFS: Clinical condition associated with immune activation. *Lancet* 1991; 338:707–712.

19. Linde A, Andersson B, Svenson SB, et al: Serum levels of lymphokines and soluble cellular receptors in primary EBV infection and in patients with CFS. *J Infect Dis* 1992; 165:994–1000.

20. Lloyd A, Hickie I, Brockman A, et al: Cytokine levels in serum and CSF in patients with CFS and control subjects. *J Infect Dis* 1991; 164:1023–1024.

21. Patarca R, Klimas NG, Lugtendorf S, et al: Dysregulated expression of tumor necrosis factor in CFS: Interrelations with cellular sources and patterns of soluble immune mediator expression. *Clin Infect Dis* 1994; 18:S147–S153.

22. DeFreitas E, Hilliard B, Cheney PR, et al: Retroviral sequences related to human T-lymphotropic virus type II in patients with CFIDS. *Proc Natl Acad Sci USA* 1991; 88:2922–2926.

23. Denys EH, Norris FH: Amyotrophic lateral sclerosis: impairment of neuromuscular transmission. *Arch Neurol* 1979; 36:202–205.

24. Reiners K, Herdmann J, Freund J: Altered mechanisms of force genation in lower motor neuron disease. *Musc Nerve* 1989; 12(8):647–659.

25. Slonim AE, Goans PJ: Myopathy in McArdle's syndrome. *N Engl J Med* 1985; 312(6):355–359.

26. Sabina RL, Swain JL, Olanow CW, et al: Myoadenylate deaminase deficiency. Functional and metabolic abnormalities associated with disruptions of the purine nucleotide cycle. *J Clin Invest* 1984; 73:720–730.

27. Dalakas MC: Pathogenetic mechanisms of post-polio syndrome: morphological, electrophysiological, virological, and immunological correlations. *Ann NY Acad Sci,* 1995; 753:167–185.

28. Bruno RL, Cohen JM, Galski T, Frick NM: The neruoanatomy of post-polio fatigue. *Arch Phys Med Rehabil* 1994; 75(5):498–504.

29. Ptacek LJ, Johnson KJ, Griggs, RC: Genetics and physiology of the myotonic muscle disorders. *New Engl J Med* 1993; 328:482–489.

30. Friedman J, Friedman H: Fatigue in Parkinson's Disease. *Neurology* 1993; 43:2016–2018.

31. Fisk JD, Pontefract A, Ritvo PG, Archibald CJ, Murray TJ: The impact of fatigue on patients with multiple sclerosis. *Can J Neurol Sci* 1994; 21(1):9–14.

32. Freal JE, Kraft GH, Coryell SK: Symptomatic fatigue in multiple sclerosis. *Arch Phys Med Rehabil* 1984; 65:135–138.

33. Krupp LB, Alvarez LA, LaRocca NG, Scheinberg L: Clinical characteristics of fatigue in multiple sclerosis. *Arch Neurol* 1988; 45:435–437.

34. Murray TS: Amantadine therapy for fatigue in multiple sclerosis. *Can J Neurol Sci* 1985; 12:251–254.

35. Krupp LB, La Rocca N: Fatigue in neurologic disorders. Annual meeting, American Academy of Neurology, April 12–19, 1996.

36. Ettinger, AB: *Fatigue in Epilepsy,* reported by Krupp LB, ibid.

37. Sharpe M, Hawton K, Seagroatt V, Pasvol G: Follow up of patients presenting with fatigue to an infectious diseases clinic. *Br Med J* 1992; 305:147–152.

38. Belza BL, Henke CJ, Yelin EH, Epstein WV, Gilliss CL: Correlates of fatigue in older adults with rheumatoid arthritis. *Nurs Res* 1993; 42:93–99.

39. Katon WJ, Buchwald DS, Simon GE, et al: Psychiatric illness in patients with chronic fatigue and those with rheumatoid arthritis. *J Gen Intern Med* 1991; 6:277–285.

40. Krupp LB, LaRocca NC, Muir J, Steinberg AD: A study of fatigue in systemic lupus erythematosus. *J Rheumatol* 1990; 17:1450–1452.

41. Krupp LB, Schwartz JE, Jandorf L: Fatigue in Lyme disease, in Coyle PK (ed): *Lyme Disease.* St. Louis, Mosby Year Book, 1993.

42. Kjerulff KH, Langenberg DM: A comparison of alternative ways of measuring fatigue among patients having hysterectomy. *Med Care* 1995; 33(4 Suppl):AS156–163.

43. Broughton RJ, Ogilvie RD (eds): *Sleep, Arousal, and Performance.* Boston: Birkhauser-Boston Inc, 1992.

44. Dinges DF: Are you awake? Cognitive performance and reverie during the hypnopompic state, in Bootzin R, Kihlstrom J, Schacter D (eds): *Sleep and Cognition.* Washington, DC: American Psychological Association, 1990.

45. Dinges DF, Kribbs NB: Performing while sleepy: effects of experimentally-induced sleepiness. in Monk T (ed): *Sleep, Sleepiness and Performance.* Chichester, UK: John Wiley and Sons Ltd, 1991.

46. Horne JA: A review of the biological effects of total sleep deprivation in man. *Biol Psych* 1978; 7:55–102.

47. Krupp LB, Coyle PK, Sliwinski M: Fatigue in the elderly, in Park M, Sage J (ed): *Practical Neurology of the Elderly.* New York: Marcel Decker, 1996.

48. Dinges DF: Probing the limits of functional capability: The effects of sleep loss on short-duration tasks, in

Broughton RJ, Ogilvie R (eds): *Sleep, Arousal and Performance: Problems and Promises.* Boston: Birkhauser-Boston, 1992.

49. Dinges DF, Broughton RJ (eds): *Sleep and Alertness: Chronobiological, Behavioral, and Medical Aspects of Napping.* New York: Raven Press, 1989.

50. Graeber RC: Aircrew fatigue and circadian rhythmicity, in Weiner EL, Nagel DC (eds): *Human Factors in Aviation.* New York: Academic Press, 1988.

51. Krupp LB, LaRocca NC, Muir-Nash J, et al: The fatigue severity scale applied to patients with multiple sclerosis and systemic lupus erythematosus. *Arch Neurol* 1989; 46:1121–1123.

52. Straus SE, Dale JK, Tobi M, et al: Acyclovir treatment of the CFS: lack of efficacy in a placebo-controlled trial. *New Engl J Med* 1988; 319:1692–1698.

53. Petajan, JH, Gappmaier E, White AT, et al: Impact of aerobic training on fitness and quality of life in multiple sclerosis patients. *Ann Neurol* 1996 39:432–441.

54. Stewart AL, Hays RD, Ware JE: The MOS short form general health survey: Reliability and validity in a patient population. *Med Care* 1988; 26:724–735.

55. Elnicki DM, Shocklor WR, Brick JE, et al: Evaluating the complaint of fatigue in primary care (Comment). *Am J Med* 1993; 95(1):117.

56. Buchwald D, Pascualy R, Bombardier C, Kith P: Sleep disorder in patients with chronic fatigue. *Clin Infect Dis* 1994; 18(Suppl 1):S68–S72.

57. Dinges DF, Orne MT, Orne EC: Sleepiness during sleep deprivation: the effects of performance demands and circadian phase. *Sleep* 1984; 13:189.

58. Giancario T, Kapen S, Saad J: Analysis of sleepiness and fatigue in multiple sclerosis. *Ann Neurol* 1987; 22:187.

59. Krupp LB, Jandorf L, Coyle PK, Mendelson WB: Sleep in chronic fatigue syndrome. *J Psychosom Res* 1993; 37:325–331.

60. Whelton CL, Salit I, Moldofsky H: Sleep, EBV infection, musculoskeletal pain, and depressive symptoms in CFS. *J Rheumatol* 1992; 19:939–943.

61. Scheffers MK, Johnson R Jr, Grafman J, et al: Attention and short-term memory in CFS patients. *Neurology* 1992; 42:1667–1675.

62. Beck AT, Ward CH, Mendelson M: An inventory for measuring depression. *Arch Gen Psych* 1961; 4:561–571.

63. Radloff LS: CES-D scale: A self-report depression scale for research in the general population. *Appl Psychol Meas* 1977; 1:385–401.

64. Weinshenker BG, Penman M, Bass B: A double-blind, randomized, crossover trial of pemoline in fatigue associated with multiple sclerosis. *Neurology* 1992; 42:1468–1471.

65. Canadian MS Research Group: A randomized controlled trial of amantadine in fatigue associated with multiple sclerosis. *Can J Neurol Sci* 1987; 14:273–278.

66. Krupp LB, Coyle PK, Doscher C, et al: A comparison of

amantadine, pemoline, and placebo in the treatment of MS fatigue. *Neurology* 1993; 43:A281.

67. Krupp LB, Sliwinski M, Masur DM, et al: Impact of fatigue treatment on cognitive functioning in MS. *Ann Neurol* 1993; 34:248.

68. Polman CH, Bertelsmann FW, van Loenen AC, Koetsier JC: 4-Aminopyridine in the treatment of patients with multiple sclerosis. *Arch Neurol* 1994; 51:292–296.

69. McNair DM, Lorr M, Droppleman LR: *Profile of Mood States (POMS)*. Educational and Industrial Testing Service, San Diego, CA, 1992.

70. Spielberger CD: Trait-state anxiety and motor behavior. *J Motor Behav* 1971; 3:265–279.

71. Paterson PY, Swanborg RH: Demyelinating diseases of the central and peripheral nervous systems, in Santon M (ed): *Immunological Diseases*, 4th ed, vol II. Boston: Little Brown, 1988.

72. Barnett LA, Fujinami RS: Molecular mimicry: a mechanism for autoimmune injury. *FASEB J* 1992; 6:840–844.

73. Fujinami RS: Molecular mimicry: Virus modulators of the immune response, in McKendall RR, Stroop WA (eds): *Handbook of Neurovirology*. New York:, Marcel Dekker, 1994.

74. Li R, Linan MJ, Stein MC, Faustman DL: Reduced expressions of peptide-loaded ALA class I molecules on multiple sclerosis lymphocytes. *Ann Neurol* 1995; 38:147–154.

75. Waxman SG: Ion channels and nerve conduction. Adrian Lecture. The X International Congress of EMG and Clinical Neurophysiology, Kyoto, Japan, 1995.

76. Kent-Braun JA, Sharma KR, Miller RG, Weiner MW: Postexercise phosphocreatine resynthesis is slowed in multiple sclerosis. *Muscle & Nerve* 1994; 17:835–841.

77. Schwartz J, Jandorf L, Krupp LB: The measurement of fatigue: A new scale. *J Psychosom Res* 1993; 37:753–762.

78. Petajan JH, Gappmaier E: Effect of rest and passive stretch on quadriceps muscle stiffness in spastic paresis. Abstract, American College of Sports Medicine, 1993.

79. Montgomery EB Jr: Basal ganglia pathophysiology. *Neurol For* 1995; 6(1):12–14.

80. Filion M, Tremblay L: Effects of dopamine agonists on the spontaneous activity of globus pallidus neurons in monkeys with MPTP-induced parkinsonism. *Brain Res* 1991; 547:152–161.

81. Miller WC, DeLong MR: Parkinsonian symptomatology. An anatomical and physiological analysis. *Ann NY Acad Sci* 1988; 515:287–302.

82. Bergman H, Wichmann T, Karmon B, DeLong MR: The primate subthalmic nucleus. II. Neuronal activity in the MPTP model of Parkinsonism. *J Neurophysiol* 1994; 72(2):507–520.

83. Lenz FA, Vitek JL, DeLong MR: Role of the thalamus in Parkinsonian tremor: evidence from studies in patients and primate models. *Stereotact Func Neurosurg* 1993; 60:94–103.

84. Van Hilten JJ, Weggeman M, Van der Velde EA, et al: Sleep, excessive daytime sleepiness, and fatigue in Parkinson's disease. *J Neuro Trans* 1993; 5:235–244.

85. Rinne JO, Roytta M, Paljarvil et al: Selegiline (deprenyl) treatment and death of nigral neurons in Parkinson's disease. *Neurology* 1991; 41:859–861.

86. Smith DL, Alchtar AJ, Garraway WM: Motor function after stroke. *Age & Aging* 1985; 14:46–48.

87. Bonita R, Beaglehole R: Recovery of motor function after stroke. *Stroke* 1988; 19:1497–1500.

88. Kotila M, Waltimo O, Niemiln, et al: The profile of recovery from stroke and factors influencing outcomes. *Stroke* 1984; 15:1039–1044.

89. Lees RS: The natural history of carotid artery disease. *Stroke* 1984; 15:603–604.

90. Fromisano R, Burbanti P, Catarci T, et al: Prolonged muscular flaccidity: Frequency and association with spatial neglect after stroke. *Acta Neurol Scand* 1993; 88:313–315.

91. Reding MJ, Potes E: Rehabilitaion outcome following initial unilateral hemispheric stroke. Life table analysis approach. *Stroke* 1988: 19:1354–1358.

92. Schneider R, Gantier JC: Leg weakness due to stroke: Site of lesions, weakness patterns and causes. *Brain* 1994; 117:347–354.

93. Gresham GE, Phillips TF, Wolf PA, et al: Epidemiologic profile of long term stroke disability: The Framingham Study. *Arch Phys Med Rehab* 1979; 60:487–491.

94. Marshall J, Thomas DJ: Vascular disease, in Arbury AK, McKhann GM, McDonald WI (eds): *Diseases of the Nervous System: Clinical Neurobiology* Philadelphia: WB Saunders, 1986.

95. Duncan PW, Goldstein LB, Horner RD, et al: Similar motor recovery of upper and lower extremities after stroke. *Stroke* 1994; 25:1181–1188.

96. Wade PT: *Measurement in neurological rehabilitation*. Oxford: Oxford University Press, 1992, p. 171.

97. Andres PL, Hedlund W, Finison LJ, et al: Quantitative motor assessment in amyotrophic lateral sclerosis. *Neurology* 1986; 36:937–941.

98. Fugl-Meyer AR, Jaasko L, Leyman L, et al: The post-stroke hemiplegic patient. I. A method for evaluation of physical performance. *Scand J Rehab Med* 1975; 7:13–31.

99. Collen FM, Wade DT, Bradshaw CM: Mobility after stroke: reliability of measures of impairment and disability. *Int Disabil Stud* 1990; 12:6–9.

100. Mahoney FI, Barthel DW: Functional evaluations: The Barthel Index. *Md Med J* 1965; 14:61–65.

101. Katz S, Ford AB, Moskowitz RW, et al: Studies of illness in the aged. The Index of ADL: A standardized measure of biological and psychosocial function. *JAMA* 1963; 185:914–919.

102. Goldstein LB, Matchar DB, Morgenlander JC, Davis JN: Influence of drugs on the recovery of sensorimotor function after stroke. *J Neuro Rehab* 1990; 4:137–144.

103. Goldstein LB, Davis JN: Physicians prescribing patterns following hospital admissions for ischemic cerebrovascular disease. *Neurology* 1988; 38:1806–1809.

104. Feeney DM, Gonzalez A, Law WA: Amphetamine, haloperidol and experience interact to affect the rate of recovery after motor cortex injury. *Science* 1982; 217:855–857.

105. Horda DA, Sutton RL, Feeney DM: Amphetamine-induced recovery of visual cliff performance after bilateral visual cortex ablation in cats: Measurement of depth perception thresholds. *Behav Neurosci* 1989; 103:574–584.

106. Horda DA, Feeney DM: Haloperidol blocks amphetamine induced recovery of binocular depth perception after bilateral visual cortex ablation in the cat. *Proc West Pharmacol Soc* 1985; 28:209–211.

107. Walker GL, Cardenas DD, Guthrie MR, et al: Fatigue and depression in brain-injured patients correlated with quadriceps strength and endurance. *Arch Phys Med Rehabil* 1991; 72(7):469–472.

108. McLean A, Dikmen SS, Temkin NR: Psychosocial recovery after head injury. *Arch Phys Med Rehab* 1993; 74(10):104–106.

109. Campbell KB, Suffreld JB, Deacon DL: The electrophysiological assessment of cognitive disorder in closed head-injured outpatients. *Electroenceph Clin Neurophysiol* 1990; 41(Suppl):202–215.

110. Packer TL, Martins I, Krefting L, Bronwer B: Activity and post-polio fatigue. *Orthopedics* 1991; 14(11):1223–1226.

111. Berlly MH, Strauser WW, Hall KM: Fatigue and postpolio syndrome. *Arch Phys Med Rehabil* 1991; 72(2):115–118.

112. Rodriguez AA, Agre JC: Physiological parameters and perceived exertion with local muscle fatigue in postpolio subjects. *Arch Phys Med Rehab* 1991; 72(5):305–308.

113. Rodriguez AA, Agre JC, Black PO, Franke TM: Motor unit firing rates in postpolio and control subjects during submaximal contraction. *Am J Phys Med Rehabil* 1991; 70(4):191–194.

114. Borg K, Borg J, Edstrom L, Grimby L: Effects of excessive use of remaining muscle fibers in prior polio and LV lesion. *Muscle & Nerve* 1988; 11:1219–1230.

115. Barry WH, Peeters GA, Rasmussen CAR, Cunningham MJ: Role of changes in [Ca++] in energy deprivation contracture. *Circ Res* 1987; 61:726–734.

116. Dalakas MC, Sever JL, Madden DL, et al: Late post-poliomyelitis muscular atrophy: clinical virological and immunological studies. *Rev Infect Dis* 1984; 6:S562–S567.

117. Sharief MKR, Hentgas R, Ciardi M: Intrathecal immune response in patients with the post-polio syndrome. *New Engl J Med* 1991; 325:748–755.

118. Leon-Monzon ME, Dalakas MC: Detection of poliovirus antibodies and poliovirus genome in patients with the post-polio syndrome. *Ann NY Acad Sci* 1995; 753:167–185.

119. Leon-Monzen MM, Agboatwalla M, Dinsmore S, et al: Comparison of antibodies to the poliomyelitis virus in patients with acute paralytic poliomyelitis, post-polio syndrome, and ALS. *Ann Neurol* 1991; 30:301–302.

120. Bruno RL, Cohen JM, Galski T, Frick NM: The neuroanatomy of post-polio fatigue. *Arch Phys Med Rehabil* 1994; 75(5):498–504.

121. Petajan JH, Currey K: Late onset muscle weakness and atrophy from undiagnosed poliomyelitis. AAEE 34th Annual Soc. Proceedings, San Antonio, TX, 1987.

122. Wiechers DO, Hubbel SL: Late changes in the motor unit after acute poliomyelitis. *Muscle & Nerve* 1981; 4:524–528.

123. Wiechers DO: Reinnervation after acute poliomyelitis, in Halstead LS, Wiechers DO (eds): *Research and Clinical Aspects of the Late Effects of Poliomyelitis*, Vol 23. White Plains, NY: March of Dimes.

124. Berily MH, Strauser WW, Hall KM: Fatigue in postpolio syndrome. *Arch Phy Med Rehab* 1991; 72:115–118.

125. Chetwynd J, Botting C, Hogan D: Postpolio syndrome in New Zealand: a survey of 700 polio survivors. *NZ Med J* 1993; 106:406–508.

126. Clark K, Dinsmore S, Grafman J, Dalakas MC: A personality profile of patients diagnosed with post-polio syndrome. *Neurology* 1994; 44:1809–1811.

127. Agre JC, Rodriguez AA: Neuromuscular function in polio survivors. *Orthopedics* 1991; 14(12):1343–1347.

128. Packer TL, Martins I, Krefting L, Brouwer B: Activity and post-polio fatigue. *Orthopedics* 1991; 14(11):1223–1226.

129. Chen MK: The epidemiology of self-perceived fatigue among adults. *Preventive Med* 1986; 15:74–81.

130. Lewis G, Wessely S: The epidemiology of fatigue: More questions than answers. *J Epidem Comm Health* 1992; 46:92–97.

131. Abbey SE, Garfinkel PE: Chronic fatigue syndrome and the psychiatrist. *Can J Psychiatr* 1990; 35:625–633.

132. Strauss SE, Tosato G, Armstrong G, et al: Persisting illness and fatigue in adults with evidence of Epstein-Barr virus infection. *Ann Intern Med* 1985; 102:7–16.

133. Sumaya CV: Serologic and virologic epidemiology of Epstein-Barr virus: relevance to CFS. *Rev Infect Dis* 1991; 13(S):S19–S25.

134. Tobi M, Morag A, Ravid Z, et al: Prolonged atypical illness associated with serological evidence of persistent Epstein-Barr virus infection. *Lancet* 1982; 1:61–64.

135. Holmes GP, Kaplan JE, Gantz NM, et al: CFS: a working case definition. *Ann Intern Med* 1988; 108:387–389.

136. Straus SE: Editorial: Defining the CFS. *Arch Intern Med* 1992; 152:1569–1570.

137. Fukuda K, Straus SE, Hickie I, et al: The chronic fatigue syndrome: A comprehensive approach to its definition and study. *Ann Intern Med* 1994; 121:953–959.

138. Hickie I, Lloyd A, Wakefield D, Parker G: The psychiatric status of patients with the CFS. *Br J Psychiatr* 1990; 156:534–540.

139. Lane TJ, Manu P, Matthews DA: Depression and somatization in the CFS. *Am J Med* 1991; 91:335–344.

140. Manu P, Matthews DA, Lane TJ: Panic disorder among patients with chronic fatigue. *So Med J* 1991; 84:451–456.

141. Manu P, et al: Screening for somatization disorders in patients with chronic fatigue. *Gen Hosp Psychiatr* 1989; 11:294–297.

142. Millon C, Salvato F, Blaney N, et al: A psychological assessment of CFS/chronic Epstein-Barr virus patients. *Psych Health* 1989; 3:131–141.

143. Deluca J, Johnson SK, Beldowicz D, Natelson BH: Neuropsychological impairment in chronic fatigue syndrome, multiple sclerosis, and depression. *J Neurol Neurosurg Psychiatr* 1995; 58(1):38–43.

144. Packer TL, Sauriol A, Brouwer B: Fatigue secondary to chronic illness: postpolio syndrome, chronic fatigue syndrome, and multiple sclerosis. *Arch Phys Med Rehab* 1994; 75(10):1122–1126.

145. Wood GC, Bentall RP, Gopfert M, et al: The differential response of chronic fatigue, neurotic, and muscular dystrophy patients to psychological stress. *Psychol Med* 1994; 24(2):357–364.

146. Krupp LB, Sliwinski M, Masur D, et al: Cognitive functioning and depression in patients with chronic fatigue syndrome and multiple sclerosis. *Arch Neurol* 1994; 51:705–710.

147. Edwards RH, Gibson H, Clague JE, Helliwell T: Muscle histopathology and physiology in chronic fatigue syndrome. *Ciba Found Symp* 1993; 173:102–131.

148. Lloyd AR, Gandevia SC, Hales JP: Muscle performance, voluntary activation, twitch properties and perceived effort in normal subjects and patients with the CFS. *Brain* 1991; 114:85–98.

149. Stokes MJ, Cooper RG, Edwards RHT: Normal muscle strength and fatiguability in patients with effort syndromes. *Br Med J* 1988; 297:296–1017.

150. Wassif WS, Sherman D, Salisbury JR, Peters TJ: Use of dynamic tests of muscle function and histomorphometry of quadriceps muscle biopsies in the investigation of patients with chronic alcohol misuse and chronic fatigue syndrome. *Am Clin Biochem* 1994; 31:462–468.

151. Roberts L, Byrne E: Single fiber EMG studies in chronic fatigue syndrome: a reappraisal. *J Neurol Neurosurg Psychiatr* 1994; 57(3):325–326.

152. Komaroff AL, Wang SP, Lee J, Grayston JT: No association of chronic chlamydia pneumoniae infection with CFS. *J Infect Dis* 1992; 165:184.

153. Shafran SD: Review: The CFS. *Am J Med* 1991; 90:730–739.

154. Bode L, Komaroff AL, Ludwig N: No serologic evidence of Borna disease virus in patients with CFS. *Clin Infect Dis* 1992; 15:1049.

155. Holmes GP, Kaplan JE, Steward JA, et al: A cluster of patients with chronic mononucleosis-like symptoms. *JAMA* 1987; 257:2297–2302.

156. Komaroff AL, Bell DS, Cheney PR: Absence of antibody to Mycoplasma fermentens in patients with chronic fatigue syndrome. *Clin Infect Dis* 1993; 17(6):1074–1075.

157. Monian FA: Simultaneous measurement of antibodies to Epstein-Barr virus, human herpes virus 6, herpes simplex virus types 1 and 2, and 14 enteroviruses in chronic fatigue syndrome: Is there evidence of activation of a nonspecific polyclonal immune response? *Clin Infect Dis* 1994; 19(3):448–453.

158. Masuda A, Nozoe SI, Matsuyama T, Tanaka H: Psychobehavioral and immunological characteristics of adult people with chronic fatigue and patients with chronic fatigue syndrome. *Psychosom Med* 1994; 56(6):512–518.

159. Natelson BA, Ellen SP, Braonain PJ, et al: Frequency of deviant immunological test values in chronic fatigue patients. *Clin Diag Lab Immunol* 1995; 2(2):238–240.

160. Patarca R, Limas NG, Lugtendorf S, et al: Dysregulated expression of tumor necrosis factor in chronic fatigue syndrome: Interrelations with cellular sources and patterns of soluble immune mediator expression. *Clin Infect Dis* 1994; 18(Suppl 1):S147–S153.

161. Levy JA: Viral studies of chronic fatigue syndrome. *Clin Infect Dis* 1994; 18(Suppl 1):S117–S120.

162. Lloyd A, Gandevia S, Brockman A, et al: Cytokine production and fatigue in patients with chronic fatigue syndrome and healthy control subjects in response to exercise. *Clin Infect Dis* 1994; 18(Suppl 1):S142–S146.

163. Demitrack MA, Dale JK, Straus SE, et al: Evidence for impaired activation of the hypothalamic-pituitary-adrenal axis in patients with CFS. *J Clin Endocrinol Metab* 1991; 73:1224–1234.

164. Krupp LB, Mendelson WB, Friedman R: An overview of CFS. *J Clin Psychiatr* 1991; 52:403–410.

165. Matthews DA, Manu P, Lane TJ: Evaluation and management of patients with chronic fatigue. *Am J Med Sci* 1991; 302:269–277.

166. Grafman J, Schwartz V, Dale JK, et al: Analysis of neuropsychological functioning in patients with chronic fatigue syndrome. *J Neurol Neurosurg Psychiatry* 1993; 56:684–689.

167. Wessely S, Powell R: Fatigue syndromes: a comparison of chronic "postviral" fatigue with neuromuscular and affective disorders. *J Neurol Neurosurg Psychiatr* 1989; 52:940–948.

168. Manu P, Lane TJ, Matthews DA, et al: Alpha-delta sleep in patients with a chief complaint of chronic fatigue. *So Med J* 1994; 87(4):465–470.

169. Moldofsky A: Fibromyalgia, sleep disorder and chronic fatigue syndrome. *Ciba Found Symp* 1993; 173:262–279.

170. Bou-Holaigah Issam, Rowe PC, Kan J, Calleins H: The relationship between neurally mediated hypotension and the chronic fatigue syndrome. *JAMA* 1995; 274:961–967.

171. Bell DS: Chronic fatigue syndrome update: Findings now point to CNS involvement. *Post Grad Med* 1994; 96(6):73–76, 79–81.

172. Schwartz RB, Komaroff AL, Gavada BM, et al: SPECT imaging of the brain: comparison of findings in patients with chronic fatigue syndrome, AIDS dementia complex, and major unipolar depression. *Am J Roentgeno* 1994; 162(4):943–951.

173. Behan PO, Behan WMH, Horrobin D: Effect of high doses of essential fatty acids on the postviral fatigue syndrome. *Acta Neurol Scand* 1990; 82:209–216.

174. Gantz NM, Holmes GP: Treatment of patients with CFS. *Drugs* 1989; 38:855–862.

175. Jacobson W, Saich T, Borysiewicz LK, et al: Serum folate and chronic fatigue syndrome. *Neurology* 1993; 43:2645–2647.

176. Lloyd A, Hickie I, Wakefield D, et al: A double-blind, placebo-controlled trial of intravenous immunoglobulin therapy in patients with CFS. *Am J Med* 1990; 89:561–568.

177. Peterson PK, Shepard J, Macres M, et al: A controlled trial of intravenous immunoglobulin G in CFS. *Am J Med* 1990; 89:554–560.

178. Cotton P: Treatment proposed for CFS: research continues to compile data on disorder. *JAMA* 1991; 266:2667–2668.

179. Goodnick PJ, Sandoval R: Psychotropic treatment of chronic fatigue syndrome and related disorders. *J Clin Psychiatr* 1993; 54(1):13–20.

180. Newsom-Davis J, et al: Function of circulating antibody to acetylcholine receptors in myasthenia gravis: Investigation by plasma exchange. *Neurology* 1978; 28:266–271.

181. Lindstrom JM, Lambert BH: Content of acetylcholine receptor and antibodies bound to receptor in myasthenia gravis, experimental autoimmune myasthenia gravis, and Eaton-Lambert syndrome. *Neurology* 1978; 28:130–135.

182. Nicklin J, Karni Y, Wiles CM: Shoulder abduction fatigability. *J Neurol Neurosurg Psychiatr* 1987; 50:423–427.

183. Sanjak M, Paulson D, Sufit R, et al: Physiologic and metabolic response to progressive and prolonged exercise in amyotrophic lateral sclerosis. *Neurology* 1987; 37:1217–1220.

184. Argov Z, Bank WI: Phosphorous magnetic resonance spectroscopy (^{31}PMRS) in neuromuscular disorders. *Ann Neurol* 1991; 30:90–97.

185. Zochodne DW, Thompson RT, Driedger AA, et al: Metabolic changes in human muscle denervation: topical ^{31}PNMR spectroscopy studies. *Mag Res Med* 1988; 7:373–383.

186. Allen GM, Gandevia SL, Veering IR, et al: Muscle performance, voluntary activation and perceived effort in normal subjects and patients with prior poliomyelitis. *Brain* 1994; 117:661–670.

187. Sharma KR, Kent-Braun J, Mynhier MA, et al: Excessive muscular fatigue in the postpoliomyelitic syndrome. *Neurology* 1994; 44:642–646.

188. McCardle B: Myopathy due to a defect in muscle glycogen breakdown. *Clin Sci* 1951; 10:13–33.

189. Mommaerts WFHM, Illingworth B, Pearson CM, et al: A functional disorder of muscle associated with the absence of phosphorylase. *Proc Natl Acad Sci USA* 1959; 45:791–797.

190. Ross BD, Radda GK, Gadian DG, et al: Examination of a case suspected of McCardle's syndrome by ^{31}P nuclear magnetic resonance. *New Engl J Med* 1981; 304:1338–1343.

191. Wiles CM, Jones DA, Edwards RHT: Fatigue in human metabolic myopathy. *Ciba Found Symp* 1981; 82:264–282.

192. Tarui S, Okuno G, Ikura Y, et al: Phosphofructokinase deficiency in skeletal muscle: A new type of glycogenosis. *Biochem Biophys Res Commun* 1965; 19:571–576.

193. Fishbein WN, Armbrustmacher VW, Griffin JL: Myoadenylate deaminase deficiency: A new disease of muscle. *Science* 1978; 299:545–548.

194. Dimauro S, Trevisan C, Hays A: Disorders of lipid metabolism in muscle. *Muscle Nerve* 1980; 3:369–373.

195. Luft R, Ikkos D, Palmieri G, et al: A case of severe hypermetabolism of nonthyroid origin with a defect in the maintenance of mitochondrial control: A correlated clinical, biochemical and morphological study. *J Clin Invest* 1962; 41:1776–1804.

196. Morgan-Hughes JA, Darvenzia P, Kahn SA: A mitochondrial myopathy characterized by a deficiency in reducible cytochrome 6. *Brain* 1989; 100:612–640.

197. Kuiach S, McComas AJ: Transient hyperpolarization of noncontracting muscle fibers in anaesthetized rats. *J Phys* 1992; 454:609–618.

198. Duchateau J, Hainaut K: Electrical and mechanical changes in immobilized human muscle. *J Appl Phys* 1987; 62:2168–2173.

199. Miller RL, Green AT, Moussavi RS, et al: Excessive muscle fatigue in patients with spastic paraparesis. *Neurology* 1990; 40:1271–1274.

200. Hayslip B Jr, Kennelly KJ, Maloy RM: Fatigue, depression, and cognitive performance among aged persons. *Exp Aging Res* 1990; 16(3):111–115.

201. Cupido CM, Hicks AL, Martin J: Neuromuscular fatigue diring repetitive stimulation in elderly and young adults. *Eur J Appl Physiol* 1992; 65(6):567–572.

202. Hicks AL, Cupido M, Martin J, Dent J: Twitch potentiation during fatiguing exercise in the elderly: The effects of training. *Eur J Appl Physiol* 1991; 63(3–4):278–281.

203. Dustman RHT, Ruhling RO, Russell EM, et al: Aerobic exercise training and improved neuropsychological function of older individuals. *Neurobiology* 1984; 5:35–42.

204. Crosby LJ: Factors which contribute to fatigue associated with rheumatoid arhritis. *J Adv Nurs* 1991; 16(8):978–981.

205. Rudick RA, Miller D, Clough JD, et al: Quality of life in multiple sclerosis: comparison with inflammatory bowel disease and rheumatoid arthritis. *Arch Neurol* 1992; 49:1237–1242.

206. Belza BL, Henke CJ, Yelin EH, et al: Correlates of fatigue in older adults with rheumatoid arthritis. *Nurs Res* 1993; 42(2):93–99.

207. Tack BB: Self-reported fatigue in rheumatoid arthritis: A pilot study. *Arthritis Care Res* 1990; 3(3):154–157.

208. Wysenbeck AJ, Leibovici L, Weinberger A, Guedj D: Fatigue in systemic lupus erythematosus. Prevalence and relation to disease expression. *Br J Rheumatol* 1993; 32(7):632–635.

209. Calin A, Edmunds L, Kennedy LG: Fatigue in ankylosing spondylitis: Why is it ignored? *J Rheumatol* 1993; 20(6):991–995.

210. Calabrese LH, Davis ME, Wilke WS: Chronic fatigue syndrome and a disorder resembling Sjögren's syndrome: Preliminary report. *Clin Infect Dis* 1994; 18(Suppl 1): 528–531.

211. St. Claire EW: New deveopments in Sjögren's syndrome. *Curr Opin Rheumatol* 1993; 5(5):604–612.

212. Dhalla Z, Bruni J, Sutton J: A comparison of the efficacy and tolerability of controlled-release carbamazepine with conventional carbamazepine. *Can J Neurol Sci* 1991; 18(1):66–68.

213. Schroeder D, Hill GH: Postoperative fatigue: a prospective physiological study of patients undergoing major abdominal surgery. *Aus NZ Surg* 1991; 61:774–779.

214. Kjerulff KH, Langenberg PW: A comparison of alternative ways of measuring fatigue among patients having hysterectomy. *Med Care* 1995; 33(4 Suppl):S156–S163.

215. Schroeder D, Hill GL: Predicting postoperative fatigue: improtance of preoperative fatigue. *World J Surg* 1993; 17(2):226–231.

216. Petersson B, Wernerman J, Waller SO, et al: Elective abdominal surgery depresses muscle protein synthesis and increases subjective fatigue: Effects lasting more than 30 days. *Br J Surg* 1990; 77(7):796–800.

217. Zeiderman MR, Welchew EA, Clark RL: Changes in cardiorespiratory and muscle functions associated with the development of postoperative fatigue. *Br J Surg* 1990; 79(5):576–580.

218. Newsholme EA, Blomstrand E, Ekblom B: Physical and mental fatigue: Metabolic mechanisms and importance of plasma amino acids. *Br Med Bull* 1992; 48(3):477–495.

219. Petersson B, von-der Declsen, Vinnars E, Wernerman J: Long-term effects of postoperative total parenteral nutrition supplemented with glycylglutamine on subjective fatigue and muscle protein synthesis. *Br J Surg* 1994; 81(10):1520–1523.

220. Jakeways MS, Mitchell V, Hashim IA, et al: Metabolic and inflammatory responses after open or laparoscopic cholecystectomy. *Br J Surg* 1994; 81(1):127–131.

221. Hill AG, Finn P, Schroeder D. Postoperative fatigue after laparoscopic surgery. *Aust NZ J Surg* 1993; 63(12):946–951.

222. Schulze S, Thorup J: Pulmonary function, pain, and fatigue after laparoscopic halecystectomy. *Eur J Surg* 1993; 159(6–7):361–364.

223. Zeiderman MR, Welchew EA, Clark RL: Influence of epidural analgesia on postoperative fatigue. *Br J Surg* 1991; 78(12):1457–1460.

224. Passchier J, Rupreht J, Keonders ME, et al: Patient controlled analgesia (PCA) leads to more postoperative

225. Christensen T, Kehlet H: Postoperative fatigue. *World J Surg* 1993; 17(2):220–225.

226. Pick B, Molloy A, Hinds C, et al: Postoperative fatigue following coronary artery bypass surgery: Relationship to emotional state and to catecholamine response to surgery. *J Psychosom Res* 1994; 38(6):599–607.

227. Hilgers A, Krueger GR, Lembke U, Ramon A: Postinfectious chronic fatigue syndrome: Case history of thirty-five patients in Germany. *In Vivo* 1991; 5(3):201–205.

228. Buchwald D, Freedman AS, Ablashi DV, et al: A chronic posinfectious fatigue syndrome associated with benign lympho-proliferation, B-cell proliferation, and active replication of herpesvirus-6. *J Clin Immunol* 1990; 10(6): 335–344.

229. McGuire TA: Recurrent upper respiratory infection, persistent paravertebral thoracolumbar muscle spasm, and fatigue associated with chronic active Epstein-Barr virus infection. *Md Med J* 1991; 40(7):595–596.

230. Okano M, Thiele GM, Purtilo DT: Severe chronic active Epstein-Barr virus infectious syndrome and adenovirus type 2 infection. *Am J Pediatr Hematol Oncol* 1990; 12(2):168–173.

231. Morrison LO, Behan WH, Behan PO: Changes in natural killer cell phenotype in patients with post-viral fatigue syndrome. *Clin Exp Immunol* 1991; 83(3):441–446.

232. Gold D, Bowden R, Sixbey J, et al: Chronic fatigue:. A prospective clincal and virological study. *JAMA* 1990; 264(1):48–53.

233. Steere AC, Taylor E, McHugh GL, Logigian EL: The overdiagnosis of Lyme disease. *JAMA* 1993; 270(22): 2683.

234. Falger PR, Schouten EG: Exhaustion: Psychological stressors in the work environment and acute myocardial infarction in adult men. *J Psychosom Res* 1992; 36(8): 777–786.

235. Chavalitsakulchai P, Shahnavaz H: Musculoskeletal discomfort and feeling of fatigue among female professional workers: The need for ergonomic consideration. *J Hum Ergo-Tokyo* 1991; 20(2):257–264.

236. Sakamoto K, Nishida K, Zhou L, et al: Characteristics of physiological tremor in five fingers and evaluations of fatigue of fingers in typing. *Am Physiol Anthropol* 1992; 11(1):61–81.

237. Hammarskjold E, Harms-Ringdahl K: The effect of arm-shoulder fatigue on carpenters at work. *Eur J App Physiol* 1992; 64(5):402–409.

238. Kilbom A, Hagg GM, Kall C: One handed load carrying—cardiovascular, muscular and subjective indices of endurance and fatigue. *Eur J Appl Physiol* 1992; 65(1):52–58.

239. Hansson GA, Stromberg C, Larsson B, et al: Electromyographic fatigue in neck/shoulder muscles and endurance in women with repetitive work. *Ergonomics* 1992; 35(11):1341 –1352.

240. Jensen BR, Schibye B, Sogaard K, et al: Shoulder muscle load and muscle fatigue among industrial sewing-machine operators. *Eur J Appl Physiol* 1993; 67(5):467–475.

241. Theriault R: *How to Tell When You're Tired: A Brief Examination of Work*. New York: W.W. Norton, 1995.

242. Baker K, Olson J, Morisseau D: Work practices, fatigue, and nuclear power plant safety performance. *Hum Fact* 1994; 36(2):244–257.

243. Brown IP: Driver fatigue. *Hum Fact* 1994; 36(2):298–314.

244. Paley MJ, Tepas DI: Fatigue and the shift worker: Firefighters working on a rotating shift schedule. *Hum Fact* 1994; 36(2):269–284.

245. Sparks DJ: Questionnaire survey of masters, mates, and pilots of a State Ferrier System of health, social, and performance indices relevant to shift work. *Am J Ind Med* 1992; 21(4):507–516.

246. Rosekind MR, Gander PH, Dinges DF: Alertness management in flight operations: Strategic napping. *SAE Technical Paper Series* #912138, 1991.

247. Makowska Z, Kluge G, Sprusinska B: The influence of occupational and non-occupational factors on chronic fatigue in women. *Pol J Occup Med Environ Health* 1992; 5(4):323–333.

248. Brodsky CM: Depression and chronic fatigue in the workplace:. Workman's compensation and occupational issues. *Prim Care* 1991; 18(2):381–396.

Chapter 24

NUTRITION AND DIET IN NEUROLOGIC REHABILITATION

Hillel M. Finestone
Linda S. Greene-Finestone

Awareness of the multiple nutritional issues and problems encountered during the rehabilitation process has great strategic value. The methodology of nutritional assessment and therapy will be addressed through broad overview first, and then with respect to specific disease states.

The nutritional status of neurorehabilitation patients is vulnerable for a host of reasons. Alterations in metabolic rate and food intake, the presence of dysphagia, impaired mobility, changes in bladder and bowel control, decreased level of consciousness, and depression are among the many factors that may lead to under- or overnutrition.

Over the past 15 years, recognition of the numerous consequences and associations of nutritional status has sparked interest in the nutritional management of patients undergoing rehabilitation. Malnutrition is defined as a deficiency or excess of one or more nutrients and/or energy (calories). Undernutrition is highly prevalent in neurorehabilitation patients. Newmark reported that 56 percent (20/36) of rehabilitation patients with neurological disease (stroke, spinal cord injuries, degenerative neurological process, and peripheral neuropathy) were malnourished.[1] This prevalence compared to 38 percent (5/13) among the remaining patients (trauma, chronic obstructive pulmonary disease, miscellaneous). Nutritional status and serum albumin (a nutrition-sensitive marker) subsequently have been used to predict functional outcome and complication rates in general and stroke rehabilitation patients.[2–4] Prolonged length of stay also has been reported in malnourished stroke rehabilitation patients.[3]

NUTRITIONAL ASSESSMENT OF THE NEUROREHABILITATION PATIENT

The purpose of the nutritional assessment is to evaluate nutritional status and establish baseline data. It is used to identify nutrient imbalances, excesses, deficiencies, and the extent of any existing malnutrition. From this data, patients' nutritional goals can be determined and therapy alternatives recommended. The goal is to attain and maintain normal nutritional status (sufficiency of energy and nutrients) in order to reduce the risk of complications associated with malnutrition and promote a high level of health.

The development of malnutrition is a staged process. Dietary inadequacy of nutrient(s) progresses from decreased levels in tissue and body fluids to reduced functional level in tissues and diminished activity in nutrient-dependent enzymes. This further progresses to functional change, clinical symptoms, and anatomical signs.[5]

The nutritional assessment can take different forms ranging from a simple and brief screening process to a comprehensive evaluation. A cost-effective nutritional screening incorporates routine tests such as complete blood count and the SMA-12. Screening can be done by a dietetic technician and interpreted by a clinical dietitian, who would also perform the nutritional assessment when a nutritional problem requiring intervention is identified. Nutritional screening usually requires: primary diagnosis and diet order, percent of usual weight, percent of ideal weight, rate of growth in children, change in appetite or ability to eat, food allergies or intolerances, medications, serum albumin, and other selected biochemical data (e.g., iron indices, cholesterol, total lymphocyte count).[6] The majority of patients at risk for nutritional insufficiency will be identified by these data. The in-depth assessment is based on medical history and dietary information, as well as biochemical, anthropometric, and/or clinical measurements. Common indices of malnutrition that are utilized in the neurorehabilitation population are described in Table 24-1. Each test has its limitations and indications for use. Tests are most effectively used in combination, and/or repetitively. Texts such as that of Gibson and Hopkins offer comprehensive descriptions of parameters of the nutritional assessment.[7,8]

The medical history provides information on past and present medical problems, procedures, and medications that may have nutritional implications. A diet history may include observation of the patient's current intake, and various techniques of dietary recall or record to estimate prior food consumption. Although dietary intake sometimes may appear to be adequate, certain drugs, dietary components or disease states can affect ingestion, absorption, transportation, utilization, or excretion of nutrients.[7]

The physical examination can reveal clinical signs of obvious protein-energy malnutrition, such as muscle wasting or minimal fat stores. Muscle wasting, with or without edema, may be apparent even in the obese protein-malnourished patient.[9] Other clinical signs of malnutrition include alopecia, beading of ribs, hair dyspigmentation, and "flag sign" (bands of depigmented and normal hair reflecting periods of poor and relatively good protein intake).

Anthropometric measurements are useful in the estimation of fat and protein stores, especially if serial measurements are performed. Weight may be measured as percent of usual weight; percent of reference weight based on height, body frame, and age; Body Mass Index (weight [kg]/height [m²]); or rate of weight change. Normative measures are readily available in the Metropolitan Life Insurance Tables, National Health and Nutrition Examination Survey (NHANES) I,II and Canadian Standardized Test of Fitness.[8,10–13] Height of children should be measured using a stadiometer or flat wall-mounted tape with a head-board. Heels, buttocks, shoulders, and head should contact the wall. In children who cannot stand, recumbent length may be measured using a measuring board. Height may be measured indirectly in people who cannot stand. The measurement of knee height, arm span, and summation of body parts are indirect methods of estimating height.[8,14] Head circumference for age is useful as an index of chronic protein energy malnutrition in children under the age of two. Abnormally low measurements may also reflect intrauterine growth retardation and microcephaly of non-nutritional origin. Subcutaneous fat may be measured indirectly using skinfold calipers and comparing measurements to norms for healthy individuals of similar age and sex. The somatic protein compartment can be estimated by the calculation of mid-arm muscle circumference from mid-arm circumference and tricep skinfold measures.

Biochemical tests may be used to estimate visceral protein. Serum albumin, transferrin, thyroxine-binding pre-albumin and retinol-binding protein have highly varying half-lives, and therefore, sensitivities to changes in protein status (see Table 24-1). Laboratory methods of estimating muscle mass include the Creatinine-Height Index. This measures the elaboration of creatinine, which is proportionate to muscle mass. The usefulness of 3-methyl histidine excretion, which approximates muscle turnover, is more limited because of the lack of interpretable standards.

Immunocompetence can be an index of protein energy malnutrition. The immune response is reduced in nutritional depletion and reversed with repletion.[15] In patients who are not critically ill, total lymphocyte count is useful as a screening parameter, reflecting immune function and T-cells.[16] Delayed cutaneous hypersensitivity testing, reflecting cell-mediated immunity, involves an intradermal injection of an antigen to which the patient likely has been exposed. Reaction may vary from reactive-swelling around the injection site in a healthy individual to anergy in the malnourished. Delayed hypersensitivity is not recommended for routine nutritional assessments.

DIAGNOSIS OF MALNUTRITION

Traditional Method

Protein energy malnutrition (PEM) can take different forms (Table 24-2). In the marasmic form, total energy intake is inadequate regardless of whether energy comes from protein, carbohydrate, or fat. Marasmus is characterized by catabolism of fat and muscle tissue (somatic protein). In chronically ill patients, this may occur with prolonged reduction of food intake. Those on prolonged clear fluid diets or hypocaloric intravenous infusion of 5 percent dextrose are at risk.[7] These individuals appear extremely thin and weak. Cellular immunity is also im-

Table 24-1

Selected indices of malnutrition in adults

Compartment	Indices	Depletion			Indications	Practical limitations
		Mild	Moderate	Severe		
Fat and protein	Percent desirable body weight (actual weight/desirable weight) × 100	80–90	70 < 80	≤69	Appropriate parameter for healthy populations	Frame size must be estimated using elbow breadth or wrist circumference/weight ratio
					Metropolitan Life Insurance Tables (MLIT)—based on disease-free insured population, and weight associated with lowest mortality rate	MLIT findings not representative of entire age 25–59 population; elderly not included
	Percentile desirable body weight	10 < 25	5 < 10	≤5	National Health Examination Survey (NHANES I, II) standards presented as percentiles according to age and frame size; identifies risk of depletion and obesity	NHANES I,II—weight not associated with longevity, morbidity, or mortality
						Loss of body parts must be considered
	Percent usual body weight (actual weight/usual weight) × 100	85–90	75 < 85	≤74	More useful with ill populations in assessing weight change	May rely on patient memory
					Will not overlook depletion in the obese	
	Percent weight loss per - 1 month	5.0	5.0	>5.0	Severity and significance of weight loss are assessed	Allowances must be made for amputations
	- 3 months	7.5	7.5	>7.5		Lack of specificity regarding body compartments
	- 6 months	10.0	10.0	>10.0		
	$\left(\dfrac{\text{usual} - \text{actual weight}}{\text{usual weight}}\right) \times 100$					
Subcutaneous fat stores	Triceps, biceps, subscapular, and suprailiac skinfold measurements (percent of standard) = (actual measurement/standard) × 100	>90	60–90	<60	Standards and percentile tables should be demographically similar to population surveyed	Requires trained personnel, standardized techniques and proper calipers to minimize errors
	Percentile	5–15	5–15	<5	Serial measurements can document depletion and repletion	Accuracy is affected by age and muscularity of subject
					More beneficial with large populations than with individual hospital patients	Reliability is improved with testing multiple sites as fat distribution is not uniform
Somatic protein stores	Midarm muscle circumference (MAMC) MAMC (cm) = midarm circumference (cm) − (3.14 × triceps skinfold [cm])				Standards and percentile tables should be demographically similar to population surveyed	Muscle mass evaluation at a single site may not be indicative of total muscle mass
	Percent of standard = (actual measurement/standard) × 100	>90	60–90	<60	Serial measurements allow subject to serve as own standard	Measurement error present
	Percentile	5–15	5–15	<60	More beneficial with large populations than with individual hospital patients	In presence of protein-energy malnutrition, values may be within normal limits
	Creatinine-height index (CHI) Percent CHI = 100 × (actual 24-hour creatinine excretion/expected 24-hour creatinine excretion)	80 < 90	60 < 80	<60	Indicator of lean body mass as urinary creatinine excretion is proportionate to muscle mass and released at a constant rate in those with normal renal function	Accurate 24-hour urine collection required
						Daily variations and ingestion of meat may influence results
						May not be accurate in the elderly as creatinine excretion declines with age
						Standards based on medium body frame
						Steroids, tobramycin sulphate, Mandol® may decrease results
Visceral protein stores	Serum albumin (g/L)	28 < 35	21 < 28	<21	Levels correlate with degree of malnutrition, morbidity, and mortality	Relatively large body pool
					Inexpensive prognostic indicator	Hypoalbuminemia not specific to visceral protein depletion; other causes: liver disease, infection, nephrotic syndrome, postoperative states, metabolic stress, fluid imbalances, zinc deficiency, malabsorptive states
					Half-life of approximately 20 days, therefore useful for long-term monitoring	

Table 24-1

Selected indices of malnutrition in adults (Continued)

Compartment	Indices	Depletion			Indications	Practical limitations
		Mild	Moderate	Severe		
	Serum transferrin (TF) (mg/dL)	150 < 200	100 < 150	<100	Shorter half-life, 8–10 days, therefore more sensitive to acute changes compared to albumin. May be calculated from total iron binding capacity (TIBC), e.g., Grant equation: TF = 0.87 TIBC (mg·dL) + 10	Other causes of low transferrin levels: chronic infection, acute metabolic stress, uremia, nephrotic syndrome, increased iron stores, liver disease, overhydration, iron overload, vitamin A deficiency
	Thyroxine-binding prealbumin (TBPA) (mg/dL)	10 < 15	5 < 10	<5	Sensitive indicator, especially in acute stages of protein energy malnutrition. Useful for measuring short-term changes. Half-life = 2–3 days	Other causes of low TBPA levels: acute metabolic stress, postsurgery, altered nitrogen and energy balance, liver disease, infection, dialysis, inflammation
	Retinol-binding protein (g/L)	<0.3	<0.3	<0.3	Reflects acute changes in protein malnutrition. Half-life approximately 12 hours	Limited use in renal failure. Other causes of low levels: Vitamin A or zinc deficiency, acute metabolic stress, postsurgery, liver disease, cystic fibrosis, hyperthyroidism
Immunocompetence	Total lymphocyte count (mm³) = percent lymphocytes × $\frac{\text{white blood cells}}{100}$	1500 < 1800	900 < 1500	<900	Screening parameter in noncritical patients. Correlated with albumin in predicting morbidity and mortality in postoperative patients	Levels increase with infection, leukemia, tissue necrosis. Levels decrease with cancer, metabolic stress, steroid therapy postsurgery, radiotherapy, chemotherapeutic agents, immunosuppressive medications and other drugs

American Dietetic Association: *Handbook of Clinical Dietetics,* 2nd ed. New Haven: Yale University Press, 1992.

Hopkins B: Assessment of nutritional status, in Gottschlich MM, Matarese LE, Shronts EP (eds): *Nutrition Support Dietetics—Core Curriculum, American Society for Parenteral and Enteral Nutrition.* Silver Springs, MD: 1993, pp. 15–65.

Ontario Dietetic Association and Ontario Hospital Association: *Nutrition Care Manual.* Don Mills, Ontario: Ontario Hospital Association, 1989.

Table 24-2

Indicators of protein and energy malnutrition

Condition	Deficit	Indicators				
		Body weight	Body fat	Somatic protein	Visceral protein	Immune function
Marasmus	Energy	↓	↓	↓	Slightly ↓ or WNL	↓
Kwashiorkor	Protein	↓	WNL	WNL	↓	↓
Marasmic Kwashiorkor	Protein and energy	↓	↓	↓	↓	↓

↓ = decreased; WNL = within normal limits.

Reprinted with permission from Hopkins B: Assessment of nutritional status, in Gottschlich MM, Matarese LE, Shronts EP (eds): *Nutrition Support Dietetics Core Curriculum.* Silver Spring, MD, Aspen, 1993.

paired. Adequate nutritional support is indicated to improve prognosis.[17]

Protein malnutrition, kwashiorkor-like, also is found in hospitalized patients. It tends to develop from an acute inadequate intake of protein and energy concomitant with hypercatabolism of protein induced by metabolic stress (e.g., trauma or sepsis).[6,7] Protein is used as a source of energy and the visceral protein pool is depleted (Table 24-2). Edema, loss of vigor, reduced immune function and secondary infection, stunted growth in children and changes in hair may be found. Despite short-term weight loss, some of these patients still may be obese. Aggressive nutritional support is required to improve prognosis.[17]

Marasmic kwashiorkor (combined PEM), occurs when a marasmic (chronically starved) patient is exposed to metabolic stress (trauma, surgery, acute illness).[8] All indicators are low (Table 24-2) and edema is evident.[6] Treatment is difficult and the prognosis is poor owing to high risk of infection and poor wound healing.[7,17]

Subjective Global Assessment

This technique of nutritional assessment is derived from the patient's history and physical examination (see Table 24-3). Weight loss over time, dietary intake relative to usual intake, persistent gastrointestinal symptoms and functional capacity, or energy level are evaluated. Aspects of physical exam include evaluation of subcutaneous fat, muscle wasting, edema, and ascites. Based on this information, patients are classified as (1) well nourished; (2) moderately, or suspected of being, malnourished; or (3) severely malnourished. The subjective global assessment correlates highly with results of nutritional assessment based on objective parameters. Interrater agreement following training has been very high (91 percent).[18] Clinicians should undergo training to ensure the reliability and reproducibility of assessments. This technique is especially useful in clinical situations where non–nutrition-related factors affect nutritional or biochemical parameters.[9]

Overnutrition

Degree of adiposity can be assessed by weight and skinfold measurements. Measurements are compared to normal values that depend on culturally accepted standards varying according to age and sex. A percentage of ideal weight between 110–120 percent represents overweight, >130 percent signifies obesity, and >200 percent, morbid obesity.[8] The Quetelet or Body Mass Index (BMI) classifies overweight or obesity according to health risk. Appropriate BMI for those 19–34 years and >35 years is 19–25 kg/m^2 and 21–27 kg/m^2, respectively. BMI between 25 or 27–30 kg/m^2 represents low risk from overweight, while 30–35 and 35–40 kg/m^2 represent moderate and high risk, respectively, from obesity. BMI >40 kg/m^2 represents very high risk for illness from severe or morbid obesity.[19] Skinfold measurements >120 percent of standard skinfold indicates obesity and percentile values >85 indicate a risk for obesity.[8]

NUTRITIONAL STRATEGIES

The major diet strategies for patients undergoing rehabilitation for neurological disease fall into five areas: (1) energy (calorie)-reduced diet; (2) high-energy, high-protein diet; (3) high-fiber diet; (4) dysphagia diets; (5) enteral feeding.

The Energy-Reduced Diet

Weight gain and obesity are observed in patients with neurological and neuromuscular disorders, such as multiple sclerosis and spinal cord injury. They tend to occur in patients whose mobility and, consequently, energy requirements are reduced. Obesity adversely affects functions such as transfers and ambulation and places additional physical demands on caregivers.

Obesity is treated by a reduction in energy intake. This generally requires a low-fat diet in adults. Nutrient requirements remain age-appropriate. Nutritional needs for growth must be accounted for in children and adolescents. Physical activity should be increased when possible. Behavior modification, such as serving food on a smaller plate and serving smaller portions, instructing the patient to eat slowly (as it takes approximately 20 minutes to feel a sense of satiety), identifying and developing strategies to deal with contributing factors such as boredom or depression, and increasing activity appropriate to the medical condition may help the patient reduce energy intake. Medications, such as antidepressants and steroids, also should be evaluated as to their adverse import on weight and fluid balance.[20]

High-Energy, High-Protein Diet

In patients demonstrating inadequate weight gain, excessive weight loss, malnutrition, or skeletal trauma, nutrition of high-energy, high-protein, and nutrient den-

Table 24-3
Features of subjective global assessment

(Select appropriate category with a checkmark, or enter numerical value where indicated by "#")

A. History
    1. Weight change
        Overall loss in past 6 months: amount = # _____ kg, % loss = # _____
        Change in past 2 weeks: _____ increase,
                              _____ no change,
                              _____ decrease.

    2. Dietary intake change (relative to normal)
        _____ no change,
        _____ change   _____ duration = # _____ weeks.
                              _____ suboptimal solid diet,   _____ full liquid diet
                              _____ hypocaloric liquids,   _____ starvation.

    3. Gastrointestinal symptoms (that persisted for >2 weeks)
        _____ none, _____ nausea, _____ vomiting, _____ diarrhea, _____ anorexia.

    4. Functional capacity
        _____ no dysfunction (e.g., full capacity),
        _____ dysfunction _____ duration = # _____ weeks.
                              _____ type: _____ working suboptimally,
                                            _____ ambulatory,
                                            _____ bedridden.

    5. Disease and its relation to nutritional requirements
        Primary diagnosis (specify) _____

        Metabolic demand (stress):   _____ no stress,   _____ low stress,
                                          _____ moderate stress,   _____ high stress.

B. Physical (for each trait specify: 0 = normal, 1+ = mild, 2+ = moderate, 3+ = severe).
    # _____ loss of subcutaneous fat (triceps, chest)
    # _____ muscle wasting (quadriceps, deltoids)
    # _____ ankle edema
    # _____ ascites

C. SGA rating (select one)
    _____ A = Well nourished
    _____ B = Moderately (or suspected of being) malnourished
    _____ C = Severely malnourished

Reprinted with permission from Detsky AS, McLaughlin JR, Baker JP, Johnson N, Whittaker S, Mendelson RA, Jeejeebhoy KN: What is subjective global assessment of nutritional status? *J Ent Nut* 1987; 11:8–13.

sity should be offered in a form that is convenient and attractive for consumption. Patients requiring this type of diet include those with traumatic brain injury, stroke, or spinal cord injury. The rationale behind this diet is that the augmented protein intakes supply amino acids required for the building, maintenance, and repair of body tissue. Supplemental energy is required to spare protein from being utilized as a source of energy. At the same time, the energy level should be appropriate to maintain body weight or promote weight gain.[9]

The normal adult protein requirement is 0.8 g/kg/day.[21] For patients requiring protein repletion, intakes in the range of 1.5–2.0 g/kg/day are recommended in the absence of renal or hepatic insufficiency.[6] To allow for the proper utilization of protein, the diet should contain 600 kJ (150 kcal) of non-protein energy for every gram of available nitrogen (or 6.25 g protein).

For inpatients, effort should be made to provide a pleasant atmosphere and offer appealing food. Six small meals and small snacks or nutritional supplements may augment energy intake. The drinking of large quantities of fluids before or during meals should be discouraged. Evaluate whether medications, dysphagia, or depression are contributing factors. Food intake should be monitored, and nutritional risk assessed.[20]

High-Fiber Diet

Constipation may be associated with neurologic impairments such as Alzheimer's disease, spinal-cord injury, multiple sclerosis, and Parkinson's disease. Hydration should be assessed. Fluid intake should be recorded and urine output and color noted. Fluid intake of 1,200–2,000 cc (six to eight 8-ounce glasses) should be encouraged, provided there is no medical reason for fluid restriction.[20] When commercial fiber supplements such as psyllium are used, additional fluids are recommended. Dietary sources of insoluble fiber are particularly effective in increasing fecal bulk.[22] The clinical dietitian can advise on sources of dietary fiber to be increased and prunes or prune juice should be included. Stool softeners, such as docusate sodium, along with judicious use of oral and rectal laxatives, are helpful adjuncts in the treatment of constipation. Exercise opportunities should be provided. Attention to the urge to defecate and the establishment of a routine schedule for toileting should be encouraged. Constipation may be a side effect of certain medications, such as anti-depressants or narcotic preparations.[20]

Dysphagia Diets

The word dysphagia is derived from the Greek *dys,* meaning difficult, and *phagein,* meaning to eat. If not diagnosed and treated, it can lead to loss of the basic pleasure of eating, death caused by aspiration pneumonia, and impaired nutritional status.[23,24] In a study by Sitzmann, of 43 patients admitted with a primary diagnosis of dysphagia and an etiology of neurologic dysfunction, 80 percent exhibited dysphagia-induced starvation as evidenced by significant rate of weight loss and markedly abnormal anthropometric exams.[23] Over 70 percent exhibited visceral protein depletion. In these patients, untreated dysphagia resulted in the development of malnutrition.

Dysphagia has been observed in those with vary-

ing central neurological dysfunction conditions, including stroke, traumatic brain injury, amyotrophic lateral sclerosis, and Parkinson's disease.[25–29] In this chapter, the focus of dysphagia discussion will be on the dysphagia diet. The pathophysiology, diagnosis, and treatment of dysphagia are covered extensively in Chapter 29.

Prescription and Implementation The approach to the treatment of dysphagia often is a multidisciplinary one.[24,30] Warning signs of dysphagia are listed in Table 24-4. Suspected cases should be referred to the speech-language pathologist (SLP) who has specialized training in the recognition of dysphagia and the treatment of swallowing disorders. Based on the results of the bedside assessment and/or the video fluoroscopic examination (modified barium swallow), in which a variety of food and liquid consistencies are used, the physician and therapist make diet recommendations.[24]

The clinical dietitian assesses the patient's nutritional status, determines the energy and protein requirements, and helps the patient adapt to the prescribed diet modifications. Together with the SLP, the patients' progress is followed in order to allow a smooth progression to the highest diet level possible while achieving or maintaining adequate nutritional status.[24] Nursing staff may assist or supervise patients at mealtimes. This can be done in a common dining room in order to enhance the social atmosphere and allow for regular

Table 24-4
Warning signs of dysphagia

Reluctance to eat certain food consistencies or any food at all

Marked slowness in chewing or eating

Fatigue during meals

A "gurgly" voice or frequent throat clearing

Complaints of food "sticking" in the throat

"Pocketing" of food in the cheek

Drooling

Unexplained respiratory symptoms

Coughing or choking during attempts to eat. (caveat: Aspiration very commonly occurs *without* coughing. The presence or absence of the *gag* reflex does not indicate whether the *swallowing* reflex is intact)

Pardoe EM. Development of a multistage diet for dysphagia. Copyright The American Dietetic Association. Reprinted by permission from the *Journal of the American Dietetic Association* 1993; 93:568–571.

monitoring of patients' progress. The occupational therapist (OT) can perform a mealtime evaluation in order to screen for feeding difficulties. The OT can provide adaptive equipment to assist with mechanical aspects of feeding. The physical therapist can help determine, along with the OT, any requirements for external support during feeding or the modified barium swallow procedure. The radiologist is responsible for performing the modified barium swallow and interpreting it together with the SLP. Pre-evaluation findings of others on the swallowing team allow the radiologist to focus the procedure.[30]

The Diet Patients with neurologic disorders commonly exhibit conditions that necessitate dietary modifications. Table 24-5 describes these conditions, their dietary considerations, and rationale for dietary change.

Characteristics of the dysphagia diet include texture modification of food and/or fluids. Foods may be chopped, minced, or pureed, whereas fluids may be "thickened." Examples of food and fluid consistencies are found in Table 24-6. An example of a multistage dysphagia diet is shown in Table 24-7. Solid foods are assigned to one of five groups that progress from the

Table 24-5

Dietary considerations for dysphagia in patients with neurologic disorders

Condition	Dietary consideration	Rationale
Slow/weak/uncoordinated pharyngeal peristalsis	Include highly seasoned, flavorful, aromatic foods Add sugar, spices	Maximize stimulus for swallow
	Serve food at either very warm or very cold temperatures	Maximize stimulus for swallow
	Include highly textured foods such as diced cooked vegetables, finely chopped raw vegetables in gelatin base, diced canned fruit	Maximize stimulus for swallow
	Maintain semisolid consistencies that form a cohesive bolus	Need to avoid consistencies that will tend to fall apart in the pharynx
	Avoid sticky or bulky foods	Reduce risk of airway obstruction
	Be cautious with thin liquids (water, juices, milk), iced tart juices, or crushed popsicles—banana and vanilla melt slowest (flavor and temperature may stimulate reflex)	They are difficult to control, unpredictable, and may spill into pharynx prior to swallow reflex
	Medium or spoon-thick liquids may be substituted	
	Thicken thin liquids with nonfat dry milk powder, fruit flakes or commercial thickeners	
	Small frequent meals	Minimize fatigue, optimize food temperature and total nutrient intake
Weakened or poor oral-muscular control	Maintain semisolid consistencies that form a cohesive bolus. Avoid slippery, sticky foods	Requires less oral manipulation, purees are difficult to control
	Avoid thin liquids (see above description of thin liquids and recommendation)	See above rationale
	Small frequent meals	Minimize fatigue, optimize total nutrient intake
Reduced oral sensation	Position food in most sensitive area	Maximize sensation possible
	Do not mix textures (e.g., vegetable soup)	Maximize sensation possible
	Use colder temperatures	Maximize sensation possible
	Use highly seasoned, flavorful foods	Maximize sensation possible
Crycopharyngeal dysfunction	Maintain liquid-pureed diet if no other contraindications present	Liquids and purees will pass into the esophagus more easily
Decreased laryngeal elevation	Limit diet to medium spoon-thick liquids, soft solids	Thin liquids easily penetrate larynx
	Avoid sticky or bulky foods or food that will fall apart	Reduce risk of airway obstruction
Decreased vocal cord closure	Avoid thin liquids	Easy, quick laryngeal penetration
	Avoid foods that will fall apart	Reduce risk of small pieces entering larynx after the swallow

Source: Megan S, Veldee RD, and Miller, RM, PhD: Seattle Department of Veterans Affairs Medical Centre, Seattle.

©1992, The American Dietetic Association. Adapted with permission from *Handbook of Clinical Dietetics.*

Table 24-6

Examples of foods and fluid consistencies

Consistency	Food Examples
Semisolids that form a cohesive bolus	Hot cereals, quiches, egg, tuna or meat salad, ground meats with gravy, moist, soft meat or fish loaf, soft cheeses, aspic, canned fruit, custard, pudding, finger gelatin, whipped gelatin, cheesecake with sauce
Spoon-thick liquids	Frozen products,[a] gelatin desserts, pudding, yogurt, pureed fruit
Medium-thick liquids	Blenderized or cream soups, eggnog, nectar, milk shakes or malts, high-protein or high-calorie commercial supplemental formulae
Thin liquids	Water, broth, milk, chocolate milk, coffee, tea, hot chocolate, fruit juices, soda, alcoholic beverages, standard commercial supplemental formulas, vegetable juice
Foods that fall apart	Plain ground meats, dry crumbly breads, crackers, plain rice, thin hot cereals, cooked peas or corn, plain chopped raw vegetables and fruits, thin pureed foods (such as applesauce)
Sticky or bulky foods	Peanut butter, fresh white bread, plain mashed potatoes, bran cereals, refried beans, raw vegetables and fruits, bananas, chunks of plain meats

[a] Frozen products such as frozen juices, popsicles, ice chips, ice cream and sherbet would be restricted if they are allowed to melt to thin liquid in the mouth, thereby becoming a hazard to swallowing.

©1992, American Dietetic Association, *Handbook of Clinical Dietetics,* 2nd ed. Used by permission.

Table 24-7

Main features of solid-food dysphagia diet

Five categories that progress in swallowing difficulty from easiest to most difficult

Stage 1	All pureed foods, smooth hot cereals, strained soups thickened to pureed consistency, creamed cottage cheese, smooth yogurt, and puddings
Stage 2	All foods in previous stages plus soft moist whole foods such as pancakes; finely chopped tender meats, fish, and eggs bound with thick dressing; soft cheeses (e.g., American); noodles and pasta; tender cooked leafy greens; sliced ripe banana; soft breads; soft moist cakes
Stage 3	All foods in previous stages plus eggs any style, tender ground meats bound with thick sauce, soft fish, whole soft vegetables, drained canned fruits
Stage 4	All foods in previous stages plus foods with solids and liquids together (e.g., vegetable soup), all whole foods except hard and particulate foods such as dry breads, tough meat, corn, rice, apples
Stage 5	Regular diet

Pardoe EM: Development of a multistage diet for dysphagia. Copyright The American Dietetic Association, Reprinted by permission from the *Journal of the American Dietetic Association* 1993; 93:568–571.

easiest stage (pureed), to the most difficult to swallow (regular diet).[24]

The dysphagia diet must meet the patient's individual needs, depending on degree and site of the oral–pharyngeal impairment and the patient's own tolerance and preference. This type of dysphagia diet is adequate nutritionally, as long as the patient consumes normal quantities of food at each meal. If oral intake is limited, the dysphagia diet should be complemented by high-energy, high-protein foods. If oral intake remains insufficient, the use of tube feedings should be considered seriously. Vitamin, mineral, and/or commercial supplements may be offered orally or by tube feeding. Patients may begin the diet at any stage and progress by more than one category at a time according to swallowing ability and tolerance.[24] Reassessment is essential in order to upgrade the oral diet as necessary. The diet should have as many normal characteristics as possible, both for psychological reasons and to enhance palatability.[31] This diet has a tendency to be low in fiber, making constipation a concern. Fiber supplementation may be necessary.

Liquids are grouped separately into thin, medium-thick, and spoon-thick categories (Table 24-6) as their ability to be swallowed is *independent* of ability to swallow solids. For some patients, thin fluids pass through the swallowing tract too quickly to be detected. Thicker fluids can be sensed more readily but they can accumulate in the back of the pharynx and spill into the trachea. Thin liquids may be thickened with starch, other food

Table 24-8
Dysphagia diet: general guidelines for the patient

1. Follow American or Canadian Dietetic Association Guidelines for food selection.

2. Eat small, frequent meals instead of three large meals to improve meal tolerance.

3. Follow each meal with oral cleaning to prevent mouth sores and to avoid swallowing any remaining unchewed food.

4. Determine, with the therapist, the best head and/or body posture for swallowing.

5. Sit upright during food ingestions and do not lie down for at least 15–30 minutes afterward. Avoid large snacks 1 to 2 hours before sleep.

6. Place food in middle of mouth or on the unaffected side, if applicable.

7. Concentrate and chew food slowly. Ingest foods in small mouthfuls (one half to one teaspoon).

8. Avoid washing food down with liquids.

9. Use liquid thickeners if thin fluids are to be avoided. The dietitian can advise on this.

10. Check the form of medication being used (e.g., liquid, crushed, or whole pills) to ensure that it complies with the swallowing regime.

Adapted with permission from *Ontario Dietetic Association–Ontario Hospital Association Nutrition Care Manual,* 1989.

Table 24-9
Baseline daily fluid requirements in adults and paediatric patients

Patient group	Fluid requirements
Children (<16 years)	
0.5–3 kg	120 mL/kg
3–10 kg	100 mL/kg
10–20 kg	1,000 mL plus 50 mL/kg each kg over 10 kg
>20 kg	1,500 mL plus 20 mL/kg each kg over 20 kg
Adults	
Young active (16–30 years)	40 mL/kg
Average adult (25–55 years)	35 mL/kg
Older patients (56–65 years)	30 mL/kg
Elderly (>65 years)	25 mL/kg

Source: Blackburn GL, Bell SJ, Mullen JL (eds): *Nutritional Medicine, Case Management Approach.* Philadelphia: W.B. Saunders, 1989, p. 180. Reprinted with permission.

ingredients such as skim milk powder, pureed fruit, infant cereals or commercial thickening agents. Thickened fluids are suitable for patients unable to tolerate any normal liquids. These fluids must maintain the consistency of a puree until swallowed.[24] General guidelines for the dysphagia diet are found in Table 24-8.

The adequacy of hydration should be verified by monitoring fluid balance and serum electrolyte levels. Fluid requirements and general guidelines are discussed in the following (see Table 24-9). If fluid intake is insufficient, despite efforts to provide thickened fluids, hydration may need to be supplemented by nasogastric or gastrostomy tube, or intravenous infusion.

Enteral Nutrition

This section will focus on tube feeding as a method of nutritional support for patients with a functional gastrointestinal (GI) tract. Neurologic conditions that may require tube feeding include stroke, traumatic brain injury, motor neuron diseases, and demyelinating diseases

and conditions associated with dysphagia. Tube feeding is contraindicated in patients with a malfunctioning gastrointestinal tract. Symptoms such as gastric or intestinal obstruction, paralytic ileus, intractable vomiting, or severe diarrhea usually preclude its use.

Enteral feeding generally is preferred over parenteral feeding because it is more physiologic, and promotes the maintenance of gastrointestinal tract integrity and the intestinal mucosal barrier to bacteria.[9] Large quantities of energy can be provided enterally without fluid overload. Central venous catheter and associated septic complications can be avoided. Enteral feeding is also lower in cost than parenteral nutrition.

The type of tube feeding and the route of access chosen are based on medical factors, prognosis for recovery, and the length of time that the tube feeding is expected to be used. Figure 24-1 provides an algorithm for determining the optimal type of feeding, by taking into account adequacy of oral intake, anticipated duration of enteral support, and risk of aspiration.

Classification of Enteral Diets   Tube feedings vary in energy density, osmolarity, lactose content, molecular form of substrate, and cost. A clinical dietitian should be consulted to advise on the optimum formulation to meet the patient's nutritional needs.

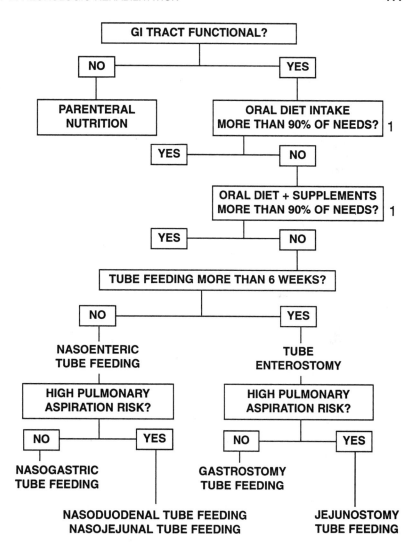

Figure 24-1
Determining the optimal feeding mode

1. Demonstrated by daily calorie counts

Enteral diets can be described as complete or supplementary. Complete formulations, if taken in adequate quantities, provide the nutrient and energy requirements for most individuals. Enteral feeding may be categorized as follows.

Polymeric This is the most common category of enteral formula employed in the neurologically impaired. These formulas are appropriate for the patient with a functional gastrointestinal tract. Typically they contain intact protein, polyunsaturated fatty acids with or without medium-chain triglycerides, glucose oligosaccharides, or starch. These formulas are complete provided sufficient volume is administered (see Table 24-10 for examples).

Subcategories of the polymeric group include standard, high-nitrogen, fiber-supplemented, concentrated, milk-based and commercial or home-made

Table 24-10

Characteristics of selected polymeric tube feedings

Polymeric tube feeding	Osmolality mOsm/kg water	Energy Kcal/kJ per mL	Protein g/100 mL	Fiber g/100 mL	Volume to meet 100% of RDA[a]	Volume to meet 100% of RNI[b]	Lactose free	Suitability for oral feeding
Standard								
Ensure (Ross)	450	1.1/4.5	3.7	0	1,887	1,650	Yes	Yes, flavored
Isocal (Mead Johnson)	305	1.0/4.2	4.2	0	1,179	1,250	Yes	Yes, flavored
Nutren (Clintec)	300[c]–390	1.0/4.2	4.0	0	1,500	1,500	Yes	Yes, flavored
Resource (Sandoz)	430	1.1/4.5	3.7	0	1,890	1,650	Yes	Yes, flavored
High Nitrogen								
Ensure High Protein (Ross)	475	1.0/4.2	6.1	0	1,321	1,000	Yes	Yes, flavored
Isocal HN (Mead Johnson)	270	1.0/4.2	5.0	0	1,000	1,250	Yes	Yes, bland
Isosource VHN (Sandoz)	300	1.0/4.2	6.2	1.0	1,250	1,250	Yes	Yes, flavored
Fiber-Supplemented								
Ensure with fiber (Ross)	480	1.1/4.6	4.0	1.4	1,530	1,525	Yes	Yes, flavored
Isocal with fiber (Mead Johnson)	300	1.0/4.2	4.2	1.4	1,179	1,250	Yes	Yes, bland
Jevity (Ross)	310	1.1/4.5	4.4	1.4	1,321	1,410	Yes	No
Nutren with fiber (Clintec)	303[c]–412	1.0/4.2	4.0	1.4	1,500	1,500	Yes	Yes, flavored
Concentrated								
Ensure plus (Ross)	690	1.5/6.3	5.5	0	1,420	1,550	Yes	Yes, flavored
Nutren 1.5 (Clintec)	410[c]–590	1.5/6.3	6.0	0	1,000	1,000	Yes	Yes, flavored
Nutren 2.0 (Clintec)	710	2.0/8.4	8.0	0	750	750	Yes	Yes, flavored
Resource Plus (Sandoz)	600	1.5/6.3	5.5	0	1,400	1,550	Yes	Yes, flavored
Milk-Based								
Meritene Powder[d] (Sandoz)	690	1.1/4.4	6.9	0	1,250	1,180	No	Yes, flavored
Sustacal Liquid (Mead Johnson)	710	1.0/4.2	6.1	0	1,080	1,000	No	Yes, flavored
Read-to-Use Blenderized								
Complete-Modified (Sandoz)	300	1.1/4.5	4.2	.4	1,500	1,600	Yes	No
Vitaneed (Sherwood Medical)	300	1.0/4.2	4.0	.8	1,500	N/A	Yes	No

[a] Recommended Daily Allowance: Food and Nutrition Board, National Research Council: *Recommended Dietary Allowances,* 10th ed. Washington, DC: National Academy of Sciences, 1989.

[b] Recommended Nutrient Intake for Canadians: Health Canada: Recommended Nutrient Intake for Canadians, Report of the Scientific Review.

[c] Refers to unflavored.

[d] Based on 32.4 g Meritene power in 240 mL Vitamin D fortified whole milk.

blenderized formulas. Examples of commercial formulae within each subgroup are given in Table 24-10. This list is by no means comprehensive and values reflect the content of formulas based on manufacturers' information available at the time of publication.

Blenderized regular food (meat, fruits, vegetables, cereal, oil) is labor intensive and poses a high contamination risk. Nutrient composition is variable. Blenderized feedings may be lactose-containing (milk added) or lactose-free (excluding milk). They supply trace elements and natural sources of fiber. However, because of their high viscosity, they require large-bore feeding tubes (>12 French). Commercially blenderized

feeds are bacteriologically safe and provide consistent nutritional composition. They are generally higher in cost than other polymeric feeding formulas.

Many polymeric tube feeds are palatable for oral use as well. They may be flavored, unflavored, or bland. Because their viscosity is low, small-bore feeding tubes may be used. Their nutritional content is standardized. They are sterile prior to opening and, once open, are bacteriologically safe, provided that protocols for handling are followed. Osmolality varies from iso-osmolar (300 mOsm/kg water) to high-level osmolar (~700 mOsm/kg water) in some of the concentrated formulas and milk-based formulas. The energy content of tube-feedings generally is 1 kcal or 4.2 kJ/mL. Concentrated formulas, supplying up to 2.0 kcals or 8.4 kJ/mL, are indicated in those with fluid restrictions or limited formula tolerance. Fiber generally is lacking in the standardized feeds, but variations with added fiber are available to promote normal bowel function. This type of formula is useful for long-term feeding. High nitrogen polymeric formulas are indicated in the presence of malnutrition, a catabolic state, or in those with, or at risk for, pressure sores.

Partially Hydrolyzed (or Elemental) Formulas These formulas contain protein in amino acid and/or peptide form, carbohydrate as glucose oligosacchorides, and fat as long- or medium-chain fatty acids. This type of feeding may be indicated in situations of gut malfunction, including malabsorption, short-bowel syndromes, chronic pancreatitis, or bile-salt deficiency.[6,9] Examples include Vital HN® (Ross) and Vivonex TEN® (Sandoz).

Modular, or Combined Modular, Protein, Carbohydrate, or Fat Products These feeds can be used to enhance an existing formula or they can be combined to produce a complete formula for those with specialized nutrient, fluid, and/or electrolyte needs.[6] Malnourished patients or those in a catabolic state may benefit by the addition of a protein supplement. Examples include Promod® (Ross) and Casec® (Mead Johnson).

Specialized Formulas These are available for rehabilitation patients with impaired renal function, compromised pulmonary function, or for diabetics.

Routes of Access Feeding modes may be classified into nasoenteric and enterostomy types. Figure 24-2 illustrates the location of these sites. Nasoenteric feeding includes the following routes: nasogastric (tube from nose to stomach), nasoduodenal (tube from nose through pylorus and into duodenum), and nasojejunal (tube from nose through pylorus and into jejunum, usually placed fluoroscopically).[6] Nasogastric feedings generally are safe, particularly when there is no evidence of reflux or aspiration. Enterostomies can be inserted surgically or percutaneously. Common routes include

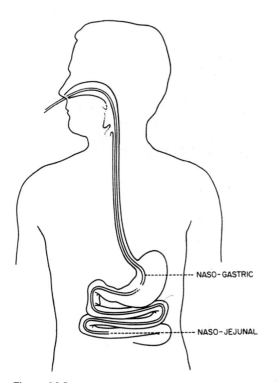
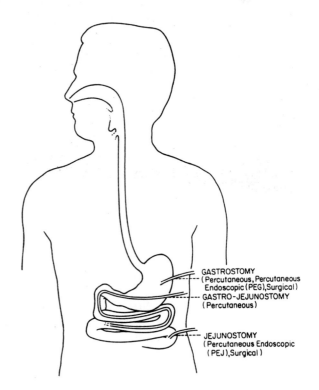

Figure 24-2
Common enteral feeding access routes

gastrostomy and jejunostomy. A gastrostomy involves tube placement in the stomach. Tube sizes, pliability, and techniques vary. Jejunostomy involves the creation of a jejunal stoma that can be catheterized intermittently by needle catheter placement or direct tube placement. Percutaneous endoscopic gastrostomy (PEG) or jejunostomy (PEJ) are procedures in which the feeding tube is inserted percutaneously under endoscopic guidance into the stomach or jejunum. The tube is secured by rubber "bumpers" or an inflated balloon catheter. Often it is performed with local anesthesia by a gastroenterologist or surgeon. When altered level of consciousness or dysfunction of cranial nerves IX, X, and XII is present, feedings should be delivered distal to the pylorus.[32] Percutaneous gastro-jejunostomy involves the percutaneous insertion of a guidewire and subsequent feeding catheter into the jejunum, via the stomach. This is performed by a radiologist, and only local anesthetic is required.

Methods of Enteral Feeding Administration Continuous drip feedings are delivered by gravity drip, or by infusion pump for better volume accuracy and tolerance. They are administered at a constant rate, reducing the possibility of pulmonary aspiration. Continuous feeding at night frees the patient from cumbersome equipment during rehabilitation therapy.

Intermittent infusions are divided feedings, infused at intervals four to six times throughout the day. They can be given by gravity drip over 30–60 minutes or by infusion pump. This type of feeding frees patients from tube-feeding equipment between feedings, so it is convenient for those undergoing active rehabilitation and those on home tube feeding. Also it is used for the non–critically ill patient. A cyclic method of intermittent infusion may be used wherein the tube feeding is administered at a high infusion rate over 8–16 hours. This may be helpful in the transition from tube feeding to oral diet, with tube feeding delivered at night and oral diet ingested by day.[32] This method allows for uninterrupted rehabilitation during the day.

Bolus feedings involve the rapid delivery of a feeding into the gastrointestinal tract by syringe or funnel. It is suited to the rehabilitation patient, those on home tube feeding, and the non–critically ill patient. Feeding is done over a short period (usually less than 15 minutes).

The risk of pulmonary aspiration can be reduced, but not eliminated, by implementation of a protocol that includes confirmation of tube placement in the upper duodenum and elevating the head to >30° during feeding and for at least 1 hour after feeding. Blue food coloring can be added to feedings (1 mL/500 mL feeding) to detect possible aspiration. Feedings should begin at a slow, continuous rate, advancing the rate every 8–12 hours until the desired volume is achieved. Gastric residuals should be verified every 4 hours. If they exceed 150 mL, feedings should be held for 2 hours, and the residual rechecked. Excessive residual may be a sign of obstruction or functional gastroparesis. If this continues, the feeding program should be re-evaluated, and an alternate route or formula considered.

Tube-Feeding Complications Adverse reactions associated with tube feeding are relatively few and usually can be detected and controlled through proper monitoring. Complications associated with tube feeding largely fall into mechanical, gastrointestinal, and metabolic categories. Mechanical complications include tube blockages and local skin infections at the site of tube insertion. Gastrointestinal complications, such as cramping and diarrhea, are seen frequently, but are rectified easily by reassessing the metabolic characteristics of the formula. Metabolic complications often are related to inadequate monitoring of fluid and electrolyte balance, blood sugars, and renal status. Table 24-11 describes potential adverse reactions, their causes, and possible management strategies.

Home Tube Feeding[34] General considerations include caregiver assessment, compatibility of the tube feeding with home-life schedule, and type of follow-up required. Formula selection will depend on the nutritional adequacy of the formula, tolerance of the feedings, form of tube feeding, cost, and availability. Equipment considerations include type of pump or gravity drip set, need for accessories, cost, and ease of administration.

Written patient instructions should be provided, including proper care of feeding and equipment, rate and strength of feedings, time of administration, position for feeding, temperature of formula, maximum hanging time, maximum time to keep open formulas, amount of fluids to flush between feedings, and tube and ostomy care.

Parenteral Nutrition Support

Parenteral nutritional support may be indicated in the acute phase of neurological impairment. This type of nutrition may be administered to the traumatic brain-injured and the spinal-cord-injured patient if paralytic

Table 24-11
Possible adverse reactions to tube feeding

Problem	Possible causes	Management strategy
Mechanical complications		
Tube displacement	Coughing, vomiting	Replace tube and confirm placement
	Dislodgement by patient	Replace tube; restrain patient if necessary; consider alternate feeding route
	Inadequate taping of tube	Position tube properly and tape correctly
Tube obstruction or clogging	Improperly crushed medication	Use liquid medications when possible
	Medications mixed with incompatible formulas	Follow drug nutrient interaction guidelines and flush tube before and after addition of medication
	Formula residue adhering to tube; failure to irrigate properly	Flush tube with 20–50 mL water before starting and after stopping feeding. Flush tube at least every 4 hours during continuous infusion[a]
Gastric retention, aspiration pneumonia	Delayed gastric emptying	Reposition tube into small intestine
	Patient lying flat during infusion	Elevate head of bed to 30° or more during and for 2 hours after infusion
	Displaced feeding tube	Monitor and confirm tube placement before feeding
Nasopharyngeal irritation; mucosal erosion; otitis media	Large-bore vinyl or rubber feeding tubes for prolonged time periods	Consider use of soft, small-bore feeding tubes or feeding by tube enterostomy
	Improper positioning or placement	Position tube properly and tape correctly; choose tube of correct size for patient
	Decreased salivary secretions owing to lack of chewing; mouth breathing	Keep mouth and lips moist. Allow chewing of sugarless gum, gargling, or sucking on anesthetic lozenges if appropriate
Skin irritation, excoriation and infection at ostomy site[b]	Leakage of gastric or intestinal secretions from stoma site; site is portal of entry for bacteria	Use appropriate enterostomal therapy. Ensure ostomy catheter anchored via retention device to avoid dislodgement. Treat infection with local and systemic antibiotics—a tube change may also be required
Gastrointestinal complications		
Nausea and vomiting; cramping; distension	Improper location of tube	Periodically confirm tube position
	Rapid increase in rate, volume, or concentration	Return to slower rate and advance by smaller increments. Advance only when tolerated at current rate.
	High osmolality	Dilute to isotonic strength if gastric residuals are consistently high. Increase concentration over several days. Consider change to isotonic formula
	Delayed gastric emptying	Check gastric residuals every 4–6 hours on continuous feedings or prior to each bolus. Monitor for drugs or disease states that may influence gastric or intestinal motility[c]
	Lactose intolerance	Change to lactose-free formula
	Cold formula	Warm to room temperature before use
	Obstruction	Stop formula feeding immediately
	Excessive fat in formula	Switch to lower-fat formula. Reduce fat in modular feedings
Constipation	Inadequate fiber or fluid intake	Monitor intake and output, add free water if intake is not greater than output by 500–1,000 mL/day. Use formula with added fiber
	Medications	Evaluate medication side effects; suggest stool softener or bulk-forming laxative
	Inactivity	Increase patient activity if possible

Table 24-11
Possible adverse reactions to tube feeding (Continued)

Problem	Possible causes	Management strategy
Diarrhea, defined as passage of more than 200 g of stool per 24 hours or the passage of liquid stools	Protein-energy malnutrition, decreased oncotic pressure owing to serum albumin below 3.0 g/dL	Use isotonic or elemental formula at slow rate initially. If severe, suggest antidiarrhea therapy or parenteral nutrition
	Infectious origin, microbial contamination of formula	Confirm with stool, blood, or formula culture. Review tube-feeding handling and infection-control procedures
	Malabsorption of fat or other nutrients	Evaluate for pancreatic insufficiency, use pancreatic enzyme replacements if indicated. Change to low-fat or elemental formula
	Bolus feeding, dumping syndrome	Change to continuous feeding or decrease bolus volume and increase frequency of feeding
	Hyperosmolar formula	Reduce rate and increase gradually, dilute formula or change to isotonic product
	Medications	Consider antidiarrheal agents such as Kaopectate, paregoric, or Lomotil. Change to fiber-containing formula
Metabolic complications		
Hyperosmolar dehydration	Administration of hypertonic formula with inadequate water	Initiate hypertonic feedings at reduced rates, dilute or consider use of isotonic formula
Fluid overload or overhydration	Refeeding of patients with PEM, common in patients with cardiac, renal, or hepatic disease	Restrict fluids, use concentrated formula
	Prolonged use of over-dilute formula	Advance formula concentration as tolerated
Hyponatremia	Congestive heart failure, cirrhosis, hypoalbumenemia, edema, ascites	Apply diuretic therapy; restrict fluids. Use concentrated formula
	Excess gastrointestinal losses	Monitor serum levels and hydration status and replace sodium as needed
Hypernatremia	Dehydration	Assure adequate fluid intake
Hypokalemia	Acidosis, insulin administration, diarrhea, marked malnutrition, diuretic therapy	Monitor electrolytes daily, supplement potassium as needed
Hyperkalemia	Renal insufficiency	Perform frequent biochemical monitoring. Use formula containing low levels of potassium
Other serum electrolyte or mineral abnormalities	Various	Monitor serum levels regularly, making individual adjustments as needed
Essential fatty acid (EFA) deficiency	Formula with low levels of EFA used over prolonged time periods	Provide a minimum of 4% of the caloric intake from EFAs. Add 5 mL safflower oil daily
Glucose tolerance, hyperglycemic hyperosmolar nonketotic coma	Diabetes mellitus or temporary insulin resistance caused by trauma or sepsis	May need to stop feeding and to rehydrate patient. Monitor blood sugar frequently, making adjustments in insulin dose. Avoid formulas high in simple sugars
Increased respiratory quotient, excess CO_2 production, respiratory insufficiency	Overfeeding of calories, especially in the form of carbohydrates	Reduce the respiratory quotient by balancing the calories provided from fat, protein, and carbohydrate. Increase the percentage of calories provided as fat by using high-fat formula or adding modular fat.

[a] The authors' facility uses a solution of 1 tablet sodium bicarbonate (300 mg) and 1 pancreolipase capsule mixed with 5–15 cc of water. The solution must be infused via a 5–10 cc syringe to generate adequate pressure. Marcaud SP, Stegall KS: Unclogging feeding tubes with pancreatic enzyme. *JPEN* 1990; 14:198–200.

[b] Ideno KT: Enteral nutrition, in Gottschlich MM, Matarese LE, Shronts EP (eds): *Nutrition Support Dietetics–Core Curriculum, American Society for Parenteral and Enteral Nutrition.* Silver Springs, MD: 1993, pp. 71–103.

[c] A nuclear medicine gastric emptying study may be helpful.

©1992, The American Dietetic Association. Adapted with permission from *Handbook of Clinical Dietetics.*

ileus or gastrointestinal intolerance persists more than 2 to 3 days after injury. In the transition from the acute to the sub-acute phase, parenteral nutrition may be used together with enteral support, until the desired strength and volume of enteral support is reached. Thereafter, in the rehabilitation phase, parenteral support seldom is required.

Fluid Requirements

Fluid requirements are affected by obligatory and facultative components. The obligatory component includes insensible losses through the skin, lungs, and feces. These can vary markedly, increasing under conditions of high temperature, high altitude, and dry air. The facultative component represents the amount of water required for fluctuating body needs as well as the maintenance of a tolerable renal salute load.[9]

General guidelines for the determination of fluid requirements are found in Table 24-9. Fluid requirements also should take into account effects of age, disease, and medical treatment. Fluid requirements are increased above normal in the setting of fever, diarrhea, vomiting, excessive sweating, fistula drainage, and during administration of hyperosmolar formulae.[35]

Effect of Changes in Mental Status on Eating-Related Behavior

Mental status changes occur frequently in the rehabilitation setting, particularly after traumatic brain injury and stroke. These changes may alter patients' ability to remember how to eat (apraxia), interfere with their response to feelings of satiety and hunger, and have a direct bearing on their activity level. These in turn, impact on nutritional requirements and nutritional status.[20] Table 24-12 describes some common eating-related behavior changes and practical interventions.

STROKE AND NUTRITION

Nutritional Consequences of Stroke

There is some evidence of increased protein catabolism following acute stroke. Mountokalakis and Dellos compared nitrogen loss, expressed as urea-creatinine ratio, in stroke and pre- and postsurgical patients.[36] Although the ratio rose significantly in both groups, only those of the stroke patients exceeded the upper limit of normal. The stroke group's rating reached its peak between days

4 and 10. These results suggest that more attention be given to ensuring adequate protein and energy intake in the stroke patient in order to improve protein sparing and reduce nitrogen loss.

Dysphagia is prevalent in the stroke population, with a reported incidence of 49 percent on entry to the rehabilitation service.[25] Other neurological deficits, such as upper-extremity paresis or paralysis, disorientation, depression, apraxia, agnosia, communication impairment, right and left disorientation, and visual neglect or denial of the paralyzed extremity, can contribute to decreased nutritional intake and subsequent malnutrition.[37] Table 24-13 describes interventions for secondary deficits that directly affect food intake. Table 24-12 describes strategies for dealing with eating-related behavior problems in stroke patients.

Prevalence of Malnutrition

A Swedish study determined that 16 and 22 percent of acute stroke patients were malnourished on hospital admission and discharge, respectively.[38] Male sex, advanced age, infection, and treatment with cardiovascular drugs significantly predicted undernutrition on discharge (median hospital stay = 16.5, range = 12–42 days). Among those patients with severe stroke and hospital stays greater than 3 weeks, 56.3 percent were malnourished at some point.[39] Among stroke rehabilitation patients, 60 percent (9/15) suffered from malnutrition of the marasmus (protein-energy) or kwashiorkor (protein) types.[1]

A study of 49 stroke patients by Finestone et al. determined that malnutrition, as assessed using anthropometric and biochemical parameters, was present in almost half (49 percent) of stroke patients on rehabilitation admission.[25] Malnutrition decreased among the remaining patients at 1-month, 2-month, and 2- to 4-month follow-up (see Table 24-14). Although overall prevalence and severity of malnutrition declined over time, in some individual cases patients who were adequately nourished became malnourished and severity increased. In this study, malnutrition was very high despite these patients being on a rehabilitation service of a tertiary-care hospital where radiologic swallowing studies, a swallowing team, dietitians, and enteral feedings were available readily. Significant predictors of malnutrition on entry to rehabilitation service included the need for tube feedings during acute hospital care and histories of prior stroke and diabetes mellitus. Tube feedings, received by 29 and 14 percent of stroke patients on acute and rehabilitation admission, respectively, were

Table 24-12

Practical interventions for eating-related behavior problems in individuals with neurologic impairment[a]

Behavior problem	Interventions
Attention-concentration deficit/ forgets to eat	Remind patient to eat and drink; discuss foods available. Verbally direct client through each step of the eating process. Place utensils in hand.
Combative/throws food	Identify provocative agent/remove. Feeder stands/sits on nondominant side. Provide unbreakable dishes, cups with suction holders. Give one food at a time. Reward appropriate behavior.
Eats too fast	Seat with role models. Set utensils down between bites. Offer food items separately. Offer foods that take time to chew. Use smaller utensil/cup.
Eats too slowly	Monitor eating pace; provide verbal cues; "chew," "take another bite." Serve first to allow ample meal time. Use insulated dishes to maintain proper temperatures. Alter texture if patient has difficulty chewing.
Forgets to swallow	Tell patient to swallow. Observe or feel for swallow before offering next mouthful. Stroke upward on patient's larynx. Check for remaining food at end of meal.
Inappropriate emotional expression	Engage in conversation. Ignore emotional display. Provide quiet environment. Reassure that continuing meal may help gain control.
Paces (won't sit to eat)	Sit beside patient at table. Change dining location. Gerichair for meals only. Aerobic exercise before meals. Several small meals daily to offset calories expended by pacing. Finger foods to eat while walking.
Chews constantly/overchews food	Tell patient to stop chewing after each bite. Serve soft foods to reduce need to chew. Offer small bites. Carefully remove food from mouth if patient is unable to swallow it.
Spits	Evaluate chewing/swallowing ability. Tell client not to spit; provide napkin. Place away from others who would be offended. Develop a behavior-modification strategy.
Will not wake up or get up to eat	Ask why. Discuss meal time preference; arrange more appropriate nap time. Evaluate medication for possible cause. Evaluate nutritional adequacy of total daily food intake. Have client wash face, brush teeth. Develop a contract identifying patient's mealtime preferences and facility's responsibility.
Refuses to eat	Try placing a small amount of food on lower lip.

[a] Primarily stroke, Alzheimer's disease, traumatic brain injury.

Adapted with permission from *Consultant Dietitians in Health Care Facilities: Dining Skills: Practical Skills for the Caregivers of Eating-Disabled Older Adults.* Chicago, American Dietetic Association, 1994.

effective in improving nutritional status. On admission to the rehabilitation service, those who were malnourished were significantly more likely to require tube feedings. Subsequent to this, prolonged tube-feeding administration (>1 month) led to adequate nutritional status in all inpatients and home tube-fed outpatients.

Functional Implications of Malnutrition

Poor nutrition has been found to predict lower functional status outcome and reduced functional improvement rate in stroke patients undergoing rehabilitation. Using the Modified Barthel Index (MBI), a functional assessment scale,[40,41] Aptaker et al. determined that serum albumin, a nutrition-sensitive marker, was associated positively with higher functional mobility and degree of improvement, decreased complication rate, and higher self-care scores.[4]

Finestone et al. explored the relationship between MBI scores and malnutrition in stroke patients on a rehabilitation service.[3] The MBI scores of the malnourished were consistently lower than those of the adequately nourished, at all times evaluated. Malnutrition on admission to rehabilitation was significantly related to lower MBI scores 1 month later. All patients scoring in the dependent range at 1 month had been malnour-

Table 24-13

Interventions for secondary medical complications affecting food intake in patients with stroke

Upper extremity hemiparesis or paralysis	Teach patient to use unaffected hand, even if paralyzed one has been dominant
	Consult occupational therapist, use assistive devices to assist in eating skills, when appropriate
	Provide opportunities for feeding rehabilitation for as long as progress is noted
	Encourage self-feeding; provide finger foods
	Prevent fatigue
	Maintain human dignity
Disorientation	Give clear, repeated, slow-paced instructions and demonstrations
Altered level of consciousness	Encourage participation of family
	Review medications (antipsychotic and sedative anticholinergis can impair mental status)
	Be nonjudgmental of changes in personality
Altered emotional behavior, e.g., depression, irascibility, lability, indifference	Reassure with word or touch
	Medications, e.g., antidepressants like methylphenidate, have the side effect of appetite suppression
	Oral supplements may be helpful
	Tubefeeds may be helpful in those who refuse to eat
	Lability may not reflect actual emotion
Dysphagia	Dysphagia evaluaton, consult speech-language pathologist, clinical dietitian
	Implement dysphagia diet and/or tube feeding
Apraxia	Break down tasks into a familiar set of small steps
	Monitor quantity eaten
	Continually encourage eating
Visuospatial perceptual deficits	Give directions and discussions on unaffected side
	Depending on level of cognition, present food within visual field or train patient to rotate tray to bring attention to the previously "hidden food" and purposefully look to side of "blind spot"
	Remediation and computer-controlled audiovisual-based rehab programs can be useful for improving feeding skills
Denture ill-fit because of facial paralysis or gum shrinkage during denture removal	Dental consultation
	New set of dentures, if necessary
	In meantime, liquid complete nutritional formula and/or soft, puree diet
Obesity	Reduced-energy diet, because excess weight can interfere with mobility and long-term outcome
Decubitus ulcers	Adequate energy and protein

Consultant Dietitians in Health Care Facilities/American Dietetic Association: *Mental Status, Nutrition Care for Specific Diseases. Practical Interventions for the Caregivers of the Eating-Disabled Older Adult*. Chicago: American Dietetic Association, 1994, pp. 109–122, 147–172.

Nelson RA, Millikan CH, Stollar C, Stone DB: Nutrition and the stroke patient, in Gastineau CF (ed): *Dialogues in Nutrition*. Bloomfield, NJ: Health Learning Systems Inc., 1979, pp. 1–6.

Arego DE, Koch S: Malnutrition in the rehabilitation setting. *Nutr Today* 1986; July/August, 28–31.

ished on admission for rehabilitation. The mean length of stay of malnourished rehabilitation patients was 48.3 days compared to 24.1 days for the adequately nourished group ($p = 0.006$). This contributed to the malnourished group's significantly reduced functional improvement rate (MBI score improvement by discharge/length of stay).

Increased dietary intake has been associated with improved functional outcome. In one report, Allison et al. described dysphagic stroke patients with recurrent aspiration pneumonia and/or nasogastric tube dislodgement whose response to rehabilitation was poor 4–6 months post-stroke.[42] When nutritional intake increased owing to gastrostomy tube feeding, improve-

Table 24-14
Prevalence and degree of malnutrition in stroke patients on the rehabilitation service

Nutritional status	Rehab admission (n = 49), %	Rehab–1 month (n = 32), %	Rehab–2 months (n = 9), %	2–4 month follow-up (n = 42), %
Malnourished-total	49 (24)	34 (11)	22 (1)	19 (8)
Mild	14 (7)	13 (4)	22 (1)	5 (2)
Moderate	19 (9)	13 (4)	0 (0)	10 (4)
Severe	16 (8)	9 (3)	0 (0)	5 (2)

Finestone HM, Greene-Finestone LS, Wilson ES, Teasell RW: Malnutrition in stroke patients on the rehabilitation service and at follow-up: Prevalence and predictors. *Arch Phys Med Rehabil* 1995; 75:310–316. Reprinted with permission.

ments in weight and serum albumin (into the normal range) and improved response to physiotherapy were noted.

Nutritional Assessment and Treatment

Given the functional implications of nutritional deprivation, metabolic management during rehabilitation is an imperative. Nutritional status must be monitored by routine ongoing nutritional screenings or assessments that include body weight, traditional biochemical indices, or standardized subjective measures. (See Table 24-3 for subjective global assessment.)

Adequate nutrition should be provided to prevent the development of malnutrition. Little is known of the metabolic demands and subsequent nutritional needs of patients with stroke. The clinical dietitian should consider food consistency, medical status, age, activity level, food preferences, and ethnic background when planning the diet. Periodic calculations of energy and protein intake ("calorie counts"), performed by a clinical dietitian or dietary technician, are indicated for those suspected of poor intake. A high-energy (calorie), high-protein diet is recommended for the malnourished or those at risk of malnutrition.

In those suspected of dysphagia, a swallowing assessment should be performed in order to establish recommendations for modifications to food and fluid consistencies. A modified barium swallow study may be required if there are serious aspiration concerns. Regular communication with team members regarding dietary treatment is essential to the progress and upgrading of the dysphagia diet. Regular observation for dehydration and fluid balance are particularly important.

If nutritional consumption is inadequate, or if the risk of aspiration is high, enteral nutrition should be provided until such time as the swallowing and gag reflex return, and oral intake is adequate. During the transition from enteral to oral intake, both types of feedings may be provided. The enteral portion of nutrition can be gradually decreased as the oral portion is increased. The adequacy of the oral intake should be verified by calorie counts.

TRAUMATIC BRAIN INJURY AND NUTRITION

Advances in emergency, intensive, and acute care over the past 15–20 years have contributed to the increased survival of patients with traumatic brain injury, and consequently demand for rehabilitation has increased. Greater understanding of the body's response to trauma and stress, its requirements for nutritional substrates and new modes of their delivery have also helped to improve outcome. Nutritional therapy of the brain-injured population must take into account heterogeneous patient characteristics and nutritional needs.[43]

Nutritional Consequences of Traumatic Brain Injury

After traumatic brain injury, aggressive therapy is necessary to manage and prevent the development of metabolic, cardiovascular, pulmonary, and renal disturbances that interfere with neurological recovery.[33]

Traumatic brain injury patients exhibit strong metabolic responses to brain trauma. These responses largely have been studied in the acute and post-acute phases (0–21 days), although there is evidence that many of these changes have not returned to normal levels by day 21.[44] The sequelae of acute metabolic responses after brain injury remain a paramount concern during the rehabilitation process.

The acute-phase response is characterized by a number of fairly typical metabolic events.

Increased mean nitrogen excretion and negative nitrogen balance are sustained until day 18 ± 8 (range 9–29), 18–21, and 22 or more in adults.[44–46] In children and adolescents, negative nitrogen balance is sustained for at least 8–14 days.[47]

Increased oxygen consumption can be seen, with a high degree of variability with regard to degree and duration.

Increased measured energy expenditure (MEE) in adults, using indirect calorimetry, averages 1.40 times predicted energy expenditure levels (PEE) as determined by the Harris-Benedict equation.[46–49] Young et al. reported that mean MEE/PEE ratio peaked at 1.50 ± .09 on day 1 after traumatic brain injury, and then declined to 1.16 ± .05 by day 22 in patients who are not treated with steroids.[46] Bruder et al. reported that mean energy expenditure of unsedated, spontaneously breathing, severely traumatic brain-injured patients was 1.34 times higher than predicted at 18 ± 8 days. Patients with abnormal motor activity (decerebrate, decorticate, muscle rigidity, fine motor tremors) have displayed mean MEE levels 1.91 times PEE.[50] Ranges between 2.60 and 3.00 MEE/PEE also have been reported for these patients.[46] In contrast, flaccid patients have exhibited mean MEE approximately at predicted levels (1.08 times PEE).[50] Patients paralyzed by pancuronium bromide display MEE/PEE ratios between 1.00 and 1.25.[51] The hypermetabolic and hypercatabolic response is evident in those with severe and moderately severe traumatic brain injury (Glasgow Coma Scale ratings <4 and 8–14, respectively) and those with and without corticosteroid treatment for traumatic cerebral edema.[44,46,48] Mean MEE is reported to be 1.3 times greater than PEE in children and adolescents.[47]

Significant weight loss is a common metabolic occurrence after brain injury. Young et al. reported a mean weight loss of 7.1 ± 2.7 kg (15.6 ± 5.9 lb) in adults by the third week following traumatic brain injury, amounting to approximately 10 percent of total body weight.[46] Weight loss in children and adolescents has been reported to range from .9 to 11.8 kg (2–26 lbs) by day 14.[47] Weight loss often persists until metabolism normalizes.[33]

After traumatic brain injury, levels of the negative acute-phase reactant serum albumin commonly are depressed. Levels often remain below normal by at least day 14 in children and adolescents and by day 21 in adults.[45–47]

Trace mineral metabolism also can be affected. Serum levels of zinc have been reported to be depressed on acute admission, but normalize by day 21. Copper levels rise and remain elevated by day 21.[44]

Special attention must be given to fluid and electrolyte balance.[33,47] The syndrome of inappropriate antidiuretic hormone (SIADH) secretion results in increased antidiuretic hormone and hyponatremia, with excessive fluid retention. Diabetes insipidus, a result of hypothalamic injury and antidiuretic hormone insufficiency, leads to increased urinary output, hypernatremia, dehydration and hypotension.

Nutritional status and therapy in the traumatic brain-injured rehabilitation population is just beginning to attract serious investigative interest. Brooke et al. retrospectively evaluated the nutritional stature of 53 patients admitted to a rehabilitation service following traumatic brain injury. Mean and minimum acute hospital stays were 201 and 28 days, respectively. Fifty-six percent were dysphagic, 60 percent were below 90 percent of their ideal body weight, with a mean weight loss (premorbid minus rehabilitation admission weight) of 13.2 kg (29 lbs). Hypoalbuminemia (<35 g/L) was evident in 31 percent of subjects. Body weight alone (< or >90 percent ideal) was not significantly related to functional status. The method used to measure functional status was not standardized. Further research is necessary to explore the predictive value of a malnutrition composite index in relation to functional outcome.

Nutritional Assessment of the Traumatic Brain-Injured Patient

Apart from exceptions such as chronic alcoholics, nutritional status prior to injury is assumed to be normal. Therefore, the goal of nutritional therapy is to prevent the development of malnutrition. In children, sufficient nutrition must be provided to support growth.

During the first 2 weeks after traumatic brain injury, levels of traditional nutritional assessment parameters, such as serum albumin, total lymphocyte count, and transferrin are not useful in studying the adequacy of nutritional support. These numbers typically continue to decline, despite adequate nutritional intake.[33] Nitrogen excretion and balance may not be effective early indicators either. Despite adequate nutritional intake, nitrogen excretion peaks at approximately

7–14 days post-injury, regardless of when nutrient administration is started.[44,46,51] Anthropometric changes, such as skinfold measurements and mid-arm muscle circumference, change slowly and malnutrition may be advanced by the time these changes occur. Although their value is limited in the acute phase, they can still serve as useful baseline measures. Nutritional parameters should be monitored prospectively to determine whether progress in therapy occurs.

Until the body metabolism after injury returns to normal, subjective global assessment and body weight can be useful in assessing nutritional status.[18] Weight changes, however, may not be accurate until after the second week of injury, because of the confounding effects of intravenous fluids, water, and sodium retention following trauma. Determination of serum proteins with short turnover rates, such as prealbumin or retinol-binding protein, can be used to reflect adequacy of energy and protein intake. There is evidence that retinol-binding protein levels increase along with protein and energy supplementation during the first 2 weeks after injury.[46] After approximately 3 weeks, traditional nutritional indices can become most useful in assessing nutritional status.[53]

Estimating Nutritional Requirements The objective for energy intake is to fully replace depleted energy stores. If this is not accomplished, protein is wasted and used as an energy source. Overfeeding is not desirable, as it can result in hyperglycemia, uremia, and increased CO_2 production.[53] Energy requirements depend on whether the patient's metabolic rate and urinary urea nitrogen or total nitrogen excretion and nitrogen balance have normalized. Energy expenditure also is affected by abnormal motor activity and posturing responses to pain, being lowest in those with brain death or with the use of neuromuscular blockers, hypnotic agents, or barbiturates (below predicted levels). Because of the high variability, it is recommended that resting measured energy expenditure (MEE) be determined by indirect calorimetry. Early on, this should be done once or twice weekly until the metabolic rate has normalized. When the patient has become more stabilized, indirect calorimetry may be done biweekly until enteral or parenteral nutrition is no longer needed.[54] MEE frequently is multiplied by a factor of 1.2 to account for extra demands imposed by therapy and minor procedures.[33,55]

If indirect calorimetry is not available, energy requirements must be estimated. During the acute stage, Magnuson suggests multiplying the Harris-Benedict equation by a stress factor of 1.4–1.75.[54] If the patient exhibits posturing, poor pain control, seizures or infections, the expenditure will be toward the upper limit of this range. Energy needs may be estimated by multiplying the Harris-Benedict equation by an activity factor plus or minus a stress, or injury factor, depending on stage of recovery. The activity factor may vary from 1.1 to 1.5, depending on whether the patient is sedentary (confined to wheelchair or bed) or actively pacing. The stress factor would depend on the degree and type of injury sustained, the presence of concomitant orthopedic injuries, and the need for surgery.[56] During rehabilitation, a stress factor of 1.2–1.5 has been suggested, unless the patient is in an advanced stage of recovery.[57] The adequacy of this estimation can be verified by monitoring weight and energy intake (calorie counts).

Protein needs normally are .8 g/kg/day.[21] Weekly nitrogen balance studies are recommended during the acute period. If nitrogen balance has not been reached, 1.75–2.0 g of protein/kg with adequate energy should be administered to achieve positive nitrogen balance, provided the patient has normal renal function.[33,54] In the postacute rehabilitation phase, protein needs of patients in need of repletion can be estimated at 1.2–1.5 g/kg/day.[57]

Nutritional Treatment of the Traumatic Brain-Injured Patient

Early initiation of nutritional supplementation should be emphasized so as to reduce the severity of nutritional depletion by the time the patient reaches active rehabilitation. A high-protein, high-energy diet is indicated for those demonstrating an increased metabolic rate. When the patient's cognition or arousal state is poor, or when there is dysphagia and danger of aspiration, nutritional support should be delivered either enterally or parenterally. Enteral feeding generally is preferred over the parenteral route.

In the acute phase of traumatic brain injury, it is sometimes possible to deliver more energy and protein by the parenteral than the enteral route. Contributing to this is poor tolerance of gastric and duodenal enteral feeding.[58,59] This phenomenon has been related to impaired gastric emptying, increased cranial pressure, severity of injury, and medications used in treatment, chiefly narcotics and barbiturates.[33,53,54,58–60]

Early feeding by percutaneous jejunostomy or percutaneous gastrojejunostomy, except for patients in barbiturate coma, can be tolerated by most.[33,61–63] Advancing the rate of formula slowly over 72 hours enhances tolerance. Continuous infusion beginning at 25–50 cc/hour of full-strength feeds is begun and advanced by 25 cc every 12 hours until energy replacement level is achieved. The goal rate can reach 100–150 cc/hour in some adults. Nocturnal continuous enteral feeding works well for traumatic brain-injury patients, allowing for greater participation in the rehabilitation program. Alternatively, success using bolus feedings delivered via a gastrostomy tube has been reported.[64] If SIADH is present and fluid restriction is necessary, a concentrated enteral formula can be selected (see Table 24-8).

MULTIPLE SCLEROSIS AND NUTRITION

Nutritional Relationships

The relationship between nutrition and multiple sclerosis (MS) has been studied primarily in terms of the relationship of dietary fat intake to MS attacks. High saturated fatty acid intake and MS incidence and prevalence have been the focus of many clinical and epidemiological investigations. Swank suggested that decreases in incidence of multiple sclerosis in Norway during the World War II German occupation could be attributable to a reduction in dietary fat during the war.[65] Farmers, who consumed more butter, appeared to experience more multiple sclerosis attacks than fishermen consuming fish liver, but the difference was not statistically significant. The theory advanced was that butterfat was a more potent precipitating agent of multiple sclerosis than fish liver oil. The suggested mechanism was that small blood vessels, occluded by aggregations of erythrocytes, platelets, and chylomicrons, produced hypoxemia, leading to the formation of multiple sclerosis plaques. Further epidemiological work supported the hypothesis that a diet high in saturated fat is associated with a high incidence and prevalence of multiple sclerosis.[66]

Attention shifted to the possible influence of diet on the lipid constitution of myelin. One hypothesis proposed that white matter containing abnormal plaques, as well as white matter without obvious disease, would be biochemically abnormal as a result of deficient intake and subsequent delivery of essential fatty acids. This situation would result in the formation of myelin with abnormal lipid content, vulnerable to agents that do not damage normal myelin.[67] Levels of polyunsaturated fats in general, and the proportion of elements of the lecithin fraction (including arachidonic acid [20:4] and linoleic acid [18:2]) in particular, were reduced in unaffected brains (by imaging criteria) of multiple-sclerosis patients compared to normal brains.[68] Other studies, however, found no consistent differences.[69,70] Wide variations between individual multiple-sclerosis brains suggested that "unaffected" white matter has been subjected to some degeneration of myelin owing to an abnormality of lipid metabolism.

Nutritional Therapy

Clinical trials have been performed by Swank that show that fat intake of less than 120 grams of saturated fat per day reduces expected disability, death rate, and relapse rate.[71] This study did not have an adequate control group and therefore its results are inconclusive. A double-blind, randomized control trial was conducted to determine whether linoleic acid supplementation was beneficial.[72] This trial was based on the premise that essential fatty acids exert prolonged immunosuppressant action.[73] Essential fatty acids can inhibit experimental allergic encephalomyelitis in the animal model. Although the precise mechanism is unknown, arachidonic acid, formed from linoleic acid via linolenic acid, and a precursor of prostaglandins, is known to have immunosuppressant effects. Results of the effects of linoleic acid supplementation on the clinical course of multiple sclerosis suggested less frequent, less severe, and shorter duration relapses, but no evidence of a reduction in overall clinical deterioration.[72] Further trials by Bates et al. and Paty et al. have not shown any overall outcome differences between treated and non-treated subjects.[74,75] Re-analysis of three double-blind studies has demonstrated that treated patients with little or no disability deteriorated significantly less than controls.[76] However, relapse severity and duration, not frequency, were reduced. The clinical significance of this effect has been questioned frequently.

Robust clinical outcome studies that show a benefit from dietary therapy do not exist. A well-balanced diet, adequate nutrients, and weight control are recommended. Vitamin supplementation and/or gluten elimination have no known place in treatment.[66] Constipation is a frequent complication of those that are more immobilized by MS, and can be remediated often by a high-fiber diet.

SPINAL-CORD INJURY AND NUTRITION

Nutritional Consequences of Spinal-Cord Injury

Spinal-cord-injured (SCI) patients lose weight in the acute phase, in spite of apparently adequate nutritional intake.[77] Anemia also has been reported.[78] Studies on

SCI patients performed 3 weeks to months after the initial injury reveal that approximately 50 percent are malnourished.[79] Peiffer has shown that quadriplegics have a higher incidence of abnormal nutritional parameters compared to paraplegics.[80] Kearns et al., studying SCI patients up to 4 weeks after injury, has demonstrated that many features of the adaptive response to SCI are qualitatively similar to those seen in immobilized patients in general. These include skeletal muscle atrophy and nitrogen and calcium wasting. Nitrogen, 3-methylhistidine (skeletal muscle and bone metabolites), and calcium excretion, however, were two- to tenfold greater in SCI patients than other immobilized patients.

Energy metabolism and weight change during rehabilitation after SCI have been subject to limited study. Peiffer found that SCI patients in the early rehabilitation phase of their treatment required up to 54 percent fewer calories than would be predicted by most standard formulae, based on populations of "normal" subjects.[80] The drop in energy expenditure related to nonuse of muscles appeared to be a greater factor in the net assessment of energy requirements than the increased energy expenditure required for the SCI patient to use braces or crutches to walk.[85] Cox et al. determined that in the rehabilitation phase of treatment, quadriplegics need 22.7 kcal/kg/day and paraplegics, 27.9 kcal/kg/day.[77]

The SCI group studied by Peiffer consumed substantially in excess of their energy needs and gained an average of 1.7 kg/week. These data have been confirmed by Cox, suggesting that levels of ideal body weight should be set lower for spinally injured patients than for normal subjects.[77] One recommendation suggests that weight guidelines be set at 4.5 kg (10–15 lbs) and 9 kg (15–20 lbs) below the Metropolitan Life Insurance Table's ideal body weights for paraplegics and quadriplegics, respectively.[10]

Nutritional Therapy

Avoid overfeeding during rehabilitation of the SCI patient. Prevention of obesity should be emphasized, as subsequent weight loss is difficult. Enteral feeds may be required early on if swallowing problems or anorexia are encountered. In the face of malnutrition, protein-losing pressure sores, and accentuation of a negative nitrogen balance owing to infection or metabolic stress secondary to surgery, a high-protein, high-energy diet would be required.[86] High fluid intakes of 2,500–3,000 cc per day are recommended for the prevention of urinary infection and calculi.

The patient who overeats to compensate for lost pleasures may need counseling to promote feelings of self-worth.[87] If overeating leads to inappropriate weight gain and obesity, a reduced-energy diet may be required.

PARKINSON DISEASE AND NUTRITION

Nutritional Consequences of Parkinson Disease

The patient with Parkinson disease (PD) often is at a higher risk for malnutrition owing to the presence of factors such as diminished appetite, depression, dementia, dysphagia, and delayed gastric emptying.[29,88] Dyskinesia may impair feeding and eating.

Diet has been weakly implicated in the pathogenesis of PD. Epidemiologic studies have found a lower prevalence of PD in mainland China and Nigeria.[89] The potential importance of diet also has been highlighted by studies linking the Parkinson-dementia-motor-neuron disease complex of Guam to consumption of cycad or "false palm."[90] Carter and Nutt have speculated that diets deficient in free radical scavengers (vitamins C and E, selenium, beta carotene, and methionine) conceivably may predispose to the development of PD, but there is little data to support this claim.[29]

The gastrointestinal side effects of nausea, vomiting, anorexia, and constipation can be seen with virtually all anti-Parkinson drugs, including anticholinergics, levodopa, amantadine, and bromocriptine. Nausea and anorexia usually subside with time. Taking levodopa with food sometimes can alleviate these symptoms. At the same time, delayed gastric emptying, a possible manifestation of the volume and composition of meals, plays a role in the absorption of levodopa. Levodopa is absorbed in the small intestine. The enzyme aromatic acid decarboxylase is present in the stomach mucosa and if levodopa remains in the stomach, it can become decarboxylated, no longer able to enter the brain and affect central dopaminergic mechanisms.[91] Domperidone, a peripheral dopamine-blocking agent that has a gastric propulsive action, potentially can alleviate some of the intractable gastrointestinal side effects and improve levodopa absorption. Gradually increasing dietary fiber will help to relieve constipation.

There is an abundance of literature concerning the interaction of levodopa, the mainstay of pharmacologic treatment of PD, and dietary protein ingestion. Levodopa is a large, neutral amino acid. Its passage through biological membranes depends on the same system that transports other neutral amino acids, including valine, leucine, isoleucine tyrosine, tryptophan, and phenylalanine. Competition between dopamine and these amino acids at the blood-brain barrier limits levodopa's entry into the brain. The two factors that determine the amount of levodopa entering the brain are the levodopa plasma concentrates and the summed concentrations of the large neutral amino acids.[92] Dietary protein, a rich source of these amino acids, therefore has been discussed in terms of its negative effects on PD. Some patients do note a worsening of their symptoms after a protein-laden meal.

Nutritional Therapy

Pincus and coworkers have advocated protein restriction and redistribution diets (protein <10 g/day with the majority consumed at the evening meal) for PD patients, particularly those with "end stage" disease.[93] Juncos et al. suggested that only protein in excess of recommended daily allowances (0.8 gm of protein/kg of body weight/24 hours) diminishes levodopa responsiveness in patients with advanced disease.[94] Eight PD subjects failed to convincingly demonstrate the superiority of a low-protein diet.[95] Berry et al. concluded that PD patients can eat balanced 5:1 carbohydrate-to-protein ratio diets and still maintain a stable plasma levodopa to large neutral amino acid ratio.[92]

At present, the best nutritional advice is to ensure adequate overall nutritional intake, while being prudent with dietary protein. Meals with extremely high protein content should be avoided, and protein intake should be distributed evenly over three or four daily meals. Greater protein restriction (low-protein meals or restricting protein ingestion to the evening hours) may be useful in patients with troublesome fluctuations in response to levodopa, but caution should be exercised because of the risk of undernourishment.[29] More severe forms of PD leading to dementia, difficulty with self-feeding, and dysphagia may require high-energy supplementation, dysphagia diets, and even enteral feeding.

AMYOTROPHIC LATERAL SCLEROSIS AND NUTRITION

Nutritional Consequences of Amyotrophic Lateral Sclerosis

Amyotrophic lateral sclerosis (ALS) is a progressive disease of unknown etiology affecting the anterior horn cells and pyramidal tracts with or without concomitant involvement of the bulbar motor nuclei and corticobulbar tracts. Weakness, muscle wasting and fasciculations, hyperactive tendon jerks, and absence of sensory loss are features of the disease.[96,97] In a large subset of patients, dysphagia and choking on foods, drinks, and saliva results in dehydration, malnutrition, additional weakness, emaciation, and pneumonia.[28]

Nutritional Therapy

Important first-line measures involve the diet, ensuring high levels of protein ingestion, high-energy foods so that a desirable weight and nutritional status is attained and maintained. Dysphagia diets may be prescribed when swallowing becomes problematic.

Pharyngeal exercises and swallow education are helpful. Medications such as atropine, an anticholinergic, can be taken one-half hour before meals to decrease saliva and facilitate swallowing.[98]

Cricopharyngeal myotomy occasionally is indicated to improve food transit through the pharynx.[99] When aspiration is suspected or oral intake is inadequate, nasogastric feedings initially can be prescribed. They are, however, uncomfortable, inconvenient, and unattractive. Percutaneous endoscopic gastrostomy (PEG) and gastrojejunostomy can be used to provide adequate nutrition if the patient will be tube fed for more than 6 weeks. Studies have not conclusively shown a prolongation of life with these procedures, but patient compliance and acceptance is quite high.[28]

Seizures and Nutrition

Medications are the first line of therapy in the child or adult with epilepsy. Surgery is a relatively new option for treatment of intractable seizures.

Nutritional Therapy

In children who have not responded to medication, the ketogenic diet often is recommended.[100] The ketogenic diet is estimated to be 33–50 percent effective and must be adhered to rigidly.[101] It is most successful for 2- to 5-year-olds, but it has helped others between ages 7 months to 38 years.[102] The individual must fast for 24–72 hours and then the diet is started. Minimal carbohydrate intake is allowed and a ketotic state is induced. Ketogenic diets are categorized according to their ratio (by weight) of fat to carbohydrate plus protein (usually 4:1 or 3:1). Supplemental vitamins, minerals, and trace elements are included in the diet.[103] A medium-chain triglyceride (MCT) sometimes is used and allows for liberalization of carbohydrate and fat intake.[104] The ketogenic diets have been effective in controlling the atonic-akinetic drop attacks of the Lennox-Gastaut syndrome, atypical absences, myoclonic seizures, partial seizures, and tonic-clonic seizures.[105]

In summary, the ketogenic diet can be implemented to help control certain types of childhood seizures, usually in institutionalized settings, when medication control is inadequate.

ALZHEIMER'S DISEASE AND DEMENTIA AND NUTRITION

Nutrition Consequences of Alzheimer's Disease

Alzheimer's disease (AD) is a progressive, irreversible degenerative disease of the brain. A nutritional factor causing AD has not been found. Various studies have indicated, however, that nutrition deficits can occur in terms of dietary and biochemical indices, among the elderly.[106,107] Energy-type malnutrition, manifested as low body weight and reduced adipose tissue, was present in 50 percent of a group of institutionalized patients.[108] Demented patients, unable to eat independently and exhibiting forgetfulness, disorientation, problems pacing, and agitation behaviors are at risk of malnutrition.[20,109,110] Other feeding problems include food refusal (active rejection of food by either ceasing to feed oneself or by refusing to open one's mouth when spoon fed) and difficulties in chewing and swallowing.[111] Behavior problems affecting food intake and strategies for intervention are found in Table 24-12.

Nutritional Therapy

Studies have not shown that improving specific aspects of a patient's diet, with lecithin, for example, will improve the patient's dementia.[112] Current evidence also does not support an important role for orally ingested aluminum in the development of Alzheimer's disease.[113,114] Therefore, no evidence-based medical recommendations can be made with respect to cooking implements. Weight loss is common and therefore attention to adequate nutrition is essential.[108] Providing high-calorie, high-energy meals at the same time, in the same place, and limiting food choices are recommended. Constipation is seen frequently and the implementation of a high-fiber diet can help. Attention to visuospatial impairment by rotating the patient's plate, is also suggested. As the patient's cognition declines, various verbal reminders to chew and swallow, cutting up food in small pieces, as well as the thickening of fluids may become important. Table 24-10 describes some common behaviors affecting food intake and offers intervention suggestions. Enteral feeds may be required during the period when the AD patient has lost the ability for self-care.[115]

CHRONIC PAIN AND NUTRITION

Dietary therapy in the management of chronic pain has long been discussed, but minimally studied. Travell and Simons have emphasized that nutritional inadequacies, particularly of the water-soluble vitamins B_1, B_6, B_{12}, C, and folic acid and certain elements, such as calcium, iron, and potassium, constitute perpetuating factors in patients with myofascial pain syndromes.[116] They have indicated that vitamin inadequacies apparently increase the irritability of myofascial trigger points (TPs) by impairing the energy metabolism needed for the contraction of muscles and increasing irritability of the nervous system. The affected muscles behave as though neurofeedback mechanisms are perpetually sensitizing TPs and the TP-referred phenomena are intensified. Vitamin inadequacies become a deficiency when the effects of impaired function of essential enzymes are grossly apparent and can be established by laboratory evidence. To date, clinical evidence supporting Travell and Simons' claims is lacking. Therefore, recommendations with regard to specific vitamin injections or other supplements cannot be made.

Nutritional manipulation of brain neurotransmitters for the treatment of chronic pain often has been discussed, but it too lacks much scientific validity despite numerous testimonies. Although transcutaneous nerve stimulation, antidepressant medications, physical therapy, and biofeedback have been used alone or in combination for pain relief, diet therapy has generated some discussion recently.[117] Tryptophan, an essential amino acid that cannot be made in the body, appears in the blood as a result of protein ingestion and protein breakdown. Serotonin is a neurotransmitter that has been linked to pain perception. High serotonin levels appear to potentiate morphine analgesia.[118,119] Serotonin antagonists decrease the pain threshold. Tryptophan can be converted to serotonin by neurons in the brain. The formation and concentration of this neurotransmitter is influenced by dietary ingestion. A high-protein diet causes a decrease in the ratio of tryptophan to other large neutral amino acids (tyrosine, phenylalanine, valine, leucine, isoleucine, and methionine), thereby decreasing tryptophan uptake at the brain-blood barrier. A high-carbohydrate meal has the opposite effect and increases the concentrations of tryptophan and serotonin in the brain.

Human studies include those by Sicuteri, Sternbach, DeBenedittis, and Moldofsky et al.[120–123] Oral forms of tryptophan were administered to headache, musculoligamentous, deafferentation, and fibromyalgia pain patients. Results were variable. A large percentage of headache, deafferentation, and central pain patients anecdotally improved. The musculoskeletal pain patients had marginal to no improvement.

Tryptophan was available without prescription at drug and health food stores for many years, but the Food and Drug Administration recalled tryptophan supplements after they were linked to eosinophilia–myalgia syndrome, a painful muscle and blood disorder.

In summary, although tryptophan has been implicated as a pain treatment, a convincing body of evidence to support its use as a dietary supplement does not exist. Phenylalanine and leucine are other neutral amino acids used in the treatment of chronic painful disorders, but evidence of their effectiveness also is mainly anecdotal. As our knowledge of neurotransmitters in pain perception grows, so will our understanding of the role of diet in the pathophysiology and treatment of chronic pain disorders.

CONCLUSION

Almost every neurological disease or injury that requires rehabilitation has the potential to affect, or be affected by, nutrition and diet. There is evidence that approximately half of neurorehabilitation patients are malnourished. The clinical goal is to prevent, or to identify and treat inadequate nutritional and feeding states. The consequences of malnutrition can include poorer functional outcome, prolonged hospitalization, and poor quality of life.

Nutritional care of the neurorehabilitation patient is a relatively new field. There is much room for further evaluation of the dietary needs of specific groups, optimal methods of assessment, nutritional delivery, and therapy. In the meantime, specific attention to nutritional issues is warranted in order to help patients achieve their full rehabilitation potential.

REFERENCES

1. Newmark SR, Sublett D, Block J, Geller R: Nutritional assessment in a rehabilitation unit. *Arch Phys Med Rehabil* 1981; 62:279–282.
2. Glenn MB, Carfi J, Belle SE, Ahn JH, Gordon WA, Myer PA, Miron-Bernstein S, Ragnarsson KT: Serum albumin as a predictor of course and outcome on a rehabilitation service. *Arch Phys Med Rehabil* 1985; 66:294–297.
3. Finestone HM, Greene-Finestone LS, Wilson ES, Teasell RW: Prolonged length of stay and reduced functional improvement rate in malnourished stroke rehabilitation patients. *Arch Phys Med Rehab,* 1996; 77:340–345.
4. Aptaker RL, Roth EJ, Reichhardt G, Duerden ME, Levy CE: Serum albumin level as a predictor of geriatric stroke rehabilitation outcome. *Arch Phys Med Rehab* 1994; 75: 80–84.
5. Sahn DE, Lockwood R, Scrimshaw NS: Methods for the evaluation of the impact of food and nutrition programmes. *Measuring Impact of Nutrition Intervention on Physical Growth.* Tokyo, Japan: United Nations University, 1984, pp. 65–93.
6. American Dietetic Association: *Handbook of Clinical Dietetics,* 2nd ed. New Haven: Yale University Press, 1992.
7. Gibson RS: *Principles of Nutritional Assessment.* New York: Oxford University Press, 1990, pp. 5–8, 307–308.
8. Hopkins B: Assessment of nutritional status, in Gottschlich MM, Matarese LE, Shronts EP (eds): *Nutrition Support Dietetics—Core Curriculum, American Society for Parenteral and Enteral Nutrition.* Silver Springs, MD: 1993, pp. 15–65.
9. Ontario Dietetic Association and Ontario Hospital Association: *Nutrition Care Manual.* Don Mills, Ontario: Ontario Hospital Association, 1989.
10. Metropolitan Life Insurance Ideal Weights for Height, 1983. *Source:* 1979 Build Study, Society of Actuaries and Association of Life Insurance Medical Directors of America, Philadelphia, Recording and Statistical Corporation, 1980.
11. Frisancho AR: New standards of weight and body composition by frame size and height for assessment of nutritional status of adults and the elderly. *Am J Clin Nutr* 1984; 40:808–819.
12. Fitness and Amateur Sport, Canadian Standardized Test of Fitness, Operations Manual. Minister of State, Fitness and Amateur Sport, Canada, 1986.
13. Garrow JS, Webster J: Quetelet's index (W/H^2) as a measure of fatness. *Int J Obesity* 1985; 8:147–153.
14. Chumlea WC, Roche AF, Steinbaugh ML: Estimating stature from knee height for persons 65–90 years of age. *J Am Geriatr Soc* 1985; 33:116–120.
15. Law DK, Dudrick SJ, Abdou NI: Immunocompetence of patients with protein-calorie malnutrition: The effects of nutritional repletion. *Ann Intern Med* 1973; 79:545–550.
16. Meakins JL, Pietsch JB, Bubernick O, Kelly R, Rode

H, Gordon J, MacLean LD: Delayed hypersensitivity: Indicator of acquired failure of host defenses in sepsis and trauma. *Ann Surg* 1977; 186:241–250.

17. Haider M, Haider SQ: Assessment of protein-calorie malnutrition. *Clin Chem* 1984; 30(8):1286.

18. Detsky AS, McLaughlin JR, Baker JP, Johnston N, Whittaker S, Mendelson RA, Jeejeebhoy KN: What is subjective global assessment of nutritional status? *J Parent Ent Nutr* 1987; 11(1):8–13.

19. Bray GA: Pathophysiology of obesity. *Am J Clin Nutr* 1992; 55:488S–494S.

20. Consultant Dietitians in Health Care Facilities/American Dietetic Association: *Mental Status, Nutrition Care for Specific Diseases. Practical Interventions for the Caregivers of the Eating-disabled Older Adult.* Chicago: American Dietetic Association, 1994, pp. 109–122, 147–172.

21. WHO (World Health Organization): Energy and protein requirements. Report of a joint FAO/WHO/UNV Expert Consultation. Technical Report Series 724. Geneva: World Health Organization, 1985, p. 206.

22. Wrick KL, Robertson JB, Van Soest PJ, Lewis BA, Rivers JM, Roe DA, Hackler LR: The influence of dietary fiber source on human intestinal transit and stool output. *Am Inst Nutr* 1983; 1464–1479.

23. Sitzmann JV: Nutritional support of the dysphagic patient: methods, risks, and complications of therapy. *J Parent Ent Nutr* 1990; 14:60–63.

24. Pardoe EM: Development of a multistage diet for dysphagia. *J Amer Diet Assoc* 1993; 93:568–571.

25. Finestone HM, Greene-Finestone LS, Wilson ES, Teasell RW: Malnutrition in stroke patients on the rehabilitation service and at follow-up: Prevalence and predictors. *Arch Phys Med Rehabil* 1995; 76:310–316.

26. Veis SL, Logeman JA: Swallowing disorders in persons with cerebrovascular accident. *Arch Phys Med Rehabil* 1985; 66:372–375.

27. Winstein CJ: Neurogenic dysphagia: frequency, progression and outcome in adults following head injury. *Phys Ther* 1983; 63:1992–1997.

28. Mathus-Vliegen LMH, Louwerse LS, Merkus MP, Tytgat GNJ, Vianney deJong JMB: Percutaneous endoscopic gastrostomy in patients with amytrophic lateral sclerosis and impaired pulmonary function. *Gastrointest Endosc* 1994; 40:463–469.

29. Carter JH, Nutt JG: Dietary issues in the treatment of Parkinsonism, in Koller WC, Paulson G (eds): *Therapy of Parkinson's Disease,* 2nd ed. New York: Marcel Dekker, 1995, pp. 442–461.

30. Bach DB, Pouget S, Belle K, Kilfoil M, Alfieri M, McEvoy J, et al: Integrated team approach to the management of patients with oropharyngeal dysphagia. *J Allied Health (Fall)* 1989; 459–468.

31. Nelson RA, Millikan CH, Stollar C, Stone DB: Nutrition and the stroke patient, in Gastineau CF (ed): *Dialogues in Nutrition.* Bloomfield, NJ: Health Learning Systems Inc., 1979, pp. 1–6.

32. Ideno KT: Enteral nutrition, in Gottschlich MM, Matarese LE, Shronts EP (eds): *Nutrition Support Dietetics— Core Curriculum.* American Society for Parenteral and Enteral Nutrition. Silver Springs, MD: 1993, pp. 71–103.

33. Hester DD: Neurologic impairment, in Gottschlich MM, Matarese LE, Shronts EP (eds): *Nutrition Support Dietetics—Core Curriculum.* American Society for Parenteral and Enteral Nutrition, Silver Springs, MD: 1993, pp. 229–241.

34. Chicago Dietetic Association Staff and South Suburban Dietetic Association Staff: *Manual of Clinical Dietetics,* 3rd ed. American Dietetic Association, 1988.

35. Health Canada: *Nutrition Recommendations, The Report of the Scientific Review Committee.* Minister of Supply and Services, Canada, 1990.

36. Mountokalakis T, Dellos C: Protein catabolism following stroke (letter). *Arch Intern Med* 1984; 144:2285.

37. Buelow JM, Jamieson D: Potential for altered nutritional status in the stroke patient. *Rehabil Nsg* 1990; 15(5): 260–263.

38. Axelsson K, Asplund K, Norberg A, Alafuzoff I: Nutritional status in patients with acute stroke. *Acta Med Scand* 1988; 224:217–224.

39. Axelsson K, Asplund K, Norberg A, Eriksson S: Eating problems and nutritional status during hospital stay of patients with severe stroke. *J Amer Diet Assoc* 1989; 89:1092–1096.

40. Fortinsky RH, Granger CV, Seltzer GB: Functional status measures in a comprehensive stroke program. *Arch Phys Med Rehabil* 1977; 58:555–561.

41. McDowell I, Newell C: *Measuring Health: A Guide to Rating Scales and Questionnaires.* New York: Oxford University Press, 1987, pp. 49–54.

42. Allison MC, Morris AJ, Park RHR, Mills PR: Percutaneous endoscopic gastrostomy tube feeding may improve outcome of late rehabilitation following stroke. *J Roy Soc Med* 1992; 85:147–149.

43. Yankelson S: Traumatic brain injury, in DJ Gines (ed): *Nutrition Management in Rehabilitation.* Rockville, MD: Aspen Publishers, 1990.

44. Young AB, Ott LG, Beard D, Dempsey RJ, Tibbs PA, McClain CJ: The acute-phase response of the brain-injured patient. *J Neurosurg* 1988; 69:375–380.

45. Bruder N, Dumont JC, Francois G: Evolution of energy expenditure and nitrogen excretion in severe head-injured patients. *Crit Care Med* 1991; 19(1):43–48.

46. Young B, Ott L, Norton J, Tibbs RN, Rapp R, McClain C, Dempsey R: Metabolic and nutritional sequelae in the non-steroid treated head injury patient. *Neurosurgery* 1985; 17(5):784–790.

47. Phillips R, Ott L, Young B, Walsh J: Nutritional support and measured energy expenditure of the child and adolescent with head injury. *J Neurosurg* 1987; 67:846–851.

48. Clifton GL, Robertson CS, Grossman RG, Hodge S, Foltz R, Garza C: The metabolic response to severe head injury. *J Neurosurg* 1984; 60:687–696.

49. Harris JA, Benedict FG: A Biometric Study of Basal Metabolism in Man. Publication No. 297. Washington: Carnegie Institute, 1919.

50. Fruin AH, Taylon C, Pettis MS: Caloric requirements in patients with severe head injuries. *Surg Neurol* 1986; 25:25–28.

51. Clifton GL, Robertson CS, Sung CC: Assessment of nutritional requirements of head-injured patients. *J Neurosurg* 1986; 64:895–901.

52. Brooke MM, Barbour PG, Cording LG, Tolan C, Bhoomkar A, McCall GW, Lyons C, Hudson J, Johnson SJ: Nutritional status during rehabilitation after head injury. *J Neur Rehab* 1989; 3(1):27–33.

53. Clifton GL, Turner H: Nutrition and parenteral therapy, in Wilkins R, Rengachary S (eds): *Neurosurgery Update I: Diagnosis, Operative Techniques and Neuro-oncology.* Toronto: McGraw-Hill, 1990, pp. 207–213.

54. Magnuson B, Hatton J, Zweng TN, Young B: Techniques and procedures: Pentobarbital coma in neurosurgical patients: Nutrition considerations. *Nutr Clin Pract* 1994; 9:146–150.

55. Ott L, Young B, Phillips R, McClain C: Brain injury and nutrition. *Nutr Clin Pract* 1990; 5:68–73.

56. Long CL, Schaffel N, Geiger JW, Schiller WR, Blakemore WS: Metabolic response to injury and illness: Estimation of energy and protein needs from indirect calorimetry and nitrogen balance. *J Parent Ent Nutr* 1979; 3(6):452–456.

57. Greene-Finestone LS, Hornick J: Traumatic head injury and stroke rehabilitation: Implications of malnutrition and strategies for nutritional support. Telemedicine Canada, Dietitian's Series, Faculty of Medicine, University of Toronto and Toronto Hospital, March 1995.

58. Norton JA, Ott LG, McClain C, Adams L, Dempsey RJ, Haack D, Tibbs PA, Young AB: Intolerance to enteral feeding in the brain-injured patient. *J Neurosurg* 1988; 68:62–66.

59. Young B, Ott L, Twyman D: The effect of nutritional support on outcome from severe head injury. *J Neurosurg* 1987; 67:668–676.

60. Ott L, Young B, Phillips R, McClain C, Adams L, Dempsey R, Tibbs P, Ryo UY: Altered gastric emptying in the head-injured patient: Relationship to feeding intolerance. *J Neurosurg* 1991; 74:738–742.

61. Graham T, Zadrozny D, Harrington T: The benefits of early jejunal hyperalimentation in the head-injured patient. *Neurosurgery* 1989; 25:729–735.

62. Borzotta AP, Pennings J, Papasadero B, Paxton J, Mardesic S, Borzotta R, Parrott A, Bledsoe F: Enteral versus parenteral nutrition after severe closed head injury. *J Trauma* 1994; 37(3):459–468.

63. Kirby D, Clifton G, Turner H, et al: Early enteral nutrition after brain injury by percutaneous endoscopic gastro-jejunostomy. *JPEN* 1991; 15:298–302.

64. Kiel MK: Enteral tube feeding in a patient with traumatic brain injury. *Arch Phys Med Rehabil* 1994; 75:116–117.

65. Swank RL: Treatment of M.S. with low fat diet. *AMA Arch Neurol Psychol* 1953; 69:91–103.

66. Bates D: Dietary supplementation in MS, in Clifford FR, Jones R (eds): *Multiple Sclerosis: Immunological, Diagnostic and Therapeutic Aspects*, vol 3: Current Problems in Neurology. London: John Libbey, 1987, pp. 179–188.

67. Mathews WB: Dietary treatment, in Mathews WB, Compston A, Allen IV, Martyn CN (eds): *McAlpine's Multiple Sclerosis*. London: Churchill Livingstone, 1991, pp. 275–278.

68. Baker RWR, Thompson RHS, Zilkha KJ: Fatty acid compositions of brain lecithins in multiple sclerosis. *Lancet* 1963; 1:26–27.

69. Gerstl B, Tavastjerna MG, Hayman RB, Eng LF, Smith JK: Alternations in myelin fatty acids and plasmalogens in multiple sclerosis. *Ann NY Acad Sci* 1965; 122:405–416.

70. Arnetoli G, Pazzagli A, Amaducci L: Fatty acid and aldehyde changes in choline and ethanolamine-containing phospholipids in the white matter of multiple sclerosis brains. *J Neurochem* 1969; 16:461–463.

71. Swank RL, Dugan BB: Effect of low saturated fat diet in early and late cases of multiple sclerosis. *Lancet* 1990; 336:37–39.

72. Millar JHD, Zilkha KS, Langman MJS, Wright HP, Smith AD, Belin J, et al: Double blind trial of lineolate supplementation of the diet in multiple sclerosis. *Br Med J* 1973; 1:765–768.

73. Mertin J, Meade CJ: Relevance of fatty acids in multiple sclerosis. *Br Med Bull* 1977; 33:67–71.

74. Bates D, Fawcett PRN, Shaw DA, Weightmann D: Polyunsaturated fatty acids in the treatment of acute remitting multiple sclerosis. *Br Med J* 1978; 2:1390–1391.

75. Paty DW, Cousin HK, Read S, Adlaka K: Linoleic acid in multiple sclerosis: failure to show any therapeutic benefit. *Acta Neurol Scand* 1978; 58:53–58.

76. Dworkin RH, Bates D, Millar JHD, Paty DW: Linoleic acid and multiple sclerosis: a reanalysis of three double blind trials. *Neurology* 1984; 34:1441–1445.

77. Cox SAR, Weiss SM, Posuniak EA, Worthington P, Prioleau M, Heffley G: Energy expenditure after spinal cord injury: An evaluation of stable rehabilitating patients. *J Trauma* 1985; 25:419–423.

78. Huang C, DeVivo MJ, Stover SL: Anemia in acute phase of spinal cord injury. *Arch Phys Med Rehab* 1990; 71:3–7.

79. Greenway RM, Houser H, Lindan O, et al: Long term changes in gross body composition of paraplegic and quadriplegic patients. *Paraplegia* 1970; 7:301.

80. Peiffer SC, Blust P, Leyson JFJ: Nutritional assessment of the spinal cord patient. *J Am Diet Assoc* 1981; 78:501–505.

81. Shizgal HM, Rosa A, Leduc B: Body composition in quadriplegic patients. *J Parent Ent Nutr* 1986; 10(4):364–368.

82. Lee BY, Agarwal N, Corcoran L, Thoden WR, Del Guercio LR: Assessment of nutritional and metabolic status of paraplegics. *J Rehab Res* 1985; 22:11.

83. Kaufman HH, Rowlands BJ, Stein DK, Kopaniky DR, Gildenberg PL: General metabolism in patients with acute

paraplegia and quadriplegia. *Neurosurgery* 1985; 16: 309–313.

84. Kearns PJ, Thompson JD, Werner PC, Pipp TL, Wilmot CB: Nutritional and metabolic response to acute spinal cord injury. *J Parent Ent Nutr* 1992; 16:11–15.

85. Fisher SV, Gullickson G: Energy cost of ambulation in health and disability: A literature review. *Arch Phys Med Rehabil* 1978; 59:124–133.

86. Agarwal N, Lee BY: Nutrition in spinal cord injured patients, in Lee BY, Ostrander LE, Cochen G, Shaw WW (eds): *The Spinal Cord Injured Patient: Comprehensive Management.* Toronto: W.B. Saunders, 1991.

87. Zejdlik CP: Maintaining optimal nutrition, in: *Management of Spinal Cord Injury,* 2nd ed. Boston: Jones and Bartlett, 1992, pp. 331–352.

88. Waxman MJ, Durtee D, Moore M, Morantz RA, Koller W: Nutritional aspects and swallowing function of patients with Parkinson's Disease. *Nutr Clin Pract* 1990; 5: 196–199.

89. Schoenberg BS, Osuntokun BO, Adeuja AO, Bademosi O, Nottidge V, Anderson DN, Haerer AF: Comparison of the prevalence of Parkinson's Disease in black populations in the rural United States and in rural Nigeria: Door to door community studies. *Neurology* 1988; 38:645–646.

90. Spencer PS: Guam ALS/Parkinsonism-dementia: A long latency neurotoxic disorder caused by "slow toxins" in food? *Can J Neurol Sci* 1987; 14:347–357.

91. Rivera-Calimlin L, Dujovne CA, Morgan JP, Lasagna L, Biachine JR: Absorption and metabolism of l-dopa by the human stomach. *Eur J Clin Invest* 1971; 1:313–320.

92. Berry EM, Growdon JH, Wurtman JJ, Caballero MD, Wurtman RJ: A balanced carbohydrate: Protein diet in the management of Parkinson's Disease. *Neurology* 1991; 41:1295–1297.

93. Karstaedt PJ, Pincus JH: Protein redistribution diet remains effective in patients with fluctuating Parkinsonism. *Arch Neurol* 1992; 49:149–151.

94. Juncos JL, Fabbrini G, Mouradian MM, Serrati C, Chase TN: Dietary influences on the anti Parkinsonian response to levodopa. *Arch Neurol* 1987; 44:1003–1005.

95. Croxson S, Johnson B, Millac P, Pye I: Dietary modification of Parkinson's Disease. *Eur J Clin Nutr* 1991; 45:263–266.

96. Williams DB, Windebank AS: Motor neuron disease (amyotrophic lateral sclerosis). *Mayo Clin Proc* 1991; 66:54–82.

97. Louwerse LS, Sillevis Smitt PAE, DeJong JMBV: Differential diagnosis of sporadic amyotrophic lateral sclerosis, progressive spinal muscular atrophy and progressive spinal bulbar palsy in adults, in DeJong JMBV (ed): *Handbook of Clinical Neurology: Diseases of the Motor System.* New York: Elsevier Science Publishers, 1991, pp. 383–423.

98. Caroscio J: Amyotrophic lateral sclerosis, in Caroscio JT (ed): *A Guide to Patient Care.* New York: Thieme Medical Publishers, 1986, pp. 123–134.

99. Loizou LA, Small M, Dalton GA: Cricopharyngeal myotomy in motor neuron disease. *J Neurol Neurosurg Psych* 1980; 43:42–45.

100. Kinsman SL, Vining EPG, Quaskey SA, Mellits D, Freeman JM: Efficacy of the ketogenic diet for intractable seizure: Review of 58 cases. *Epilepsia* 1992; 3(6):1132–1136.

101. O'Donohoe NV: The MCT-based ketogenic diet, in O'Donohoe NV (ed): *Epilepsies of Childhood, Appendix I,* 3rd ed. Toronto: Butterworth Heinemann, 1994.

102. Dodson WE, Prensky AL, DeViVo DC, Goldring S, Dodge PR: Management of seizure disorders: Selected aspects. Part II *J Pediat* 1976; 89:695–703.

103. Dodson WB, Pellock JM: Other antiepileptic therapies, in Dodson WG, Pellock JM (eds): *Ketogenic Diet, in Paediatric Epilepsy: Diagnosis and Therapy.* New York, Demos Publications, 1993, pp. 339–342.

104. Dreyfus PM: Diet and nutrition in neurologic disorders, in Shils M (ed): *Modern Nutrition in Health and Disease.* Philadelphia: Lea and Febiger, 1988.

105. Sills MA, Forsythe WI, Haidukewych D: The medium chain triglyceride diet and intractable epilepsy. *Arch Dis Child* 1986; 61:1168–1172.

106. Vir SC, Love AHG: Nutritional status of institutionalized and noninstitutionalized aged in Belfast, Northern Ireland. *Am J Clin Nutr* 1979; 32:1937–1947.

107. Munro HN: Overview: Nutritional status of the aged, in Corkin S (ed): *Alzheimer's Disease: A Report of Progress, in Aging,* vol 19. New York: Raven Press, 1992.

108. Sandman PO, Adolfsson R, Nygren C, Hallman G, Winblad B: Nutritional status and dietary intake in institutionalized patients with Alzheimer's Disease and multi-infarct demential. *J Am Gerontol Soc* 1987; 35:31–38.

109. Stahelin HB, Hofer HO, Vogel M, Held C, Seiler WO: Energy and protein consumption in patients with senile dementia. *Gerontology* 1983; 29:145–148.

110. Volicer L, Seltzer B, Rheaume Y: Progression of Alzheimer-type dementia in institutionalized patients: A cross-sectional study. *J Appl Gerontol* 1987; 6:125–128.

111. Volicer L, Fabiszewski K, Rheaume Y, Lasch K: Management of advanced Alzheimer dementia: Promoting optimal nutritional status, in Volicer L, Fabiszewski K, Rheaume Y, Lasch Y (eds): *Clinical Management of Alzheimer's Disease.* Gaithersburg, MD: Aspen Publishers, 1988.

112. Kushnir SL, Ratner JT, Gregoire PA: Multiple nutrients in the treatment of Alzheimer's Disease. *J Am Ger Soc* 1987; 3(5):476–477.

113. Graves AB, White E, Koepsell TD, et al: The association between aluminum containing products and Alzheimer's disease. *J Clin Epidemiol* 1990; 43:35–44.

114. Wettstein A, Aeppli J, Gautschi K, et al: Failure to find a relationship between mnestic skills of octogenarians and aluminum in drinking water. *Int Arch Occup Environ Health* 1991; 63:97–103.

115. Miziniak H: Persons with Alzheimer's: Effects of nutrition and exercise. *J Ger Nurs* 1994; 20(10):27–32.

116. Travell JG, Simons DG: *Myofascial Pain and Dysfunction: The Trigger Point Manual.* Baltimore: Williams & Wilkins, 1983, pp. 114–144.

117. Bonica JJ, Maggio G: Nutrition and pain, in Bonica JJ (ed): *The Management of Pain,* 2nd ed. Philadelphia: Lea & Febiger, 1990, pp. 1838–1849.

118. Berger S: Nutrition, in Warfield CA (ed): *Principles and Practice of Pain Management.* Toronto: McGraw-Hill, 1993.

119. Akil H, Liebeskind JC: Monaminergic mechanisms of stimulation-produced analgesia. *Brain Res* 1975; 94:279.

120. Sicuteri F, Anselmi B, Fanciullaci M: The serotonin (5-HI) theory of migraine. *Adv Neurol* 1974; 4:383–394.

121. Sternbach RA: Effects of altering brain serotonin activity on human chronic pain, in Bonica JJ, Albe-Fessard D (eds): *Advances in Pain Research and Therapy,* vol. 1. New York: Raven Press, 1986, pp. 601–606.

122. DeBenedittis G, DiGiulio AM, Massei R, Villani R, Panerai AE: Effects of 5-hydroxytryptophan on central and deafferentation chronic pain: A preliminary clinical trial, in Bonica JJ, Lindblom U, Iggo A (eds): *Advances in Pain Research and Therapy.* New York: Raven Press, 1983, pp. 295–304.

123. Moldofsky H, Warsh JJ: Plasma tryptophan and musculoskeletal pain in non-articular rheumatism ("fibrositis syndrome"). *Pain* 1978; 5:65.

124. Food and Nutrition Board, National Research Council: *Recommended Dietary Allowances,* 10th ed. Washington, DC: National Academy of Sciences, 1989.

125. Health Canada: Recommended Nutrient Intake for Canadians, Report of the Scientific Review Committee, Minister of Supply and Services Canada, 1990.

126. Marcaud SP, Stegall KS: Unclogging feeding tubes with pancreatic enzyme. *JPEN* 1990; 14:198–200.

127. Arego DE, Koch S: Malnutrition in the rehabilitation setting. *Nutr Today* 1986; July/August, 28–31.

Chapter 25

NEUROREHABILITATION AND SEXUAL FUNCTION AFTER SPINAL CORD INJURY

Allen D. Seftel
Melissa D. Reigle
Donald R. Bodner

There are approximately 300,000 people in the United States with spinal cord injury, and an additional 14,000 to 15,000 new cases occur each year. It has been estimated that 1.5 billion dollars are spent annually in the United States to treat individuals with spinal cord injury.[1] The most frequent age of injury is 19 years, with the mean age being 26 years. Spinal cord injuries occur more frequently in men than women. Such an injury can change an individual's ability to walk, control the bowels and bladder, and in the case of a male, can alter his ability to achieve an erection or ejaculate. It requires that an individual learn not only to cope with the physical injury, but also to adapt to a new sexual self.

Rehabilitation success is a subjective measure encompassing many perspectives. In the case of neurologic injury, success may be measured by the amount of neurologic function regained, by the ability to perform activities of daily living, by re-entry into the work force, or by a subjective sense of well-being. Great progress has been made in the urologic management of the individual with spinal cord injury. At one time, renal failure was the leading cause of death of spinal cord injury patients. This is no longer the case. With a more normal life expectancy, in part secondary to better urologic care, emphasis has shifted to improving the quality of life. Urologic goals remain to preserve kidney function, prevent bladder and kidney infections, and avoid catheters whenever possible. With greater success in accomplishing these goals, sexual concerns have emerged as an important component of rehabilitation.

Sexual education, a need of all SCI patients, is best accomplished during the initial rehabilitation through a team approach, including a psychologist or psychiatrist (or both), urologist, and physiatrist. Because spinal cord injury typically involves young adults, sexuality is a very important concern. Many have not yet married nor found a regular partner. The ability to achieve erections, ejaculate, and achieve orgasm is important to most men and the ability to achieve orgasm and pregnancy is important to most women. Education should be provided to the individual, family members, and caregivers about what physical changes occur as a result of the injury and what treatment options are available.

NORMAL SEXUAL FUNCTION

Sexual function in males and females is divided into three main categories: libido, potency, and fertility. The sexual response cycle for men has been described as beginning with erection, followed by ejaculation or orgasm and finally with involution.[2] The female response cycle begins with an excitement phase, followed by a plateau phase, then orgasm, and finally resolution. The neurologic pathways for both sexes are similar. A brief description of libido will be followed by an in-depth discussion of the physiology of erection and ejaculation and the means for restoring either after spinal cord injury.

Libido refers to sexual desire or drive. Libido is determined in men by both psyche and the androgen status. Androgens are governed by the hypothalamic-pituitary-gonadal axis. The hypothalamus acts as the control center for the reproductive axis, receiving messages from both the testis and central nervous system. It then releases gonadotropin-releasing hormone (GnRH) in a pulsatile fashion. This stimulates the release of luteinizing hormone (LH) and follicle-stimulating hormone (FSH) from the anterior pituitary. Episodic release of LH and FSH stimulate Leydig and Sertoli cell metabolism in the testis. This axis is a closed-loop feedback system. Testosterone is secreted by the Leydig cells in response to LH pulses. The biologic effects of testosterone include regulation of the axis, spermatogenesis, sexual maturation, and preservation of sexual drive. Testosterone may also have a positive effect on the corpus caversonal tissue. Androgen deficiency resulting from pituitary disease or from primary testicular failure may result in loss of libido.

NEUROLOGIC MECHANISM OF ERECTION

In order for erections to occur, there must be adequate arterial inflow without venous leakage, providing an adequate steady state to provide a firm erection. These erection-producing vascular changes are controlled by complex neurologic pathways in a tightly controlled hormonal milieu. The pelvic parasympathetic nerve fibers, originating in the second through fourth sacral (S2–S4) roots, are responsible for the sacral reflex arc, which in turn provides parasympathetic enervation to the urinary bladder and nerve fibers to the penis that are responsible for reflex erections. Reflex erections are those produced by direct stimulation of the penis. They are mediated by the parasympathetic nervous system and require the sacral reflex arc (S2–S4) to be intact. Sensory stimuli travel via the dorsal nerve of the penis, which joins the pudendal nerve and then travels to the spinal cord. Efferent enervation to the penis travels via the pudendal nerve, which enters the penis at the cavernosal nerve. Reflex erections are generally preserved with spinal cord injury above the L2 vertebral level, thus preserving the S2–S4 nerve roots.[3]

Psychogenic erections, in contrast to reflex erections, are those produced by thoughts, and are speculated to originate from cerebral impulses that travel down the lateral columns of the spinal cord primarily via the thoracolumbar portion of the cord, and perhaps via the sacral roots as well.[3] Psychogenic erections are produced by thoughts and erotic stimuli and are mediated through the sympathetic nervous system. They require thoracolumbar nerve routes to be intact and occur independently of direct stimulation of the penis. Psy-

chogenic erections often are lost after injury to the thoracolumbar or cervical portion of the spinal cord.

ERECTILE PHYSIOLOGY

The field of erectile physiology has exploded over the past decade, ushered in by the demonstration that nitric oxide (NO) was the main mediator of penile erection. The challenge ahead is to understand the pathophysiology of erectile dysfunction as it relates to the recognized disease processes associated with erectile dysfunction (ED), and also to relate these concepts to the SCI male.

Erection is a neurovascular phenomenon that may be divided into two local events. First, there is neurally mediated vasorelaxation of the penile resistance arteries, the cavernosal and helicine arteries, as well as the trabecular smooth muscle that surrounds the lacunar spaces. This permits an increase in blood flow and pressure through the internal pudendal arterial system into the penis. The second event is activation of the corpus cavernosum trabecular smooth muscle (cavernosal smooth muscle) that surrounds the lacunar spaces to trap the blood that has entered into the penis. Blood under systemic blood pressure is now transmitted through the dilated cavernosal and helicine arteries and the relaxed trabecular walls, and expands the cavernosal smooth muscle against the tunica albuginea. This compresses the plexus of subtunical venules, reduces lacunar space venous outflow, and elevates lacunar space pressure, making the penis rigid.[4] The pressure in the lacunar space during an erection is the result of the equilibrium between the perfusion pressure in the cavernosal artery, helicine artery, and the resistance to blood outflow through the compressed subtunical venules.

With respect to the neurogenic component, pelvic parasympathetic cholinergic nerves arising from the sacral plexus, S2–S4, were historically thought to be responsible for the vasodilation of the penile cavernosum and erection.[4] However, vasodilation was recently found not to be directly owing to the action of cholinergic nerves, but rather to nonadrenergic-noncholinergic (NANC) nerves.[5] Cholinergic nerves appear to serve to augment relaxation by inhibition of adrenergic nerves and potentiate relaxation.[6–8] It has been readily demonstrated that rabbit and human corpus cavernosum contracted with an alpha–adrenergic agonist relaxes to electrical field stimulation in the presence of atropine, hence the term nonadrenergic-noncholinergic. It has been demonstrated subsequently that this relaxation was mediated through NO and cyclic GMP (cGMP).[6,9–11] These investigators demonstrated that NANC nerves appeared to release NO directly, through a nonendothelium-dependent mechanism.[5,12] Soon after, NO release and cGMP formation as a mechanism for human and rabbit cavernosal endothelium-dependent vasodilation was demonstrated as well.[13] In addition, it has been demonstrated that injection of an NO synthesis inhibitor in vivo into the primate, cat, rabbit, or rat prevented penile erection.[14] These compelling data strongly support NO as the main mediator of penile erection.

NITRIC OXIDE

Nitric oxide is a neurotransmitter produced from intracellular L-arginine in a reaction catalyzed by the enzyme nitric oxide synthase (NOs). NO is ubiquitous and has many regulatory functions, including regulation of blood pressure and prevention of platelet aggregation.[15] However, NO is a short-lived molecule with a half-life of a few seconds and therefore attention has been devoted toward characterizing NO formation at the level of its synthesis.[16] This has been accomplished by examining the enzyme responsible for NO synthesis, NOs. NOs has several isoforms: a constitutive neuronal isoform (nNOs) originally identified in rat brain and a constitutive endothelial isoform (eNOs) independently identified in bovine aortic endothelial cells.[17–19] In addition, there is an inducible isoform, iNOs, that is synthesized in response to various pathogens or other noxious stimuli.[16] nNOs has been described in the human and rat penis by immunohistochemistry and NADPH staining.[20] iNOs has been identified in the rat penis after being induced by exogenous substances such as LPS.[21] We have identified eNOs in the human penis. The following presents a review of eNOs and nNOs function with respect to their roles in erectile function.

eNOs

Clinically, the endothelial isoform of cNOs (eNOS) appears to have a regulatory role in blood-pressure maintenance, as evidenced by the recent identification of mutant homozygous transgenic mouse model deficient in eNOs that is hypertensive.[22] Furthermore, acetylcholine-mediated endothelium-dependent relaxation is absent in the blood vessels of these mice.[22] This suggests that eNOs may regulate basal vessel tone, and that nonendothelial isoforms of NOs may be involved in regulating blood pressure. Moreover, a reduced expression of eNOs has been identified in the lungs of patients with

pulmonary hypertension, and that the reduction paralleled the severity of the hypertension.[23] These studies clearly suggest that eNOs and by inference its product (NO) may play a role in the pathogenesis of vascular diseases; its role recently has also been applied to penile pathophysiology.

eNOS was first identified in bovine aortic endothelial cells, and appears to play a key role in the transduction of signals from the bloodstream to the underlying smooth muscle to produce vasorelaxation.[24,25] This isoform of cNOs is regulated by physiologic concentrations of calcium, via calmodulin.[19,26] eNOS is greater than 90 percent particulate, that is, membrane-bound, in endothelial cells.[26] The solubilized enzyme has a molecular mass of 135–150 kDa. Others have recently shown that the N-terminal end undergoes myristoylation, and that this modification is necessary for membrane association.[27] The cytosolic form of eNOS does not appear to have the N-myristoylation consensus sequence, suggesting that a loss of the myristate moiety may be important for subcellular translocation.[28] Interestingly, it appears that N-terminal myristoylation is not regulated at the level of agonists. Investigators have demonstrated that eNOS undergoes palmitoylation, which is dynamically regulated at the level of agonists such as bradykinin.[29] Although it had been originally thought that eNOS phosphorylation was an important component of its subcellular movement, it has been demonstrated that in transiently transfected endothelial cells deficient in the N-myristoylation moiety, eNOS undergoes serine phosphorylation despite restriction to the cytosol.[26] Finally, eNOS has been localized to the Golgi in cultured endothelial cells and intact blood vessels.[30] The importance of eNOs localization and changes in its biochemistry are, at this time, ill-defined.

Immunohistochemistry of Human Corpus Cavernosum

We have identified eNOs in the human penis via immunhistochemistry and electron microscopy. Tissue was procured at the time of penile prosthesis surgery under an approved protocol. Adjacent paraffin-embedded tissue sections were processed for immunocytochemical localization of eNOS and nNOS using a commercially available antibody. The tissue was permeablilized with 0.2 percent Triton X-100 in PBS and treated with methanol/hydrogen peroxide to reduce background staining. The primary antisera (polyclonal) were used at a concentration 5 μg/mL in PBS/0.3 percent Triton X-100 (Tx). After the incubation period, tissue sections were rinsed

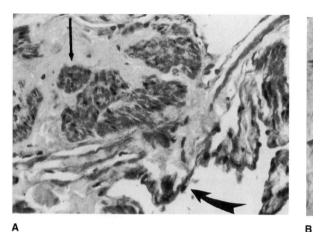

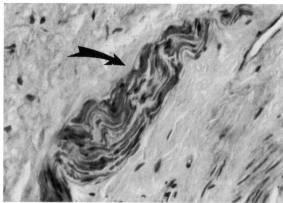

A

B

FIGURE 25-1

Immunohistochemical staining for eNOS using a commercially available polyclonal antibody (Trans-duction Labs, Lexington, KY). A. Staining of human cavernosal tissue for eNOS. Large arrows show endothelial staining. Small arrows show staining of smooth muscle. B. nNOS staining in nerves only (large arrow) with a lack of staining of smooth muscle, demonstrating specificity of eNOS polyclonal antibody.

thoroughly in PBS/0.3 percent Tx and processed for avidin-biotin localization of reaction product. The tissue was counterstained with hematoxylin to define morphological features of the tissue. Control tissue was included in staining protocols in which no primary antiserum was used. The tissue was then examined to determine if staining was completely blocked by this procedure. The staining revealed the presence of eNOS in the endothelium and the smooth muscle cells.

The staining of nNOS was specific to nerve bundles; there was no discernible staining of the endothelium or smooth muscle. The negative control revealed no staining (Figure 25-1). These data suggest that the polyclonal antibody is specific for eNOS and nNOS in human penile tissue and therefore allows for immunohistochemical identification of these enzymes.

Electron Microscopy

The postembedding immunogold procedure was used as described by Bates.[31] In brief, human cavernosal tissue blocks were fixed in 4 percent paraformaldehyde and 0.05 percent glutaraldehyde in 0.1 M cacodylate buffer for 3 h at 4°C. Samples were rinsed in cacodylate buffer and postfixed for 1 min at 4°C in 0.05 percent osmium tetroxide in cacodylate buffer. Blocks were rinsed in distilled water, dehydrated through a graded acetone series and embedded in Spurr resin. Thin sections (80

nm) were cut using a Reichert Ultracut E Ultramicrotome and collected on nickel grids. Grids were submerged in 10 percent aqueous hydrogen peroxide for 15 min, rinsed with distilled water and transferred to 0.05M ammonium chloride for 15 min, and again rinsed with distilled water. Grids were treated with heat-treated normal goat serum (1 : 30 in 0.05M tris buffered saline and 0.1 percent bovine serum albumin) for 30 min and incubated with anti-eNOS monoclonal antibody overnight at 4°C (1 : 25, Transduction Laboratories, mouse IgG_1). Grids were rinsed briefly in TBS/BSA and incubated in goat anti-mouse gold secondary antibody (10 nm, 1 : 25 BioCell) for 1 h. Grids were fixed with 2 percent aqueous glutaraldehyde and counterstained with uranyl acetate and lead citrate. Sections were examined using a JEOL 100CX transmission electron microscope. Controls for specificity included omission of the primary antibody and preadsorption of the primary antibody with human endothelial cell lysate, both of which resulted in the elimination of labeling. Using the immunogold technique, and the monoclonal antibody, EM demonstrated specific deposition of eNOS in the endothelium and smooth muscle (Figure 25-2). Confirmation of staining was produced via negative staining with pre-adsorbed controls. Ultrastructural sectioning revealed the presence of eNOS in the endothelial cell membrane, consistent with earlier reports of its particulate distribution. In addition, eNOS was

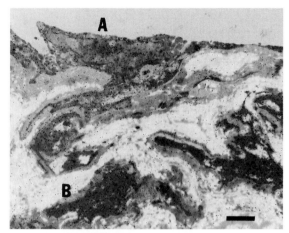
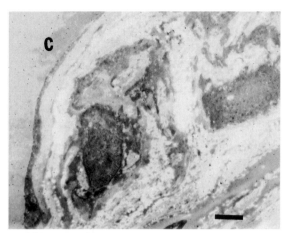

FIGURE 25-2
Electron microscopic section of eNOS in human corpus cavernosum smooth muscle cell (reduced from ×8,000) with monoclonal antibody (Transduction Labs, Lexington, KY) demonstrates staining in the endothelial cell (A) and smooth muscle cell (B), but no staining in the preadsorbed section (C).

present in the endothelial cell cytosol and nucleus, the smooth-muscle cell membrane, cytosol, and nucleus. Interestingly, eNOS was identified throughout the cytosol. There was no staining noted in mitochondria or Golgi. There was no discernible staining of eNOS in the intercellular matrix, between the endothelial cell and smooth muscle cell (Figures 25-1 and 25-2).

nNOs

nNOs, like eNOs, is calcium/calmodulin dependent. The neural isoform of cNOs (nNOs), originally identified in rat brain, has more recently been identified in skeletal muscle.[32,33] Its specific location in neural tissue has prompted several lines of investigation into its function. One role for nNOs has been that of behavioral changes.[34] Most notably, mutant homozygous mice deficient in nNOs have been found to be behaviorally aggressive. In addition, nNOs presence may predispose to a widening of focal cerebral infarction, in that transgenic homozygous nNOs mutant mice are protected against further cerebral ischemia.[35] This suggests that nNOs may have a role in spinal-cord or neurologic injury. Furthermore, NO synthesis inhibitors are also protective versus cerebral infarction, suggesting that NO has a critical role in the progression of cerebral ischemia.[36] There is emerging data suggesting that a deficiency in nNOs is associated with the neuromuscular disorder Duchenne's muscular dystrophy.[37] Thus, these

data circumstantially suggest that nNOs may play a role in various neurologic phenomena, and suggest a role for nNOs in the neurogenic component of the erection mechanism. Burnett et al. described nNOs in the human and rat penis, and Garban et al. described a decrease in nNOs activity with aging.[38,39]

nNOs in Spinal Cord Injury Spinal cord injury, both paraplegia and quadriplegia, are associated with erectile dysfunction. It is well known that men with SCI respond to minimal amounts of vasoactive agents injected intracavernosally. This would suggest that nNOs activity may be decreased in these men, in that they cannot initiate an erection and that the remainder of the erectile mechanism is intact. More work is needed in this area to understand the pathophysiology of nitric oxide in the SCI male.

iNOs

The inducible, calcium-independent form of NOs has yet to be identified in the human penis. Garban et al. described iNOs in the rat penis after induction by lipopolysaccharide (LPS). The role of iNOs in the normal erectile mechanism is unclear. Recently, Rajfer et al. have described the use of gene therapy via upregulation of iNOs to treat erectile dysfunction in the rat.[40] The theory is that there is a global difference in NO expression with ED. The restoration of NO activity is the goal. iNOs is placed genetically into the penile tissue via liposomes. This is an exciting and novel area of research that has great applicability to the therapy of erectile dysfunction. In men with SCI, one could imagine that significant upregulation of NO might allow a reflexogenic erection or a psychogenic erection to become a full rigid erection, given a sufficient quantity of NO.

In sum, these data point toward NO as the main mediator of penile erection. The enzymes responsible for NO synthesis, eNOs, nNOs, and iNOs, are just now being understood.[41]

NO Activity on Effector Tissue

The potential signaling pathways by which NO induces relaxation recently has been described in vascular smooth muscle cells. Regulation of K^+ transport mechanisms by humoral and osmotic stimuli is of primary importance for excitable cells, transepithelial transport systems, and for cell-volume regulation in contractile cells.[42,43] In contractile tissue, such as vascular smooth muscle, regulation of potassium transport mechanisms is thought to play a critical role in the control of vascular tone at the cellular level. Vasoactive agents have been recently found to regulate K^+ flux pathways in vascular smooth muscle cells, in particular the $Na^+/K^+/Cl^-$ cotransporter and certain K^+ channels.[45–49] It has been suggested that a change in electrical properties of contractile cells leads to the modulation of cell tone thereby leading to contraction. One mechanism by which endothelium-dependent release factor (EDRF)/NO induces its vasorelaxant effect is that of changes in membrane potential.[49] Initial work by Chen and Suzuki demonstrated that muscarinic agonist-induced endothelium-dependent release was responsible for the hyperpolarization seen in vascular smooth muscle cells from intralobular pulmonary arteries.[49] Although regional vascular vasodilatory differences have been described for acetylcholine (ACh), the relaxing properties of ACh have been presumed to be the release of NO.[50,51] Moreover, additional findings by Tare et al. clearly demonstrated that when smooth muscle cells exposed to ACh, arterial smooth muscle cells from uterine arteries underwent a membrane hyperpolarization and relaxation as measured by tension.[47] These findings also illustrated that the effect was abolished through the use of N^G-monomethyl-L-arginine (L-NMMA), an inhibitor of NO biosynthesis. We have recently demonstrated that in mesangial cells fluorescent indicators for potassium can be used to measure rapid changes in $[K^+]_i$, and that sodium nitroprusside (SNP), ACh, and bradykinin

induce a transient decrease in $[K^+]_i$ and induce a transient membrane hyperpolarization.[52] Moreover, this change in $[K^+]_i$ and membrane potential is through a Ba^{2+}/TEA-sensitive K^+-conductive pathway, and the effect on $[K^+]_i$ and membrane hyperpolarization is mediated through the release of NO. Using rabbit cavernosal smooth muscle cells in culture, we have also found similar results. We have demonstrated that NO induces a change in $[K^+]_i$ and with a concomitant membrane potential that might be related to changes in contractility and be responsible for the relaxation seen in erection.[53]

K conductance occurs through K^+ channels. Christ et al. have shed light into the various types of K channels; there are several types of K^+ channels in the human corpus cavernosum. His group has found that there is a decrease in the TEA sensitivity of the K_{Ca} channel, the predominant channel in the cavernosum, with diabetes and other vascular diseases. Further, this group has demonstrated that there are gap junctions that exist in the cavernosum, and that these specialized channels allow for rapid communication between the cavernosal cells.[54] Thus, these cells may allow the rapid intracellular spread of the ACh-induced membrane hyperpolarization to produce the significant, rapid, and coordinated vasodilation seen with erection.

In summary, normal physiology of penile erection, in part, appears to intimately involve nitric oxide synthesis and activity via cGMP, membrane hypolarization, and K-channel activity.

NO Is Not the Main Mediator of Penile Erection

The penis is in a state of contraction for the majority of its life, and only becomes erect at specific times and for specific purposes. Thus, some authorities believe that the main impetus toward erection is the counteraction of the contraction mechanism, which permits the vasodilation to ensue. It is felt that adrenergic nerves and other endothelial vasoactive agents, such as endothelin and angiotensin, play a strict regulatory role in the maintenance of the contracted state. Neural stimulation "switches" these contractile agents off and allows for vasodilation.[55] This is a controversial area in the field of erectile physiology.

NERVE REGENERATION

Although the pathophysiology of erectile dysfunction is now being investigated, gene therapy and nerve regeneration offer new and exciting possibilities for the treatment of the neurogenically impaired. Gene therapy was discussed earlier. Nerve regeneration is a new and exciting area. Nerve transection owing to surgical intervention or trauma was thought to be irreversible. Recent work has demonstrated the feasibility of neoneuronal regrowth.[56] This raises the possibility that nerve regeneration or regrowth may be in the offing.

EJACULATORY FUNCTION

Gross Anatomy

Ejaculation is mediated through the sympathetic nervous system and the thoracolumbar portion of the spinal cord. Ejaculation includes emission, bladder neck closure, and antegrade ejaculation. Although the neurologic pathways for vaginal lubrication and orgasm in the female are less well described, the sacral parasympathetics are thought to be responsible for reflex lubrication and the thoracolumbar sympathetics are thought to be responsible for psychogenic lubrication.[57] Smooth muscle contraction of the uterus, fallopian tubes, and paraurethral glands is thought to be mediated by the thoracolumbar sympathetics. Contraction of the striated pelvic-floor muscles, the analogue of antegrade ejaculation is mediated through the sacral parasympathetics and the somatic efferents.

Ejaculation is a highly complex and coordinated event. There are three distinct phases of the ejaculatory process: emission, bladder neck closure, and antegrade ejaculation. Emission is the initial deposition of the seminal fluid components into the posterior urethra. During emission, bladder neck closure occurs to prevent reflux of semen into the bladder during the ejaculatory phase. This closure, coupled with contraction of the external urethral sphincter, creates a closed space in the posterior urethra as the emission phase continues. Ejaculation results from the forceful expulsion of this trapped seminal fluid in an antegrade direction to exit the urethral meatus. Seminal fluid consists of spermatozoa from the vas/ampulla (10 percent), fructose-rich seminal vesicle secretions (70 percent), and prostatic fluid (20 percent). Orgasm is a short-lived cortical experience and occurs concurrent with emission and ejaculation.[58]

True ejaculation is the forceful propulsion of seminal fluid from the posterior urethra through the penile meatus. Electromyographic studies indicate that it is accomplished with rhythmic contractions of the striated bulbocavernosus, ischiocavernosus, and associated pelvic-floor muscles, concomitant with closure of the bladder neck and coordinated and rhythmic relaxation of the external sphincter.[59] In man, three to seven contractions of the involved musculature at 0.8-second intervals usually occur during the normal ejaculatory cycle. From the sacral cord grey matter (S2–S4), somatic efferents arise and journey via the motor division of the pudendal nerve to innervate the different striated muscle groups, as well as the outer muscle group of the external sphincter mechanism. Sacral parasympathetics travel via the pelvic nerve to innervate the inner muscle group of the external sphincter. Afferent sensory stimuli from the seminal vesicle, prostate, and vas are relayed to the cord through the pelvic splanchnics. Genital skin afferents course through the sensory division of the pudendal nerve.

There is a putative ejaculatory reflex center located between T12 and L2. This center is believed to be responsible for the coordination and integration of the neural input from above (higher cerebral centers) and from below (sensory fibers) and then for the proper sequencing of the efferent outflow through, first, the thoracolumbar sympathetics (emission) and then through the sacral somatics (antegrade ejaculation). This center is therefore responsible for the ejaculatory reflex and is highly influenced by cortical and/or genital sensory input.

Effect of Spinal Cord Injury on Sexual Function

After spinal cord injury, the ability to achieve erections and ejaculate can be affected. Talbot reported that only 20 percent (40 of 186) men after spinal cord injury were able to have intercourse.[60] Bors and Comarr reported their findings on carefully questioning 529 men with spinal cord injury and correlating the ability to achieve erections and to ejaculate with their level and completeness of injury. Patients with complete lower motor neuron injuries (injury to the cauda equina or conus medullaris that disrupt the sacral reflex arc) were generally not able to obtain any erection. In the event that an erection could be obtained, it was psychogenic in nature.[61] Patients with complete or incomplete upper motor neuron injuries, on the other hand, were generally able to obtain reflex erections. However, the erections were often not satisfactory for coitus.

Comarr subsequently reported on 150 patients (115 with upper motor neuron lesions and 35 with lower motor neuron injuries).[62] Ninety-four percent of the patients with upper motor neuron lesions were able to obtain spontaneous erections; 92 percent could obtain an erection by direct external stimulation, whereas only 22 percent were able to achieve psychogenic erections. Patients with lower motor neuron lesions fared worse. None of these 35 patients was able to achieve reflex erections. Only 11 percent achieved spontaneous erections and 26 percent noted psychogenic erections. Sixty-two percent of the patients in this series attempted coitus and 43 percent considered themselves successful. In regards to ejaculation, 9 percent of individuals with upper motor neuron injuries could ejaculate (only 1 percent if the injury was complete), whereas 17 percent of those with lower motor neuron injuries could ejaculate. One must be careful not to make definite predictions of sexual function based solely on the level and completeness of injury, but a general trend has emerged.

PATIENT EVALUATION

A careful history, including a sexual history, should be obtained from a patient and his partner during rehabilitation. Although an individual with spinal cord injury can have problems obtaining or maintaining an erection on a neurologic basis, psychologic factors may contribute significantly to erectile dysfunction. Patients are best assessed by the urologist and the psychologist or psychiatrist who is experienced in dealing with individuals with spinal cord injury. The team approach provides for better patient care. It is important to inquire into the patient's sexual history and any problems experienced prior to injury. A careful evaluation of the actual injury may help explain an erection problem. A quadriplegic patient with a simultaneous pelvic fracture may lose his ability to achieve reflex erections on the basis of the pelvic fracture. Many of the medications commonly used to manage the neurogenic bladder, such as the anticholinergic medications (probanthene, oxybutynin chloride), can not only give the patient a dry mouth, but may lead to erectile dysfunction. The alpha blockers used commonly to treat bladder-outlet obstruction symptoms from either an enlarged prostate or bladder-sphincter dyssynergia occasionally can lead to hypotension and inhibit ejaculation.

Physical examination should carefully document the neurologic level and completeness of injury. The presence of rectal tone, perineal sensation, and the bulbocavernous reflex should be tested, along with reflexes and sensation in the lower extremities. Preservation of pinprick sensation in the perineum and along the shaft of the penis and scrotum is frequently indicative that the patient will regain reflex and psychogenic erections and the ability to ejaculate. In addition to the physical examination, serum blood levels of testosterone, FSH, LH, and prolactin should be obtained as a baseline prior to instituting therapy, if erection or ejaculation difficulties occur.

Initial Management

During the initial rehabilitation, the patient with spinal cord injury is instructed in the normal physiology of erection and ejaculation and the effects of injury on sexual function. The patient is encouraged to experiment with his partner when he goes home for passes during acute rehabilitation. The bladder should be emptied prior to intercourse to avoid the embarrassing reflex loss of urine during intercourse. Individuals on intermittent catheterization should catheterize the bladder immediately prior to intercourse. If the bladder is managed with a chronic indwelling catheter, the catheter can be folded on itself and covered with a condom or removed prior to intercourse. Individuals with reflex voiding should attempt suprapubic tapping to elicit a bladder contraction prior to intercourse. If an individual has poor leg function where pelvic thrusting may not be possible, assuming the down position may provide a practical alternative. Individuals with spinal cord injury can achieve reflex erections that are short-lived. These erections can often be sustained by providing direct stimulation to the penis.

Ejaculatory Failure

Ejaculatory failure is a common problem among those with spinal cord injury. Patients with complete upper motor neuron lesions rarely ejaculate during coitus, in general, whereas 29 percent of incomplete upper motor neuron lesion patients may experience coital orgasm. In contrast, 17 percent of complete and 60 percent of incomplete lower motor neuron lesion patients may have at least the emission phase of the ejaculatory event intact and experience a dribbling, weak "ejaculation." As a group, spontaneous fertility rates are poor, ranging from 1 to 10 percent, depending on the level and nature of the lesion.[63] To compound the difficulty involving delivery of semen (ejaculation), many studies have demonstrated impairments in spermatogenesis in some spinal-cord-injured patients. Theories to explain the testicular dysfunction include scrotal hyperthermia owing to the loss of normal testicular thermoregulatory mechanisms, chronic epididymitis/orchitis, and other non-specific factors.[64] Whereas no consistent pattern of abnormal spermatogenesis has been noted, testicular biopsies have revealed hypospermatogenesis, maturation arrest, tubular atrophy, interstitial fibrosis, and Leydig cell hyperplasia.[65] However, many patients retain an adequate level of sperm production, making conception an achievable goal.

TREATMENT

Treatment of ejaculatory failure and infertility has included a wide range of both nonspecific and specific therapeutic options. In an effort to reduce scrotal temperature and possibly improve spermatogenesis, patients have been told to keep the knees apart when sitting, wear underwear with a scrotal slit, and prop the scrotum up onto the thighs when sitting. No objective evidence exists to support these recommendations.

Ejaculatory failure is the major cause of infertility in these patients. In attempts to induce ejaculation by direct stimulation of the ejaculatory coordination center and/or the spinal sympathetic outflow, intrathecal pharmacotherapy with neostigmine has been employed with limited success. Injected via lumbar puncture, neostigmine will not traverse the blood-brain barrier. However, severe hypertension due to autonomic dysreflexia requires intensive and continuous monitoring, and actually caused the death of one patient. This led to a general disinterest in this technique in recent years.

Initially popularized by Brindley in some of his pioneering work, vibratory stimulation applied to the frenular undersurface of the glans penis may result in normal antegrade ejaculation.[64] This is a reflexogenic event in which vibratory tactile stimuli from the penile area enter the cord through sacral roots and travel cephalad to the ejaculatory coordination center in the upper thoracolumbar cord. Here, the rapid sequence of sympathetic outflow from T10–L3 is generated to induce emission, followed by the precisely timed efferent outflow from S2–S4 to stimulate contractions of the perineal musculature and create antegrade semen flow. The bladder neck and external sphincter act in a coordinated fashion as well, indicating that this reflex recapitulates the normal ejaculatory sequence. Therefore, it is applicable only in patients with an intact and functional lower thoracolumbosacral cord segment. In general, patients with lesions below T12 will be unsuccessful using vibratory stimulation.[66] In ideal circumstances the patient and his spouse are able to use vibratory stimulation coupled with self insemination of the resultant semen to achieve pregnancy. It is not suited for those patients still in spinal shock. Reporting on 81 spinal-cord-injury patients, Brindley found this technique successful in 59 percent of patients, with seven pregnancies reported.[64] Autonomic dysreflexia may complicate this therapy, but is easily controlled with supportive measures and sublingual nifedipine (10 mg). Using a portable, commercially available massage unit, Oates et al. reported successful induction of ejaculation in 52 percent of patients overall; 75 percent in cervical cord, 62 percent in thoracic cord (above T12), and 0 percent in lumbar cord (below T12) injured patients.[67] Therefore, vibratory stimulation always should be tried as the first option because of its ease and simplicity.

Rectal probe electroejaculation (RPE) has been used in veterinary medicine since the 1930s. This technique and its use to induce ejaculation in spinal-cord-injured patients is gaining popularity in the United States. The basic concept involves the direct electrical stimulation with resultant contraction and discharge of the structures responsible for the elaboration of the constituents of semen during the normal emission process, that is, seminal vesicles, vasal ampullae, and prostate. Therefore, the result is really no more than electrically induced emission and there is no true antegrade ejaculation component since the perineal musculature does not rhythmically contract following deposition of the seminal fluid into the posterior urethra. This is the primary physiologic difference between rectal probe electroejaculation and vibratory induction of ejaculation.

RPE can be performed in the lithotomy or lateral decubitus position, with systemic blood pressure monitored throughout the procedure. The probe is made of polyvinyl chloride with electrodes placed internal to this coating. The probe incorporates a temperature monitoring device to alert the operator should the probe temperature reach levels at which tissue damage could occur. The probe is connected to a stimulator, and an average of 30 stimulations of 15 volts and 315 mamps are delivered in a sine wave summation fashion (Figure 25-3). The bulbous and pendulous portions of the urethra are milked and the posterior urethra and bladder are catheterized following stimulation to recover all the seminal fluid delivered into the posterior urethra. The semen is then processed appropriately and prepared for spousal intrauterine insemination and/or other advanced reproductive techniques, such as in vitro fertilization. Obviously, the procedure is timed to be coincident with ovulation or oocyte retrieval, and coordination between the urologist and gynecologist/reproductive endocrinologist must be superb.

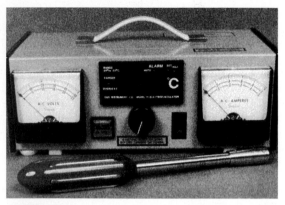

FIGURE 25-3
Rectal Probe Electroejaculation Equipment (Model 12): The stimulator box is connected by insulated cable (not shown) to the hand-held rectal probe. The electrodes that will deliver the current to the ejaculatory structures are seen on the outer surface of the probe. (Developed by SWJ Seager, D.V.M. and presently distributed by National Rehabilitation Hospital, Fertility Center, Washington, D.C. Reprinted with permission.)

The seminal quality, in terms of sperm number and motility, is used to assess which procedure might be most applicable to achieve conception. Using a new simplified probe along with a computer-based stimulator, Perkash et al. achieved seminal emissions in 13 of 17 spinal-cord-injury patients, and partial emission in the remainder.[68] Lerner et al. report that RPE was successful in 71 percent of their spinal-cord population with resultant sperm counts in the normal range, although the sperm motility was depressed to moderately low levels.[69] Recoverable sperm density and motility did improve in successive ejaculates. Bennett et al. reported the first pregnancies in the United States and currently quote a 40 percent pregnancy rate utilizing this technique in combination with proper spousal management.[70] Microsurgical epididymal sperm aspiration coupled with in vitro fertilization is applicable for those refractory cases in which semen cannot be obtained via stimulatory methods, as mentioned earlier.[71]

SPERM BANKING AND MICROSCOPIC EPIDIDYMAL SPERM ASPIRATION

As new improvements in the technique of in vitro fertilization have been realized, such as intracytoplasmic sperm injection (ICSI), pregnancy is now easily accomplished with only a few, or even no viable sperm.[72] Thus techniques such as microscopic epididymal sperm aspiration (MESA) with baking of sperm, as well as banking of sperm obtained at the time of vibratory or rectal probe ejaculation, become viable options for fertility for the SCI male.

MANAGEMENT OF ERECTILE DYSFUNCTION

Impotence is defined as the inability to obtain and sustain an erection that is satisfactory to complete the sexual act. Although many individuals with spinal cord injury do not require any intervention, being aware of the changes that can occur to sexual function after spinal cord injury and the treatment options available is an important component of the education provided during rehabilitation.

In the past, erections were restored in spinal cord injury patients by the use of external appliances placed over the penis. These devices increased the rigidity of the penis, permitting penetration. The only alternative was the placement of a penile prosthesis. Penile prostheses are cylinders that are surgically implanted. They may be semirigid or inflatable. However, because of the lack of sensation and more frequent urinary tract infections from the neurogenic bladder, SCI patients are at higher risk for erosion or infection of the prosthesis, approaching 20 percent compared to 1 to 9 percent in the general population.[73–75] Results have been better when the prosthesis was placed for the purpose of keeping an external urinary collection device in place rather than for sexual function.[76] The explanation for these improved results may be owing either to better patient selection or to the fact that no pressure is being applied to the tip of the glans penis, where the tip of the prostheses is located when the external condom catheter is used. Placement of penile prostheses is expensive, irreversible, and can be complicated by infection or erosion. With improvement in the noninvasive treatment options for erectile dysfunction in patients with spinal cord injury, penile prostheses generally are reserved for those individuals who fail less invasive treatment options or who require a prosthesis to help keep a condom catheter in place.

There is no evidence to support the use of yohimbine or other psychotropic agents to improve erections in patients with spinal cord injury. Since many noninvasive methods have proven effective, they are favored when intervention is required.

VACUUM ERECTION DEVICES

Devices for creating erections are not new.[77] They work on a mechanical basis, using a cylinder placed about the penis and a pump mechanism. This allows blood to be drawn into the corpora to produce tumescence. A constriction band is placed at the base of the penis and a pump is used to create a vacuum of air within the cylinder. Nadig reported that 91 percent of 35 patients studied with a vacuum device used in combination with a constricting band achieved an erection and 80 percent of these men were satisfied with the erection. Because of the constricting band, the temperature of the penis was noted to drop an average of 0.96°C over 30 minutes. Most subjects did not report this to be a problem.[78] Turner et al. evaluated 36 non-spinal-cord-injured patients with one such device, and noted that 7 (19 percent) dropped out within 6 months.[79] Dropout was attributed to retardation of ejaculation from the constricting band. There has been limited experience reported using vacuum devices in patients with spinal-cord injury. Lloyd reported that of 13 SCI patients using the Erecaid, 90 percent achieved satisfactory erections.[80] When manual dexterity is impaired, a partner can be taught to use the device. Newer electrical devices are available that require less manual dexterity. Vacuums may be difficult for some men to uses and have been reported to cause penile trauma, if improperly used.[81] They may be somewhat cumbersome, can cause the erect penis to bend at the constricting band and are not accepted by all patients.[82]

INTRACAVERNOSAL INJECTION OF VASOACTIVE MEDICATIONS

Intracorporal injection of vasoactive medications to produce erections was first reported by Michal and colleagues in 1977 when they accidentally injected papaverine, a smooth muscle relaxant, into the corpora cavernosa of the penis during a revascularization procedure and produced an erection.[83] Virag and Brindley reported that Intra corporal injection of papaverine produced an erection satisfactory for intercourse.[84,85] In 1985, Virag reported that sustained erections lasting up to 18 hours occurred in 42 of 227 patients who were given 80 mg of papaverine, with 15 of the patients requiring aspiration of the corpora of blood to end the erection.[86] Zorgniotti and LeFleur were the first to report intracavernosal self injection as a treatment for impotence, and 59 of 62 patients had successful erections.[87]

Sidi reported results of intracavernosal injection of vasoactive medications in 100 patients.[88] Of the 17 patients with neurologic impotence, all achieved satisfactory erections and four of the 17 had sustained erections. Bodner et al. reported their experience in 20 men with spinal cord injury treated with intracavernosal injection therapy.[89] Of the 20 patients, 19 achieved satisfactory erections and three patients had sustained erections lasting greater than 4 hours. Wyndaele reported results with intracavernosal injection therapy in 12 individuals with spinal cord injury and emphasized the need to begin with a low doses of medication to prevent the complication of priapism.[90] In subsequent series reporting results of SCI patients treated with injection therapy, the drop-out rate was approximately 40 percent at 1 year and the injection frequency was approximately two times per month.[91,92] Penile plaque formation was noted in only one of 50 patients, whereas the treatment was effective in 45 of the 50 patients.[91] The incidence of plaque formation in non-SCI men is reported to be approximately 30 percent at 1 year and is directly related to the frequency and dosage of the medication.[93] The use of Prostaglandin E1 has been less frequently associated with priapism and penile fibrosis than papaverine and phentolamine and starting with low doses of the medication has been recommended.[94,95] Limited experience has been reported specifically using Prostaglandin E1 as an intracorporeal agent in the spinal-cord-injured population.

Intracorporeal injection therapy has been very effective in treating erectile dysfunction in the spinal-cord-injury population. The risk of a sustained erection requiring intervention, the need to place a needle into the penis, and the possibility of a bruise or fibrosis from the injection site has made alternative delivery systems appealing. The use of alprostadil (Prostaglandin E1) delivered transurethrally in a double-blind, placebo-controlled study of 1511 impotent men was recently reported. Erections sufficient for intercourse were achieved in 65.9 percent of the men who had chronic organic impotence of various etiologies.[96] All groups tended to respond comparably. Neurologic patients were not examined separately. The intraurethral topical application of this medication appears less invasive than intracorporal injection and warrants further evaluation in the SCI population.

In summary, when reflex erections are inadequate for intercourse and a patient has been fully evaluated and counseled in the treatment alternatives, vacuum erection devices or intracorporal injection therapy is recommended. Success has been achieved with both treatment options with acceptable complication rates when the patient is followed closely by individuals familiar with these therapies. Further research is underway in developing less invasive delivery systems for the vasoactive medications. SCI patients should continue to benefit from these new advances. Based on the new discoveries in the physiology and the pathophysiology of erection and ejaculation, these advances make restoration of erection and ejaculation, sexual function, and fertility a realistic possibility.

REFERENCES

1. Stover SL, Fine PR, Kennedy EJ (eds): *Spinal Cord Injury: The Facts and Figures*. Birmingham, AL: University of Alabama, 1986.
2. Masters WH, Johnson VE: *Human Sexual Response*. Boston: Little, Brown, 1966.
3. Newman HF, Northup JD: Mechanism of human penile erection: an overview. *Urology* 1981; 27:399–408.
4. Krane RJ, Goldstein I, Saenz de Tejada I: Impotence. *N Engl J Med* 1989; 321:1648–1659.
5. Kim N, Azadzoi KM, Goldstein I, Saenz de Tejada I: A nitric oxide-like factor mediates nonadrenergic-noncholinergic neurogenic relaxation of penile corpus cavernosum smooth muscle. *J Clin Invest* 1991; 88:112–118.
6. Saenz de Tejada I, Blanco R, Goldstein I, Azadzoi K, de las Morenas A, Krane RJ, Cohen R: Cholinergic neurotransmission in human corpus cavernosum. I. Responses of isolated tissue. *Am J Physiol* 1988; 254:459–467.
7. Blanco R, Saenz de Tejada I, Goldstein I, Krane RJ, Wotiz HH, Cohen, RA: Cholinergic neurotransmission in human corpus cavernosum. II. Acetylcholine synthesis. *Am J Physiol* 1988; 254:468–472.
8. Saenz de Tejada I, Kim N, Lagan I, Krane RJ, Goldstein I: Regulation of adrenergic activity in penile corpus cavernosum. *J Urol* 1989; 142:1117–1121.
9. Ignarro LJ, Bush PA, Buga GM, Wood KS, Fukuto JM, Rajfer J: Nitric oxide and cyclic GMP formation upon electrical field stimulation cause relaxation of corpus cavernosum smooth muscle. *Biochem Biophys Res Commun* 1990; 170:843–850.
10. Rajfer J, Aronson WJ, Bush P, Dorey F, Ignarro L: Nitric oxide as a mediator of relaxation of the corpus cavernosum in response to nonadrenergic, noncholinergic neurotransmission. *N Engl J Med* 1992; 326:90–94.
11. Bush PA, Gonzalez NE, Ignarro LJ: Biosynthesis of nitric oxide and citrulline from L-arginine by constitutive nitric oxide synthase present in rabbit corpus cavernosum. *Biochem Biophys Res Commun* 1992; 186:308–314.
12. Trigo-Rocha F, Aronson WJ, Hoheenfellner M, Ignarro LJ, Rajfer J, Lue TF: *Am J Physiol* 1993; 264:H419–H422.
13. Azadzoi KM, Kim N, Brown ML, Goldstein I, Cohen RA,
Saenz De Tejada I: Endothelium-derived nitric oxide cyclooxygenase products modulate corpus cavernosum smooth muscle tone. *J Urol* 1992; 147:220–225.
14. Holmquist F, Stief CG, Jonas U, Andersson KE: Effects of the nitric oxide synthase inhibitor NG-nitro-L-arginine on the erectile response to cavernous nerve stimulation in the rabbit. *Acta Physiol Scand* 1991; 143:299.
15. Bredt DS, Snyder SH: Nitric oxide: A physiologic messenger molecule. *Annu Rev Biochem* 1994; 63:175–195.
16. Forstermann U, Kleinert H: Nitric oxide synthase: Expression and expressional control of the three isoforms. *Arch Pharmacol* 1995; 352:351–364.
17. Janssens SP, Shimouchi A, Quertermous T, Bloch DB, Bloch KD: Cloning and expression of a cDNA encoding human endothelium-derived relaxing factor/nitric oxide synthase. *J Biol Chem* 1992; 267:14519–14522.
18. Lamas S, Marsden PA, Li GK, Tempst P, Michel T: Endothelial nitric oxide synthase: Molecular cloning and characterization of a distinct constitutive enzyme isoform. *Proc Natl Acad Sci USA* 1992; 89:6348–6352.
19. Pollock JS, Forstermann U, Mitchell JA, Warner TD, Schmidt HHHW, Nakane M, Murad F: Purification and characterization of particulate endothelium-derived relaxing factor synthase from cultured and native bovine aortic endothelial cells. *Proc Natl Acad Sci USA* 1991; 88:10480–10484.
20. Burnett AL, Lowenstein CJ, Bredt DS, Chang TSK, Snyder SH: Nitric oxide: A physiologic mediator of penile erection. *Science* 1992; 257:401–403.
21. Hung A, Vernet D, Xie Y, Rajavashisth T, Rodriguez JA, Rajfer J, Gonzalez-Cadavid N: Expression of inducible nitric oxide synthase in smooth muscle cells from rat penile corpora cavernosa. *J Androl* 1995; 16:469.
22. Huang PL, Huang Z, Mashimo H, Bloch K, Moskowitz MA, Bevan JA, Fishman MC: Hypertension in mice lacking the gene for endothelial nitric oxide synthase. *Nature* 1995; 377:239–242.
23. Giaid A, Saleh D: Reduced expression of endothelial nitric oxide synthase in the lungs of patients with pulmonary hypertension. *N Engl J Med* 1995; 333:214–221.
24. Horackova M, Armour JA, Hopkins DA, Huang MH: Nitric oxide modulates signaling between cultured adult peripheral cardiac neurons and cardiomyocytes. *Am J Physiol* 1995; 269:504–510.
25. Balligand JL, Kelly RA, Marsden PA, Smith TW, Michel T: Control of cardiac muscle cell function by an endogenous nitric oxide signaling system. *Proc Natl Acad Sci USA* 1993; 90:347–351.
26. Busconi L, Michel T: Endothelial nitric oxide synthase. *J Biol Chem* 1993; 268:8410–8413.
27. Sakoda T, Hirata K, Kuroda R, Miki N, Suematsu M, Kawashima S, Yokoyama M: Myristoylation of endothelial cell nitric oxide synthase is important for extracellular release of nitric oxide. *Mol Cell Biochem* 1995; 152:143–148.
28. Sessa WC, Barber CM, Lynch KR: Mutation of N-myristoylation site converts endothelial cell nitric oxide synthase

from a membrane to a cytosolic protein. *Circ Res* 1993; 72:921–924.

29. Robinson LJ, Busconi L, Michel T: Agonist-modulated palmitoylation of endothelial nitric oxide synthase. *J Biol Chem* 1995; 270:995–998.

30. Sessa WC, Garcia-Cardena G, Liu J, Keh A, Pollock JS, Bradley J, Thiru S, Braverman IM, Desai KM: The golgi association of endothelial nitric oxide synthase is necessary for the efficient synthesis of nitric oxide. *J Biol Chem* 1995; 270:17641–17644.

31. Bates TE, Loesch A, Burnstock G, Clark JB: Immunocytochemical evidence mitochondrially located nitric oxide synthase in brain and liver. *BBRC* 1995; 213:896–900.

32. Bredt DS, Snyder SH: Isolation of nitric oxide synthetase, a calmodulin-requiring enzyme. *Proc Natl Acad Sci USA* 1990; 87:682–685.

33. Nakane M, Schmidt H, Pollock JS, Forstermann U, Murad F: Cloned human brain nitric oxide synthase is highly expressed in skeletal muscle. *FEBS Letts* 1993; 316:175–180.

34. Nelson RJ, Demas GE, Huang PL, Fishman MC, Dawson VL, Dawson TM, Snyder SH: Behavioural abnormalities in male mice lacking neuronal nitric oxide synthase. *Nature* 1995; 378:383–386.

35. Huang Z, Huang PL, Panahain N, Dalkara T, Fishman MC, Moskowitz MA: Effects of cerebral ischemia in mice deficient in neuronal nitric oxide synthase. *Science* 1994; 265:1883–1885.

36. Nagafuji T, Sugiyama M, Muto A, Makino T, Miyauchi T, Nabata H: The neuroprotective effect of a potent and selective inhibitor of type I NOS (L-MIN) in a rat model of focal cerebral ischaemia. *Neuroreport* 1995; 6:1541–1545.

37. Brenman JE, Chao DS, Xia H, Aldape K, Bredt DS: Nitric oxide synthase complexed with dystrophin and absent from skeletal muscle sarcolemma in Duchenne Muscular Dystrophy. *Cell* 1995; 82:743–752.

38. Burnett AL, Tillman SL, Chang TS, Epstein JI, Lowenstein CJ, Bredt DS, Snyder SH, Walsh PC: Immunohistochemical localization of nitric oxide synthase in the autonomic innervation of the human penis. *J Urol* 1993; 150:73–76.

39. Garban H, Vernet D, Freedman A, Rajfer J, Gonzalez-Cadavid N: Effects of aging on nitric oxide-mediated penile erection in rats. *Am J Physiol* 1995; 268:H467–H475.

40. Garban H, Moody D, Marquez J, Magee D, Vernet T, Rajfer DJ, Gonzalez-Cadavid N: Correction of erectile dysfunction by induction of iNOs in the penis. *Int J Imp Res* 1996; 8:100(abstract A03).

41. Elabbady AA, Gagnon C, Hassouna MM, Begin LR, Elhilali MM: Diabetes mellitus increases nitric oxide synthase in penises but not in major pelvic ganglia of rats. *Br J Urol* 1995; 76:196–202.

42. Eveloff J, Warnock D: Activation of ion transport systems during cell volume regulation. *Am J Physiol* 1987; 252:F1–F10.

43. Cook N: The pharmacology of potassium channels and their therapeutic potential. *TIPS* 1989; 9:21–28.

44. Nelson M, Tatlak J, Worley J, Standen N: Calcium channels, potassium channels, and voltage dependence of arterial smooth muscle tone. *Am J Physiol* 1990; 259:C3–C18.

45. Paris S, Pouyssegur J: Growth factors activate the bumetanide-sensitive Na/K/Cl cotransport in hamster fibroblasts. *J Biol Chem* 1986; 261:6177–6183.

46. Soltoff S, Mandel L: Potassium transport in the rabbit renal proximal tubule: effects of barium, ouabain, valinomycin and other ionophores. *J Membr Biol* 1986; 94:153–161.

47. Tare M, Parkington H, Coleman A, Neild T, Dusting G: Hyperpolarization and relaxation of arterial smooth muscle caused by nitric oxide derived from the endothelium. *Nature* 1990; 346:69–71.

48. Ganz M, Kasner S, Unwin R: Nitric oxide alters cytosolic potassium in cultured glomerular mesangeal cells. *Am J Physiol* 1995; 268:F1081.

49. Chen G, Suzuki H: Some electrical properties of the endothelium-dependent hyperpolarization recorded from rat arterial smooth muscle cells. *J Physiol* 1989; 410:91–106.

50. Archer S, Huang J, Hampl V, Nelson P, Shultz J, Weir, E: Nitric oxide and cGMP cause vasorelaxation by activation of a charybdotoxin-sensitive K channel by cGMP dependent protein kinase. *Proc Natl Acad Sci USA* 1994; 91:7583–7587.

51. Bolotina VM, Soheil Najibi M, Palacino JJ, Pagano PJ, Cohen RA: Nitric oxide directly activates calcium-dependent potassium channels in vascular smooth muscle. *Nature* 1994; 368:850–853.

52. Kasner S, Ganz M: Regulation of intracellular potassium in mesangial cells: A fluorescence analysis using the dye, PBFI. *Am J Physiol* 1992; 262:F462–F467.

53. Seftel AD, Viola KA, Kasner SE, Ganz MB: Nitric oxide relaxes rabbit corpus cavernosum smooth muscle via a potassium-conductive pathway. *Biochem Biophys Res Commun* 1996; 219:382–387.

54. Fan SF, Brink PR, Melmam A, Christ G: Analysis of maxi-K+ (Kca) channel in cultured human corporal smooth muscle cells. *J Urol* 1995; 153:818.

55. Adams MA, Bantinh J, Manabe K, Morales A, Heaton JPW: The major role for nitric oxide in the penis is to regulate the vasoconstrictor actions of endothelins. *Int J Imp Res* 1996; 8, 124(abstract D07).

56. Carrier S, Zvara P, Nunes L, Kour NW, Rehman J, Lue TF: Regeneration of nitric oxide synthase-containing nerves after cavernous nerve neurotomy in the rat. *J Urol* 1995; 153:1237.

57. Griffith ER, Trieschmann RB: Sexual functioning in women with spinal cord injury. *Arch Phys Med Rehab* 1975; 56:18–21.

58. Jenkins AD, Turner TT, Howards SS: Physiology of the male reproductive system. *Urol Clin N Am* 1978; 5:437.

59. Koraitim M, Schafer W, Melchior H, Lutzeyer W: Dynamic activity of bladder neck and external sphincter in ejaculation. *Urology* 1977; 10:130.

60. Talbot HS: The sexual functioning in paraplegia. *J Urol* 1955; 73:91–100.

61. Bors E, Comarr AE: Neurologic disturbances of sexual

function with special reference to 529 patients with spinal cord injury. *Urol Surv* 1960; 10:191–222.

62. Comarr AE: Sexual function among patients with spinal cord injury. *Urol Int* 1970; 25:134–168.

63. Munro D, Horne HH Jr, Paull DP: The effect of injury to the spinal cord and cauda equina on the sexual potency of men. *NEJM* 1948; 239:903–911.

64. Brindley GS: The fertility of men with spinal injuries. *Paraplegia* 1984; 22:337.

65. Leriche A, Berard E, Vauzelle JL, Minaire P, Girard R, Archimbaud JP, Bourret J: Historical and hormonal testicular changes in spinal cord patients. *Paraplegia* 1977; 15:274–279.

66. Beretta G, Chelo E, Zanollo A: Reproductive aspects in spinal cord injured males. *Paraplegia* 1989; 27:113.

67. Oates RD, Staskin DR: *Vibratory stimulation of ejaculation in the spinal cord injured male.* Presented at American Fertility Society 45th Annual Meeting. San Francisco, Nov. 1989.

68. Perkash I, Martin DE, Warner H, Speck V: Electroejaculation in spinal cord injury patients: Simplified new equipment and technique. *J Urol* 1990; 143:305.

69. Lerner BD, Hellerstein DK, Meacham RB, et al: *Rectal probe electroejaculation in anejaculatory men.* Presented at American Fertility Society 46th Annual Meeting. Washington, DC. Oct. 1990.

70. Bennett CJ, Seager SW, Vasher EA, McGuire EJ: Sexual dysfunction and electroejaculation in men with spinal cord injury: Review. *J Urol* 1988; 139:453.

71. Ayers JWT, Moinipanah R, Bennett JC, et al: Successful combination therapy with electroejaculation and in vitro fertilization: Embryo transfer in the treatment of a paraplegic male with severe oligoasthenospermia. *J Urol* 1988; 49:1089.

72. Mulhall JP, Burgess CM, Cunningham D, Carson R, Harris D, Oates RD: Presence of mature sperm in testicular parenchyma of men with nonobstructive azoospermia: Prevalence and predictive factors. *Urology* 1997; 49:91.

73. Collins KP, Hackler RH: Complications of penile prostheses in the spinal cord injury population. *J Urol* 1988; 140:984–985.

74. Rossier AB, Fam BA: Indications and results of semirigid penile prostheses in spinal cord injury patients: long term follow up. *J Urol* 1989; 131:59–62.

75. Steidle CP, Mulcahy JJ: Erosion of penile prosthesis: A complication of urethral catheterization. *J Urol* 1989; 142:736–739.

76. Perkash I, Kabalin JN, Lennon S, et al: Use of penile prostheses to maintain external condom catheter drainage in spinal cord injured patients. *Paraplegia* 1992; 30:327.

77. Lederer O: May 8, 1917. Surgical device. US patent number 1,255,341.

78. Nadig PW, Ware JC, Blumoff R: Noninvasive device to produce and maintain an erection-like state. *Urology* 1986; 27:126–131.

79. Turner LA, Althof SE, Levine SB, et al: Treating erectile dysfunction with external vacuum devices: Impact upon sexual, psychological and marital functioning. *J Urol* 1990; 144:79–82.

80. Lloyd EE, Toth LL, Perkash I: Vacuum tumescence: An option for spinal cord injured males with erectile dysfunction. *SCI Nurs* 1989; 6:25–28.

81. Meinhardt W, Lyeklama A, Nijeholt AAB, Kropman RF, Zwartendijk J: The negative pressure device for erectile disorders: When does it fail? *J Urol* 1993; 149:1285–1287.

82. NIH Consensus Development Panel on Impotence. *JAMA* 1993; 270:83–90.

83. Michal V, Kramer R, Pospichal J: Arterial epigastrico cavernous anastomosis for the treatment of sexual impotence. *World J Surg* 1977; 1:515–520.

84. Virag R: Intracavernous injection of papaverine for erectile failure (Letter). *Lancet* 1982; 2:938.

85. Brindley GS: Cavernosal alpha-blockade: A new technique for investigating and treating erectile impotence. *Br J Psychiatry* 1983; 143:332–337.

86. Virag R: About pharmacologically induced prolonged erection. (Letter). *Lancet* 1985; 2:519.

87. Zorgniotti AW, LeFleur RS: Auto-injection of the corpus cavernosum with a vasoactive drug combination for vasculogenic impotence. *J Urol* 1985; 133:39–41.

88. Sidi AA, Chen KK: Clinical experience with vasoactive intracavernous pharmacotherapy for treatment of impotence. *World J Urol* 1987; 5(3):156–159.

89. Bodner DR, Lindan R, Leffler E: The application of intracavernous injection of vasoactive medications for erection in men with spinal cord injury. *J Urol* 1987; 138:310–311.

90. Wyndaele JJ, De Meyer JM, De Sy WA, et al: Intracavernous injection of vasoactive drugs: One alternative for treating impotence in spinal cord injury patients. *Paraplegia* 1986; 24:271–275.

91. Bodner DR, Frost F, Leffler E: The role of intracorporeal injection of vasoactive medications for restoration of erection in the SCI male: A three year follow up. *Paraplegia* 1992; 30:118–120.

92. Lloyd KL, Richards JS: Intracorporeal injections in spinal cord injury: Two year follow up. *Am Spinal Cord Inj Assoc* Abstracts Dig. 1990; 68.

93. Levine SB, Althof SE, Turner LA, et al: Side effects of self-administration of intracavernous papaverine and phentolamine for the treatment of impotence. *J Urol* 1989; 141:54–57.

94. Chen J, Godschalk P, Katz PG, Mulligan T: The lowest effective dose of prostaglandin E1 as treatment of erectile dysfunction. *J Urol* 1995; 153:80–81.

95. Godschalk MF, Chen J, Katz PG, Mulligan T: Prostaglandin E1 as treatment for erectile failure in elderly men. *J Am Ger Soc* 1994; 42:1263–1265.

96. Padma-Nathan H, Hellstrom WJG, Kaiser FE, Labasky RF, Lue TF, Wolfram EN, Norwood PC, Peterson CA, Shabsigh R, Tam PY, Place VA, Gesundheit N: Treatment of men with erectile dysfunction with transurethral alprostadil. *NEJM* 1997; 336:1.

Part IV

THERAPEUTIC INTERVENTION IN NEUROLOGIC REHABILITATION

Chapter 26

ORTHOTICS IN NEUROLOGIC DISEASE

Robin Soffer
Mindy Lipson Aisen

The practice of neurorehabilitation requires careful attention to all aspects of the patient's condition. The goal of this clinical discipline is to arrest the disease process, improve damaged nervous system function, restore the ability to perform activities of daily living, and prevent and treat the medical or surgical complications of chronic neurologic impairment. A knowledge of orthotics as a discipline can be indispensible.

Orthoses are external devices for the limbs and spinal column that serve to correct position, protect joint alignment, and enhance functional adaptation. Orthoses can be static or dynamic, mechanical or power-driven. Fundamental knowledge of the potential benefits, limitations, and complications of orthoses can be important for patients to reach full rehabilitation potential.

Principles of orthotic prescription, focusing on the needs of the neurologically impaired, basic definitions and terminology, and an overview of the methods and materials employed in orthosis manufacture are provided. The specific issues encountered in different classes of neurologic diseases also are reviewed.

BASIC DEFINITIONS, TERMINOLOGY, AND CONCEPTS

Orthotics is the discipline that addresses the principles involved in the design and construction of devices to aid or improve the function or position of movable body parts. The devices are called *orthoses,* of which there are numerous types with varied indications. Individual orthosis prescriptions are best achieved through the joint efforts of an involved physician, an occupational or physical therapist, and a professional who designs and produces orthoses, the orthotist. Certified orthotists are knowledgeable about the properties of materials available, body mechanics, movement patterns, and anatomy. By convention, orthoses are named for the joints they cover and the force and support exerted there. Examples are KAFO (knee-ankle-foot orthosis) or TLSO (thoraco-lumbo-sacral orthosis).

Orthotic devices were first used to splint fractures. Subsequently, their use expanded to include corrective and protective roles for orthopedic injuries and deformities. The use of orthotics in substitutive and assistive capacities in patients with weakness of neurologic origin is a relatively recent development. The adaptation of orthotic devices for neurologic conditions has required that attention be paid to normal and pathologic motor patterns, and basic biomechanical principles. In addition to weakness, aberrations in motor function include spasticity, abnormal reflexes, and involuntary movement. Perceptual disturbances must also be considered. Neurologic functioning affects and is affected by the design of the orthosis. Proper prescription of orthoses requires an understanding of standardized nomenclature and patterns of motor impairment common to specific neurologic conditions.

Orthoses are used for supplementation and substitution, protection and correction. Modern braces use a combination of biomechanical principles. They rely on force systems and neurophysiologic principles to assist muscle control and decrease tone by using reflexes, postures, and pressure. Forces may be created and applied, for instance, by increasing the bulk of plastic on one side of a brace to facilitate a reflex.[1] A set of forces may be applied in multiple places on a limb to inhibit a posture. Some systems strive to facilitate useful reflexes, others to diminish counterproductive ones, with the goal of promoting functional movement.

Joints may be incorporated into an orthosis to assist or modify motion. The inclusion of a stop, a mechanical brake, in the joint can serve to augment or limit movement under different circumstances.

449

MATERIALS AND MANUFACTURE

Historically, orthoses were made from leather straps and metal supports. Metals are traditional materials, and include stainless steel, aluminum, and titanium magnesium alloys. Steel is inexpensive, easily molded, strong, and rigid. It is also very heavy. Steel is used in prefabricated orthotic joints, cables and motors. Aluminum is much lighter, but has poor resistance to fatigue at high load levels and is more often used in bracing the upper limb. Titanium alloys are lightweight and as strong as steel, but more costly.

Metal-and-leather combinations produce a durable system that permits the incorporation of joints if needed, at the cost of bulk and weight. Furthermore, the forces applied by such orthoses are confined to relatively focal areas of skin from strap contact, resulting in a higher potential for skin breakdown or local discomfort. Metal-and-leather orthoses may be the optimal choice in the setting of limb edema, because they are not form-fitting. If the brace is subjected to heavy use, they are especially useful.

Plastic orthoses are any synthetic materials that can be hardened or molded.[2–4] Plastic braces are lightweight and strong, and can be used to create complex shapes. Braces made of plastic can insert into the patient's own shoes, are custom-molded to permit a better distribution of forces over skin contours, and are water-resistant. Flexibility and rigidity are controlled by the thickness and shaping of the plastic. The extent to which a plastic orthosis envelops a joint, known as its "trimline," affects degree of flexibility and the amount of support provided, which varies among patients.[5] Though joints can be incorporated into plastic orthoses, often the flexibility of the material alone is adequate to permit limited joint motion.

There are many types of plastic available for use in orthotics, and differences in mechanical properties determine which one is most appropriate in each case. Thermoplastics are hard at lower temperatures and soften at higher ones. They can be molded and remolded. Low temperature thermoplastics soften at 180°F, and can be formed directly on a body segment. These include polypropylene, the most rigid and most widely used thermoplastic for lower extremity orthoses. Thickness varies from 3 to 6 mm and increases with the age and size of the patient, and the need for greater stiffness.[5]

The second commonly used thermoplastic is co-polymer plastic, made from a combination of polypropylene and the more flexible polyethylene. It is of inter-mediate rigidity, but more durable than polypropylene. Polyethylene is used for nonweight-bearing or total circumference orthoses, or as a closure panel. These braces are translucent. Transparent plastics are also available that allow better inspection of the underlying skin.

A third type of thermoplastic is elastomere, derived from urethane rubber. Although more flexible, permitting a more dynamic splint, elastomere offers less support than other thermoplastics.

Compared to thermoplastics, thermosetting plastics are light and strong, but can be rigid and brittle. They develop a permanent shape when formed and cannot be reheated and reshaped. The advantage of thermosetting plastics is that they can be laminated, pigmented, drilled, and riveted to create joints. Because of their strength, they are especially helpful when transverse rotational forces must be limited.

Newer materials allow the fabrication of lightweight devices that provide enormous durability, strength, and rotational stability. These include Kevlar, the substance from which bulletproof vests are made and composites of braided carbon fiber bonded with epoxy resin. Alternatively, thermosetting plastics can be laminated with carbon fiber to increase strength. Such materials are particularly useful for the ambulatory patient with chronic, profound spasticity or weakness.

Plastic orthoses can be either custom-molded or mass-produced in uniform sizes. Plastic braces produced in bulk are less expensive, and readily available, but may not be suitable for specific bracing needs. No matter what bracing material is selected, design consistency is desirable when replacements are necessary over the duration of a lifetime on an ongoing basis.

Complex dynamic orthoses are sometimes required under some circumstances. Such devices may be power-assisted, using electricity or cables and hydraulics, or incorporate functional electrical stimulation to augment forces generated by weak or paralyzed muscle groups.

GENERAL PRINCIPLES OF PRESCRIPTION

Although the orthotist designs and builds the brace, the rehabilitation physician prescribes it, and must recognize complications and order revisions when necessary. The neurological impairments that are most amenable to therapy with bracing are weakness, spasticity, and tremor.[2,4,6,7]

Orthoses necessarily apply rotational forces to limb segments around the anatomic joint. Rotational forces are not possible unless there are at least three points of contact between the device and limb. Care must be taken when choosing the pressure points to seek anatomic sites with muscle and fat tissue. Skin breakdown can be avoided by using a long lever arm and increasing the area over which pressure is applied. Brace and anatomic joints should be aligned to minimize shearing forces.[2,8]

In neurologic disease orthotic devices are generally applied to distal limb portions. This is owing to a combination of factors. First, weakness in neurologic disease is often greatest distally. Second, distal strength and preservation of motion may be more important for "real-life" activities. Finally, proximal limb bracing is cumbersome and can limit range of motion across joints that allow movement in multiple planes, leading to loss of function. Furthermore, distally placed braces often improve proximal limb control through transmitted mechanical forces.

Appropriate prescription requires an understanding of movement patterns in the normal case as well as in the case of the particular pathology affecting the patient.[9–11] The clinician must be familiar not only with the characteristic neurological deficits (sensory impairment, neglect, weakness, fatiguability, tone changes), but with the temporal pattern of illness (progressive, static, improving, relapsing). These principles determine the type of brace, design features, and the need for long-term follow-up.

Orthoses impede some movements while aiding others, and decisions must be made individually as to whether a brace will improve the overall function.[2,12] For example, joint stabilization may be enhanced by heavier metal braces at the expense of function. Goals must be considered carefully, with an eye to compromises when necessary for the sake of improved function.

A brace usually will be most effective when the patient and family have realistic expectations. Satisfaction and compliance will be limited if the orthosis fails to save energy or makes real-life tasks more difficult. The ideal brace must be comfortable and easy to don and doff. Aesthetics also are important, including appearance, as well as ease of maintenance.

Orthoses must be cost-effective in order to recommend routine prescription. Most expenses relate to the orthotist's time, the expense of materials and manufacture (including casting), and follow-up. The addition of joints, modifications, or adjustments for tone reduction to a plastic AFO can increase cost substantially. Custom long leg braces used for paraplegic ambulation are especially costly. To justify the expense, braces must signifi-

cantly improve quality of life and functional independence.

COMMONLY PRESCRIBED BRACES

Nearly all braces are assistive (as in upper-extremity orthoses in spinal-cord injury) or protective (as in resting hand splints to prevent deformity in stroke). The most commonly prescribed braces are those that assist ambulation: ankle-foot orthoses (AFO) and knee-ankle-foot orthoses (KAFO).

AFOs brace the ankle and compensate for foot drop resulting from weak ankle dorsiflexion.[13] They also prevent injury to the ankle or to the knee by preventing excessive plantar flexion and resultant genu recurvatum. AFOs also help overcome quadriceps weakness and knee buckling. Figure 26-1 shows two types of AFOs, the posterior leaf spring (PLS) and a solid-ankle AFO. The former is flexible and allows some degree of motion

Figure 26-1

A solid ankle-foot orthosis (AFO) contrasted with a posterior leaf spring (PLS).

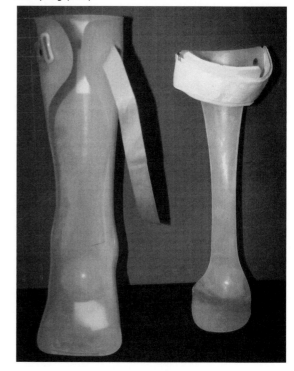

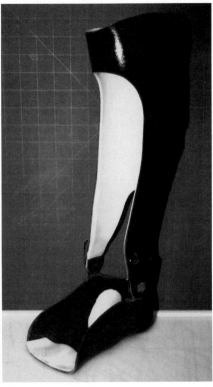

Figure 26-2
A knee-locking floor reaction splint with a double-action (adjustable) ankle joint. It is fabricated from a Kevlar carbon-fiber composite.

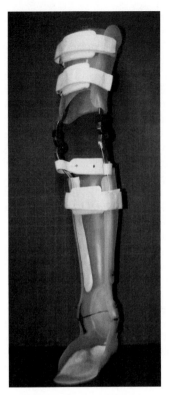

Figure 26-3
A knee-ankle-foot orthosis (KAFO) with posterior offset knee joints, drop-locks, and an articulated ankle.

around the joint for the individual with mild weakness and with adequate mediolateral stability. The PLS provides a spring-like force that pushes the foot back into dorsiflexion following "toe-off."[14] The solid-ankle AFO is used for the patient who requires rigid support owing to weakness, spasticity, or mediolateral instability.[7]

Spasticity is another neurologic symptom that may be improved by the use of the AFO.[1,7] Increased extensor tone at the hip and knee can help ambulation in the setting of paresis. On the other hand, excessive soleus tone produces plantar flexion and supination at the ankle that can adversely affect walking. This can impair gait by interfering with toe clearance, promote lateral weight bearing and ankle injury, and drive the knee into hyperextension.[2] A rigid AFO that corrects equinovarus, dorsiflexes the foot, and decreases tone can be especially helpful here.

AFOs can alter knee biomechanics either favor-

ably or unfavorably. By rigidly fixing the ankle in dorsiflexion, APOs can be used to prevent or correct genu recurvatum. Alternatively they can assist knee stability, by placing the ankle joint in a slightly plantar-flexed position and causing a minor degree of knee hyperextension. Figure 26-2 shows a knee-locking floor reaction splint. For those using such devices, frequent assessments of skin and knee-joint integrity, particularly if sensory perception is impaired, are mandatory.

With severe quadriceps weakness knee support for stability and ligamentous protection may be required. The KAFO, shown in Figure 26-3, is useful in this setting. Mediolateral as well as anterior-posterior control is provided at the ankle and knee joints. Other long leg braces include Craig-Scott hip-knee-ankle-foot orthoses (HKAFOs), shown in Figure 26-4. These very durable braces are used almost exclusively by paraplegics who advance their legs by using abdominal musculature as "hip-hikers." For some, the weight of these

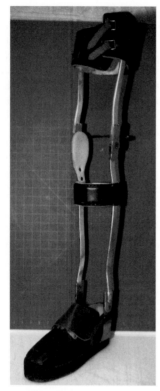

Figure 26-4
A Craig-Scott brace.

braces may render the gait pattern inefficient, and may therefore be of limited usefulness. The energy requirements for this form of ambulation may become so great that the bracing with long leg braces is useless.

The commonly used upper-limb braces are dorsal and volar wrist supports, thumb post splints, mobile arm supports, and slings. The specific indications for these braces are covered in the sections that follow.

SPECIFIC NEUROLOGIC CONDITIONS IN WHICH ORTHOSES ARE INDICATED

Stroke

Substantial functional return in the upper extremity after stroke is far less likely than for the lower extremity for most stroke types.[15–18] Bracing the upper limb after

stroke is recommended for protective and corrective reasons, rather than assistive. In the lower extremity, orthoses are used for correction of abnormal joint pain owing to increased extensor tone, protection of joints from injury due to weakness or altered tone, and restoration of ambulation.

Upper Extremity Bracing in Stroke Therapeutic bracing of the arm after stroke is useful in the prevention of shoulder-joint complications, reducing contractures distally, and limiting hand edema. Of the few stroke patients that regain use of their affected upper extremity most have a limb that serves as a gross functional assist for the unaffected limb. Because upper-extremity orthoses limit range of motion and limb use, they are used most often to maintain correct posture and joint alignment.

Upper-extremity orthoses also are useful in the prevention of shoulder subluxation, and injuries to articular structures and soft tissues (including the rotator cuff) owing to trauma and abnormal posture.[19,20] The relationship between mechanical injury and the development of sympathetically maintained pain following stroke is controversial. The risk of shoulder subluxation leading to sympathetically nucleated pain by soft-tissue injury must be counterbalanced against the risk of shoulder immobilization leading to frozen-shoulder syndrome.

The primary classes of devices used are shoulder support systems consisting of slings, wheelchair lap boards, troughs, wrist and hand splints, and foam wedges.[21] Shoulder supports should elevate and externally rotate the scapulae, while maintaining proper alignment of the glenohumeral joint. Common slings include vertical humeral cuff slings, "figure 8" clavicular slings and Bobath slings with axillary roll. Supplemental support for the humerus may be provided in ambulatory patients by providing distal support to the thumb and wrist with a sling. When seated, proper positioning is achieved with a clear lap board, with or without an armed trough, to prevent internal humeral rotation and pectoralis major shortening.

Wrist-hand orthoses help maintain a neutral position, reduce flexor tone, and prevent development of contractures. They are constructed of thermoplastics, secured with Velcro straps, and apply pressure to the forearm, wrist, and digits or palm. Fingers generally rest on a platform, although forearm contact may be dorsal or volar. Palm contact is avoided, as it may increase flexor tone.[22] When a hand-wrist splint is not used, a firm cone placed in the hand may prevent finger contracture.

Avoiding contractures is important to hygiene and skin integrity as well as appearance.

Edema owing to disuse and gravity can be reduced or eliminated with compression gloves, elevation of the distal limb with a foam wedge on the lap board or armrest, or, when in bed, with pillows. In extreme cases intermittent compression pumps are used.

Lower-Extremity Bracing in Stroke The most commonly prescribed lower extremity brace is the AFO.[23] The vast majority of stroke patients will regain the ability to walk, generally with assistive devices.[24] Lower-extremity bracing can improve speed and reduce energy consumption for the stroke patient. The typical hemiplegic gait is slow and energy-consuming, even at slower walking speeds. Bracing may be needed to correct weakness, abnormal posturing, disinhibited reflexes, reduced range of motion, and loss of fine motor control.

The pattern and degree of muscle weakness and spasticity determine the components of the orthotic prescription. When tibialis anterior weakness and foot drop are present, for example, toes make initial floor contact. A PLS may provide adequate ankle support if mediolateral ankle stability is not impaired. However, a PLS does not resist dorsiflexion significantly, and cannot be used to compensate for quadriceps weakness.

If exaggerated hip-knee flexion enables the toes to clear the floor on gait swing-through, an AFO may not be needed. If the exaggerated compensatory movements are not adequate, a flexible AFO that assists dorsiflexion can improve toe clearance. When excessive ankle dorsiflexion during stance phase owing to soleus weakness is present, knee buckling occurs. If the quadriceps are weak, compensatory knee hyperextension occurs. This can lead to arthropathy and ligamentous damage over time. A rigid AFO that limits dorsiflexion may be indicated in this setting.

AFOs that assist dorsiflexion are insufficient when toe drag is owing to hip and knee flexor weakness. Even if bracing encompasses the knee (as with a KAFO), functional ambulation may not result because proximal weakness leads to excessive circumduction and trunk deviations to advance the limb.[25]

Although increased extensor tone in the hemiplegic patient often permits weight-bearing, excessive ankle inversion and plantar flexion may require suppression with an AFO. Plantar flexion, whether owing to spasticity or contracture, will interfere with dorsiflexion as weight is transferred to that leg, resulting in knee hyperextension. A rigid AFO set in dorsiflexion will eliminate knee hyperextension and improve stride. When knee hyperextension occurs, the 'knee cage' is a useful device that permits flexion but prevents recurvatum.

Ankle inversion promotes weight-bearing over the lateral plantar surface of the foot. Rigid plastic AFOs with anterior trim lines, as well as certain metal and leather AFOs (with double uprights with or without a T-bar or shoe-insert arch supports) will prevent inversion. Lesser degrees of mediolateral stability can be attained with air-cast AFOs.

Excessive toe flexion owing to spasticity or contracture can make weight-bearing painful, and lead to orthopedic deformities. This can be prevented with a foam pad under the toes in some cases.

Multiple Sclerosis

In contrast to stroke, multiple sclerosis (MS) requires special consideration because of its highly variable nature, with progression over time with or without interval improvements, and its ability to cause multifaceted symptoms.[26] These include not only weakness and sensory loss, but cognitive decline, ataxia, tremor, visual disturbances, difficulty communicating owing to dysarthria, incontinence, and fatiguability. Despite recent therapeutic advances, it is likely that MS treatment will have a continued emphasis on symptomatic treatment and rehabilitation. The variability and potentially progressive nature of this disease, as well as its long duration, must influence orthotic prescription.

Lower-Extremity Bracing in MS Lower-extremity bracing and other assistive devices are often prescribed to improve gait. Some symptoms, especially fatigue and spasticity, manifested as dragging of the lower limbs, may be amenable to bracing. As with stroke, upper-motor neuron signs of spasticity and weakness may cause toe drag or foot drop during the swing phase of gait, or ankle inversion and poor push-off. AFOs are useful for correction of excessive plantar flexion and ankle inversion, and improve toe clearance. The optimal brace must be simple to put on and remove. Polypropylene AFOs are favored over metal-and-leather exoskeleton AFOs because of their lighter weight.

Individual prescription is influenced by considerations similar to those discussed for stroke. Gait observation is necessary to observe patterns of weakness, spasticity, and joint instability in different phases. Often the AFO is constructed to provide a limited amount of dorsiflexion (5–10 degrees) to permit toe clearance during the swing phase of gait. Plantar flexion and heel-strike should not be limited so that the knee is not thrown into flexion, causing it to buckle. A slightly dorsiflexed position of the AFO is recommended to reduce the tendency for the knee to hyperextend during early stance phase. When substantial quadricep weakness is present, knee buckling may be avoided by modifying the shoe in such a fashion as to move the site of force applied on heel-strike anteriorly. Occasionally, knee cages or KAFOs are needed to protect the knee from capsule and ligamentous damage owing to repetitive hyperextension.

Upper-Extremity Bracing in MS   Many deficits occur that can impair upper extremity function in MS. Pyramidal and cerebellar dysfunction commonly impair both fine and gross motor function of the upper extremity. The fluctuating nature of MS may make complex orthoses less appropriate than for other neurologic conditions. Nevertheless, sophisticated tremor-dampening splints have shown promise experimentally.[6]

Wrist cock-up splints are often used to functionally position the hand and prevent injury. It is possible to modify such splints to attach utensils and writing implements.[27,28] Wrist splinting in extension can facilitate functional finger flexion through tenodesis.

Spinal-Cord Injury

Spinal-cord injury (SCI) rehabilitation requires prescription adaptive devices, trunk or cervical braces, and mobility aids.[29,30] Spine-stabilizing orthoses are used acutely after injury. Upper-extremity and lower-extremity braces can play an essential role in assisting function in activation of daily living and ambulation.

The SCI patient arrives on the rehabilitation unit with axial bracing prescribed during acute care in place. The rehabilitation physician must supervise the ongoing use of the device, monitoring brace adjustments and weaning, and thus must have an understanding of the relative merits of different braces, their potential complications, and proper use and withdrawal.

Neck Braces   There are a variety of neck braces that stabilize and immobilize the cervical spine.[31] The need for stabilization is greatest immediately following the injury or surgery. Weaning depends on radiographic evidence of healing and stability, and typically occurs 2–3 months later. The commonly used devices are the halo traction system, which provides nearly complete immobilization, and the Philadelphia collar, which limits flexion and extension but permits rotation.

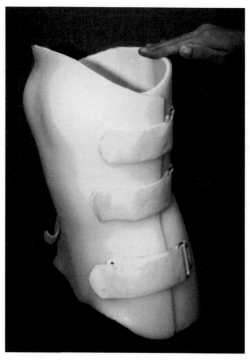

Figure 26-5
A bivalve thoraco-lumbral-sacral orthosis (TLSO), used for support and stabilization after thoraco-lumbar spine injuries.

Thoracic and Lumbar Braces   Back braces are required during many phases of care following spinal-cord injury. In the acute stage, the purpose is to offer support until there is x-ray evidence of fusion.[2] After the fusion has solidified, weaning can be instituted. Spine stability is reached 4–6 months after injury or surgery.

Bracing after spine stability is reached can help prevent back deformities, such as scoliosis, particularly in growing children.

Body jackets, made of molded plastic with padding (Figure 26-5), are commonly used. The anterior and posterior sections are bivalved, and attached with Velcro. Potential complications include skin breakdown, respiratory compromise, and exacerbation of disordered thermoregulation.

Arm Braces and Orthoses   Upper extremity braces are used during the acute and chronic phases after spinal-cord injury. In the acute stage, splints are used protectively. In the subacute phase, splinting promotes residual limb function by proper positioning of the hand and arm to ready them for grasp, and substitution to facilitate grasp. The level of the injury will determine what can realistically be achieved with bracing. With a C5 lesion, shoulder movement and elbow flexion will be preserved, allowing proper position of the hand, but no grasp, either actively or using tenodesis. Preserved C6 function permits active wrist extension, allowing tenodesis grasp.

To understand the role of bracing in the quadriplegic hand, the effects of wrist position on normal hand function must be discussed. The wrist extends during finger flexion and flexes during finger extension, through a range of 20–30 degrees. This mechanically reduces the amount of voluntary contraction required to produce hand motion. If finger flexors are weak, setting the wrist in extension facilitates grasp. If the stressors are weak, splint in a neutral or slightly flexed position.

Four major categories of arm and hand braces used in quadriplegia are counter-balanced overhead slings, mobile arm supports, wrist splints, and hand splints. Counterbalanced overhead slings require some C5 function to place the limb and are primarily used for therapeutic exercise.

Mobile arm supports (MAS), also known as balanced forearm orthoses, require attachment to a wheelchair or regular chair.[32] These facilitate gravity-eliminated elbow flexion and extension, and are most often used in the C5–6 quadriplegic. Modified MAS devices, which are spring-loaded at the shoulder can help with actions such as shoulder abduction. Distal attachments can be added to position or support forearm and hands. Activities of daily living, such as self-feeding, may be facilitated. The distal arm piece is designed to be lateralized for function, and is not interchangeable.

Dynamic wrist splints enhance tenodesis. An external power source will be required for patients with C5 or higher lesions. Activation of these devices is controlled by a switch that the patient controls by elbow or shoulder movement. Simple mechanical splints, such as the tenodesis splint, pull the fingers into flexion as the wrist extends by a string attached to the volar wrist surface, improving tenodesis in the patient with C6 function.

Static wrist extension splints facilitate tenodesis and prevent flexion injuries. Wrist splints also protect against overstretching of extensors and may be used at night to prevent contractures. They can also be combined with thumb post splints to promote better finger flexion and grasp. Thumb post splints are small braces that fit over the thumb to overcome laxity or weakness of the carpal-metacarpal or metacarpal-phalangeal joints. The splint places the thumb in a position to meet the first two fingers, serving as a "post" against which the fingers can operate.

Lower-Extremity Braces Prescription of leg braces requires attention to the level of injury, the neurological function below the injury, and the underlying goal of bracing. Orthoses are used for joint protection, therapeutic standing, and functional ambulation. The higher the level of injury, the greater number of joints which will need to be braced. Alternating leg movement in patients with thoracic lesions may require a reciprocating gait orthosis (RGO) system, which consists of long leg braces connected by a cable system and a body plate.

With lesions below L3, hip flexion, abduction, and some degree of knee extension will be preserved. If quadriceps weakness is present, KAFOs with knee locks may be prescribed. Knee locks release the knees into flexion for sitting, and may be activated manually or by pressure from the chair surface. Plastic or metal-leather exoskeleton orthoses, such as the Craig Scott brace, are often used. For others, AFO modified floor-reaction boots may be appropriate.

Lesions below L4–L5 produce weakness limited to the ankle. For these individuals, the AFO is most appropriate. Substantial support generally is required, and solid-ankle AFOs set in a small degree of dorsiflexion are often recommended. Laminated materials containing carbon fiber can enhance strength and durability if heavy use is expected.

Ambulation The need to walk and stand is expressed often after spinal-cord injury. This can be a challenging goal. There are theoretical advantages and disadvantages to modified orthotic standing or walking after SCI. The relative benefits and risks for therapeutic bracing are listed in Table 26-1.

Standing frames offer a less costly alternative to dynamic walking braces, with many of the same benefits, where ambulation is not a realistic long-term goal. Selection of patients for prescription of ambulation orthotics should be done with care. As a rule of thumb, children who have not reached skeletal maturity have significant ambulation potential with complete lesions below T6. For adults and children who are mature in growth, this level is at or below T10. In general, younger age and incomplete nature of lesions are factors associated with a higher rate of continued use of the ambulation devices after discharge. Higher or more complete lesions, significant impairment of proprioception, poor motivation, spasticity, and discomfort from the devices tend to be

Table 26-1
Possible advantages and disadvantages of therapeutic bracing

Possible advantages	Disadvantages
Psychological health	Tremendous energy expenditure (400–1300% increase)
Lower incidence of pressure sores, owing to less sitting	Overuse of upper extremities when using walkers, crutches, and canes, leading to pathologic strain on upper extremity joints and ligaments
Improved bowel evacuation	
Facilitation of ADL related to standing	Expense
Maintenance of residual muscle functions	Frequent maintenance needs
Prevention of lower-extremity contractures	Amount of time needed for training, use, and maintenance
Enhancement of cardiopulmonary function	Threat to skin integrity from brace pressure
Diminished incidence of osteoporosis	

Sources: Fisher LR, McLellan DL: Questionnaire assessment of patient satisfaction with lower limb orthoses from a district hospital. *Pros Orth Int* 1989; 13:29–35. Fisher SV, Gullickson G: Energy cost of ambulation in health and disability: A literature review. *Arch Phys Med Rehab* 1978; 59:124–133. Merkel KD, Miller NE, Westbrook PR, Merritt JL: Energy expenditure of paraplegic patients standing and walking with two knee-ankle-foot orthoses. *Arch Phys Med Rehab* 1984; 65:121–124.

associated with poor orthotic acceptance following discharge.[33–37]

Functional electrical stimulation (FES) uses electrical stimulation to peripheral nerves below the level of injury to generate muscle contractions that can be used for standing and walking. FES can be coupled with orthotic devices in selected spinal-cord-injury patients with leg weakness to assist in reaching these goals.[38–40] Isokinetic strengthening must precede FES-orthotic assisted standing in order to prepare the muscles and bones for weight-bearing.

FES may serve as an adjunct to voluntary upper extremity exercises to achieve better aerobic conditioning than might otherwise be obtained through upper-extremity or lower-extremity exercises alone.

Once isokinetic strengthening and conditioning have been achieved FES is applied to bilateral gluteal, hamstring, and quadriceps muscles.[40–43] Muscle fatigue, electrode failure, and skin infections at the stimulation site may limit use. Preserved sensation below the injury can be a barrier to successful use of FES because electrical stimulation can be quite painful.

Most FES systems have control, feedback, and interface components. The controller regulates the amount of stimulation and spatial and temporal sequences of muscle stimulation. Various parameters may be used for feedback in addition to or instead of EMG, in order to modify the intensity of the stimulation and initiate the next stimulation in the sequence. Interface

with the patient muscle usually is through surface electrodes connected to stimulators that provide current.

PERIPHERAL NEUROPATHIES

The protective, corrective, and substitutive roles of orthoses can be applied to optimize the function of those with peripheral neuropathy.[44,45] Supplemental rehabilitation modalities, such as functional adaptation, sensory re-education, range of motion, and, occasionally, tendon transfers may be necessary.[46,47] Wearing time must be increased gradually. Monitoring for skin breakdown, vasomotor changes and comfort are required.

Splints may be static or dynamic. The former serve to protect the limb, position it properly and prevent stretch injuries. Dynamic splints permit unidirectional active movement of the weakened limb.[44]

Bracing Contractures

Orthotics play an important role in the prevention and management of contractures. For more extensive discussion, see Chapter 19.

Contracture and overstretching injury prevention is paramount when there is reversible paralysis.[46,47] Range of motion exercises and proper bracing may serve to effectively prevent some contractures from developing. Footboards and splints may prevent gastrocnemius and soleus contractures, and bed boards may prevent hip flexor and shoulder flexor contractures. If contractures develop, dynamic and static orthoses can offer gentle, prolonged stretching. Adjustable, padded, and hinged dynamic splints can be fabricated for nighttime use. Meticulous angle adjustment, skin inspection, and a gradual increase in wearing time are essential. Some dynamic splints permit active functional movement in one direction against resistance, while providing stretch in the opposite direction. This tension must be continuously readjusted as recovery progresses to optimize function and return.

Commonly Occurring Neuropathies

Radial Nerve   Most commonly, active wrist and metacarpal phalangeal joint extension are impaired, which reduces grasp and release.[46] Static splints with 30-degree wrist extension, and metacarpal phalangeal extension bars prevent overstretching and maintain the hand in a functional position. Dynamic splints permit active wrist extension, which results in passive finger flexion using tenodesis, permitting grasp. Static splints support wrist extension; in the active dynamic state they support metacarpal phalangeal extension and facilitate finger flexor movements.

Ulnar Nerve   Motor impairments involve wrist flexion, metacarpal phalangeal, and fourth- and fifth-digit proximal and distal interphalangeal joints; abduction and adduction of all fingers; and thumb abduction.[4] Sensory loss occurs in digits four and five. When there is significant ulnar motor involvement, prevention of metacarpal phalangeal joint hyperextension contracture is important. This can be accomplished with a lumbrical bar over digits four and five (static), with or without a dynamic interphalangeal extension assist. If the injury is longstanding and metacarpal phalangeal joint hyperextension and contracture have developed, a splint that applies a flexion force across the metacarpal phalangeal joint may be indicated to prevent progression and provide corrective forces. Wrist immobilization is required immediately after surgical repairs of traumatic lesions.

Median Nerve Lesions   Grasp is often reduced by impairment of thumb abduction and opposition and index and middle finger flexion. Hand function is also impaired by reduced sensation of the palmar and first through fourth digits. When there is significant weakness, splinting can prevent contracture and assist func-

tion. Splinting is also useful to aid in decompression in milder, primarily sensory disturbances (carpal tunnel syndrome). Static splints that maintain the wrist in neutral or from 20- to 30-angle extension with the fingers unrestricted, can be worn at night, and as tolerated by day. The more volar coverage the splint provides, the greater the protection offered, but the greater the restriction of hand function.[44,46,48]

When significant motor deficits are present, a static splint to prevent contracture between the first metacarpal and the thumb, usually employing a C-bar and an opponens bar, is useful. If the wrist is not immobilized, tenodesis can assist weakened finger flexion.

Brachial Plexus   Motor and sensory deficits may be proximal, distal, or mixed. For closed traumatic injuries, initial treatment usually is nonsurgical. Splinting goals include prevention of contractures, maintenance of joints in functional or neutral position, reduction of edema, and prevention of further nerve compression. Aggressive range-of-motion exercises and skin inspection also are required.[49]

In upper and total plexus injuries, shoulder slings may reduce edema, prevent shoulder subluxation, and secondary rotator cuff injury. Static hand splints prevent metacarpal phalangeal joint contractures and maintain the wrist and hand in neutral position. Even if innervation of the hand is intact, proximal weakness will reduce function owing to lack of ability to place and stabilize the hand. A mobile arm support can increase upper extremity use from the seated position. This is more successful when there is some proximal function.

Flail arm splints can be fabricated for those without any movement. These are activated by a cable controlled by the mobile intact shoulder. They offer proximal support to prevent shoulder subluxation as well as distal attachments and appliances to facilitate use of the injured arm when both hands are being used.

Lumbar Plexus and Femoral Nerve Lesions[45,48,50] Impaired hip flexion and knee extension with knee buckling during ambulation are the most commonly observed abnormalities. When motor function is severely impaired, plastic KAFOs improve knee extension by limiting ankle dorsiflexion and placing the foot in slight plantar flexion. In cases of bilateral lesions, plastic KAFOs with metal knee hinges can be used in order to permit knee flexion when sitting. For milder cases of quadriceps weakness, a cane or crutch may suffice in place of an orthosis.

Sciatic and Peroneal Nerve Lesions[45,51] Most commonly, ankle dorsiflexion and foot eversion are impaired. Weakness of knee extension, ankle plantar flexion, and foot inversion may be present. Bracing should be directed toward the prevention of falls and improvement of a gait rendered inefficient by lateral ankle instability and impaired toe clearance. This can be accomplished with either an AFO or PLSO. AFOs are preferred if there is reduced mediolateral ankle stability. If weakness is expected to improve, adjustability of the brace is important. Metal-leather AFOs may be more adjustable, but have some disadvantages discussed earlier. An overly rigid AFO can hinder plantar flexion. Knee hyperextension leading to genu recurvatum and traumatic arthropathy also may result if the ankle is overly rigid.

Polyneuropathies[2–8,47,52] Splinting should address functional impairments and proper anatomical alignment of affected joints. When sensory loss is severe, splints may cause disturbances of skin integrity and careful monitoring is necessary. Repeated modifications may be expected in progressive and reversible neuropathies. General principles regarding ease of application and removal, weight, bulk, and cosmesis apply.

Care of the Neuropathic Foot[53,54]

The foot is at risk in peripheral neuropathies owing to both sensory and motor deficits. Sensory loss may lead to foot injuries, including ulcers, neuropathic arthropathy ("Charcot joints"), and osteomyelitis. Injuries often are slow to heal even with proper treatment. Imbalances in calf and intrinsic foot musculature classically produce a high arched foot with the plantar aponeurosis contracture of pes cavus. This is typically accompanied by hammer toes, metatarsal phalangeal hyperextension, and interphalangeal joint flexion. A reduction in plantar surface-ground contact during ambulation results, which can be aggravated by coexisting foot drop, metatarsal calluses, foot pain, and fatigue.

For the insensate foot, frequent inspection is clearly important. Barefoot ambulation should be avoided, and shoes with a close heel fit, wide toe areas, and soft leather are recommended. If areas of incipient change are noted, the use of inserts that spread pressure and force over the entire foot and pad bony prominences should be prescribed. If the foot slides once the insert is placed, blisters may develop at the margins. Custom-molded insoles (total contact orthoses) worn in a shoe of extra depth may be required. Metatarsal heel bars, rocker bars, and rigid heels on the sole may prevent recurrent metatarsal head ulcers. Rocker-bottom shoes and heel cushions assist push-off when plantar flexion is weak.

Pes cavus can be treated with active and passive stretching, shoe modification, or ankle-foot orthoses. Shoe inserts or metatarsal bars are sufficient for many. When significant dorsiflexion weakness is present and insufficient to oppose plantar flexion forces, ankle-foot orthoses are useful. When pes cavus is owing to a non-progressive disorder, such as polio, surgical correction by tendon transfer may be necessary. When foot deformities, such as pes cavus predispose to pressure ulcers, surgical correction may be advised.

Charcot joints owing to peripheral neuropathy usually develop first in the feet.[47,55] Lateral deviation and pronation of the foot, collapse of the arch, and excessive weight-bearing by the talus are common. In extreme cases, varus and valgus deformity cause the malleoli to be weight-bearing surfaces. The use of supports and orthotics to normalize foot position can prevent or arrest the process that leads to Charcot joints.

Once a Charcot joint has developed, reduced ambulation and foot orthoses are recommended. Either a rigid AFO, to immobilize the ankle, or a patellar tendon weight-bearing orthosis that reduces distal weight bearing can prevent further damage and preserve ambulatory function.

NEUROMUSCULAR DISEASES

Orthotic prescription for neuromuscular dysfunction is a dynamic process that requires long-term follow-up and reevaluation. Joint and spinal deformities and contractures are common.

Corrective surgery must be coordinated diligently with orthotic intervention.

Spinal Muscular Atrophy (SMA)

Bracing may be extremely helpful in the milder forms of SMA with onset after infancy. Orthotic intervention should be directed toward devices that promote standing and walking, and delay or arrest the development of scoliosis

Standing and walking can be achieved and improved by the use of KAFOs. If the degree of weakness precludes KAFO use, devices incorporating a standing platform, trunk supports, and large wheels mounted on a frame may permit standing and independent mobility.

Scoliosis may be retarded by thoracolumbar spinal orthoses, but surgery generally is required for curves that exceed 340 degrees.

Postpolio Syndrome

Postpolio syndrome causes increasing limb and respiratory weakness, fatigue, pain, and progressive joint dysfunction.[57] Affected muscle groups may or may not have been involved at the time of the original viral paralytic illness. The recommendation that rehabilitation treatment should avoid exhausting exercise is controversial.[58] Orthotic devices can improve the efficiency of energy expenditure during exercise, correct gait abnormalities, and prevent further injury to already injured joints. Gentle stretching, strengthening, and aerobic exercises are important adjuncts to rehabilitative care.[59,60] Old braces that have been used for many years, perhaps since the acute polio infection, should be reevaluated, altered, or replaced.[61,62] Proper padding and positioning must be used on crutches and canes to avoid compression neuropathies.

Duchenne Muscular Dystrophy (DMD)

Duchenne muscular dystrophy is the most common and rapidly progressive of the dystrophies. The rehabilitation management of DMD encompasses most, if not all, of the therapeutic issues that arise in the other, less common, dystrophies. Limb and truncal weakness leads to compensatory postures. The child with DMD rapidly develops a striking gait pattern. This is characterized by toe walking with equinocavovarus posture (anterior greater than posterior calf weakness). Achilles tendon, triceps surae, and thigh flexion contractures soon follow. Gait and stance are wide-based. Quadriceps, iliopsoas, and tensor fascia latae weakness combine with hamstring contractures to displace the body's center of gravity anteriorly during walking. To compensate, lumbar lordosis and posteriorly held shoulders develop. Toe walking causes the knees to lock in spite of quadriceps weakness, a useful compensation.[63,64] As weakness and contractures progress, falling becomes more frequent, until ambulation is lost.

Skillful use of orthotics and surgery can stabilize contractures, support fragile joints, and facilitate naturally occurring compensatory biomechanical adjustments.[64,65] Bracing and corrective surgery offer psychological advantages, preserve muscle strength, and slow the progression of contractures and scoliosis. The adverse impact of progressive scoliosis on pulmonary function can be considerable. Gains in ambulation can be prolonged.

Bracing is appropriate when falls become more frequent, but ambulation is difficult when the quadriceps have less than antigravity power. If anterior lower extremity compartment weakness is present, an AFO set in 5–10 degrees equinus can be used to reduce steppage gait, but not eliminate the genu recurvatum that toe walking promotes. Both plastic and metal AFOs can be used. Metal braces provide more support and adjustability, at the expense of versatility and weight. Chronic and progressive genu recurvatum, a cause of knee pain and chondromalacia, can be prevented by orthotic augmentation of knee support. A Swedish knee cage or AFO in slight dorsiflexion can be especially useful for this.

Eventually, more substantial knee and ankle support are necessary. This can be obtained by using a KAFO.[66,67] These are typically made of polypropylene with lightweight steel side supports with hinges or locks at the knees, and are lighter than the traditional metal and leather exoskeleton KAFO. As proximal weakness progresses, a reciprocal gait orthosis may permit continued standing and ambulation.[66] Achilles-tendon release surgery may be required before brace fitting, in order to reduce ankle deformity and ensure that the heel is firmly in contact with the shoe.

Adjustive surgical interventions may be necessary to optimize function and improve overall biomechanical efficiency of the gait cycle. Iliotibial band release can prevent a wide-base gait that interferes with hip elevation through the swing phase. Hamstring-contracture release permits extension sufficient to activate knee locks.[68] Shorter patients and those with relatively preserved tensor fascia latae, gluteal, and hamstring strength benefit the most from such treatment.

Regular and periodic orthotic reevaluation is necessary, especially during skeletal growth. If the top of the KAFO falls more than 1 inch below the gluteal folds, the patient will begin to obtain support by sitting on the thigh band and will develop lumbar kyphosis.

As DMD progresses, walking becomes impossible, in spite of the best surgical and orthotic interventions. Nevertheless, braces may still be useful for transfers, slowing of contracture development, and improved seated posture. To prevent plantar flexion and inversion contractures of the foot, molded polythene splints lined with sheepskin to prevent pressure sores are useful.

When the child is wheelchair-bound, the beneficial effects of gravity and the locking of posterior facet joints by lumbar lordosis are lost.[64,65,69] These factors, in conjunction with the underlying weakness of the patient and growth spurts, can result in rapid progression of scoliosis. This leads to pulmonary compromise and pain. Preventive efforts are necessary, although not always effective.

Wheelchair design and modification such as narrow seats, side pads, molded seat inserts, and special cushions (J-backs, J-seats) have been widely used, but their effectiveness is unproven. The benefits of trunk and body braces and jackets are unclear. Body jackets can be uncomfortable and limit ventilation as well as trunk and limb function. When body jackets are used, they should be introduced very gradually, with initial periods of wear of up to 30 minutes. The goal is for the child to wear the jacket whenever upright.

Neck support, when necessary, should be provided to prevent flexion-extension injuries. Philadelphia collars and rubber-coated metal frame braces with open design are used. Properly designed wheelchairs with head rests are also important.

Upper-extremity weakness can be compensated for with mobile arm supports, with or without distal attachments.[70] These serve to support the forearms for gravity-eliminated and some gravity-assisted movements. Intellectual impairment, although common in DMD, is not a barrier to using such devices. Contractures or weakness of *both* the shoulder girdle and the neck and trunk muscles may interfere with the effective use of mobile arm supports.

Robotic arms have also been used effectively in DMD.[71,72] A control panel, in the form of a multi-button touch pad, sip- and- puff, chin control, joy stick, voice control, or head-position lever can be used to activate the device. The patient controls a robotic arm, that in turn moves the patient's own arm in multiple functional positions. Complicated movement sequences can be stored in the control unit. Wheelchair power units typically power the robotic arms. These devices have limited ability to lift or reach, and lack fine movements.

Other Dystrophies

In Duchenne's muscular dystrophy the course is rapidly progressive, culminating in death by the third trimester of life. The other dystrophies such as Becker's muscular dystrophy, facioscapulohumeral dystrophy (FSH) and limb-girdle dystrophy have a slower, more chronic disease pattern, justifying a more aggressive rehabilitation approach.[2]

Affected muscle groups and thus orthotic and surgery needs will differ slightly depending on the particular dystrophy. Contractures and scoliosis are considerably less common in all but Becker's muscular dystrophy. For a more detailed discussion, see Chapter 10.

ASSISTIVE DEVICES FOR WALKING

Canes, crutches, and walkers are often prescribed to enhance ambulation by providing support and stability for patients at risk for falling owing to many different types of deficits. Cognitive status, hand grip, lower and upper extremity strength, balance, and coordination help to determine the proper aid.

A single cane supports 20–25 percent of body weight.[73] The top of the cane should ideally be at the top of the greater trochanter, maintaining elbow flexion at less than 30 degrees. Adding a forearm cuff can increase support to 40–50 percent of body weight.

Canadian crutches have cuffs above and below the elbow to compensate for triceps weakness. A platform cane has a horizontal platform that cradles the forearm, and is useful for patients with distal arm and hand weakness insufficient to bear weight.

Additional stability can be provided with a widened base of support by a four-footed (quad) cane. It is particularly useful for severely hemiparetic patients, and available in small and large base forms. With more extreme instability, the hemiwalk can be recommended.

If neurologic impairment precludes cane ambulation, a walker may be used. Wheeled walkers are prescribed for patients with upper extremity ataxia, because they do not have to be lifted from the floor. Walker height should be adjusted to allow the user to stand erect with shoulders erect and elbows flexed at a 20-degree angle. For maximum stability, the walker should be held about 10 inches in front of the patient.

REFERENCES

1. Lima D: Overview of the causes, treatment, and orthotic management of lower limb spasticity. *J Prosthet Orthot* 1989; 2(1):33–39.
2. Aisen ML (ed): *Orthotics in Neurorehabilitation.* New York: Demos Publications, 1992.
3. Murphy EF, Burstein AH: Physical properties of materials, including solid mechanics, in *Atlas of Orthotics,* 2nd ed. St. Louis: CV Mosby, 1985, pp. 6–33.
4. Redord JB: Materials for orthotics, in Redford JB (ed): *Orthotics Etcetera,* 3rd ed. Baltimore: Williams & Wilkins, 1986, pp. 52–79.

5. Stills M: Thermoformed ankle-foot orthoses, in *Selected Reading: A Review of Orthotics and Prosthetics.* Washington, DC: The American Orthotic and Prosthetic Association, 1980, pp. 305–316.

6. Aisen ML, Arnold A, Baiges I, Maxwell S, Rosen M: The effects of mechanical damping loads on disabling action tremor. *Neurology* 1993; 43:1346–1350.

7. Kaplan N: Effect of splinting on reflex inhibition and sensorimotor stimulation in treatment of spasticity. *Arch Phys Med Rehab* 1962; 43:566–568.

8. Fishman S, Berger N, Edelstein JE, Springer WP: Lower-limb orthoses, in *Atlas of Orthotics,* 2nd ed. St. Louis: CV Mosby, 1985, pp. 199–237.

9. Dietz V, Quintern J, Boos G, Berger W: Obstruction of the swing phase during gait: Phase-dependent bilateral leg muscle coordination. *Brain Res* 1986; 384(1):166–169.

10. Inman RP: Disability indices, the economic costs of illness, and social insurance: The case of multiple sclerosis. *Acta Neurol Scand* (suppl) 1984; 70:46–55.

11. New York University Medical Center: *Lower Limb Orthotics.* New York: University Medical Center, 1981, pp. 179–191.

12. Corcoran PJ, Jebsen RH, Brengelmann GL, Simons BC: Effects of plastic and metal leg braces on speed and energy cost of hemiparetic ambulation. *Arch Phys Med Rehab* 1970; 51:69–77.

13. Lehmann JF: Lower Limb Orthosis, in Redford JB (ed): *Orthotics Etc.* 3rd. ed. Baltimore: Williams & Wilkins, 1986, pp. 278–351.

14. Perry J, Montgomery J: Gait of the stroke patient and orthotic indication, in Brandstater ME, Basmajian JV (eds): *Stroke Rehabilitation.* Baltimore: Williams & Wilkins, 1987, p. 254.

15. Adams GF, McComb SG: Assessment and prognosis in hemiplegia. *Lancet* 1953; 266–269.

16. Gowland C: Management of the hemiplegic upper limb, in Brandstater ME, Basamajian JV (eds): *Stroke Rehabilitation.* Baltimore, Williams & Wilkins, 1987; 221–222.

17. Gowland C: Recovery of motor function following stroke: Profile and predictions. *Physiother Can* 1984; 34:77–84.

18. Joshi J, Singh N, Varma SK: Residual motor deficits in adult hemi-plegic patients. Proceedings World Conference for Physical Therapy, Seventh International Conference, Montreal, Quebec, June 1974.

19. Moodie NB, Brisbin J, Morgan AMG: Subluxation of the glenohumeral joint in hemiplegia evaluation of supportive devices. *Physiother Can* 1986; 38:151–157.

20. Williams R, Taffs L, Minuk T: Evaluation of two support methods for the subluxated shoulder of hemiplegic patients. *Phys Ther* 1988; 68(8):1209.

21. Smith RO, Okamoto GA: Checklist for the prescription of slings for the hemiplegic patient. *Am J Occup Ther* 1981; 35:9–95.

22. Charait S: A comparison of volar and dorsal splinting of the hemiplegic hand. *Am J Occup Ther* 1968; 22:319–321.

23. Reding MJ, McDowell F: Stroke rehabilitation. *Neurol Clin* 1987; 5(4):615–622.

24. Reding MJ, Potes E: Rehabilitation outcome following initial unilateral hemispheric stroke. *Stroke* 1988; 19(11):1354–1358.

25. Wijesinha C: Hemiplegia and bracing. *Med J Aust* 1979; 2:77.

26. Smith CR, Scheinberg LC: Symptomatic treatment and rehabilitation in multiple sclerosis, in Cook SD (ed): *Handbook of Multiple Sclerosis.* New York: Marcel Dekker, 1990, pp. 327–350.

27. Long C, Schutt AH: Upper extremity orthotics, in Redford JB (ed): *Orthotics Etcetera,* 3rd ed. Baltimore: Williams & Wilkins, 1985, pp. 198–277.

28. Long C, Redford JB: Upper limb orthotics, in Jahss MH (ed): *Disorders of the Foot,* vols 1 and 2, 2nd ed. Baltimore: Williams & Wilkins, 1982, pp. 190–282.

29. Guttman L: *Spinal Cord Injuries: Comprehensive Management and Research,* 2nd ed. London: Blackwell Scientific Publications, 1976, pp. 223–229.

30. Staas WE Jr, et al: Rehabilitation of the spinal-cord injured patient, in DeLisa JA (ed): *Rehabilitation Medicine: Principles and Practice.* Philadelphia: J.B. Lippincott, 1988.

31. Johnson RM, Hart DL, Simmons EF, et al: Cervical orthoses. *J Bone Joint Surg* 1977; 59-A:332–339.

32. Malick MH, Meyer CMH: *Manual on Management of the Quadriplegic Upper Extremity.* Pittsburgh, PA: Harmarville Rehabilitation Center, 1978, 79–88.

33. Edberg E: Paralytic dysfunction IV: Bracing for patients with traumatic paraplegia. *Phys Ther* 1967; 47:818–823.

34. Heinemann AW, Magiera-Planey R, Schiro-Geist C, Gimines G: Mobility for persons with spinal cord injury: An evaluation of two systems. *Arch Phys Med Rehab* 1987; 68:90–93.

35. Hussey RW, Stauffer ES: Spinal cord injury: Requirements for ambulation. *Arch Phys Med Rehab* 1973: 54:544–547.

36. Kaplan LI, Grynbaum BB, Rusk HA, et al: A reappraisal of braces and other mechanical aids in patients with spinal cord dysfunction: Results of a follow-up study. *Arch Phys Med Rehab* 1966; 47:393–405.

37. Mikelberg R, Reid S: Spinal cord lesions and lower extremity bracing: An overview of follow-up study. *Paraplegia* 1981; 19:379–385.

38. Cybulski GR, Penn RD, Jaeger RJ: Lower extremity functional neuromuscular stimulation in cases of spinal cord injury. *Neurosurgery* 1984; 15:132–146.

39. Peckham PH: Functional electrical stimulation: current status and future prospects of applications to the neuromuscular system in spinal cord injury. *Paraplegia* 1987; 25:279–288.

40. Turk R, Obreza P: Functional electrical stimulation as an orthotic means for the rehabilitation of paraplegic patients. *Paraplegia* 1985; 23:344–348.

41. Graupe D, Kohn KH, Basseas SP: Control of electrically stimulated walking of paraplegics via above- and below-

lesion EMG signature identification. *IEEE Trans Auto Cont* 1989; 34:130–138.

42. Winchester P, Carollo J, Habasevich R: Physiologic costs of reciprocal gait in FES-assisted walking. *Paraplegia* 1994; 32:680–686.

43. Philips CA: Functional electrical stimulation and lower extremity bracing for ambulation exercise of the spinal cord injured individual: A medically prescribed system. *Phys Ther* 1989; 69:842–849.

44. American Academy of Orthopedic Surgeons: *Atlas of Orthotics: Biomechanical Principles and Application*, 2nd ed. St. Louis: CV Mosby, 1985.

45. Podesta Z, Sherman MF: Knee bracing. *Orthop Clin No Am* 1988; 19(4):737–745.

46. Berger AR, Schaumberg HH: Rehabilitation of focal nerve injuries. *J Neurorehab* 1988; 2:65–91.

47. Berger AR, Schaumberg HH: Rehabilitation of peripheral neuropathies. *J Neurorehab* 1988; 2:25–36.

48. Calditz JC: Splinting peripheral nerve injuries, in Jahss MH (ed): *Disorders of the Foot*, vols 1 and 2. Philadelphia: W.B. Saunders, 1982, pp. 647–657.

49. Fishman S, Berger N, Edelstein JE, Springer WP: Upper-limb orthoses, in *Atlas of Orthotics,* 2nd ed. St. Louis: CV Mosby, 1985, pp. 163–198.

50. Hsu JD, Imbus CE: Pes cavus, in Jahss MH (ed): *Disorders of the Foot*, vols 1 and 2. Philadelphia: W.B. Saunders, 1982, pp. 463–485.

51. Brond PW: The insensitive foot, in Jahss MH (ed): *Disorders of the Foot*, vols 1 and 2. Philadelphia: W.B. Saunders, 1982, pp. 1266–1286.

52. Milgram JE: Padding and devices to relieve the painful foot, in Jahss MH (ed): *Disorders of the Foot*, vols 1 and 2. Philadelphia: W.B. Saunders Co, 1982, pp. 1703–1732.

53. Demopoulos JT: Orthotics and prosthetic management of foot disorders, in Jahss MH (ed): *Disorders of the Foot*, vols 1 and 2. Philadelphia: W.B. Saunders, 1982, pp. 1783–1813.

54. Lehmann JF: Lower limb orthotics, in: Jahss MH (ed): *Disorders of the Foot*, vols 1 and 2, 2nd ed. Baltimore: Williams & Wilkins, 1982, pp. 190–282.

55. Borderlon RL: Management of foot problems. *Orthop Clin N Am* 20(4):751–757.

56. Granata C, et al: Promotion of ambulation of patients with spinal muscular atrophy by early fitting of knee-ankle-foot orthoses. *Dev Med Child Neurol* 1987; 29:221–224.

57. Halstead LS, Rossi CD: Post-polio syndrome: clinical experience with 132 consecutive patients, in Halstead LS, Wiechers DO (eds): *Late Effects of Poliomyelitis*. Symposia Foundation, Miami, FL, 1985, pp. 13–26.

58. Peach PE: Overwork weakness with evidence of muscle damage in a patient with residual paralysis from polio. *Arch Phys Med Rehab* 1990; 71:248–250.

59. Agre JC, Rodriguez AA, Sperling KB: Symptoms and clinical impressions of patients seen in a postpolio clinic. *Arch Phys Med Rehab* 1989; 70:367–370.

60. Twist DJ, Ma DM: Physical therapy management of the patient with post-polio syndrome: A case report. *Phys Ther* 1986; 66:1403–1406.

61. Cosgrove JL, et al: Late effects of poliomyelitis. *Arch Phys Med Rehab* 1987; 68:4–7.

62. Waring WP, et al: Influence of appropriate lower extremity orthotic management on ambulation, pain, and fatigue in a postpolio population. *Arch Phys Med Rehab* 1989; 70:371–375.

63. Siegel IM, Glantz RH: Orthopedic rehabilitation for standing and walking in selected neuromuscular disease. *J Neurol Rehab* 1988; 2:131–136.

64. Vignos PJ, Archibald KC: Maintenance of ambulation in childhood muscular dystrophy. *J Am Med Assoc* 1963; 184:89–110.

65. Vignos PJ: Rehabilitation in progressive muscular dystrophy, in Licht SH (ed): *Rehabilitation and Medicine.* New Haven, CT: Elizabeth Licht, 1968.

66. Hyde SA, Scott OM, Goddard CM, Dubowitz V: Prolongation of ambulation in Duchenne Muscular Dystrophy by appropriate orthoses. *Physiotherapy* 1982; 68:105–108.

67. Siegel IM: Plastic-molded knee-ankle-foot orthoses in the treatment of Duchenne muscular dystrophy. *Arch Phys Med Rehab* 1975; 56:322.

68. Spencer GE: Orthopaedic care of progressive muscular dystrophy. *J Bone Joint Surg* 1967; 49-A:1201–1204.

69. Harris SE, Cherry DB: Childhood progressive muscular dystrophy and the role of physical therapy. *Phys Ther* 1974; 54:4–12.

70. Chyatte SB, Long C, Vignos PJ: The balanced forearm orthosis in muscular dystrophy. *Arch Phys Med Rehab* 1965; 46:633–636.

71. Shramowiat M, Bach JR, Bocobo C: Functional enhancement of patients with Duchenne Muscular Dystrophy with the use of robot-manipulator trainer arms. *J Neurol Rehab* 1989; 3:129–132.

72. Shramowiat M, Bach JR, Bocobo C: Functional enhancement of patients with Duchenne muscular dystrophy with the use of robot-manipulator trainer arms. *J Neurol Rehab* 1989; 3:129–132.

73. Kemenentz HL: Wheelchairs and other motor vehicles for the disabled, in Redford JB (ed): *Orthotics, Etcetera*, 3rd ed. Baltimore: Williams & Wilkins, 1986, pp. 464–517.

Chapter 27

PRINCIPLES OF WHEELCHAIR DESIGN AND PRESCRIPTION

R. Lee Kirby

The wheelchair is arguably the most important therapeutic tool in rehabilitation, equivalent in importance to vaccination in preventive medicine or antibiotics in curative medicine. A wheelchair is a medical device in the form of a chair on wheels, the principal purpose of which is to minimize a disability of locomotion (getting from one point to another).[1,2] In 1992, there were 1,072,000 wheelchair users in the United States (4.2 per 1000 population).[3] Manual rear-wheel-drive wheelchairs represent the majority of prescription wheelchairs and are the focus of this chapter. Customized-seating, stand-up, stair-climbing, and racing wheelchairs are specialized topics that are beyond the scope of this chapter.[4,5] The main body of the chapter deals with the components of manual wheelchairs (listed in Table 27-1), followed by brief discussions of wheelchair safety and the prescription process.

COMPONENTS

Frame

In considering the ease with which a wheelchair can be transported in a vehicle (one of the most important issues to be considered in making the decision about a wheelchair frame), one needs to consider the vehicle in which the chair will be transported, where in the vehicle the chair will be placed (trunk, front seat, rear seat, or roof), the size and weight of the components after the chair has been broken down and/or folded for transport, and the attributes of the person who will be loading the wheelchair (often someone other than the user).

In a folding-frame wheelchair, the folding usually takes place by means of an X-shaped cross-brace connecting the two side frames (Figure 27-1). Folding the wheelchair reduces its width for storage or transporta-tion. For someone who uses a wheelchair only intermittently, it is useful to be able to fold the wheelchair and store it compactly.[6] A folding wheelchair can be narrowed slightly with the user in the wheelchair (e.g., to get through a tight doorway) using an optional wheelchair narrower available on some wheelchairs. The flexibility of the folding frame also leads to a more comfortable ride and makes it more likely that all four wheels will remain in contact with uneven terrain. However, because a folding chair can deform downhill when on a side slope or in the direction of a lean, stability is reduced somewhat. On side slopes or when leaning to the side, the chair may even inadvertently fold up, causing a lateral tip. Some of the flexibility of a folding wheelchair can be eliminated by clips on the superior tube on the side frame that capture and restrain the seat rails when the chair is in the open position, and by modifications of the cross-brace.

A rigid frame (Figures 27-2 and 27-3) is strong, light, attractive, and requires little maintenance. The rigidity provides a responsive feel to wheelchair propulsion and turning, with the applied forces not being dampened by the chair flexing. The rigidity also allows more precise alignment of components (e.g., of the toe angle of the rear wheels). However, the ride over rough terrain may be less comfortable, with every crack in the sidewalk transmitted to the user. An increasing number of wheelchairs therefore have some form of suspension to smooth the ride. Cantilever-style frames have some inherent suspension in comparison with box frames.[7] Because there is no flexibility in a rigid-frame wheelchair, one wheel may be off the ground (caster "float") if the terrain is uneven.[7] Rigid frames that have crossbars at the level of the superior frame eliminate the option of using a drop seat. For transportation, the size and weight of the largest component can often be reduced by removal of the rear wheels and by folding the

Table 27-1

Important component considerations in manual wheelchairs

Frame	Front Rigging
Folding	Length
Rigid	Height
Weight	Fixed
Material	Flip-up
	Swing-away
Seat	Removeability
Sling	Elevating
Rigid	Footrests
Width	Restraints
Depth	Wedge shape
Height	Knee-flexion angle
Position	
Seat-plane angle	Rear Wheels
Seat belt	Diameter
Clothing guard	Spokes
Cushion	Hubs and bearings
	Axle type
Backrest	Axle position
Sling	Propulsion
Rigid	Handrims
Height	Tires
Angle	Wheel locks
Chest strap	Grade aids
Recline	Camber
Tilt	Toeing error
Push-handles	
	Casters
Armrests	Diameter
Height	Base footprint
Removability	Tires
Length	Trail
Wraparound	Flutter
	Stems
	Wheelbase
	Pin locks
	Antitippers
	Rear
	Forward
	Carriers
	Content
	Location

backrest forward. The method that the wheelchair user uses to transfer to and from the wheelchair is a key consideration in prescription, because many rigid-frame wheelchairs have fixed front rigging that interferes with standing transfers.[6,8]

The weight of the wheelchair is an important consideration. Lightweight wheelchairs make it easier for the user to overcome the initial inertia when starting to roll and to propel the wheelchair on inclines. Lightweight chairs also are easier to lift into a car. Although there are no widely accepted weight criteria for making such distinctions, the terms "standard,", "lightweight" (under about 32 lbs) and "ultralight" (under about 25 lbs) are commonly used to distinguish the extent to which the manufacturer has been able to minimize the weight. Regrettably, these terms have been used as a shorthand way to convey other information. For instance, lightweight wheelchairs usually have the most modularity and adjustability of components. Ultralight wheelchairs, designed for special purposes (e.g., tennis), have often achieved their low weights by sacrificing adjustability. The weight of the wheelchair will be affected by the materials used, as well as by the size, number, and complexity of the components. The frame constitutes a major proportion of the weight of most manual wheelchairs. Although lighter wheelchairs tend to be less stable,[9] this is more often due to the way in which the wheelchair is set up (e.g., to optimize performance) than to weight alone.[9]

Most wheelchair frames are made of metal, in tubular form. The strength:weight ratios of some of the newer materials (e.g., titanium) are permitting chairs to be manufactured that are both light and strong. Steel is still the most commonly used material, and comes in various types (e.g., "common," stainless, chrome-moly). Steel is strong, inexpensive, and easy to repair, but heavy and prone to rust. Aluminum also comes in different grades. It is light, strong, relatively inexpensive, and does not rust. However, it nicks easily and can develop burrs that can cut the hands. Surface treatment or coating is needed to prevent oxidation from staining the hands. Specialized equipment and skills are needed to weld it. Titanium is light and strong, but expensive and difficult to repair. Composite materials (plastic, carbon fiber) around a foam core are the newest addition to the list of materials used to construct wheelchairs. These materials are light, attractive, and shock-absorbent. However, they are expensive, weakened by drilling or attaching features to them, and the surface finish can be easily chipped.

Seat

Sling seats (Figure 27-1) are inexpensive and allow the wheelchair to be folded easily. However, they tend to roll the hips into internal rotation. A flat rigid surface (Figure 27-4) under the cushion is preferable. It should be removeable (or hinged) if the wheelchair is to be folded.

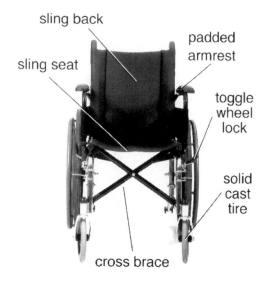
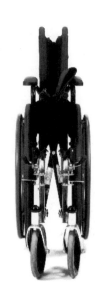

sling back

padded armrest

sling seat

toggle wheel lock

solid cast tire

cross brace

Figure 27-1

*Front view of a folding wheel-
chair, open on the left and folded
on the right.*

The seat width of the wheelchair is the distance between the outside borders of the seat rails.[10] The relevant user dimension is his or her width at the level of the lower pelvis and greater trochanters. Problems can be encountered if the user is wider and/or the wheelchair is narrower above this level. Some wheelchairs have a backrest width different from the seat width.[10,11]

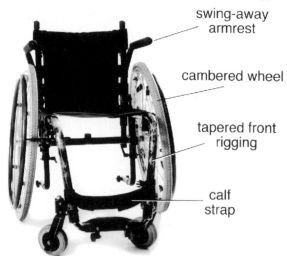

Figure 27-2

Front view of a rigid-frame wheelchair of the cantilever type.

swing-away armrest

cambered wheel

tapered front rigging

calf strap

When deciding on seat width, one should allow for winter clothing, anticipated weight change, orthoses, prostheses, and objects that the user may wish to carry between the body and clothing guard. About 1 in. of lateral clearance on either side between the user and the wheelchair components is the usual standard. Seats that are too wide for the user interfere with propulsion (because the user must reach out and over the armrests and wheels to reach the handrims) and make it difficult to get through narrow doors. Wide seats also can force the user to lean to one side to obtain support from an armrest, causing asymmetrical posture and uneven pressure under the buttocks. If the seat is too narrow, sores can develop on the posterolateral aspects of the greater trochanters from pressure by the seat rails, the hips may be rolled into internal rotation, clothing or thigh tissue may drag on the wheels, and the lateral stability of the wheelchair is reduced.[12]

The seat depth of the wheelchair is the distance along the seat plane between its intersections with the back and leg planes.[10] The relevant user dimension is from the back of the buttocks to the back of the bent knee. The seat length is the fore-aft dimension of the supporting surface. There should be 2 to 3 in. between the front edge of the seat and the back of the knee. Seat depth can be varied in some wheelchairs by moving the backrest forward or back, but it is important to remember that stability is affected by the fore-aft position of the person on the seat.[13] Seat depth also is af-

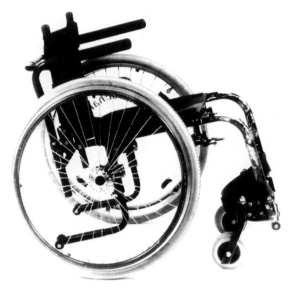

Figure 27-3
Side view of a rigid-frame wheelchair.

fected by the backrest style (i.e., sling vs rigid). If the seat is too short and the thighs are unsupported, the area over which forces are distributed is reduced and the pressure under the buttocks is increased. A long seat makes propulsion with the legs and sit-to-stand transfers more difficult, by preventing the knees from flexing under the seat. Seats that are too long can also cause pressure sores in the popliteal space or may force the user to slide the buttocks forward into a slumped (lumbar-kyphotic) position. Similarly, calf supports can prevent the user from positioning the sacrum against the backrest, causing a slumped posture. By leaning on one of them, the front of the seat rails can be used to provide trunk stability while reaching forward.

The seat surface height of the wheelchair (usually about 20 in.) is measured from the floor to the front end of the loaded seat (115 mm from the midline).[10] The relevant user dimension is the leg length, measured from the bottom of the heel (with the shoe on) to the popliteal fold behind the bent knee. Long legs necessitate higher seats (or an altered knee angle), because the footrests need to clear the ground by at least 2 in. The effective seat height includes the height of the compressed cushion. There should be about 1 in. of vertical clearance between the anterior seat margin and the corresponding thigh, to avoid edge pressure. Drop hooks (Figure 27-4) can be used to lower a rigid seat surface below the level of the side rails, but caution

needs to be taken that the frame components (e.g., the folding cross-brace) do not cause pressure ulcers. Alternatively, the seat height can be reduced by raising the rear-wheel axle or using a rear wheel with a smaller diameter.

Seat height affects the ability to reach high objects (e.g., public telephones), the ability to reach low objects (e.g., a dropped book), eye contact with standing people, the ability to get the knees under surfaces in the environment (e.g., sinks, table tops) and stability (a lower chair is more stable).[12] If, however, only the back of the chair is lowered (e.g., by raising the axle position), the resulting rearward tilt offsets this stability-enhancing effect. Seat height also affects the ability to use one or both feet to propel the wheelchair. Because this is most commonly the case for users with hemiplegia, such wheelchairs are commonly referred to as "hemi height" (about 2 in. lower than usual).

The relationship of the arms to the rear wheels for propulsion also is affected by seat height. A rule of thumb is that, with the hand on the handrim at its highest point, the elbow should be flexed about 60 to 80° (with full elbow extension being 0°).[14] Sit-to-stand transfers are easier if the seat is high, but floor-to-chair transfers are easier if the seat is low. A user on a low seat will have more difficulty in lateral transfers, having to lift

Figure 27-4
Folding wheelchair with the sling seat and the back replaced.

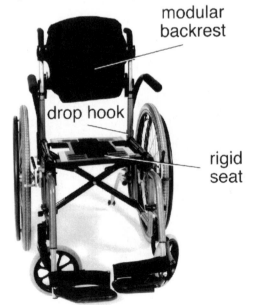

modular
backrest

drop hook

rigid
seat

higher to get over the wheel or having to move farther forward to get around the wheel.

Some wheelchairs allow the entire seat position relative to the frame to be adjusted, in the horizontal or vertical directions. A forward seat position increases rear stability and reduces forward stability.[15]

The seat-plane angle is the angle of the seat plane relative to the horizontal and is positive if the front is higher, as is usually the case (by 1 to 4°).[10] This angle may be accentuated ("dunking" the seat) to reduce spasticity, to reduce the tendency for the user to slide forward on the seat, and to reduce lumbar lordosis. However, an increased seat-plane angle makes transfers more difficult and puts more weight on the ischial tuberosities, unless the angle is so steep that the body is suspended by the back and thighs.

If a seat belt is used, it should be based near the intersection of the seat and backrest frames. A variety of closure styles are available—buckle, velcro, snap, magnet. Auxiliary straps are sometimes used to control thigh position. A seat belt may help a user to remain properly positioned in the seat (e.g., if he or she slides forward because of weakness or spasticity), but it reduces the ability to relieve pressure on sitting surfaces by pushups or weight shifts and creates a risk of strangulation if the user slips down under the belt.[16]

A clothing guard (Figure 27-5) keeps the clothing from being rubbed by the rear wheel. It may be based on the seat or be part of the armrest. The space between the clothing guard and the body is convenient for carrying objects.

Virtually all personal wheelchairs should be fitted with a removable cushion for pressure distribution, shock absorption, and/or positioning. Very flexible cushions should be supported fully by the seat surface, so that they do not fold over the seat margins and affect the seat depth. The cushion should be removable, so a high-friction undersurface or velcro is needed to prevent slippage. In choosing the cushion materials (e.g., foam, air, gel), their distribution, and the shape of the cushion, one needs to consider such issues as sensibility, pressure distribution, the presence of spasticity/flaccidity, and incontinence. For instance, a user with adductor spasticity may benefit from a slight pommel between the thighs, whereas a user with flaccidity, whose knees rest apart, may benefit from lateral support. Decisions about the cushion should be made early, because the dimensions of the compressed cushion affect a number of wheelchair dimensions (e.g., backrest, armrest, and seat height). If the cushion is thick, it may need to be undercut (or beveled) in front if knee flexion beyond 90° is needed (e.g., for propulsion, transfers).

Backrest

In comparing a sling to a rigid backrest, the sling backrest is less expensive and more portable. The backrest should curve around the trunk, enclosing about 30 percent of the trunk depth.[11] A number of different materials are used, and some have adjustable tension. For the occasional user who needs or prefers to enter the chair from the rear, a zipper or snaps in the sling-backrest upholstery are available to permit entry. Better support is available as an option in some chairs and as an add-on (Figure 27-4) in others.

The backrest height of the wheelchair is measured in the midline from the rear of the seat plane to the top of the supporting surface, but the effective backrest height must take into consideration the height of the compressed cushion. The relevant dimension for users who propel their own wheelchairs is from the sitting surface to the inferior angle of the scapula. The upper border of the backrest should be 1 to 2 in. lower than the scapulae, to minimize irritation from rubbing them during propulsion. Higher backrests (sometimes with an added headrest) provide more support and more area for pressure distribution for the user who does not propel the wheelchair independently or who uses a recliner. Backrests that do not extend above the lumbar region are increasingly common and are surprisingly

Figure 27-5
Side view of a folding wheelchair, illustrating its desk-length armrests and toggle wheel locks.

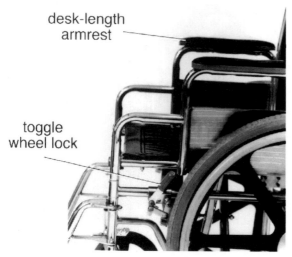

desk-length armrest

toggle wheel lock

well-tolerated if the lumbar area is supported. Such low backrests have the advantage of permitting greater freedom of upper body and trunk movement. Padding the backrest uprights (or "canes") throughout their vertical length provides comfort, reduces the likelihood of pressure lesions if the user habitually leans to one side, and decreases the likelihood of damage to the radial nerve owing to pressure between the cane and the back of the arm.[17]

The backrest angle is the angle of the backrest plane relative to vertical, positive if the top of the backrest is behind the bottom.[10] The angle of the backrest is commonly tilted back about 8° from vertical (and, therefore, approximately 95° from the seat plane).[18] The backrest canes may have an additional rearward angulation that begins part way up, to provide appropriate support for both the lumbar and thoracic spines. Some alteration in the backrest angle can be achieved by changing the upholstery or by replacing it with an adjustable back support.

When users of lightweight wheelchairs increase the seat-plane angle and reduce the angle between the backrest and seat planes, this position is sometimes referred to as "squeeze" (Figure 27-3). A relatively forward inclination of the backrest like this can assist the user in applying force to the wheels, by preventing the trunk from being pushed backwards. For the user with weak trunk muscles, an increased backrest angle can decrease the likelihood of falling forward onto the lap. This must be balanced against the desirability of being more upright to improve the ability to function on a work surface. A chest strap can prevent the user with trunk weakness from pitching forward when decelerating or reaching forward. However, there is a risk of accidental strangulation if the user slides down.[16]

Some backrest frames allow an assistant to recline them, partially or fully (to the horizontal position) (Figure 27-6). Reclining the backrest reduces the pressure on the ischial tuberosities, in proportion to the extent of the recline. Being able to lie back without having to get out of the wheelchair can be useful for the user who has orthostatic hypotension. However, as the user is extended, spasticity is sometimes triggered. Furthermore, because the mechanical axis of the recliner usually is below and behind the anatomical axis of the user's hip joint (the surface marking for which is the greater trochanter), there are shear forces produced because of the relative movement of the chair and user's backs.[19] Most powered recliners now have shear compensators for this reason, but manually reclined wheelchairs do not. The movement of the trunk and head backwards

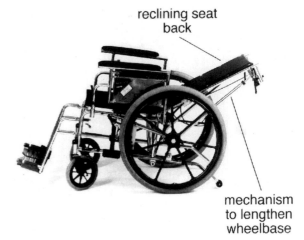

Figure 27-6
Reclining wheelchair. Note the rearward displacement of the rear-wheel axle.

moves the center of gravity (CG) of the chair-occupant combination back, lowering the rear stability.[20] Therefore, manual wheelchairs that are intended to be reclined have their rear axles offset posteriorly. Because this makes them more awkward to propel independently, some wheelchair models (e.g., as in Figure 27-6) couple the offset of the axle to the extent of recline.

The seats of some manual wheelchairs can be tilted backwards by an assistant (Figure 27-7). Tilt (or "tilt-in-space") is a change in the entire seat's position or attitude rather than a change in the wheelchair user's posture (relative position of body parts). Tilt obviates

Figure 27-7
Tilt-in-space wheelchair. Elevating legrests (of the telescoping type) are also shown in their lowered positions.

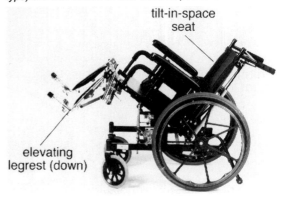

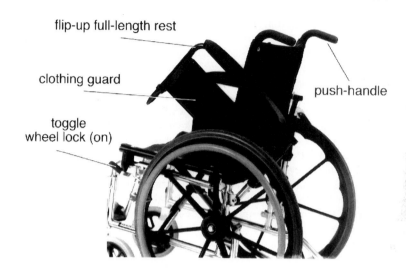

flip-up full-length rest

clothing guard

push-handle

toggle
wheel lock (on)

Figure 27-8
*Rear-oblique view of a folding
wheelchair, illustrating a flip-up
full-length armrest, an attached
clothing guard, a push-to-lock
toggle wheel lock, and push-
handles.*

the shear problem of recliners, is less likely to induce spasticity and, like reclining, reduces the pressure on the ischial tuberosities in proportion to the extent of the tilt. Although tilt lowers rear stability, some chairs with tilt functions have a compensatory mechanism (with the seat moving forward as it tilts back) to reduce the effect of the tilt on stability.[20] Users of unmodified wheelchairs can achieve the advantages of rear tilt by performing a wheelie and leaning against a fixed object or on antitippers with sufficient range.

Many manual wheelchairs have push-handles at the top of the backrest canes (Figure 27-8), to allow an assistant to push the wheelchair, to help lift it (e.g., up a curb), to brake it (e.g., while descending ramps or stairs), to pull it backwards, and to tip the wheelchair (with the assistant's foot on the tipping lever). Push-handles also provide some protection in a full rearward tip. By hooking an arm around them, they are often used for leaning. For wheelchair users who can walk short distances, the push-handles can allow the wheelchair to serve as a wheeled walker. The height of the push-handles should be appropriate to the person pushing the wheelchair. The rubber covering the handles can become loose and pull off at an inopportune moment.

Armrests

Armrests serve a number of useful purposes. In addition to providing a place to rest the arms during inactivity, they can reduce glenohumeral subluxation in users with flaccid shoulder muscles, position the arm (e.g., by a trough in which to rest a paretic arm), simplify pushups

(to relieve pressure on the ischial tuberosities), assist repositioning in the chair (for the user who slides forward), provide something for the user to push on during transfers or hold onto while leaning, and be used to restrict the extent to which the hips abduct. The disadvantages of armrests are that they add weight, add overall width (except wrap-around armrests), and can interfere with reaching the wheels for propulsion, limit the extent to which the user can reach and lean to the side, or cause compression neuropathy of the ulnar nerve at the elbow.

The armrest height is measured as the perpendicular distance from the seat plane (12 cm forward of the back plane) to the top of the armrest.[10] The effective armrest height needs to take the height of the compressed cushion into consideration. The relevant user dimension is from the sitting surface to the bottom of the bent elbow. The armrest should be 1 in. higher. The armrest should support the forearm without necessitating elevation or depression of the shoulder girdle, or leaning to one side. Variable-height armrests are useful for the user who may benefit from having higher armrests during specific activities (e.g., sit-to-stand transfers).

It should be possible to remove the armrests, pivot them back (Figure 27-8), or swing them to the side (Figure 27-2), to allow side transfers and closer access of the user to a table. Most wheelchairs are not intended to be lifted by their armrests. The armrests should either come off easily or not at all when upward forces are applied to them. Completely removable armrests can be mislaid and, if dropped, can be deformed enough to prevent them from fitting well into their receptacles on the frame.

The armrest length is the length of the surface available to support the arm, measured as the distance between the back plane and the front of the armrest, parallel to the seat plane.[10] Desk-length armrests (Figure 27- 5) eliminate the forward third of the armrest. They allow a closer approach to a desk or table, but may not provide enough length to be useful for sit-to-stand transfers. This limitation can be circumvented if the armrests are reversible. In the reversed position the missing section allows better access of the arms to the wheels for propulsion, but eliminates any lateral support of the trunk through the armrests. A few wheelchairs have armrests with a downward slope in front that can allow closer access to a desk or table. Full-length armrests (Figure 27-8) may be needed for transfers (sit-to-stand), for users whose posture or anatomy do not allow them to reach back enough to use desk-length armrests, and for those who need a base for trays that attach to the armrests.

The rear attachment of the wrap-around armrest is behind the frame (Figure 27-9) rather than beside it. This allows the rear wheels to be placed closer to the frame, narrowing the outside width of the wheelchair without narrowing the seat width. However, wrap-around armrests are not reversible and can be difficult to relocate once removed.

Front Rigging

The term "front rigging" includes the footrests (the components on which the feet rest), the legrests (any components that support the legs) and the footrest hangers (the structures that support the footrests and legrests) (Figure 27-10). The purposes of the front rigging are to keep the feet off the floor, to optimize the sitting posture and weight distribution, to provide a surface against which the wheelchair user can apply force to prevent him- or herself from falling forward out of the wheelchair when leaning forward or coming to a sudden stop, to provide protection for the feet and legs when bumping into objects, to apply force (e.g., to open a door), and to limit the extent of forward tipping.[21,22]

The farther forward the footrests protrude, the greater the turning circle, the lower the approach angle (leading to the footrests scraping on incline transitions), and the more likely the wheelchair is to tip over forward if the user puts much weight through the footrests.

The footrest height affects the ground clearance (the lowest point on the footrests), which should be at least 2 in. above the floor to avoid being caught on obstacles and incline transitions. The footrest-to-seat distance is measured from the rear support point of the footrest to the seat plane.[10] The effective distance should take into consideration the height of the compressed cushion. If the footrests are too high, the thighs are lifted from the seat, increasing the pressure on the ischial tuberosities. If the footrests are too low (or removed), the front edge of the seat will bear more weight than appropriate (with the potential for pressure ulceration under the distal thighs) and there will be no support for forward leans.

Fixed footrests (Figure 27-2) have the advantage of being light and durable. They may be needed to resist spasticity. However, they interfere with standing transfers, cannot be easily removed for transport or to propel the chair with the feet, and cannot be replaced by elevating footrests. Flip-up footrests (Figure 27-10) permit sit-to-stand transfers and allow the wheelchair to be folded. Some flip-up footplates with heel loops need to have the heel loop bowed forward (Figure 27-10) to allow the footplate to flip up fully (and thereby avoid tripping the user or injuring the user's leg).

By removing the feet from them and releasing a lock, swing-away footrests (Figure 27-11) can be swung to a different position. The new position usually is to

Figure 27-9

Rear-oblique view of an amputee adaptor to offset the axle of the rear wheel (although the rear axle is in its original position in this figure). The attachment of the rear post of the wraparound armrest behind the frame and a rear antitipper are also shown.

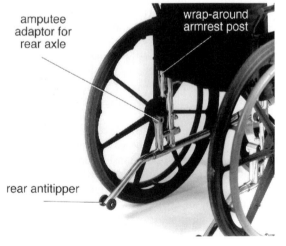

amputee adaptor for rear axle

wrap-around armrest post

rear antitipper

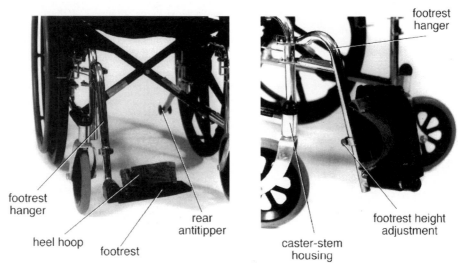

Figure 27-10
Front view of a swing-away removable flip-up footrest and heel loop. On the left the footrest is down and the heel loop bows back in the functional position. On the right the footrest is up, the heel loop having been bowed forward out of the way.

the side, but some can swing inward out of the way. Generally swing-away footrests are a better way than flip-up footrests to clear the area between the casters for a sit-to-stand transfer, assuming that there is enough room for the footrests to swing. They also allow the wheelchair to be brought closer to an object. However,

Figure 27-11
Front-oblique view illustrating a swing-away footrest, swung laterally. The left footrest has been removed.

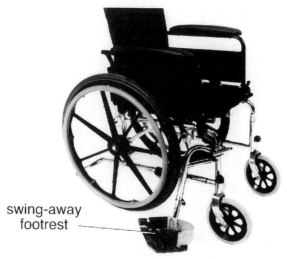

some release mechanisms are difficult to use and the attachment base and/or the release mechanism of some swing-away footrests protrude into the space occupied by the legs (Figure 27-1), with injury to the skin a common result.

Most swing-away footrests are also removable, but there are removable footrests that cannot be swung away. Being able to remove the footrests is useful if there is limited space for turning in the user's environment. The advantages and disadvantages of removable footrests are similar to those for swing-away footrests. Removability also permits the wheelchair to be reduced in dimension and weight for transport and storage. Furthermore, the wheelchair can be adjusted easily for individual user needs (e.g., removing one footrest for a user who needs to use one foot to assist with propulsion, or adding an elevating footrest). However, it is important that footrests not be free to lift off unexpectedly, as when the occupied wheelchair is being carried up stairs. Removing the footrests habitually can cause problems owing to damage of the feet or pressure sores under the distal thighs. Footrests can be removed permanently if the user has an amputation and does not use prostheses. This allows closer access, tighter turns, and a lighter chair, compensating for some of the disadvantages of posteriorly offset rear axles. However, the user also loses the footrests in their capacity as forward antitippers.

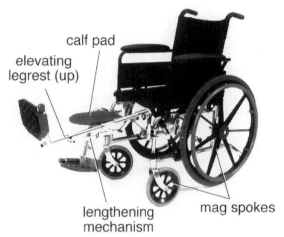

calf pad

elevating legrest (up)

lengthening mechanism

mag spokes

Figure 27-12
Front-oblique view illustrating an elevating legrest and some of its components.

Elevating footrests (Figure 27-12) are an option whereby the footrest can be positioned at any angle between the usual resting position and one where the leg is horizontal. They are useful for users with edema, a recent fracture, inability to flex the knee fully, or at risk of knee-flexion contractures. Most reclining wheelchairs are equipped with elevating footrests. Elevating footrests decrease maneuverability by lengthening the wheelchair. Elevating the footrests decreases forward stability, both because the CG is altered and because footrests serve as forward antitippers.[23] This latter effect can lead to a violent yawing tip when only a single footrest is elevated. There can be relative movement between the elevating footrest and the user if the axes of the mechanical and anatomical joints are not co-linear. If the leg is always elevated, such shear is not a problem. Some elevating footrests minimize shear by either a gooseneck attachment (to raise the mechanical axis) or a telescoping mechanism (Figure 27-12) that lengthens the footrest as it is elevated.

Usually only a single footrest angle is available, intended to support the foot in a position with the ankle neutral with respect to dorsiflexion–plantarflexion and inversion–eversion. Customization is commonly necessary. The user's forefoot usually protrudes past the end of the footrest. Full-length footrests are available when toe protection is a priority. Plastic impact guards or corner rollers can be used to prevent the outer corner of the footplate from being caught on (or damaging) objects struck. These guards can also be used to push doors open.

Heel loops (Figure 27-10) are commonly used to keep the heels from moving behind the footplates where they can be damaged by, or interfere with, caster swivel. In some designs, the heel loops can interfere with flipping the footrests up fully. Also, users with insensitive feet sometimes rest them on the posts that support the heel loops, causing pressure ulcers. Toe loops can be used to keep the feet from slipping (or being pulled by spasticity) off the front of the footplates. A calf strap (Figure 27-2) (or an H strap) can be used as an alternative or in addition to heel loops, but it needs to be undone to allow the footrests to be swung away or removed. A calf pad can be used instead of a calf strap on elevating footrests (Figure 27-12) to support the weight of the leg. A trough can be used to maintain the leg in a neutral position.

Some manufacturers provide models that are narrower in front, a wedge (or tapered) configuration of the front rigging (Figure 27-2). This permits tighter cornering, holds the legs together, and makes the chair look less bulky. However, this type of front rigging may aggravate hip deformities (e.g., chronic or recurrent dislocation of the hip), may produce pressure lesions on the lateral aspects of the lower legs, may interfere with side transfers (if the legs are tightly jammed in place), and may interfere with floor-to-seat transfers if the pelvis is too wide for the user to sit on the footrests.

The extent to which the user's knees are flexed while sitting in the wheelchair varies from wheelchair to wheelchair, and is sometimes adjustable (e.g., with elevating footrests). In the usual clinical terms, the position in which the thigh and leg are a straight line is defined as 0° of knee flexion and full flexion is about 140°. The commonly referred to "hanger angle" (e.g., 60 or 70°) uses the same definition. However, in describing the corresponding wheelchair angle between the leg and seat planes, the International Organization for Standardization (ISO) defines full extension as 180°.[10] These differences need to be kept in mind when interpreting wheelchair specifications.

Some wheelchairs set the knees in flexion of >90° (Figure 27-3). This has several intended effects, including tighter turns, closer access to objects, protection of the feet, ease of transport of the wheelchair, and inhibition of spasticity. Also, by bringing the limb segments closer to the yaw axis, turns can be faster (analogous to a spinning skater who speeds up when bringing the arms closer to the body). However, users with long legs may be difficult to accommodate with the knees in a hyperflexed position. Also, this position may necessitate a small caster diameter and caster trail to avoid having the caster swiveling into the footrests/heels when changing direction. Furthermore, the footrests cannot serve as forward antitip devices unless they extend beyond the casters. In addition, the hyperflexed posture may occlude the circulation and may cause pressure lesions under the points where pressure is applied to achieve the hyperflexed position.

Rear Wheels

The usual diameter of the rear wheels is 24 in., but 20 to 26 in. wheels are readily available. Increasing the diameter of the wheels raises the seat height, reduces rolling resistance, eases obstacle climbing, and allows a given force at the handrim to induce more propulsive moment (torque). The tradeoff is that larger wheels increase the overall length of the wheelchair and make lateral, anterolateral, and floor-to-chair transfers more difficult.

Wire-spoked wheels are light, strong, and inexpensive, but need to be checked regularly. Tightening selective spokes can true a warped wheel. Radially oriented spokes (Figure 27-3) provide rigidity to the wheel, whereas cross-laced spokes (Figure 27-13) make a wheel more flexible and tolerant of side impacts (e.g., in sports). Spoke guards can be added to protect the spokes from side impacts. Wire spokes are needed for the attachment of small-diameter handrims. Molded plastic

Figure 27-13

Rear view of a one-arm-drive wheelchair. In this design, both handrims are on the side of the functional arm. The left-wheel handrim is connected to the axle of the left wheel by the accordion-like mechanism shown, that permits the wheelchair to be folded.

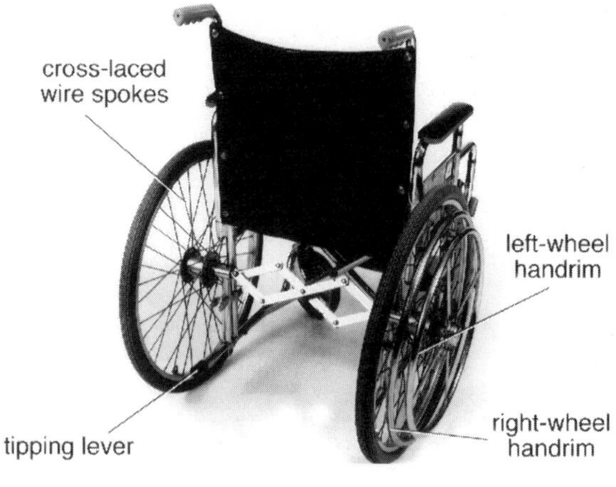

cross-laced
wire spokes

left-wheel
handrim

right-wheel
handrim

tipping lever

("mag") spokes (Figure 27-12) require no maintenance but do not allow a wheel to be trued, and many are heavy (up to 1 lb heavier per wheel than a wire-spoked wheel).[8]

Most hubs and bearings are now of good quality, low in friction, and sealed from the elements. If the wheel can be rocked from side to side, the bearings probably need to be replaced.[12] Fixed threaded axles allow the wheel to be adjusted closer to or farther away from the frame, for instance, to compensate for the lost distance between the upper wheels that accompanies an increase in camber. Quick-release axles are essential if the user wishes to break a chair down quickly for transportation. However, they are expensive and require some dexterity (more so to put the wheel back on than to take it off). Quad attachments are available for users with weak hands.[12,24]

Many wheelchairs allow the rear-wheel axle positions to be adjusted in the vertical and/or horizontal directions. The position of the rear wheel axle is defined with respect to the intersection of the back and seat planes.[10] The axle position profoundly affects a number of stability, performance, and maneuverability parameters. For instance, raising the axle tilts the wheelchair backwards, reduces rear stability, increases forward stability, and toes out a cambered wheel. Moving the axle back increases rear stability, decreases the ease of doing wheelies, limits the ability of a wheelchair user or an attendant to lift the front wheels, reduces traction, lengthens the wheelbase, increases rolling resistance, and increases downhill-turning tendency.[25,26]

Some chairs provide a much more rearward position of the axle (either built into the frame or as an optional adaptor [Figure 27-14]) to compensate for the loss of rear stability that accompanies amputation.[27] Moving the rear wheels back, however, makes it more awkward for the user to position the hands on the wheels for propulsion and increases the overall length of the wheelchair.

A conventionally equipped wheelchair can be self-propelled with two hands, with one hand and one or two feet, or just with one or two feet. If a foot is regularly used for propulsion, the footrest should be removed. For users with only one functional arm and no functional lower extremities, one-arm-drive mechanisms are available for some wheelchairs. One common type has both handrims on the same side (Figure 27-13); the handrim that propels the contralateral wheel is of slightly smaller diameter and is connected to the opposite axle. Another option is a lever-like mechanism (Figure 27-14); the user cranks the lever forward and back to propel the wheelchair.

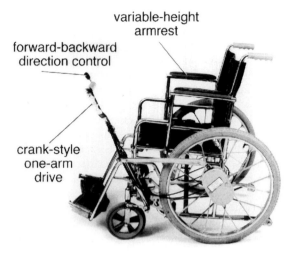

Figure 27-14
One-arm-drive wheelchair of the crank type.

Handrims (Figure 27-15) are usually slightly smaller in diameter than the rear wheels (e.g., 20 in. for a 24-in. wheel) and attached to the wheel rims. When smaller-diameter handrims (e.g., 12 in.) are used, they are usually fastened to the spokes. They are useful for users who travel at higher wheel speeds, with the smaller handrim being analogous to the smaller sprockets in a multiple-geared bicycle. Handrims add to the overall width of the chair. The distance between the handrim and the wheel rim is adjustable in some wheelchairs. If a user does not use the handrim on one or both sides (e.g., because the wheelchair is propelled by the feet or by an attendant), the handrims can be removed to narrow the chair. Chrome is a popular material, but may be difficult to grip when wet. Aluminum is easier to grip when the handrims are wet, but has other limitations noted earlier. Plastic or foam coating improves the grip, protects the metal, and is less cold in winter. Wrapping surgical hose in a spiral pattern around the handrims is a convenient and effective way to increase the grip, usually on a temporary basis.[28] Optional handrims are available with projections, for the individual who needs the extra grip. These are available as vertical, oblique, or horizontal lugs, usually covered by rubber, although knobs are available. However, the oblique and horizontal projections increase the chair width. Also, projections are only of any use for the user who propels the chair very slowly (e.g., the person with high quadriplegia).[28] One set of lugs is usually at a different position than the other, rendering the arm position asymmetrical. Most users who are weak and slow enough to need these accessories would be more functional in a powered wheelchair.

Solid tires are durable and need little maintenance. However, they are less likely to be perfectly round, more likely to come off the rim, and can be deformed by long periods of sitting with the wheel locks

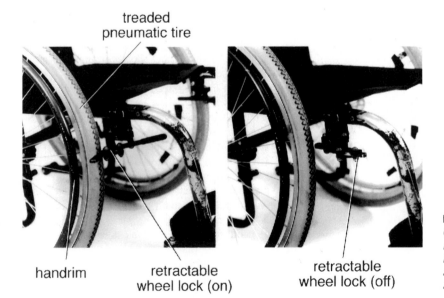

Figure 27-15
Close-up front-oblique view of a rigid-frame wheelchair, illustrating a retractable wheel lock, on and off. A treaded pneumatic tire and a handrim are also shown.

on.[12] Pneumatic tires (Figure 27-15) provide a cushioned ride and better traction on soft surfaces. However, they are susceptible to puncture and gradually lose air, so the pressure should be checked at least monthly. The amount of pressure within the manufacturer's recommended pressure range affects the ease of rolling on hard surfaces and the rate of tire wear (higher pressure is better), as well as the sense of cushioning and the ease of rolling on soft surfaces (lower pressure is better). The Schraeder valve is easier to use and more directly compatible with air-pressure sources at service stations. Athletes may prefer the narrow, lighter Presta valve that, although it requires more dexterity, is easier to use with a hand pump.[24] Foam inserts (and other options) can be used to prevent punctures, but these may add weight to the tire and eliminate some of the advantages of the pneumatic tire. For off-road purposes, wide "all-terrain" tires with deep treads are available. Treaded tires last longer and have better traction on soft surfaces, but pick up dirt. Sophisticated pneumatic tires (e.g., light high-pressure [100–200 PSI] "sew ups") are available for wheelchair athletes, to reduce rolling resistance. However, these are more expensive and usually require replacement when punctured. "Semipneumatic" tires have thick rubber walls with a small central air channel that is not under pressure. They combine some of the advantages of solid and pneumatic tires. As for tire color, darker tires last longer but gray tires have more grip and do not stain the floor.

Wheel locks maintain the wheelchair in a stationary position (like the parking brake on a car), to avoid rolling unintentionally when resting on an incline or when pushing or pulling an object in the environment. They are not intended to be used as brakes to slow the wheelchair while moving, although some users have the skill to partially apply the locks for this purpose. This practice wears the tires rapidly and has the danger, if the lock is inadvertently put into the "full on" position, of bringing the wheelchair to a rapid stop and pitching the user forward out of the chair. Toggle locks (Figure 27-5) have largely supplanted lever locks. Toggle locks work through a linkage mechanism, and may be push-to-lock or pull-to-lock. The push-to-lock version is more commonly used, because more force is required to apply the locks than to release them and the user can lean forward to add body weight when pushing. For the user with reach or strength insufficient to apply and release the locks, removable extensions can be added to the brake handles. However, the extensions need to be moved through a greater arc and can interfere with side transfers.

High-mount locks attach to the upper side-frame of the chair. This position is the most common because the locks are readily accessible. However, the thumbs can be jammed against the locks during wheel propulsion and the locks can interfere with side transfers. Low-mount locks attach to the bottom tube of the side frame (if there is one). Although they are more difficult to reach, the thumbs cannot be jammed during propulsion. Longer locks may be needed to reach from the side frame to the tire if the rear wheel is cambered. Retractable (or scissor) locks (Figure 27-15) are often used in this position. In addition to being out of the way when not on, they provide a narrower wheelchair for transport when the rear wheels have been removed. For optimum wheel-lock function, pneumatic tires must be maintained at a consistent pressure. If the rear wheels are moved (e.g., backward), the wheel locks also need to be moved. As counterintuitive as it may seem, the rear stability of a wheelchair with the wheel locks on is less than with the brakes off.[29,30] This is primarily due to the different axes of rotation in the two situations—at the wheel–ground interface with the locks on and at the level of the rear-wheel axles with the locks off.[15] Grade aids are optional attachments that, when engaged, keep the wheel from rolling back while permitting forward movement. This is useful when ascending an incline. However, they need to be adjusted carefully to function properly.

Camber is present when the distance between the tops of the rear wheels is less than the distance at the bottoms (Figure 27-2). The angle of each wheel should be measured independently. Usually 3 to 9°, the extent of camber can be altered by using washers to build up under the lower bolts on the axle-adjustment plate, or by the use of pre-set camber bars. Camber provides a natural angle for the arms to address the wheels during propulsion, protects the user's hands from doorways or from other players in sports, reduces downhill-turning tendency on side slopes, and increases ease of turning. Increasing the extent of camber induces many mechanical effects—including lengthening the wheelbase, tilting the wheelchair backward, toe-out, altering the caster-stem angle and the caster-trail distance—that may necessitate compensation.[29,31] Camber increases lateral stability and, unless compensations are made, also increases forward and reduces rear stability, owing to some of the noted effects that are coupled to camber angle.[29,31] Camber increases the wear on the wheel bearings and slightly increases rolling resistance.[12] Because there is a wider track, the wheelchair user may experience more difficulty in tight spaces. A cambered wheel, even if perfectly aligned when all four wheels are on the ground, will toe out during a wheelie, in proportion to the wheelie angle. Reverse camber is rarely intentional and serves no useful purpose.

The rear wheels are "toed in" when the fronts of the rear wheels are closer to each other than the backs; the opposite is "toed out." Because this can be asymmetrical, each wheel should be measured independently, relative to the sagittal plane. Asymmetrical toeing can cause the wheelchair to deviate to one side persistently. If the wheelchair has an axle-adjustment plate, toeing error can be eliminated by adding washers under the front or back bolts. If the axle is housed in a tube of fixed alignment, the tube can be rotated. Symmetrical toeing error (of as little as 2°) increases the rolling resistance dramatically.

Casters

Casters 8 in. in diameter are common in standard-weight wheelchairs (Figure 27-10). Many users of lightweight wheelchairs prefer 5-in. diameter casters (Figure 27-2). "Roller-blade" casters (2- to 3-in. diameter) are appropriate only for sport applications or when there is very little weight distribution on the casters. The effect of the casters on performance increases as the proportion of the weight on them increases (i.e., as the CG moves forward). The smaller the caster, the more likely it is to become jammed in cracks or grooves (e.g., an elevator door). Forward stability increases as a function of the caster diameter.[32] Small, hard casters transmit forces from encountered obstacles to a greater extent than larger, softer ones. This can lead to an uncomfortable ride and shortens the life of the wheelchair.

Usually the casters are attached to the outside of the wheelchair frame (Figures 27-2 and 27-14), but, even so, the caster tracks are inside the rear-wheel tracks. In the lightweight chairs that permit it, the casters can be set inside the frame. Some lightweight chairs use only a single midline caster. Narrowing the wheelchair in front allows tighter turns, but also reduces lateral stability and the room available for the feet.

Many of the issues discussed for the rear wheels apply equally to the casters (e.g., the effect of diameter on rolling resistance, tire issues) and will not be repeated. However, the freedom of the casters to swivel (making turns possible) provides some additional issues to consider. For instance, caster trail is the distance on the ground between two points: one obtained by dropping a vertical from the caster axle, the other by projecting the caster-swivel axis to the ground.[31] The

greater the trail, the greater is the diameter that must be kept free (of the rear wheels, footrests, and heels) if the caster is to swivel freely.

Caster flutter (or "shimmy") is the tendency for the casters to oscillate from side to side at certain speeds.[12,24,33] This can be annoying, increase rolling resistance, cause an unintentional change in direction, and cause the chair to track poorly.[7] There are a number of factors to check if the shimmy is problematic: caster-stem verticality, tension in the caster-swivel axle, caster roundness, and damage to the caster forks. To decrease shimmy at normal rolling speeds, one can reduce the size and weight of the caster, increase the caster trail, or increase the proportion of the weight on the casters.

With any swivel caster, it is important that the caster stem (and therefore the axis around which the swivel occurs) is vertical. If not, the caster axle will be lower at one swivel extreme than the other. This may cause the wheelchair to "settle" after the wheelchair has come to a halt. When starting up, there may be some resistance to overcome to get the caster stem "uphill."

In some lightweight chairs, the casters can be set in different fore-aft positions on the chair frame. If the casters are set farther back, the wheelbase is shorter (so the chair is more maneuverable in turning) and more room is created for the heels and footrests. However, the casters may hit the rear wheels when they swivel; more weight is then put on the front wheels, the forward stability of the chair decreases and, because the wheelchair can be tilted backwards by moving the casters back, rear stability can be reduced as well.

Optional pin locks can fix the caster swivel in a variety of positions. Wheelchair stability increases when the caster is swung and locked in the direction of a transfer (e.g., anteriorly or to the side).[34] On ascent of a curb, after the casters have been popped up onto the curb, the wheelchair should be backed up slightly to swing the casters forward. This has the effect of reducing the extent to which the wheelchair is tipped backwards and the likelihood of tipping over backwards when powering the rear wheels up onto the curb. Caster locks help to maintain this advantage until the whole chair is up on the curb.

Antitippers

Rear antitippers are available as an option on many wheelchairs (Figure 27-9). Of the types of floor contact, a wheel is superior to a post (being less likely to bring the chair to a stop if the antitippers make contact while the chair is moving). A caster with a swivel is ideal if turns are intended while the wheelchair is tipped back onto the antitippers. Most antitippers have a limited range of adjustability and, when adjusted in a way that makes them effective in preventing full rear tips, interfere with maneuverability (e.g., by "grounding out" during incline transitions or by preventing the wheelchair from being tipped back sufficiently to get the casters up a curb). For this reason, many wheelchair users remove them or adjust them into ineffective positions.[35] If the antitipper permits the wheelchair to be tipped back sufficiently to allow the chair to remain stably balanced on the antitippers and rear wheels, the user will have some of the advantages of a tilt-in-space wheelchair or of those who can perform wheelies.

Forward antitippers are available as optional attachments on a small number of wheelchairs. The footrests usually are positioned forward and low enough to function as forward antitippers. Some manufacturers provide rollers or wheels under the footrests for this reason (Figure 27-2). If a wheelchair allows the user to balance while tipped forward onto the footrests and casters, with the rear wheels off the ground, the skilled user (with quick-release axles) may be able to change the rear wheels of the chair without getting out of the chair.[24]

Wheelchair Carriers

Carriers come in a variety of sizes and styles. Most common is a knapsack hung from the push-handles. Other common locations are a pouch under the front of the seat or a briefcase carrier on the footrests. Special-purpose carriers (that sit on the tipping levers) are available for devices like canes and crutches. The carrier should be in a position that makes it possible for the wheelchair user to reach it easily. Added loads can affect stability.[36,37] To raise rear stability, the footrest position would be the first choice of location; to lower rear stability, the high-rear position would be used. To raise forward stability, the low-rear position would be preferred, whereas to lower forward stability, the footrest position would be used. To minimize the effect that added loads have on stability, the lap or low-anterior positions would be appropriate.

WHEELCHAIR SAFETY

The long-term use of wheelchairs can adversely affect the health of users owing to chronic or repetitive stresses—for instance, affecting shoulders, peripheral nerves, and skin.[17,19,42–46] Also there have been a number of reports of acute injuries.[16,47–56,57] In the United States, there are about 50 wheelchair-related deaths per year and over 36,000 wheelchair-related injuries per year that are serious enough to cause the injured person to seek attention at an emergency department.[16,55] The majority of these deaths and injuries are because the wheelchair users tip over and/or fall from their chairs. Of noninstitutionalized users of manually propelled wheelchairs who have used their wheelchairs for a decade, about half of them will have sustained injuries caused by tipping accidents.[58] This underlines the importance of proper wheelchair prescription, adjustment, and training.

THE PRESCRIPTION PROCESS

The goal of prescription is to assist the user to obtain (and learn to use) the wheelchair with the best possible combination of comfort, support, safety, and performance that the user can afford. This is a challenging exercise because of the bewildering (and constantly changing) array of options available, the constraint that tradeoffs are frequently necessary (e.g., between safety and performance), and the fact that a change in one wheelchair feature often alters a number of others.

The steps that follow should fully involve the user (and, if appropriate, the family or other caregivers). For their first wheelchairs, the limited experience of users will mean that they will need to rely heavily on the clinical team. As users develop more experience, they are able to participate more fully in the process.

The clinical team needs to obtain information about the user's impairments, diagnoses, prognosis, variances from the usually expected natural history (e.g., owing to a complication like heterotopic ossification limiting hip flexion), disabilities, and handicaps. The overall goals of wheelchair use will need to be determined, as well as the specific activities and settings in which the wheelchair will be used. Because tradeoffs often will be necessary, priorities need to be established.

Then the clinical team can develop a list of the ideal wheelchair and seating features for this user. A team member will measure the dimensions of the user that are relevant to the corresponding wheelchair dimensions.[10,18,59,60] The dimensions should be measured bilaterally (because asymmetries are common)[4] and with the user sitting on a cushion like the one being prescribed.[4] The local wheelchair dealers then compare the ideal-feature list and the user dimensions with what is available from a reputable manufacturer in the user's price range. The user should test drive the chair, with a member of the clinical team present.

When the most appropriate wheelchair has been decided on and purchased, the chair is adjusted to optimize safety and performance, and the user is trained in the use and maintenance of the wheelchair. Because of natural delays in the prescription process, much of the user's training will have already been completed in another wheelchair. It is important nevertheless to instruct the user in the idiosyncrasies of the actual wheelchair to be used. Finally, after the user has used the wheelchair for a few months, the situation should be reviewed and adjustments made.

REFERENCES

1. *Food, Drug and Cosmetic Act,* Pub. L. No. 75-717, 52 Stat. 1040 (1938), as am. 21 U.S.C. 301–392 (1982).
2. *Medical Device Amendments,* Pub. L. No. 94-295, 90 Stat. 540 (1976).
3. Disability Statistics Abstract. *People with Disabilities in Basic Life Activities in the U.S.* Disabilities Statistics Program, University of California, San Francisco, No. 3, April 1992.
4. Bergen AF, Presperin J, Tallman T: *Positioning for function. Wheelchairs and other assistive technologies.* Valhalla, NY: Valhalla Rehabilitation Publications, Ltd., 1990.
5. Cooper RA: Racing chair lingo: Talking the talk to win the race. *Sports 'n Spokes,* March/April 1995, pp. 71–77.
6. Leonard RB: To fold or not to fold. *TeamRehab Report.* March/April 1992, pp. 30–32.
7. Cooper RA: High-tech wheelchairs gain the competitive edge. *IEEE Engineering in Medicine and Biology.* December 1991, pp. 49–55.
8. Sullivan M: Lightweight wheelchairs and you. *Action Digest.* July/August 1992, pp. 10–12.
9. Loane TD, Kirby RL: Static rear stability of conventional and lightweight variable-axle-position wheelchairs. *Arch Phys Med Rehabil* 1985; 66:174–176.
10. International Organization for Standardization: *Wheelchairs—Part 7: Seating and wheel dimensions.* 1992, ISO/TC 173/SC 1, ISO/DIS 7176-7. 1992-12-10.
11. Brubaker C: Ergonometric considerations. Choosing a wheelchair system. *J Rehabil Res Dev* 1990; (suppl)2:37–48.
12. Thacker JG, Sprigle SH, Morris BO: *Understanding the Technology when Prescribing Wheelchairs.* Charlottesville, VA: University of Virginia, Rehabilitation Engineering Centre, 1992.
13. Hamilton EA, Strange T, Luker C: Modification of standard 8BL chair for use of double amputees. *Rheumatol Rehabil* 1976; 15:24–25.
14. van der Woude LHV, Veeger D-J, Rozendal RH, Sargeant TJ: Seat height in handrim wheelchair propulsion. *J Rehabil Res Dev* 1989; 26:31–50.
15. Majaess GG, Kirby RL, Ackroyd-Stolarz S, Charlebois P: Effect of seat position on the static and dynamic rear and forward stability of occupied wheelchairs. *Arch Phys Med Rehab* 1993; 74:977–982.
16. Calder CJ, Kirby RL: Fatal wheelchair-related accidents in the United States. *Am J Phys Med Rehab* 1990; 69:184–190.
17. Hardigan JD, Connolly TJ: Is "wheelchair wrist drop" a new syndrome to watch for? *Geriatrics* 1990; 45:63–71.
18. Axelson P: Chair & chair alike. *Sports 'n Spokes.* March/April 1995, pp. 26–61.
19. Warren CG, Ko M, Smith C, Imre JV: Reducing back displacement in the powered reclining wheelchair. *Arch Phys Med Rehab* 1982; 83:447–449.
20. Kirby RL, Loane TD, MacLeod DA: Effect of the tilt-in-space and reclining functions of a powered wheelchair on its static stability. *Clin Invest Med* 1992; 15(Suppl):A129 (abstract 786).
21. Kirby RL, Chari VR: Prostheses and the forward reach of sitting lower-limb amputees. *Arch Phys Med Rehab* 1990; 71:125–127.
22. Chari VR, Kirby RL: Lower limb influence on sitting balance while reaching forward. *Arch Phys Med Rehab* 1986; 67:730–733.
23. Kirby RL, Atkinson SM, MacKay EA: Static and dynamic forward stability of occupied wheelchairs: Influence of elevating legrests and forward stabilizers. *Arch Phys Med Rehab* 1989; 70: 681–686.
24. Denison I, Shaw J, Zuyderhoff R: *Wheelchair Selection Manual: The Effect of Components on Manual Wheelchair Performance.* Vancouver, BC: The British Columbia Rehabilitation Society, 1994.
25. Brubaker CE, McLaurin CA, McClay IS: Effects of side slope on wheelchair performance. *J Rehab Res Dev* 1986; 23:55–57.
26. Kauzlarich JJ, Collins TJ: Performing a wheelchair wheelie balance, in de Groot G, Hollander AP, Huijing PA, van Ingen Schenau GJ (eds): *Biomechanics XI-A.* Amsterdam:. Free University Press, 1988, pp. 507–512.
27. Kirby RL, Xu HY, Baird CR, Sampson M, Ackroyd-Stolarz S: Static stability of wheelchairs occupied by amputees: a computer simulation study. *Proc 7th World Congress of ISPO* 257, 1992.
28. Lehmann JF, Warren CG, Halar E, Stonebridge JB, DeLateur BJ: Wheelchair propulsion in the quadriplegic patient. *Arch Phys Med Rehab* 1974; 55:183–186.
29. Trudel G: Effect of rear-wheel camber on wheelchair stability. MSc Thesis, Dalhousie University, August 18, 1994.
30. Cooper RA, Stewart KJ, VanSickle DP: *Evaluation of Methods for Determining Static Stability of Manual Wheelchairs.* Sacramento, CA: California State University, 1992.
31. Trudel G, Kirby RL, Bell AC: Mechanical effects of rear-wheel camber on wheelchairs. *Assistive Technology* 1995; 7:79–86.
32. Kirby RL, MacLean AD, Eastwood BJ: Influence of caster

diameter on the static and dynamic forward stability of occupied wheelchairs. *Arch Phys Med Rehab* 1992; 73: 73–77.

33. Kauzlarich JJ, Bruning T, Thacker JG: Wheelchair caster shimmy and turning resistance. *J Rehab Res Dev* 1984; 20(BPR 10-40):15–29.

34. Kirby RL, Atkinson SM: Influence of caster position on the static forward stability of an occupied wheelchair. *Clin Invest Med* 1988; (abs)II:C100.

35. Kirby RL, Thoren F, Ashton B, Ackroyd-Stolarz SA: Effect of the position of rear antitippers on safety and maneuverability. *Arch Phys Med Rehab* 1994; 75:525–534.

36. Loane TD, Kirby RL: Low anterior counterweights to improve static rear stability of occupied wheelchairs. *Arch Phys Med Rehab* 1986; 67:263–266.

37. Kirby RL, Ashton BD, Ackroyd-Stolarz SA, MacLeod DA: Adding loads to occupied wheelchairs: effect on static rear and forward stability. *Arch Phys Med Rehab* 1996; 77:183–186.

38. Bayley JC, Cochran TP, Sledge CB: The weight-bearing shoulder: The impingement syndrome in paraplegics. *J Bone Joint Surg* 1987; 69-A:676–678.

39. Pentland WE, Twomey LT: The weight-bearing upper extremity in women with longterm paraplegia. *Parapelgia* 1991; 29:521–530.

40. Sie IH, Waters RL, Adkins RH, Gellman H: Upper extremity pain in the post rehabilitation spinal cord injured user. *Arch Phys Med Rehabil* 1992; 73:44–48.

41. Silfverskiold J, Waters RL: Shoulder pain and functional disability in spinal cord injury users. *Clin Orthop Rel Res* 1991; 272:141–145.

42. Wylie EJ, Chakera TMH: Degenerative joint abnormalities in users with paraplegia of duration greater than 20 years. *Paraplegia* 1988; 26:101–106.

43. Davidoff G, Werner R, Waring W: Compressive mononeuropathies of the upper extremity in chronic paraplegia. *Paraplegia* 1991; 29:17–24.

44. Gellman H, Chandler DR, Petrasek J, Sie I, Adkins R, Waters RL: Carpal tunnel syndrome in paraplegic users. *J Bone Joint Surg* 1988; 70-A:517–519.

45. Salcido R, Farrage JR Jr, Lindsey RM, Akchison JW: Painful compression of the lateral antebrachial cutaneous nerve in C5-C6 quadriplegia. *Arch Phys Med Rehab* 1992; (abst)73:960.

46. Hobson DA: Comparative effects of posture on pressure and shear at the body-seat interface. *J Rehab Res Dev* 1992; 29:21–31.

47. Bloomquist LE: Injuries to athletes with physical disabilities: Prevention implications. *Phys Sports Med* 1986; 14: 97–105.

48. Curtis KA, Dillon DA: Survey of wheelchair athletic injuries: common patterns and prevention. *Paraplegia* 1985; 23: 170–175.

49. Ferrara MS, Davis RW: Injuries to elite wheelchair athletes. *Paraplegia* 1990; 28:335–341.

50. Dudley NJ, Colter DHG, Mulley GP: Wheelchair-related accidents. *Clin Rehab* 1992; 7:9–14.

51. Gray B, Hfu JD, Furumafu J: Fractures caused by falling from a wheelchair in users with neuromuscular disease. *Devel Med Child Neurol* 1992; 34:589–592.

52. Nilsen R, Nygaard P, Bjorhott PG: Complications that may occur in those with spinal cord injuries who participate in sport. *Paraplegia* 1985; 23:152–158.

53. Notthev WM: A review of long-bone fractures in users with spinal cord injuries. *Clin Orthop Rel Res* 1981; 155:65–70.

54. Paulson SM, Hatrani C, Long C: Splenic rupture and splenectomy due to fall from wheelchair. *Arch Phys Med Rehab* 1983; 64:180–181.

55. Ummat S, Kirby RL: Nonfatal wheelchair-related accidents reported to the National Electronic Injury Surveillance System. *Am J Phys Med Rehab* 1994; 73:163–167.

56. Becker DG, Washington V, Devlin PM, Zook JE, Edlich RF: Injury due to uncontrolled acceleration of an electric wheelchair. *J Emerg Med* 1991; 9:115–117.

57. Hays RM, Jaffe KM, Ingman E: Accidental death associated with motorized wheelchair use: A case report. *Arch Phys Med Rehab* 1985; 66:709–710.

58. Kirby RL, Ackroyd-Stolarz SA, Brown MG, Kirkland SA: Wheelchair-related accidents caused by tips and falls among non-institutionalized users of manually propelled wheelchairs in Nova Scotia. *Am J Phys Med Rehab* 1994; 73:319–330.

59. Axelson P, Minkel J, Chesney D: *A Guide to Wheelchair Selection: How to Use the ANSI/RESNA Wheelchair Standards to Buy a Wheelchair.* Washington, DC, Paralyzed Veterans of America, 1994.

60. Wilson AB, Jr: *How to Select and Use Manual Wheelchairs.* Topping, VA: Rehabilitation Press, 1992.

Chapter 28

AUGMENTATIVE AND ALTERNATIVE COMMUNICATION OPTIONS FOR PERSONS WITH NEUROLOGIC IMPAIRMENT

David R. Beukelman
Joanne Lasker

The communication disorders that result from neurologic impairments are diverse in their nature and severity. Patients with a variety of etiologies may experience such severe communication disorders that they are unable to meet their daily communication needs as a result of neuromotor, neurolinguistic, or cognitive impairments. For those with amyotrophic lateral sclerosis, Parkinson's disease, and Huntington's disease, the communication disability becomes more severe as the disease or syndrome progresses. For those with brain-stem or cortical strokes, the communication disorder remains essentially stable for extended periods of time. Persons with traumatic brain injury may recover functional speech within months of their injury, while others recover speech very gradually over months to years until they reach a stable plateau.

For many individuals with the most severe communication disorders, communication strategies other than natural speech are required for them to meet their daily communication needs. This collection of strategies and options is referred to as augmentative or alternative communication (AAC). The changing course of a specific neurological impairment often dictates the type of intervention provided. This chapter summarizes the clinical decision making needed to provide AAC services to persons with neurologic impairments. Because each etiology presents somewhat different challenges, this chapter is organized according to etiology. Extensive descriptions of technology will not be included in this chapter.

Historical Context

During the past 25 years, the availability of AAC for persons with neurologic impairments has expanded considerably. Initially, a considerable amount of effort was focused on meeting the communication needs of individuals with severe cerebral palsy who were unable to speak functionally. The first group of these individuals to be served were those who could not speak because of severe physical impairment, but who were literate and able to spell their message using alternative access strategies to operate typewriters and computers. Soon, AAC systems for patients with degenerative diseases, such as amyotrophic lateral sclerosis (ALS), were developed. Many of the communication strategies that had been developed for cerebral palsy were modified to be implemented in ALS. The methods of interfacing or allowing the patient to control the electronic equipment were modified in consideration of the inexorably progressive deterioration of movement. However, the preservation of literacy skills in ALS supported the use of writing-based communication systems.

Recently, efforts have been made to address the communication needs of persons with linguistic and cognitive impairments. Many of these systems are not based on letter-by-letter spelling skills, but on coding of messages using photos and icons that require less linguistic ability than letter-by-letter spelling. These interventions require careful linguistic and cognitive assessment of the potential users in order to select technology that can be operated and matched to a specific deficit profile.

483

Meeting Communication Needs

AAC intervention decisions for patients with neurologic diseases are usually guided by a "Communication Needs" model. Rather than attempting to develop an AAC system that will replace all of the natural speech and handwriting functions that have been lost as a result of the cognitive, language, or motor impairments associated with neurologic disease, clinicians usually recommend strategies that meet the communication needs of individuals so that they can participate effectively and maintain as many of their family, education, employment, and social memberships as possible.

Multimodal AAC Systems

Rarely are the communication needs of patients with severe communication disorders met with a single AAC device. A multimodal approach to AAC is usually necessary to accommodate an individual's communication needs in a variety of contexts and with a variety of listeners. Some communicate through residual natural speech or low-technology options (eye gaze, yes/no signals), especially when the listeners are familiar and the messages are quite predictable. Persons with ALS use low techology options to communicate immediate needs and to converse with family members.[1] However, electronic communication systems may be needed to communicate detailed information. When persons with neurologic impairments are involved in community activities, such as school, job training, employment, and social settings, they usually encounter listeners who are unfamiliar with them and with their disability. In these contexts, communication options that provide more understandable message transmission and greater independence are preferred for effective communication.

Service Delivery

AAC intervention usually requires a four-phase intervention process. The first phase involves careful analysis of communication needs. The participation of the patient, caregivers, school or work colleagues, and peers may be required. The second phase involves the selection of an AAC system. During the third phase, the patient is taught to efficiently use an AAC system. Finally, during the fourth phase, follow-up services are provided to maintain the AAC system and to modify the system as the patient's communication needs or capabilities change. As the individual's communication needs, capabilities, and skills change, adjustments to the communication intervention must keep pace.

The decision to provide AAC services to individuals with neurologic speech and language disorders has been somewhat controversial in the medical community. Usually, these concerns revolve around issues of natural skill development and duration of technology use. When AAC intervention and restoration of natural speech are viewed as two mutually exclusive treatment goals, there can be a tendency to select an AAC option and ignore efforts to establish or reestablish natural speech. At other times, there may be pressure to focus exclusively on the natural speech and ignore a patient's immediate communication needs.

Effective communication intervention programs view AAC and natural speech as parts of a multimodal communication approach. Natural speech is used to meet some needs, whereas AAC fulfills functions that are unachievable through natural speech. As natural speech improves or deteriorates, the balance shifts between the use of AAC and natural speech. A second area of concern relates to the financial, emotional, and treatment costs of acquiring and maintaining an AAC system. Many people in the medical community are hesitant to recommend AAC for patients with neurologic disorders because they believe that the patient may not use the technology for an extended period of time. This occurs when life expectancy is limited or when rapid recovery is expected.

ACQUIRED MOTOR-CONTROL IMPAIRMENTS

Amyotrophic Lateral Sclerosis (ALS)

Amyotrophic lateral sclerosis (ALS) is a rapidly progressive degenerative disease that often results in severe functional communication limitations owing to bulbar dysfunction. Nearly 75 percent of persons with ALS are unable to speak at the time of their deaths.[2] An even larger number experience such severe functional communication difficulties that they are unable to meet all of their daily communication needs using natural speech. Because of the prevalence of severe communication disorders in this population, AAC strategies have become routine. The overall goal of the AAC intervention strategy is to provide appropriate augmentative services to meet communication needs in the face of progressive neuromuscular impairment.

The progression of the motor speech disorder experienced in ALS is dependent on the pattern of neurological pathology. Those individuals with primarily brain-stem (bulbar) ALS symptoms experience such severe communication disorders early in their disease progression that they require AAC systems at a time when they may still be able to walk and drive. However, persons with primarily spinal involvement may be able to communicate quite effectively using their natural speech, even as their ability to walk, drive, and feed themselves is deteriorating.

Staging AAC Interventions

A framework to stage the communication disorders of persons with ALS and to guide communication interventions has been developed.[3]

Stage 1 involves persons with ALS who are able to meet their daily communication needs through natural speech. Many of these individuals demonstrate no or minimal signs of dysarthria. No active speech and language therapy or AAC intervention is needed for these individuals. Intervention is limited to confirming the normalitys of speech and answering questions about future communication needs.

Intervention Stage 2 is characterized by a detectable speech disturbance. Speech symptoms, such as reduced loudness and imprecision of articulation, become worse with fatigue. Changes in speech intelligibility may be more noticeable to unfamiliar listeners than to daily communication partners familiar with their style of speaking. In this stage, persons with ALS and their families usually benefit from some instruction regarding environmental and interactional strategies. Competing background noise should be reduced or eliminated if possible. In addition, some individuals need specific instruction to establish the topic or context of a message before proceeding with the discussion. The ability of a listener to understand a message improves considerably if the topic of the discussion is known to the listener up front. Finally, some patients require the assistance of a portable voice amplifier at this stage.

Intervention Stage 3 is reached when there is a reduction in speech *intelligibility*. The need for frequent repetition of spoken language is now apparent. Behavioral modifications, such as slower speaking rate, and energy conservation strategies, so that speech is not further degraded by fatigue, often are useful. Palatal lifts for excessive nasal discharge and hypernasality caused by weakness of the velopharyngeal mechanism may be required.

Intervention Stage 4 is distinguished by a reduction in speech intelligibility that is so severe that AAC support is needed. Generally, the AAC interventions in this stage will be to support and augment natural speech and to resolve communication breakdowns. For example, persons with sufficient hand movement to point at the letters on an alphabet board may use alphabet or icon supplementation in this stage.

During Stage 4, persons with ALS will learn to use their AAC systems with those listeners who have particular difficulty understanding their natural speech and in situations or contexts in which it is difficult for them to speak functionally. These are often contexts that are noisy or filled with distractions. Typically at this stage, speech is not sufficiently intelligible to be functional over the telephone. It may be necessary to provide systems for written communication.

During Intervention Stage 5 useful speech is lost. Natural speech can only be used for simple answers, or not at all. A simple yes/no system can be used during mealtime. Rapid eye-gaze systems can be used to indicate preferences, identify needs and choices, and communicate when a more advanced system is not available, or when the user is too fatigued to operate the high-tech system.

Unique AAC Intervention Issues

Timing Implementation of an AAC system should be considered when the rate of natural speech is 50 percent of the habitual rate. Considering that adults read sentences aloud at a rate of approximately 190 words a minute, AAC intervention for persons with ALS should be considered when their natural speaking rate reaches approximately 100 words a minute. Typically, persons with ALS teach themselves to reduce speaking rate in order to preserve intelligibility. Therefore, a significant reduction in spontaneous speech often occurs prior to loss of intelligibility.

Because of the progressive nature of ALS, it is not uncommon for persons with ALS to use multiple AAC approaches. For example, an individual with primary bulbar ALS may need an AAC system that employs a typing interface with speech output. However, as the disease progresses, keyboard typing on a traditional keyboard may be impossible. Alternative switches to support interfaces with the AAC system may be required. Individuals with differing motor-control disabilities require different AAC strategies. For example, for persons with primarily spinal ALS, hand control is insufficient to support keyboard typing by the time an AAC system is needed.

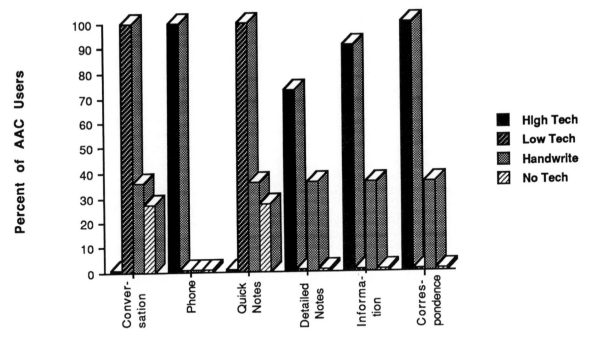

Figure 28-1
AAC system use patterns for 11 persons with ALS.

Use of Multiple AAC Approaches

Interviews with 11 individuals unable to speak owing to ALS were conducted to determine patterns of strategic AAC use (Figure 28-1).[1] Most ALS subjects used their low-technology (yes/no, eye gaze, communication board) approaches for conversation with familiar people, for brief instructions, and for emergency needs. High-technology electronically based systems are more useful for phone conversations, detailed instructions, brief instructions with unfamiliar listeners, and letter writing. A variety of AAC approaches can be used successfully to promote successful communication.

Successful use of AAC systems in ALS has a high degree of variability in relation to longevity. Given a bimodal survival peak, this is not unexpected. Of those individuals who use AAC systems successfully, approximately one third of them use the systems for less than 1 year. The remaining two thirds use their AAC systems for more than 2 years.[4]

Given the protean nature of the disease pattern and the relatively short length of time that many of these individuals use these systems, the ALS group leads to unusual service-delivery considerations. Generally the most successful intervention networks share several characteristics. First, an equipment bank allows individuals with ALS to have access to a variety of different AAC equipment as their disease progresses. Given that the use duration is relatively short, the ability to provide AAC from an equipment bank is the most cost-effective way to meet the needs of these patients.

Ongoing contact and follow-up care of the ALS patient and his support system is critical. Access to high-grade technical support is also essential.

MULTIPLE SCLEROSIS

Multiple sclerosis (MS) is a progressive disease of the white matter of the central nervous system. Symptoms depend on the location of the lesions. Therefore, the nature of the communication disorder is not consistent from person to person. Fully one third of those with MS exhibit functionally significant dysarthria.[5] Approximately 4 percent of persons with MS report that they are sufficiently impaired so that they cannot be understood by others.[6]

Unique AAC Issues

MS presents several unique AAC intervention issues. The use of AAC applications in MS is developing. Efforts at successful intervention have been limited by associated visual and coordination deficits.[7,8] AAC techniques rely extensively on the visual presentation of communication options. Given the visual impairments that are common in the MS population, many visually based systems cannot be used. In order to compensate for visual impairment, some MS interventions have utilized auditory scanning technology. In auditory scanning, the letters and words that are available to the individual using the AAC system are spoken aloud or through an earphone, and the individual is able to select from spoken options.

Intention tremor present in many individuals with MS can complicate use of AAC systems by interfering with motor control. For some, tremor intensity is worsened by the anxiety associated with system use.

PARKINSON'S DISEASE

Parkinson's disease (PD) is a progressive degenerative disorder in which motor-speech disorders are common. The range of severity of motor-speech involvement is variable. However, within this population there are many whose natural speech is so impaired that they are unable to meet their daily communication needs. Yorkston et al. stage persons with PD according to their communication performance.[3]

Before speech intelligibility is reduced, changes in vocal quality and loudness are seen. As motor speech deteriorates, a marked reduction in loudness, increased monotony, increased breathiness of voice, imprecise consonants, and alterations in speaking rate are seen. Speech cadence may become rapid. Short rushes of speech are often embedded within a normal speaking rate. Voice amplification systems are most helpful for low-volume speech where cadence is normal.

Several types of devices are available for those whose speech is significantly impaired. A pacing board in which a finger is placed in a segment of the board each time a word is spoken can be useful for some. The use of alphabet supplementation is another helpful strategy.

Some with PD are unable to be understood in daily communication contexts. Portable typing systems have been successfully used by many. These systems require that an individual be able to activate a standard keyboard with or without a keyguard in single-finger-typing fashion. The use of speech output AAC systems has not been widely advocated in PD.

GUILLAIN-BARRÉ SYNDROME

The predominant communication disorder observed in patients with Guillain-Barré syndrome is flaccid dysarthria or anarthria resulting from weakness. Many persons with Guillain-Barré syndrome are severely communicatively impaired during their paralysis. In fact, many are unable to speak at all and require AAC strategies on a temporary basis. Since neurologic recovery is the rule, the need for long-term AAC services is uncommon. Eye-pointing devices, switch-control scanners, and the electrolarynx have all been tried with success.[9,10]

The implementation of a consistent communication system allows patients with Guillain-Barré syndrome to participate more effectively in their medical care and in emotional support opportunities.

HUNTINGTON'S DISEASE

The movement and cognitive disorders associated with Huntington's disease result in a number of functional limitations that impact speech. Hyperkinetic involuntary contractions of muscle may affect any aspect of the speech mechanism, including respiration, phonation, and articulation. The speech impairment associated with Huntington's disease may vary considerably from person to person. For some, choreatic movements may be restricted primarily to the lower extremities without obvious speech disorder. For others, speech is so impaired that AAC strategies are required.

Successful use of high-technology AAC has been limited. The nature of motor and cognitive impairments and the relentless progression of symptoms are chiefly responsible. Several principles should be considered when AAC is being evaluated.[3] Select simple systems that take advantage of all skills and do not demand a great deal of new learning. Initiate training before speech intelligibility is severely impaired. Early practice is useful to establish the techniques and develop procedural memory.

AAC Options

Alphabet Boards   Alphabet boards can be used to spell messages on a letter-by-letter basis or to supplement speech. Letters must be enlarged to accommodate choreathetotic pointing.

The development of choice-making systems often is effective. Icons are presented to the patient, and choices are made by pointing or directing eye-gaze toward the symbol. Usually, minimal training is required to prepare medical and support staff to utilize such a system.

The choices offered can be displayed on small communication boards. These displays contain vocabulary and messages that are appropriate to a single topic or event. Individul display boards may be developed that are activity-specific.

CEREBRAL PALSY

Communication disorders represent a major disability for those with cerebral palsy (CP). AAC can be extremely useful for some. Given the wide range of motoric, cognitive, language, and sensory deficits known to occur in CP, the range of AAC strategies is extensive. AAC is usually delivered through a system approach that is coordinated at an early age by the public schools or a developmental preschool, and later modified to meet adult, vocational rehabilitation, or family needs. During the preschool years, it is critical that children have access to communication options that will allow them to meet their wants and needs, to develop social relationships with their families, and to acquire language skills. Readiness for participation in school is important as well. During the school years, a child with CP an AAC system that permits the communication of personal needs, conversation, language and literacy learning, and classroom participation.

BRAIN-STEM STROKE

Patients with brain-stem stroke often experience severe impairments in oral motor control, rendering them incapable of meeting basic communication needs. Depending on the location and extent of the lesion, associated problems may include extensive loss of motor control of the upper and lower extremities, swallowing, ventilatory function, and extraocular muscles. Successful AAC interventions have been used even in the locked-in syndrome, with spastic quadriparesis and aphonia. Several detailed descriptions of AAC devices for severe communication disorders fol-

lowing brain-stem stroke have been reported.[9,11] The basic strategic objectives and modalities are similar to those described earlier for ALS with progressive bulbar dysfunction.[12]

SPINAL-CORD INJURY

The communication disorder experienced by persons with spinal-cord injury depends on the level of their injury. Those who are not ventilator-dependent are usually able to meet conversational needs without specialized equipment or instruction. High quadriplegics who require ventilatory support usually are able to achieve natural speech with the adaptation of their ventilatory system to provide flow of air through the larynx.

Impaired writing is present in most persons after cervical spinal-cord injury. One- and two-finger typing can be facilitated by simple hardware adaptations to their computer systems. Usually these adaptations are designed to eliminate dual keystrokes by adding software programs or components that allow dual keystrokes (control plus letter) to be operated in sequential fashion. In addition, the communication rate for "single-finger" typists can be enhanced by computer-supported writing adaptations that allow word retrieval with an abbreviated code or selection from a cue list that is presented simultaneously on the screen.

When the level of spinal-cord injury is high, many quadriplegics are unable to control a keyboard or modified keyboard with their hands. A mouth stick can be effective for some with limited writing needs. Rate enhancement strategies (see the preceding) can be used to reduce the number of keystrokes and fatigue.

Recently, a number of technological innovations have become available for those with high quadriplegia. A keyboard emulator can be used to translate switch closures into morse code. Typically, the interface that is most efficient and least fatiguing is a "sip'n puff switch" in which the sips control the dits and the puffs control the dahs. The positive and negative pressures generated by the user to operate sip'n puff switches can be efficiently created using buccal musculature. Keyboard emulation using morse code allows the individual to operate a wide range of traditional word processing, spreadsheet, and data-basing software. For those who commit the time to learn morse code and become fluent in it, typing rates from 30 to 40 words per minute are possible, a rate similar to a nonprofessional typist.[9] Recently, reliable and accurate speech recognition technology has become available to enhance computer access for the quadriplegic. In the past, the accuracy of these systems had been problematic.

TRAUMATIC BRAIN INJURY (TBI)

As knowledge about head injury increases, cognitive-communicative deficits associated with each stage of the recovery process have become better understood. A shift has occurred in the implementation of AAC strategies. Previously, AAC devices were considered late in the recovery process, when the neurologic picture had reached a plateau. Typically, AAC systems were given to those who exhibited severe, persistent anarthria or dysarthria. The dynamic nature of recovery complicated device selection. Cognitive limitations present in the earlier stages of recovery precluded the use of complex AAC approaches. The eventual recovery of many from major head injury obviated the need for an expensive technological tool to improve speech. Recently, emphasis has shifted to promoting optimal function early in the rehabilitation process. Rehabilitation teams have recognized the importance communication plays in cognitive recovery, social participation, education, employment, and emotional health.

Three strategies can be especially useful for people attempting to communicate with marginally intelligible speech, as is often seen in those with traumatic brain injury: topic identification, supplemented speech, and portable voice amplification. In topic identification, the subject informs communication partners of the topic of conversation or semantic context verbally or by pointing to an AAC array. In speech supplementation, the first letters of the spoken words are identified by pointing to an alphabet board as the word is spoken. Both topic identification and supplemented speech allow conversation partners to limit their word retrieval search, so that, if a word is not completely understood, they have some idea of what is being said. Portable voice amplifiers may be helpful, especially in noisy settings, for individuals with hypophonia.

In the early phase of recovery after TBI, AAC interventions often focus on consistent command following and indicating preference through the use of simple switches, beepers, or environmental controls. In the middle phase, AAC may help to compensate for verbal and cognitive deficits. In the late phases of recovery, high-technology AAC can serve as a substitute for those who remain severely dysarthric.

During the past 20 years, AAC has had an important impact on persons with severe communication disorders due to neurologic disease. As the AAC knowledge and technical base has grown, AAC applications have become more available for people of all ages. As technology and computer science advance, widespread application of these devices will enhance independence and quality of life for those with neurologically based communication impairments.

REFERENCES

1. Mathy P, Brune P: Using personal computers as AAC devices. Presented at the RESNA 1993 Annual Conference, Las Vegas, NV, 1993.
2. Saunders C, Walsh T, Smith M: Hospice care in motor neuron disease, in Saunders C, Teller J (eds): *Hospice: The Living Idea*. London: Edward Arnold Publishers, 1981.
3. Yorkston K, Miller R, Strand E: *Management of Speech and Swallowing Disorders in Degenerative Disease*. Tucson, AR: Communication Skill Builders, 1995.
4. Sitver M, Kraat A: Augmentative communication for the person with amyotrophic lateral sclerosis. *ASHA* 1982; 24:783.
5. Darley F, Brown J, Goldstein N: Dysarthria in multiple sclerosis. *J Speech Hearing Res* 1972; 15:229–245.
6. Beukelman D, Kraft G, Freal J: Expressive communication disorders in persons with multiple sclerosis: A survey. *Arch Phys Med Rehab* 1985; 66:675–677.
7. Porter P: Intervention in end stage of multiple sclerosis: A case study. *Aug Alt Communun* 1989; 5:125–127.
8. Honsinger M: Midcourse intervention in multiple sclerosis: An inpatient model. *Aug Alt Commun* 1985; 5:71–73.
9. Beukelman D, Yorkston K, Dowden P: *Communication Augmentation: A Casebook of Clinical Management*. Austin, TX: Pro-ed, 1985.
10. Fried-Oken M, Howard J, Roach S: Feedback on AAC intervention from adults who are temporarily unable to speak. *Aug Alt Commun* 1991; 7:43–50.
11. Beukelman D, Yorkston K: A communication system for the severely dysarthric speaker with an intact language system. *J Speech Hear Dis* 1977; 42:265–270.
12. Culp D, Ladtkow M: Locked-in syndrome and augmentative communication, in Yorkston K (ed): *Augmentative Communication in the Medical Setting*. Tucson: Communication Skill Builders, 1992.

Chapter 29

SPEECH THERAPY AND DISORDERS OF DEGLUTITION

Richard D. Zorowitz

Researchers have studied swallowing and disorders of deglutition far longer than one might expect. In 1824, Magendie first enumerated the events of swallowing by dividing them into stages based on the anatomical regions of the mouth, pharynx, and esophagus.[1] In the latter part of the century, Falk and Kronecker studied the movements of the mouth and pharynx, and supported the notion that the act of swallowing required the coordinated contraction of the oral musculature.[2] During the same year, Kronecker and Meltzer confirmed the mechanism of swallowing using two balloons placed in the pharynx and esophagus.[3] They concluded that liquids and semi-solids are propelled into the esophagus by the actions of the mouth muscles.

Until this time, swallowing research was performed without the benefit of dynamic images. The first fluorographic images of swallowing were obtained in 1898 using subnitrate of bismuth as the inert opaque vehicle with which boluses were mixed.[4] Studies performed on geese, cats, dogs, horses, and humans demonstrated that the total time for deglutition was variable, depending on the consistency. Fluorographic studies later demonstrated the upward movement of the hyoid bone and downward movement of the epiglottis to cover the larynx.[5] Barclay further elaborated on the fluorographic observations of deglutition, and correctly observed that the epiglottis did not fold down during swallowing, nor did the posterior pharyngeal wall contract.[6] The technique of recording fluorographic studies on film for analysis finally came into being in 1936.[7] Cinefluorography and, later, videofluorography are responsible for much of the knowledge of the anatomy and physiology of deglutition.

Swallowing, in fact, requires a series of interdependent, coordinated muscle contractions that break down food boluses and transport them from the oral cavity to the stomach. The process of deglutition requires six cranial nerves, four cervical nerves, and over 30 pairs of muscles. Diagnosis and treatment of dysphagia requires a knowledge of the normal anatomy and physiology of swallowing as well as the disease processes and associated mechanisms that cause dysphagia. An understanding of the evaluation of the dysphagia heightens the suspicion of swallowing difficulties in appropriate patient populations and decreases the risk of debilitating complications, such as malnutrition and aspiration pneumonia. Recognition of treatment options allows the clinician to provide the patient with the most optimal nutritional support while the patient practices strategies that improve deglutition and maximize oral caloric intake. An awareness of the course of recovery, prognosis, and ethical issues of dysphagia in various disease states helps to confirm the treatment plan and serves to reassure the patient that he or she is receiving the best possible dysphagia therapy for the condition.

ANATOMY AND PHYSIOLOGY

Normal deglutition consists of four phases: (1) oral preparatory; (2) oral; (3) pharyngeal; and (4) esophageal. A list of the muscles, their innervations and functions, and the phases in which they are associated is found in Table 29-1. Some of the structures of the pharynx are displayed in Figures 29-1 and 29-2.

During the oral preparatory phase (Figure 29-3A), food is manipulated in the mouth and masticated if necessary. Mastication involves a repeated cyclical pattern of rotary lateral movement of the labial and mandibular musculature. Some food normally falls into the pharynx during this phase.[8] Once broken down into particles, food is collected into a bolus and held anterolaterally by the tongue against the palate. The oral activity required for appropriate bolus size and consistency

Table 29-1
Muscles involved in swallowing

Muscle	Nerve	Stage	Action
Temporalis	V	OP	Elevates, retracts mandible
Masseter	V	OP	Elevates mandible
Pterygoideus medialis	V	OP	Elevates, protracts mandible
Pterygoideus lateralis	V	OP	Depresses, protracts mandible Moves mandible laterally
Obicularis oris	VII	OP,O	Opens, closes, protracts lips
Zygomaticus major	VII	OP,O	Elevates mouth angle upward, backward
Levator labii superioris	VII	OP,O	Elevates upper lip, mouth angle
Depressor labii inferioris	VII	OP,O	Depresses lower lip
Levator anguli oris	VII	OP,O	Elevates mouth angle
Depressor anguli oris	VII	OP,O	Depresses mouth angle
Mentalis	VII	OP,O	Elevates, protracts lower lip
Risorius	VII	OP,O	Retracts mouth angle
Buccinator	VII	OP,O	Flattens, retracts cheek, mouth angle
Hyoglossus	XII	OP,P	Depresses tongue
Genioglossus	XII	OP,P	Depresses, protrudes tongue
Musculus uvulae	IX,X,XI	O	Elevates uvula
Palatoglossus	IX,X,XI	O	Elevates posterior tongue Narrows fauces
Levator veli palatini	IX,X,XI	P	Elevates soft palate
Tensor veli palatini	V	P	Stretches soft palate
Mylohyoideus	V	P	Elevates tongue base, mouth floor, hyoid bone; depresses mandible
Digastricus	V	P	Elevates hyoid bone, tongue base
Geniohyoideus	XII,C1	P	Elevates hyoid bone, tongue
Stylohyoideus	VII	P	Elevates hyoid bone, tongue base
Thyrohyoideus	XII,C1	P	Depresses larynx, hyoid bone Elevates thyroid cartilage
Styloglossus	XII	P	Elevates, retracts tongue
Palatopharyngeus	IX,X,XI	P	Narrows oropharynx Elevates pharynx
Stylopharyngeus	IX	P	Elevates, dilates pharynx
Salpingopharyngeus	IX,X,XI	P	Elevates nasopharynx
Aryepiglotticus	IX,X	P	Tilts epiglottis downward
Cricoarytenoideus lateralis	IX,X	P	Closes glottis, approximates vocal folds
Thyreoarytenoideus	IX,X	P	Closes glottis, shortens vocal folds
Constrictor pharyngeus superioris	IX,X,XI	P	Compresses pharynx
Constrictor pharyngeus intermedius	IX,X,XI	P	Compresses pharynx
Constrictor pharyngeus inferioris	X,XI	P	Compresses pharynx
Cricopharyngeus	X	P	Closes upper esophageal sphincter

OP, oral preparatory stage; O, oral stage; P, pharyngeal stage.

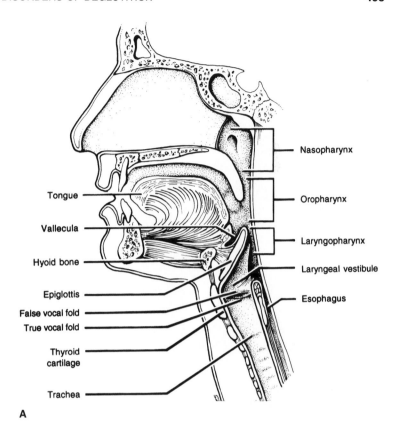

Nasopharynx

Oropharynx

Laryngopharynx

Laryngeal vestibule

Esophagus

Tongue

Vallecula

Hyoid bone

Epiglottis

False vocal fold

True vocal fold

Thyroid cartilage

Trachea

Figure 29-1
Lateral view of the pharynx. A. Schematic view.

A

requires complex sensory input such as taste, touch temperature, and proprioception.[9]

During the oral phase (Figure 29-3B), the tongue propels food posteriorly until the pharyngeal swallow is triggered in the area of the anterior faucial arches. A labial seal is maintained to prevent food or liquid from leaking from the mouth. Tension of the buccal musculature prevents food from falling into the lateral sulci between the mandible and the cheek. The tongue elevates sequentially in an anterior–posterior direction and propels the bolus into the pharynx.[10] The oral phase lasts approximately 1 second.

During the pharyngeal phase (Figures 29-3C through 29-E), the pharyngeal swallow is triggered and moves the bolus through the pharynx. The pharyngeal swallow is triggered primarily at the anterior faucial arches so that posterior movement of the bolus is not interrupted.[11,12] The velum is elevated and retracted, and the velopharyngeal port is completely closed to prevent material from entering the nasal cavity. The true vocal folds, false vocal folds, and aryepiglottic folds

close to prevent material from entering the trachea. The larynx and hyoid bone elevate and move forward, causing the cricopharyngeus muscle to stretch and the pharynx to shorten through elevation of the hypopharynx.[13,14] The tongue pushes posteriorly and downward into the pharynx, and pushes the bolus through the pharynx into the esophagus. Pharyngeal contraction causes a stripping action that minimizes pharyngeal residue.[15] The pharyngeal phase may last approximately 1 second when swallowing liquids, but may be longer in normal adults for solid consistencies.

During the esophageal phase (Figure 29-3F), peristalsis moves the bolus into the stomach. The peristaltic wave begins at the superior end of the esophagus when the pharyngeal swallow begins, and progresses in sequential fashion caudally to the gastroesophageal sphincter. The gastroesophageal sphincter then relaxes, allowing the bolus to enter the stomach.

Swallowing must interact with ventilation so that eating and drinking does not result in a bolus violating the larynx and trachea. Swallowing usually interrupts

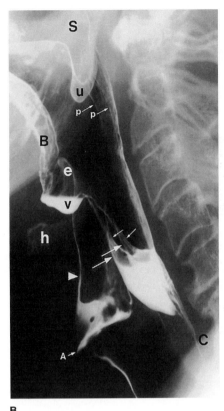

B

Figure 29-1 *(Continued)*
B. Radiographic view. The soft palate (S) elevates to appose the posterior pharyngeal wall (u, representing the uvula). The paired palatopharyngeal folds, or posterior tonsillar pillars (p) course from the lateral portion of the mid-soft palate to the lateral pharyngeal walls, forming the posterior border of the tonsillar fossae. Phonation widens the oropharynx and separates the tip of the epiglottis (e) from the base of the tongue (B). The valleculae (v) are overlapped. The aryepiglottic folds (small white arrows) curve posteriorly, and the anterior walls of the piriform sinuses bow anteriorly (large white arrows). Barium coats the anterior wall of the laryngeal vestibule (arrowhead), extending to the anterior commissure of the larynx (A). The upper esophageal sphincter (C) is actively contracted, and the hyoid bone (h) is in its resting position. (Radiograph and text courtesy of Stephen E. Rubesin, M.D., Department of Radiology, University of Pennsylvania School of Medicine).

the expiratory phase of ventilation, and the completion of expiration occurs at the conclusion of the swallow.[16] There is a positive correlation between the expiration-onset-to-swallow-onset interval and the duration of the total interrupted expiration. If a swallow is initiated

during the inspiratory phase of ventilation, a short expiration usually follows the completion of the swallow. Tidal volume may increase in the breaths following the swallow.[17] Simultaneous recording of ventilatory patterns and videofluorography may be performed to relate the feeding ventilatory pattern to sounds elicited during swallowing.[18]

The organization of the swallowing motor sequence depends on the activity of a neural network known as the swallowing center. The swallowing center is divided into three levels: (1) the afferent level, or the input arm; (2) the efferent level, or the output arm; and (3) the organizing level, which is the interneuronal network that programs the motor sequence of swallowing.

The afferent level consists of sensory receptors of the faucial arches, tonsils, soft palate, tongue base, and posterior pharyngeal wall, which transmit messages to the swallowing center through cranial nerves VII, IX, and X.[19] The fibers of the superior laryngeal nerve carry impulses to the swallowing center through the solitary tract.[20]

The efferent level consists of fibers carried through cranial nerves V, VII, IX, X, and XII.[21] Some have associated cranial nerve V with mastication rather than deglutition and cranial nerve VII with only a small proportion of neurons that participate in deglutition. Others have defined the efferent level of swallowing as the trigeminal and hypoglossal nuclei along with the nucleus ambiguus.[22]

The organizing level of swallowing is thought to be located in two regions of the pontine reticular formation: (1) dorsal, including the nucleus of the solitary tract and adjacent reticular formation; and (2) ventral, corresponding to the lateral reticular formation above the nucleus ambiguus. The dorsal portion appears to initiate and organize the swallowing motor sequence. The ventral portion distributes the motor impulses to the various motor neurons involved with swallowing. In animals, stimulation of the solitary tract or its nucleus in the cat, rat, or sheep can elicit a swallow.[23,24]

In addition to the brain stem swallowing center, a cortical swallowing center has been described just anterior to the orbital gyrus. In animals, single-pulse stimulation of the cortical center causes rhythmic activation of the ipsilateral nucleus of the solitary tract, but the frequency of deglutition decreases rapidly. The cortical center is thought to receive information from the contralateral cortical center and oropharyngeal and laryngeal receptors. Its purpose is not well understood but may be important for repeated swallowing or initiation of the motor sequence of deglutition.

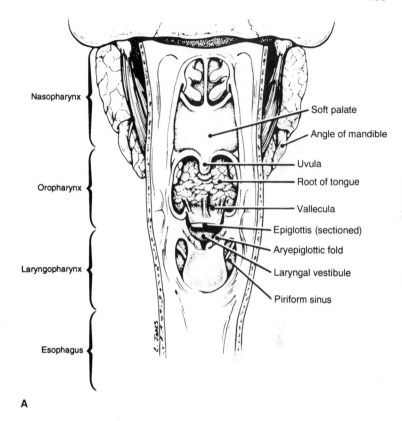

Nasopharynx

Oropharynx

Laryngopharynx

Esophagus

Soft palate

Angle of mandible

Uvula

Root of tongue

Vallecula

Epiglottis (sectioned)

Aryepiglottic fold

Laryngal vestibule

Piriform sinus

Figure 29-2
Anteroposterior view of the pharynx.
A. Schematic view.   **A**

PATHOPHYSIOLOGY

Dysphagia affects one or more stages of deglutition, and may result in aspiration or penetration of a bolus into the laryngotracheal tract. Some define penetration as active entry of a bolus into the trachea (e.g., during swallowing) and aspiration as passive entry into the trachea (e.g., during inhalation). In this text, penetration denotes entry of a bolus by any means into the laryngeal vestibule, and aspiration designates entry of a bolus into the trachea.

Subjects with neurologic disease most commonly have oral stage abnormalities.[25,26] Weakness or incoordination of the lips, cheeks, or tongue may result in oral leakage, pocketing in the lateral sulci, or premature spillage into the pharynx. Premature spillage into the pharynx may result in aspiration before the pharyngeal swallow can be initiated (Figure 29-4). Abnormal tongue thrusting may be indicative of a weak posterior tongue. Severe cognitive deficits may be associated with decreased interest in swallowing and absence of initiating the swallow. Although the pharyngeal phase may be normal in these cases, overall abnormal oral functions are correlated with abnormal pharyngeal functions and defective opening of the cricopharyngeus.[27]

Many significant problems may occur in the pharyngeal stage of swallowing. Nasopharyngeal reflux suggests soft-palate or superior-pharyngeal dysfunction. Reduced elevation of the larynx and pharynx may be owing to impaired hyoid bone elevation or thyrohyoid or palatopharyngeal dysfunction. Defective closure of the laryngeal vestibule may cause aspiration during the pharyngeal swallow (Figure 29-5). Pharyngeal constrictor weakness may produce residue of the bolus in the valleculae or piriform sinuses, which may be subsequently aspirated after the swallow (Figure 29-6). Failure of the cricopharyngeus muscle to open may be owing to impaired relaxation or distensibility, hypertrophy or hyperplasia, or fibrosis (Figure 29-7).

Anatomic or physiologic abnormalities are associated with esophageal dysfunction. A Zenker's diverticulum may be located in the midline or may be of the Killian-Mamieson type when located laterally and inferior to the cricopharyngeus muscle insertion on the cri-

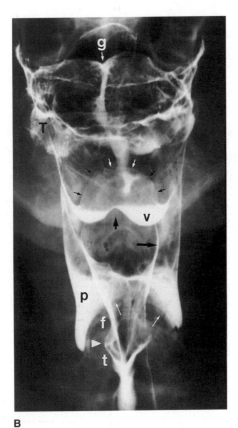

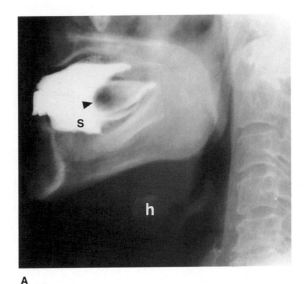

A

Figure 29-3
Phases of deglutition. A. Oral preparatory phase. The barium bolus is held in the mouth in the anterior and lateral sublingual sulci and on top of the tongue. The tongue (ovoid lucency identified by arrowhead) is just about to collect the barium from the sublingual sulci (s). The hyoid bone is positioned well below the mandible.

B

Figure 29-2   *(Continued)*
B. Radiographic view. The right tonsillar fossa (T) and central groove of the tongue (g) are seen in profile. The median gloss-oepiglottic fold (medium-size black arrow) divides the retroglot-tic space into the two cup-shaped valleculae (v). The epiglottis (tip outlined by small arrows) rises above the valleculae. The inner margin of the left aryepiglottic fold (large black arrow) is coated by aspirated barium. The right vocal fold (t), laryngeal vestibule (arrowhead), and false vocal fold (f) are shown in relationship to the hypopharynx. The lower hypopharynx remains collapsed except during swallowing. The piriform sinus (p) lies along the anterior wall of the mid-hypopharynx, which appears as an inverted U (long white arrows). (Radiograph and text courtesy of Stephen E. Rubesin, M.D., Department of Radiology, University of Pennsylvania School of Medicine).

coid cartilage (Figure 29-8).[28] Absent or weak esophageal peristalsis may be a sign of scleroderma or may be associated with "nutcracker" esophagus (Figure 29-9). Esophageal webs, rings, or strictures often cause obstructions that are most pronounced while swallowing solids. Gastroesophageal reflux commonly are associ-

ated with hiatal hernia but have been observed in conjunction with cricopharyngeal dysfunction (Figure 29-10).[29] Achalasia is characterized by reduced relaxation of the gastroesophageal junction ("bird-beak" narrowing) and absent esophageal peristalsis (Figure 29-11).

Disruptions of the swallowing centers or nervous system pathways can result in dysphagia. Swallowing difficulties occur in a variety of neuromuscular disorders (Table 29-2). However, dysphagia research has been undertaken in some of the more common conditions.

Stroke

Up to 45 percent of acute stroke survivors may have dysphagia, and up to 55 percent of these demonstrate evidence of aspiration.[30–33] Although dysphagia may be associated with lesions of the cortical hemispheres or brain stem, symptoms may differ with lesion site. Cortical lesions may result in contralateral reductions in labial and lingual strength, range of motion, and sensation; delayed pharyngeal swallow; and contralateral reductions in pharyngeal strength.[34,35] Subjects with left hemi-

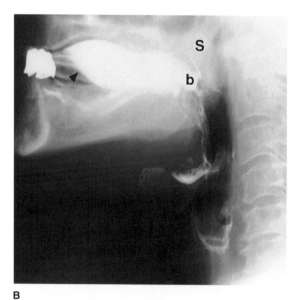

B

Figure 29-3 *(Continued)*
B. Early oral phase. The tongue tip (arrowhead) has collected the barium from the sublingual sulci and is beginning to rise to appose the hard palate. The bolus is beginning to pass the palatoglossal folds (anterior tonsillar pillars). The soft palate is beginning to rise, and an air gap still is seen between the mid-soft palate (S) and the posterior pharyngeal wall.

sphere lesions tend to have longer pharyngeal transit durations, whereas those with right hemispheric lesions have longer pharyngeal stage durations and higher incidences of laryngeal penetration and aspiration of liquid.[36] Brainstem lesions may result in reduced labial, lingual, and buccal strength, range of motion, and sensation; absence or delay of the pharyngeal swallow; reduced pharyngeal strength, reduced laryngeal adduction and elevation; and cricopharyngeal dysfunction.[37,38] Even subjects with periventricular white matter changes may demonstrate increases in the combined duration of the oral and pharyngeal stages.[39]

Stroke survivors who aspirate acutely tend to have combined large- and small-vessel disease, resulting in multifocal lesions. Patients with bilateral cranial nerve dysfunction are at the greatest risk of aspiration, and dysphonia is the most common symptom associated with aspiration. Patients with brain stem strokes may have cranial nerve IX abnormalities, vocal fold weakness, and severe dysarthria.[40] Up to 40 percent of dysphagia stroke survivors may aspirate silently, and these patients may express fewer subjective complaints and have a weaker cough.[41,42]

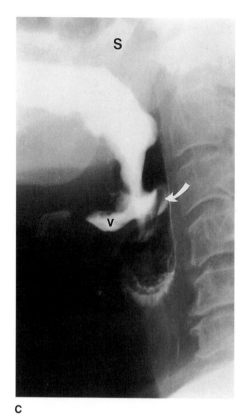

C

Figure 29-3 *(Continued)*
C. Early pharyngeal phase. The bolus has spilled into the valleculae (v). The soft palate is apposed to the posterior pharyngeal wall, sealing the nasal passages. The epiglottis (curved arrow) is beginning to tilt posteriorly. The pharynx has elevated and is broader in the anterior-posterior diameter (compare with B.), indicating pharyngeal shortening and elevation. The laryngeal vestibule is partially closed, and the upper esophageal sphincter is still closed.

Traumatic Brain Injury

Approximately 26 to 30 percent of patients who suffer a traumatic brain injury are diagnosed with a swallowing disorder.[43–45] Traumatic brain injury may cause a hypermetabolic state that makes nutritional support more necessary to support life.[46] However, patients below a Ranchos Los Amigos scale of 4 usually are not capable of eating.[47] The most common swallowing disorders observed in this population include a delayed or absent pharyngeal swallow, reduced tongue control, and pharyngeal weakness.[48] As in stroke, apraxia or abnormal movements may prevent the bolus from properly pass-

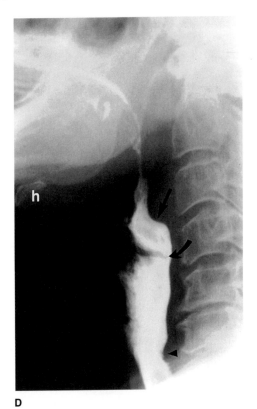

D

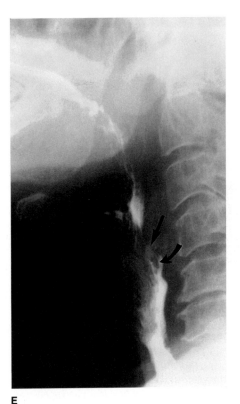

E

Figure 29-3   *(Continued)*
D. Midpharyngeal phase. The bolus is passing through the mid- and lower hypopharynx and the upper esophageal sphincter. The epiglottis (curved arrow) is tilting further inferiorly. The posterior pharyngeal contraction wave (straight arrow) represents sequential contraction of the superior, middle, and inferior constrictor muscles and is seen in the lateral view as a forward bulge of the posterior pharyngeal wall that progresses inferiorly. The upper esophageal sphincter (arrowhead) is incompletely opened. The hyoid bone has elevated and moved forward beneath the mandible.

Figure 29-3   *(Continued)*
E. Late pharyngeal phase. The bolus has passed nearly completely through the pharynx. The epiglottis (curved arrow) has inverted completely. The posterior pharyngeal contraction wave (straight arrow) clears the pharynx of residual bolus.

ing through the pharynx.[49] Full oral intake usually does not occur until the patient reaches Ranchos Los Amigos level 6, at which time patients display more appropriate behavior.

Even as cognitive status improves, the traumatic brain injury patient may exhibit behavioral problems that limit the ability to use or participate in compensatory swallowing techniques.[50] Attentional deficits tend to have a greater negative influence than do memory deficits.[51] The presence of primitive reflexes or neglect of a bolus may increase the risk of aspiration if not closely monitored. Impulsive patients may attempt to ingest large amounts of food into the mouth at one time.[52] High-level cognitive deficits such as sequencing or organizing feeding activities may affect the ability of the patient to select appropriate foods or self-monitor rates of feeding or compensatory strategies. Memory deficits may cause the patient to forget when he or she ate last or prevent the patient from learning skills needed to eat safely. Even mild problems may keep the patient from being able to feed him- or herself independently.

Multiple Sclerosis

Bronchopneumonia is a leading direct cause of death in patients with multiple sclerosis (MS). Although a link with dysphagia has not been demonstrated, clinically unsuspected aspiration associated with dysphagia has

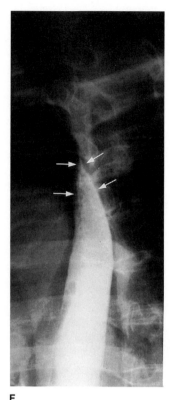

F

Figure 29-3   *(Continued)*
F. Esophageal phase. A normal peristaltic wave appears as an inverted V (arrows) that progresses inferiorly. The contraction wave is mediated by skeletal muscle above the level of the aortic arch, and smooth muscle fibers produce a true peristaltic wave below the aortic arch. (Radiographic illustrations and text courtesy of Stephen E. Rubesin, M.D., Department of Radiology, University of Pennsylvania School of Medicine).

been correlated with a significantly higher risk of pneumonia.[53] Swallowing dysfunction may occur in up to 55 percent of patients with multiple sclerosis.[54] The duration of the disease correlates with the presence of symptoms, which are related to oral–motor function and airway protection.[55]

Brain Tumors

Dysphagia is a common symptom in patients both before and after resection of a brain tumor. Up to 14.5 percent of patients with primary brain tumors complained of swallowing difficulties, whereas 75 percent of patients who underwent resection of basal skull tumors

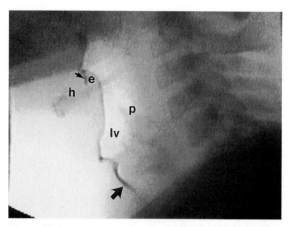

Figure 29-4
Aspiration before the swallow. As a result of poor lingual control, a liquid bolus spills into the vallecula (small arrow), through the laryngeal vestibule (lv), and into the trachea (large arrow). The hyoid bone (h) and epiglottis (e) remain in their resting positions, and the laryngeal vestibule remains open. The hypopharynx (p) ends at the contracted cricopharyngeus muscle.

aspirated during videofluorographic swallowing studies.[56,57] Level of alertness strongly correlates with both quality of swallowing function and ability to compensate for swallowing difficulties.

Extrapyramidal Diseases

Parkinsonism is the most common extrapyramidal disease associated with dysphagia. Early studies of patients

Figure 29-5
Aspiration during the swallow. Because of pharyngeal weakness reflected by partial deflection of the epiglottis (long arrow), a portion of a liquid bolus enters into the trachea (t) through the laryngeal vestibule and the true vocal folds (short arrow). The remainder of the bolus successfully passes into the esophagus (e). Note that the hyoid bone (h) is in its most elevated position.

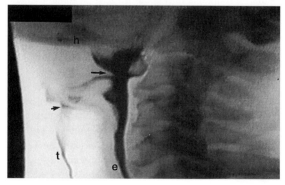

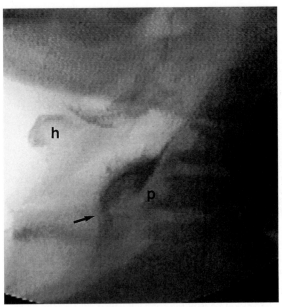

Figure 29-6
Aspiration after the swallow. Owing to pharyngeal weakness, a portion of a liquid bolus pools in the piriform sinuses (p) and spills over the aryepiglottic fold into the trachea (t). Note that the hyoid bone (h) is in its resting position.

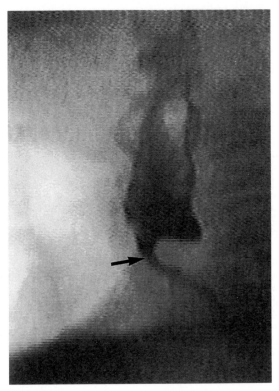

Figure 29-7
Cricopharyngeal dysfunction. The cricopharyngeus muscle does not relax, resulting in a "bar" (arrow) that prevents much of this liquid bolus from passing into the esophagus.

with Parkinsonism have described increased transit times throughout all stages, lingual dysfunction, pharyngeal residue, esophageal reflux, and tertiary esophageal contractions.[58] Aspiration may occur in up to 46 percent of patients, and is seen more commonly with liquid swallows than with solids or semi-solids.[59] In ambulatory patients, abnormal bolus formation, piecemeal deglutition, and reflux are significant symptoms, but pulmonary infection is not readily seen.[60] However, swallowing disorders may be identified in many asymptomatic patients.[61] Dysphagia may occur both in patients with and without dementia.[62] Dysphagia may decrease when appropriate medications are given.[63]

The manifestations of swallowing problems in Huntington's disease, on the other hand, has not been studied as much. Patients with hyperkinetic Huntington's disease may exhibit rapid lingual chorea, incoordinated pharyngeal swallow, multiple swallows per bolus, prolonged laryngeal elevation, an inability to stop respiration, and frequent eructations.[64] In contrast, patients with rigid-bradykinetic Huntington's disease may demonstrate mandibular rigidity, slow lingual chorea, and coughing and choking on foods and liquids. In the earlier

stages of the disease, compensatory techniques benefit many of these patients.

Motor-Neuron Diseases

Dysphagia in motor-neuron diseases is best represented by amyotrophic lateral sclerosis (ALS) and Guillain-Barré syndrome (GBS). Common symptoms include weakness of the lingual, palatal, and pharyngeal muscles.[65] Guillain-Barré syndrome also has been associated with achalasia.[66] Dysphagia also has been reported in progressive bulbar palsy, in which atrophy and fasciculations of the tongue, dysarthria, dysphagia, and excessive accumulations of secretions were observed.[67]

Post-Polio Syndrome

More recently, dysphagia has become recognized as a late complication of poliomyelitis. Most patients will

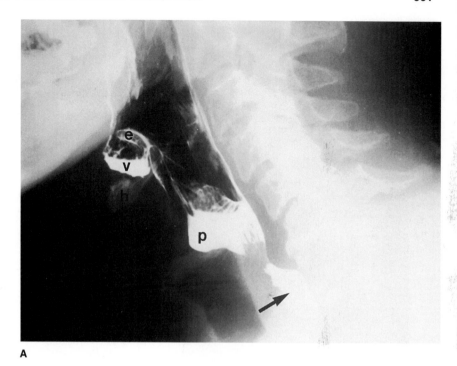

Figure 29-8
Zenker's diverticulum. This abnormality is located in the midline just inferior to the cricopharyngeus muscle in the cervical esophagus (arrows). A. Lateral view. B. Anteroposterior view (v, vallecula; e, epiglottis; p, piriform sinus).   **A**

experience clinical or subclinical dysfunction in the muscles of deglutition.[68] Electromyographic studies demonstrate decreased recruitment and increased amplitude of muscle action potentials.[69] Diagnostic studies show evidence of weakened oral and pharyngeal musculature, prolonged oral transit time, silent aspiration without responsive cough, delayed pharyngeal swallow, unilateral pharyngeal residue, esophageal dysmotility, and gastroesophageal reflux.[70,71] Oropharyngeal function usually deteriorates slowly, with new symptoms corresponding to the severity of dysfunction.

Neuromuscular Junction Diseases

Dysphagia may the first symptom in conditions such as myasthenia gravis.[72] Swallowing may be normal at the beginning of a day or meal, and may worsen as the day or meal progresses. The oral musculature becomes progressively weaker and slower. Tongue atrophy and persistent dysphonia may be observed in late stages of the disease.[73] Nasal regurgitation may reflect gradual incompetence of the velopharyngeal port, and pharyngeal residue may be associated with loss of pharyngeal tone. The injection of acetylcholinesterase inhibitor medications helps to assist the diagnosis of myasthenia gravis and to evaluate the efficacy of treatment.

Muscle Diseases

Both denervative and inflammatory diseases may be responsible for symptoms of myogenic dysphagia. However, symptoms may be varied depending on the disease.[74] Difficulties in mastication and bolus formation are seen in the muscular dystrophies (MD) and spinal muscular atrophy (SMA). Limitations in mouth opening are noted in SMA. Pharyngeal transit times are prolonged in polymyositis, dermatomyositis, limb-girdle muscular dystrophy (LGMD), and SMA. Associated characteristics include macroglossia in Duchenne muscular dystrophy (DMD) and xerostomia in polymyositis and dermatomyositis. The cricopharyngeus muscle usually opens briefly but adequately, but cricopharyngeal myotomy may be indicated in a subpopulation of patients with partial pharyngeal weakness.[75] The overall prevalence of dysphagia in facioscapulohumeral muscular dystrophy (FSHMD), MD, SMA, polymyositis, and dermatomyositis may be as high as 34.9 percent.

EVALUATION

History

The evaluation of dysphagia begins with a focused history. If the subject cannot give a history owing to altered

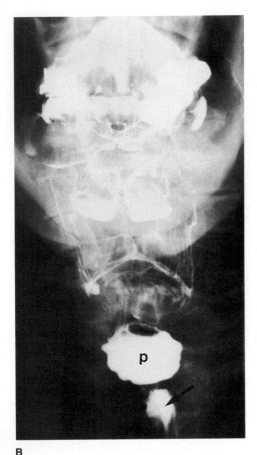

B

Figure 29-8.   (*Continued*)

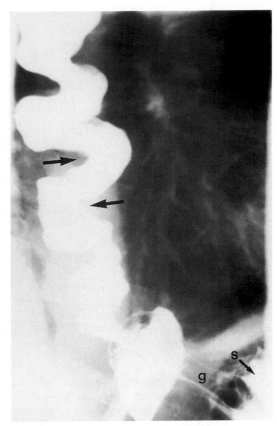

Figure 29-9
"Nutcracker" esophagus. The corkscrew appearance of the lower esophagus (arrows) is characteristic of diffuse esophageal spasm (g, gastroesophageal junction; s, stomach).

mental status or speech-language disorder, information may come from a health professional, family member, or medical record. Chief complaints related to dysphagia are found in Table 29-3.

Consistencies and temperatures of foods may influence symptoms. Subjects with neurogenic dysphagia tend to have liquid dysphagia since muscles are weakened or uncoordinated.[76] Subjects with complaints of obstruction may have strictures, webs, or tumors. Subjects with esophageal abnormalities may complain of solid or liquid dysphagia.[77] Cold liquids may reduce primary esophageal peristalsis or produce esophageal spasm or myotonus.

Attention should be paid to the subject's medical and surgical history. Neurologic conditions are a major source of dysphagia. Medical problems, such as diabetes, thyroid disease, chronic obstructive pulmonary disease,

or cancer, should be noted, as these can contribute directly or indirectly to a swallowing problem. Head and neck surgery or radiation therapy can significantly change the anatomy or physiology of the swallowing mechanism. Medications can cause dry mouth (diuretics, anticholinergics), weaken muscles (antispasmodics), cause extrapyramidal symptoms (neuroleptics), acidify gastric secretions (aspirin, vitamin C, tetracycline, $FeSO_4$), weaken esophageal motility (calcium-channel blockers, nitrates), or cause reflux (beta-adrenergics, theophylline, ethanol, tobacco).

Physical Examination

The physical examination concentrates on areas of interest identified from the history. It serves to better identify

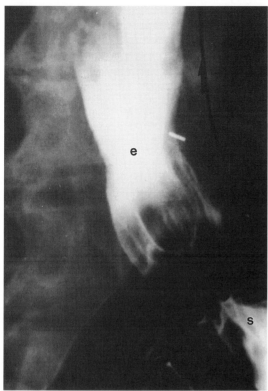

Figure 29-10
Gastroesophageal reflux. Although the bolus in this picture appears to be emptying from the esophagus (e) into the stomach (s), it is in fact refluxing from the stomach all the way to the cricopharyngeus muscle.

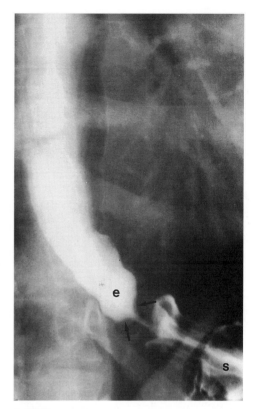

Figure 29-11
Achalasia. The esophagus has the characteristic "bird-beak" appearance (arrows) where the gastroesophageal junction (g) does not relax (s, stomach).

the etiology of the problem; determine whether, what, and how the subject may be fed orally; and decide on the necessity for further testing. The examination begins with a review of vital signs, especially weight, to determine whether the subject is capable of supporting him- or herself nutritionally. All structures that can be visualized easily, such as teeth and the oral mucosa, should be inspected and palpated for abnormal lesions or masses.

The remainder of the examination merely is a focused neurologic assessment. All oral and facial muscles should be tested for strength, range of motion, and coordination. Sensation of the face and intraoral structures should be evaluated. The presence of pathologic reflexes, such as the bite and suck, should be determined. The gag reflex should be tested for response and symmetry. However, as the gag reflex is highly variable even among healthy people, it should be considered abnormal if asymmetrical, if a history of normal gag reflex is

known, or if other cranial nerve dysfunction is present. A brief mental status examination should evaluate comprehension, praxis of oral structures, and visual–perceptual skills to determine the ability to compensate for potential problems.

The final portion of the physical examination involves a clinical evaluation of swallowing. If there is possible risk of aspiration, test swallows should be performed with consistencies that carry a relatively low risk of aspiration. Nasogastric tubes should be removed to normalize the oropharyngeal mucosa. Palpation of the tongue and larynx over the neck is helpful in assessing the speed and smoothness of the swallow. Coughing, signs of aspiration, or nasal regurgitation should be noted. If a tracheostomy is present, the trachea should be suctioned and the cuff should be deflated during testing. The use of methylene blue-dyed water may be used to increase the suspicion of aspiration, but suggests aspiration on only one consistency of liquid.

Table 29-2
Examples of neuromuscular conditions causing dysphagia

Upper Motor Neuron
  Stroke
  Traumatic brain injury
  Parkinsonism
  Huntington's disease
  Alzheimer's disease
  Neurosyphilis
  Encephalitis
  Meningitis
  Spinocerebellar degeneration
  Olivopontocerebellar atrophy
  Progressive supranuclear palsy

Lower Motor Neuron
  Poliomyelitis
  Amyotrophic lateral sclerosis (ALS)
  Guillain-Barré syndrome
  Polyneuritis

Neuromuscular Junction
  Myasthenia gravis
  Botulism
  Eaton-Lambert syndrome

Muscle
  Polymyositis
  Dermatomyositis
  Muscular dystrophies (Duchenne [DMD], limb-girdle
    [LGMD], myotonic [MD], facioscapulohumeral
    [FSHMD])
  Spinal muscular atrophy (SMA)
  Scleroderma and collagen vascular diseases
  Achalasia
  Metabolic myopathy

Table 29-3
Symptoms of dysphagia

Dry mouth

Drooling

Nasal regurgitation

Vomiting

Difficulty with phlegm

Postnasal drip

Globus (obstruction)

Odynophagia (pain in throat, chest, or stomach)

Exhaustion after eating or drinking

Change in voice

Dyspnea

Coughing or choking while eating or drinking

Mouth odor

Heartburn

Chest pain

Weight loss

Videofluorographic Swallowing Study (VFSS)

Only 42 percent of subjects who aspirate may be identified by clinical examination.[78] When a clinical examination cannot identify the nature of a swallowing problem, VFSS still is considered the "gold standard" for the diagnosis of dysphagia. The study can be divided into two sections: oropharyngeal and gastroesophageal. The oropharyngeal portion usually is viewed in the lateral plane to better identify structures, but anteroposterior views may identify problems of pharyngeal asymmetry. The fluoroscopy unit maintains a stationary view of the oropharyngeal cavity, whereas calibrated and functional amounts of different liquids and solids mixed with barium preparations are swallowed. Liquids are given in thin (water), thick (nectar), or thickened (milkshake

or honey) consistencies that optimize oral control of swallowed boluses and prevent aspiration by premature spillage of boluses into the pharyngeal cavity or by incoordination or weakness of the pharyngeal musculature. Calibrated amounts, such as the teaspoon, are utilized in order to minimize the amount of potential aspiration that may occur in high-risk patients, and to determine the amount per bolus a patient may attempt in functional situations. Solids typically are presented as purees (pudding or barium paste) and cookie, but other foods that replicate swallowing difficulties also may be attempted. VFSS should identify the etiology of dysphagia before compensatory measures are undertaken. The order of presentation of consistencies and amounts reflect the patient's ability to tolerate the procedure (i.e., endurance and level of alertness). Compensatory strategies (see Direct Methods) are incorporated one at a time to systematically evaluate the efficacy of each technique. Pharyngeal residue in the valleculae, reduced hyoid elevation, deviant epiglottic function, and delayed pharyngeal swallow are independent predictors of aspiration.[79]

The esophagus and gastroesophageal junction usually are not studied in many patients. The patient may be studied in the sitting, standing, or prone positions, but a traditional prone view with gravity eliminated will accentuate obstructions or dysmotility. An inspection of the lower portion of the upper gastrointestinal tract may identify lesions that can refer symptoms to the pharynx.[80] A complete study of the mouth, pharynx, and esophagus is necessary in patients with dysphagia of unknown origin. However, no studies have correlated known neurological diseases causing oropharyngeal dysphagia with associated esophageal dysfunction.

Fiberoptic Endoscopic Evaluation of Swallowing (FEES)

FEES provides information about the pharyngeal stage of swallowing when VFSS cannot be performed adequately.[81] A fiberoptic laryngoscope is passed nasally to view portions of the swallowing mechanism directly. The integrity of the palate, pharynx, and vocal folds may be visualized. Sensation of the pharyngeal cavity may be assessed. Boluses of different consistencies and sizes may be introduced to visualize pharyngeal residue and laryngeal penetration and aspiration. Although FEES is not as sensitive as VFSS in detecting aspiration, it is an excellent method to screen subjects for swallowing abnormalities.[82]

Pulmonary Function Tests

Three factors are required for effective airway clearance.[83] First, the mucociliary system secretes approximately 100 cc of mucus per day and propels trapped particles upward from the lower respiratory tract. Second, alveolar macrophages trap and deposit particles during mucociliary transport and carry them out of the respiratory system through the lymphatic system. Finally, coughing assists in facilitating aspirate and secretion clearance when inspiratory volume, glottic closure, and intrathoracic pressure are adequate.

Pulmonary function tests are the most sensitive determinant of the ability to clear the airway of aspirated material. Tidal volume (TV), vital capacity (VC), maximum inspiratory pressure (MIP), and maximum expiratory pressure (MEP) most commonly are used for daily or periodic monitoring. MIP is an indirect measure of airway resistance and is the most sensitive indicator of ventilatory muscle compromise.[84] Since TV requires minimal effort, reductions in TV occur only when ventilatory impairment is severe.

Manometry

Manometry involves the placement of a catheter containing intraluminal solid-state transducers into the pharynx and esophagus. The catheter obtains pressure readings while the subject swallows. Although the diagnostic yield of VFSS is high, manometry complements VFSS by quantitating the pressures of the pharynx, cricopharyngeus muscle, and esophagus.[85] It is a cost-effective method of diagnosing pharyngeal and esophageal dysfunction in connective tissue disease, noncardiac chest pain, achalasia, and gastroesophageal reflux disease.[86] The technique has been used to demonstrate a significant decrease in relaxation and negative opening pressures of the cricopharyngeus muscle during the aging process.[87] Simultaneous contractions and incomplete lower esophageal sphincter relaxation have been observed in patients with oculopharyngeal muscular dystrophy.[88] Combining manometry with videofluorography ("manofluorography") assists in visualizing the transport of a bolus while measuring pharyngeal and esophageal walls pressures.[89] This is especially useful in studying cricopharyngeal dysfunction because measurement of intrabolus pressures is dependent on the position of the sensor.[90]

Ultrasonography

Ultrasonography to examine the oral cavity was first introduced in the early 1980s.[91] Initially, the transducer was placed submentally with the beam aimed cephalad toward the tongue.[92] The anteroposterior movement of the tongue was well visualized, although the posterior aspect of the tongue often disappeared from the image when it made contact with the posterior pharyngeal wall. However, it is now possible to examine the tongue, hyoid bone, and larynx during swallowing.[93] The hyoid bone is recognized as a high echogenic area that can be identified as it elevates during a swallow. Laryngeal motion can be monitored using an externally applied pressure transducer whose tracing is incorporated into the video image. Ultrasound is useful in diagnosing tongue incoordination and thrusting in children.[94] It can be combined with endoscopy to diagnose submucosal or extramural lesions missed with endoscopy alone.[95] Ultrasound is a radiation-free technique, but cannot provide an overall picture of the swallowing mechanism.

Scintigraphy

Scintigraphy uses radionuclide imaging to monitor a radioactive bolus during and after a swallow.[96] The patient swallows a bolus of Tc-99m sulfur colloid, and pictures are taken up to several hours later to determine the percentage of the bolus that ascends the esophagus and enters the trachea.[97] Scintigraphy is more sensitive in identifying the flow dynamics and quantification of aspirated material than VFSS. It can be combined with 24-hour pH-manometry to test the temporal association between pain, esophageal reflux, and esophageal dysmotility in patients with noncardiac chest pain.[98]

Electromyography (EMG)

EMG is an important clinical and research tool in studying patients with dysphagia.[99] Analysis of individual muscle-action potentials provides information to localize neuropathology and to develop a differential diagnosis. Concentric, monopolar, or hooked-wire electrodes may be inserted into the various muscles. Combined electrophysiological and mechanical methods have been described in measuring laryngeal movements and related submental EMG activity during swallowing.[100] EMG of the facial, lingual, and palatal muscles, along with the blink reflex, have been used to observe the sucking-swallowing reflex, in normal and abnormal newborns and infants.[101] EMG studies of patients with scleroderma have uncovered two types of disorders: those with disorganized myoelectric hyperactivity consistent with diffuse esophageal spasm, and those with a marked decrease in myoelectric activity consistent with classic findings in scleroderma.[102] Pharyngeal EMG is a technically difficult procedure, and is usually not performed in most clinical laboratories.

Cervical Auscultation

Cervical auscultation is a relatively new technique to enhance the ability of an examiner to detect aspiration and determine specialized diet management. The pharyngeal swallow is characterized by stereotypical sounds that may be audible through a stethoscope. Abnormal sound patterns identified throughout the swallowing process are found in Table 29-4. Cervical auscultation may be a useful clinical tool when no other methods of diagnosing dysphagia are available to the clinician.[103]

TREATMENT

The goals of dysphagia therapy are twofold: (1) to maintain adequate nutritional intake; and (2) to maximize airway protection. Treatment for dysphagia begins by feeding the subject orally with those solid and liquid consistencies found to minimize risk of aspiration. Modifications of consistencies and compensatory strategies

Table 29-4
Features identified by cervical auscultation

Prior to swallow
　Abnormalities in ventilation
　　"Bubbles" in pharynx, larynx, or trachea: must test effect
　　　of "dry" swallow on bubbles
　　Stridor on inspiration, expiration
　　Grunt
　　Throat clearing
　　Cough
During swallow
　Pharyngeal swallow
　Aspiration: cough, stridor, bubbling, clearing throat
　Residual bolus in pharynx, larynx: stridor, bubbling
　Adaptation of swallow to individual bolus
After swallow
　Changes in sounds of respiration: more effortful, new sounds
　Evidence of aspiration after swallow: bubbles, stridor

are incorporated based on diagnostic studies. Treatment of dysphagia may consist of one or more approaches: dysphagia therapy (direct or indirect) by a speech-language pathologist; medical interventions; surgical interventions. Nonoral feedings may be instituted if the patient is unable to attain sufficient oral caloric intake.

Direct Therapy

Direct therapy methods consist of compensatory strategies that immediately reduce the risk of aspiration. Neck flexion (chin tuck) is a common maneuver that protects the larynx by increasing postural and epiglottic angles and pushing the anterior laryngeal wall more posteriorly, thereby narrowing the airway entrance (Figure 29-12).[104] Head rotation closes the ipsilateral pharynx, forces the bolus into the contralateral pharynx, and decreases cricopharyngeal pressures (Figure 29-13).[105] The cricopharyngeal opening diameter increases by an average of 2 mm, but the duration of cricopharyngeal opening and oropharyngeal transit time is not affected. Head tilting uses gravity to guide the bolus into the ipsilateral pharynx.

A sequence of oropharyngeal postures also may be efficacious in preventing aspiration. A supraglottic swallow involves concomitant breath holding and swallowing, to close the vocal folds and protect the trachea. Instead of exhaling, the patient opens the vocal folds with a cough to expel any residue that may have entered

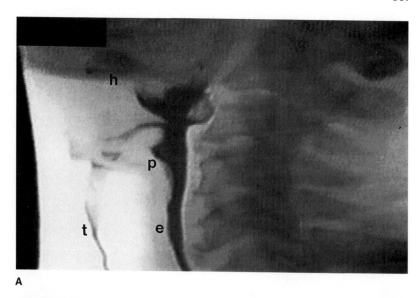

A

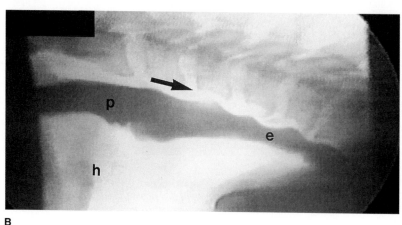

B

Figure 29-12

Neck flexion ("chin tuck"). A. In this patient, a portion of the bolus enters the trachea (t) while the remainder of the bolus passes through the hypopharynx (p) into the esophagus (e). Note that the hyoid bone (h) is in its most superior and anterior position. B. Using maximal neck flexion, the bolus successfully passes through the pharynx (p) into the esophagus. Again, the hyoid bone (h) is in its most superior and anterior position.

the laryngeal vestibule. A super supraglottic swallow adds a Valsalva maneuver in order to maximize vocal-fold closing. The Mendelsohn maneuver may be used to prolong voluntary opening of the cricopharyngeus muscle.[106] As the larynx elevates, the patient attempts to voluntarily hold the larynx at its maximal height to lengthen the duration of cricopharyngeal opening. These techniques can help a select population of patients with neurogenic dysphagia, but are difficult to teach if the patient has difficulties with comprehension (i.e., aphasia) or motor planning (i.e., apraxia).

Food consistencies and amounts may be modified as a result of diagnostic testing. Liquids may be thickened to increase oropharyngeal control and slow their passage through the oropharyngeal cavity. Solids may be cut up or pureed to decrease difficulties with mastication, improve tongue control, and maintain a cohesive bolus as they pass into the esophagus. Bolus amounts may be limited, to decrease the risk of tracheal aspiration. Temperatures and textures (e.g., carbonated beverages, sour boluses) may hasten the initiation of the oral swallow and decrease pharyngeal swallow delay.[107]

Indirect Therapy

Indirect therapy methods use facilitation and exercises to alter muscle tone, improve function of the voluntary muscles used in swallowing, and to augment the pharyn-

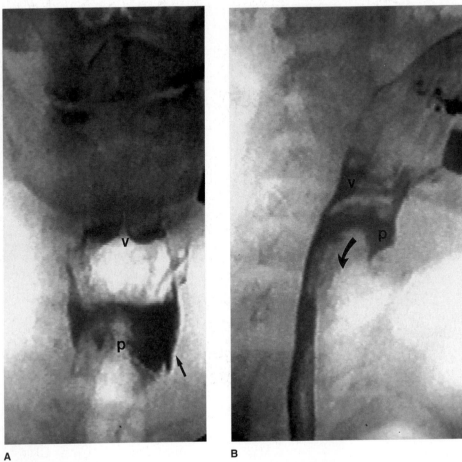

A   B

Figure 29-13
Head rotation ("head turn"). A. In this patient, a liquid bolus has pooled in the valleculae (v) and piriform sinuses (p) bilaterally. The left piriform sinus (arrow) appears larger than the right, thus suggesting more weakness. B. Using head rotation to the left, the patient is able to obliterate the left side of the pharynx and successfully divert the bolus through the right side of the pharynx (curved arrow), which is stronger and more capable of channeling the bolus into the esophagus without aspiration.

geal swallow. The speech-language pathologist may teach exercises that focus on altering tone and improving strength, range of motion, and coordination of the jaw, lips, cheek, tongue, soft palate, and vocal folds. Thermal stimulation involves icing the anterior faucial arches with a pharyngeal mirror to decrease delay of the pharyngeal swallow (Figure 29-14). Generally, indirect therapies appear to be effective when used alone or in conjunction with direct therapies.[108] However, whereas thermal stimulation appears to be effective, it has failed to demonstrate efficacy in clinical trials.[109]

Another method of indirectly facilitating the muscles of deglutition is through the use of biofeedback. Biofeedback utilizes visual, auditory, or tactile cues to modify targeted behaviors or skills. Biofeedback has been used to reeducate muscles affected in facial palsy and disorders of articulation.[110,111] In dysphagia, patients may use VFSS as visual feedback while experimenting with head positions and swallowing maneuvers.[112] More recently, EMG biofeedback utilizes the placement of a surface electrode over the anterior neck or specific muscles to measure gross motor activity during swal-

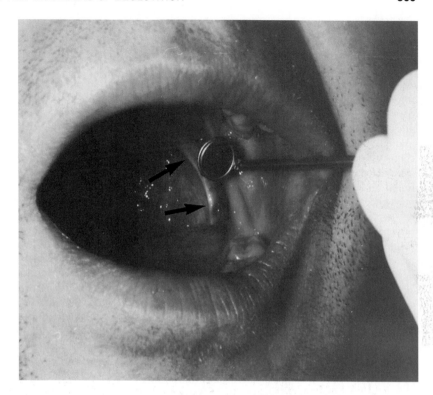

Figure 29-14

Thermal stimulation. An iced laryngeal mirror is rubbed against the anterior faucial arches (arrows), thus providing sensory stimulation to the oral cavity and theoretically facilitating the initiation of the pharyngeal swallow.

lowing trials.[113] Although electrode placement locations have been standardized, formal diagnostic and treatment protocols have not been established.[114]

Medical Interventions

Medications usually are implicated in causing dysphagia (see History). However, some of their effects actually may alleviate symptoms of swallowing disorders. Diltiazem has been used in a double-blind, crossover prospective trial to decrease noncardiac chest pain associated with strong esophageal contractions ("nutcracker esophagus").[115] The decrease in symptoms was associated with a significant decrease in contraction pressures. Isosorbide dinitrate decreased symptoms associated with achalasia in a randomized, double-blind, placebo-controlled study of patients with Chagas disease.[116] On the other hand, no significant effect was observed in a multicenter, placebo-controlled, double-blind study of glucagon and diazepam to disimpact esophageal foreign bodies.[117]

More recently, botulinum toxin type A (BOTOX®) has been used in the treatment of dysphagia. Botulinum toxin, which is purified from the anaerobe Clostridium botulinum, blocks neuromuscular conduction by binding to receptor sites on motor-nerve terminals, entering the nerve terminal, and blocking the release of acetylcholine. Botulinum toxin has been injected endoscopically into the muscles in both the upper esophageal and the gastroesophageal sphincters.[118,119] In the former, no side effects or postoperative complications were observed. In the latter, esophageal dysfunction remained unchanged, and gastroesophageal reflux was observed in one patient. Gastroesophageal sphincter pressures remained significantly reduced for 3 to 6.5 months after injection. Botulinum toxin therapy may be useful as a noninvasive alternative to cricopharyngeal myotomy or gastroesophageal dilatation, or could be used preoperatively to test the efficacy of these more invasive procedures.

Surgical Interventions

Surgical interventions sometimes are required to normalize swallowing physiology or to bypass abnormal lesions or masses in the upper digestive tract. Cricopharyngeal myotomy relieves upper esophageal sphincter spasm by incising the muscle.[120] Zenker's diverticula may be resected or suspended to minimize their effect. Cervical osteophytes causing dysphagia may be resected, but treatment is controversial. Esophageal dilatation may be required for achalasia, webs, or strictures.

Glottic insufficiency may occur because of an anatomical deficiency, mechanical impairment, or uncompensated neuromuscular disability.[121] When symptomatic the paralyzed vocal cord may be moved toward the midline through surgical means. Early in the twentieth century, vocal-cord medialization was accomplished by injecting paraffin, but was stopped when paraffin was found to cause granuloma formation.[122] Teflon has been injected into the larynx during direct laryngoscopy or percutaneously through the cricothyroid membrane.[123,124] However, once injected, Teflon is very difficult to remove from the larynx. Because of this, reversible vocal-cord medialization techniques have been developed. In these, a window is created in the thyroid ala, and the paralyzed vocal cord is medialized using cartilage or alloplastic material.[125,126] Surgical intervention should not be considered until maximal spontaneous recovery of the swallowing mechanism has occurred.

Nonoral Feedings

Subjects with persistent dysphagia may be fed nonorally or with a combination of oral and nonoral methods. Approaches for nonoral feedings depend upon alterations in the anatomy and physiology of the individual patient. *Esophagostomy* may be indicated in subjects in whom other placements are contraindicated or to control pharyngeal secretions.[127] However, its use in dysphagic subjects is limited.

Nasogastric tubes may be placed immediately in debilitated or unconscious subjects. Radiographs usually are taken after placement to insure that the tip of the tube lies in the stomach. Some clinicians prefer to let the tip of the tube migrate past the pyloric sphincter into the duodenum so that gastroesophageal reflux is less problematic. Nasogastric tubes are convenient for short-term use, but discomfort, bleeding, and irritation are common complications that limit their use.

Gastrostomy is the most common approach for long-term nonoral feeding. Placement of a gastrostomy tube can be performed with little risk of complication either surgically under general anesthesia or endoscopically (percutaneous endoscopic gastrostomy [PEG]) under local anesthesia. The tube is located away from the head, reducing the risk of morbidity attributable to nasogastric tubes, and causes little mortality.[128] As the stomach acts as a reservoir, feedings may be adminis-

tered either continuously or by bolus. The latter method is advantageous since feedings can coincide with mealtime and bedtime, and a feeding pump is not necessary for regulating the rate of administration. A small but significant risk of gastroesophageal reflux exists, especially in patients with a history of hiatal hernia or gastroesophageal incompetence. To prevent reflux, feedings usually are given while the patient sits vertically, and chlorpromazine or cisapride are given to facilitate gastric emptying. A histamine-blocking agent may be given to decrease gastric pH, and omeprazole may be given to decrease gastroesophageal reflux.

Jejunostomy is indicated in subjects with known reflux and aspiration. Placement of a jejunostomy must be completed under general anesthesia.[129] Unlike gastrostomy tubes, jejunostomy feedings must be administered continuously by pump to prevent discomfort caused by distention of the gastrointestinal tract. However, small boluses up to approximately 240 cc may be given without a pump.

Nonoral feedings should be gauged to meet both the caloric and fluid requirements of the patient. Once the caloric requirements of the patient are calculated, the free water content of the feed should be calculated and supplemented with enough fluid to satisfy bodily needs. Free water in the initial feeding helps to decrease osmolar load and prevent the occurrence of diarrhea. The strength of the feed may be increased as long as the patient remains asymptomatic. If oral caloric intake increases, the nonoral feeding accordingly may be reduced. A calorie count should be undertaken to determine whether nonoral feedings may be discontinued.

RECOVERY AND PROGNOSIS

Recovery of swallowing function depends upon the condition with which it is associated. Patients with potential for recovery, such as after stroke or traumatic brain injury, may require from 3 weeks to 6 to 9 months or longer for swallowing function to normalize.[130] They should be assessed frequently as compensatory strategies are mastered or symptoms decrease. After stroke, many patients followed up to 270 days following discharge from rehabilitation tolerated normal oral caloric intake, but some required partial or total nonoral supplementation. Swallowing dysfunction assessed 1 and 6 months post-stroke is associated with hospital readmission and death.[131]

Subjects with static or progressive conditions such as amyotrophic lateral sclerosis, multiple sclerosis, muscular dystrophy, Parkinsonism, or post-polio syndrome should be evaluated periodically or when new symptoms of dysphagia occur. New compensatory strategies or nonoral feeding techniques should be considered as appropriate.

ETHICAL ISSUES

The institution and withdrawal of nonoral feedings represents a major ethical issue and controversy in the treatment of patients with dysphagia. Providing nutrition nonorally sometimes can represent extraordinary rather than ordinary means of prolonging life.[132] Therefore, the indications for beginning or stopping nonoral feedings must be seriously considered. Patients who refuse or are unable to feed orally should be subject to a full evaluation of the alimentary canal to rule out reversible forms of dysphagia.[133] The assessment should include many of the components of the dysphagia evaluation described in this chapter. The risks and benefits of nonoral feedings as well as the procedure to insert a feeding tube should be analyzed closely to determine how quality of life will be affected. The use of alternative methods of feeding or hydration (e.g., total parental nutrition, intravenous fluids, medications) should be contemplated to minimize discomfort or pain if enteral feedings are not pursued. The consequences of starting or stopping nonoral feedings must be considered, since implementing a change in management later may require legal proceedings.

Table 29-5
Who makes the decision to start or stop nonoral feedings?

Patient
  Oral consent or refusal
  Advance directive

Health care surrogate
  Durable power of attorney
  Health-care proxy
  Family member
  Guardian

Physician

Hospital
  Ethics committee
  Administrator

State
  Court system

Finally, the decision to initiate or terminate nonoral feedings should be made in conjunction with the patient's wishes. The American Neurological Association has listed the sources from which guidance in making decisions for patients with persistent vegetative state may be sought, but these may applied to dysphagic patients as well (Table 29-5).[134] The patient or his or her designee should express his or her wishes before the need for an emergent decision becomes necessary. The physician likewise should discuss his or her rationale for treatment options at his or her earliest convenience. Since morals, ethics, and decisions in medical care greatly vary among medical professionals, a consensus among the patient, family, friends, and health care providers will solidify the prerequisites of initiating and withdrawing nonoral feedings, thereby establishing guidelines that are in the best interest of the patient.

REFERENCES

1. Magendie F: *An Elementary Compendium of Physiology; for the Use of Students* (Milligan E, trans.). Philadelphia: J. Webster, 1824.
2. Falk F, Kronecker H: Über den mechanismsus der schluckbewegung. *Arch für Physiologie (Leipzig)* 1880; ii:296–297.
3. Kronecker H, Meltzer S: Über der vorgänge beim schlucken. *Arch für Physiologie (Leipzig)* 1880; ii: 446–447.
4. Cannon WB, Moser A: The movements of the food in the oesophagus. *Am J Phys* 1898; 1:435–444.
5. Mosher HP: X-ray study of movements of the tongue, epiglottis, and hyoid bone in swallowing, followed by a discussion of difficulty in swallowing caused by retropharyngeal diverticulum, post-cricoid webs, and exostoses of cervical vertebrae. *Laryngoscope* 1927; 37(4):235–262.
6. Barclay AE: The normal mechanism of swallowing. *Proceedings of the Staff Meetings of the Mayo Clinic* 1930; 5(36):251–257.
7. Janker R: Roentgen cinematography. *AJR* 1936; 36: 384–390.
8. Linden P, Tippett D, Johnston J, et al: Bolus position at swallow onset in normal adults: preliminary observations. *Dysphagia* 1989; 4:146–150.
9. Doty RW: Handbook of physiology. Section 6: Alimentary canal. Volume IV: *Motility*. Washington DC: American Physiological Society, 1968, pp. 1861–1902.
10. Logemann JA: *Evaluation and Treatment of Swallowing Disorders*. San Diego: College-Hill, 1983.
11. Jean A, Car A: Inputs to the swallowing medullary neurons from the peripheral afferent fibers and the swallowing cortical area. *Brain Res* 1979; 178:567–572.

12. Lederman M: The 17th Knox lecture, delivered 21 June 1974. The oncology of breathing and swallowing. *Clin Radiol* 1977; 28:1–14.

13. Jacob P, Kahrilas PJ, Logemann JA, Shah V, Ha T: Upper esophageal sphincter opening and modulation during swallowing. *Gastroenterology* 1989; 97(6):1469–1478.

14. Palmer JB, DuChane AS: Rehabilitation of swallowing disorders due to stroke. *Phys Med Rehab Clin N Am* 1991; 2(3):529–546.

15. Kahrilas PJ, Logemann JA, Lin S, Ergun GA: Pharyngeal clearance during swallowing: A combined manometric and videofluoroscopic study. *Gastroenterology* 1992; 103(1):128–136.

16. Nishino T, Yonezawa T, Honda Y: Effects of swallowing the pattern of continuous respiration in human adults. *Am Rev Respir Dis* 1985; 132:1219–1222.

17. Smith J, Wolkove N, Colacone A, Kreisman H: Coordination of eating, drinking, and breathing in adults. *Chest* 1989; 96:578–582.

18. Selley WG, Ellis RE, Flack FC, Bayliss CR, Pearce VR: The synchronization of respiration and swallow sounds with videofluoroscopy during swallowing. *Dysphagia* 1994; 9(3):162–167.

19. Donner MW: Swallowing mechanism and neuromuscular disorders. *Sem Roentgenol* 1974; 9(4):273–282.

20. Miller AJ: Characteristics of the swallowing reflex induced by peripheral nerve and brain stem stimulation. *Exp Neurol* 1972; 34:210–222.

21. Hellemans J, Pelemans W, Vantrappen G: Pharyngo-esophageal swallowing disorders and the pharyngo-esophageal sphincter. *Med Clin N Am* 1981; 65(6):1149–1171.

22. Jean A: Brainstem organization of the swallowing network. *Brain Behav Evol* 1984; 25:109–116.

23. Kessler JP, Jean A: Identification of the medullary swallowing regions in the rat. *Exp Brain Res* 1985; 57:256–263.

24. Holstege G, Graveland G, Bijker-Biemond C, Schuddeboom I: Location of motoneurons innervating soft palate, pharynx, and upper esophagus. Anatomical evidence for a possible swallowing center in the pontine reticular formation. *Brain Behav Evol* 1983; 23:47–62.

25. Horner J, Massey EW, Riski JE, Lathrop DL, Chase KN: Aspiration following stroke: clinical correlates and outcome. *Neurology* 1988; 38:1359–1362.

26. Dantas RO, Dodds WJ, Massey BT, Kern MK: The effect of high- vs. low-density barium preparations in the quantitative features of swallowing. *AJR* 1989; 153:1191–1195.

27. Dodds WJ: The physiology of swallowing. *Dysphagia* 1989; 3:171–178.

28. Ekberg O, Nylander G: Lateral diverticula from the pharyngoesophageal junction area. *Radiology* 1983; 146:117–122.

29. Ekberg O: The cricopharyngeus revisited. *Br J Radiol* 1986; 59:875–879.

30. Barer DH: The nature history and functional consequences of dysphagia after hemispheric stroke. *J Neurol Neurosurg Psychiatr* 1989; 52:236–241.

31. Gordon C, Hewer RL, Wade DT: Dysphagia in acute stroke. *Br Med J* 1987; 295:411–414.

32. Veis SL, Logemann JA: Swallowing disorders in persons with cerebrovascular accident. *Arch Phys Med Rehab* 1985; 66(6):372–375.

33. Alberts MJ, Horner J, Gray L, Brazer SR: Aspiration after stroke: Lesion analysis by brain MRI. *Dysphagia* 1992; 7:170–173.

34. Miller RM, Groher ME: The evaluation and management of neuromuscular and mechanical swallowing disorders. *Dyarthr Dysphon Dysphag* 1982; 1:50–70.

35. Leopold NA, Kagel MC: Swallowing, ingestion, and dysphagia: A reappraisal. *Arch Phys Med Rehabil* 1983; 64:371–373.

36. Robbins J, Levine RL, Maser A, Rosenbek JC, Kempster GB: Swallowing after unilateral stroke of the cerebral cortex. *Arch Phys Med Rehabil* 1993; 74(12):1295–1300.

37. Silbiger ML, Rikielney R, Donner MW: Neuromuscular disorders affecting the pharynx: Cineradiographic analysis. *Invest Radiol* 1967; 2(6):442–448.

38. Kilman WJ, Goyal RK: Disorders of pharyngeal and upper esophageal sphincter motor function. *Arch Int Med* 1976; 136(5):592–601.

39. Levine R, Robbins J, Maser A: Periventricular white matter changes and oropharyngeal swallowing in normal individuals. *Dysphagia* 1992; 7:142–147.

40. Horner J, Buoyner FG, Alberts MJ, Helms MJ: Dysphagia following brain-stem stroke: Clinical correlates and outcome. *Arch Neurol* 1991; 48:1170–1173.

41. Logemann JA: *Evaluation and Treatment of Swallowing Disorders.* San Diego: College-Hill Press, 1983.

42. Horner J, Massey EW: Silent aspiration following stroke. *Neurology* 1988: 38:317–319.

43. Winstein CJ: Neurogenic dysphagia: Frequency, progression, and outcome in adults following head injury. *Phys Ther* 1983; 63(12):1992–1997.

44. Field LH, Weiss CJ: Dysphagia with head injury. *Brain Injury* 1989; 3(1):23–26.

45. Cherney LR, Halper AS: Recovery of oral nutrition after head injury in adults. *J Head Trauma Rehab* 1989; 4(4):42–50.

46. Ott L, McClain C, Young B: Nutrition and severe brain injury. *Nutrition* 1989; 5(2):75–79.

47. Groher ME: *Dysphagia: Diagnosis and Management,* 2nd ed. Boston: Butterworth, 1992.

48. Lazarus C, Logemann JA: Swallowing disorders in closed head trauma patients. *Arch Phys Med Rehab* 1987; 68:79–84.

49. Avery-Smith W, Dellarosa DM: Approaches to treating dysphagia in patients with brain injury. *Am J Occup Ther* 1994; 48(3):235–239.

50. Tippett DC, Palmer J, Linden P: Management of dysphagia in a patient with closed head injury. *Dysphagia* 1987; 1:221–226.

51. Neumann S: Swallowing therapy with neurologic patients: Results of direct and indirect therapy methods in 66 patients suffering from neurological disorders. *Dysphagia* 1993; 8:150–153.

52. Adamovich BB, Henderson JA, Auerbach S: *Cognitive Rehabilitation of Closed Head Injured Patients: A Dynamic Approach.* San Diego: College-Hill Press, 1985.

53. Ekberg O, Hildersfors H: Defective closure of the laryngeal vestibule: frequency of pulmonary complications. *AJR* 1985; 145:1245–1249.

54. Daly DC, Code CF, Anderson HA: Disturbances of swallowing and esophageal motility in multiple sclerosis. *Neurology* 1962; 12:250–256.

55. Herrera W, Zeligman BE, Gruber J, et al: Dysphagia in multiple sclerosis: Clinical and videofluoroscopic correlations. *J Neurol Rehab* 1990; 4(1):1–8.

56. Newton HB, Newton C, Pearl D, Davidson T: Swallowing assessment in primary brain tumor patients with dysphagia. *Neurology* 1994; 44(10):1927–1932.

57. Jennings KS, Siroky D, Jackson CG: Swallowing problems after excision of tumors of the skull base: diagnosis and management in 12 patients. *Dysphagia* 1992; 7(1):40–44.

58. Blonsky ER, Logemann JA, Boshes B, Fisher HB: Comparison of speech and swallowing function in patients with tremor disorders and in normal geriatric patients: A cinefluorographic study. *J Gerontol* 1975; 30(3):290–303.

59. Stroudley J, Walsh M: Radiological assessment of dysphagia in Parkinson's disease. *Br J Radiol* 1991; 64(766): 890–893.

60. Wintzen AR, Badrising UA, Roos RA, Vielvoye J, Liauw L, Pauwels EK: Dysphagia in ambulant patients with Parkinson's disease: Common, not dangerous. *Can J Neurol Sci* 1994; 21(1):53–56.

61. Robbins JA, Logemann JA, Kirshner HS: Swallowing and speech production in Parkinson's disease. *Ann Neurol* 1986; 19:283–287.

62. Bine JE, Frank EM, McDade HL: Dysphagia and dementia in subjects with Parkinson's disease. *Dysphagia* 1995; 10(3):160–164.

63. Wang SJ, Chia LG, Hsu CY, Lin WY, Kao CH, Yeh SH: Dysphagia in Parkinson's disease. Assessment by solid phase radionuclide scintigraphy. *Clin Nucl Med* 1994; 19(5):405–407.

64. Kagel MC, Leopold NA: Dysphagia in Huntington's disease: A 16-year retrospective. *Dysphagia* 1992; 7(2): 106–114.

65. Dworkin JP, Hartman DE: Progressive speech deterioration and dysphagia in amyotrophic lateral sclerosis: Case report. *Arch Phys Med Rehab* 1979; 60(9):423–425.

66. Firouze M, Keshavarizian A: Guillain-Barré syndrome and achalasia: two manifestations of a viral disease or coincidental association? *Am J Gastroenterol* 1994; 89(9): 1585–1587.

67. Progressive bulbar palsy: a case report of a type of motor neuron disease presenting with oral symptoms. *Oral Surg Oral Med Oral Pathol* 1990; 69(2):182–184.

68. Sonies BC, Dalakas MC: Dysphagia in patients with the post-polio syndrome. *N Engl J Med* 1991; 324(17):1162–1167.

69. Driscoll BP, Gracco C, Coelho C, et al: Laryngeal function in postpolio patients. *Laryngoscope* 1995; 105(1):35–41.

70. Coelho CA, Ferrante R: Dysphagia in postpolio sequelae: report of three cases. *Arch Phys Med Rehab* 1988; 69(8):634–636.

71. Buchholz D, Jones B: Dysphagia occurring after polio. *Dysphagia* 1991; 6:165–169.

72. Khan OA, Campbell WW: Myasthenia gravis presenting as dysphagia: clinical considerations. *Am J Gastroenterol* 1994; 89(7):1083–1085.

73. De Assis JL, Marchiori PE, Scaff M: Atrophy of the tongue with persistent articulation disorder in myasthenia gravis: report of 10 patients. *Auris Nasus Larynx* 1994; 21(4):215–218.

74. Willig TN, Paulus J, Lacau St Guily J, Beon C, Navarro J: Swallowing problems in neuromuscular disorders. *Arch Phys Med Rehab* 1994; 75(11):1175–1181.

75. St Guily JL, Perie S, Willig TN, Chaussade S, Eymard B, Angelard B: Swallowing disorders in muscular diseases: functional assessment and indications of cricopharyngeal myotomy. *Ear Nose Throat* 1994; 73(1):34–40.

76. Linden P, Siebens AA: Dysphagia: Predicting laryngeal penetration. *Arch Phys Med Rehab* 1983; 64:281–284.

77. Jones B, Donner MW: How I do it: Examination of the patient with dysphagia. *Dysphagia* 1989; 4:162–172.

78. Splaingard ML, Hutchins B, Sutton LD, Chadhuri G: Aspiration in rehabilitation patients: Videofluoroscopy vs. bedside clinical assessment. *Arch Phys Med Rehab* 1988; 69:637–640.

79. Perlman AL, Booth BM, Grayhack JP: Videofluoroscopic predictors of aspiration in patients with oropharyngeal dysphagia. *Dysphagia* 1994; 9(2):90–95.

80. Buchholz DW, Marsh BR: Multifactorial dysphagia—looking for a second, treatable cause. *Dysphagia* 1986; 1:88–90.

81. Langmore SE, Schatz K, Olsen N: Fiberoptic endoscopic examination of swallowing safety: A new procedure. *Dysphagia* 1988; 2:216–219.

82. Langmore SE, Schatz K, Olsen N: Endoscopic and videofluoroscopic evaluations of swallowing and aspiration. *Ann Otol Rhinol Laryngol* 1991; 100:678–681.

83. Hoffman LA: Ineffective airway clearance related to neuromuscular dysfunction. *Nurs Clin North Am* 1987; 22(1):151–166.

84. Griggs RC, Donohoe KM, Utell MJ, et al: Evaluation of pulmonary function in neuromuscular disease. *Arch Neurol* 1981; 38:9–15.

85. Olsson R, Castell JA, Castell DO, Ekberg O: Solid-state computerized manometry improves diagnostic yield in pharyngeal dysphagia: simultaneous videoradiography and manometry in dysphagia patients with normal barium swallows. *Abd Image* 1995; 20(3):230–235.

86. Johnston PW, Johnston BT, Collins BJ, Collins JS, Love

AH: Audit of the role of oesophageal manometry in clinical practice. *Gut* 1993; 34(9):1158–1161.

87. Dejaeger E, Pelemans W, Bibau G, Ponette E: Manofluorographic analysis of swallowing in the elderly. *Dysphagia* 1994; 9(3):156–161.

88. Castell JA, Castell DO, Duranceau CA, Topart P: Manometric characteristics of the pharynx, upper esophageal sphincter, esophagus, and lower esophageal sphincter in patients with oculopharyngeal muscular dystrophy. *Dysphagia* 1995; 10(1):22–26.

89. Olsson R, Nilsson H, Ekberg O: Simultaneous videoradiography and computerized pharyngeal manometry—videomanometry. *Acta Radiol* 1994; 35(1):30–34.

90. Olsson R, Nilsson H, Ekberg O: An experimental manometric study simulating upper esophageal sphincter narrowing. *Invest Rad* 1994; 29(6):630–635.

91. Sonies BC, Shawker TH, Hall TE, Gerber LH, Leighton SB: Ultrasonic visualization of tongue motion during speech. *J Acoust Soc Am* 1981; 70:683–686.

92. Shawker TH, Sonies BC, Stone M: Sonography of Speech and Swallowing, in Sanders RC, Hill M (eds): *Ultrasound Annual 1984*. New York: Raven Press, 1984.

93. Shawker TH, Sonies B, Hall TE, Baum BF: Ultrasound analysis of tongue, hyoid, and larynx activity during swallowing. *Invest Radiol* 1984; 19(2):82–86.

94. Fuhrmann RA, Diedrich PR: B-mode ultrasound scanning of the tongue during swallowing. *Dento-Maxillo-Facial Radiol* 1994; 23(4):211–215.

95. Lorenz R, Jorysz G, Classen M: The value of endoscopy and endosonography in the diagnosis of the dysphagic patient. *Dysphagia* 1993; 8(2):91–97.

96. Muz J, Mathog RH, Rosen R, Miller PR, Borrero G: Detection and quantification of laryngotracheopulmonary aspiration with scintigraphy. *Laryngoscope* 1987; 97:1180–1185.

97. Silver KH, Van Nostrand D: The use of scintigraphy in the management of patients with pulmonary aspiration. *Dysphagia* 1994; 9(2):107–115.

98. Schwizer W, Borovicka J, Fried M, Inauen W: Motility disorders and assessment methods of the esophagus. *Motilitat Untersuchung Osophagus (suppl)* 1993; 54:8–14.

99. Palmer JB, Tanaka K, Siebens AA: Electromyography of the pharyngeal musculature: technical considerations. *Arch Phys Med Rehab* 1989; 70:283–287.

100. Ertekin C, Pehlivan M, Aydogdu I, et al: An electrophysiological investigation of deglutition in man. *Muscle Nerve* 1995; 18(10):1177–1186.

101. Renault F, Raimbault J: Facial, lingual, and pharyngeal electromyography in children: a method to study sucking and swallowing disorders and their pathophysiology. *Neurophysiol Clin (France)* 1992; 22(3):249–260.

102. Bortolotti M, Pinotti, Sarti P, Barbara L: Esophageal electromyography in scleroderma patients with functional dysphagia. *Am J Gastroenterol* 1989; 84(12):1497–1502.

103. Zenner PM, Losinski DS, Mills RH: Using cervical auscultation in the clinical dysphagia examination in long-term care. *Dysphagia* 1995; 10(1):27–31.

104. Shanahan TE, Logemann JA, Rademaker AW, Pauloski BR, Kahrilas PJ: Chin-down posture effect on aspiration in dysphagic patients. *Arch Phys Med Rehabil* 1993; 74(7):736–739.

105. Logemann JA, Kahrilas PJ, Kobara M, Vakil NB: The benefit of head rotation on pharyngoesophageal dysphagia. *Arch Phys Med Rehab* 1989; 70(10):767–771.

106. Kahrilas PJ, Logemann JA, Krugler C, Flanagan E: Volitional augmentation of upper esophageal sphincter opening during swallowing. *Am J Phys (Gastrointest Liver Physiol)* 1991; 260(23):G450–G456.

107. Logemann JA, Pauloski BR, Colangelo I, Lazarus C, Fujiu M, Kahrilas PJ: Effects of a sour bolus on oropharyngeal swallowing measures in patients with neurogenic dysphagia. *J Speech Hear Res* 1995; 38(3):556–563.

108. Neumann S, Barolome G, Buchholz D, Prosiegel M: Swallowing therapy of neurologic patients: correlation of outcome with pretreatment variables and therapeutic methods. *Dysphagia* 1995; 10(1):1–5.

109. Rosenbek JC, Robbins J, Fishback B, Levine RL: Effects of thermal application on dysphagia after stroke. *J Speech Hear Res* 1991; 34(6):1257–1268.

110. Brown DM, Nahai F, Wolf S, Basmajian JV: Electromyographic biofeedback in the reeducation of facial palsy. *Am J Phys Med* 1978; 57(4):183–190.

111. Dratzer A: Clinical EMG feedback in motor speech disorders. *Arch Phys Med Rehabil* 1984; 65:481–484.

112. Logemann JA, Kahrilas PJ: Relearning to swallow after stroke—application of maneuvers and indirect biofeedback: a case study. *Neurology* 1990; 40:1136–1138.

113. Bryant M: Biofeedback in the treatment of a selected dysphagic patient. *Dysphagia* 1991; 8:140–144.

114. O'Dwyer NJ, Quinn PT, Guitar BE, Andrews G, Neilson PD: Procedures for verification of electrode placement in EMG studies of orofacial and mandibular muscles. *J Speech Hear Res* 1981; 24:273–288.

115. Cattau EL Jr., Castell DO, Johnson DA, Spurling TJ, Hirszel R, Chobanian SJ, Richter JE: Diltiazem therapy for symptoms associated with nutcracker esophagus. *Am J Gastroenterol* 1991; 86(3):272–276.

116. Ferreira-Filho LP, Patto RJ, Troncon LE, Oliveira RB: Use of isosorbide dinitrate for the symptomatic treatment of patients with Chagas' disease achalasia. A double-blind, crossover trial. *Brazil J Med Biol Res* 1991; 24(11):1093–1098.

117. Tibbling I, Bjorkhoel A, Jansson E, Stenkvist M: Effect of spasmolytic drugs on esophageal foreign bodies. *Dysphagia* 1995; 10(2):126–127.

118. Schneider I, Thumfart WF, Potoschnig C, Eckel HE: Treatment of dysfunction of the cricopharyngeal muscle with botulinum A toxin: Introduction of a new, non-invasive method. *Ann Otol Rhinol Laryngol* 1994; 103(1):31–35.

119. Rollan A, Gonzalez R, Carvajal S, Chianale J: Endoscopic

intrasphincteric injection of botulinum toxin for the treatment of achalasia. *J Clin Gastroenterol* 1995; 20(3): 189–191.

120. Blakley WR, Garety EJ, Smith DE: Section of the cricopharyngeus muscle for dysphagia. *Ann Surg* 1968; 96: 745–760.

121. Blitzer A: Approaches to the patient with aspiration and swallowing disabilities. *Dysphagia* 1990; 5:129–137.

122. Bruning W: Über eine neue behandlungsmethode. *Verh Deutsche Laryngol* 1911; 18:93–151.

123. Arnold GE: Vocal rehabilitation of paralytic dysphonia. *Arch Otolaryngol* 1962; 76:358–368.

124. Ward PH, Hanson DG, Abemayor E: Transcutaneous Teflon injection of the paralyzed vocal cord: a new technique. *Laryngoscope* 1985; 95:644–649.

125. Smith GW: Aphonia due to vocal cord paralysis corrected by medial positioning of the affected vocal cord with a cartilage autograft. *Can J Otolaryngol* 1972; 1:295–298.

126. Isshiki N, Okamura H, Ishikawa T: Thyroplasty type I (laryngeal compression) for dysphonia due to vocal cord paralysis or atrophy. *Act Otolaryngol* 1975; 80:465–473.

127. Skolnik EM, Tenta LT, Massair FS: Pharyngo-esophagostomy. *Arch Otolaryngol* 1966; 84:534–537.

128. Rozier A, Ruskone Fourmestraux A, Rosenbaum A, Delvigne JM, Besancon F, Meininger V: Place de la gastrostomie endoscopique percutanee dans la sclerose laterale amyotropique. *Revue Neurol (France)* 1991; 147(2):174–176.

129. Liffman KE, Randall HT: A modified technique for creating a jejunostomy. *Surg Gynecol Obster* 1972; 134:663–664.

130. Logemann JA: *Recovery of Swallowing after Brainstem (Medullary) Stroke. Swallowing and Swallowing Disorders: From Clinic to Laboratory.* Evanston, IL: Continuing Education Programs of America, October 4–5, 1991.

131. Barer DH: The natural history and functional consequence of dysphagia after hemispheric stroke. *J Neurol Neurosurg Psychol* 1989; 52(2):236–241.

132. Watts DT, Cassel CK: Extraordinary nutritional support: A case study and ethical analysis. *J Am Geriatr Soc* 1984; 32(3):237–242.

133. Groher ME: Ethical dilemmas in providing nutrition. *Dysphagia* 1990; 5:102–109.

134. ANA Committee on Ethical Affairs: Persistent vegetative state: report of the American Neurological Association Committee on Ethical Affairs. *Ann Neurol* 1993; 33(4):386–390.

Chapter 30

APHASIA REHABILITATION

Steven L. Small

BASIC ISSUES

Speech and Language

Speech Speech is a complex activity that involves a large sequence of parallel computations involving the conceptualization of an idea in conjunction with a communicative goal, and its formulation into a grammatically structured sequence of specific words, each consisting of an interacting set of ordered sounds. The production of these sound sequences involves organizing a parallel interacting sequence of neural commands to specific muscles of the mouth, which must then execute without error the graded parallel and sequential muscle movements that lead to the target utterance. Breakdown can occur at any stage of the speech process.

The first stage of this overall process, the development of the communicative idea and selection of sentence structure and words that embody meaning, is the essence of language. The second stage of this process consists of organizing a sequence of neural signals from the telencephalon to coordinate the proper sequence of secondary neural signals from the brain stem that signal the muscles of articulation to produce the movements and air flow that make the sounds. This coordination of cortical signals is called speech praxis. Activation of brain-stem motor nuclei that innervate the muscles of articulation leads to bulbar speech. This, of course, requires the normal function of peripheral nerves that innervate these muscles. Finally, normal functioning in bulbar musculature is crucial to normal speech.

Speech Planning An important component of speech dysfunction that often accompanies aphasia is thought to reflect impairments in the timing and sequential coordination of telencephalic signals. Such apraxia of speech is poorly understood, difficult to diagnose, and controversial. A unifying neuropathological substrate has never been identified, although recent neuroimaging data suggest a role for the insular cortex of the dominant hemisphere.[1]

Speech Motor A large number of muscles are involved in the production of speech, including the muscles of the larynx, pharynx, velum, tongue, lips, and face. Cortical signals from the primary motor cortex descend to the lower pons (facial nerve [VII] nucleus) and medulla (motor nuclei for glossopharyngeal [IX], vagal [X], and hypoglossal [XII]) to innervate the brain-stem nuclei that provide signals to these muscles. Damage to the descending signals, the nuclei, or the muscles themselves can produce articulation problems, or dysarthria. By definition, dysarthria does not involve the conceptualization of the communicative message and thus is fundamentally different from aphasia. The distinction between the two is not always easy to make. Distinguishing apraxia of speech from dysarthria can be even more challenging.

Language To a linguist, language is a set of symbols and rules. The rules determine how the symbols may be combined to make larger symbols and symbol structures, eventually leading to meaningful sentences and discourse. Language also incorporates the mechanisms for producing and understanding symbol structures, with capacity limits. The time course, memory requirements, and intermediate codes for language processing are as important.[1a]

Although it is beyond the scope of this chapter to provide a tutorial on language, a number of basic aspects of language will be discussed in order to provide perspective for the discussion of rehabilitation. For more complete discussions of general linguistics, the psychology of language, and the neurology of language, the reader is referred to the major textbooks in the field.[2–4]

Language Levels Language processing can be divided into a number of levels based on the nature of component processes and an approximation of the order in which these component processes must be performed to produce or understand language.

PHONOLOGY At the phonological level are processes for turning the sound stream into recognizable units of spoken language for purposes of comprehension, or for turning words into articulated sound for purposes of production. The intermediate steps in these transformations are thought to use codes that distinguish linguistically important elements of sound called phonemes. Each consonant or vowel in a language may take a number of different pronunciations; for example, the letter "c" can sound like "k" or like "s," and each pronunciation is considered a phoneme. Since the same phoneme will sound quite different depending on the other sounds that must be spoken before and after it in actually producing an utterance, the actual instances of phonemes are given another name and referred to as phones. A syllable is a pair or triplet of phonemes, including exactly one vowel (V) and one or two consonants or consonant clusters (C) in the patterns CV, VC, or CVC.

Many patients with aphasia have problems at the phonological level of processing. Patients who make errors in speech commonly substitute one phoneme or one syllable for another, a problem that relates to phonological processing. Likewise, although less obviously, patients can misinterpret particular phonemes or syllables and hear an unintended word, thereby misinterpreting what is being said.

Syntax Whereas phonological processing is a phenomenon of syllables and words, the construction of sentences from individual words requires application of structure building operations. An important part of linguistic communication is to produce and understand meaningful sentences. Language production involves organizing words into sequences that convey information, whereas language interpretation entails the decoding of ordered sequences into meaningful messages. Syntax (grammar) is the use of word order, word affixes, and specialized functional words to give intended meaning to collections of words. In English, word order plays the most important role in syntactic processing, whereas in other languages with richer systems of affixation (e.g., Italian, German), word order plays a less of a role, with word affixes proportionately more important.[5]

Syntactic impairments are not uncommon in aphasia. Some observers believe that grammatical processing problems are characteristic of patients with damage to the frontal part of the left peri-Sylvian region, and have dubbed this disorder agrammatism. Such patients more easily say and understand single meaningful words, called content words or open-class words, than they do the small function words or closed-class words. Function words do not denote objects, actions, or locations, but rather play a role similar to word affixes and word order in guiding sentence production or interpretation. Function words form a closed class, since they are relatively fixed in the language, whereas content words form an open class, with new words constantly being added to the set. A less common syndrome, called paragrammatism, involves grammatical processing problems from damage to the posterior (temporoparietal) portion of the left peri-Sylvian region. Although there are postulated theoretical differences between the two syndromes, functional data distinguishing the two syndromes remain inconclusive.[6,7]

Semantics Semantics is meaning, and conveying meaning is the essence of communication. Words have meanings and the study of word meanings is called lexical semantics. Sentences have a different form of meaning—conveying entire "thoughts" or statements—and the study of these meanings is called sentential semantics. Meanings of words can be understood in terms of synonyms and antonyms that place these words into a particular place in the meaning space of all words.[8] The meanings of sentences, on the other hand, are built up from a combination of the meanings of the individual (content) words in the sentence, the syntactic aspects of word order, function words, and word affixes, and the higher linguistic context (i.e., the entire conversation or discourse).

Lexical semantic processing often is disrupted in aphasia. Many patients with stroke cannot find the names of objects and actions that they understand visually and functionally. Some substitute an unintended word for a word with a related meaning. Many patients with Alzheimer's disease cannot provide the names of objects, and sometimes provide the name of a higher order category instead (e.g., "animal" for "dog"). These are lexical semantic deficits. Patients with agrammatism sometimes cannot distinguish the subject from the object of a sentence, particularly if word order is somewhat uncommon (e.g., in a passive sentence) and the subject and object words both represent things able to perform actions (e.g., animals, machines). This is a problem of syntax and sentential semantics.

Language Channels Language processing includes an input channel and an output channel. Until the advent of functional neuroimaging, information about these channels corresponded to directly observable behaviors, the only data from which the language system of the brain could be studied.

Input   The input channel is concerned with receptive communication, which in the linguistic mode corresponds to language comprehension. The input channel in humans consists of perceptual systems and the brain processes that manipulate these input perceptions to form meanings. To what extent input processes are modular, that is, functionally encapsulated and isolable from output processes, is unknown. However, in the early stages of input processing, it is not unreasonable to consider intput processes separately. The earliest parts of this input system include the eyes and ears and the first brain nuclei that coordinate these inputs. Spoken sounds and written text must first be processed as perceptual data. Secondary stages of the input system, which probably occur in the cerebral cortex, recognize these percepts as linguistically meaningful tokens, and begin to process them as necessary to build up lexical phonological and semantic structures, followed by encodings of sentence meanings.

The anatomical and physiological structure of this system has yet to be worked out, including the nature of feedback within the system from higher-order cortical processes to basic perceptual processes. It is becoming clearer that the complexity of the input system is far greater than anyone anticipated, and that many processes are occurring simultaneously in various regions of the brain. We have investigated this distributed processing in the input system with functional magnetic resonance imaging. The widespread participation of many left peri-Sylvian regions during sentence reading in a young normal right-handed subject is discussed later.

Output   The output channel is concerned with expressive communication, which in the linguistic mode corresponds to language production. The output channel consists of the brain processes that bring sentence meanings into particular sequences of words and their sound and/or graphic structures, and the basic motor systems that ultimately produce the utterance.

Language Modality   For each processing channel, there are two distinct language modalities, corresponding to linguistic representations as sound or as writing. Language disturbances commonly affect both modalities, although there are many interesting cases of impairments to one or another modality. Since the spoken word constitutes the basis of the linguistic system, and

reading and writing are superimposed (developmentally) on highly organized and structured linguistic systems, speaking and understanding impairments have a more fundamental theoretical role.

Speaking and Understanding   Producing and understanding oral speech requires mechanisms for encoding and decoding auditory waveforms, and mechanisms for encoding and decoding the words and sentences that constitute the message. Since oral speech is in many ways the backbone of language—it is learned first and in some cases exclusively—it is thought to be the architectural foundation of all neural circuits involved in language. Patients with disorders of spoken-language production and comprehension usually have concomitant problems in the written modality, reinforcing the ontogenetic coupling of these two neuroanatomical systems.

Consequently, aphasia is defined in terms of impairments in speaking and understanding, and the preponderance of treatment approaches are aimed directly at this form of communication. To the extent that these two modalities share underlying mechanisms, such as lexical retrieval and sentence syntax and semantics, treatment does not need to be modality-specific. When the language deficit is inextricably entwined with modality-specific problems, such as apraxia of speech, an integrated approach might be preferable.

Reading and Writing   Analogously, producing written language requires neural and motor mechanisms for encoding a message in letters and visual words and performing the somatic motor movements to write or type the visual product. Understanding written language requires distinguishing particular visual stimuli as linguistic, and then decoding them into letters, words, and sentences. Disorders of reading and writing frequently accompany aphasia, and this overlap suggests a significant degree of common underlying neural substrate for language processing from the two modalities. The manifestation of a writing disorder that is disproportionate to the degree of impairment in speaking is considered dysgraphia (or agraphia). The analogous reading disorder is called dyslexia (or alexia).

Most current theories suggest that the unit of processing for reading is the individual word. It seems that word reading occurs through two parallel routes of neural processing. One route involves direct translation of visual word shapes into word meanings, which are then incorporated into higher-order encodings of the verbal messages. The other route begins with the visual perception of letters (not the whole word), and constructs a phonological encoding of the word, from which the word meaning can be accessed and used in comprehension.

The psychological evidence for the existence of two routes comes from studies of words that differ in frequency of occurrence and regularity of spelling. Words with unusual spellings (e.g., "yacht") can be read quickly if they are well known. Words that are very infrequent but have normal spellings (e.g., "lurch") are read more slowly than frequent words with unusual spellings, but both can be read fairly easily. Furthermore, it is possible to read strings of letters that follow the normal spelling rules but are not words (called pseudowords) simply by sounding them out (e.g., "korb").

Neurological evidence also points to the existence of two word-reading routes. Following stroke, some patients have relative loss of word-reading ability in one or another of these pathways.[9] Many patients with aphasia cannot read entire words without decomposing them into parts. With neurological involvement of the neural connections from the primary visual cortices to the left peri-Sylvian language areas, patients decompose words into letters and then recombine the letters into words. A characteristic feature of these letter-by-letter readers is that reading is much slower than normal and takes an amount of time directly proportional to word length. Letter-by-letter reading is also called pure alexia (dyslexia) or alexia without agraphia and was first described by Déjerine.[9a]

Patients with surface dyslexia, by contrast, decompose words by applying letter-to-sound rules. The reliance of these readers on these rules is most apparent in their reading of irregularly spelled words, which they pronounce according to phonetic rules (e.g., "yacht" pronounced to rhyme with "thatched"). A contrasting group of patients with phonological dyslexia are unable to decompose words at all. Although these patients are perfectly able to read irregularly spelled words that were known to them before their stroke, they cannot read pseudowords or infrequent words. Some patients with phonological dyslexia also make reading errors in which they substitute a word with a similar or related meaning for the word they are trying to read. When such errors are present, these patients are said to have deep dyslexia rather than phonological dyslexia.

Communication *Linguistic* Speech and written language are not the only possible means of communication, nor the only means commonly used. Another type of language, based on hand positions and their move-

ments in space, or sign language, is used throughout the world for linguistic communication among the hearing-impaired. Most signers in the United States use American Sign Language (ASL), which has a well-studied history and evolution, with specific relationships to other sign languages in the world. The most important characteristic of ASL for our purposes is its fundamental character as a true language, not an iconic system. This is discussed in a later section.

Linguistic utterances encompass more than specific words and syntactic structures. Both individual words and larger sentences are uttered with variability in tonal quality. Oral speech contains tonal aspects at the levels of both the individual word and the sentence. This aspect of speech is called stress or prosody, and it gives each utterance a particular cadence that can convey crucial information from the speaker to the hearer. Non-native speakers often fail to produce the stress patterns of a language, making their speech more difficult to understand.

An interesting literature has suggested that the neurobiological substrate of prosody is found in the opposite peri-Sylvian region from language, and thus patients with aphasia can have relatively spared prosody, even in the face of markedly impaired word and sentence production.[10] An amusing story was conveyed to me about a father with severe aphasia marked by very poor production and comprehension. Father and son had frequently shared jokes, and the son claimed he had heard all of the father's jokes many times. One weekend day several months after his stroke, the father began to address his son using a stream of unintelligible sounds. The son instantly recognized the prosody, and discerned precisely which joke the father was recounting, and the two enjoyed a hearty laugh together. This formed the basis of a strong relationship, with prosody contributing significantly to shared communication.

Other adjuncts to words and sentences are also commonly used for communicative purposes. Many aspects of the head and face play an adjunctive role in linguistic communication, and in the absence of language, can themselves have communicative roles. Examples include facial expression, eye contact and movements, head position and movements, and the static and dynamic positions of the hands, arms, and trunk. Experienced politicians and actors exploit these nonverbal movements in gestures that reinforce or give nuance to their verbal messages.

Nonlinguistic Prosodic and gestural schemes are most commonly used as adjuncts to linguistic communication because language is the easiest, most efficient, and precise method of communication available. In the aphasic patient, however, gestures and prosody can take on more prominence. In a mild or moderate aphasia, gesture and other motor movements can very nearly compensate for the loss of precision in word and sentence production caused by the brain lesion. In a more severe aphasia, when production is severly limited, these nonlinguistic modalities may be the mainstay of communicative effort. Behavioral therapeutic methods to harness these skills to expand the communicative repertoire of such patients have been used with some success.[11,12]

Anatomy of Language

History In 1861, Pierre Paul Broca presented a paper to the Anatomical Society of Paris discussing autopsy findings on a patient with a language disorder. Broca found a large brain lesion in the left frontotemporal region, and postulated a role for this region in the physiology of language. Although neurologists prior to Broca had suspected and even published similar arguments, Broca is generally acknowledged as the initiator of the modern study of language and the brain through the method of clinicopathological correlation (CPC) (lesion analysis or neuropsychological localization).[13–15] Following this work, a number of additional papers were published on the brain mechanisms of language, including those by Wernicke, Lichtheim, Grashey, and Freud. These discussions generally described a left peri-Sylvian cortex with specialized centers for different channels ("motor" and "sensory" centers), and for different modalities ("written" and "spoken" centers for each channel). The centers described by these so-called "diagram-makers" were meant to be distinct anatomical regions, and their models have much in common with those of contemporary box-and-arrows modelers.

The diagrams of these 19th-century anatomists of language form the basis of the most popular contemporary diagnostic scheme for aphasia. The anatomical diagram of Lichtheim is shown in Figure 30-1, with each center labeled with a letter designating its role in the overall scheme.[16] Disorders of language were viewed in terms of damage to these centers per se or to the connections between them. We will discuss each in turn, since this system of aphasia diagnosis is still used today by many practitioners. The inherent problems of this system are described later.

Region M (motor speech codes) plays a principal

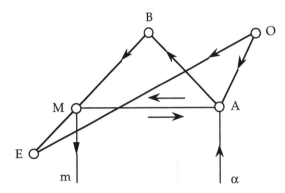

Figure 30-1
Lichtheim Model: Each letter signifies an anatomical "center." The particular centers of this model by Lichtheim are described in the text.

role in speech production and articulation, and damage to this area leads to an aphasia characterized by deficits in these areas. Spontaneous speech and writing and repetition are impaired, but comprehension is spared. Currently, this sort of deficit is called Broca's aphasia. Region A (input phonological codes) plays its main role in auditory and visual comprehension, and thus damage to region A leads to problems with understanding of written and spoken language, repetition, and reading. In current terminology, this aphasia is called Wernicke's aphasia. The connection between areas A and M was thought to be important for repetition of language utterances, and lesions to this pathway produce difficulties of which repetition is the most severe. This form of aphasia is now called conduction aphasia. Damage to both A and M leads to a profound language deficit called global aphasia.

Lesions in pathways to and from Region B (semantic knowledge) lead to deficits similar to those just described, but sparing the connection between M and A leaves repetition relatively uninvolved. Damage to the connection from A to B leads to problems with comprehension, and is called transcortical sensory aphasia, whereas damage to the B-to-M connection leads to production problems and is called transcortical motor aphasia. The combination of these two problems is called transcortical mixed aphasia (also called isolation of the speech area, since the primary language regions A and M are disconnected from the semantic store).

Since the CPC method relies both on clinical evaluation and anatomical evaluation, it was less clear how the patients of these early investigators differed in their behavior than in their anatomical lesions. Some psychologists and physiologists in the second half of the 19th century were developing methods for fine-grained functional dissection, whereas anatomists were studying anatomical lesion location. The psychologist Donders described the division of simple functional tasks (e.g., arm movement) into a large number of component subparts, and attempted to determine the temporal characteristics of each component by subtracting from the time required to perform the large-scale task the time to perform collections of subcomponents.[17] This subtraction method is at the heart of contemporary neuroimaging. At the turn of the century, the physiologist Ferrier described larger-scale functions in terms of more narrowly defined functions, but also attempted to localize each small component in a particular brain area.[18]

These three influences led to the current CPC method in neuropsychology, which involves careful psychological evaluation of a patient and then careful anatomical description of the brain region affected. The goal is to construct task relationships and subdivisions such that each subtask unambiguously implicates a particular brain locus, and the entire collection of tasks and subtasks characterizes a common language function. Significant progress has been made with this method, although some of its assumptions may be invalid and significant paradigmatic changes may be underway in the study of brain and language.[19,20]

Hemispheric Specialization   In most people, the two cerebral hemispheres have relative specialization, with the left hemisphere taking predominant responsibility for many varieties of language functions. This left specialization—"dominance for language"—is true for about 95 percent of right-handed people and about 60 percent of left-handers, with most of the remainder having an analogous asymmetry in the other direction. In people without brain injury from, for example, neonatal stroke or infection, functional symmetry is unusual. In contrast to the relative specialization for language in the left hemisphere, areas of the right hemisphere seem relatively specialized for other types of cognitive functioning, including spatial awareness and aspects of nonlinguistic sound processing such as music, although some advanced musical processing seems lateralized to the left hemisphere.[21–23]

Attempts have been made to determine the anatomical and physiological substrate of this asymmetry. This has not been so easy, as despite these functional differences, the two hemispheres generally are very symmetrical anatomically and seem to have the same low-level physiological representations. One potentially important anatomical difference has been found in the volumes of human cortical regions. The planum temporale (tPT), a brain region that forms part of superior temporal gyrus and is part of the region traditionally thought to be important for language function, is larger on the left than the right in the majority of people.[24–25] This finding seems to be present neonatally beginning at or before 30 weeks gestation.[26] The functional significance of this finding remains the subject of significant inquiry.

Localization   The localization approach has taught us that patients with slow and effortful spontaneous speech accompanied by relatively good comprehension ability tend to have lesions in the frontotemporal region. Patients with normally paced speech that may include phoneme substitutions (that may reach the point of predominantly unrecognizable words) along with poor comprehension tend to have lesions in the temporoparietal regions. In lesions involving primarily the whitematter tracts, with relative sparing of the cortex, aphasic patients have sparing of the ability to repeat words and phrases, whereas there is a predominance of cortical involvement when repetition is involved. Although a number of behavioral syndromes have been tentatively correlated with specific brain areas, these prevalent descriptions are misleading and of questionable value in localization or rehabilitation.

Anatomical Variability   The anatomical variability among the brains of different individuals constitutes one of the main difficulties in devising a standardized anatomical/behavioral scheme for aphasia. In the ideal scenario for localization, a particular location in the brain would correlate with a particular function, and rehabilitation measures could simultaneously address recovery of behavior and recovery or reorganization of anatomically localized neural circuits. This idealized approach might have more relevance at the present time to somatic sensory and motor functioning than to language, since the anatomical underpinnings of the sensorimotor systems seem to be more encapsulated and better understood. In relation to language, this inference is problematic, for two main reasons. First, the brains of different individuals are quite different anatomically. Second, the localization of function in the brain is very imprecise, probably because of a failing in our current notions of functions that might localize and of locations that might encode functionally important neurological tasks.

Anatomical variability in the brain has been demonstrated in several different ways. It can be seen by gross anatomical inspection that there are tremendous differences in gyral anatomy even at this low-resolution macroscopic level.[27] By direct cortical stimulation with electrical current, many neurosurgical research studies have demonstrated wide variability in the cortical regions required to perform both sensorimotor and cognitive tasks. This was noted in the earliest and most prominent cortical stimulation study of this century, which produced a famous map of the motor "homunculus" but also ironically led to the mistaken interpretation that the motor cortex could be captured by a map representing a fixed standard rather than an idealized average.[28] Recent studies using the method of direct cortical stimulation have demonstrated substantial variability in structure–function relationships both in motor cortex encodings of simple motor tasks and in left peri-Sylvian encodings for object naming.[29–31] Additional evidence on variability comes from a widely used stereotactic atlas of the human brain that has its greatest application in the standardization of images from multiple individuals into a single template. The most recent version of this atlas shows that the central sulcus has a remarkably different course from one person to the next, thus leading necessarily to significant differences in the location of sensory and motor codes in the pre- and postcentral gyri.[32] The earlier version of this atlas illustrates the same individual variability for the location and course of the Sylvian (lateral) fissure, around which are located most of the neural structures that process language.[27]

Large-Scale Functions Neurological localization of function has two fundamental requirements—a notion of function and a notion of location. We have already seen that the notion of location is complex because of the anatomical variability among individuals. Unfortunately, the concept of function is perhaps even more ambiguous. Historically, language functions of the brain were classified into a number of broadly defined categories, including comprehension, production, naming, and repetition. Most aphasia tests incorporate subparts aimed at assessing performance on these tasks (as will be described later) and language impairments typically are described and classified in terms of these categories.

The main problem is that there is scanty evidence that these tasks relate directly to cognitively or neurobiologically important functions. As cognitive neuroscientific theories improve, increasing numbers of cognitive tasks appear to have neurobiological correlates, particularly in vision and spatial reasoning.[33–34] The situation is less optimistic for language, although functional

neuroimaging ultimately may provide evidence on this question.[35,37] What this means for therapy is that treatment decisions must continue to be made on the basis of behavioral symptoms and neurological site and type of lesion, but not on the basis of a presumed relationship between location and symptom complex.

Truisms and Questions As described, the commonly held beliefs about the anatomy of language date from the pioneering work of Broca, Wernicke, Lichtheim, and others in the second half of the 19th century.[24,38,39] Their work led to the general notions that (a) the left peri-Sylvian region is anatomically responsible for most of the neural mechanisms of language; (b) the codes and processes of the language output channel are anatomically instantiated by structures in and around the opercula of the left inferior frontal gyrus; and (c) the analogous codes and processes for the language input channel are anatomically centered around the posterior aspect of the superior temporal gyrus.

These generalizations have led to the predominant aphasia-classification schemes currently in use. Since the 19th century, much research has been done within the CPC method, and some of the finer functional structure of these areas has been determined. Unfortunately, this has made the anatomical localization of function more rather than less muddled. One line of research has been to challenge the specific role of the frontal operculum as the seat of language production. One finding was that patients with damage to this region demonstrated certain problems with language comprehension, possibly related to complex grammatical structures.[40,41] The behavioral data have been supplemented by both direct cortical stimulation, demonstrating a role for this region in language comprehension, and by functional neuroimaging.[42] Both PET and fMRI have demonstrated that the frontal operculum is important for a variety of tasks, including verbal working memory and certain motor tasks.[43,44]

In general, increasing evidence is being accrued to challenge the concept that small regions of the brain are specifically responsible for the intuitively determined language functions such as comprehension or naming. This is not to say that brain regions do not have specific functions, or that there are not neural circuits to perform these classically determined functions. It simply appears that the homomorphic relationship between historically important brain regions and functions has broken down. The same problem holds for other brain regions, such as the thalamus, basal ganglia, and the inferior parietal lobule, and other functions.[19] A new approach to localization recognizes the existence of distributed anatomical circuits, interactivity among regions, and different types of functions.[45,46] Examples include the role of the distributed circuits of the left temporal lobe in encoding word meanings and the role of the hippocampus in intermediate encoding of memories prior to integration into cortical memory circuits.[47,48]

Distributed Representations By using functional magnetic resonance imaging (fMRI), it is possible to demonstrate that certain brain locations are important for the performance of specific large-scale language tasks (e.g., comprehension), but that these areas alone are not responsible for carrying out the tasks. Rather, the areas of traditional importance in the study of aphasia seem to be the anatomical cornerstones of more distributed networks that are involved in task performance (i.e., they are less variably involved). For example, a dozen or more discrete areas of involvement that differ to some extent from individual to individual make up the distributed processing for sentence comprehension in normal subjects.[35,49] A single case in which this pattern changed with aphasia has been reported, although it is not yet clear whether there are regularities in the nature of this change and whether or not the changes can be influenced and measured in the context of rehabilitation.[35,50]

Figure 30-2 shows the areas of activation (present in a single left parasagittal plane) in sentence reading by a normal subject. The words of the sentence were presented to this subject one at a time, with 250 ms available to read each word. A small number of discrete regions throughout the left peri-Sylvian region seems to participate in this task (at this rate). Since sentence reading is a complex activity, involving many aspects of language processing, each area of involvement requires further study as to the nature of the tasks in which it participates. The combination of this neuroimaging approach with predictive distributed computer models might ultimately lead to new functional localization concepts in language.

Implications for Recovery The anatomy and physiology of the normal language system in the brain constrain the possible courses of its recovery after damage. For example, if the frontal operculum were completely responsible for speech articulation, it would not be possible for someone with (theoretically) complete destruction of this region (and only this region) to speak. Although some patients certainly do not recover the ability

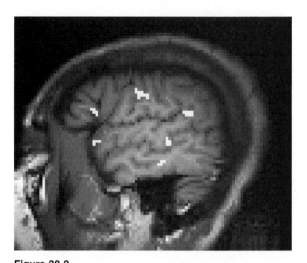

Figure 30-2

fMRI of sentence reading (single left parasagittal slice): Words were presented one at a time for 250 msec each, with each subset of eight to 10 words followed by a period. At the end of each sequence, subjects were asked to determine if the sentence was meaningful. Most of the sentences were meaningful. In a control task, subjects viewed sequences of images that looked like text, but were not (false font strings). Comparison of the two tasks shows the left hemisphere brain regions involved in reading sentences. Note that many peri-Sylvian regions are participating, including parts of areas traditionally thought important for language comprehension and production.

to articulate, these patients ordinarily have large regions that extend from the frontal operculum to other cortical and subcortical regions of the frontal lobe, including the insula.[51]

No Single Region Is Completely Responsible The presence of neural circuits that are both computationally and spatially distributed means that no one brain region is completely responsible for any specific language function. On the other hand, there is little evidence to support the position that the entire brain participates in every task.[52] A large lesion might damage so much of the distributed circuit responsible for a particular task that recovery of that task would be unlikely to occur regardless of type or quantity of therapeutic intervention. By contrast, very small lesions affecting parts of the same circuit might lead to easy and rapid spontaneous recovery, independent of therapy. These lesions might occur frequently and subclinically.[53] Since the vast majority of lesions seen by neurologists fall in between these two situations, the therapeutic implications of distributed language circuits on the intermediate case must be addressed.

Adaptability in Representations The hope for these lesions of intermediate size is that the regional neural circuitry can be manipulated to compensate for the lost neural tissue. There is considerable evidence that the brain regions encode function in a dynamic manner, with constant remodeling and reshaping. In animal models, it has been possible to perform electrophysiological mapping of areas of the primary sensory and motor cortex before, during, and after altered behavior aimed to augment or reduce the functional responsibility of parts of these cortical regions. With practiced motor activity of certain fingers, the volume of motor cortical tissue dedicated to those fingers increased.[54] Repetitive peripheral nerve stimulation led to reorganization of the primary sensory cortex (SI) dedicated to the stimulated appendage.[55] When two fingers were tied together and used as a single digit, the functional organization of SI changed to encode the new structure as a single digit, losing the previous cortical encoding of the inner surfaces of the two fingers.[56] Amputation of a finger led to reorganization of SI, with loss of the cortical encoding of the missing finger, and increase in size of the areas responsible for the adjacent fingers.[57]

In humans, slow-growing tumors can become quite large before affecting function at all. Using fMRI, three patients were recently reported with vascular malformations in the cerebral cortex prior to stereotactic radiosurgery. None of these patients had noticeable functional deficits, even one with a lesion affecting the inferior frontal gyrus. Only by careful testing was a very mild dysnomia discovered. In these patients, functional activation uniformly occurred at a location adjacent to the region that would be expected to be involved in the target task.[58] In therapy for aphasia, it would be desirable to intervene in such a way to exploit this natural reorganization ability of the distributed cortical representations. Although current therapies may act in this way, there has not yet been experimental verification of such a brain–behavior interaction.

Physiology and Pharmacology of Language

This section reviews the existing data on brain chemistry and pharmacotherapy following both experimental stroke in animal models and stroke in humans. Of course, the animal data characterize systems other than

language, but are relevant to language because of similarities in basic neuronal system architecture of the cerebral cortex. The pharmacological studies in humans originate from studies of both motor and language rehabilitation. The combined results of this research constitutes a degree of future promise for drug therapy of aphasia.

Experimental Stroke The concentrations of catecholamines in the rat and cat brainstem and the subcortex of the rat are decreased following cerebral cortical infarction. After the acute phase following rat unilateral cortical infarction (40 days), there remain decreases in ipsilateral norepinephrine concentrations in the cortex and brain stem, and decreases in ipsilateral brain stem (but not cortical) dopamine concentrations.[59–62] This catecholamine deficit may result from right cortical but not left cortical infarction.[63] Such experimental stroke also causes widespread depression of glucose utilization in the cortex on both sides, the ipsilateral red nucleus, and the locus ceruleus bilaterally.[64]

The postulated role of monoamines in stroke recovery led to a number of therapeutic studies in animal models, as summarized in Table 30-1. In studies of recovery of function in animal models, the duration of spontaneous recovery from a motor cortex lesion in a rat is about 2 weeks, and for a cat, spontaneous recovery takes several months.[65] A single dose of dextroamphetamine (*d*-amphetamine), which augments postsynaptic catecholamines, including norepinephrine and dopamine, led to accelerated recovery in a beam walking task in rats with unilateral motor cortex ablation.[65,66] A single dose of haloperidol, a dopamine antagonist, blocked the amphetamine effect. When given alone, haloperidol delayed spontaneous recovery and phenoxybenzamine, an α-adrenergic antagonist, reproduced the deficits in recovered animals. Paradoxically, treatment with intraventricular norepinephrine, but not dopamine, reproduced the beneficial effect of *d*-amphetamine.[67] Analogous results have been obtained with *d*-amphetamine therapy of motor system injury in the cat.[68,69]

These motor system results generalize to the visual system.[70] Bilateral ablation of the primary visual cortex of the cat causes impairment of visual depth perception. When given both visual experience and dextroamphetamine, such cats demonstrate marked improvement in function. The effect was not seen when the dextroamphetamine was unaccompanied by visual experience or when the visual experience was accompanied by saline instead of active drug.

Table 30-1

Drugs used in experimental studies of aphasia pharmacotherapy and their pharmacologic effects

Drug	Neurotransmitter	Effect
Amphetamine	Norepinephrine, dopamine	Increased release from storage
Apomorphine	Dopamine	Agonist
Bromocriptine	Dopamine	Agonist
Caffeine	Unknown (?adenosine)	CNS stimulation
Chlordiazepoxide	γ Aminobutyric acid (GABA)	Potentiation of inhibition
Haloperidol	Dopamine	Antagonist
Meprobamate	Unknown (?opiate)	CNS depression
Methylphenidate	Norepinephrine, dopamine	Release from storage sites
Phenoxybenzamine	Norepinephrine (α)	Antagonist
Propanolol	Norepinephrine (β)	Antagonist
Selegiline	Dopamine	Blocks metabolic breakdown
Sodium amytal	γ Aminobutyric acid (GABA)	Potentiation of inhibition
Tranylcypromine	Norepinephrine, epinephrine	Blocks metabolic breakdown

As the locus ceruleus is the origin of diffuse noradrenergic arborizations throughout the cortex, the role of the LC in stroke recovery was studied.[64] Following experimental stroke, there was widespread cerebral cortical depression of glucose utilization, which could be accelerated by prior ablation of the LC. Dextroamphetamine could reverse this metabolic depression, which was exacerbated by haloperidol administration, and reverse the effects of LC damage.

Animal models thus suggest that endogenous and exogenous catecholamines, particularly norepinephrine, acting through α receptors, play an important role in recovery from stroke. These data also suggest that the effect of catecholamine augmentation therapy depends on concomitant experience. Thus motor recovery following stroke, while facilitated by pharmacotherapy, depended on the presence of motor practice, just as visual recovery depended on visual experience.

History of Aphasia Pharmacotherapy In an early case report, Linn describes two aphasic patients with language disorders from traumatic brain injury.[71] The patients had language testing before and after the injection of intravenous amobarbital sodium. Although language performance of the first patient improved, he attributed the result to improved attention and "energy." The second patient went from a state of near mutism to a markedly improved state, which endured

only when the drug was administered. Unfortunately, the patient eventually developed tolerance to the treatment, and the conclusion was that sodium amytal impacts the "psychological component" present in organic disease.

The most realistic explanation for improvement in these patients with traumatic brain lesions relates to the short-acting anticonvulsant properties of amobarbital. One could speculate that the beneficial effect of this drug in the alleviation of aphasia following brain trauma was the direct result of stopping ongoing partial seizures in the left temporal lobe. Aphasic seizures constitute a well documented form of partial epilepsy.[72–74]

A carefully controlled clinical study involving 27 hospitalized patients with aphasia failed to replicate Linn's finding.[75] Comprehensive language and cognitive testing of these patients before and after administration of intravenous amobarbital found that although many patients felt that they were more fluent during the amobarbital infusion, no patient showed objective improvement in function.

West and Stockel selected 29 patients with right hemiparesis and aphasia from stroke for a double-blind placebo-controlled crossover study of meprobamate therapy combined with behavioral speech therapy.[76] In each 6-month cycle, a patient had one 3-month period of meprobamate plus speech therapy and another of placebo plus speech therapy. General physical and neurological examinations, laboratory evaluations, and comprehensive language and cognitive measures were performed before and after four such cycles. After careful statistical analysis, the authors determined that the medication did not produce better results than speech therapy alone. Although this double blind crossover study produced valid results for a subpopulation of patients with aphasia, eligibility required a right hemiparesis, excluding many patients with aphasia.

Sarno et al. studied the effects of hyperbaric oxygen on sixteen chronic aphasic patients with right hemiplegia and aphasia from left-hemisphere stroke.[77] Comprehensive neurological and cognitive evaluation before and after treatment with hyperbaric air or hyperbaric oxygen failed to show improvement in auditory comprehension or functional communication during or following therapy.

Augmentation of Brain Dopamine Studies of brain catecholamines in animals following stroke led to an analogous study in humans. In this study, it was found that the concentration of catecholamines in the human cerebrospinal fluid is decreased following cerebral cortical infarction.[78] This theoretical motivation and a number of empirical speculations have led to studies aimed at augmenting these transmitters in the brains of patients following stroke.

Several studies have examined the role of dopamine. Albert and his colleagues described a case suggesting that the dopamine agonist bromocriptine helped restore speech fluency in a patient with transcortical motor aphasia resulting from stroke.[79,80] The patient was tested before treatment with bromocriptine, during treatment, and then following cessation of treatment. Fluency improved when the patient was taking bromocriptine and evaporated following cessation of the drug. This case is particularly difficult to interpret, given the lack of many specific neurological details and of careful controls on the evaluation process. The absence of an underlying basal ganglia disorder was never documented, and the possiblity of a placebo effect or performance variability was not discussed.

Another case report failed to find a similar benefit from bromocriptine in a man with transcortical motor aphasia from ischemic stroke.[81] Multiple baselines for testing and withdrawal periods were used to study this patient, who showed no improvement in language performance, despite his perception to the contrary. The authors concluded that a placebo effect may be responsible for the apparent improvement in language function seen in some patients.

Recently, two patients with "left frontoparietal infarcts" and "nonfluent aphasia" were treated with bromocriptine for 3 months in an escalating dose, and underwent comprehensive language testing prior to therapy and monthly during therapy.[82] Both patients improved markedly in speech fluency and not in other aspects of language function. The presence of multiple baselines, with lack of improvement in language measures other than fluency, gives this study some weight. However, its value is limited by certain design flaws, including inability to rule out placebo effects and lack of any withdrawal phase.

A prospective open-label trial of bromocriptine in treatment of nonfluent aphasia studied seven patients with left-frontal ischemic infarctions and a nonfluent aphasia.[83] Every 2 weeks, the dose of bromocriptine was escalated and then de-escalated, with language and neuropsychological testing before and during treatment. Statistical analysis of behavioral measures correlated improvement with escalating doses and deterioration with declining doses of the drug in patients with moderate aphasia. Severely impaired patients did not improve. The open-label nature of this study, with few controls, no withdrawal periods, and improvement in all baselines diminishes the generalizability of these results.

Augmentation of Brain Catecholamines with Amphetamine An early study of aphasia pharmacotherapy focused on the amphetamine-related drug methylphenidate and the benzodiazepine chlordiazepoxide. In this double-blind placebo-controlled crossover study, a language battery was performed 1 hour after drug (or placebo) administration.[84] Statistical analysis of the data revealed no difference in language performance between any of the conditions for the patients as a group.

Recently, Walker-Batson et al. reported a study of six patients with ischemic cerebral infarction, all in the distribution of the left middle cerebral artery. All patients were aphasic, and were evaluated by the Porch Index of Communicative Ability.[85,86] Each patient took dextroamphetamine every 4 days, (about) an hour prior to a session of speech and language therapy, for a total of 10 sessions. When evaluated after this period, the patients performed at significantly above 100 percent of their expected levels, according to the PICA norms. Of potential significance was the fact that the two studies showing beneficial effects of dextroamphetamine—this study and a controlled study of motor rehabilitation—share the common feature of evaluating the drug as an enhancement to behavioral or physical therapy, rather than as a monotherapeutic panacea.[85,87]

Our group has performed two studies of aphasia pharmacotherapy using the method of single-subject experimental design in patients with stroke[87a] and one in a patient with primary progressive aphasia (PPA).[99,108] One stroke patient received dextroamphetamine and the other received selegiline hydrochloride. The patient with PPA received dextroamphetamine. In no case did pharmacotherapy alone help the patients, and only in the patient with progressive disease was there a suggestion that pharmacotherapy plus therapy was more helpful than therapy alone (which helped in all cases).

Problems with Studies   Pharmacotherapy of aphasia has been tried intermittently for many years. The early studies, motivated by intuitive behavioral and physiological rationales, demonstrated little success. The first concept was that "patients with aphasia speak more easily when they are relaxed," leading to studies of the barbiturates.[75] Although this therapy was reported to work in one or two patients, possibly owing to the anticonvulsant properties of amobarbital, prospective study failed to show benefit. A similar rationale, "to condition [aphasic patients] physiologically and psychologically" with meprobamate yielded similar results.[76]

Another therapeutic rationale, motivated by the many aphasic patients with cerebrovascular disease, concerned cerebral perfusion and blood oxygenation. Investigators postulated that decreased tissue oxygen from vascular thrombosis or embolism might inhibit language recovery, and that hyperbaric oxygen therapy might improve aphasia rehabilitation. This theory did not hold up in a carefully designed study.[77]

Recent animal studies of experimental stroke and stroke recovery, with functional injury to motor or visual systems, have suggested that pharmacological augmentation of brain catecholamine concentrations can greatly accelerate the beneficial effects of practice. Dextroamphetamine was the most successful agent used in these studies, and helped motor recovery when coupled with exercise and visual recovery when accompanied by visual experience. A study of intraventricular norepinephrine and dopamine suggested that the beneficial effect of dextroamphetamine was owing to its ability to increase postsynaptic norepinephrine rather than dopamine.

These animal models provide a different sort of therapeutic rationale than has been present previously for the pharmacological treatment of aphasia. In particular, these studies provide evidence that certain neurochemical defects are present after stroke, even in brain areas not thought to be injured during the acute event. These studies focused on the catecholamines, and led to subsequent animal and human studies of stroke recovery, both physical and cognitive aspects, with exogenous augmentation of brain catecholamine concentrations.

The studies of human pharmacotherapy with dextroamphetamine and bromocriptine are difficult to interpret for several reasons. Although not all studies fail on all counts, the studies as a whole are marked by a myriad of problems, summarized in Table 30-2.

Implications for Recovery *Avoiding Negative Agents*   One important consequence of this research into the pharmacology of aphasia is the realization that drugs are not only potential therapeutic adjuncts, but that they can also serve as inhibitors of successful recovery. If some pharmacological manipulation appears to play a role in accelerating or improving recovery, then the opposite manipulation could delay or prevent recovery. With this in mind, several investigators have performed retrospective studies of medication use during aphasia rehabilitation and made some important findings.

Since hypertension is an important risk factor for cerebrovascular disease, patients with stroke frequently require medications to reduce blood pressure. The earliest study on the effects of inadvertent pharmacological interference with aphasia recovery was motivated by the fact that some of these agents, particularly catecholamine antagonists, might be expected to disturb stroke recovery. A retrospective review of the medications of 32 patients presenting for language evaluation following stroke showed that the 19 patients taking medicines performed more poorly on the Porch Index of Communicative Ability (PICA) than the 13 who were not taking medicines.[86,88] This study was poorly controlled and the results cannot be easily accepted, yet it was important for recognizing the effect of drugs on rehabilitative outcome.

Recently, however, a well-controlled study has been conducted to address the issues raised in this pre-

Table 30-2
Limitations of current studies of aphasia pharmacotherapy

Anatomical definitions of aphasia	Patient selection
	Placebo effects and controls
Functional definitions of aphasia	Concomitant and related illness

Table 30-3

Drugs with potentially deleterious effects on stroke recovery

Benzodiazepines	Phenothiazines
Clonidine	Phenytoin
Haloperidol	Prazosin

liminary work. One initial observation in this research was that over 80 percent of all patients were taking some medicine at the time of their stroke, and that 65 percent were taking multiple medications. Included in this list were such drugs as α-adrenergic blockers and benzodiazepines, which are known to impede stroke recovery in animal studies. A study was undertaken to assess the potentially deleterious effects on human stroke recovery of several drugs that seemed problematical in animal studies.[89] A total of 96 patient records were reviewed and patients were grouped on whether or not they were taking one of the predetermined deleterious drugs shown in Table 30-3. Statistical analysis revealed that, whereas patient demographics and stroke severity were similar between groups, motor recovery time was significantly shorter in the group that was not taking one of these drugs. Drugs that potentially interfere with catecholaminergic or GABAergic function, or are thought to delay recovery by empirical study (i.e., the drugs in Table 30-3), ought to be avoided if possible during aphasia rehabilitation.

Supplementing Pharmacological Lack Since they are marked by design problems that limit interpretation of the results, existing studies are ambiguous about the potential beneficial effect of increased central nervous system catecholamines on human motor recovery and aphasia rehabilitation. In the realm of motor system recovery, both human and animal studies suggest that dextroamphetamine can facilitate recovery when combined with practice. Weaker evidence also suggests that when coupled with practice in oral communication, increasing brain norepinephrine and/or dopamine might facilitate improvement in speech and language impairments after stroke. Only with carefully designed and well-controlled studies can the promise of pharmacotherapy be rigorously evaluated.

Psychology of Language

History The lesion-analysis method for the study of language and the brain requires correlation between the site of an anatomical lesion and a measure of behavioral performance. With these two components, it is possible to build a conception of the functional anatomy of the brain for language. Psychology thus represents a crucial part of the story, and one that has been a focus of investigation since Broca. As concepts of anatomy and physiology have advanced, so have the methods of psychological inquiry and knowledge of mental processes. The works of Donders and Ferrier were particularly influential late in the 19th century for the methods of process description and subcomponent analysis.[17,18] The advent of computers led to another revolution in the study of cognition, with the information-processing method reaching prominence.[90]

Both computer models and componential models of modular processing became commonplace, and language processing was thought to involve symbol manipulation by computational processes.[91] Psychological studies attempted to quantify aspects of linguistic rule application, lexical retrieval, and similar componential tasks. More recently, these studies have changed with the new characterization of the elemental psychological processes involved in language as highly parallel nonsymbolic "connectionist" processes.[92] Now psychological studies aim to identify components of distributed connectionist circuits or of spreading activation networks.[93,94] Psychological testing methods for neuropsychology now make use of both modularity concepts to identify apparently dissociated functions and connectionist concepts to identify aspects of parallel circuits.[95,96]

Performance Variability Performance variability is a constant feature of aphasia, and one that complicates therapy and the assessment of efficacy in individual patients. Patients differ in their language abilities at different times.[97] Just as speech errors in normal adults can be increased substantially by certain manipulations, such as increasing speaking rate or adding intoxicants (e.g., ethanol), so error patterns in patients with aphasia can be changed by environmental conditions.[94] Manipulations known to alter performance include fatigue, intoxications, particularly ethanol and prescription drugs, illness, anxiety, stress, and physical exhaustion. Attempts to use performance variability to therapeutic advantage include the pharmacological interventions discussed later in this chapter.[98,99]

This variability makes careful evaluations of treatment efficacy difficult. Multiple-baseline single-subject experimental design is a powerful but cumbersome method that helps eliminate variability as a confound in treatment research.[100] Both individual assessments of patient progress in aphasia therapy and research studies on new treatments that do not take into account performance variability in some way must be viewed with skepticism.

Resource Limitations Successful language performance depends on the proper sequencing of information over time and the ability to build up utterances from small component parts. This holds true both for comprehending and producing utterances. The construction process requires that (a) particular time constraints be met in sequencing the information; and (b) linguistic-structure building can take place with intermediate results retained long enough to contribute to the final output utterance or interpretation of an input utterance. Both time and space (memory) are limited resources, and are to some degree interdependent.[101,102] With enough space, the temporal constraints can be minimized, and with enough time, the memory limits can be minimized. Although normal language users have surplus capacity in time and space, patients with brain damage have less "cerebral reserve" capacity. This affects a variety of cognitive functioning (and other types of cortically mediated functioning, such as complex sensory and motor performance), but is particularly evident in language processing. Many patients with aphasia comprehend well at slow rates, but quite poorly at fast rates. Some patients who have problems repeating long fragments of speech will repeat an initial part of the fragment or paraphrase the whole fragment. Resource limitations can be used as a partial explanation for a wide variety of language disorders.

Neurology of Language Rehabilitation

Causes of Aphasia Although many types of brain insult produce language disturbances, the most common by far is ischemic or hemorrhagic stroke. Ischemic damage almost anywhere in the left hemisphere is likely to disrupt some circuit of importance to language performance, as is certain damage to the right peri-Sylvian cortex. Even infarcts in the distribution of the posterior cerebral arteries can cause language disturbances by affecting inferior temporal structures and occipitotemporal structures. Overall, an estimated two million people live in the United States with previous strokes, and about 40 percent of them have some impairment in language.[103,104] With almost a million Americans with aphasia from stroke alone, there is tremendous motivation for advances in therapy.

The second most common cause of aphasia next to stroke is dementia. The prevalence of dementia in the U.S. population over the age of 65 is about 10 to 15 percent, with over two million cases of Alzheimer's disease (AD) alone.[105,106] Most patients with AD have some degree of language impairment.[107] Therapy for the language impairments of dementia are not so much aimed at cortical reorganization as in remediating the chronic disease process itself (specifically if possible) and in compensating for the language and memory problems. We have used a combination of pharmacotherapy and lexical training to improve lexical semantic functioning (transiently) in one patient with a focal dementia and a conversational method (i.e., PACE) in a second such patient.[99,108–110]

In young people, an important cause of aphasia is traumatic head injury. Although it is much less prevalent than stroke or dementia, head injury has special importance because it primarily affects young adults. Recovery has been unpredictable and variable, with therapeutic goals similar to those in stroke. Other causes of aphasia include neoplasms, vascular malformations, and surgically induced lesions. Treatment for aphasia accompanying brain tumors begins with specific treatment for the tumor, followed by the same aphasia therapy methods applicable for stroke. Postoperative aphasia also is treated similarly to stroke, with rapid spontaneous improvement in the first few weeks. Neurological dysfunction following stereotactic radiotherapy, including aphasia, can spontaneously recover over an extended period of time (as long as 1 year) following surgery.[111]

Neuropathology As can be seen throughout this volume, one feature of neurological rehabilitation is that the etiology of damage to the nervous system has an important impact on the preferred method of intervention. Although this holds for language disorders, etiology plays an additional role in aphasia diagnosis and treatment. Since the behavioral classification of aphasia, upon which certain specific therapies are based, was derived in the study of patients with stroke, it does not readily hold for patients with language disturbances from other causes. This has led some investigators, particularly non-neurologists, to apply the term "aphasia" solely to language disturbances that occur after stroke, rather than to the gamut of neurogenic language disorders. In this chapter, we use the broader definition, which necessitates some comment about aphasia classification and neuropathology.

Although the standard tools of aphasia diagnosis can be used to evaluate patients with all neurological causes of aphasia, the focus must be on the individual symptoms and signs of the tested patients, rather than the diagnostic labels that might be invoked to classify them. Patients with traumatic head injury have a variety of cognitive deficits caused by a combination of brain contusion and axonal shearing, as described in Chapter 7 in this volume. Although language is often affected in head injury, more commonly it is supportive systems that are affected primarily, with language affected secondarily, and with language-specific deficits uncommon. Thus patients will have difficulty with such skills as concentration, attention, and verbal memory, but not so much with processing at the phonological, lexical, or sentential levels of language use.

Implications for Recovery   The rehabilitation of patients with aphasia depends not only on the location of the neurological damage and its extent, but also on the specific pathogenesis of the underlying process. Certain patients with aphasia will have spontaneous improvement in their condition (e.g., stroke, trauma), whereas others will have progression (e.g., dementia, neoplasm). Although no patient will remain static, some patients, particularly those with longstanding stable disease (e.g., old stroke, previous head injury, or treated cancer) can have relatively minimal change in condition over time. In the early stage of disease, rehabilitative goals must be adjusted to the particular circumstances of the illness and its dynamics. Thus a patient with AD might not embark on a 6-month program of word training, despite marked lexical semantic deficits, whereas this might be the most appropriate course for a patient with similar symptoms recovering from herpes simplex encephalitis (HSE). A patient with AD, on the other hand, might benefit from learning about the disease process and mechanisms for compensating.

Knowledge of the underlying deficit is important for another reason. Success or failure in meeting rehabilitative goals can be a valuable index of disease progression or remission. Thus, if a patient with treated cancer begins to have difficulty with previously intact language tasks or begins to have more difficulty responding to treatment, the treating physician should look for tumor regrowth, radiation necrosis, or chemotherapeutic side effect. A patient with presumed AD who is able to employ numerical processing skills normally, perhaps as part of therapy, might have a primary progressive aphasia or frontotemporal dementia instead.[112] Even in a patient with relatively fixed deficit from stroke,

rehabilitative difficulties could arise from any number of concomitants of stroke, such as hypertension, diabetes mellitus, extracranial vascular disease (e.g., arterial nephrosclerosis), or new cerebrovascular events. Certainly intermittent seizures, which occur following stroke, head injury, HSE, and neoplasm, could lead to unexplained rehabilitation failure.

The particular distribution of disease also provides insight into plausible anatomical patterns of recovery, and can help guide the development of rehabilitative goals. Although stroke leads to the best-defined fixed lesions, even aspects of stroke are sometimes difficult to gauge, since diaschisis and radiographically silent lesions lead to damage remote from the principal site of the lesion. HSE involves the limbic system, with extension into the medial and inferior temporal lobes. AD also affects these structures, but less severely early on, and with ultimate extension over time posteriorly into the superior temporal and parietal regions. In these cases, focusing during rehabilitation on memory systems to compensate for language impairments often is not helpful. Knowing the pathogenesis of particular disease states helps determine the extent of injury and the paths of progression and potential recovery.

The treatment of neoplastic language deficits depends on the type of tumor and its dynamic properties. Glial neoplasms infiltrate the brain parenchyma, spreading along axonal pathways, and cause subtle degrees of cognitive impairment (e.g., concentration) even without neuroimaging evidence of spread. When more aggressive, these tumors involve the corpus collosum and can cause disconnection syndromes (e.g., splenial lesions leading to reading impairments). These tumors cause marked focal deficits when they become large, but can be associated with subtle cognitive deficits early. Metastatic lesions can lead to focal cognitive deficits early, partly owing to vasogenic edema. Following aggressive oncological therapy, we have had the most success in language therapy of patients with neoplasm by both working on functional communication and helping them identify possible cognitive concomitants of tumor recurrence.

In traumatic brain injury, patients can have severe focal deficits from contusion. Although language can be affected in brain contusion, this is made uncommon by the anatomy of language processing. With language centered around the peri-Sylvian region, typical coup-contrecoup injury does not affect language. Even without contusion, such patients commonly have "axonal shearing" in the white-matter pathways, and consequent cognitive deficits in complex integrative cognitive processing. Patients with mild head injury not uncommonly have subtle deficits of this type.[113] Reliance on strategic cognitive mechanisms to overcome language processing difficulties may not be helpful in such patients.

APPLIED ISSUES

Early Aphasia Therapy

There are a number of early reports of aphasia therapy. In 1880, Mills reported a single case of aphasia in which a patient "benefited from training which was largely of the patient's own initiation and conducted by himself.[114,115] In a subsequent case, Mills reported several additional cases, in which treatment consisted of rote training of different aspects of language processing. His approach was based on "Wylie's physiological alphabet," and encouraged production of a variety of different phonemic forms. One use of this approach, an antecedent of current developmental methods, was called the "Mother's Method," in which words were prompted by the first letter, beginning with the same bilabial words repeated by children learning language for the first time (e.g., "mama," "papa"). Mills reports great success of his treatment.

In this book *Aphasiology,* Lecours and his colleagues report on some early efforts of therapy in the French literature, beginning with the efforts in 1886 by Ch. Féré, who wrote on the "re-education" of patients with aphasia.[116,117] Lecours points out that with these few exceptions, treatment of aphasia did not gain widespread acceptance until World War II.

Does Aphasia Therapy Work?

The value of behavioral treatment of aphasia has been difficult to assess quantitatively or qualitatively for a number of substantive reasons. First, following stroke, most patients will have some degree of functional recovery from language impairments without any intervention. Second, all patients with aphasia exhibit severe performance variability, such that skills may seem to improve dramatically from one session to the next, but then revert back at a third session. Third, lessons learned in the clinic are sometimes only applied while the patient is in that particular clinic or interacting with a single particular therapist. Fourth, abilities and approaches vary among therapists.

Efficacy of Speech Therapy In addition to substantial empirical data, academic speech pathologists have provided a significant literature on the philosophical questions surrounding the efficacy of aphasia therapy. There are three reasons commonly discussed to address why the efficacy question is problematical in its own right: (1) There are over a hundred studies addressing the efficacy of aphasia therapy, far more than for many other medical therapies, the majority of which attest to the benefit of therapy.[118,119] (2) A traditional belief among many medical practitioners, part of a difficult-to-eradicate "folk mythology," is that spontaneous recovery accounts for all language improvement after stroke.[119,120] (3) Last, the question is impossible to answer because it is poorly crafted. The important question to ask is how a particular treatment for a particular pathology fares in relation to a quantifiable outcome measure.

Outcome studies on the effects of specific therapeutic approaches (e.g., melodic intonation therapy [MIT]) or specific aphasia subtypes (e.g., a BDAE classification of Broca Aphasia) are badly needed.[121,122] In fact, this form of proof has led the Therapeutics Committee of the American Academy of Aphasia to accept MIT as a treatment for this specific group of patients.[123]

The question of efficacy for aphasia treatment is confounded by a number of factors. One source of confusion is the issue of remediation versus eradication. Aphasia therapy is not a cure for aphasia. Compensatory strategies may provide essential skills to improve quality of life and independence without impacting aphasia at all. There is, nevertheless, ample evidence that frequent sessions of aphasia therapy over a long period of time can lead to continued improvement.[124]

The issue of spontaneous recovery of function has been misunderstood by many critics of aphasia therapy. After a stroke, some degree of functional recovery in multiple modalities is the rule, with or without therapy. The aphasia characteristics of a patient can improve dramatically over the first weeks and even months after a stroke. However, the presence of spontaneous recovery has nothing whatsoever to do with the effectiveness of aphasia therapy. For an analogy, consider the many people who recover spontaneously from heart attacks each year. Vasodilators, sympathetic blockers, and cardiac rehabilitation are integral to standard treatment and are aimed at specific physiological goals such as increasing regional perfusion or augmenting collateral circulation. Similarly, in aphasia treatment, researchers are examining such questions as the effectiveness of mapping therapy to improve grammatical production in patients with damage to the inferior frontal gyrus. For some reason, the efficacy of "aphasia therapy" has been the subject of much invective not found in other fields.[125,125a,126]

How to Design an Interpretable Study of Aphasia Treatment

The effectiveness of particular therapies for symptoms of language disturbance in selected individuals can be assessed by group studies or single-subject studies. For data from group studies to be interpretable, the studies must be well controlled, with random assignment to treatment and no-treatment groups. They must be controlled for age, etiology, severity, and type of aphasia. They must employ the same treatment regimen for all enrollees, and be analyzed with proper statistical methods.[119] Single-subject experimental studies must be conducted with the same degree of control, including careful assessment of baseline performance on a variety of measures, some that are expected to be improved by therapy and others that are not; consistency of treatment over time; repeated assessment of all measures (those expected to improve and others that are not); and control periods that are exactly like treatment periods in all possible respects other than the presence of treatment.[127]

Group Studies

Many group studies have been conducted, but most have not met the design requirements that would lead to interpretable results. While it is beyond the scope of this chapter to examine each study, several common methodological pitfalls should be highlighted. For example, an important study often cited to demonstrate the lack of efficacy of aphasia therapy failed to control for a number of selection criteria, failed to provide the same treatment to all subjects (many of whom had minimal treatment), and failed to use the appropriate statistical analysis.[119,128] The controversy surrounding efficacy and group studies led to the development of a multicenter study of the effectiveness of aphasia therapy, supported by the Veterans Administration.[129] Rather than depriving some patients of therapy, the study delayed therapy for a portion of patients. This carefully designed study showed significant benefit to patients who received 8 to 10 hours of standardized treatment per week for 12 weeks compared to those who did not receive treatment.

Single-Subject Experimental Designs

Single-subject experimental design has been used to evaluate a number of different therapeutic interventions.[130] Since they are inexpensive to conduct and can be performed well by following a number of specific guidelines, single-subject studies are commonly employed in assessment of efficacy of specific interventions. Good single-subject designs have been conducted on particular methods for the treatment of agrammatism, verb generalization, and pharmacotherapy.[99,100,108,131]

Meta-analysis

In recent years, the effectiveness of aphasia therapy has been addressed in several large meta-analysis studies.[118,132,135] They bear out the fact that existing studies from which subjects were enrolled lacked important information in the majority of cases. They also suggest that aphasic patients with stroke who are treated by speech/language pathologists have better outcomes than patients who do not receive such treatment. The effect of treatment exceeds that of spontaneous recovery alone.[133]

Goal Setting in Aphasia Rehabilitation

Outcome Measures in General

Aphasia rehabilitation, like other forms of medical treatment, is subject to critical evaluation regarding the endpoint. This leads to three important questions: (1) What is the purpose of the intervention? (2) How much is the cost and what is the expected gain? (3) When has treatment been completed? These are issues that society at large must face, for it can be costly to patients and to society to implement "therapies" of minimal benefit, or worse yet, of distinct harm.

When therapy is finished is a difficult issue for many therapists, who believe the old adage that "learning is a lifelong experience." In some patients therapy can be useful for a prolonged period. In others a natural endpoint is reached when the cost outweighs the possibility of incremental gains.

Language Assessment

The direct assessment of language ability is the first step for many therapists planning to direct and evaluate therapy. Unfortunately, language ability is not easily and unambiguously measured, nor is improvement. Nonetheless, aphasia constitutes a deficit of language, and assessment of language ability is an integral part of virtually all aphasia rehabilitation programs.

A number of testing instruments for aphasia focus on language performance. Most of these tests evaluate language ability at a relatively gross level, characterized by spontaneous speech, comprehension, repetition, naming, reading, and writing. Most evaluative tools also delve into subtypes of these language performance skills, subclassifying ability hierarchically. For example, in repetition, a patient might be asked to repeat words, nonwords, phrases, short simple sentences, and long complex sentences. Naming ability might be tested on naming to tactile, visual, or auditory modalities, and within each modality, by different stimulus types, such as in the visual modality including actual objects, black-and-white pictures, or color pictures.

The most commonly used tests of language ability in aphasia (in the United States) are the Western Aphasia Battery (WAB) and the Boston Diagnostic Aphasia Examination (BDAE).[122,134] These have both been evaluated in large numbers of patients and are well standardized. Additional tests for types of language ability that are commonly in use include the Boston Naming Test (BNT) for naming, and the Token Test or its more psychometrically sophisticated version the Revised Token Test (RTT) for comprehension.[135–137] Certain specialized instruments originally devised for research purposes are increasingly used clinically, such as the Philadelphia Comprehension Battery, a valuable aid in the assessment of comprehension at both the word and sentence levels.[138] An important test for general language ability that has desirable psychometric properties and is thus used in many research settings to assess language improvement is the Porch Index of Communicative Ability (PICA).[86]

Communication Ability Communication ability is different from language ability, and there have been many advocates for using communication ability, rather than language ability, as the preferred outcome measure in aphasia. Good communication can exist without using language. A patient who enters a supermarket, and without speaking a single intelligible word, communicates needs to the supermarket staff, or without understanding a single spoken word, arrives at the answers to particular questions, has communicated successfully. The focus of asphasia rehabilitation need not be language to the exclusion of functional communication. The emphasis of this functional communication movement is on the practical aspects of human interaction. Although the first evaluative tool for functional communication was devised in 1969, purely linguistic methods drove most clinical aphasia programs until about a decade later.[139]

A new evaluation instrument, the test of Communicative Abilities in Daily Living (CADL), and a new treatment program, Promoting Aphasics Communicative Effectiveness (PACE), were devised based on the functional perspective. With functional methods, patients are evaluated and treated to improve interactions in real world contexts. Additional emphasis is placed on aspects of pragmatic linguistic abilities, such as turn-taking, maintaining eye contact, maintaining topic, and asking relevant questions.[140–143]

Brain Function Now that it is possible to measure brain activity during the course of language performance, it should soon be possible to use brain activity measures as a yardstick for recovery. Such measures address the anatomical substrate of recovery, and thus are relevant only in the context of some concomitant measure of behavior. However, if brain activity measures can be obtained in a manner that has objectivity and consistent replicability, combining anatomical and behavioral measures could have some distinct advantages over measures of function (language tests) or anatomy (imaging tests) alone.

Although there are currently few functional neuroimaging studies demonstrating the anatomical substrate of recovery, there is a great deal of enthusiasm for this method as a future research goal.[144] Some tantalizing evidence has emerged from positron emission tomography (PET) and functional magnetic resonance imaging (fMRI) that brain reorganization after stroke can be measured and correlated with behavioral performance. The work in PET has shown apparent reorganization in both motor function and language.[145–147] Recently, differences by fMRI in the brain encodings for the mechanisms of sentence understanding in normal and aphasic women have been demonstrated.[35,36]

Attention and Variability Performance variability is a vexing problem in aphasia therapy and assessment. Maximizing performance consistency is a legitimate goal of aphasia therapy. Most of the efforts to address this performance parameter have focused on attention, the ability to direct one's mental efforts to competing stimuli, both externally and internally generated.

Although attention is a complex and sometimes controversial topic, with a number of different definitions and theoretical bases, it is generally agreed that an individual has only a limited amount of attention to allocate to any given stimulus field. Patients with aphasia are thought to have fewer processing "resources," including attention, than people without aphasia.[101] In addition, patients with aphasia are less able to shift and divide attention among competing stimuli.[148]

In addition to difficulties with selective attention to externally generated perceptual stimuli, patients with aphasia have difficulties allocating attention away from internally generated stimuli that do not typically disturb normal people. One aspect of performance variability in aphasic language performance is its interaction with human physiology. Fatigue, infection, constipation, and other physiological states adversely affect language performance in patients with aphasia.[149] Minimizing adverse internal physiological stimuli may improve language performance in some aphasic patients.[108]

Functional Classification of Language Disorders

The classical approach to aphasia diagnosis involves testing the main categories of language function: spontaneous speech, comprehension, repetition, naming, reading, and writing. Each of these categories has been divided into subparts, and all of the standardized tests of aphasia incorporate subtests to assess many aspects of each general behavior. By combining performance across these subtests, the standardized tests arrive at an assessment for each category, and the pattern of performance across categories leads to a specific behavioral classification.

Spontaneous Speech Spontaneous speech is commonly tested in a number of ways. An ideal way to evaluate spontaneous speech is to tape-record some informal discussion with a patient and then to analyze the patient's language production in terms of specific parameters. Another way to do this is to ask a patient to describe some event or to describe the goings-on in a picture. Several pictures are commonly used for this purpose, the most famous of which is probably the "Cookie Theft" picture of the Boston Diagnostic Aphasia Examination (BDAE). The most important parameters to measure in speech production are the ability to start and complete utterances, grammatical richness, and speed. When spontaneous speech is normal, the aphasia patient is considered fluent. When aphasia is characterized by impaired spontaneous speech, the term nonfluent is used.

Comprehension The ability to comprehend speech is tested by two methods, interrogative and imperative. By asking questions to which the answers are known (interrogative) or by requesting the performance of some commands (imperative), the initial assessment of language comprehension is begun. By altering the lexical, syntactic, and semantic complexity of the sentences, such questions and commands can serve to assess sentence comprehension in a graded fashion. The simplest sentences must be short, active, and declarative, containing only simple words that are acquired early in life and used frequently. The most complex sentences should contain more complex words that are used infrequently, and involved sentence structures containing relative clauses or embedded components.

In some cases, patients with aphasia will perform very poorly on tests of sentence comprehension, yet still demonstrate an ability to perform a degree of processing capability in the input channel. For these patients, tests of single-word comprehension can reveal remarkable strengths. The easiest way to test for the understanding of single-words is to ask the patient to match words with pictures. A collection of four object pictures can be placed in front of the patient and a word spoken or written. The patient is asked to match the word with the correct picture.[150] In assessing subcomponents of the word or picture recognition processes, these pictures can be manipulated to include objects that look similar or have names that are pronounced similarly, have different frequencies of occurrence or spelling patterns. This same picture-matching approach can be successfully used in tests of sentence comprehension.[138]

Repetition According to some theories, such as the Wernicke/Lichtheim approach outlined earlier, a linguistic string can be repeated by using solely phonological (input and output) processes and phonological memory systems, without requiring comprehension of the string itself. On the other hand, repetition often leads to attempts at comprehension of the target string and recoding for production. In most cortical lesions of the left peri-Sylvian region, deficits in comprehension or production of spoken language are accompanied by repetition errors. Focal cortical lesions in this region can impair spontaneous speech and comprehension, while sparing repetition. In strokes involving primarily the subcortical white matter, repetition can be relatively impaired, compared to comprehension or verbal fluency.

Repetition of single words and longer phrases and sentences can be tested by several methods using different stimulus types, including words, nonwords, phrases, and sentences. Each of these stimulus types requires different subsets of the input and output mechanisms. One variable of particular importance in repetition is memory. For repetition, input words (or other strings) must be retained for some period of time prior to output processing. This retention process is sometimes called auditory verbal short-term memory. Repetition ability can be degraded by impairment of auditory verbal short-term memory, proportionate to the length of the linguistic string.

Naming Naming tasks require providing a single word label for a stimulus. The most common stimulus type is a physical object or a picture of a physical object, although a variety of different stimuli are used to examine different functional components of the main task. The neural circuits to perform naming are highly distributed in the brain, including much of the left peri-Sylvian cortex and probably areas of the homologous structures in the right hemisphere.[30,151,152] This distributed representation reflects the complexity of the naming process. Naming the object in a picture requires early visual processing, complex visual recognition, interaction between visual and verbal semantic coding mechanisms, word selection, phonological encoding, and articulation.[153,154]

Although naming can be tested in any modality and with a variety of stimuli, the most common method is visual presentation of small physical objects or pictures of objects. Pictures can be full-color photographs, black-and-white photographs, complete drawings, or even line drawings. The actual objects can also be named by tactile recognition, characteristic features or sounds, or even prose descriptions.

Reading and Writing Reading and writing are complex tasks that are commonly affected in aphasia. In examining reading, patients should be tested on two related but different tasks, reading aloud and reading for comprehension. In both reading and writing, stimuli can be graded in linguistic complexity. For reading aloud, patients should be tested on single words, phrases, and larger texts. Certain reading tasks demonstrate functional dissociations. Careful testing should include reading of function words and content words, high- and low-frequency words, and words with regular and irregular spellings. Since reading for comprehension can be relatively preserved even when reading aloud is marked by errors, this task also should be tested.

Performance in writing spontaneously and to dictation can also differ depending on the types of stimuli presented. As in repetition, memory can come into play in writing to dictation, and can lead to graded performance depending on the size of the target. Stimulus types include words, nonwords, phrases, and sentences.

Symptoms of Aphasia Although evaluation of aphasia has generally been in terms of performance success

or failure, in reality it is the nature of the errors made during performance that is the most revealing, both for understanding the patient's condition and for prescribing therapy. Therapy based on the nature of errors produced during performance of functional tasks has been a popular and successful approach to therapy. This section surveys the different symptoms that have been considered important in aphasia and mentions therapeutic programs aimed at ameliorating them.

Fluency Fluency generally refers to the rate and apparent ease of spontaneous speech.[155] Various metrics are used to quantify fluency, including (a) amount of speech per unit time; (b) phrase length; (c) "effort" required; and (d) amount of prosody. Nonfluent patients have a decreased volume and rate of output, use shorter phrases, and seem to take considerable effort to speak. Content words are used to a greater degree than function words. Poor clarity of articulation is common. Patients with fluent aphasia have normal to increased volume and rate of speech and normal prosody. Speech is well articulated and seems to flow with ease. Impairments in fluency are generally more common in aphasias involving the frontal cortex than in those involving the posterior structures.

Paraphasia Errors in language production are called paraphasias and encompass a variety of different behaviors. Paraphasias generally are more common in aphasias involving the temporal and parietal cortex than in those involving the frontal lobe. Substitutions of one syllable for an intended syllable are called phonemic (literal) paraphasias and are common in aphasia. One of the most interesting aspects of phonemic paraphasias is that they always follow the combination rules of the speaker's language, or its phonotactic constraints. This is one way that errors of praxis or errors of articulation can be distinguished from linguistic errors. Substitution of an entire word for another intended word is called a semantic (verbal) paraphasia. These substituted words often are related semantically to the target word. Substitution of a nonword for an intended word is called a neologism. Speech filled with many paraphasias and neologisms is considered jargonaphasia.

Perseveration Some patients will become locked on certain outputs, such as individual words or even phrases. Patients taking a picture-naming test, for example, may provide the same name for a number of successive pictures, or repeat a name after a sequence of other correct (or errorful) names. Sometimes words are repeated when they are of the same semantic category as the intended word, so that a favorite word might be used to name every similar object. After discussing his physician granddaughter, a patient performed a naming test and called every animate object in the test "doctor," including Mickey Mouse, Ronald Reagan, and Shirley Temple. This type of repetition is called perseveration. Sometimes patients can perseverate on an entire phrase rather than a single word. Perseveration is not restricted to language output, and also occurs in somatic motor activity on verbal commands.

Stereotypy Occasionally a single word (or syllable or nonword) is used in many communicative roles. This is a form of perseveration in which one word is used instead of many intended words, with the entire process called stereotypy. The stereotype is often a word commonly used by the person before the onset of the language disturbance or a word used only in emotionally charged situations, such as a curse word. This use of stereotypes can be embarrassing or confusing. Just as with other production errors, understanding the speech of such patients must rely on prosody, gesture, facial expression, and similar cues.

Agrammatism and Paragrammatism Deficits in language that involve syntax problems are not uncommon with aphasias that involve neurological lesions to the frontal lobe. Such patients may have particular problems producing or understanding sentences that have complex grammatical structures, such as those in the passive voice or containing relative clauses. Sometimes the output of such patients has a paucity of function words or other inflectional elements of language. The speech of such patients is sometimes called "telegraphic."[156] When such deficits occur in the context of frontal lesions, the behavior is called agrammatism. A less common syndrome involving grammatical errors in copious speech output occurs with temporal and parietal lesions and is called paragrammatism.

Aphasia Tests *General Tests of Aphasia* Both the WAB and the BDAE provide quantitative indices of language ability along each of the dimensions of language function discussed, as well as a summary index of aphasia severity.[122,134] These tests also provide an aphasia diagnosis according to the Wernicke/Lichtheim scheme, and this behavioral classification can be used to aid in cerebral localization of the lesion (to the extent that this is possible) and to choose a treatment method or direct therapy. The quantitative measures also can be used to follow recovery. The Porch Index of Communicative Ability (PICA) has particularly good psychometric properties, and has widespread use in research settings and significant use in clinical settings as well.[86] The Aachen Aphasia Test also has desirable metrical properties, and the recently introduced English-language version may soon become popular.[157]

Naming: The Boston Naming Test Since a naming impairment, or dysnomia, is a prominent feature of most cases of aphasia, naming is a fundamental part of the assessment of aphasia. Although aphasia recovery can change the characteristics of a patient's language functioning, including its diagnostic label according to the WAB or BDAE, a dysnomia (and sometimes only a dysnomia) typically persists. The Boston Naming Test (BNT) is a widely used test for assessment of naming.[135] The BNT tests picture naming and uses a collection of black-and-white drawings of objects that have variable word and image frequencies.[158] Although this test has a limited stimulus type in a single modality, it has wide applicability in aphasia recovery from stroke as well as aphasia progression in dementia.

Auditory Comprehension: The Token Test The Token Test is probably the most widely used test for auditory comprehension.[124,136] The test materials consist of a number of large and small "tokens" (three-dimensional geometric shapes, such as pyramids and cubes) of different colors, and the test consists of various commands to the subject to manipulate the tokens. By using syntactic structures of graded complexity in these commands, comprehension can be readily tested. Simple commands ask the subject to identify single, easily identified tokens, and the more complex commands require specific manipulations of multiple tokens with shared or different properties. These can require many levels of comprehension, including lexical semantics, sentential syntax, and short-term memory. A psychometrically validated version of this test, the Revised Token Test, is often used in research settings.[137]

Important Tests in Other Languages Whereas the BDAE and WAB are commonly used in the United States, they are obviously inapplicable in countries where English is not the predominant language. Tests with similar goals in terms of quantification and aphasia diagnosis within the Wernicke/Lichtheim system exist in a number of other languages. The best known of these tests is the Aachen Aphasia Test (AAT), mentioned previously because its English language edition (currently undergoing standardization) gives it practical as well as theoretical importance in this country.[157,159] The AAT was developed by a well-respected aphasia research team at Aachen and is widely used throughout the German-speaking world. The Milan Aphasia Test has a similar following in Italy for similar reasons. The aphasia research groups from Montréal and Toulouse collaborated on a general test for native French speakers, called the Protocole Montréal-Toulouse d'Examen Linguistique de l'Aphasie.[160] Three comprehensive standardized language tests are commonly in use in Japan.[161]

Functional Communication Tests   The concept of functional communication assessment and therapy grew out of the notion that the measure of ability and the goals of rehabilitation would be better served by focusing on the everyday communicative needs of patients with aphasia rather than an abstract measure of linguistic competence or performance. These approaches focus attention on natural conversation and informational exchange in real-world contexts. The initial proposal for a functional communication approach was accompanied by an assessment instrument called the Functional Communication Profile, which is still in use in a number of clinics.[139,162] Another commonly used test for functional communication is the test of Communicative Abilities in Daily Living (CADL).[140] CADL tests patients on tasks common to everyday experience; they are given as many of the actual contextual cues as possible, and assessed on their ability to communicate (with or without explicit verbalization) during the simulation. CADL tests different abilities than linguistic assessment procedures, and possibly ones that are more relevant to the quality of aphasia recovery. The American Speech, Language, and Hearing Association (ASHA) has introduced a new instrument for the Functional Assessment of Communication Skills (ASHA-FACS), which attempts a more comprehensive evaluation of functional communication.[163]

Other Tests Useful in Assessment of Aphasia

Reading and Writing   Although examinations of reading and writing are included in the most commonly used general aphasia profiles, there do exist specialized measures for these skills in particular. Reading ability can be evaluated using the Reading Comprehension Battery for Aphasia (RCBA), which tests reading at the word, phrase, and sentence level.[164,165] It does not test nonwords. It also tests functional reading (menus, phone books) in such a way that the patient must dem-

onstrate knowledge of what is read in a practical context. The Discourse Comprehension Test tests auditory comprehension with questions about stated and impled main points, and can be used as a reading battery, with stimuli that are longer than RCBA.[166]

Writing is usually tested using the standard comprehension aphasia batteries, since no specific writing batteries are in general use. These tests evaluate writing through a written picture description task. Although this is the extent of most clinical evaluations, many clinics, including ours, use individualized measures after an initial screening procedure yields a gross category of reading impairment.

General Cognition and Dementia   General cognitive abilities are very difficult to test in patients with language disturbances, since the vast majority of cognitive functions tested on standard evaluative measures rely on language to a significant extent. Even when a task may not rely on knowledge of syntax or semantics, it may depend on an ability to retain temporarily or to recall in the longer term symbolic information. Various types of short-term memory depend on symbolic codes, which in turn are intertwined in an incompletely understood manner with verbal or linguistic codes.

The most common rapid screening test for general cognitive abilities in the Mini-Mental State Examination (MMSE), which includes a simple question in each of a number of different cognitive categories.[167] Many of these questions, even when not explicitly designed to test language, rely on aspects of language performance (e.g., symbolic memory), and so a number of MMSE questions are not reliable in patients with aphasia. Since components of the language-processing system are so fundamental to general cognition, patients with aphasia commonly do poorly on these tests, giving a potentially misleading impression of their general intellectual functioning. This test is appealing to researchers, particularly in the study of dementia, because of its interrater reliability and correlation with more extensive measures. Consequently it is a widely used instrument.

Nonlinguistic Functions   Visual and spatial information processing can be tested straightforwardly in aphasic patients, and by using specific (rather than general) measures, reliable information can be obtained. The most commonly used test of nonlinguistic cognitive function is the evaluation of Raven's Coloured Progressive Matrices, in which subjects must analyze the features of complex visual patterns.[168] The Benton Visual Discrimination Test is a test of spatial judgments.[169] Patients with aphasia who have good cognitive functioning (outside of the obvious language deficits) ordinarily perform well on these tests. Since the neurological lesions of patients with aphasia often encompass regions that participate in functions other than language, specific tests of such abilities often are helpful in understanding the span of abilities that might be harnessed for compensatory processing. Commonly used tests that do not depend on language per se include the Wisconsin Card Sorting Test for ability to adapt to changing environmental demands, the Stroop task for evaluating visual attention, and the Trails tests for concentration and attention.[170–172] The block design subcomponent of the WAIS-R is useful for testing visuospatial problem solving.[173] Drawing is often tested with a clock face set at "ten past eleven," which has been widely used and consequently has associated normative data. Although aphasic patients often have difficulty with memory for symbolic information, such as sequences of single digits or words, a visual analog of such information can be tested with sequences of finger movements across an array of blocks (which can be numbered for the tester, thus providing a direct analogy with digit span tests).

General Approaches to Rehabilitation

Behavioral Manipulation The behavioral treatment approach for a particular patient can be motivated by a variety of different factors. This can derive from (a) a formal behavioral evaluation according to a standardized method (e.g., BDAE); (b) a careful symptomatic evaluation; (c) an assessment of cognitive strengths; (d) performance variability; or (e) assessment of communication abilities of family and friends. Certainly, expert therapists demonstrate an ability to tailor behavioral therapy to particular individuals, based on a combination of these and other factors.

Impressions on the ideal duration of therapy vary considerably. At the Aphasia Center in Milan, where treatment decisions are made by the clinician without consideration of cost, each patient is treated daily for 6 months prior to any decision of efficacy for that patient.[124] With demonstration of progress, treatment continues in 3-month blocks until such time as progress can no longer be demonstrated. After careful patient selection, the Aachen aphasia group performs nine treatment sessions per week for 6 to 8 weeks.[174] In the United States, treatment decisions cannot be made without consideration of cost, and consequently, treatment duration is significantly shorter.

Stimulation The stimulation approach has been the predominant approach to the treatment of aphasia in the United States since the late 1960s.[175–177] The underlying assumptions of this approach are that patients with aphasia share many similarities in behavioral impairment regardless of site or size of neurological lesion. Although these assumptions have undergone some serious argument since the method was first proposed, the method has been successful and remains a cornerstone of therapy in many settings. The stimulation method involves the "organized presentation of controlled, intensive, and adequate stimuli to the patient for the purpose of eliciting target responses."[161] The theoretical underpinning of this approach is that selective reinforcement of patient responses can lead to specialized brain reorganization to facilitate language performance.

Syndrome- and Symptom-Based Approaches In contrast with general stimulation methods, there are approaches specifically designed to remedy particular subtypes of aphasia (typically according to the Wernicke/Lichtheim classification) or particular symptoms of aphasia (e.g., paraphasia, perseveration). Thus, instead of treating the diverse population of patients with aphasia as sharing the same underlying disorder, with similar treatment required for all, these syndrome- or symptom-based approaches treat subgroups of aphasic patients differently. One successful symptom-based approach is the method of Treatment of Aphasic Perseveration (TAP), an approach specifically tailored to remediation of the particular symptom complex of perseveration.[178]

Several syndrome-based methods were developed at the Boston Aphasia Center and are based on the aphasia diagnosis of the BDAE. Visual Action Therapy (VAT) is aimed at those with global aphasia, and uses gestures as precursors to reestablishment of referential communication. Melodic intonation therapy (MIT) is aimed at patients with Broca's aphasia, who have difficulty with spontaneous speech and speech fluency.[11,121] This method makes use of prosody to improve language output. A program to treat patients with Wernicke's aphasia also has been developed.[179] MIT and VAT are discussed further in the following.

Neurobiology REORGANIZATION There is increasing evidence that behavioral interventions of various kinds can influence the anatomical structure of the brain. This has been best seen in studies of the motor system, where a relative increase in the use of one muscle group compared to another can lead to motor cortical changes reflecting this change. In one experiment, animals underwent amputation of a single digit in one hand and subsequently underwent physiological study.[57] Over time using the revised hand, these animals developed cortical reorganization reflecting the new functional situation: The somatosensory regions allocated to the amputated digit were completely taken over by the cortical representations for the neighboring digits. This study was pioneering and very important, as it demonstrated convincingly that behavior could influence cortical structure in adult animals.

Subsequent experiments by the same group extended this result to the study of anatomical organization following stroke. In these studies, animals were given experimental cortical lesions and subsequently trained on behavioral tasks to attempt to influence reorganization of cortical anatomy. They found that indeed cortical reorganization occurs adjacent to the damaged areas, providing tantalizing data for neurobiological approaches to rehabilitation.[180]

Although these results were obtained in sensorimotor systems, they give hope that cognitive reorganization could occur and lead to neuroanatomical changes supporting compensatory strategies that are known to play a part in aphasia recovery.[6] Many aphasia treatment approaches are based on the development of such compensations, although as of yet there are no approaches based on the explicit reorganization of the anatomical substrate. Although stimulation methods aim to develop general compensation strategies, other methods, such as melodic intonation therapy, aim to develop specific compensation strategies for specific deficits. With the advent of functional neuroimaging, we should soon be able to develop behavioral approaches to alter neuroanatomical organizations in a favorable way.[144]

ADAPTATION It has been recognized that the behavior of a patient with a focal brain lesion, for example, from a vascular insult, reflects less on the function of the damaged region than on the function of the entire brain when it is missing that region. This is a subtle but important distinction, and bears on rehabilitative approaches, particularly in language and cognition. The language performance of a patient with a frontal infarction typically involves slow speech initiation and production of few words, particularly function words, as well as other problems. Does this mean that the damaged region is responsible for faster speech initiation and function word production? Or does it mean that whereas this region of the brain might contribute

something to the performance of these complex tasks, performance actually reflects the adaptive behavior of the entire organism (and especially the brain) in the presence of the damage? The behavioral implications change from restoration of lost function to improving the functional adaptation to damage.

MELODIC INTONATION THERAPY Melodic Intonation Therapy (MIT) is the only method of aphasia rehabilitation approved by the American Academy of Neurology (AAN) Committee on Therapeutics.[121] MIT is predicated on the fact that most aphasia occurs via damage to the left peri-Sylvian cortex, with sparing to the right peri-Sylvian regions that have primary responsibility for the intonational and melodic aspects of language and for some aspects of music.[10,22,23] Since a major methodological approach to aphasia therapy is to harness spared brain areas to perform or to compensate for damaged brain regions, the idea of using melody to bolster verbal communication is well-motivated theoretically. Basically, the method couples words with song, in an incremental manner. As pointed out by the AAN committee, it has been shown to be of value in patients with aphasia characterized by poor spontaneous speech; choppy, slow, effortful speech with a relative loss of inflectional morphemes (typical of Broca's aphasia); and not in other types of aphasia. Although many such patients have frontotemporal lesions, lesion location does not enter into the eligibility criteria for this method.

Cognitive Psychology **THEORETICALLY MOTIVATED THERAPY** Although there exist frameworks for therapy based on specific theories in neuropsychology and psycholinguistics, there are several reasons why such approaches do not have widespread applicability and use. An important reason is that cognitive neuropsychology has only indirect relationships to therapy.[181] The problem is that the choice of therapy "cannot be made in the absence of an equally rich theory of the modifications that a damaged cognitive system may undergo as a function of different forms of intervention."[182]

Thus, although there do exist several aphasia treatment approaches based on theories about the cognitive architecture of the language system of the brain, they might not be expected to have great efficacy. In fact, there are several such methods that do seem effective, but they do not apply to the vast majority of patients with aphasia. Although therapeutic approaches in general ought to be tailored to specific patterns of language impairments and to particular individuals, that limits significantly the utility of the fine-grained, theory-driven method. In these cases, the patterns of impairment are very specific.

On the other hand, there are approaches to the development of new therapeutic techniques that are driven by careful theoretical (neuropsychological) analysis. Just as a finding of decreased cortical catecholamines in the brain after stroke motivated one type of therapeutic intervention, so a finding of impaired thematic role assignment or lexical network activation has motivated others. Ultimately, a theory of aphasia rehabilitation must take into account all these different levels of analysis to form a unifying approach.

REBUILDING LEXICAL NETWORKS   Many researchers view the lexicon in terms of networks of word meanings and use a metaphor of "activation" to explain the invocation of one word meaning over another in the right context.[3] Certainly the activation metaphor has been of tremendous value, particularly the context of "spreading activation," whereby the involvement of one word in some language task leads to automatic involvement of related words.[183] Words that are the most related are thought to become involved both faster and to a stronger degree than less-related words. This concept and computer models that have been used to instantiate it formally have been successful in explaining a variety of phenomena in lexical semantics, particularly speed of lexical access and lexical semantic priming.[183,184]

The metaphor of spreading activation can be used as a basis of therapy of lexical semantic deficits in patients with aphasia. This method, termed Lexical-Semantic Activation/Inhibition Treatment (L-SAIT) uses a patient-generated cueing hierarchy and an antonym/synonym word retrieval task.[185,185a] The synonyms and antonyms of lists of adjectives, nouns, and prepositions can be taught in order to build up the lexical associations needed for successful spreading activation.

MAPPING SENTENCE FORM TO MEANING   Certain patients with aphasia who had been thought to have grammatical-processing deficits instead have problems with mapping sentence form to meaning.[41,186,187] Two types of mapping problems are described: (a) loss of lexical information about the thematic structure associated with particular verbs; and (b) loss of rules by which thematic roles are assigned to verb argument structures, particularly when they are not in their standard locations in the sentence.[188] Although the concept of mapping applies both to sentence production and comprehension, the order of preserved and impaired processes differs.

Therapy based on mapping involves either relearning the thematic structures associated with verbs or relearning the rules by which thematic roles are assigned to sentence structures.[125,125a] A total of 10 patients have been treated by a number of investigators in six different studies with therapy based on the mapping hypothesis.[188] Tremendous benefit has occurred for individual patients. In all cases, generalization occurred for untreated exemplars of treated predicates. Generalization from comprehension to production or vice versa occurred in about half the patients, as did generalization from treated exemplars to untreated exemplars within a single channel (i.e., comprehension or production). The treatment successes with mapping therapy suggest that behavioral interventions that are motivated by specific cognitive theory not only can be successful, but also can contribute to the theory itself.

Pragmatics   **SPEECH-ACT THEORY**   An important contribution to the study of discourse was the development of speech-act theory, which had a large impact on cognitive science in the 1970s, and continues to be influential.[189] In this theory, linguistic behaviors are performed within the context of specific communicative goals. Suppose, for example, a person at the Philadelphia train station wants to get a train to Pittsburgh. If he asks an information agent near a train to Washington, "Is this the train to Pittsburgh?" a number of responses are possible.[190] One answer could be "no," but this would reflect an ignorance or purposeful ignoring of the goal of the questioner, who wants information about the train to Pittsburgh. A more appropriate answer would be "No, the train to Pittsburgh is at platform 10 and leaves in 5 minutes." This would recognize that the questioner was performing a speech act, a linguistic utterance with a specific intent that may not be explicitly evident from analysis of the words of the utterance alone. Recognizing and understanding speech acts is a fundamental aspect of human linguistic communication.

PROMOTING APHASICS COMMUNICATIVE EFFECTIVENESS (PACE)   Following the original exposition of speech-act theory, therapeutic progress was made by focusing on speech acts, despite linguistic impairments.[109,141,191] Instead of focusing on the production and recognition of specific types of words or higher-order linguistic structures, PACE aims at improving "communicative effectiveness." It does so by placing patients with aphasia into actual communication situations with other people, rather than into the instructive environment of therapist and patient. Considering the difficulties of transferring linguistic gains from the clinical speech-therapeutic setting into the actual communicative life of aphasic patients, the PACE approach has a logical appeal. Furthermore, by emphasizing communication over speech and language, patients are encouraged to use whatever aspects of verbal or nonverbal strategies can get their message across and achieve their communicative goals.

PACE is becoming a mainstay of behavioral therapy for all types of patients, including those with acute and chronic aphasia. Since the focus is on communicative effectiveness, and inherently encourages strategies of all kinds, the etiology or site of damage does not matter for successful employment of PACE. Furthermore, the PACE can be naturally combined with other therapeutic methods, including symptom-specific or lesion-specific behavioral methods or other modalities. PACE has been successsfully used in a patient with a focal degenerative process involving the left temporal lobe and insula as well as many patients with stroke.[110] PACE is commonly used throughout the world, for functional treatment of aphasic communication.[192]

Sign Language   American Sign Language (ASL) and other languages of the deaf throughout the world have been evaluated as possible solutions to aphasic language impairments. After all, a prominent feature of many patients with aphasia is profound impairments in oral speech, with severe articulation problems getting in the way of language production. In fact, in patients with neurological damage restricted to brain structures subserving speech motor mechanisms (e.g., with bulbar dysfunction from brain-stem infarction), the use of ASL might be considered. The reason ASL is not a valid alternative in patients with aphasia is that ASL shares a large number of common features of articulated languages. Thus, speaking patients who are aphasic following cerebral infarction would be aphasic in ASL as well, since all of the levels of language present in spoken languages are present in ASL, including syntax, semantics, and even phonology. Components of particular words in ASL, called handshapes, are analogous to the phonemes of spoken languages.

The neurobiology of sign languages are beginning to be investigated, using the same methods that have been applied to other languages. These include lesion analysis, cortical stimulation, and functional neuroimaging with PET and fMRI.[193] What has been learned is truly amazing. Recent pioneering work has demonstrated that despite a degree of right-hemisphere specialization for many types of spatial processing in most people, there remains a relative left-hemisphere specialization for ASL. This is surprising, since many of the temporal aspects of spoken speech are replaced in ASL with a spatial component. Many of the brain structures thought to be important for spoken language production and comprehension are involved in the processing of ASL as well. There is obviously a direct consequence of this exciting research on aphasia treatment: Sign languages such as ASL are not appropriate tools for treatment of aphasia.

Gesture   NONLINGUISTIC SIGN   On the other hand, there do exist systems of sign that do not have the complex characteristics of language, that is, phonological, morphological, and syntactic structures. In general, systems of icons, including both systems of hand signs and other nonlinguistic pictorial signs, might be useful communicative adjuncts for aphasic patients. Since gesture plays a significant adjunctive role in unimpaired communication, it is a natural consideration as an aid to patients with impaired language.

VISUAL ACTION THERAPY   Visual Action Therapy (VAT) is a therapy based on gestural communication was devised for patients with the most severe forms of aphasia.[11] The authors of VAT present four rationales for gestural communication, including the independence of gesture from vocalization; the relative lack of need for fine motor control; the relative unilateral brain control of gesture; and its ability to be visually monitored. The method teaches patients to associate hand gestures with physical objects and ultimately to be able to use these gestures communicatively when the objects are no longer present. The staged approach uses real objects, different varieties of pictures of the objects, and action pictures illustrating use of the objects. Patients manipulate the objects, associate the objects and the object manipulations with the pictures, and associate each of these with gestures. The VAT program is indicated for patients with severe aphasias involving both input and output language systems (global aphasia), and in these patients, seems to help.[11]

Iconic Communication   VIC   There are a number of reasons to believe that an iconic communication system might be useful to patients with aphasia, including the possibility that they could invoke mechanisms mediated in the cerebral hemisphere contralateral to that dominant for language.[194,195] Iconic systems have made their way into experimental treatment protocols for patients with severe "global" aphasia. These studies have demonstrated communication benefit to patients from using these systems.[12,196] The method of Visual Communication (VIC) uses stacks of index cards containing different types of representational figures, and involves selecting cards of the appropriate types (following certain combination rules of "VIC grammar") to create iconic utterances.

C-VIC Although these iconic methods are not in significant use in clinical settings, a computer-based VIC (C-VIC) has led to a commercial iconic communication product. There is every reason to believe that computer technology will ultimately have a role in both the treatment of aphasia and the augmentation of communication ability in patients with aphasia. The C-VIC system is a first step in that direction. It is predicated on the notion that despite impairments in verbal memory and verbal symbol processing, many patients with aphasia have spared ability to perform visual image processing.

C-VIC was incorporated into a Macintosh-based computer program and a number of studies conducted. Patients were able to learn the computer interfaces and use the system to produce utterances in the iconic vocabulary and grammar of C-VIC.[197] The role of this system as a therapeutic tool to help improve other forms of communication is less clear.

Formal Linguistics **GRAMMAR** The dominant theory among researchers in linguistics over the past half-century has emphasized linguistic structures and formal grammars. The most successful of these formal grammatical theories was originally devised in the 1960s as Transformational Grammar and has been continuously refined and reshaped since that time.[198,199] A recent reshaping of this theory has been called Government and Binding (GB) Theory after two of the theoretical concepts that play a prominent role in the theory.[200] The basic premise of these grammatical theories is that all languages of the world share certain common features, called universal grammar (UG), but that they differ in the particular ways that these features are instantiated. Presumably, the existence of UG reflects the presence across all people of unique and dedicated neural structures for language.[201] Much research has focused on the primitive operations of UG, which are thought to reflect universals regarding languages in general, and by implication, the neurobiological instantiation of language in the brain.

There remains significant controversy about the existence of universal grammar and about its relationship to the brain. Even more controversy surrounds the postulate that GB theory accurately reflects the primitive operations of UG. Although some researchers have attempted to demonstrate the specific loss of particular primitive grammatical operations in aphasia, others have disputed the very existence of a specialized cognitive mechanism dedicated to language.[202,203] With the existence of substantial evidence that linguistic impairments in aphasic patients do not break down in an isomorphic fashion with the primitive operations of GB, many argue that regardless of the accuracy of the concept of universal grammar, the operations of GB theory are not relevant to the neurobiological mechanisms of language.

TREATMENT OF WH-MOVEMENT Sentences containing the so-called "wh" words (e.g., "who," "what," "which," "where") are interrogative sentences in which the "wh" word substitutes for a sought-after thematic role. In some of these cases, the sought-after role is the direct object of the verb, in which case the "wh" word takes a different position in the interrogative sentence (the first word of the sentence) than it would in the declarative version of the sentence (after the verb). Thus, in the question "What did the boy play?" the word "what" is in the first position and substitutes for the word "game," which is in the last position in the declarative sentence "The boy played the game." In the syntactic theory of GB, the declarative version of the sentence is viewed as the norm (or deep structure or d-structure), and the interrogative "wh" sentence viewed as a transformation of this norm (or surface structure or s-structure). Thus, the word "moves" from it normal position in the transformation from a "deep" to a "surface" representation. The original location (i.e., in the "deep" structure) continues to have a special significance, or a "trace" of the "moved" word.

An inability of some patients with aphasia to understand "wh" questions and yet to understand their declarative counterparts is thus viewed by GB theorists as a breakdown in "wh-movement." An attempt to treat this breakdown has been investigated in two patients with aphasia characterized by poor fluency and grammatical processing difficulties, with comprehension skill superior to verbal-production ability.[100] The treatment method consisted of a stepwise approach to teaching the patients about the "movement" of the word from the underlying "deep" structure to its ultimate (and poorly understood) "surface" structure. During treatment, the patient manipulated index cards illustrating different intermediate structures in the "movement" process. Although each patient only saw sentences using one "wh" word and one sentence structure, learning carried over from one word to the other and from one complex structure to simpler structures.[100] This is an important result since the generalization of treatment effects is a major therapeutic goal that is difficult to achieve. Whether linguistic theory can be used as the basis for more widely applicable therapeutic methods has yet to be demonstrated.

Pharmacology The existing research in pharmacotherapy has been discussed in detail in the first section of this chapter. Currently, no pharmacological methods have proven effective in aphasia rehabilitation, despite many great hopes by many investigators.[98] The future may hold some such agents, possibly to be used adjunctively with behavioral methods. Furthermore, new functional imaging methods such as fMRI may ultimately help us uncover the neurobiological substrate of recovery and methods of affecting its course.[35,144]

Prognosis of Aphasia

Factors that Influence Recovery Every patient with aphasia and all of their family members want an assessment of prognosis. Prognosis for functional communication is typically better than prognosis for normal speech and auditory comprehension. Some patients and families are realistic about this and others are not. Since the entire language-rehabilitative effort depends to some degree on the prior probabilities for aspects of recovery, and since patients and families need realistic information, having hard data about prognosis is crucial.

A multivariate statistical analysis of aphasia recovery from stroke made important contributions to our knowledge of factors that influence recovery.[204] Selection required new unilateral ischemic or hemorrhagic stroke with impaired language functioning at the time of hospital discharge. Fifty such patients were enrolled in the study. The variables examined included age, sex, involved hemisphere, etiology of infarction, length of hospital stay, race, presence of hemiplegia, Western Aphasia Battery Aphasia Quotient (AQ), and previous history of stroke.[134] Patients were considered completely recovered if they had an AQ ≥93.8 at 3 months poststroke. The analysis of these data using a multiple linear logistic regression model demonstrated that a shorter hospital stay or a young age (age ≤69) were independently and strongly associated with recovery. Male gender, right hemisphere infarction, hemorrhagic

etiology, and lack of hemiplegia were also associated with recovery, but not as strongly as were short hospital stays and younger age.

Expectations The expectations for language recovery in stroke thus depend on a number of specific factors, and these can be used to tailor therapy and advise patients and families about what to expect.[205,206] While patients with cerebral hemorrhages are at grave risk from the acute process, their language recovery on average may be better than patients with ischemic infarcts.[207] More severe strokes make for more difficult recovery. This can be demonstrated with total volume of infarct as seen on CT and by the presence of concomitant deficits in other areas.[208,209] The role of age is less clear, although in the study described above, patients who were above the mean in age did more poorly.[204,205] Certainly children can have significant recovery from large lesions.[210] Whereas adults generally do not have such extensive recovery, it may be that age does not affect prognosis for recovery except for the very young or the very old.[211,212]

Gender differences are not yet clear in aphasia recovery, despite the increasingly popular postulates about sexual dimorphism of the brain and the greater likelihood of bilateral language representations in women compared to men.[213,214] Another group that has been postulated to have a higher degree of bilateral encodings for language comprises left-handers.[215] In fact, this group may have better language recovery from stroke than right-handers.[216]

Of course, etiology affects prognosis, and this has been demonstrated formally in the case of ischemic and hemorrhagic infarction, where patients with hemorrhage are more likely to have full recovery.[204] In progressive neurological conditions such as dementia, the prognosis depends on factors having to do with the type of cellular process causing the problem and the overall rate of progression of the disease. Language recovery in the context of neoplasms can be very good if successful treatment of the cancer is achieved, and the effects of treatment have not been damaging in their own right. Language recovery from traumatic head injury can be dramatic, or similar to hemorrhagic infarction if cerebral contusion is the cause of the aphasia.[206] If a general cognitive impairment is present, then assessment of prognosis is very complex. Finally, as mentioned previously the role of depression in aphasia rehabilitation needs emphasis. Not only is depression a common concomitant of stroke, but it seems to be more common with left-hemisphere stroke than right-hemisphere stroke, and adversely affects recovery.[217–222] Others have disputed this assertion.[223]

Time Course Expectations for recovery include not only the amount of recovery but also the time frame in which this recovery can be expected. Most aphasiologists agree that the majority of spontaneous recovery takes place in the first 3 months following stroke.[206,209,224] Although there is historical precedent for extending this period to 6 months, there is also evidence that the greatest proportion of recovery is actually complete by 2 months or even earlier.[225,226] It is important to realize, however, that some aphasic patients continue to improve well past this early period, sometimes in dramatic fashion.[205] Of course, rehabilitative interventions aid recovery, both in concert with the inherent homeostatic mechanisms that lead to neural reorganization and independent of these mechanisms. In the well-designed VA Cooperative study, delaying therapy did not alter the overall value of the intervention.[129]

POSTSCRIPT: SUMMARY AND CONCLUSIONS

Many patients with injury to the cerebral cortex manifest communication problems, and some cannot use language effectively.

Aphasia recovery continues throughout the life of the patient and the benefits of rehabilitative intervention may continue. With the advent of new imaging methods, it may soon be possible to find therapeutic methods that can be shown to affect neural reorganization. If correlation can be made between neuroanatomical and positive linguistic change, even better methods of treatment can be developed in the future.

ACKNOWLEDGMENTS

The author gratefully acknowledges the support of the National Institute on Deafness and other Communication Disorders (NIDCD) of the National Institutes of Health under grants K08-DC-00054 and R01-DC3378. I am particularly grateful for the generous help with the manuscript provided by Audrey Holland and Margie Forbes, who have helped me clarify and state clearly the views expressed. The erroneous views that remain are those that I stubbornly refused to correct despite their excellent critiques. Finally, I would like to dedicate this chapter to Kathy Pollak of the College of General Studies of the University of Pennsylvania, who helped me move from the abstract study of computational linguistics to the research and care of people with language disorders.

REFERENCES

1. Dronkers NF: A new brain region for coordinating speech articulation. *Nature* 1996; 384:159–161.
1a. Marr D: *Artificial Intelligence —A Personal View.* Artificial Intelligence Laboratory: Massachusetts Institute of Technology, 1976.
2. Bolinger D: *Aspects of Language.* New York: Harcourt, Brace & World, 1968.
3. Fodor JA, Bever TG, Garrett MF: *The Psychology of Language.* New York: McGraw-Hill, 1974.
4. Caplan D: *Language: Structure, Processing, and Disorder.* Cambridge, MA: MIT Press, 1992.
5. Bates E, Friederici A, Wulfeck B: Grammatical morphology in aphasia: Evidence from three languages. *Cortex* 1987; 23:545–574.
6. Kolk H, Heeschen C: Agrammatism, paragrammatism, and the management of language. *Lang Cog Proc* 1992; 7:89–129.
7. de Bleser R: From agrammatism to paragrammatism: German aphasiological traditions and grammatical disturbances. *Cog Neuropsychol* 1987; 4:187–256.
8. Miller GA, Fellbaum C, Kegl J, Miller K: Wordnet: An electronic lexical retrieval system based on theories of lexical memory. *Revue Québécoise de Linguistique* 1988; 17:181–211.
9. Friedman R: Acquired alexia, in Boller F, Grafman J (eds): *Handbook of Neuropsychology:* vol 1. Amsterdam: Elsevier, 1988, pp. 377–391.
9a. Déjerine J: Contribution à l'étude anatomo-pathologique et clinique des differentes variétés de cécité verbale. *Comptes Rendus Hebdomodaires des Séances et Mémoires de la Société de Biologie* 1892; 4((Series 9)), 61–90.
10. Ross ED: The aprosodias: Functional-anatomic organization of the affective components of language in the right hemisphere. *Arch Neurol* 1981, 38:561–569.
11. Helm-Estabrooks N, Fitzpatrick PM, Barressi B: Visual action therapy for global aphasia. *J Speech Hear Dis* 1982; 47:385–389.
12. Gardner H, Zurif E, Berry T, Baker E: Visual communication in aphasia. *Neuropsychologia* 1976; 14:275–292.
13. Dax M: Lésions de la moitié gauche de l'encéphale coincident avec l'oublie des signes de la pensée, *Gazette Hebdomaire de la Médicine et de Chirurgie* 1865; 33:259.
14. Damasio H, Damasio AR: *Lesion Analysis in Neuropsychology.* New York: Oxford University Press, 1989.
15. Kertesz A: *Localization in Neuropsychology.* New York: Academic Press, 1983, p. 527.
16. Lichtheim L: On aphasia. *Brain* 1885; 7:433–484.

17. Donders FC: On the speed of mental processes. *Acta Psychologica* 1868/1969; 30:412–431.

18. Ferrier D: *Functions of the Brain.* London: Smith, Elder, 1876.

19. Craver CF, Small SL: Subcortical aphasia and the attribution of functional responsibility to parts of distributed brain processes. *Brain Lang* 1995, in press.

20. Kuhn TS: *The Structure of Scientific Revolutions.* Chicago: University of Chicago Press, 1962.

21. Newcombe F, Ratcliff G: Disorders of visuospatial analysis, in Boller F, Grafman J (eds): *Handbook of Neuropsychology,* vol. 2. Amsterdam: Elsevier, 1989, pp. 333–352.

22. Zatorre RJ, Evans AC, Meyer E, Gjedde A: Lateralization of phonetic and pitch discrimination in speech processing. *Science* 1992; 256:846–849.

23. Schlaug G: In vivo evidence of structural brain asymmetry in musicians. *Science* 1995; 267:699–701.

24. Wernicke C: *Der Aphasische Symptomenkomplex.* Breslau: Cohn & Weigert, 1874.

25. Galaburda AM, LeMay M, Kemper TL, Geschwind N: Right-left asymmetries in the brain: Structural differences between the hemispheres may underlie cerebral dominance. *Science* 1978; 199:852–856.

26. Damasio AR, Geschwind N: The neural basis of language. *Ann Rev Neurosci* 1984; 7:127–147.

27. Talairach J, Szikla G, Tournoux P: *Atlas d'Anatomie Stereotaxique du Telencephale.* Paris: Masson, 1967.

28. Penfield W, Boldrey E: Somatic motor and sensory representation in the cerebral cortex of man as studied by electrical stimulation. *Brain* 1937; 60:389–443.

29. Uematsu D, Lesser R, Fisher RS, et al: Motor and sensory cortex in humans: Topography studied with chronic subdural stimulation. *Neurosurgery* 1992; 31:59–71.

30. Ojemann G, Ojemann J, Lettich E, Berger M: Cortical language localization in left, dominant hemisphere: An electrical stimulation mapping investigation in 117 patients. *J Neurosurg* 1989; 71:316–326.

31. Gordon B, Hart J, Lesser R, et al: Individual variations in Perisylvian language representation. *Neurology* 1990; 40(suppl 1):172.

32. Talairach J, Tournoux P. *Co-Planar Stereotaxic Atlas of the Human Brain: 3D Proportional System: An Approach to Cerebral Imaging.* New York: Georg Thieme Verlag, 1988.

33. Schneider W, Casey BJ, Noll DC: Functional MRI mapping of stimulus rate effects across visual processing stages. *Hum Brain Map* 1994; 1:117–133.

34. Colby CL: Ventral intraparietal area of the macaque: Anatomic location and visual response properties. *J Neurophysiol* 1993; 69:902–914.

35. Small SL, Noll DC, Schneider W, Perfetti CA, Thulborn K, Hlustik P: FMRI of sentence processing in normal and aphasic women. *Proc Third Ann Meet Soc Mag Reson* 1995; 3:1339.

37. Small SL, Noll DC, Perfetti, CA, Schneider W: Functional magnetic resonance imaging of sentence processing: The role of grammaticality and stimulus rate (extended abstract). *Brain Lang* 1995; 51:80–83.

38. Broca PP: Nouvelle observaton d'aphémie produite par une lesion de la partie postérieure des deuxième et troisième circonvolutions frontales. *Bull Soc Anat Paris* 1861; 6:398–407.

39. Lichtheim L: Ueber aphasie. *Deut Arch f Klin Med* 1884; 36:204–268.

40. Heilman KM, Scholes RJ: The nature of comprehension errors in Broca's, conduction, and Wernicke's aphasics. *Cortex* 1976; 12:258–265.

41. Schwartz MF, Saffran EM, Marin OSM: The word order problem in agrammatism I: Comprehension. *Brain Lang* 1980; 10:249–262.

42. Schäffler L, Luders HO, Dinner DS, Lesser RP, Chelune GJ: Comprehension deficits elicited by electrical stimulation of Broca's area. *Brain* 1993; 116 (pt 3):695–715.

43. Cohen JD, Forman SD, Braver TS, Casey BJ, Servan-Scheiber D, Noll DC: Activation of prefrontal cortex in a non-spatial working memory task with functional MRI. *Hum Brain Mapping* 1994; 1:293–304.

44. Fox PT: Broca's area: Motor encoding in somatic space. *Behav Brain Sci* 1995; 18:344–345.

45. Damasio AR, Damasio H, Tranel D, Brandt JP: Neural regionalization of knowledge access: preliminary evidence. *Cold Spring Harbor Symposia on Quantitative Biology,* vol LV. Cold Spring Harbor, NY: Cold Spring Harbor Laboratory Press, 1990, pp. 1039–1047.

46. McClelland JL: *The Case for Interactionism in Language Processing.* Hillsdale, NJ: LEA, 1987.

47. Small SL, Hart J, Jr., Nguyen T, Gordon B: Distributed representations of semantic knowledge in the brain. *Brain* 1995; 118:441–453.

48. O'Reilly RC, McClelland JL: Hippocampal conjunctive encoding, storage, and recall: Avoiding a trade-off. *Hippocampus* 1994; 4:661–682.

49. Small SL, Noll DC, Perfetti CA, Xu B, Schneider W: Activation of left frontal operculum and motor cortex with functional MRI of language processing (abstract). *Soc Neurosci Abs* 1994; 20:6.

50. Small SL, Noll DC, Perfetti CA, Xu B, Schneider W: Using functional magnetic resonance imaging to determine the architecture of language processing in normal and impaired subjects (abstract). *Neurology* 1995; 45(suppl 4):A372.

51. Dronkers NF, Redfern BB, Shapiro JK: The third left frontal convolution plays no special role in the function of language: Marie's quadrilateral space revisited (abstract). *30th Annual Meeting of the Academy of Aphasia.* Toronto, Ontario: 1992, pp. 1–2.

52. Lashley KS: In search of the engram. *Symposia for the Society for Experimental Biology,* no. 4. Cambridge, England: Cambridge University Press, 1950.

53. Maria G, Ferriero G, Migliozzi S, Cantone G, Lombardi E: Malattia di binswanger. Quadri tomografici e correlati clinici. *Clinica Terapeutica* 1993; 143:499–506.

54. Nudo RJ, Jenkins WM, Merzenich MM: Repetitive micro-stimulation alters the cortical representation of movements in adult rats. *Somato Motor Res* 1990; 7:463–483.

55. Jenkins WM, Merzenich MM, Ochs MT, Allard T, Gu'ic-Robles E: Receptive-field changes induced by peripheral nerve stimulation in SI of adult cats. *J Neurophysiol* 1990; 63:82–104.

56. Allard T, Clark SA, Jenkins WM, Merzenich MM: Reorganization of somatosensory area 3b representations in adult owl monkeys after digit syndactyly. *J Neurophysiol* 1991; 66:1048–1058.

57. Merzenich MM, Nelson RJ, Stryker MP, Cynader MS, Schoppmann A, Zook JM: Somatosensory cortical map changes following digit amputation in adult monkeys. *J Comp Anat* 1984; 224:591–605.

58. Witt TC, Konziolka D, Baumann S, Noll DC, Small SL, Lunsford LD: Pre-operative cortical localization with functional MRI for use in stereotactic radiosurgery. *Stereotac Funct Neurosurg* 1996; 66:24–29.

59. Cohen HP, Woltz AG, Jacobson RL: Catecholamine content of cerebral tissue after occlusion or manipulation of middle cerebral artery in cats. *J Neurosurg* 1975; 43:32–36.

60. Brown RM, Carlson A, Ljungren BL, Seisjö BK, Snider SR: Effect of ischemia on monoamine metabolism in the brain. *Acta Scand Physiol* 1974; 90:789–791.

61. Robinson RG, Shoemaker WJ, Schlumpf M: Time course of changes in catecholamines following right hemisphere cerebral infarction in the rat. *Brain Res* 1980; 181:202–208.

62. Robinson RG, Shoemaker WJ, Schlumpf M, Valk T, Bloom FE: Effect of experimental cerebral infarction of rat brain on catecholamines and behavior. *Nature* 1975; 255:332–334.

63. Robinson RG: Differential behavioral and biochemical effects of right and left hemisphere cerebral infarction in the rat. *Science* 1979; 205:707–710.

64. Feeney DM, Sutton RL, Boyeson MG, Hovda DA, Dail WG: The locus coeruleus and cerebral metabolism: Recovery of function after cortical injury. *Physiol Psychol* 1985; 13:197–203.

65. Feeney DM, Gonzalez A, Law WA: Amphetamine, haloperidol, and experience interact to affect rate of recovery after motor cortex injury. *Science* 1982; 217:855–857.

66. Goldstein LB, Miller GD, Cress NM, Tyson AG, Davis JN: Studies of an animal model for the recovery of function after stroke (abstract). *Ann Neurol* 1988; 22:159–160.

67. Boyeson MG, Feeney DM: The role of norepinephrine in recovery from brain injury (abstract). *Ann Meet Soc Neurosci* 1984; 10:68.

68. Feeney DM, Hovda DA: Amphetamine and apomorphine restore tactile placing after motor cortex injury in the cat. *Psychopharmacology* 1983; 79:67–71.

69. Hovda DA, Feeney DM: Amphetamine with experience promotes recovery of locomotor function after unilateral frontal cortex injury in the cat. *Brain Res* 1984; 298:358–361.

70. Feeney DM, Hovda DA: Reinstatement of binocular depth perception by amphetamine and visul experience after visual cortex ablation. *Brain Res* 1985; 342:352–356.

71. Linn L: Sodium amytal in treatment of aphasia. *Arch Neurol Psychiatry* 1947; 58:357–358.

72. Wells CR, Labar DR, Solomon GE: Aphasia as the sole manifestation of simple partial status epilepticus. *Epilepsia* 1992; 33:84–87.

73. Lesser RP: Aphasia as the initial manifestation of epilepsy. *Mayo Clin Proc* 1991; 66:325–326.

74. Rosenbaum DH, Siegel M, Barr WB, Rowan AJ: Epileptic aphasia. *Neurology* 1986; 36:822–825.

75. Bergman PS, Green M: Aphasia: Effect of intravenous sodium amytal. *Neurology* 1951; 1:471–475.

76. West R, Stockel S: The effect of meprobamate on recovery from aphasia. *J Speech Hear Res* 1965; 8:57–62.

77. Sarno MT, Sarno JE, Diller L: The effect of hyperbaric oxygen on communication function in adults with aphasia secondary to stroke. *J Speech Hear Res* 1972; 15:42–48.

78. Meyer JS, Stoica E, Pascu I, Shimazu K, Hartman A: Catecholamine concentrations in CSF and plasma of patients with cerebral infarction and haemorrhage. *Brain* 1973; 96:277–288.

79. Albert ML, Bachman DL, Morgan A, Helm-Estabrooks N: Pharmacotherapy for aphasia. *Neurology* 1988; 38:877–879.

80. Albert ML: Aphasia is now treatable. *Hosp Prac* 1988; 23:31–38.

81. MacLennan DL, Nicholas LE, Morley GK, Brookshire RH: The effects of bromocriptine on speech and language function in a man with transcortical motor aphasia. *Clin Aphasiol* 1991; 21:145–155.

82. Gupta SR, Mlcoch AG: Bromocriptine treatment of non-fluent aphasia. *Arch Phys Med Rehab* 1992; 73:373–376.

83. Sabe L, Leiguarda R, Starkstein SE: An open-label trial of bromocriptine in nonfluent aphasia. *Neurology* 1992; 42:1637–1638.

84. Darley FL, Keith RL, Sasanuma S: The effect of alerting and tranquilizing drugs upon the performance of aphasic patients. *Clin Aphasiol* 1977; 7:91–96.

85. Walker-Batson D, Devous MD, Curtis S, Unwin DH, Greenlee RG: Response to amphetamine to facilitate recovery from aphasia subsequent to stroke. *Clin Aphasiol* 1991; 21:137–143.

86. Porch BE: *Porch Index of Communicative Ability,* vol 1. *Theory and Development.* Palo Alto, CA: Consulting Psychologists Press, 1967.

87. Crisostomo EA, Duncan PW, Propst M, Dawson DV, Davis JN: Evidence that amphetamine with physical therapy promotes recovery of motor function in stroke patients. *Ann Neurol* 1988; 23:94–97.

87a. McNeil MR, Doyle PJ, Spencer, KA, Goda AJ, Flores, D., & Small, S. L. A double blind, placebo controlled study of pharmacological and behavioral treatment of lexical semantic deficits in aphasia. *Aphasiology,* submitted.

88. Porch B, Wyckes J, Feeney DM: Haloperidol, thiazides, and some antihypertensives slow recovery from aphasia (abstract). *Ann Meet Soc Neurosci* 1985; 11:52.

89. Goldstein LB, Investigators SiASS: Common drugs may influence motor recovery after stroke. *Neurology* 1995; 45:865–871.

90. Newell A, Simon HA: *Human Problem Solving.* Englewood Cliffs, NJ: Prentice-Hall, 1972.

91. Fodor JA: *Modularity of Mind: An Essay in Faculty Psychology.* Cambridge, MA: MIT Press, 1983.

92. Feldman JA, Ballard D: Connectionist models and their properties. *Cog Sci* 1982; 6:205–254.

93. Seidenberg MS, McClelland JL: A distributed, developmental model of word recognition and naming. *Psychol Rev* 1989; 96:523–568.

94. Dell GS: A spreading-activation theory of retrieval in sentence production. *Psychol Rev* 1986; 93:283–321.

95. Shallice T: *From Neuropsychology to Mental Structure.* Cambridge, MA: Cambridge University Press, 1988.

96. Plaut DC: *Connectionist Neuropsychology: The Breakdown and Recovery of Behavior in Lesioned Attractor Networks: School of Computer Science.* Pittsburgh, PA: Carnegie Mellon University, 1991.

97. Crisman LG: *Response Variability in Naming Behavior of Aphasic Patients.* Pittsburgh, PA: University of Pittsburgh, 1971.

98. Small SL: Pharmacotherapy of aphasia: A critical review. *Stroke* 1994; 25:1282–1289.

99. McNeil MR, Small SL, Masterson RJ, Fossett T: Behavioral and pharmacological treatment of lexical-semantic deficits in case of primary progressive aphasia (extended abstract). *Brain Lang* 1994; 47:469–473.

100. Thompson CK: A neurolinguistic approach to sentence production treatment and generalization research in aphasia, in Cooper JA (ed): *Aphasia Treatment: Current Approaches and Research Opportunities,* vol 2. Bethesda, MD: National Institutes of Health, U.S. Public Health Service, 1993, pp. 117–134.

101. McNeil MR, Odell K, Tseng C-H: Toward the integration of resource allocation into a general theory of aphasia. *Clin Aphasiol* 1991; 20:21–39.

102. Just MA, Carpenter PA: A capacity theory of comprehension: Individual differences in working memory. *Psychol Rev* 1992; 99:122–149.

103. Robinson MK, Toole JF: Ischemic cerebrovascular disease, in Joynt R (ed): *Clinical Neurology.* Philadelphia: J.B. Lippincott, 1989, pp. 1–64.

104. Benson DF, Geschwind N: The aphasias and related disturbances, in Joynt R (ed): *Clinical Neurology.* Philadelphia: J.B. Lippincott, 1989, pp. 1–28.

105. Karp HR, Mirra SS: Dementia in adults, in Joynt R (ed): *Clinical Neurology.* Philadelphia: J.B. Lippincott, 1989, pp. 1–74.

106. Strub RL, Black FW: *Neurobehavioral Disorders: A Clinical Approach.* Philadelphia: F.A. Davis, 1988.

107. Bayles KA, Boone DR, Kaszniak AW, Stern LZ: Language impairment in dementia. *Arizona Med* 1982; 34:308–311.

108. McNeil MR, Small SL, Masterson RJ, Fossett T: Behavioral and pharmacological treatment of lexical-semantic deficits in case of primary progressive aphasia. *Am J Speech Lang Pathol* 1995; 4:76–87.

109. Wilcox MJ, Davis GA: *Promoting Aphasic Communication Effectiveness.* Atlanta, GA: American Speech and Hearing Association. 1979.

110. Forbes MM, Small SL: A PACE approach to enhancing functional communication in primary progressive aphasia. *Brain Lang* 1994; 47:530–532.

111. Lunsford LD, Kondziolka D, Flickinger JC, et al: Stereotactic radiosurgery for arteriovenous malformations of the brain. *J Neurosurg* 1991; 75:512–524.

112. Holland AL, McBurney DH, Moossy J, Reinmuth OM: The dissolution of language in Pick's disease with neurofibrillary tangles: A case study. *Brain Lang* 1985; 24:36–58.

113. Levin HS, Eisenberg HM, Benton AL: *Mild Head Injury.* New York: Oxford University Press, 1989.

114. Mills CK: A case of aphasia. *Med Bull* (Philadelphia) May, 1880.

115. Mills CK: Treatment of aphasia by training. *J Am Med Assoc* 1904; 43:1940–1949.

116. Lecours AR, Lhermitte F, Bryans B: *Aphasiology.* London: Baillière Tindall, 1983.

117. Féré C: La rééducation des aphasiques. *Revue Générale de Clinique et de Thérapeutique* 1886; 785.

118. Greenhouse JB, Fromm D, Iyengar S, Dew MA, Holland AL, Kass RE: *The Making of a Meta-Analysis: A Case Study of a Quantitative Review of the Aphasia Treatment Literature.* Pittsburgh, PA. Carnegie-Mellon University; 1986.

119. Holland AL, Wertz RT: Measuring aphasia treatment effects: Large-group, small-group, and single-subject studies, in Plum F (ed): *Language, Communication, and the Brain.* New York: Raven Press, 1988, pp. 267–273.

120. Hartman J, Landau WM: Comparison of formal language therapy with supportive counseling for aphasia due to acute vascular accident. *Arch Neurol* 1987; 44:646–649.

121. Sparks R, Helm N, Albert M: Aphasia rehabilitation resulting from melodic intonation therapy. *Cortex* 1974; 10:303–316.

122. Goodglass H, Kaplan E: *The Assessment of Aphasia and Related Disorders.* Philadelphia: Lea & Febiger, 1972.

123. Anonymous: Assessment: Melodic intonation therapy. Report of the Therapeutics and Technology Assessment Subcommittee of the American Academy of Neurology. *Neurology* 1994; 44:566–568.

124. Basso A: Therapy for aphasia in Italy, in Holland AL, Forbes MM (eds): *Aphasia Treatment: World Perspectives.* San Diego, CA: Singular Publishing Group, 1993, pp. 1–24.

125. Mitchum C, Haendiges A, Berndt R: Treatment of thematic mapping in sentence comprehension: Implications

for normal processing. *Cognitive Neuropsychology* 1995; 12:503–547.

125a. Schwartz MF, Saffran EM, Fink R, Myers J, Martin N: Mapping therapy: A treatment programme for agrammatism. *Aphasiology* 1994; 8(1):19–54.

126. Benson DF: Aphasia rehabilitation. *Arch Neurol* 1979; 36:187–189.

127. Barlow DH, Hersen M: *Single Case Experimental Designs: Strategies for Studying Behavior Change*. New York: Pergamon Press, 1984.

128. Lincoln NB, McGuirk E, Mulley GP, Lendrem W, Jones AC, Mitchell JR: Effectiveness of speech therapy for aphasic stroke patients. A randomised controlled trial. *Lancet* 1984; 1:1197–1200.

129. Wertz RT, Weiss DG, Aten JL, et al: Comparison of clinic, home, and deferred language treatment for aphasia: A Veterns Administration cooperative study. *Arch Neurol* 1986; 43:653–658.

130. Howard D: Beyond randomised controlled trials: The case for effective case studies of the effects of treatment in aphasia. *Br J Dis Commun* 1986; 21:89–102.

131. Kearns KP, Salmon S: An experimental analysis of auxiliary and copula verb generalization in aphasia. *J Speech Hear Dis* 1984; 49:152–163.

132. Whurr R, Lorch MP, Nye C: A meta-analysis of studies carried out between 1946 and 1988 concerned with the efficacy of speech and language therapy treatment for aphasic patients. *Eur J Dis Commun* 1992; 27:1–17.

133. Robey RR: The efficacy of treatment for aphasic persons: A meta-analysis. *Brain Lang* 1994; 47:582–608.

134. Kertesz A: *The Western Aphasia Battery*. New York: Grune and Stratton, 1982.

135. Kaplan E, Goodglass J, Weintraub S: *Boston Naming Test*. Philadelphia: Lea & Febiger, 1983.

136. De Renzi E, Vignolo LA: The token test: A sensitive test to detect receptive disturbance in aphasics. *Brain* 1962; 85:665–678.

137. McNeil MR, Prescott TE: *Revised Token Test*. Austin, TX: Pro-Ed, 1978.

138. Schwartz MF, Saffran EM, Marin OSM: Philadelphia Comprehension Battery. Philadelphia: Temple University, 1985.

139. Sarno MT: *The Functional Communication Profile: Manual of Directions*. New York: Institute of Rehabilitation Medicine: New York University Medical Center, 1969.

140. Holland AL: *Communicative Activities in Daily Living*. Baltimore: University Park Press, 1980.

141. Davis GA, Wilcox MJ: Incorporating parameters of natural conversation in aphasia, in Chapey R (ed): *Language Intervention Strategies in Adult Aphasia*. Baltimore: Williams & Wilkins, 1981, pp. 169–194.

142. Armstrong EM: Aphasia rehabilitation: A sociolinguistic perspective, in Holland AL, Forbes MM (eds): *Aphasia Treatment: World Perspectives*. San Diego: Singular Publishing Group, 1993, pp. 263–290.

143. Damico J: Clinical discourse analysis: A functional approach to language assessment, in Simon CS (ed): *Communication Skills and Classroom Success: Assessment of Language-Learning Disabled Students*. San Diego: College Hill Press, 1993.

144. Dobkin BH: Neuroimaging correlates of recovery, in Couch JR, Good DC (eds): *American Academy of Neurology—Course in Neurorehabilitation of the Stroke Patient*, vol 320. Seattle, WA: American Academy of Neurology, 1995, pp. 39–48.

145. Weiller C, Chollet F, Friston K, Wise RJS, Frackowiak RSJ: Functional reorganization of the brain in recovery from striatocapsular infarction in man. *Ann Neurol* 1992; 31:463–472.

146. Weiller C, Ramsey SC, Wise RJS, Friston K, Frackowiak RSJ: Individual patterns of functional reorganization of the human cerebral cortex after capsular infarction. *Ann Neurol* 1993; 33:181–189.

147. Weiller C, Christian O, Rijntjes M, et al: Recovery from Wernicke's aphasia: A positron emission tomography study. *Ann Neurol* 1995; 37:723–732.

148. Tseng C-h, McNeil MR, Milenkovic P: An investigation of attention allocation deficits in aphasia. *Brain Lang* 1993; 45:276–296.

149. McNeil MR: Aphasia: Neurological considerations. *Topics Lang Dis* 1983; 3:1–19.

150. Warrington EK, McCarthy R: Category specific access dysphasia. *Brain* 1983; 106:859–878.

151. Joanette Y, Goulet P, Le Dorze G: Impaired word naming in right brain damaged right handers: Error types and time-course analyses. *Brain Lang* 1988; 34:54–64.

152. Hart J Jr, Gordon B: Neural subsystems for object knowledge. *Nature* 1992; 359:60–64.

153. Small SL, Hart J Jr, Gordon B: Automated Boxology: A Modular Connectionist Approach to Modelling with Application to Picture Naming (extended abstract). Annual Meeting of the Academy of Aphasia. Toronto, Canada, 1992.

154. Small SL, Holland AL: Towards a Computational Model of Picture Naming. Annual Meeting of the Academy of Aphasia. Rome, Italy, 1991.

155. McNeil MR: Current concepts in adult aphasia. *Int Rehab Med* 1984; 6:128–134.

156. Benson DF: *Aphasia, Alexia, and Agraphia*. New York: Churchill Livingstone, 1979.

157. Huber W, Poeck K, Willmes K: The Aachen aphasia test, in Rose FC (ed): *Progress in Aphasiology*. New York: Raven Press, 1984.

158. Brookshire RH, Nicholas LE: Relationship of word frequency in printed materials and judgments of word frequency in daily life to Boston naming test performance of aphasic adults. *Clin Aphasiol* 1995; 23:107–120.

159. Huber W, Weniger D, Poeck K, Willmes K: Der Aachener aphasie-test, Aufbau und Überprüfung der Konstruktion. *Nervenartz* 1980; 51:475–482.

160. Nespoulous JL, Lecours AR, Lafond D, et al: *Protocole Montréal-Toulouse d'Examen linguistique de l'aphasie*.

Centre de Recherche du Centre Hospitalier Côte-des-Neiges, 1986.

161. Sasanuma S: Aphasia treatment in Japan, in Holland AL, Forbes MM (eds): *Aphasia Treatment: World Perspectives*. San Diego: Singular Publishing Group, 1993, pp. 175–198.

162. Taylor ML: A measurement of functional communication in aphasia. *Arch Phys Med Rehab* 1965; 46:101–107.

163. ASHA: *ASHA-FACS: Functional Assessment of Communication Skills*. Rockville, MD: American Speech, Language, and Hearing Association, 1995.

164. LaPointe LL, Horner J: *Reading Comprehension Battery for Aphasia*. Austin, TX: Pro-Ed Publishers, 1979.

165. Van Demark AA, Lemmer EC, Drake ML: Measurement of reading comprehension in aphasia with the RCBA. *J Speech Hear Dis* 1982; 47:288–291.

166. Brookshire RH, Nicholas LE: *Discourse Comprehension Test*. Tucson, AZ: Communication Skill Builders, 1993.

167. Folstein MF, Folstein SE, McHugh PR: "Mini-mental state": A practical method for grading the cognitive state of patients for the clinician. *J Psychiat Res* 1975; 12:189–198.

168. Raven JC: *The Ravens' Coloured Progressive Matrices*. Beverly Hills: Western Psychological Services, 1956.

169. Benton A, Hannay HJ, Varney NR: Visual perception of line direction in patients with unilateral brain disease. *Neurology* 1975; 25:907–910.

170. Berg EA: A simple general technique for measuring flexibility in thinking. *J Gen Psychiatr* 1948; 39:15–22.

171. Perret E: The left frontal lobe in man and the suppression of habitual responses in verbal categorical behavior. *Neuropsychologia* 1974; 12:323–330.

172. Reitan R: Investigation of the validity of Halstead's measures of biological intelligence. *Arch Neurol Psychiatr* 1955; 48:475.

173. Wechsler D: *Wechsler Adult Intelligence Scale—Revised*. New York: The Psychological Corporation, 1981.

174. Huber W, Springer L, Willmes K: Approaches to aphasia therapy in Aachen, in Holland AL, Forbes MM (eds): *Aphasia Treatment: World Perspectives*. San Diego: Singular Publishing Group, 1993, pp. 55–86.

175. Duffy JR: Schuell's stimulation approach to rehabilitation, in Chapey R (ed): *Language Intervention Strategies in Adult Aphasia*. Baltimore: Williams & Wilkins, 1985, pp. 187–214.

176. Shuell HM, Jenkins JJ, Jimenez-Pabon E: *Aphasia in Adults: Diagnosis, Prognosis, and Treatment*. New York: Harper & Row, 1964.

177. Peach RK: Clinical intervention for aphasia in the United States of America, in Holland AL, Forbes MM (eds): *Aphasia Treatment: World Perspectives*. San Diego: Singular Publishing Group, 1993, pp. 335–369.

178. Helm-Estabrooks N, Emery P, Albert ML: A new approach to aphasia rehabilitation. *Arch Neurol* 1987; 44:1253–1255.

179. Helm-Estabrooks N, Albert ML: *Manual of Aphasia Therapy*. Austin TX: Pro-Ed Publishers, 1991.

180. Jenkins WM, Merzenich MM: Reorganization of neocortical representations after brain injury: A neurophysiological model of the bases of recovery from stroke. *Progr Brain Res* 1987; 71:241–266.

181. Holland AL: Cognitive neuropsychological theory and treatment for aphasia: Exploring the strengths and limitations, in Lemme ML (ed): *Clinical Aphasiology 22*, vol 21. Austin, TX: Pro-Ed Publishers, 1994, pp. 275–282.

182. Caramazza A: Cognitive neuropsychology and rehabilitation: An unfulfilled promise?, in Seron X, Deloche G (eds): *Cognitive Approaches in Neuropsychological Intervention*. Hillsdale, NJ: LEA, 1989, pp. 383–398.

183. Collins AM, Loftus EF: A spreading activation theory of semantic processing. *Psychol Rev* 1975; 82:407–428.

184. Collins AM, Quillian MR: Retrieval time from semantic memory. *J Verbal Learn Verbal Behav* 1969; 8:240–247.

185. Linebaugh C: Lexical retrieval problems: Anomia, in LaPointe LL (ed): *Aphasia and Related Neurogenic Language Disorders*. New York: Thieme Medical Publishers, 1990, pp. 96–112.

185a. McNeil MR, Doyle PJ, Spencer KA, Goda AJ, Flores D, Small SL: Lexical semantic activation inhibition (LSAIT): A single subject multiple baseline study. *Brain Lang* 1996; 55(1):112–115 (extended abstr).

186. Saffran EM, Schwartz MF, Marin OSM: The word order problem in agrammatism II: Production. *Brain Lang* 1980; 10:263–280.

187. Saffran EM, Schwartz MF: "Agrammatic" comprehension it's not: Alternatives and implications. *Aphasiology* 1988; 2:389–394.

188. Marshall J: The mapping hypothesis and aphasia therapy. *Aphasiology* 1995; 9:517–539.

189. Searle J: *Speech Acts: An Essay in the Philosophy of Language*. London: Cambridge University Press, 1969.

190. Allen JF, Perrault CR: Analyzing intention in utterances. *Artif Int* 1980; 15:143–178.

191. Wilcox MJ, Davis GA: Speech act analysis of aphasic communication in individual and group settings. *Clin Aphasiol* 1977; 7:166–174.

192. Holland AL, Forbes MM: *Aphasia Treatment: World Perspectives*. San Diego: Singular Publishing Group, 1993.

193. Corina DP, Vaid J, Bellugi U: The linguistic basis of left hemisphere specialization. *Science* 1992; 255:1258–1260.

194. Hatta T: Recognition of Japanese Kanji in the left and right visual fields. *Neuropsychologia* 1977; 15:685–688.

195. Sasanuma S: Kana and Kanji processing in Japanese aphasics. *Brain Lang* 1975; 9:298–306.

196. Velletri-Glass A, Gazzaniga M, Premack D: Artificial language training in global aphasia. *Neuropsychologia* 1973; 11:95–103.

197. Steele R, Weinrich M, Wertz RT, Kleczewska MK, Carlson GS: Computer-based visual communication in aphasia. *Neuropsychologia* 1989; 27:409–426.

198. Chomsky N: *Syntactic Structures*. The Hague: Mouton and Company, 1957.

199. Chomsky N: *Aspects of the Theory of Syntax.* Cambridge, MA: MIT Press, 1965.

200. Chomsky N: *Lectures on Government and Binding.* Dordrecht: Foris, 1981.

201. Pinker S: *The Language Instinct: How the Mind Creates Language.* New York: William Morrow and Company, 1994.

202. Grodzinksy Y: Language deficits and theory of syntax. *Brain Lang* 1986; 27:135–159.

203. Blackwell A, Bates E: Inducing agrammatic profiles in normals: Evidence for the selective vulnerability of morphology under cognitive resource limitation. *J Cog Neurosci* 1995; 7:228–257.

204. Holland AL, Greenhouse JB, Fromm D, Swindell C: Predictors of language restitution following stroke: A multivariate analysis. *J Speech Hear Res* 1989; 32:232–238.

205. Holland AL: Recovery in aphasia, in Boller F, Grafman J (eds): *Handbook of Neuropsychology,* vol 2. Amsterdam: Elsevier Science Publishers, 1989, pp. 83–90.

206. Kertesz A, McCabe P: Recovery patterns and prognosis in aphasia. *Brain* 1977; 100:1–18.

207. Rubens AB: The role of changes within the central nervous system during recovery of aphasia, in Sullivan M, Kommers MS (eds): *Rationale for Adult Aphasia Therapy.* Lincoln, NE: University of Nebraska Press, 1977, pp. 28–43.

208. Knopman DS, Selnes OA, Niccum N, Rubens AB: Recovery of naming in aphasia: Relationship to fluency, comprehension, and CT findings. *Neurology* 1984; 34:1461–1470.

209. Wade DT, Hewer RL, David RM, Enderby PM: Aphasia after stroke: Natural history and associated deficits. *J Neurol Neurosurg Psychiatr* 1986; 49:11–16.

210. Aram DM, Ekelman BL, Rose DF, Whitake RHA: Verbal and cognitive sequelae following unilateral lesions acquired in early childhood. *J Clin Exp Neuropsychol* 1985; 7:55–78.

211. Basso A, Capitani E, Vignolo LA: Influence of rehabilitation on language skills in aphasic patients: A controlled study. *Arch Neurol* 1979; 36:190–196.

212. Holland AL, Bartlett C: Some differential effects of age on stroke-produced aphasia, in Ulatowska HK (ed): *The Aging Brain: Communication in the Elderly.* San Diego: College Hill Press, 1985, pp. 141–155.

213. Small SL, Hoffman GE: Neuroanatomical lateralization of language: Sexual dimorphism and the ethology of neural computation. *Brain Cog* 1994; 26:300–311.

214. Shaywitz BA, Shaywitz SE, Pugh KR, et al: Sex differences in the functional organization of the brain for language. *Nature* 1995; 373:607–609.

215. Gloning I, Gloning K, Haub G, Quatembe R: Comparison of verbal behavior in right-handed and non right-handed patients with anatomically verified lesion of one hemisphere. *Cortex* 1969; 5:43–52.

216. Smith A: Objective indices of severity of chronic aphasia in stroke patients. *J Speech Hear Dis* 1971; 36:167–207.

217. Starkstein SE, Bryer JB, Berthier ML, Cohen B, Price TR, Robinson RG: Depression after stroke: The importance of cerebral hemisphere asymmetries. *J Neuropsychiatr Clin Neurosci* 1991; 3:276–285.

218. Downhill JR Jr, Robinson RG: Longitudinal assessment of depression and cognitive impairment following stroke. *J Nerv Ment Dis* 1994; 182:425–431.

219. Robinson RG, Kubos KL, Starr LB, Rao K, Price TR: Mood disorders in stroke patients: Importance of location of lesion. *Brain* 1984; 107:81–93.

220. Benson DF: Psychiatric aspects of aphasia. *Br J Psychiatr* 1973; 123:555–566.

221. Morris PL, Raphael B, Robinson RG: Clinical depression is associated with impaired recovery from stroke. *Med J Aust* 1992; 157:239–242.

222. Robinson RG, Starr LB, Kubos KL, Price TR: A two-year longitudinal study of post-stroke mood disorders: Findings during the initial evaluation. *Stroke* 1983; 14:736–741.

223. Agrell B, Dehlin O: Depression in stroke patients with left and right hemisphere lesions. A study in geriatric rehabilitation in-patients. *Aging* 1994; 6:49–56.

224. Culton GL: Spontaneous recovery from aphasia. *J Speech Hear Res* 1969; 12:825–832.

225. Butfield E, Zangwill OL: Re-education in aphasia: A review of 70 cases. *J Neurol Neurosurg Psychiatr* 1946; 9:75–79.

226. Pashek GV, Holland AL: Evolution of aphasia in the first year post-onset. *Cortex* 1988; 24:411–423.

Chapter 31

CLINICAL ASPECTS AND TREATMENT OF NEUROPSYCHIATRIC DISTURBANCES IN PATIENTS WITH CHRONIC NEUROLOGIC DISORDERS

Moises Gaviria
Kevin Furmaga

Neuropsychiatric disturbances of chronic neurologic disease, defined as psychiatric disturbances including mood, anxiety, psychotic and personality syndromes, and neurobehavioral disturbances associated with "organic" etiologies, are poorly delineated in psychiatric nosology. For example, depression is a normal psychological response to a medical disability. However, stroke patients often develop depressive signs and symptoms as a direct neurobiological consequence of an ischemic brain lesion. Because disorders of emotion, behavior, thought, and cognition can severely impede physical rehabilitation efforts, recognizing and treating neuropsychiatric syndromes can optimize recovery in the neurological patient.

Most neuropsychiatric disorders can be classified under the system established in the Diagnostic and Statistical Manual for Mental Disorders, Fourth Edition (DSM-IV).[1] There are three general categories that are applicable to the neurological patient: (1) mood disorder due to a general medical condition; (2) personality change due to a general medical condition; and (3) psychotic disorder due to a general medical condition (Table 31-1). The specific diagnosis is based on the presence of requisite clinical signs and symptoms and the identification of a specific etiological neurological condition.

Cerebrovascular accidents, head trauma, and degenerative central nervous system inflammatory and infectious disorders cause a great number of neuro-psychiatric syndromes. Although they have different pathophysiologies, these neurologic entities can cause a variety of similar neuropsychiatric disturbances, reflective chiefly of the location and distribution of lesion load.

Ischemic vascular disease can produce focal or diffuse lesions in cortical, subcortical, and brain stem areas of the brain, resulting in the full spectrum of neuropsychiatric disorders. Because stroke is the most common neurological disorder associated with the psychiatric disturbances likely to be encountered in a rehabilitation setting, it provides an ideal paradigm for the discussion of the clinical aspects and treatment of neuropsychiatric disorders in patients with neurological disease. The spectrum of neuropsychiatric disorders also has been reported after ischemic or hemorrhagic brain lesions caused by brain injury.

In addition to their association with focal cerebrovascular disease, neuropsychiatric disorders also can be associated with vascular dementia, even in the observance of major cognitive dysfunction.[2]

Cognitive disturbances are defined as impairments in memory, language, calculation, praxis, visuospatial skills, abstraction, or executive functions. The term vascular dementia is more encompassing than multi-infarct dementia (MID), since dementia may be associated with hemorrhagic stroke or a single infarct as in the angular gyrus of the dominant hemisphere.[3]

Table 31-1
DSM-IV diagnostic criteria

Mood Disorder Due to a General Medical Condition

A prominent and persistent disturbance in mood predominates in the clinical picture and is characterized by either (or both) of the following:

Depressed mood or markedly diminished interest or pleasure in all, or almost all, activities

Elevated, expansive, or irritable mood

There is evidence from the history, physical examination, or laboratory findings that the disturbance is the direct physiological consequence of a general medical condition

The disturbance is not better accounted for by another disorder (e.g., Adjustment Disorder with Depressed Mood in response to the stress of having a general medical condition)

The disturbance does not occur exclusively during the course of a delirium

The symptoms cause clinically significant distress or impairment in social, occupational, or other important areas of functioning

Personality Change Due to a General Medical Condition

A persistent personality disturbance that represents a change from the individual's previous characteristic personality pattern

There is evidence from the history, physical examination, or laboratory findings that the disturbance is the direct physiological consequence of a general medical condition

The disturbance is not better accounted for by another disorder (including other mental disorders owing to a general medical condition)

The disturbance does not occur exclusively during the course of a delirium and does not meet criteria for a dementia

The disturbance causes clinically significant distress or impairment in social, occupational, or other important areas of functioning

Specific Type

Labile: If the predominant feature is affective lability

Disinhibited: If the predominant feature is poor impulse control (e.g., sexual indiscretions)

Apathetic: If the predominant feature is marked apathy and indifference

Paranoid: If the predominant feature is suspiciousness or paranoid ideation

Other: If the predominant feature is not one of the preceding (e.g., personality change associated with a seizure disorder)

Combined: If more than one feature predominates in the clinical picture

Unspecified

Psychotic Disorder Due to a General Medical Condition

Prominent hallucinations or delusions

There is evidence from the history, physical examination, or laboratory findings that the disturbance is the direct physiological consequence of a general medical condition

The disturbance is not better accounted for by another mental disorder

The disturbance does not occur exclusively during the course of a delirium

---

SOURCE: Adapted from the American Psychiatric Association.[1]

NEUROPSYCHIATRIC SYNDROMES

The following section provides a clinical description of the neuropsychiatric disturbances commonly associated with neurological diseases. Using ischemic cerebrovascular disease as a paradigm, the location of cortical or subcortical damage associated with each neuropsychiatric syndrome is discussed.

Depression

Poststroke depression manifestations may include depressed mood, diurnal mood variation, and loss of energy, appetite, weight, and sex drive. Delayed sleep onset or early-morning awakening, suicidal ideation, poor concentration, social withdrawal, and irritability are common. Starkstein and colleagues[4] found depression occurs in patients with cortical and subcortical strokes, and correlates with left anterior basal ganglion infarcts, or left and right thalamic infarcts. Depression strongly correlates with lesion proximity to the left frontal pole, whereas dysthymia correlates with right or left posterior parietal and occipital regions.[5] Recent magnetic resonance imaging analysis indicates that concentration difficulty may be associated with lesions of the rostral body of the corpus callosum.[6]

Unipolar Mania and Bipolar Mood Disorder

Organic mania is characterized by episodes of elation, hyperactivity, insomnia, pressured speech, grandiosity, and flight of ideas. A clear distinction between organic and "nonorganic" mania is difficult. Mania can be caused by right hemispheric lesions in the thalamus, perithalamic region, basitemporal lobe, or inferior medial frontal lobe anterior to the third ventricle.[7] Alternating episodes of depression and mania (bipolar mood disorder) are associated with subcortical lesions involving right head of the caudate and thalamus, whereas the presence of mania alone has been linked to lesions in the right orbitofrontal and right basitemporal cortex.

Catastrophic Reaction

Catastrophic reaction, uniquely associated with organic brain disease, is characterized by restlessness, hyperemotionality, sudden outbursts of tears, irritation, anger toward the examiner, coprolalia, anxiety displacement, aggressive behavior, refusal to continue examination, objections to evaluation, and tendency to brag or be anxiously expectant.[8] No specific lesion pattern has been described to date.

Abulia

Fisher defines abulia as a loss of spontaneous activity and speech, accompanied by apathy. Indifference to failure, lack of interest in family and friends, anhedonia, and lack of concern about physical difficulties or illness is common.[9] Abulia characteristically is seen after lesions of the right inferomedial frontal cortex, particularly known to occur after stroke and head injury.

Akinetic Mutism

Bilateral infarction of the anterior medial frontal cortex (cingulate gyri) produces akinetic mutism in which patients make no effort to communicate verbally or gesturally, and maintain an empty, noncommunicative facial expression.[10] Movement is limited to tracking moving targets with the eyes and body, and arm movements connected with daily routines, such as eating, pulling up bedclothes, and going to the bathroom. Spontaneous speech and movement are not observed.

Disinhibition

Psychosocial disinhibition syndrome is characterized by impulsive and inappropriate behavior, often with a jocular affect.[11] Emotional lability, poor judgment and insight, distractibility, euphoria, and tactless and irritable behavior are common. Lesions of the inferomedial subcortical white matter bilaterally are the rule.

Psychosis

Delusional or psychotic thinking, paranoia, and extreme agitation can be observed after either right or left hemispheric injuries involving the temporoparietal region or subcortical white matter.[12] Capgras syndrome, the conviction that someone familiar has been replaced by an identical-appearing imposter, and Fregoli syndrome, the belief that familiar persons are disguised as others, are associated with right-hemispheric lesions. Delusions after stroke often resemble idiopathic psychiatric disorders such as schizophrenia. However, organic hallucinations usually are visual, whereas schizophrenic hallucinations usually are auditory.[13]

Hallucinations

Visual hallucinations may occur after any lesions between the geniculate body and occipital cortex. Lesions of the optic radiations and geniculocalcarine cortex can produce formal and informal visual hallucinations, depending on location. Rarely, midbrain lesions cause diurnal peduncular hallucinosis, typically appearing in the evening.

Pathological Laughing and Crying

Frequent, rapidly vacillating episodes of uncontrolled laughing and crying and emotional incontinence, unconnected to internal states of feeling are known as pseudobulbar affect. Bifrontal subcortical white matter lesions are the rule.

Confabulation

The fabrication of material in response to questioning, and/or spontaneous, untruthful conversation characterize the confabulatory state. Primarily associated with basal forebrain disease, confabulations often appear to be generated as memory-gap fillers or actual, organically based fantasies.[14]

Pharmacological Management of Selected Neuropsychiatric Sequelae

Patients with neuropsychiatric syndromes associated with neurological disease often benefit from treatment with psychotropic medications. We will utilize the ischemic cerebrovascular disease paradigm to dicuss the pharmacological treatment of these disorders. Effective neuropsychopharmacologic management can enhance participation in rehabilitation programs and activities of daily living, and result in an overall improvement in quality of life. On the other hand, factors such as advanced age, brain injury, medical comorbidity, and polypharmacy can place this patient population at increased risk for adverse drug effects that slow or delay recovery. Pharmacotherapy should not be the only approach when devising a treatment plan, but should complement nonpharmacologic strategies.

A presumptive neuropsychiatric diagnosis often is based on the temporal relationship between signs or symptoms and an acute brain event. The existence and location of an identifiable brain lesion are diagnostic features that help distinguish neuropsychiatry from psychiatry. Since similar clinical presentations, regardless of etiology, may share common neurobiological mechanisms, medications that are effective in the treatment of psychiatric disorders often are employed in the management of neuropsychiatric complications during rehabilitation.

There are relatively few published clinical trials that adequately assess the efficacy and safety of the agents used for the treatment of the neuropsychiatric complications of neurologic disorders. Current pharmacotherapeutic approaches largely are based on cumulative clinical experience from published case reports and demonstrated efficacy in psychiatric or neurologic patients with similar symptoms. As a result, the benefits and risks of a given medication in a specific patient are unpredictable. Although no medications are approved specifically for the treatment of the emotional, behavioral, and thought disorders that can result from neurological disease, some broad pharmacotherapeutic guidelines for their safe and efficacious use have emerged from published clinical data. Desirable therapeutic outcomes can be optimized and the risk of a severe adverse drug event can be minimized if the clinician employs a cautious and systematic approach to drug selection and dosing.

Depression

Antidepressants enhance the transmission of serotonergic, noradrenergic, and dopaminergic neurons associated with the limbic and frontal regions of the brain. Advances in biological psychiatry support the hypothesis that depressive syndromes are caused by a functional downturn in these neurotransmitter systems. Brain-damage models that have demonstrated depletion of cortical catecholamines following focal ischemic brain lesions in rats point to similar central neurotransmitter dysfunction in poststroke depression.[15] Consequently, it is not surprising that antidepressants treat depression associated with stroke and other neurological diseases effectively.

There has been a dramatic increase in the number of available antidepressants with enhanced pharmacologic selectivity for the neurobiological targets believed to subserve major depression. Although improvements in drug design have led to agents that are better tolerated with fewer serious side effects, clinical efficacy is not significantly different among the various classes of antidepressants (Table 31-2).

Only a few published studies have assessed the efficacy and safety of antidepressants in poststroke depression (Table 31-3). The agents evaluated include selected members of the tricyclics (TCAs), second-generation, and serotonin-selective reuptake inihitor (SSRIs) classes.[16–19] Currently there are no data concerning the newest antidepressants, venlafaxine (Effexor) and nafazadone (Serzone), in this patient population. Although not classified as an antidepressant, the psychostimulant methylphenidate has been evaluated and has demonstrated effectiveness in patients suffering from poststroke depression.[20–22]

Antidepressants differ in their effects on central neurotransmitter systems. The older class of agents, represented by the tricyclic antidepressants (TCAs), increase synaptic concentrations of serotonin and/or norepinepherine through blockade of presynaptic reuptake. Chronic dosing of TCAs causes changes in postsynaptic receptors leading to enhanced postsynaptic serotonin neurotransmission.[23]

Unfortunately, the pharmacologic actions of these agents is not limited to the therapeutic targets described. Their lack of pharmacologic selectivity is responsible for a number of adverse effects that can occur at subtherapeutic doses.[24] Central nervous system injury and ad-

Table 31-2

Selected antidepressant medications: dosing and therapeutic plasma concentrations

Antidepressant	Starting dose (mg)	Dosage range (mg/day)	Therapeutic plasma concentration (mg/mL)
Tricyclics			
Amitriptyline	25 QHS	50–300	60–200
Desipramine	25 QD	50–300	125–250
Doxepin	25 QHS	75–300	110–250
Imipramine	25 QD	50–300	180
Nortriptyline	25 QHS	50–200	50–150
Second Generation (Heterocyclics)			
Amoxapine	50 QHS	100–600	180–600
Bupropion	100 QD	300–450	180–600
Maprotiline	25 QD	50–300	200–400
Trazadone	50 QHS	50–600	800–1600
SSRIs			
Fluoxetine	10 QAM	10–80	—
Paroxetine	10 QD	10–50	—
Sertraline	50 QD	50–200	—
Newer Agents			
Nafazadone	50 QD	100–600	—
Venlafaxine	25 BID	75–375	

Table 31-3

Published studies evaluating antidepressants and psychostimulants in poststroke depression

Drug	Design	n	Responders: drug (%)	Responders: placebo (%)	p Value	Drug withdrawal (%)	Placebo withdrawal (%)	Reference
Nortriptyline	DB, PC	39	11/11 (100)	0/15 (0)	0.006	6/17 (35)	7/22 (32)	14
Trazodone	DB, PC	?	NA	NA	<.05	6(?)	6(?)	16
Citalopram	DB, PC	45	12/18 (67)	3/20 (15)	<.05	6/24 (25)	1/21 (5)	17
Imipramine + mianserin vs desipramine + mianserin	DB, NP	20	Imipramine 8/10 (80)	Desipramine 0/5 (0)	<0.01	2/10 (20%)	5/10 (50%)	15
Methylphenidate	P, O	10	8/10	NA	NA	0	NA	18
Methylphenidate	R, O	25	13/25 (52%)	NA	NA	(0)	(0)	19
Methylphenidate	R, O	10	7/10 (70)	NA	NA	3/10 (30%)	NA	20

NA = Data not available; DB = double blind; PC = placebo controlled; P = prospective; O = open; R = retrospective.

vanced age increase the risk for adverse anticholinergic effects, especially urinary retention, confusion, and memory impairment. These same factors increase neurological patient susceptibility to sedation that is mediated via histamine blockade. However, sedation may be therapeutic in patients with anxiety or who suffer from insomnia. Older patients and those with congestive heart failure are more likely to develop orthostatic hypotension owing to TCA blockade of alpha$_1$-adrenergic receptors, increasing the risk of falls and hip fractures. Because TCAs' slow conduction through the A-V node (via sodium fast-channel blockade), they are contraindicated in patients with cardiac conduction abnormalities, including second- or third-degree heart block or bundle-branch block. These agents also possess arrythmogenic activity that can lead to ventricular arrhythmias in susceptible patients.

Therapeutic drug monitoring is recommended when patients are elderly, experiencing adverse effects, not responding to therapy, are noncompliant, or are receiving multiple medications that may result in a drug interaction.[25] Therapeutic plasma concentrations have been established only for nortriptyline, imipramine, and desipramine. Routine monitoring is not recommended for patients receiving other antidepressants. Since only steady-state concentrations are useful clinically, patients should receive treatment with a fixed TCA antidepressant dose for at least 1 week before blood levels are obtained, and 12 hours after the last dose. Depressed patients should be switched to an antidepressant from a different class if there is no response at therapeutic plasma concentrations. Weekly dose titration should continue in nonresponders with subtherapeutic levels if they are not experiencing serious side effects.

Trazadone is the only second-generation antidepressant that has been studied in stroke patients. The varying side effect profile of this antidepressant class has some advantages compared to the TCAs in selected patients. For example, trazadone lacks significant cardiac conduction and proarrhythmic effects, but can cause significant orthostatic hypotension. Its sedating effects may be beneficial in patients with anxiety or insomnia, and its lack of anticholinergic activity is desirable in patients prone to urinary retention.

The serotonin selective reuptake inhibitors enhance serotonin neurotransmission via presynaptic mechanisms that include serotonin reuptake blockade and augmentation of serotonin release.[23] Because the SSRIs are highly selective for the serotonin system, they do not appear to cause significant cardiovascular or anticholinergic side effects. Also, they cause less sedation

than most TCAs and second-generation agents. However, nausea and sexual dysfunction are common problems associated with SSRI administration. Because of their inhibitory actions on the cytochrome P450 enzyme system, the SSRIs can slow the clearance of some hepatically metabolized medications. This effect can last several weeks after discontinuing an SSRI antidepressant. Drugs known to interact with this class of antidepressant should be used with caution and at decreased doses.

Citalopram, an SSRI not available in the United States, was shown to be safe and effective for the treatment of poststroke depression.[19] Because all agents in this class share the same pharmacologic mechanism of action, the findings of this study probably can be generalized to all SSRIs. Efficacy studies for approved SSRIs in organic depression are needed in order to justify their widespread use.

The newest antidepressants, venlafaxine and nafazadone, have not been evaluated in the treatment of poststroke depression. Venlafaxine is a selective inhibitor of presynaptic norepinepherine and serotonin reuptake.[26] As a result of its pharmacologic selectivity, it is less likely to cause the anticholinergic and cardiovascular side effects seen with the TCAs. However, higher doses (>300 mg/day) are associated with increases in blood pressure and therefore should be used with caution in patients with hypertension. Nafazadone's antidepressant effects appear to be mediated via blockade of the serotonin receptor subtype 5HT$_{2a}$, and presynaptic serotonin reuptake inhibition at higher doses.[27] Although it has a side effect profile similar to the SSRIs, it is less likely to cause sexual dysfunction.

Several open trials have reported that methylphenidate has a rapid and beneficial effect on mood, motivation, and cognition in depressed stroke patients.[20–22] This mild psychostimulant is believed to improve mood through its ability to enhance central dopaminergic, noradrenergic, and serotonergic function. Methylphenidate can cause nervousness and insomnia. However, these effects can be controlled in most patients by reducing the dose and scheduling administration before late afternoon. Although side effects of methylphenidate include cardiac arrhythmia, hypertension, and hypotension, it has been used safely in cardiac patients.

In general, most antidepressants, as well as methylphenidate, appear to be effective treatments for depression associated with cerebrovascular disease. However, the small number of patients studied and the design of the trials do not permit definite conclusions concerning relative safety or efficacy of the agents involved.

Onset of improvement occurs 10 to 12 days after beginning treatment with the antidepressants, and within 72 hours following initiation of methylphenidate. A full therapeutic response with antidepressants may require 2 to 4 weeks of treatment. The optimum duration of treatment also is unclear. Epidemiologic data indicate that if not treated, depressive symptoms persist for up to 2 years following stroke in up to 30 to 40 percent of patients.[28] One strategy is to treat the patient with an effective agent for at least 6 months followed by a gradual dosage decrease over 2 to 4 weeks before discontinuation. Should signs and symptoms of depression recur, treatment can be reinstated.

Given the comparable efficacy of available agents, antidepressant selection should be based on minimizing the potential for medication side effects related to the patient's age, other medical conditions, and potential medication interactions. Currently, the SSRIs appear to be the antidepressants of first choice. They have a favorable side effect profile, do not require therapeutic drug monitoring, and there is extensive experience with their use in a variety of patient populations.

Apathy, Abulia, and Akinetic Mutism

The lack of motivation or initiative that characterizes apathy often is a feature of neuropsychiatric syndromes such as depression, dementia, or delirium. When apathy occurs as an isolated symptom, usually it is associated with lesions involving the frontal cortical or basal ganglion regions of the brain. Apathy is classically linked with damage to the medial frontal cortex, caudate nucleus, and globus pallidus. Evidence suggests that structural or functional lesions that disrupt dopamine neurotransmission between the frontal cortex and these basal ganglia structures can result in apathetic behavior.

Pharmacological strategies that enhance central dopaminerigic neurotransmission can be effective in the specific treatment of apathy and akinetic mutism. A number of case reports and small series have reported clinical improvement in a variety of brain disorders using dopamine agonists or psychostimulants (Table 31-4).[29-31] Adverse effects associated with the use of dopamine agonist strategies include nausea, hypotension, hypertension, psychosis, delirium, agitation, and dystonias.

Aggression

Aggression in the neurological patient is a heterogenous syndrome that lacks a satisfatory definition. Associated features include disinhibition impulsiveness, and irritablility. Dysregulation of brain systems that regulate mood (limbic), arousal (brain stem), perception (cortical association areas), planning abilities (frontal lobes), or behavioral inhibition (orbital frontal lobes) have been implicated in aggressive behavior. Aggressive patients often can be managed through environmental changes and behavioral protocols that reduce stress and somatosensory stimulation. When these approaches fail, a number of pharmacological strategies can be used safely in the aggressive patient with neurological disease. Medications found to be effective in neuropsychiatric aggression include agents that increase central serotonergic tone, agents that decrease central noradrenergic tone, mood stabilizers, and agents that increase central GABAergic tone (Table 31-5).[32-43]

Antipsychotic medications traditionally have been the drugs of choice for the treatment of aggressive

Table 31-4
Pharmacologic treatment of apathy

Drug	Typical dose	Mechanism
Bromocriptine	2.5–60 mg/day in divided doses	Direct D_2 agonist
Carbidopa/levodopa (Sinemet)	300–1200 mg/day levodopa equivalent in two to four divided doses	Indirect dopamine agonists
Amantadine	100 mg BID	Indirect dopamine agonists
Selegiline	5 mg QD-BID	MAO-B inhibitor
Methylphenidate	2.5–30 mg/day in divided doses	Psychostimulant
Amphetamine	5–20 mg/day in divided doses	Psychostimulant

Table 31-5

Pharmacologic management of aggressive behavior

	Dose	Mechanism of action
Beta Blockers		
Propranolol (Inderal)	200–800 mg/day in divided doses	Beta-adrenergic blockade
Pindolol (Visken)	20–60 mg/day in divided doses	
Nadolol (Corgard)	80–320 mg/day in divided doses	
Metoprolol (Lopressor)	100–400 mg/day, dose BID	
Serotonin Agonists		
Buspirone (BuSpar)	30–120 mg, dose BID to QID	Direct serotonin agonist
Paroxetine (Paxil)	20–60 mg/day	SSRI
Fluoxetine (Prozac)	20–60 mg/day	SSRI
Mood Stabilizers/Anticonvulsants		
Carbamazepine (Tegretol)	600–1600 mg/day in three divided doses (8–12 mcg/mL)	Anticonvulsant/mood stabilizer
Sodium Divalproex (Depakote)	1000–3000 mg/day in three divided doses (50–100 mcg/mL)	Anticonvulsant/mood stabilizer/ GABA agonist
Lithium carbonate	600–1200 mg/day in two to three divided doses (0.6–1.2 mEq/L)	Mood stabilizer/Serotonin agonist

behavior, regardless of etiology. Long-term use of antipsychotics is appropriate if aggression is associated with dangerous psychotic symptomatology. However, their pharmacologic actions place the neurological patient at increased risk for extrapyramidal and anticholinergic side effects, cognitive impairment, and oversedation. Short-term use of antipsychotic agents, either alone or in combination with a benzodiazepine, is preferable for the restraint of the violent patient at risk of harming him- or herself or others. However, their side-effect profile makes them poor choices for the long-term management of aggression. Both neuroleptic agents and benzodiazepines have been shown to retard recovery after stroke in experimental models.[44,45]

Psychotic Symptoms

There are limited data on the use of antipsychotic agents in the treatment of psychotic symptoms caused by neurological disease. Special consideration must be given to neurological patients when choosing an antipsychotic. Brain-injured patients are more susceptible to the anticholinergic and sedating effects of these agents.

Currently available antipsychotics can be classified as either low-potency, high-potency, or atypical (Table 31-6). Low-potency agents tend to be highly sedating, and are associated with high risk of anticholinergic and cardiovascular side effects. In addition, they can significantly lower the seizure threshold. High-potency agents pose a lower risk for the side effects associated with low-potency agents. However, high-potency drugs place the neurological patient at increased risk for extrapyramidal side effects, such as parkinsonism, akathesia, and tardive dyskinesia. The two atypical antipsychotic agents currently available, clozapine and risperidone, are least likely to cause extrapyramidal side effects, and vary with regard to anticholinergic, cardiovascular, and seizure threshold-lowering properties.[46,47]

High-potency agents tend to be safer in neurological patients. The routine use of anticholinergic agents, such as benztropine, to prevent extrapyramidal side effects increases the risk for anticholinergic toxicity and sedation. The atypical antipsychotic risperidone may be the agent of choice in the future for neurological patients. Its lack of anticholinergic activity, very low risk for extrapyramidal side effects, and lower tendency toward seizure potentiation gives it advantages over other antipsychotic drugs. Recent data indicate that resperidone is safe and effective in patients with severe brain injury and psychotic symptoms.[48] The risk of orthostatic

Table 31-6
Selected antipsychotic agents

Antipsychotic	Dosage range (mg/day)	Sedation	Anticholinergic	Cardiovascular	EPSP
Low Potency					
Thioridazine (Mellaril)	300–800	High	High	High	Low
High Potency					
Fluphenazine (Prolixin)	2.5–80	Low	Low	Low	Very high
Haloperidol (Haldol)	2.5–100	Very low	Very low	Very low	Very high
Atypical					
Clozapine (Clozaril)	50–900	High	High	High	Very low
Risperidone (Risperdal)	0.25–6	Moderate	Very low	High	Very low

hypotension is minimized when the medication is introduced gradually.

Mania

Data are limited concerning the use of safe and effective agents for the treatment of mania owing to brain injury. Lithium carbonate, antipsychotic agents, benzodiazepines, and mood-stabilizing anticonvulsants are the agents shown to be effective for the acute and chronic management of mania in patients with bipolar disorder.[49] However, brain injury places the neurological patient at increased risk for drug toxicity. Currently, the safest agents for the treatment of mania after brain injury appear to be the mood-stabilizing anticonvulsants divalproex sodium and carbamazepine. A number of small controlled clinical trials and case reports supports the use of divalproex as the agent of choice for the treatment of secondary mania. Carbamazepine is a less well-evaluated alternative. Desired doses and serum concentrations are similar to those used for the treatment of aggressive behavior (Table 31-5).

Pathological Laughing and Crying

Limited published data on the pharmacologic management of pathological laughing and crying indicate that the tricyclic antidepressants and serotonin-selective reuptake inhibitors can be effective.[50,51] Dosing and clinical safety considerations are similar to the use of these agents in the treatment of depression.

SUMMARY

This chapter has focused on the neuropsychiatric sequelae of neurological disease, with emphasis on appropriate pharmacological management. However, medications should not be viewed as the only option. Psychological and behavioral approaches involving neurological patients and their families can greatly benefit patients with neurologic disabilites and psychiatric illness, often negating the need for psychopharmacologic management. Psychotherapy and/or behavioral-modification strategies are essential components of any rehabilitation program serving patients with neuropsychiatric disturbances. Medications should be viewed as adjunctive treatment that can facilitate patient recovery.

REFERENCES

1. American Psychiatric Association: *Diagnostic and Statistical Manual of Mental Disorders,* 4th ed. Washington DC: American Psychiatric Press, 1994.
2. Krasuski JS, Gaviria M: Neuropsychiatric sequelae of ischemic cerebrovascular disease: Research and diagnostic implications. *Neurol Res* 1994; 16:241–250.

3. Cummings JL, Bensen DF: *Dementia: A Clinical Approach*, 2nd ed. Boston: Butterworth-Heinmann, 1992.

4. Starkstein SE, Pearlson GD, Boston JD, et al: Mania after brain injury: A controlled study of causative factors. *Arch Neurol* 1987; 44:1069–1073.

5. Robinson RG, Starr LV, Kubos KL, et al: A two-year longitudinal study of poststroke mood disorders: Findings during the initial evaluation. *Stroke* 1983; 14:736–741.

6. Baumgardner TL, Singer HS, Dencklin MB, Rubin MA, Rubin BS, Abrams MT, Colli MJ, Reiss AL: Corpus callosum morphology in children with Tourette syndrome and attention deficit hyperactivity disorder. *Neurology* 1996; 47:477–482.

7. Starkstein SE, Boston JD, Robinson RG: Mechanisms of mania after brain injury: 12 case reports and review of the literature. *J Nerv Ment Dis* 1988; 176:87–100.

8. Goldstein K:. *The Organism: A Holistic Approach to Biology Derived from Pathological Data in Man*. New York: American Books, 1939.

9. Fisher CM: Abulia minor vs agitated behavior. *Clin Neurosurg* 1984; 31:9–31.

10. Damasio AR, Van Hoesen G: Emotional disturbances associated with focal lesions of the limbic frontal lobe, in Heilman KM, Satz P (eds): *Neuropsychology of Human Emotion*. New York: Guilford, pp. 85–110.

11. Tucker GL: Regional syndromes. *J Neuropsychiatr Clin Neurosci* 1993; 5:260–264.

12. Hier DB, Mondlock J, Caplan LR: Behavioral abnormalities after right hemisphere stroke. *Neurology* 1983; 33:337–344.

13. Hier DB, Mondlock J, Caplan LR: Recovery of behavioral abnormalities after right hemisphere stroke. *Neurology* 1983; 33:345–350.

14. Davison C, Kelman H: Pathological laughing and crying. *Arch Neurol Psychiatr* 1939; 42:595–643.

15. Berlyne N: Confabulation. *Br J Psychiatr* 1972; 120:31–39.

16. Finklestein S, Campbell A, Stoll AL, et al: Changes in cortical and subcortical levels of monoamines and their metabolites following unilateral ventrolateral cortical lesions in rats. *Brain Res* 1983; 271:279–288.

17. Lipsey JR, Robinson RG, Pearlson GD, et al: Nortriptyline treatment of poststroke depression: A double-blind study. *Lancet* 1984; Feb 11; 1(8372):297–300.

18. Lauritzen L, Bendsen BB, Vilmar T, et al: Poststroke depression: Combined treatment with imipramine or desipramine and mianserin. *Psychopharmacology* 1994; 114:119–122.

19. Reding MJ, Orto LA, Winter SW, et al: Antidepressant therapy after stroke. *Arch Neurol* 1986; 43:763–765.

20. Andersen G, Vestergaard K, Lauritzen L: Effective treatment of poststroke depression with the selective serotonin reuptake inhibitor citalopram. *Stroke* 1994; 25:1099–1104.

21. Lazarus LW, Winemiller DR, Lingam VE, et al: Efficacy and side effects of methylphenidate for poststroke depression. *J Clin Psychiatr* 1992; 53:447–449.

22. Lingam VR, Lazarus LW, Groves L: Methylphenidate in treating poststroke depression. *J Clin Psychiatr* 1988; 49:151–153.

23. Johnson ML, Roberts MD, Ross AR, et al: Methylphenidate in stroke patients with depression. *Am J Phys Med Rehab* 1992; 71:239–241.

24. Blier P, DeMontigny C, Chaput Y: Modifications of the serotonin system by antidepressant treatments: Implications for the therapeutic response in major depression. *J Clin Psychopharmacol* 1987; 7(suppl):42S–34.

25. Preskorn SH: Antidepressant drug selection: Criteria and options. *J Clin Psychiatr* 1994; 55:9(suppl A):6–22.

26. American Psychiatric Association Task Force: The use of laboratory tests in psychiatry: Tricyclic antidepressants-blood level measurements and clinical outcome. An APA Task Force Report. *Am J Psychiatr* 1985; 142:155–166.

27. Bolden-Watson C, Richelson E: Blockade by newly-developed antidepressants of biogenic amine uptake into rat brain synaptosomes. *Life Sci* 1993; 52:1023–1029.

28. Eison A, Eison M, Torrente J, et al: Nafazadone: preclinical pharmacology of a new antidepressant. *Psychopharmacol Bull* 1990; 26:311–315.

29. Robinson RG, Boldue PL, Price JR: Two-year logitudinal study of poststroke mood disorders: Diagnosis and outcome at one and two years. *Stroke* 1987; 18:837–843.

30. Muller U, Von Carmon Y: The therapeutic potential of bromocriptine in neuropsychological rehabilitation of patients with acquired brain damage. *Prog Neuropsychopharmacol Biol Psychiatr* 1994; 18:1103–1120.

31. Marin RS, Fogel BS, Hawkins J, et al: Apathy: A treatable syndrome. *J Neuropsychiatry* 1995; 7:23–30.

32. Furmaga KM, DeLeon OA, Sinha SB, et al: Psychosis in medical conditions: Response to risperidone. *Gen Hosp Psychiatr* 1997 (in press).

33. Linniola M: Low cerebrospinal fluid 5-hydroxyindolacetic acid concentrations differentiates impulsive from non-impulsive violent behavior. *Life Sci* 1983; 33:2609–2614.

34. Ratey J: Buspirone treatment of aggression and anxiety in mentally retarded patients: A multiple baseline, placebo controlled study. *J Clin Psychiatr* 1991; 42:159–163.

35. Stanislav SW, Fabre T, Crismon ML, et al: Buspirone's efficacy in organic-induced aggression. *J Clin Psychopharmacol* 1994; 14;126–130.

36. Greendyke RM, et al: Propranolol treatment of assaultive patients with organic brain disease. *J Nerv Ment Dis* 1986; 175:240–243.

37. Mattes JA: Metoprolol for intermittent explosive disorder. *Am J Psychiatr* 1985; 142:1108–1110.

38. Ratey JJ, Sorgi P, O'Driscoll GA, et al: Nadolol to treat aggression and psychiatric symtomatology in chronic psychiatric inpatients: A double-blind, placebo controlled study. *J Clin Psychiatr* 1992; 53:41–46.

39. Greendyke RM: Therapeutic effects of pindolol on behavioral disruption associated with organic brain disease: A double blind study. *J Clin Psychiatr* 1986; 47:423–426.

40. Patterson JF: A preliminary study of carbamazepine in the treatment of assaultive patients with organic brain disease. *Psychosomatics* 1987; 28:579–581.

41. Gleason RP, et al: Carbamazepine treatment of agitation in Alzheimer's outpatients refractory to neuroleptics. *J Clin Psychiatr* 1990; 51:115–118.

42. Wilcox J: Divalproex sodium in the treatment of aggressive behavior. *Ann Clin Psychiatr* 1994; 6:17–20.

43. Craft M, et al: Lithium in the treatment of aggression in mentally handicapped patients: A double blind trial. *Br J Psychiatr* 1987; 160:685–686.

44. Feeney DM, Gonzalez A, Law WA: Amphetamine, haloperidol, and experience interact to affect the rate of recovery after cortex injury. *Science* 1982; 217:855–857.

45. Schallert T, Hernandez TD, Barth TM: Recovery of function after brain damage: Severe and chronic disruption by diazepam. *Brain Res* 1986; 379:104–111.

46. Watanabe MD, Martin EM, DeLeon OA, et al: Successful methylphenidate treatment of apathy after subcortical infarcts. *J Neuropsychiatr* 1995; 7(4):502–504.

47. Ereshefsky L: Clozapine: An atypical antipsychotic agent. *Clin Pharm* 1989; 8:691.

48. Cohen LJ: Risperidone. *Pharmacotherapy* 1994; 14:253–265.

49. Eichelman B: Neurochemical and psychopharmacologic aspects of aggressive behavior, in Meltzer M (ed): *Psychopharmacology: The Third Generation of Progress*. New York: Raven Press, 1987.

50. Evans DL, Byerly MJ, Green RS: Secondary mania: Diagnosis and treatment. *J Clin Psychiatr* 1995; 56(suppl 3): 31–37.

51. Schiffer RB, Herndon RM, Rudick RA: Treatment of pathologic laughing and weeping with amitriptyline. *New Engl J Med* 1985; 312:1480–1482.

Chapter 32

PHARMACOLOGIC EFFECTS ON RECOVERY OF NEUROLOGIC FUNCTION

Larry B. Goldstein

Regardless of severity, most stroke survivors recover over time.[1-6] Optimization of the rate and degree of this recovery is one of the primary goals of post-stroke treatment. Whether intended to augment normal compensatory strategies for particular impairments or to specifically improve lost functions, the various techniques of physical therapy currently form the cornerstone for these interventions.[7-11] As with stroke, the cognitive and motor deficits following traumatic brain injury can be particularly disabling. Of patients with moderate traumatic brain injury, approximately two thirds have moderate-to-severe disabilities 3 months after the injury.[12] Physical interventions also form the primary mode of treatment aimed at facilitating recovery of the head-injured patient.

A variety of innovative therapies for the management of stroke and brain-injured patients are being explored, with novel approaches being based on the rapidly expanding knowledge of the fundamental neurobiology underlying normal recovery. One particularly fruitful avenue of clinical investigation has been based on laboratory studies showing that drugs influencing the activity of specific central neurotransmitters can modulate the recovery process. These data not only suggest that pharmacotherapy to enhance recovery of lost function may be possible, but that some commonly prescribed medications used for the treatment of coincident medical conditions in both stroke and traumatic brain injury patients may be harmful. This review focuses on neurotransmitter-related drug effects on behavioral recovery after focal injury to the cerebral cortex.

LABORATORY STUDIES OF DRUG EFFECTS ON BEHAVIORAL RECOVERY

Behavioral recovery is the ultimate target of therapeutic interventions in humans with acute stroke or traumatic brain injury. Demonstrating that a drug improves histologic damage may have no clinical significance if that improvement does not translate into a concomitant reduction of disability or handicap. Although behavioral studies are limited in their capacity to delineate mechanisms of recovery on a cellular basis, they offer the advantage of providing measurable endpoints of "clinical" importance.

Sympathomimetic and Related Drugs

More than 50 years have elapsed since the first reports of favorable effects of amphetamine administration on behavioral recovery after experimental brain injury.[13-16] In a seminal series of experiments performed 40 years after these early studies, Feeney and coworkers found that the administration of a single dose of *d*-amphetamine the day following a unilateral sensorimotor cortex injury in the rat resulted in an enduring enhancement of motor recovery.[17,18] Similar effects of amphetamine administration subsequently have been found by others.[19-21] In the rat, the effect of amphetamine is to speed the normal recovery process. However, in other species, amphetamine administration results in restitution of motor function that otherwise would be permanently lost. For example, post-lesion treatment with amphetamine enhanced motor recovery in cats that had unilateral or bilateral frontal cortex ablations.[15,22,23]

These studies of the effects of amphetamine on recovery focused on motor impairment in animal models in which an area of cerebral cortex had been surgically removed. However, the amphetamine effect extends to functional deficits that occur following focal lesions produced through a variety of mechanisms and to lesions affecting other areas of the cortex, as well as to other behaviors. Amphetamine administration enhances behavioral recovery after infarction of the barrel cortex in rats, improves motor function after middle cerebral artery occlusion in spontaneously hypertensive rats, and facilitates motor recovery after focal traumatic brain injury.[24–26] Recovery of stereoscopic vision has been demonstrated in cats that had been subjected to bilateral visual cortex ablations.[27,28] Relearning of a visual discrimination task in visually decorticated rats is enhanced by amphetamine.[29] Unlike the relatively consistent effect of amphetamine on recovery from focal lesions, experiments testing the impact of amphetamine on behavioral recovery after more diffuse, nonfocal types of brain injury have been conflicting.[30,31]

Pharmacological studies designed to elucidate the mechanism of amphetamine's effect on behavioral recovery are complicated because of the drug's diverse central and peripheral actions. Systemic administration of amphetamine may increase blood pressure and heart rate in addition to increasing regional cerebral blood flow and metabolism.[32–34] The drug also causes nonspecific behavioral arousal and hypermotility.[32] In addition, amphetamine may induce a disaggregation of brain polysomes, thereby influencing protein synthesis.[35]

The effects of other selected sympathomimetic agents have been studied in the laboratory. Phentermine, an amphetamine analog with weaker cardiovascular effects, also accelerates motor recovery in both rats and cats.[36] Similarly, phenylpropanolamine at high doses facilitates recovery in a rat hemiplegia model.[37,38] However, the administration of a single dose of methylphenidate, a piperidine derivative structurally similar to amphetamine, was initially found to have only a transient beneficial effect on locomotor function after sensorimotor cortex injury in rats.[39] The lack of effectiveness of methylphenidate was hypothesized to be owing to its short half-life. In subsequent experiments, it was found that giving intensive task-relevant experience in tight conjunction with drug administration resulted in a significant and enduring enhancement of motor recovery.[40]

Amphetamine's central actions may be mediated through dopaminergic, serotonergic, as well as through noradrenergic neurons.[41] The hypothesis that amphetamine-facilitated recovery is due to effects of the drug on norepinephrine is supported by several lines of evidence. Pretreatment with the neurotoxin DSP-4, a drug that selectively depletes central norepinephrine, slows motor recovery.[42,43] Bilateral lesions of central noradrenergic projection neurons with cell bodies located in the locus ceruleus also interfere with behavioral recovery after subsequent cortex injury.[44] Microdialysis

studies show that focal injury to the cerebral cortex results in a diffuse impairment of norepinephrine release throughout the brain.[45,46] Finally, intraventricular or cerebellar infusions of norepinephrine facilitate recovery.[47,48] Intraventricular administration of dopamine in combination with a dopamine-β-hydroxylase inhibitor or dopamine alone has no effect.[47]

Assumption of the noradrenergic hypothesis of amphetamine-facilitated recovery leads to testable hypotheses concerning the impact of other drugs. Drugs that enhance norepinephrine release or decrease its metabolism would be expected to be beneficial, whereas those that impair norepinephrine release or increase its metabolism would be expected to be detrimental. For example, although not sympathomimetic amines, both yohimbine and idazoxan (centrally acting α_2-adrenergic receptor antagonists) increase norepinephrine release and enhance motor recovery when given as a single dose after unilateral sensorimotor cortex injury.[21,49–52]

Antihypertensives

As noted, centrally acting α_2-adrenergic receptor antagonists enhance recovery in the rat hemiplegia model. Therefore it was hypothesized that a centrally acting α_2-adrenergic receptor agonist would be deleterious. In fact, when given even as a single dose the day after cortex injury, the α_2-adrenergic receptor agonist clonidine has a prolonged detrimental effect on motor recovery.[53] Repeated dosing also impairs motor recovery.[21] When given to rats that had already recovered motor function, the administration of clonidine reinstates the motor deficit.[52,54] Prazosin and phenoxybenzamine, centrally acting α_1-adrenergic receptor antagonists, are also harmful.[51–55] In contrast, propranolol, a nonselective β-adrenergic receptor antagonist, has no effect on motor recovery.[51]

Major Tranquilizers

Coadministration of haloperidol blocks amphetamine-promoted motor recovery in rats and haloperidol impairs motor recovery when given alone.[18] When given to rats that had recovered, haloperidol as well as other butyrophenones (fluanisone, droperidol) transiently reinstate the motor deficit.[56] Haloperidol administration also blocks amphetamine-facilitated recovery of stereoscopic vision in visually decorticated cats.[28,57] These detrimental effects of haloperidol initially raised concern that amphetamine may act through a dopaminergic rather than a noradrenergic mechanism. However, haloperidol has antagonist effects at noradrenergic receptors.[58–60] As previously discussed, intraventricular administration of dopamine has a nonsignificant beneficial effect on recovery from hemiplegia after sensorimotor cortex injury in rats.[47] If a dopamine-β-hydroxylase inhibitor (blocking the conversion of dopamine to norepinephrine) is given in conjunction with intraventricular dopamine, even this weak beneficial effect is blocked.[47]

Tricyclic Antidepressants

There is surprisingly little data concerning the impact of tricyclic antidepressants on recovery after cortical injury in laboratory animals. The administration of a single dose of trazodone transiently slows motor recovery in rats with sensorimotor cortex injury and reinstates the hemiparesis in recovered animals.[61] In contrast, when rats are given a single dose of desipramine, a facilitation of motor recovery is observed.[61] The mechanisms of these tricyclic antidepressant effects in animal models of hemiplegia are uncertain, but may have important clinical implications as discussed below.

Anxiolytics

The preceding sections have focused on catecholamine effects on behavioral recovery. However, other classes of centrally acting drugs affecting other neurotransmitter systems may also have potent effects on the recovery process. For example, intracortical infusion of the inhibitory neurotransmitter γ-aminobutyric acid (GABA) increases the hemiparesis produced by a small motor cortex lesion in rats.[62] Benzodiazepines are indirect GABA agonists and would be hypothesized to impair recovery. The short-term administration of diazepam permanently impedes recovery from the sensory asymmetry caused by anteromedial neocortex damage in the rat.[63–65] The long-term deleterious effect of diazepam is mimicked by short-term infusion of the GABA agonist muscimol into the sensorimotor cortex adjacent to the lesion and is blocked by coadministration of the benzodiazepine antagonist Ro 15-1788.[66,67] Ro 15-1788 alone produces a transient facilitation of recovery.[68] Anxiolytics that do not act through the GABA/benzodiazepine receptor complex may not interfere with recovery.[68] Gepirone is an anxiolytic with no activity at the benzodiazepine receptor. Chronic administration of this drug does not impair recovery from the sensory asymmetry caused by anteromedial neocortex injury in the rat.

Anticonvulsants

In addition to their anxiolytic effects, benzodiazepines also are potent anticonvulsants. The deleterious effect of GABA on motor recovery after motor cortex injury is increased by the systemic administration of phenytoin, which may act through a GABA-mediated mechanism.[69,70] Phenobarbital also delays behavioral recovery after injury to the cerebral cortex in laboratory studies.[71,72] In contrast, chronic administration of carbamazepine in anticonvulsant doses did not affect sensory recovery after anteromedial cortex injury.[68]

MK-801 is a noncompetitive N-methyl-D-aspartate (NMDA) receptor antagonist with anticonvulsant activity. The administration of MK-801 had no effect on motor recovery in rat models of hemiplegia, no effect on recovery of limb placing and facilitated recovery of the sensory asymmetry resulting from anteromedial cortex injury.[73,74] The drug had no effect on sensory function, but reinstated forelimb placing deficits in rats recovered from anteromedial cortex injury.[74] This observation led to the hypothesis that the NMDA receptor is involved in maintenance of motor "relearning" because recovery of limb placing, unlike sensory asymmetries, is dependent on practice.[74] However, NMDA antagonists interfere with the acquisition rather than retention of learned behaviors and MK-801 had no effect on rats that had recovered from hemiplegia (a behavior also dependent on practice).[73,75]

Anticholinergics

In 1942 Ward and Kennard reported that cholinergic agonists increased the rate of motor recovery after motor cortex lesions in monkeys.[76] Interestingly, the beneficial effects of cholinergic agonists were blocked by administration of phenytoin (see the preceding).[72] More recent data suggest that the anticholinergic drug scopolamine facilitates recovery when given soon after either focal traumatic brain injury or electrolytic lesions of the sensorimotor cortex, but reinstates motor deficits if given long after cortex infarction in rats.[77–80]

Trophic Agents

As discussed elsewhere in this volume, a variety of neuronal rearrangements occur after many types of brain injuries. Drugs affecting the action of central neurotransmitters can have trophic effects and thereby influence neuronal rearrangements after brain injury. For example, norepinephrine has been implicated in trophic changes in the central nervous system.[81] Norepinephrine released in the cerebral cortex from locus ceruleus projection fibers have been suggested to lead to synaptic plasticity that may encode learning.[82] Kasamatsu used changes in visual cortex ocular dominance that followed brief monocular deprivation as an index of cortical plasticity. Local perfusion of 6-hydroxydopamine blocked the effects of monocular light deprivation in kittens. Local infusion of norepinephrine reinstated plasticity in animals that were no longer sensitive to visual deprivation.

IMPLICATIONS OF LABORATORY STUDIES

The pharmacological studies reviewed in the previous sections have several important implications for both considering potential drug effects on recovery after focal brain injury in humans and for the evolving understanding of the neurobiology underlying the recovery process. However, no single hypothesis explains all of the available experimental data.

General Implications

One important implication of the laboratory experiments discussed in the preceding sections is that specific drugs can have either beneficial (e.g., amphetamine, α_2-adrenergic receptor antagonists) or detrimental (e.g., haloperidol, α_2-adrenergic receptor agonists, benzodiazepines) effects on recovery. If drugs have similar effects in humans with brain injury, then these data offer two complementary potential avenues for therapeutic intervention. First, specific agents may be given to facilitate recovery. Second, drugs that may interfere with recovery could be avoided.

A second general principle from the laboratory studies is that at least certain of the drug effects on recovery are dependent on the behavioral experience of the animal after the drug is given. Even without drug administration, task-specific post-lesion training is quite effective in enhancing motor recovery.[83–86] Post-lesion non-task-specific environmental enrichment also is effective in improving the motor deficit in these animals, albeit to a somewhat lesser degree. Feeney found that if rats were restrained rather than given motor practice after drug administration, the amphetamine effect was not observed.[18] Although the beneficial amphetamine effect on motor recovery is clearly greater in animals given motor training after drug administration, a smaller independent positive drug effect may

be observed in rats not given specific training.[85] The recovery of stereoscopic vision in visually decorticated cats also depends on visual experience after drug administration.[27,28]

A third important principle is that the same drug may have opposite effects on the animal's ultimate behavioral deficit depending on when it is given in relation to the injury.[19,87,88] For example, immediate post-ischemic administration of a benzodiazepine is neuroprotective after transient global ischemia models in the gerbil and rat.[89,90,91] However, their effects have not been well studied after focal ischemia. Other drugs, presumably acting through a GABA-ergic mechanism such as barbiturates, phenytoin, and muscimol also have neuroprotective properties.[92–97] As reviewed herein, experimental studies show that benzodiazepines, phenytoin, and barbiturates are harmful when given during the recovery period.[98] Muscimol administration also interferes with recovery.[66] Thus, for GABA-ergic agents, the timing of administration in relation to the onset of the deficit may be a critical determinant of whether the drug has a beneficial or harmful effect. Similarly, the anticholinergic scopolamine may be protective if given soon after a focal cortical lesion, but harmful if given later.[77–80] In contrast, certain drugs that influence central noradrenergic neurotransmission may have similar effects when given in either the hyperacute or recovery periods. The α_2-adrenergic receptor agonists are harmful whereas α_2-adrenergic receptor antagonists (which increase the rate of firing of central nonadrenergic neurons by blocking autoreceptors) are beneficial during recovery.[98] Selective lesions of central noradrenergic pathways aggravate ischemic damage in the rat brain and the hyperacute administration of an α_2-adrenergic receptor antagonist protects against ischemia-induced neuronal damage.[99–101]

Implications for Understanding the Neurobiology of Recovery

Processes underlying behavioral recovery may be considered in two major groups; first, processes related to the resolution of the pathologic sequellae of brain injury, and second, processes related to the brain's adaptive responses to injury.[102,103] These adaptive responses may occur rapidly or develop more slowly over time.

Diaschisis The development and resolution of pathologic sequellae of focal brain injury such as cerebral edema, local inflammation, and diaschisis may be reflected in the functional deficit.[104–108] The potential effects of certain drugs on diaschisis forms the basis of an attractive hypothesis for considering their effects on recovery after focal cortical injury.[109] Diaschisis entails a "remote functional depression" of brain regions distant from the site of primary injury. Diaschisis has been demonstrated experimentally in a variety of laboratory animal models.[110–113] In human stroke patients, diaschisis-like changes in metabolism have been demonstrated by positron-emission tomography in the noninjured ipsilateral cerebral hemisphere, the contralateral cerebral hemisphere, and the contralateral cerebellum.[114–117] Crossed cerebellar-cortical diaschisis occurs in patients with unilateral cerebellar infarction.[118] Deep hemispheric strokes can have remote effects on metabolism in both the cerebral cortex and cerebellum.[119] The observed depression of metabolic activity in distant brain regions might be the direct result of regional changes in cerebral blood flow; or, the decreased regional cerebral blood flow might be secondary to locally depressed cerebral metabolism. Drugs that prolong or worsen diaschisis would be anticipated to be detrimental, whereas those that promote the resolution of diaschisis would be anticipated to facilitate recovery. For example, amphetamine may act to reverse diaschisis.[109] It has been hypothesized that benzodiazepines might exert their detrimental effects by prolonging the diaschisis effect.[68] However, the presence of diaschisis does not add to the clinical deficit after stroke in humans.[120] Further, crossed cerebellar diaschisis does not correlate with recovery after stroke affecting the cerebral hemisphere.[121] The primary clinical manifestation of crossed cerebellar diaschisis appears to be a prolonged flaccidity associated with the hemiparesis related to stroke.[122] These observations present a challenge to the diaschisis hypothesis of recovery.

Rapid Adaptive Responses Rapid adaptive responses to brain injury may be considered as forms of relearning. However, it is often difficult to determine whether this relearning represents behavioral substitution (compensation) or specific behavioral recovery.[123] The physiologic mechanisms by which this relearning occurs remain uncertain. Lashley and Luria suggested that redundant neural networks might take over functions lost owing to brain injury.[124–126] Positron-emission tomography studies in human stroke patients show metabolic changes consistent with this phenomenon (also termed "unmasking").[127] In uninjured humans, motor movement is associated with increases in regional cerebral blood flow (rCBF) in a circumscribed region in the contralateral primary sensorimotor cortex. However, in patients recovered from stroke that had resulted in limb paresis, movement of the previously affected extremity is associated with significant changes in rCBF in widespread areas of the brain, including both the ipsilateral and contralateral sensorimotor cortex and both cerebellar hemispheres.[128–130]

It is also possible that the normal neuronal processes responsible for learning might underlie the "relearning" that occurs after brain injury. Long-term potentiation (LTP) is the best-understood putative cellular mechanism of learning and memory.[131–133] LTP occurs in diverse brain regions, including those not typically associated with memory, including hypothalamus, visual cortex, and motor cortex.[134–137] Under experimental conditions, the development of LTP is mediated by the N-methyl-D-aspartate (NMDA) subtype of glutamate receptor.[138–140] The administration of NMDA receptor antagonists block the induction of LTP and disrupt learning and memory.[141–143] Other neurotransmitters such as catecholamines, γ-aminobutyric acid (GABA), and acetylcholine can modulate the induction of LTP.[138,141–152]

Drugs that either promote the activation of redundant neural networks ("unmasking") or facilitate the induction of LTP would be anticipated to hasten recovery. In contrast, drugs that either inhibit the activation of alternative neural pathways or impair the induction of LTP would interfere with the recovery process. Interestingly, amphetamine both facilitates the induction of LTP in a dose-dependent manner and enhances memory retrieval.[153,154] Amphetamine may also facilitate "unmasking." For example, its administration results in a widespread increase in glucose metabolism following sensory activation after barrel field infarction in the rat.[155] The administration of benzodiazepines impair learning and memory and may suppress the induction of LTP.[156–159] However, unlike motor recovery after sensorimotor cortex injury, the sensory asymmetry after anteromedial cortex damage is not influenced by practice, suggesting a mechanism other than interference with "relearning."[160] Chronic administration of diazepam in anteromedial-cortex-injured rats led to a significant loss in size of the ipsilateral striatum.[161,162] Further, not all drug effects on recovery can be predicted based on their impact on the induction of LTP. β-adrenergic receptor antagonists interfere with LTP induction, but propranolol has no effect on motor recovery after sensorimotor cortex injury in rats.[51,163] In addition, we completed a series of experiments in which we were unable to demonstrate a detrimental effect of the NMDA receptor antagonist MK-801 on motor recovery after unilateral motor cortex lesions.[73] We had hypothesized that MK-801 would be detrimental because this motor recovery is highly dependent on post-lesion experience and the administration of NMDA receptor antagonists block the induction of LTP and disrupt learning and memory.[18,85,86,141,164] Our experiments suggest that if "relearning" is involved in motor recovery after cortex injury, the process is not susceptible to permanent disruption by the early administration of an NMDA receptor antagonist.

Slow Adaptive Responses The slow adaptive responses involve anatomic neuronal rearrangements that occur after many types of brain injuries.[165–171] Some of these neuronal reorganizations would be expected to be beneficial, whereas others are potentially maladaptive.[166] For a drug to enhance behavioral recovery by influencing these types of neuronal alterations, it would have to selectively facilitate the favorable rearrangements and/or retard potentially harmful ones. A variety of specific growth factors that may improve functional recovery after brain injury are under experimental study.[172] Drugs that influence central neurotransmitters may also have neuronotrophic effects.[173] For example, amphetamine administration results in reactive synaptogenesis in the frontal cortex of gerbils.[174,175]

CLINICAL DATA

The underlying pharmacology and basic principles derived from laboratory-based experiments have directly led to several clinical studies of the effects of drugs on recovery. Although small randomized studies of the effects of drugs with the potential to enhance recovery after stroke have been performed, studies designed to investigate potentially harmful drug effects cannot employ this methodology and must rely on retrospective (and therefore less fully controlled) analyses.

Amphetamine

Motivation in elderly patients refractory to rehabilitation procedures improves with amphetamine treatment.[176] This effect is likely nonspecific and due to the stimulant effects of the drug. However, several other anecdotal reports and small controlled trials suggest that treatment with amphetamine may enhance functional recovery after focal brain injury under certain conditions. These studies vary significantly with regard to patient populations, dosing regimens, and the timing of the interventions.

The first study of amphetamine's effects on recovery after stroke was carefully designed to simulate the paradigm used in the laboratory experimental studies. Eight patients with stable motor deficits were randomized to receive either a single dose of amphetamine or placebo within 10 days of carotid-distribution ischemic stroke. Motor function was measured with a reliable and validated scale, the Fugl-Meyer Assessment.[177] Within 3 hours of drug administration, all of the patients underwent intensive physical therapy (e.g., drug administration was coupled with task-specific experience). The following day, the patients' abilities to use their affected limbs were reassessed. Overall, the amphetamine-treated group had a significant improvement in motor performance, whereas there was little change in the placebo-treated group. This study was important in that it suggested that the same drug effect observed in the laboratory might occur in humans. However, because this study involved only a small group of highly selected patients, the results might not be generalizable. Because only very short-term motor recovery was measured, there were no data from the study with regard to the longer-term efficacy of amphetamine administration. It should also be noted that only two of the four patients had a "dramatic" motor improvement. (The intervention had a variable effect even in this highly select group.) Because of concern about the potential harmful effects of sympathomimetic agents in patients immediately following stroke, studies reproducing and extending this finding have been lacking. Until recently, this study provided some of the only controlled data of a beneficial effect of amphetamine treatment on motor recovery in humans.

A second, unpublished, double-blind, placebo-controlled trial of the effects of amphetamine on motor recovery in rehabilitation patients subsequently was performed.[178] This study included five amphetamine-treated and five placebo-treated patients. Drug or placebo was given once every 4 days for 10 sessions beginning 15 to 30 days after stroke. Each dose was given in tight conjunction with a session of intensive physical therapy. Motor function was again measured with the Fugl-Meyer Assessment, with the final evaluation being performed 1 week after the last dose. Patients treated with amphetamine had significantly greater improvements in motor scores compared to placebo-treated patients. Although preliminary, these results suggest that amphetamine administration combined with physical therapy may enhance motor recovery in human stroke patients, that the effect is still present at least 1 week after drug treatment is halted, and that the effect is present even when the intervention is delayed for up to 1 month after stroke.

A third, double-blind, placebo-controlled trial was negative.[179] In this study, 12 patients were given 10 mg of amphetamine daily for 14 days followed by 5 mg for 3 days. Twelve patients received placebo. Interventions began more than 1 month after the stroke and the administration of the drug/placebo was not tightly linked with physical-therapy sessions. Thus, this study varied in several significant ways from the previous trial. These differences include a different dosing regimen, a longer delay between stroke and treatment, and a lack of a tightly coupled physical-therapy regimen. These findings, although negative, will help in the design of future studies.

Speech pathologists have begun to study the effects of amphetamine on language recovery after stroke.[180,181] In one study, six aphasic patients had language function rated with the Porch Index of Communicative Ability 10 to 30 days after stroke.[181,182] Based on this initial evaluation, 6-month language scores were predicted for each patient. All patients were then given 10 mg of *d*-amphetamine followed by speech therapy every fourth day for 10 sessions. The patients actual scores after 3 months were then compared with their 6-month predicted scores. Most patients achieved or exceeded their 6-month predicted scores by the time of the 3-month evaluation.

Methylphenidate

Nonspecific stimulant medications including methylphenidate have been used in cognitively impaired brain-injured patients for many years. The drug has also been used in the treatment of post-stroke depression in patients undergoing rehabilitative therapy.[183–185] Only limited data are available concerning the drug's impact on neurological impairments.[186] This study did not find any effect of the drug on physical performance despite significant effects on cardiovascular function. However, variables shown to be important from laboratory studies and suggested from the clinical amphetamine trials previously reviewed (e.g., timing in relationship to brain injury, tight conjunction of drug administration and physical therapy) were not considered in the design of this early study.

Tricyclic Antidepressants

Clinical depression is associated with impaired recovery after stroke in humans.[187] Tricyclic antidepressants are used commonly to treat mood disorders in stroke patients. Trazodone, a drug that impairs recovery from hemiplegia in the rat, was found to improve outcome as measured with the Barthel Index in depressed stroke patients.[188] However, trazodone was given in only a single dose in the animal study and repeated dosing likely has a different effect on neurotransmitter levels. Therefore, recommendations concerning the choice of specific tricyclic antidepressants in stroke patients must await further laboratory and clinical studies.

Other Catecholaminergic Drugs

Phenoxybenzamine caused slight transient worsening of the neurologic deficit in several stroke patients, but this might be due to the hemodynamic effects of the drug.[189] One retrospective study found that both thiazide diuretics and a mixed group of antihypertensives were associated with impaired language recovery in aphasic stroke patients.[190] Propranolol, a drug that had no effect on motor recovery in experimental studies, also had no effect on language recovery in these patients. Preliminary studies indicate that the administration of bromocriptine improves fluency in certain aphasics.[191–193]

Detrimental Drug Effects in Humans

Although the previous discussion has focused on the use of drugs to enhance recovery after stroke, it is important to recognize that the laboratory studies also suggest that some drugs may be detrimental. We carried out a retrospective study of physician prescribing patterns to determine what drugs were used in the treatment of stroke patients.[194] Over 80 percent of individuals were taking at least one drug at the time of the stroke. Sixty-five percent of patients were receiving multiple drugs. Antihypertensives such as clonidine and prazosin and sedative hypnotics, including benzodiazepines, were among the most commonly prescribed agents. The number of stroke patients prescribed sedative-hypnotic agents more than doubled over the first 2 days of hospitalization (17–44%), including a doubling of the number receiving benzodiazepines (10–20%). Thus, several of the drugs that have deleterious effects on recovery of function in laboratory animals were commonly prescribed for stroke patients for the treatment of coincident medical conditions. Similarly, certain potentially detrimental drugs including dopamine receptor antagonists, benzodiazepines, and anticonvulsants are given commonly to patients with traumatic head injury.[195]

Determining whether the detrimental effects of

drugs anticipated from laboratory studies also occur in humans recovering from stroke is difficult. Largely anecdotal reports indicate that treatment with haloperidol and certain antihypertensives may interfere with language recovery in patients with aphasia following stroke.[38,190,198] We performed a retrospective study that tested the hypothesis that drugs that are harmful during recovery in laboratory animals would interfere with motor recovery in human stroke patients.[197] These potentially deleterious drugs included the antihypertensives clonidine and prazosin, neuroleptics, benzodiazepines, and phenytoin. The motor recoveries of stroke patients who received one or a combination of these drugs were compared to the recoveries of a similar group of patients who were not given any of these agents. The two groups were similar with respect to a variety of characteristics, including age, blood pressure, gender, and medical comorbidity. Motor function was measured prospectively with the Fugl-Meyer Assessment by observers who were blind to the study hypothesis. Although the results of this study need to be interpreted with caution, patients who received one or a combination of the hypothesized "detrimental" drugs at the time of stroke or during the subsequent hospitalization had significantly slower motor recoveries than a comparable group of patients who did not receive one of these drugs. A multivariate analysis indicated a significant effect of "drug group," after correcting for the contributions of other variables, including the initial severity of the deficit.

Supporting the findings of the previous study, the deleterious effect of certain drugs on motor recovery also was found in a separate cohort of patients with anterior circulation ischemic stroke.[98] These patients were control subjects in a prospective acute stroke interventional trial.[198] Nearly 40 percent of the control patients enrolled in this study received one or a combination of drugs hypothesized to impair recovery after stroke. Although the groups of patients who did or did not receive one of the "detrimental" drugs were not prospectively randomized, they were quite similar with respect to the presence of a variety of comorbid conditions and patient characteristics that could impact on the recovery process. As with the previous study, stepwise regression models indicate that drug group had an effect on outcome independent of the degree of the initial motor impairment, comorbid conditions, and other patient characteristics. Further, the most commonly prescribed of the potentially detrimental medications were benzodiazepines, and the most commonly given of these was triazolam. Although the reasons a medication was given was not recorded, triazolam was likely prescribed for its soporific effect.

Because both studies involved retrospective analyses, it cannot be certain that the reason for the administration of a given drug rather than the drug itself influenced recovery. Another limitation is that these studies did not permit an analysis of the impact of specific "detrimental" drugs, nor did they permit analyses of dose or timing effects. However, the consistency of the overall effect is noteworthy.

SUMMARY

It is clear that certain drugs influence behavioral recovery in laboratory animals with focal brain injury. These drug effects can be either beneficial or harmful to the recovery process. Importantly, similar drug effects may occur in humans. The routine use of drugs such as amphetamine to hasten recovery cannot be advocated based on the available data. Subpopulations that might benefit must be identified and issues related to the timing of the intervention and dosing schedules must be clarified through controlled trials.

In choosing drugs to treat coincident medical problems in stroke patients, this emerging pharmacology should be kept in mind. Given the available data, the use of a β-adrenergic receptor antagonist is preferable to either an α_1- or α_2-adrenergic receptor antagonist in the treatment of hypertension following stroke. Thiazide diuretics should be used cautiously. Haloperidol is potentially harmful and until the pharmacology of the effects of major tranquilizers is better understood, they should be withheld whenever possible in patients recovering from stroke. Recommendations concerning the choice of specific tricyclic antidepressants in stroke patients must await further laboratory and clinical studies. Benzodiazepines generally should be avoided. Of the anticonvulsants experimentally tested during the recovery period, the only drug not found to be harmful is carbamazepine. This drug should be considered when nonemergency treatment of seizure disorders is necessary in stroke patients. The use of specific drugs capable of enhancing recovery after stroke may be possible in the future.

REFERENCES

1. Duncan PW, Goldstein LB, Matchar D, Divine GW, Feussner J: Measurement of motor recovery after stroke. Outcome assessment and sample size requirements. *Stroke* 1992; 23:1084–1089.

2. Newman M: The process of recovery after stroke. *Stroke* 1972; 3:702–710.

3. Wade DT, Langton HR, Wood VA, Skilbeck CE, Ilsmail HM: The hemiplegic arm after stroke: Measurement and recovery. *J Neurol Neurosurg Psychiatr* 1983; 46:521–524.

4. Loewen SC, Anderson BA: Predictors of stroke outcome using objective measurement scales. *Stroke* 1990; 21:78–81.

5. Wade DT, Wood VA, Hewer RL: Recovery after stroke: The first three months. *J Neurol Neurosurg Psychiatr* 1985; 48:7–13.

6. Kinsella G, Ford B: Acute recovery patterns in stroke patients. *Med J Aust* 1980; 2:662–666.

7. Wescott EJ: Traditional exercise regimens for the hemiplegic patient. *Am J Phys Med* 1967; 46:1012–1023.

8. Bobath B: *Adult Hemiplegia: Evaluation and Treatment.* London: Heinemann, 1984.

9. Brunnstrom S: *Movement Therapy in Hemiplegia: A Neurophysiological Approach.* New York: Harper & Row, 1970.

10. Wolf SL, Binder-Macleod SA: Electromyographic biofeedback applications to the hemiplegic patient. *Phys Ther* 1983; 63:1393–1403.

11. Basmajian JV, Gowland CA, Finlayson AJ, et al: Stroke treatment: Comparison of intergrated behavioral-physical therapy vs traditional physical therapy programs. *Arch Phys Med Rehab* 1987; 68:267–272.

12. Rimel RW, Giordani MA, Barth TJ, Jane JA: Moderate head injury: completing the clinical spectrum of brain trauma. *Neurosurgery* 1982; 11:344–351.

13. Maling HM, Acheson GH: Righting and other postural activity in low-decerebrate and in spinal cats after d-amphetamine. *J Neurophysiol* 1946; 9:379–386.

14. Macht MB: Effects of d-amphetamine on hemi-decorticate, decorticate, and decerebrate cats. *Am J Physiol* 1950; 163:731–732.

15. Meyer PM, Horel JA, Meyer DR: Effects of dl-amphetamine upon placing responses in neodecorticate cats. *J Comp Physiol Psych* 1963; 56:402–404.

16. Feeney DM, Hovda DA: Amphetamine restores tactile placing after motor cortex lesions. *Fed Proc* 1980; 39:1095.

17. Feeney DM, Gonzalez A, Law WA: Amphetamine restores locomotor function after motor cortex injury in the rat. *Proc West Pharmacol Soc* 1981; 24:15–17.

18. Feeney DM, Gonzalez A, Law WA: Amphetamine, haloperidol, and experience interact to affect the rate of recovery after motor cortex injury. *Science* 1982; 217:855–857.

19. Goldstein LB: Pharmacology of recovery after stroke. *Stroke* 1990; 21 (Suppl III):III-139–III-142.

20. Dunbar GL, Lescaudron LL, Stein DG: Comparison of GM1 ganglioside, AGF2, and D-amphetamine as treatments for spatial reversal and place learning deficits following lesions of the neostriatum. *Behav Brain Res* 1993; 54:67–79.

21. Irish SL, Davis GW, Barth TM: A specific behavioral role for norepinephrine in the recovery of locomotor placing following cortical lesions in the rat. *Soc Neurosci Abstr* 1995; 21:170.

22. Hovda DA, Feeney DM: Amphetamine with experience promotes recovery of locomotor function after unilateral frontal cortex injury in the cat. *Brain Res* 1984; 298:358–361.

23. Sutton RL, Hovda DA, Feeney DM: Amphetamine accelerates recovery of locomotor function following bilateral frontal cortex ablation in cats. *Behav Neurosci* 1989; 103:837–841.

24. Hurwitz BE, Dietrich WD, McCabe PM, Watson BD, Ginsberg MD, Schneiderman N: Amphetamine-accelerated recovery from cortical barrel-field infarction: Pharmacological treatment of stroke, in Ginsberg MD, Dietrich WD (eds): *Cerebrovascular Diseases: The Sixteenth Research (Princeton) Conference.* New York: Raven Press, 1989, pp. 309–318.

25. Stroemer RP, Kent TA, Hulsebosch CE: Amphetamines permanently promote recovery following cortical infarction. *Soc Neurosci Abstr* 1994; 20:186.

26. Feeney DM, Sutton RL: Catecholamines and recovery of function after brain damage, in Stein DG, Sabel BA (eds): *Pharmacological Approaches to the Treatment of Brain and Spinal Cord Injury.* New York: Plenum, 1988, pp. 121–142.

27. Feeney DM, Hovda DA: Reinstatement of binocular depth perception by amphetamine and visual experience after visual cortex ablation. *Brain Res* 1985; 342:352–356.

28. Hovda DA, Sutton RL, Feeney DM: Amphetamine-induced recovery of visual cliff performance after bilateral visual cortex ablation in cats: Measurements of depth perception thresholds. *Behav Neurosci* 1989; 103:574–584.

29. Braun JJ, Meyer PM, Meyer DR: Sparing of a brightness habit in rats following visual decortication. *J Comp Physiol Psych* 1986; 61:79–82.

30. Dunbar GL, Hecht SA, Merbaum SL, DeAngelis MM, Stein DG: Use of gangliosides and amphetamines to promote behavioral recovery following bilateral caudate nucleus lesions, in Masland RL, Portera-Sanchez A, Toffano G (eds): *Neuroplasticity: A New Therapeutic Tool in the CNS.* Padova: Liviana Press, 1987, pp. 117–124.

31. Colbourne F, Corbett D: Effects of *d*-amphetamine on the recovery of function following cerebral ischemic injury. *Pharmacol Biochem Behav* 1992; 42:705–710.

32. Innes IR, Nickerson M: Norepinephrine, epinephrine, and the sympathomimetic amines, in Goodman LS, Gilman AG, Gilman A, Koelle GB (eds): *The Pharmacological Basis of Therapeutics.* New York: Macmillan, 1985, pp. 477–513.

33. Mathew RJ, Wilson WH: Dextroamphetamine-induced changes in regional cerebral blood flow. *Psychopharmacology* 1985; 87:298–302.

34. McCulloch J, Harper AM: Cerebral circulatory and metabolism changes following amphetamine administration. *Brain Res* 1977; 121:196–199.

35. Moskowitz MA, Weiss BF, Lytle LD, Munro HN, Wurt-

man RJ: D-amphetamine disaggregates brain polysomes via a dopaminergic mechanism. *Proc Natl Acad Sci USA* 1975; 72:834–836.

36. Hovda DA, Bailey B, Montoya S, Salo AA, Feeney DM: Phentermine accelerates recovery of function after motor cortex injury in rats and cats. *Fed Am Soc Exp Biol* 1983; 42:1157.

37. Chen MJ, Sutton RL, Feeney DM: Recovery of function after brain injury in rat and cat: Beneficial effects of phenylpropanolamine. *Soc Neurosci Abstr* 1986; 12:881.

38. Feeney DM, Sutton RL: Pharmacotherapy for recovery of function after brain injury. *CRC Crit Rev Neurobiol* 1987; 3:135–197.

39. Kline AE, Flores TP, Tso-Olivas DY, Chen MJ, Feeney DM: Effects of methylphenidate on recovery from ablation-induced hemiplegia. *Soc Neurosci Abstr* 1988; 14: 1152.

40. Kline AE, Chen MJ, Tso-Olivas DY, Feeney DM: Methylphenidate treatment following ablation-induced hemiplegia in rat: Experience during drug action alters effects on recovery of function. *Pharmacol Biochem Behav* 1994; 48:773–779.

41. Fuxe K, Ungerstedt U: Histochemical, biochemical and functional studies on central monoamine neurons after acute and chronic amphetamine administration, in Costa E, Garattini S (eds): *Amphetamines and Related Compounds.* New York: Raven Press, 1970, pp. 257–288.

42. Goldstein LB, Coviello A, Miller GD, Davis JN: Norepinephrine depletion impairs motor recovery following sensorimotor cortex injury in the rat. *Restorative Neurol Neurosci* 1991; 3:41–47.

43. Boyeson MG, Callister TR, Cavazos JE: Biochemical and behavioral effects of a sensorimotor cortex injury in rats pretreated with the noradrenergic neurotoxin DSP-4. *Behav Neurosci* 1992; 106:964–973.

44. Boyeson MG, Krobert KA, Grade CM, Scherer PJ: Unilateral, but not bilateral, locus coeruleus lesions facilitate recovery from sensorimotor cortex injury. *Pharmacol Biochem Behav* 1992; 43:771–777.

45. Goldstein LB, MacMillan V: Acute unilateral sensorimotor cortex injury in the rat blocks d-amphetamine induced norepinephrine release in cerebellum. *Restorative Neurol Neurosci* 1993; 5:371–376.

46. Krobert KA, Sutton RL, Feeney DM: Spontaneous and amphetamine-evoked release of cerebellar noradrenaline after sensorimotor cortex contusion: An in vivo microdialysis study in the awake rat. *J. Neurochem* 1994; 62:2233–2240.

47. Boyeson MG, Feeney DM: Intraventricular norepinephrine facilitates motor recovery following sensorimotor cortex injury. *Pharmacol Biochem Behav* 1990; 35: 497–501.

48. Boyeson MG, Krobert KA: Cerebellar norepinephrine infusions facilitate recovery after sensorimotor cortex injury. *Brain Res Bull* 1992; 29:435–439.

49. Goldstein LB: Amphetamine-facilitated functional recovery after stroke, in Ginsberg MD, Dietrich WD (eds): *Cerebrovascular Diseases: Sixteenth Research (Princeton) Conference.* New York: Raven Press, 1989, pp. 303–308.

50. Goldstein LB, Poe HV, Davis JN: An animal model of recovery of function after stroke: Facilitation of recovery by an α_2-adrenergic receptor antagonist. *Ann Neurol* 1989; 26:157.

51. Feeney DM, Westerberg VS: Norepinephrine and brain damage: Alpha noradrenergic pharmacology alters functional recovery after cortical trauma. *Can J Psychol* 1990; 44:233–252.

52. Sutton RL, Feeney DM: α-Noradrenergic agonists and antagonists affect recovery and maintenance of beam-walking ability after sensorimotor cortex ablation in the rat. *Restorative Neurol Neurosci* 1992; 4:1–11.

53. Goldstein LB, Davis JN: Clonidine impairs recovery of beam-walking in rats. *Brain Res* 1990; 508:305–309.

54. Stephens J, Goldberg G, Demopoulos JT: Clonidine reinstates deficits following recovery from sensorimotor cortex lesion in rats. *Arch Phys Med Rehab* 1986; 67:666–667.

55. Hovda DA, Feeney DM, Salo AA, Boyeson MG: Phenoxybenzamine but not haloperidol reinstates all motor and sensory deficits in cats fully recovered from sensorimotor cortex ablations. *Soc Neurosci Abstr* 1983; 9:1002.

56. Van Hasselt P: Effect of butyrophenones on motor function in rats after recovery from brain damage. *Neuropharmacology* 1973; 12:245–247.

57. Hovda DA, Feeney DM: Haloperidol blocks amphetamine induced recovery of binocular depth perception after bilateral visual cortex ablation in the cat. *Proc West Pharmacol Soc* 1985; 28:209–211.

58. Davis JN, Arnett CD, Hoyler E, Stalvey LP, Daly JW, Skolnick P: Brain alpha-adrenergic receptors: comparison of [3H]WB4101 binding with norepinephrine-simulated cyclic AMP accumulation in rat cerebral cortex. *Brain Res* 1978; 159:125–135.

59. Peroutka SJ, U'Pritchard DC, Greenberg DA, Snyder SH: Neuropleptic drug interactions with norepinephrine alpha receptor binding sites in rat brain. *Neuropharmacology* 1977; 16:549–556.

60. Cohen BM, Lipinski JF: In vivo potencies of antipsychotic drugs in blocking alpha 1 noradrenergic and dopamine D2 receptors: Implications for drug mechanisms of action. *Life Sci* 1986; 39:2571–2580.

61. Boyeson MG, Harmon RL: Effects of trazodone and desipramine on motor recovery in brain-injured rats. *Am J Phys Med Rehab* 1993; 72:286–293.

62. Brailowsky S, Knight RT, Blood K: γ-aminobutyric acid-induced potentiation of cortical hemiplegia. *Brain Res* 1986; 362:322–330.

63. Schallert T, Hernandez TD, Barth TM: Recovery of function after brain damage: Severe and chronic disruption by diazepam. *Brain Res* 1986; 379:104–111.

64. Hernandez TD, Kiefel J, Barth TM, Grant ML, Schallert T: Disruption and facilitation of recovery of behavioral function; implication of the γ-aminobutyric acid/benzodi-

azepine receptor complex, in Ginsberg MD, Dietrich WD (eds): *Cerebrovascular Diseases: The Sixteenth Research (Princeton) Conference.* New York: Raven Press, 1989, pp. 327–334.

65. Moratalla R, Barth TM, Bowery NG: Benzodiazapine receptor autoradiography in corpus striatum of rat after frontal cortex lesion and chronic diazepam treatment. *Neuropharmacology* 1989; 28:893–900.

66. Hernandez TD, Schallert T: Long-term impairment of behavioral recovery from cortical damage can be produced by short-term GABA-agonist infusion into adjacent cortex. *Restorative Neurol Neurosci* 1990; 1:323–330.

67. Herenandez TD, Jones GH, Schallert T: Co-administration of Ro 15-1788 prevents diazepam-induced retardation of recovery of function. *Brain Res* 1989; 487:89–95.

68. Schallert T, Jones TA, Weaver MS, Shapiro LE, Crippens D, Fulton R: Pharmacologic and anatomic considerations in recovery of function. *Phys Med Rehab* 1992; 6:375–393.

69. Brailowsky S, Knight RT, Efron R: Phenytoin increases the severity of cortical hemiplegia in rats. *Brain Res* 1986; 376:71–77.

70. Chweh AY, Swinyard EA, Wolf HH: Involvement of a GABAergic mechanism in the pharmacologic action of phenytoin. *Pharmacol Biochem Behav* 1986; 24:1301–1304.

71. Hernandez TD, Holling LC: Disruption of behavioral recovery by the anti-convulsant phenobarbital. *Brain Res* 1994; 635:300–306.

72. Watson CW, Kennard MA: The effect of anticonvulsant drugs on recovery of function following cerebral cortical lesions. *J Neurophysiol* 1945; 8:221–231.

73. Goldstein LB, Coviello A: Post-lesion administration of the NMDA receptor antagonist MK-801 does not impair motor recovery after unilateral sensorimotor cortex injury in the rat. *Brain Res* 1992; 580:129–136.

74. Barth TM, Grant ML, Schallert T: Effects of MK-801 on recovery from sensorimotor cortex lesions. *Stroke* 1990; 21(suppl III):III-153–III-157.

75. Heale V, Harley C: MK-801 and AP5 impair acquisition, but not retention, of the Morris milk maze. *Pharmacol Biochem Behav* 1990; 36:145–149.

76. Ward AA, Jr., Kennard MA: Effect of cholinergic drugs on recovery of function following lesions of the central nervous system in monkeys. *Yale J Biol Med* 1942; 15: 189–228.

77. Hayes RL, Lyeth BG, Dixon CE, Stonnington HH, Becker DP: Cholinergic antagonist reduces neurologic deficits following cerebral concussion in the rat. *J Cereb Blood Flow Metab* 1985; 5(suppl 1):S395–S396.

78. Lyeth BG, Ray M, Hamm RJ, et al: Postinjury scopolamine administration in experimental traumatic brain injury. *Brain Res* 1992; 569:281–286.

79. Saponjic RM, Hoane MR, Barbay S, Barth TM: Scopolamine facilitates recovery of function following unilateral electrolytic sensorimotor cortex lesions in the rat. *Restorative Neurol Neurosci* 1995; 8:205–212.

80. De Ryck M, Duytschaever H, Janssen PAJ: Ionic channels, cholinergic mechanisms, and recovery of sensorimotor function after neocortical infarcts in rats. *Stroke* 1990; 21(suppl III):III-158–III-163.

81. Kasamatsu T, Pettigrew JD, Ary M: Restoration of visual cortical plasticity by local microperfusion of norepinephrine. *J Comp Neurol* 1979; 185:163–182.

82. Crow TJ: Cortical synapses and reinforcement: A hypothesis. *Nature* 1968; 219:736–737.

83. Stephens J: Effects of assistance, practice, and learning rate on recovery from sensorimotor cortex lesions in rats. *Soc Neurosci Abstr* 1986; 12:1285.

84. Stephens J: Rat model for studying recovery from brain injury: Training and assistance facilitate recovery. *Phys Ther* 1986; 66:781.

85. Goldstein LB, Davis JN: Post-lesion practice and amphetamine-facilitated recovery of beam-walking in the rat. *Restorative Neurol Neurosci* 1990; 1:311–314.

86. Goldstein LB, Davis JN: Beam-walking in rats: Studies towards developing an animal model of functional recovery after brain injury. *J Neurosci Meth* 1990; 31:101–107.

87. Goldstein LB: Pharmacologic modulation of recovery after stroke: Clinical data. *J Neurol Rehab* 1991; 5: 129–140.

88. Goldstein LB: Drugs and stroke recovery. *Neurology* 1996; 46:1187–1188.

89. Schwartz RD, Huff RA, Yu X, Carter ML, Bishop M: Postischemic diazepam is neuroprotective in the gerbil hippocampus. *Brain Res* 1994; 647:153–160.

90. Johansen FF, Diemer NH: Enhancement of GABA neurotransmission after cerebral ischemia in the rat reduces loss of hippocampal CA1 pyramidal cells. *Acta Neurol Scand* 1991; 84:1–6.

91. Schwartz RD, Yu X, Katzman MR, Hayden-Hixson DM, Perry JM: Diazepam, given postischemia, protects selectively vulnerable neurons in the rat hippocampus and striatum. *J Neurosci* 1995; 15:529–539.

92. Sternau LL, Lust WD, Ricci AJ, Ratcheson R: Role for γ-aminobutyric acid in selective vulnerability in gerbils. *Stroke* 1989; 20:281–287.

93. Smith AL, Hoff JT, Nielsen SL, Larson CP: Barbiturate protection in acute focal cerebral ischemia. *Stroke* 1974; 5:1–7.

94. Boxer PA, Cordon JJ, Mann ME, et al: Comparison of phenytoin with noncompetitive *N*-methyl-D-aspartate antagonists in a model of focal brain ischemia in the rat. *Stroke* 1990; 21(suppl III):III-47–III-51.

95. Lyden PD, Lonzo L: Combination therapy protects ischemic brain in rats: A glutamate antagonist plus a γ-aminobutyric acid agonist. *Stroke* 1994; 25:189–196.

96. Lyden PD, Hedges B: Protective effect of synaptic inhibition during cerebral ischemia in rats and rabbits. *Stroke* 1992; 23:1463–1470.

97. Lyden P, Lonzo L, Nunez S: Combination chemotherapy extends the therapeutic window to 60 minutes after stroke. *J Neurotrauma* 1995; 12:223–230.

98. Goldstein LB: Sygen in acute stroke study investigators: Common drugs may influence motor recovery after stroke. *Neurology* 1995; 45:865–871.

99. Blomqvist P, Lindvall O, Wieloch T: Lesions of the locus coeruleus system aggravate ischemic damage in the rat brain. *Neurosci Lett* 1985; 58:353–358.

100. Gustafson I, Westerberg E, Wieloch T: Protection against ischemia-induced neuronal damage by the α_2-adrenoceptor antagonist idazoxan: Influence of time of administration and possible mechanisms of action. *J Cereb Blood Flow Metab* 1990; 10:885–894.

101. Gustafson I, Miyauchi Y, Wieloch TW: Postischemic administration of idazoxan, an α_2 adrenergic receptor antagonist, decreases neuronal damage in the rat brain. *J Cereb Blood Flow Metab* 1989; 9:171–174.

102. Goldstein LB: Pharmacologic enhancement of recovery, in Good DC, Couch J (eds): *The Handbook of Neurorehabilitation.* New York: Marcel Dekker, 1994, pp. 343–369.

103. Goldstein LB: Basic and clinical studies of pharmacologic effects on recovery from brain injury. *J Neurol Transplant Plast* 1993; 4:175–192.

104. Katzman R, Clasen R, Klatzo I, Meyer JS, Pappius HM, Waltz AG: Report of Joint Committee for Stroke Resources. IV. Brain edema in stroke. *Stroke* 1977; 8: 512–540.

105. Dereski MO, Chopp M, Kight RA, Chen H, Garcia JH: Focal cerebral ischemia in the rat: temporal profile of neutrophil responses. *Neurosci Res Commun* 1992; 11: 179–186.

106. Bednar MM, Raymond S, McAuliffe T, Lodge PA, Gross CE: The role of neutrophils and platelets in a rabbit model of thromboembolic stroke. *Stroke* 1991; 22:44–50.

107. Feeney DM, Baron J-C: Diaschisis. *Stroke* 1986; 17: 817–830.

108. Kempinsky WH: Vascular and neuronal factors in diaschisis with focal cerebral ischemia, in Millikan CH (ed): *Research Publications: Association for Research in Nervous and Mental Disease,* vol. XLI. Baltimore: Williams & Wilkins, 1966, pp. 92–113.

109. Feeney DM: Pharmacologic modulation of recovery after brain injury: A reconsideration of diaschisis. *J Neurol Rehab* 1991; 5:113–128.

110. Jaspers RMA, Van Der Sprenkel JWB, Tulleken CAF, Cools AR: Local as well as remote functional and metabolic changes after focal ischemia in cats. *Brain Res Bull* 1990; 24:23–32.

111. Theodore DR, Meier-Ruge W, Abraham J: Microvascular morphometry in primate diaschisis. *Microvasc Res* 1992; 43:147–155.

112. Castella Y, Dietrich WD, Watson BD, Busto R: Acute thrombotic infarction suppresses metabolic activation of ipsilateral somatosensory cortex: Evidence for functional diaschisis. *J Cereb Blood Flow Metab* 1989; 9:329–341.

113. Feeney DM, Sutton RL, Boyeson MG, Hovda DA, Dail WG: The locus-coeruleus and cerebral metabolism: Recovery of function after cortical injury. *Physiol Psych* 1985; 13:197–203.

114. Lenzi GL, Frackowiak RSJ, Jones T: Cerebral oxygen metabolism and blood flow in human cerebral infarction. *J Cereb Blood Flow Metab* 1982; 2:321.

115. Martin WRW, Raichle ME: Cerebellar blood flow and metabolism in cerebral hemisphere infarction. *Ann Neurol* 1983; 14:168–176.

116. Fiorelli M, Blin J, Bakchine S, Laplane D, Baron JC: PET studies of cortical diaschisis in patients with motor hemineglect. *J Neurol Sci* 1991; 104:135–142.

117. Tanaka M, Kondo S, Hirai S, Ishiguro K, Ishihara T, Morimatsu M: Crossed cerebellar diaschisis accompanied by hemiataxia: A PET study. *J Neurol Neurosurg Psychiatr* 1992; 55:121–125.

118. Botez MI, Leveille J, Lambert R, Boetz T: Single photon emission computed tomography (SPECT) in cerebellar disease: Cerebello-cerebral diaschisis. *Eur Neurol* 1991; 31:405–412.

119. Pappata S, Mazoyer B, Dinh T, Cambon H, Levasseur M, Baron JC: Effects of capsular or thalamic stroke on metabolism in the cortex and cerebellum: A positron tomography study. *Stroke* 1990; 21:519–524.

120. Bowler JV, Wade JPH, Jones BE, et al: Contribution of diaschisis to the clinical deficit in human cerebral infarction. *Stroke* 1995; 26:1000–1006.

121. Infeld B, Davis SM, Lichtenstein M, Mitchell PJ, Hopper JL: Crossed cerebellar diaschisis and brain recovery after stroke. *Stroke* 1995; 26:90–95.

122. Pantano P, Formisano R, Ricci M, et al: Prolonged muscular flaccidity in stroke patients is associated with crossed cerebellar diaschisis. *Cerebrovasc Dis* 1993; 3:80–85.

123. Finger S, Stein DG: Behavioral compensation and response and cue theories, in *Brain Damage and Recovery.* New York: Academic Press, 1982, pp. 303–317.

124. Lashley KS: *Brain Mechanisms and Intelligence.* Chicago: University of Chicago Press, 1929.

125. Luria AR: *Restoration of Function after Brain Injury.* New York: Macmillan, 1963.

126. Luria AR: *Higher Cortical Functions in Man.* New York: Basic Books, 1966.

127. Wall PD: Mechanisms of plasticity of connection following damage in adult mammalian nervous systems, in Bachy-Rita P (ed): *Recovery of Function: Theoretical Considerations for Brain Injury Rehabilitation.* Baltimore: University Park Press, 1978, pp. 91–105.

128. Chollet F, DiPiero V, Wise RJS, Brooks DJ, Dolan RJ, Frackowiak RSJ: The functional anatomy of motor recovery after stroke in humans: A study with positron emission tomography. *Ann Neurol* 1991; 29:63–71.

129. Weiller C, Chollet F, Friston KJ, Wise RJS, Frackowiak RSJ: Functional reorganization of the brain in recovery from striatocapsular infarction in man. *Ann Neurol* 1992; 31:463–472.

130. Weiller C, Ramsay SC, Wise RJS, Friston KJ, Frackowiak RSJ: Individual patterns of functional reorganization in

the human cerebral cortex after capsular infarction. *Ann Neurol* 1993; 33:181–189.

131. Bliss TVP, Dolphin AC: What is the mechanism of long-term potentiation in the hippocampus? *TINS* 1982; 5:289–290.

132. Bliss TVP, Lomo T: Long-lasting potentiation of synaptic transmission in the dentate area of the anaesthetized rabbit following stimulation of the perforant path. *J. Physiol* 1973; 232:331–356.

133. Bliss TVP, Gardner-Medwin AR: Long-lasting potentiation of synaptic transmission in the dentate area of the unanaesthetized rabbit following stimulation of the perforant path. *J Physiol* 1973; 232:357–374.

134. Corbett D: Long term potentiation of lateral hypothalamic self-stimulation following parabrachial lesions in the rat. *Brain Res Bull* 1980; 5:637–642.

135. Artola A, Singer W: NMDA receptors and developmental plasticity in visual neocortex, in Collingridge GL, Watkins JC (eds): *The NMDA Receptor.* Oxford: Oxford University Press, 1989, pp. 153–166.

136. Aroniadou VA, Teyler TJ: The role of NMDA receptors in long-term potentiation (LTP) and depression (LTD) in rat visual cortex. *Brain Res* 1991; 562:136–143.

137. Keller A, Iriki A, Asanuma H: Identification of neurons producing long-term potentiation in the cat motor cortex: Intracellular recordings and labeling. *J Comp Neurol* 1990; 300:47–60.

138. Swanson LW, Teyler TJ, Thompson RF: Hippocampal long-term potentiation: Mechanisms and implications for memory. *Neurosci Res Prog Bull* 1982; 20:601–769.

139. Collingridge GL, Bliss TVP: NMDA receptors—their role in long-term potentiation. *TINS* 1987; 10:288–293.

140. Wenk GL, Grey CM, Ingram DK, Spangler EL, Olton DS: Retention of maze performance inversely correlates with *N*-methyl-D-aspartate receptor number in hippocampus and frontal neocortex in the rat. *Behav Neurosci* 1989; 103:688–690.

141. Benvenga MJ, Spaulding TC: Amnesic effect of the novel anticonvulsant MK-801. *Pharmacol Biochem Behav* 1989; 30:205–207.

142. Handelmann GE, Contreras PC, O'Donohue TL: Selective memory impairment by phencyclidine in rats. *Eur J Pharmacol* 1987; 140:69–73.

143. Morris RGM, Anderson E, Lynch GS, Baudry M: Selective impairment of learning and blockade of long-term potentiation by an *N*-methyl-D-aspartate receptor antagonist, AP5. *Nature* 1986; 319:774–776.

144. Stanton PK, Sarvey JM: Blockade of norepinephrine-induced long-lasting potentiation in the hippocampal dentate gyrus by an inhibitor of protein synthesis. *Brain Res* 1985; 361:276–283.

145. Dahl D, Sarvey JM: Norepinephrine induces pathway-specific long-lasting potentiation and depression in the hippocampal dentate gyrus. *Proc Natl Acad Sci USA* 1989; 86:4776–4780.

146. Hopkins WF, Johnston D: Frequency-dependent norad-renergic modulation of long-term potentiation in the hippocampus. *Science* 1984; 226:350–352.

147. Wigstrom H, Gustafsson B: Facilitation of hippocampal long-lasting potentiation by GABA antagonists. *Acta Physiol Scand* 1985; 125:159–172.

148. Douglas RM, Goddard GV, Riives M: Inhibitory modulation of long-term potentiation: Evidence for a postsynaptic locus of control. *Brain Res* 1982; 240:259–272.

149. Douglas RM, McNaughton BL, Goddard GV: Commissural inhibition and facilitation of granule cell discharge in fascia dentata. *J Comp Neurol* 1983; 219:285–294.

150. Olpe HR, Karlsson G: The effects of baclofen and two GABA B-receptor antagonists on long-term potentiation. *Naunyn Schmiedebergs Arch Pharmacol* 1990; 342:194–197.

151. Ito T, Miura Y, Kadokawa T: Effects of physostigmine and scopalamine on long-term potentiation of hippocampal population spikes in rats. *Can J Physiol Pharmacol* 1988; 66:1010–1016.

152. Williams S, Johnston D: Muscarinic depression of long-term potentiation in CA3 hippocampal neurons. *Science* 1988; 242:84–87.

153. Gold PE, Delanoy RL, Merrin J: Modulation of long-term potentiation by peripherally administered amphetamine and epinephrine. *Brain Res* 1984; 305:103–107.

154. Altman HJ, Quartermain D: Facilitation of memory retrieval by centrally administered catecholamine stimulating agents. *Behav Brain Res* 1983; 7:51–63.

155. Dietrich WD, Alonso O, Busto R, Ginsberg MD: Influence of amphetamine treatment on somatosensory function of the normal and infarcted rat brain. *Stroke* 1990; 21(suppl III):III-147–III-150.

156. Lister R: The amnesic action of benzodiazepines in man. *Neurosci Biobehav Res* 1985; 9:87–93.

157. Roth T, Roehrs T, Wittig R, Zorick F: Benzodiazepine and memory. *Br J Clin Pharmacol* 1984; 18(suppl):45S–49S.

158. Riches IP, Brown MW: The effect of lorazepam upon hippocampal long-term potentiation. *Neurosci Letts* 1986; S42–S40.

159. Satoh M, Ishihara K, Iwama T, Takagi H: Aniracetam augments, and midazolam inhibits, the long-term potentiation in guinea-pig hippocampal slices. *Neurosci Letts* 1986; 68:216–220.

160. Schallert T, Whishaw IQ: Bilateral cutaneous stimulation of the somatosensory system in hemidecorticate rats. *Behav Neurosci* 1984; 98:518–540.

161. Schallert T, Jones TA, Lindner MD: Multi-level transneuronal degeneration after brain damage: behavioral events and effects of GABAergic drugs. *Stroke* 1990; 21(suppl III):III-143–III-157.

162. Jones TA, Schallert T: Subcortical deterioration after cortical damage: Effects of diazepam and relation to recovery of function. *Behav Brain Res* 1992; 51:1–13.

163. Dahl D, Sarvey JM: β-Adrenergic agonist induced long-lasting synaptic modifications in hippocampal dentate gy-

rus require activation of NMDA receptors, but not electrical activation of afferents. *Brain Res* 1990; 526:347–350.

164. Held JM, Gordon J, Gentile AM: Environmental influences on locomotor recovery following cortical lesions in rats. *Behav Neurosci* 1985; 99:678–690.

165. Finger S, Stein DG: *Brain Damage and Recovery.* New York: Academic Press, 1982.

166. Davis JN: Neuronal rearrangements after brain injury: A proposed classification, in Becker DP, Povlishock JT (eds): *NIH Central Nervous System Trauma Status Report.* Washington, DC: National Institutes of Health, 1985, pp. 491–501.

167. Cotman CW, Nieto-Sampedro M, Harris EW: Synapse replacement in the nervous system of adult vertebrates. *Physiol Rev* 1981; 61:684–784.

168. Lund RD: *Development and Plasticity of the Brain.* New York: Oxford University, 1978.

169. Raisman G: Neuronal plasticity in the septal nuclei of the adult rat. *Brain Res* 1969; 14:25–48.

170. Raisman G, Field PM: A quantitative investigation of the development of collateral reinnervation after partial deafferentation of the septal nuclei. *Brain Res* 1973; 50:241–264.

171. Jones TA, Schallert T: Overgrowth and pruning of dendrites in adult rats recovering from neocortical damage. *Brain Res* 1992; 581:156–160.

172. Lipton SA: Growth factors for neuronal survival and process regeneration: Implications for the mammalian central nervous system. *Arch Neurol* 1989; 46:1241–1248.

173. Lipton SA, Kater SB: Neurotransmitter regulation of neuronal outgrowth, plasticity and survival. *TINS* 1989; 12:265–270.

174. Dawirs RR, Teuchert-Noodt G, Busse M: Single doses of methamphetamine cause changes in the density of dendritic spines in the prefrontal cortex of gerbils. *Neuropharmacology* 1991; 30:275–282.

175. Dawirs RR, Teuchert-Noodt G, Molthagen M: Indication of methamphetamine-induced reactive synaptogenesis in the prefrontal cortex of gerbils (Meriones unguiculatus). *Eur J Pharmacol* 1993; 241:89–97.

176. Clark ANG, Mankikar GD: d-Amphetamine in elderly patients refractory to rehabilitation procedures. *J Am Geriatr Soc* 1979; 27:174–177.

177. Fugl-Meyer AR, Jaasko L, Leyman I, Olsson S, Steglind S: The post-stroke hemiplegic patient. I: A method for evaluation of physical performance. *Scand J Rehab Med* 1975; 7:13–31.

178. Walker-Batson D, Smith P, Unwin H, et al: *Amphetamine Paired with Physical Therapy Accelerates Motor Recovery Following Stroke: Further Evidence.* 1992, Unpublished.

179. Reding MJ, Solomon B, Borucki SJ: Effect of dextroamphetamine on motor recovery after stroke. *Neurology* 1995; 45(suppl 4):A222.

180. Homan R, Panksepp J, Mcsweeny J, et al: d-Amphetamine effects on language and motor behaviors in a chronic stroke patient. *Soc Neurosci Abstr* 1990; 16:439.

181. Walker-Batson D, Unwin H, Curtis S, et al: Use of amphetamine in the treatment of aphasia. *Rest Neurol Neurosci* 1992; 4:47–50.

182. Porch B: *The Porch Index of Communicative Ability: Administration, Scoring, and Interpretation.* Palo Alto: Consulting Psychologists Press, 1981.

183. Johnson ML, Roberts MD, Ross AR, Witten CM: Methylphenidate in stroke patients with depression. *Am J Phys Med Rehab* 1992; 71:239–241.

184. Lazarus LW, Moberg PJ, Langsley PR, Lingam VR: Methylphenidate and nortriptyline in the treatment of poststroke depression: A retrospective comparison. *Arch Phys Med Rehab* 1994; 75:403–406.

185. Lazarus LW, Winemiller DR, Lingam VR, et al: Efficacy and side effects of methylphenidate for poststroke depression. *J Clin Psychiatr* 1992; 53:447–449.

186. Larsson M, Ervik M, Lundborg P, Sundh V, Svanborg A: Comparison between methylphenidate and placebo as adjuvant in care and rehabilitation of geriatric patients. *Comp Gerontol* 1988; 2:53–59.

187. Morris PLP, Raphael B, Robinson RG: Clinical depression is associated with impaired recovery from stroke. *Med J Aust* 1992; 157:239–242.

188. Reding MJ, Orto LA, Winter SW, Fortuna IM, Di Ponte P, McDowell FH; Antidepressant therapy after stroke: A double-blind trial. *Arch Neurol* 1986; 43:763–765.

189. Meyer JS, Miyakawa Y, Welch KMA, et al: Influence of adrenergic receptor blockade on circulatory and metabolic effects of disordered neurotransmitter function in stroke patients. *Stroke* 1976; 7:158–167.

190. Porch BE, Feeney DM: Effects of antihypertensive drugs on recovery from aphasia. *Clin Aphasiol* 1986; 16:309–314.

191. Albert ML, Bachman DL, Morgan A, Helm-Estabrooks N: Pharmacotherapy for aphasia. *Neurology* 1988; 38:877–879.

192. Bachman DL, Morgan A: The role of pharmacotherapy in the treatment of aphasia. *Aphasiology* 1988; 3–4:225–228.

193. Sabe L, Leiguarda R, Starkstein SE: An open-label trial of bromocriptine in nonfluent aphasia. *Neurology* 1992; 42:1637–1638.

194. Goldstein LB, Davis JN: Physician prescribing patterns after ischemic stroke. *Neurology* 1988; 38:1806–1809.

195. Goldstein LB: Prescribing of potentially harmful drugs to patients hospitalised following head injury. *J Neurol Neurosurg Psychiatr* 1995; 58:753–755.

196. Porch B, Wyckes J, Feeney DM: Haloperidol, thiazides, and some antihypertensives slow recovery from aphasia. *Soc Neurosci Abstr* 1985; 11:52.

197. Goldstein LB, Matchar DB, Morgenlander JC, Davis JN: The influence of drugs on the recovery of sensorimotor function after stroke. *J Neuro Rehab* 1990; 4:137–144.

198. The SASS Investigation: Ganglioside GM1 in acute ischemic stroke: The SASS trial. *Stroke* 1994; 25:1141–1148.

Chapter 33

NEUROPSYCHOLOGICAL ASSESSMENT

Neil H. Pliskin
Tanis J. Ferman
Maureen Lacy
Katherine C. Wood

Clinical neuropsychology is an applied science based on empirical research that examines the relationships between brain function and behavior. Neuropsychological assessment uses standardized, objective measurements to determine the presence, nature, and severity of cognitive decline. Reliability in administration between patients and across settings is obtained through standardization of the instruments, and the determination of cognitive decline is based on comparisons to normative samples and estimates of premorbid function.

Neuropsychology has its roots in the nineteenth century with behavioral neurology, and in the early twentieth century with psychological measurement of intelligence (for detailed historical accounts see Meier).[1] Following World War II, the first neuropsychological test battery, the Halstead-Reitan Battery, was relied on to localize the neuroanatomical site or hemisphere associated with neurologic change.[2,3] Over the years, testing patients with a variety of neurological insults and diseases has greatly contributed to our understanding of brain-behavior relationships.

With the development of advanced neuroimaging techniques such as magnetic resonance imaging (MRI) and positron emission tomography (PET), the role of the clinical neuropsychologist has broadened. Neuropsychologists now are commonly called on to determine whether there is functional (i.e., cognitive) disruption in association with radiologic or neurologic evidence of brain injury. Neuropsychological evaluations are also used to determine whether there is evidence of compromised brain function secondary to systemic disease or indirect neurologic injury related to conditions such as diabetes, organ failure, organ transplant (i.e., liver, heart, kidney, lung), chronic obstructive pulmonary disease, electrical injury, and exposure to environmental or industrial toxins.[4–8] Neuropsychological evaluations are also helpful in clarifying the impact of pharmacological treatments on neurocognitive status (e.g., prophylactic anticonvulsant treatment following brain injury). Questions of differential diagnosis also are addressed with neuropsychological evaluation since clusters or patterns of neuropsychological deficits have been identified for various neurologic syndromes. Examples of such disorders include cortical and subcortical dementia, postconcussion syndrome, depression, anxiety, alcoholic dementia, and amnesic disorders.[9–21]

In the rehabilitation setting, lesion localization and diagnosis usually are well established. Therefore, the rehabilitation neuropsychologist's role in the evaluation process is to help the treatment team formulate an individualized rehabilitation plan for the patient based on a clear understanding of cognitive strengths and limitations obtained through neuropsychological evaluation.[22–26] In this chapter, the role of the clinical neuropsychologist in the rehabilitation setting will be presented along with a detailed review of the neuropsychological evaluation process.

THE NEUROPSYCHOLOGICAL EVALUATION

In a rehabilitation setting, a comprehensive neuropsychological evaluation can play an active part in treatment, from admission to postdischarge. Admission status has been shown to be highly predictive of discharge status and long-term outcome.[27] Thus, on admission a screening of the patient's cognitive status can be important for preparing and assisting staff and family members in developing realistic expectations. As the rehabilitation process begins, a more comprehensive assessment can focus on examining individual strengths and weaknesses, taking into account premorbid cognitive and personality styles to create a truly individualized treatment plan. As the patient progresses, the neuropsychologist's use of standardized batteries, which allow for valid serial testing, can be useful in documenting subtle changes in cognitive, behavioral, and emotional functioning. Often testing by other disciplines fails to assess the equivalency of alternative test forms or take into account practice effects, resulting in inaccurate reporting of treatment gains. Obtaining objective measures of cognitive functioning during a hospital stay also can be useful when questioning changes in cognitive status on subsequent admission. Often patients return for treatment owing to new functional declines (e.g., series of falls). Subsequent test data may serve as a baseline to assess cognitive decline in the future. Standardized tests take into account age-related changes and thus are more sensitive to subtle cognitive changes that may reflect brain dysfunction, such as recent onset of dementia.

Neuropsychological assessments are also often useful in determining discharge planning. Understanding the patient's severity of memory and problem-solving deficits compared to age peers may be useful in determining placement issues or need for supervision of medications. Competency and guardian evaluations often should take into account neuropsychological status. Finally, discharge assessments can be useful in providing feedback to patients and family members regarding expectations about cognitive functioning and impact on daily living. Follow-up testing in 3 to 6 months can be useful in demonstrating continuing recovery, or failure to experience gains, which may signal medical or emotional complications. Postdischarge testing also can be useful when the patient is making decisions regarding returning to work or school and in designing compensation strategies.

A comprehensive evaluation includes assessment of general intellectual abilities and specific cognitive domains, along with addressing emotional and behavioral functioning. These components are described in the following.[28,29]

NEUROPSYCHOLOGICAL DOMAINS

Estimating Premorbid Intellectual Ability

Rehabilitation is focused on returning patients to their previous level of functioning. Thus, the neuropsychologist's first goal is to provide an estimation of the individual's premorbid capabilities and determine if a decline in cognitive functioning has occurred. With a reasonable estimation of the degree of cognitive impairment, realistic treatment goals can be developed.

Along with influencing goal setting, providing an estimation of a patient's premorbid abilities may limit inappropriate or frustrating interactions. Preinjury medical and psychiatric history, as well as preinjury cognitive, vocational, and interpersonal history, is important to determine when assessing for rehabilitation.[30] Without this knowledge, team members may view patients with developmental disabilities, learning disabilities, or lower-than-average IQs as exhibiting a decline in functioning. This is especially important to consider as patients with mild traumatic brain injury have a higher frequency of learning disability and poor school attainment than the general population.[31] Thus, in order to determine whether the patient has sustained a decline and therein formulate an appropriate treatment plan, it is important to determine whether the patient was in special education classes as a child or if he or she had developmental learning or behavioral difficulties (i.e., learning disability, attention deficit disorder). Expecting these patients to improve in areas of long-standing weaknesses may prove frustrating to the patient and staff. These patients may also be viewed as unmotivated and viewed negatively by staff. At the other end of the cognitive spectrum, team members may view patients with above-average intellectual abilities, who are suffering more-subtle higher-level deficits, as intact. Thus, these patients are at risk for missing needed services if the treatment team is unaware of the patient's premorbid functioning. Estimating premorbid intellectual abilities is one step in assessing if a change in cognitive functioning has occurred and when treatment should be pursued.

Since data from premorbid testing are rarely available, it is necessary to estimate premorbid capabilities. Several approaches are currently used in clinical practice. One method relies on interviews with patient and family members, along with reviewing school or occupational records. Another uses the verbal subtests on the Wechsler Adult Intelligence Scale, Revised (WAIS-R) that examine recall of overlearned factual information and vocabulary. These subtests are most resistant to brain changes and thus are valuable in estimating premorbid IQ. Although this is a reasonable and often-used method, it is important to note that patients with memory retrieval or verbal expression deficits will obtain underestimation of preinjury abilities using this approach. A third approach involves examining performance on reading tests of irregularly spelled words, which has been shown to correlate with intellectual function and tends to be most resilient to brain injury.[32,33] Again, underestimations can occur with patients who have a primary language deficit as in cases of moderate-to-severe dementia.[34] Sensitivity of such reading tests also tends to decline at the lower end of the intellectual scale. Finally, investigators have developed regression equations to calculate an estimated premorbid IQ.[35] The advantage to this method is that it is unaffected by the patient's current illness or psychological level of distress. Variables include age, gender, years of education, profession, rural or urban residence, and race.

Along with assessing premorbid cognitive ability, a comprehensive neuropsychological evaluation may also assess an individual's premorbid emotional functioning, coping style, and other personality traits. These data may be useful in predicting how a patient may react, adapt, and eventually cope with the demands of rehabilitation, including the series of successes and setbacks many patients experience during an inpatient stay and the often-long outpatient recovery period.

Intellectual Function

It is helpful to perform a full intellectual evaluation if possible, not only to obtain an indication of current function but because intellectual testing incorporates a broad range of verbal and visual skills. Beginning an evaluation with a test of intellectual abilities informs the neuropsychologist about how the patient negotiates a wide range of tasks, and provides the opportunity to develop hypotheses regarding spared and unspared skills.[28] The Wechsler Adult Intelligence Scale (WAIS-R) scales are most frequently used to provide an index of intellectual function. (IQ scores have an average of 100 and a standard deviation of 15 points.) Factor analyses have demonstrated that the subtests fall into three clusters of skills. There is the verbal comprehension factor, a perceptual-organization factor, and a freedom from distractibility factor. If the patient is grossly aphasic, administering the verbal subtests would clearly be unhelpful; however, administering the tasks of perceptual-organization and some of the freedom from distractibility tasks would be informative regarding level of function despite language impairments. Several subtests from the WAIS-R have been shown to correlate with rehabilitation gains in self-care, ambulation, and mobility.[22]

Underestimating and overestimating intellectual abilities can be frustrating for all concerned. Underestimating a patient's abilities may occur such that expectations may be below the patient's actual level. For exam-

ple, underestimating the comprehension of an aphasic who is alert to social cues and gestural communication can be extremely distressing to the patient, and may lead to excessive restriction of participation in chores or other activities. Acknowledging and allowing the patient to utilize the spared skills may serve to increase the patient's sense of internal control, sense of self-worth, and level of independence.

Conversely, overestimating a patient's abilities following a brain injury may occur. This may result in expectations that the patient can perform at a higher level than that of which he or she is capable at that point in time. This is frequently a problem following frontal lobe injury when the patient has recovered from the overt physical manifestations of the injury, or when time has shown minimal functional improvement. Neuropsychological deficits following damage to the frontal lobe are associated with problems with planning, organization, and initiation.[36] Often times such problems result in job loss, trouble carrying out apparently simple responsibilities at home, and interpersonal difficulties. The family (and even the patient) are baffled and frustrated by the catastrophic losses incurred by the injury, and may not understand why the patient appears to be so incapable of initiating projects or performing sequences of activities (e.g., using a microwave, putting dishes away) that he or she could once do. Neuropsychological evaluation is helpful in disentangling the role of cognitive, emotional, and motivational factors following brain injury. In this example, interventions that emphasize increasing structure, instruction, and practice regarding methods of planning, organizing, and sequencing may be helpful.

Attention and Concentration

There is no single construct of attention. Selective attention refers to the ability to orient to and focus on a specific stimulus, at the exclusion of other information. Vigilance is the ability to sustain attention while preparing to detect a target, whereas concentration is the ability to sustain attention once it is focused. Interference or distractibility is the capacity to be disengaged from current focus. Distractibility can be internal (e.g., worry, depression) or external (e.g., outside noise, bright lights). Immediate attention span is sometimes referred to as working memory, and refers to the amount of information one can attempt to hold onto after being exposed to it. Divided, or joint, attention refers to focusing on multiple stimuli simultaneously and shifting attention between them. Patients with traumatic brain injury show some variability depending on whether the injury was mild, moderate, or severe, but generally exhibit deficits in attention, as do patients who have suffered a stroke, regardless of hemisphere.[23] When patients are required to actively engage in multiple hours of therapy a day, any breakdown in attentional processing can adversely affect the treatment plan. A neuropsychological assessment should provide an understanding of the type of attentional deficit, when this deficit is most likely to prove problematic for the patient, and possible treatment strategies.

Learning and Memory

Memory is a complex set of subsystems and includes declarative and procedural, working memory, recent and remote memory, and conditioning.[37] Damage to the temporal lobes or mesial temporal structures including the hippocampus usually results in a memory deficit characterized by a loss of newly learned information, such as forgetting, failure to learn over repeated trials, and poor recall and recognition.[10,10a,38] This is the expected pattern of memory deficits following dementia of the Alzheimer type. Patients with damage to the subcortical, diencephalic structures, and frontal systems, commonly occurring in traumatic brain injury, demonstrate memory disorders that involve poor organization resulting in a less efficient learning strategy, susceptibility to interference, and greater difficulty with recall than recognition, indicating problems pulling the information out of memory storage.[10,10a,39,40]

Determining the patient's premorbid learning style is helpful, but often is not possible. In such cases, the years of education can provide some indication as to whether the individual is more likely to have an efficient or less efficient premorbid learning style. Neuropsychological assessment measures the patient's ability to acquire new information (encoding), store it, and retrieve the information from storage. Verbal and visual learning and memory tasks are provided in a neuropsychological evaluation. Verbal memory may involve remote memory for facts or incidents, rote memory for digits, immediate and delayed memory for word pairs, lists, or stories. Visual memory may involve rote memory for location; incidental memory for a complex figure; and immediate, delayed, and recognition memory for visual designs. Evaluation of memory can help lateralize deficits and assist in differentiating types of memory difficulties associated with damage to cortical versus subcortical or frontal systems. Some patients, especially those with marked brain injury involving arousal, may present with problems sustaining attention and there-

fore typically have problems encoding new information. In contrast, others may be able to encode the information (e.g., subcortical involvement, frontal involvement), but have difficulty with complicated retrieval of the information from memory. Still others (e.g., mesial temporal involvement) show adequate encoding, but poor recall and recognition, indicating a rapid rate of forgetting. Although most therapists working with patients may notice memory problems interfering with learning new information, a detailed evaluation of the different types (e.g., verbal vs. visual) and stages (i.e., encoding vs. retrieval) of memory functioning can assist in designing treatment strategies (e.g., using graphic illustrations instead of written or verbal material) and compensation techniques (e.g., mnemonic devices/approaches).

Language and Communication

The anterior language centers that govern expressive language are examined by assessing verbal expression of thoughts, reading aloud, writing, fluency (the capacity to generate words pertaining to a letter or category), rate of speech, and articulation. The posterior language centers that govern receptive language are examined by assessing verbal and written comprehension. Assessment for the various types of aphasia is most often completed by the team's speech pathologist, whereas a neuropsychologist often looks for more-subtle changes in language functioning, such as deficits that may reflect dysfunction in other cognitive domains (e.g., executive functions) and brain regions (e.g., frontal lobes). Also, the neuropsychologist examines reading and writing skills in the context of current intellectual abilities and scholastic history. It may be important for the team to recognize that a certain patient is reading at the fifth grade level and will not benefit from standardized written instructions. Alerting the team to such situations will facilitate selection of the approach most likely to succeed. In such a case, for example, the team may be advised to rely on demonstration rather than written descriptions of home exercises. Finally, patients with significant language dysfunction, especially those suffering from expressive aphasia, are more likely to experience depressive symptomatology. Thus, assessment of language functioning may assist in targeting patients who are in need of psychotherapy for depression management and treatment.

Visual Perceptual and Visual Spatial Skills

Higher-order visual abilities include perception and spatial skills. Deficits in higher-order visual skills are common after right hemisphere injury but may be less appreciated because they are not as obvious as hemiplegia or aphasia. Nonetheless, deficient visual perceptual or spatial abilities cause a wide range of problems affecting self-care (e.g., shaving, buttoning a shirt) and daily living (e.g., cooking). Such deficits also may raise safety issues as these skills are needed to take medications properly, use the stove or iron, and navigate an automobile. This information may be especially important for the occupational therapist. Visual skills also may interfere with occupational duties and social interactions. These visual skills may affect one's ability to type, read, scan for certain numbers, judge distance while stationary (or moving), and find an object or person in an array. Research has shown that perceptual functioning is a significant predictor of rehabilitation outcome.[41,42] Along with strict visual perceptual and spatial problems, patients may also exhibit right-left confusion, hemi-inattention, and perceptual organizational deficits. These deficits may underlie more-noticeable problem-solving difficulties.

Sensory Evaluation

Elementary evaluation of the senses is of tremendous importance and should not be overlooked. The neuropsychologist relies on careful observation and query of the patient and family members, and review of medical evaluations regarding hearing, vision, smell, taste, and tactile abilities. It is essential that the neuropsychologist differentiate between problems of elementary sensory experience and higher-order function. Tools such as the sensory-perceptual examination, Snellen chart, tactile form discrimination, or provision of olfactory samples are commonly used to determine sensory function.

Mild or moderate hearing loss may go undetected unless queried or tested and may cause misunderstanding between staff and patients. For example, peripheral hearing deficits may impede the recovery process because patients, especially geriatric adults, fail to hear instructions or techniques, but are ashamed or embarrassed to discuss this with their therapist. The therapist in turn may assume that the patient is suffering from comprehension or memory deficits and begin interacting accordingly with the patient.

Problems with tactile discrimination may result in problems manipulating objects that can affect self-care (e.g., fastening buttons)—information that may be especially important for the occupational therapist.

Altered sense of smell has significant safety consequences regarding the ability to smell smoke or detect spoiled food. In addition, altered sense of smell suggests

that there may be additional damage to the orbitofrontal cortex and serves as a flag for disinhibition, self-monitoring deficits, and distractibility.[36] Alerting the treatment team to prepare for these potential deficits and how they may interfere with therapy may speed the recovery progress.

Visual acuity deficits are of marked importance because such problems could be mislabeled as perceptual or constructional deficits, which have different treatment implications. Assessing for extinction provides one opportunity to address whether the patient exhibits unilateral sensory neglect or hemi-inattention, which is the lack of attention to contralateral hemispace.[43] This has obvious implications regarding environmental manipulation and therapeutic intervention.

Motor Speed, Dexterity, and Grip Strength

The speed by which the hands can manipulate objects, write, or tap provides not only information regarding each hemisphere, but also speed of information processing. Motor speed measures have been identified as an important factor for postinjury employment outcome for patients with head injury and patients with epilepsy.[44] Although most neuropsychological evaluations will contain some elementary assessment of motor function, this area typically is addressed more extensively by the rehabilitation physician and occupational therapist.

EXECUTIVE FUNCTION

Executive functions refers to a broad group of skills including problem solving, planning and organization, altering behavior in response to the environment, drive, initiating activities, dividing attention, and mental flexibility. Impairments in executive functions commonly are associated with damage to the frontal lobes, which frequently occurs in closed head injuries.[45] Deficits in executive function are frustrating and may lead to problems in organizing oneself to carry out seemingly simple activities (e.g., making bed, washing clothes). Moreover, deficits in executive function are least understood or appreciated by family members or friends, who may view the patient as lazy, unmotivated, or depressed.

Awareness and self-monitoring are important components of executive function as well. Unawareness of one's disease state or cognitive deficit is a particularly important issue and a common manifestation of brain injury, particularly injury sustained to the right hemisphere or frontal lobe.[46] Unawareness can pose safety problems when activities are attempted (e.g., cooking, driving) that they are no longer capable of performing. Unawareness of problems with more-complex social skills may result in interpersonal difficulties, frustration for the patient and family, and possibly isolation. Patients with traumatic brain injury may overestimate their competency in social interactions and emotional control.[47] Such patients may also fail to engage in or benefit from rehabilitation when they do not appreciate the deficits.

Subtle deficits in executive functions may not be noticed on a rehabilitation unit, as the day-to-day functioning often becomes very routine, with the same therapies and therapist, at the same time each day. At times, these deficits may become apparent only when the person attempts to reintegrate into his or her family life and previous employment position. Thus, executive function is an important consideration in treatment planning and outcome. Heinemann et al. found, for example, that impaired problem solving and abstraction were predictive of functional outcome, length of stay, and the need for increased outpatient therapies and home services.[48] Neuropsychological assessment can detect these subtle deficits and thus prepare the patient and family for possible functional difficulties. Followup testing may be useful in assisting patients in deciding when to return to work and developing necessary compensation strategies.

Emotional and Personality Assessment

Emotional factors, including depression and anxiety, can influence cognitive performance and length of hospital stay.[18,49] Although there is much disagreement about the etiology of postconcussion syndrome, persisting postconcussion symptoms after minor or mild head injury may stem from psychological causes and personality style.[13,23,50–52] Persons who are highly driven and whose sense of self is tightly associated with intellectual pursuit and achievement are at risk for a catastrophic breakdown following a mild traumatic brain injury.[23] Other vulnerable premorbid personality styles include individuals with a tendency to be dependent, insecure, or grandiose, or have chaotic interpersonal relationships.[53]

Along with premorbid personality traits, damage to the brain can cause personality and emotional changes that affect recovery. For example, Rapport and colleagues found that behavioral impulsivity in right stroke patients predicted fall status and speed of rehabilitation. Impulsivity and personality disturbance following frontal lobe damage is especially common in brain-injured patients.

A neuropsychologist is a fully trained clinical psychologist who utilizes the clinical interview and formal tests of mood and personality to assess emotional status. In a rehabilitation setting, the evaluation of current and long-standing emotional and personality variables can prove very useful in predicting areas that may be problematic and designing effective treatment plans. However, administration of these psychological tests should be carried out with knowledge that neurologically relevant items may produce a particular pattern of performance in patients with brain injury.[55–57]

TEST SELECTION AND TIME MANAGEMENT

A proper neuropsychological evaluation integrates current and premorbid assessment and historical information. Neuropsychological test batteries, when constructed properly, assess a broad range of functions. Given the constraints of time and cost, it is necessary to be expeditious and to choose tests carefully for maximum amount of information. The range of behaviors and backgrounds for any single patient is varied, and although there are patterns associated with various neurologic syndromes, a proper neuropsychological assessment does not rely exclusively on testing, and conclusions are not derived on the basis of a single test score. Administration time may range from 2 to 8 hours, depending on the breadth of the battery. An inpatient assessment usually includes a general screening evaluation to assess general cognitive functioning. Over the course of rehabilitation, specific tests are then used to address possible areas of weaknesses and document progress. Outpatient batteries typically are more comprehensive and may be directed at specific questions, such as return to work, or etiology (i.e., psychologically or organically based).

Observation During Testing

A great deal of clinical information can be derived from examining how the patient derives solutions during test and the types of errors that are made.[58] Patients with frontal injury may demonstrate stimulus-boundedness or perseverative behavior, which has implications regarding the patient's capacity to shift attentional set. Visual problem-solving strategies that emphasize details first or the global contours of the design first have implications not only for diagnosis but for treatment. Right-hemisphere–damaged patients are more likely to break the overall pattern in a visual construction task, whereas left-hemisphere–damaged patients are more likely to miss the individual features.[59–60] Behavioral observations of test-taking behavior provide valuable information about tolerance for frustration, ability to adapt, and ability to profit from mistakes. Data concerning how the individual responds to success or failure are crucial, and provide predictive information as to which situational demands will be tolerable and which will be excessive.

WHAT TO EXPECT BACK

The Report

Report styles vary depending on the nature and extent of assessment. Comprehensive reports typically contain identifying patient information, referral question and presenting complaint, background information, mental status examination, results of testing by domain, summary, and impressions and recommendations. Brief assessments frequently omit the background information and detailed results section, but include the impressions and recommendations.

Impressions

Impressions include whether the pattern of cognitive capabilities is consistent with what would be expected given the patient's age, education, and estimated premorbid capabilities. Information regarding whether the pattern is consistent with known medical, psychiatric, or neurologic illness, including the effects of medication, should be presented.

The neuropsychological impressions section should also clearly explain the nature of the cognitive deficits. For example, distinctions in memory failure may occur at the stage of encoding, retention of information across time, or retrieval from memory. This information has important treatment implications. Specifically, patients with dementia of the Alzheimer type may show adequate immediate attention and encoding, but a rapid forgetting rate following a delay. In contrast, a patient with multiple subcortical infarcts may show mild attention impairment and mild retention problems, but difficulty retrieving the information from memory storage.

The impressions section should also summarize the patterns of strengths as well as weaknesses, and coincident emotional factors (e.g., depression or post-traumatic stress disorder), or mitigating personality variables present prior to the trauma (e.g., long-standing coping skills, social support) and following the trauma (e.g., self-awareness, depression).

Recommendations

The recommendations section includes suggestions regarding program implementation and communication with the patient, and also may include recommendations for medical consultation in various areas, if not already considered (e.g., radiologic imaging, medication consultation, psychiatric consultation, vision or hearing tests). Specifically, this section of the report is directed at providing treatment strategies that address the patient's cognitive, behavioral, and emotional functioning. Recommendations that address cognitive functioning often capitalize on the patient's strengths and assist in developing compensation strategies for weaknesses. Behavioral interventions often include addressing aggression and noncompliance by behavioral analysis and contracting with the team and the patient. Recommendations addressing emotional functioning include strategies for depression and anxiety management. Treatment of depression has been shown to facilitate speed of recovery in a rehabilitation setting.[61] Other areas that can be addressed in this section include academic and work functioning; activities of daily living; capacity to live independently, manage finances, and drive; social and interpersonal skills; verbal and nonverbal communication; safety; personality factors; competency issues; self-awareness; and match of skill level and personal and vocational goals.[30]

Specific recommendations may include suggestions of modified work schedules or work environment, or graduated work program or work hardening. Suggestions regarding living arrangements may refer to level of independence, assistance, adult day care, or structured living arrangements. Important environmental alterations may be addressed, including ways to organize the household for best cognitive maneuverability and factors concerning safety. Suggestions regarding ways to facilitate communication also may be provided. Type or level of intervention that is most likely to be successful, and the goals to be attained also should be provided in a neuropsychological assessment for rehabilitation. Suggestions regarding modality and means by which to improve the success of interpersonal therapy that may be most beneficial to the patient may be presented. For example, a patient with memory difficulties can utilize writing and monitoring to facilitate expression and recall of events in and out of the therapy room. Therapy for skills building can be facilitated from the neuropsychological evaluation, such as pain management, coping skills, social skills, and self-monitoring skills.

ADDITIONAL ACTIVITIES OF THE NEUROPSYCHOLOGIST IN THE REHABILITATION SETTING

Education: Patient, Family, and Staff

Neuropsychologists can serve as educational resources for patients, families, and staff members. Neuropsychologists should be involved in the delivery of information to the staff, patient, and family in the form of team meetings or educational support groups.

It is important for the patient to have factual information about his or her functioning in order to set realistic goals. It is important for this education not to be overlooked, but to be done in a manner that respects each individual's reaction to such knowledge. If not carried out in a careful manner, such information could create a catastrophic reaction of its own and worsen the patient's capacity to function.

Patients who present with behavioral changes following a brain injury are frequently baffling to both staff and family members, and this may result in substantial misunderstandings of the patient's level of motivation or interest in improving his or her level of functioning. The neuropsychologist's role in educating staff and family about neurobehavioral changes may be the crucial component in assisting this oftentimes-difficult population, leading to frustration on behalf of the staff, family, and patient alike. Interventions that emphasize clearly outlined rules and structure may help the patient to self-regulate. The clinical neuropsychologist is in a position to provide the patient and staff with ways to cope with problematic outbursts or aggressive behavior that uphold respect for the patient. The provision of external structure, patience, and behavioral techniques may help the family and staff members contain their own frustration with the patient's distress and noncompliance.

Therapy

The clinical neuropsychologist is in a unique position to combine knowledge of neurologic and neuropsychologic impairment with clinical psychology's tools of supportive psychotherapy. Therapy with a brain-injured patient should emphasize empathic and unconditional acceptance, and full recognition and acknowledgement of the grief and loss the brain-injured patient is experiencing. The brain-injured patient can suffer a disruption of self-identity, and may feel overwhelmed, out of control, and unable to screen out and make sense of the demands placed on him or her. The clinical neuropsychologist should recognize that cognitive and physical limitations may be confusing and humiliating, or that ability to self-reflect or self-monitor behavior may be impaired.

With growing cognitive awareness, many brain-injured patients often undergo a process of mourning that initially involves emotional shock or denial, followed by depression, eventually leading to acceptance, resolution, and adaptation.[61] Issues of blame, guilt, shame, and feelings of being punished are not uncommon after brain injury, and these feelings should be validated and openly discussed. At times, these patients may be viewed as unmotivated by the treatment team. The neuropsychologist can play a crucial role by explaining to the team how the patient's rebellion against some aspect of treatment may reflect intrapsychic needs, such as a chance to regain some control over his or her life.[62]

Alerting the treatment team to signs of learned helplessness, where the patient begins to feel he or she has no control over recovery, may be especially important. To counteract this reaction, therapists should be advised to create situations in which the patient experiences success and comfort, therein providing some reinforcement and a sense of having some control over the future. As a member of the rehabilitation team, the neuropsychologist is aware that providing structure in therapy with brain-injured patients is especially important.

Setting reasonable personal goals that are attainable and appropriate can facilitate the patient's sense of improvement and sense that he or she has some control over his or her life, rather than being a helpless victim of external forces. Information obtained from the neuropsychological evaluation, such as attention and concentration capacity, ability to learn new information presented verbally, deductive and inductive reasoning skills, and the patient's ability to benefit from feedback are pertinent aspects of therapy that can facilitate rapport and help designate the appropriate level of psychotherapy for the brain-injured patient. For example, if a patient has trouble rapidly shifting from one concept to another, then therapy can be structured in such a manner that progression into a new area is gradual. This factor may limit how many new areas are addressed in one session, or how many aspects of a therapeutic theme should be addressed at one time. It also can be discussed with the patient, who can be made more aware regarding how it feels when he or she is trying to shift mental set, and it may lessen frustration if the patient is able to recognize it when it happens.

The neuropsychologist as therapist will be knowledgeable of the patient's cognitive limitations and can modify techniques of therapy to suit the patient's needs. For example, a patient with memory difficulties can utilize techniques of writing to facilitate recall of events in therapy. Additionally, some psychotherapeutic techniques that emphasize keeping notes and monitoring one's experiences, emotions, and thoughts may be employed by the neuropsychologist doing therapy. Other tools that utilize recordkeeping can be helpful for the patient. This is particularly useful for the patient with retrieval deficits, who is better able to recall past events and experiences when cued.

Ultimately, the clinical neurophysiologist devises strategies for the patient and treatment team to promote adaptive behavior that fosters independence and enhancement of quality of life.

REFERENCES

1. Meier M: Modern clinical neuropsychology in historical perspective. *Am Psychol* 1992; 47(4):550–558.
2. Halstead W: *Brain and Intelligence*. Chicago: University of Chicago Press, 1947.
3. Reitan R: Investigation of the validity of Halstead's measure of biological intelligence. *Arch Neurol Psychiatr* 1955; 73:28–35.
4. Adrian J, Crankshaw D, Tiller J, & Stanley R: Affective, cognitive and subjective changes in patients undergoing cardiac surgery: A preliminary report. *Anaesth Int Care* 1988; 16:144–149.
5. Barclay L, Weiss E, Mattis S, Bond O, Blass J: Unrecognized cognitive impairment in cardiac rehabilitation patients. *J Am Ger Soc* 1988; 36:22–28.
6. Hart R, Kreutzer J: Renal system, in Tarter R, Van Thiel D, Edwards L (eds): *Medical Neuropsychology: The Impact of Disease on Behavior*. New York: Plenum Press, 1988, pp. 99–120.
7. Pliskin N, Meyer G, Dolske M, Heilbronner R, Kelley K, Lee R: Neuropsychiatric aspects of electrical injury: A review of neuropsychological research from Electrical injury: A multidisciplinary approach to therapy, prevention and rehabilitation. *Ann NY Acad Sci* 1994; 720:219–223.
8. Reinvang I, et al: *J Neurol Neurosurg Psychiatr* 1994; 57:614–616.
9. Delis D, Massman P, Butters N, Salmon D: Profiles of demented and amnesic patients on the California Verbal Learning Test: Implications for the assessment of memory disorders. *J Consult Clin Psychol* 1991; 3(1):19–26.
10. Troster A, Jacobs D, Butters N, Cullum M, Salmon D: Differentiating Alzheimer's disease from Huntington's disease with the Wechsler Memory Scale, Revised. *Clin Ger Med* 1989; 5(3):611–632.
10a. Troster AI, Butters N, Salmon DP, Cullum CM, Jacobs D, Brandt J, White RF: The diagnostic utility of saving scores: differentiating Alzheimer's and Huntington's diseases with logical memory and visual reproduction tests. *J Clin Exp Neuropsychol,* 1993; 15(5), 773–788.
11. Alves W, Colohan A, O'Leary T, Rimel R, Jane J: Understanding post-traumatic symptoms after minor head injury. *J Head Trauma Rehab* 1986; 1:1–12.
12. Binder L: Persisting symptoms after mild head injury: A review of the postconcussive syndrome. *J Clin Exp Neurol* 1986; 8:323–346.
13. Youngjohn J, Burrows L, Erdal K: Brain damage or compensation neurosis? The controversial post-concussion syndrome. *Clin Neuropsychol* 1995; 9(2):112–123.
14. Boone K, et al: Cognitive functioning in older depressed outpatients: Relationship of presence and severity of depression to neuropsychological test scores. *Neuropsychology* 1995; 9(3):390–398.
15. Jones R, Tranel D, Benton A, Paulsen J: Differentiating dementia from "Pseudodementia" early in the clinical course: Utility of neuropsychological tests. *Neuropsychology* 1992; 6(1):13–21.
16. Lamberty G, Bieliauskas L: Distinguishing between depression and dementia in the elderly: A review of neuropsychological findings. *Arch Clin Neuropsychol* 1993; 8:149–170.
17. Massman P, Delis D, Butters N, Dupont R, Gillin J: The subcortical dysfunction hypothesis of memory deficits in depression: Neuropsychological validation in a subgroup of patients. *J Clin Exp Neuropsychol* 1992; 14(5):687–706.
18. Gass C: MMPI-2 variables in attention and memory test performance. *Psychol Assess* 1996; 8(2):135–138.
19. Davila M, Shear P, Lane B, Sullivan E, Pfefferbaum A: Mammillary body and cerebellar shrinkage in chronic alcoholics: An MRI and neuropsychological study. *Neuropsychology* 1994; 8(3):433–444.
20. Butters N, Delis D, Lucas J: Clinical assessment of memory disorders in amnesia and dementia. *Annu Rev Psychol* 1995; 46:493–523.
21. Parkin A: Amnesic syndrome: A lesion-specific disorder? *Cortex* 1984; 20:479–508.
22. Heaton R, Pendleton M: Use of neuropsychological tests to predict adult patients' everyday functioning. *J Consult Clin Psychol* 1981; 49(6):807–821.
24. Kay T, Silver S: The contribution of neuropsychological evaluation to the vocational rehabilitation of the head injured adult. *J Head Trauma Rehab* 1988; 3:65–76.
25. Klonoff P, Costa L, Snow W: Predictors and indicators of quality of life in patient with closed head injury. *J Clin Exp Neuropsychol* 1986; 8:469–485.
26. McSweeny A, Grant I, Heaton R, Prigatano G, Adams K: Relationship of neuropsychological status to everyday functioning in healthy and chronically ill persons. *J Clin Exp Neurol* 1985; 7:281–291.

27. Alexander, MP: Stroke rehabilitation outcome: A potential use of predictive variables to establish levels of care. *Stroke* 1994; 25:128–134.

28. Spreen O, Strauss E: *A Compendium of Neuropsychological Tests.* New York: Oxford University Press, 1991.

29. Lezak M: *Neuropsychological Assessment.* New York: Oxford University Press, 1995.

30. Bergquist T, et al: Neuropsychological rehabilitation: Proceedings of a consensus conference. *J Head Trauma Rehab* 1994; 9(4):50–61.

31. Dicker B: Profile of those at risk for minor head injury. *J Head Trauma Rehab* 1992; 7:83–91.

32. Blair J, Spreen O: Predicting premorbid IQ: A revision of the national adult reading test. *Clin Neuropsychol* 1989; 3(2):129–136.

33. Nelson HE, O'Connell A: Dementia: The estimation of premorbid intelligence levels using the National Adult Reading Test. *Cortex* 1978; 14:233–244.

34. Stebbins GT, et al: Use of the National Adult Reading Test to estimate premorbid IQ in dementia. *Clin Neuropsychol* 1990; 4:64–68.

35. Barona A, Reynolds CR, Chastain R: A demographically based index of premorbid intelligence for the WAIS-R. *J Consult Clin Psychol* 1984; 52:885–887.

36. Stuss D, Gow C, Hetherington C: "No longer Gage": Frontal lobe dysfunction and emotional changes. *J Consult Clin Psychol* 1992; 60(3):349–359.

37. Butters N, Wolfe J, Martone M, Granholm E, Cermak L: Memory disorders associated with Huntington's disease: Verbal recall, verbal recognition, and procedural memory. *Neuropsychologia* 1985; 23:729–743.

38. Moss M, Albert M, Butters N, Payne M: Differential patterns of memory loss among patients with Alzheimer's disease, Huntington's disease, and alcoholic Korsakoff's syndrome. *Arch Neurol* 1986; 43:239–246.

39. Mangels J, Gershberg F, Shimamura A, Knight R: Impaired retrieval from remote memory in patients with frontal lobe damage. *Neuropsychology* 1996; 10(1):32–41.

40. Helkala E, Laulumaa V, Soinninen H, Riekkinen P: Recall and recognition memory in patients with Alzheimer's and Parkinson's disease. *Ann Neurol* 1988; 24:214–217.

41. Wade DT, Skillbeck CE, Langston HR: Predicting Barthel ADL score at 6 months after acute stroke. *Arch Phys Med Rehab* 1983; 64:24–28.

42. Andrews K, Brocklehurst JC, Richards B, Laycock PJ: The recovery of severely disabled stroke patients. *Rheumatol Rehab* 1982; 21:225–230.

43. Heilman K, Watson R, Valenstein E: Neglect and related disorders, in Heilman K, Valenstein E (eds): *Clinical Neuropsychology,* 3rd ed. New York: Oxford University Press, 1993, pp. 279–336.

44. Dikman S, Morgan SF: Neuropsychological factors related to employability and occupational status in persons with epilepsy. *J of Nervous and Mental Disorders* 1980; 168(4):236–240.

45. Levin HS, Eisenberg HM, Benton AL: *Frontal Lobe Func-* *tion and Dysfunction.* New York: Oxford University Press, 1991.

46. Anderson S, Tranel D: Awareness of disease states following cerebral infarction, dementia and head trauma: Standardized assessment. *Clin Neuropsychol* 1989; 3(4):327–339.

47. Prigatano G: Behavioral limitations TBI patients tend to underestimate: A replication and extension to patients with lateralized cerebral dysfunction. *Clin Neuropsychol* 1996; 10(2):191–201.

48. Heinemann AW, Linacre JM, Wright BD, Hamilton BB, Granger C: Prediction of rehabilitation outcomes with disability measures. *Arch Phys Med Rehab* 1994; 75:133–143.

49. Gass C: Emotional variables and neuropsychological test performance. *J Clin Psychol* 1991a; 47:153–157.

50. Jacobson RR: The post-concussional syndrome: Physiogenesis, psychogenesis, and malingering. An integrative model. *J Psychosomatic Research* 1995; 39(6):675–693.

51. Binder LM, Rohling ML: Money matters: A metaanalytic review of effects of financial incentives on recovery after closed head injury. *Am J Psychiatry* 1996; 153(1):7–10.

52. Middleboe T, Anderson HS, Birket-Smith M, Friis ML: Minor head injury: Impact on general health after 1 year. A prospective follow-up study. *Acta Neurologica Scandinavia* 1992; 85(1):5–9.

53. Kay T, Newman B, Cavallo M, Ezrachi O, Resnick M: Toward a neuropsychological model of functional disability after mild traumatic brain injury. *Neuropsychology* 1992; 6:371–384.

54. Rapport LJ, Webster JS, Flemming KL, Lindberg JW, Godlewski MC, Brees JE, Abadee PS: Predictors of falls among right hemisphere stroke patients in the rehabilitation setting. *Arch Phys Med Rehab* 1993; 74(6):621–626.

55. Alfano D, Finlayson M, Stearns G, Neilson P: The MMPI and neurologic dysfunction: Profile configuration and analysis. *Clin Neuropsychol* 1990; 4(1):69–79.

56. Wooten A: MMPI profiles among neuropsychology patients. *J Clin Psychol* 1983; 39:392–406.

57. Gass C: MMPI-2 interpretation and closed head injury: A correction factor. *J Consult Clin Psychol* 1991b; 3(1):27–31.

58. Kaplan E: A process approach to neuropsychological assessment, in Boll T, Bryant E (eds): *Clinical Neuropsychology and Brain Function: Research, Measurement and Practice.* Washington DC: American Psychological Association, 1988, pp. 129–167.

59. Ben-Yishay Y, et al: Neuropsychological rehabilitation: Quest for a holistic approach. *Semin Neurol* 1985; 5:252–259.

60. Kramer J, Kaplan E, Blusewicz M, Preston K: Visual hierarchical analysis of block design configural errors. *J Clin Exp Neuropsychol* 1991; 13(4):455–465.

61. Lazarus LW, Moberg PJ, Lansley PR, Lingam VR: Methylphenidate and nortriptyline in the treatment of poststroke depression: A retrospective comparison. *Arch Phys Med Rehab* 1994; 75:403–406.

Chapter 34

BEHAVIORAL AND PHARMACOLOGICAL MANAGEMENT OF BRAIN INJURY

Andrew Hornstein
Glenn M. Seliger

Disturbances of cognition and behavior are well recognized sequelae to traumatic brain injury (TBI). They are a prominent part of the symptomatology of nearly all patients referred to acute TBI rehabilitation units, and can range from the global unresponsiveness of the coma patient to the subtle but potentially devastating impairments of demeanor in patients with frontal lobe syndromes.[1] The clinical management of these disturbances is a challenging but critically important aspect of the neurorehabilitation of the TBI patient. In the months and years following an acute traumatic brain injury, residual cognitive and behavioral deficits are the most frequent cause for the failure to return to premorbid levels of vocational and interpersonal functioning.[2] In acute rehabilitation settings, disturbances of behavior such as aggression, impulsivity, apathy, and distractibility can markedly interfere with, and at times preclude, therapeutic interventions such as physical, occupational, or speech therapies. Thus disturbances of behavior can keep a TBI patient from achieving a level of recovery one might otherwise expect. Timely and effective management of behavioral disturbances can have a profound effect on clinical outcome.

GENERAL PRINCIPLES

There has been a marked paucity of systematic, placebo-controlled studies of the medications used to treat the cognitive and behavioral disturbances in TBI patients. The clinical utility and long-term side effects of medications in this population remain uncertain. Consequently, it is our practice to avoid pharmacological interventions if at all possible, and to utilize the variety of behavioral

techniques outlined below. However, if nonpharmacological interventions prove obviously ineffective in curtailing maladaptive behaviors or cognitive impairments, or if a patient's behavior puts him or her at imminent risk of injuring him- or herself or others, we do not hesitate to attempt a trial of medication management. With any therapy, but especially with pharmacological interventions, it is important to have clear, specific target symptoms and therapeutic end points. This can help minimize the number and dosage of medications to which patients are exposed, and thus minimizes the risk of adverse events.

MANAGEMENT OF PATIENTS WITH PERSISTENT UNCONSCIOUSNESS

Behavioral and therapeutic interventions are limited for this population. Sensory stimulation programs are frequently attempted, but their efficacies are uncertain. During the last decade, there has been increasing interest in trying pharmacologic agents to shorten or end the persistent unconsciousness of TBI patients. In general, the majority of TBI patients who remain in a state of persistent unconsciousness remain so because of severe shearing of axons, leading to a deafferentation of connections to the cortical gray matter.[3] In particular, there may be a great deal of parasagittal white matter shearing of axons transporting catecholamines from brain stem nuclei to the cortex, leading to a relative noradrenergic and dopaminergic deafferentation of frontal lobe structures.[4] A number of animal studies have demonstrated that augmentation of the catecholamine systems may result in improved neurologic functioning after brain injury.[5] There have been uncontrolled case reports of stimulants such as methylphenidate and dextroamphetamine shortening the length of coma in TBI patients.[6] Despite the lack of controlled studies, it has been common practice in many head injury rehabilitation programs to attempt a trial of a stimulant medication in persistently unconscious patients. It is our opinion that this is a reasonable therapeutic intervention, given the poor prognosis for this group of patients and the long and well-established safety of judiciously used stimulants. However, it is imperative that multicenter controlled studies be organized to determine which TBI patients, if any, benefit from such treatment.

When using stimulants, dexedrine is a good first choice, beginning at 2.5 mg per day, increasing every 1 to 2 days in 2.5-mg increments. We generally titrate the dose to a maximum of 20 mg per day in two divided doses, usually given in the morning and early afternoon. Reversible hypertension is the only significant side effect, though tachycardia and arrhythmias can occur infrequently. In elderly patients, ritalin can be used. It has fewer cardiovascular side effects than dexedrine. An initial dose of ritalin 5 mg a day is recommended, titrating the medication up to a maximum dose of 30 mg per day, usually in two or three divided doses. If there has been no clinical improvement after a few days on ritalin or dexedrine, both medications can be tapered or discontinued. In patients who respond to psychostimulants, a clinical response can persist even after the stimulant is tapered and stopped.

MANAGEMENT OF THE ACUTELY AGITATED PATIENT

Patients emerging from coma secondary to diffuse axonal injury often experience a significant period of agitated encephalopathy. Behaviors may include thrashing about, rocking, shouting, combativeness, removal of intravenous or feeding lines, motor restlessness, throwing any object at hand, and, if the patient is ambulatory, wandering about the hospital.[1,7] Agitated behavior needs to be quickly evaluated and treated to keep the patient from bringing harm to him- or herself or others.

The absence of a consistent operational definition of agitation makes it difficult to accurately determine its frequency in TBI patients and its correlation with the post-traumatic amnesia that commonly occurs after patients regain consciousness. Some authors have described post-traumatic agitation as a natural part of the recovery from closed head injury.[8] Preliminary evidence

suggests that agitation and restlessness during recovery portend a better outcome, but this has not been replicated.[9]

Trzepacz describes post-traumatic agitation as being part of the delirium that patients with significant TBI commonly experience at some point during their recovery.[10] Her analysis of the clinical descriptions and clinical course of post-traumatic amnesia closely overlaps the cognitive deficits and neuropsychiatric symptoms of delirium (Table 34-1). This formulation has the potential for clinical utility, by applying the well-established guidelines for the treatment of delirium owing to general medical or neurologic conditions to acutely agitated TBI patients.

Delirium is a common sequela for a multitude of insults to the central nervous system. It is often exacerbated by sensory deprivation, overstimulation, or pain. The identification and remediation of factors exacerbating post-traumatic delirium are the first and most important steps in managing agitation in patients emerging from coma. For example, an unrecognized or untreated source of pain can easily cause a confused and aphasic patient to become agitated. A careful examination for such things as previously unrecognized fractures, constipation, soft tissue injury, joint subluxations, heterotropic ossification, and reflex sympathetic dystrophy is essential. When a pain source is identified, the cause should be remedied, if possible, and appropriate analgesics used. In general, TBI patients tolerate narcotic analgesics prescribed for severe pain well. Oxycodone is preferred over acetaminophen with codeine or other narcotics because it is less constipating. Painful constipation is a common cause of agitation in those recovering from head injury, despite the prophylactic use of bulk laxatives. Aggressive bowel regimens, such as daily use of bulk laxatives and suppositories, may be required.

Delirium can be exacerbated by nearly any infectious or metabolic disturbance. Autonomic instability and temperature dysregulation that can occur as a result of brain injury can make early recognition of infectious causes of agitation difficult.[11] Careful assessment for

Table 34-1.
Cognitive deficits in delirium

Disorientation	Deficits in higher-order thinking
Attentional deficits	Visuoconstructional dysfunction
Memory defects	

Note: Some or all deficits may occur.

occult respiratory, urinary tract, or blood-borne pathogens may be especially rewarding. Postoperative infections in those who have undergone placement of a ventriculoperitoneal shunt, open reduction of a fracture, gastrostomy, or central or peripheral intravenous catheters are common. Low serum albumin and electrolyte imbalance, particularly the syndrome of inappropriate secretion of antidiuretic hormone, are common causes of delirium.

Many medications commonly used in those recovering from brain injury, including antiepileptic agents, anticholinergics, and antispasticity agents, are well known to have central nervous system side effects, often leading to agitation and delirium. Those with central nervous system depression are especially sensitive to the neurobehavioral side effects of medication. Every effort should be made to avoid unnecessary medication, and monitor therapeutic levels when possible of any agent that has the potential to lead to an altered mental state.

The initial step in actively managing acute posttraumatic agitation involves manipulating the patient's environment to minimize the fear and distress experienced as a result of the cognitive impairment and disorientation. Staff should be trained to maintain a calm, reassuring, sympathetic demeanor. Continual patient reorientation should be emphasized by having all staff consistently address patients by name and by repeatedly identifying themselves, their title, and their function. Clear and succinct explanations about the purpose of hospitalization and the nature of the recovery process are essential. The great majority of agitated patients can be engaged and calmed by caring professionals. The constant, one-on-one presence of concerned family members, friends, or staff is often very effective in calming agitated patients, especially when combined with orienting information, empathy, and reassurance. Such supervision is also important for preventing the patient from injuring him- or herself. For the significant majority of agitated patients, this phase of recovery is time limited. The intensive utilization of staff time in constant, one-on-one supervision of agitated patients is the most reasonable first step for behavior management before more restrictive, and possibly toxic, interventions, such as restraints or medications, are tried.

Confused and forgetful patients often experience separation anxiety, especially when they do not recall visits by loved ones. Family photographs posted on the wall of the patient's room, log books in which visitors sign in and leave personal messages, and even videotapes of visits can reassure patients and reduce agitation.

A window as a source of natural daylight can be helpful in reestablishing a normal sleep–wake cycle. Prominently posted clocks and calendars help maintain orientation. A quiet, consistent, personalized environment may be difficult to maintain in a busy hospital setting, but can be, nonetheless, a significant factor in reducing agitation.

Despite the best efforts of a committed nursing staff, many patients require some form of physical restraint to keep them from wandering away from the hospital or from possibly injuring themselves or others. This is especially true for patients with a history of alcohol abuse.[12] A spectrum of restraining techniques should be available, ranging from more to less restrictive, in order to allow patients the maximum degree of freedom consistent with their safety. Graduated, increasing degrees of freedom can also serve to reinforce adaptive, nonagitated behavior, just as increasing restraint can negatively reinforce relapses of agitated behavior. Typical restraining techniques commonly used include four-point soft restraints, full posey vest, and wheelchair seat belts.

Confused, wheelchair-bound patients can be kept from leaving their designated areas or from entering other patients' rooms by fitting their wheelchairs with attendant-controlled extension rods that are fastened to the chair backs. When extended, and when used with attendant-controlled seat belts, the rods prevent passage through doorways without supervision. Confused, ambulatory patients can be fitted with light, unobtrusive bracelets that set off an alarm when they attempt to leave designated areas.

The use of physical restraints is not without risks. Reports of injury and death from hyperthermia and strangulation have surfaced recently.[13] Nonetheless, with appropriate safety protocols and very frequent monitoring, such risks can be minimized.

Those who have emerged successfully from postcoma agitation can experience temporary relapse, often as part of a "catastrophic reaction" when overly challenged or stimulated.[14] When agitation or aggression become intermittently persistent, special interventional measures may be required. For most patients, supportive attention from a well-trained empathetic staff will ease overwhelming fear and frustration. Periods of "time out," with patients gently separated from others until they regain control of their behavior, can be used to effectively reinforce appropriate behavior while reducing overstimulation. These periods can range from the least-disruptive "nonexclusionary time out," in which patients remain within sight of others, to having the patient stay in a quiet room with close staff supervision. Use of safe, well-padded "isolation rooms," has been useful for agitated patients, but bureaucratic constraints can prevent their use in some parts of the country.[15]

Patients at risk of hurting themselves or others while acutely agitated must be quickly physically restrained by well-trained staff. During this process, clear gentle communications and reassurance are essential. Release from restraint must be predicated on a return to equanimity. From a strategic standpoint, de-escalation of agitated behavior can be encouraged by reinforcing patient involvement in behavioral management. Agitation often is a consequence of lost independence, dignity, and self-esteem. Patient participation in the management and decision-making process, with agreement on clear limits and consequences, is essential. Formal behavior-modification programs have been described as being effective in specifically designed neurobehavioral units. In the acute rehabilitation setting, where lengths of stay are relatively brief, formal behavior-modification protocols are cumbersome. For the vast majority of patients, the most effective reinforcement for adaptive behavior change is the attention and approval of family, friends, and staff.

If agitation cannot be controlled by nonpharmacological means, and precludes participation in rehabilitation, medication should be considered. Given that postcoma agitation is, for most patients, self-limited, brief courses of low-dose sedatives are effective. Good short-term results with high-potency neuroleptics such as haloperidol can be achieved when given orally, intramuscularly, or intravenously.[16] Side effects are kept to a minimum by the use of very low starting doses, with the dose titrated upward as needed. However, even with conservative dosing, side effects, such as akathisia, dystonia, excess sedation, and parkinsonian rigidity, can occur. Anticholinergic effects, such as urinary retention, gastrointestinal hypomotility, hypohidrosis with hyperthermia, and memory impairment, are also important to recognize.

There is literature suggesting that major tranquilizers that have alphameninergic and dopminergic blocking properties may worsen outcome in brain injury.[17] The newer neuroleptic risperdone is reported to have a more benign side effect profile, especially in low dosages.[18] The risk of side effects, such as neuroleptic malignant syndrome, must always be considered in the therapeutic decision-making process.

The major tranquilizer class of medications seems to work best when there is reasonably well-formed psychiatric symptomatology, such as paranoid delusions. Brief intervention with benzodiazepines can be effective in relieving agitation, with a side effect profile that compares favorably to the neuroleptics. However, benzodiazepines have been reported to worsen delirium and impair cognition.[10] Lorazepam is the agent of choice both for its relatively brief half life and its effectiveness in both oral and intramuscular forms.

Animal studies have described both neuroleptics and benzodiazepines as interfering with learning in brain-injured animals.[5] Given the critical importance of verbal and procedural learning in rehabilitation, the use of sedating agents should be kept to a minimum. Amantadine, a dopamine agonist, has been described as effective in reducing agitation in over 50 percent of those emerging from post-traumatic coma, and appears to have a relatively benign side effect profile.[18] Nonpharmacologic approaches to patients with persisting agitation or aggression will be discussed in the following.

MANAGEMENT OF PATIENTS IN ACTIVE REHABILITATION

Typically, recovery from brain trauma is characterized by spontaneous improvement in agitation. A period of post-traumatic amnesia, however, can persist for days or weeks. During this period, patients begin to recall their circumstances. They become increasingly aware of having sustained an injury, of being in a hospital, and of having to participate in various therapeutic activities. Recall of personal information, such as names of family members, gradually improves, as does day-to-day memory of hospital routines and staff. This phase of recovery corresponds to levels V and VI on the Rancho los Amigos scale, confused-inappropriate and confused-appropriate.[19] With significant structuring, patients in this phase can fully participate in a comprehensive cognitive and physical rehabilitation program.

A broad range of problematic behaviors can occur during this phase, jeopardizing recovery. The classification proposed by Eames remains a heuristically useful way of organizing maladaptive post-traumatic behaviors (Table 34-2).[20] Among the active behavior disorders, impulsive and disinhibited behaviors are the most common. Traumatic brain injuries are most commonly caused by violent acceleration-deceleration of the head, which typically causes shear injury to the orbitofrontal cortex and basal temporal lobe as they abrade against the base of the skull.[21] The orbitofrontal cortex appears to play a critical role in the assignment of emotional

Table 34-2.

Descriptive classification of behavioral disorders after brain injury

Active
  Aggressive
    Habitual
    "Short fuse"
    Explosive
    Malicious
  Impulsive
  Disinhibited
  Antisocial

Passive
  Insightless
  Driveless
  Abulic (lacking in motivation)
  Slow (a pervasive slowness)
  Anhedonic

Syndromal
  Manipulative
  Manipulative and dissociative ("hysterical")
  Ritualistic or obsessive-compulsive
  Cyclothymic
  Fantasizing or confabulating
  Paranoid

---

salience to external and internal stimuli.[22,23] Damage to this part of the brain appears to cause difficulties in modulating affective responses to both internal and external stimuli. Damage to these structures can cause profound motivational blunting, leading to passive behavior disorders listed by Eames. On the other hand, gross overreaction to external or internal stressors, sometimes referred to as a catastrophic reaction, is common after injury to the basal forebrain. Normal reactions to internal stimuli such as hunger, physical discomfort, interpersonal irritation, or sexual tension can be amplified to the level of urgency and insistence that totally disregards social norms or the needs of others.

A minority of those with brain injury display overtly aggressive behavior, either in the context of an explosive dyscontrol or rage directly attributable to the brain injury, or a premorbid antisocial personality organization. It is well established that a pattern of premorbid alcohol abuse is more common in the brain-injured than the population at large.[24] Premorbid antisocial personality disorders or attention-deficit disorders are also more highly represented in the brain-injured than the general population. Such individuals, already "disinhibited" from the perspective of empathic, socially attuned

behavior, can be highly problematic when further disinhibited by a brain injury. The management of negativistic and aggressive behavior can pose unique challenges to comprehensive rehabilitation management.

The nonpharmacological techniques for managing posttraumatic behavior disturbances can be generally categorized into three groups, behavioral, interpersonal, and psychodynamic. There is evidence from both animal and human studies that procedural and associative learning is preserved, even after extensive damage to cortical structures.[25] This fact, together with the demonstration that brain-injured patients can successfully apply learned procedures to novel, "real-life" situations, supports the use of behavior modification techniques.[26] The principles of classical and operant conditioning have been applied to well-described and, in ideal circumstances, quantified maladaptive behaviors for many years in brain injury rehabilitation.[27-29] Even those with intractable behavioral disturbances, such as uncontrollable rage attacks or consistent negativity toward rehabilitation care, have been treated with some success in specialized, long-term, closed units wherein nearly all behavior can be monitored, assessed, and subjected to either positive or negative reinforcers.[30]

Most acute rehabilitation facilities, with patients often requiring active medical care, and located in hospital settings that preclude locked doors are not suitable for formal, carefully structured behavior modification programs. However, as with the acutely agitated patient just emerging from coma, reinforcement of adaptive behavior and extinction of aggressive or impulsive behavior can often be achieved.[31] The importance of clear, consistent, enthusiastic praise by staff cannot be overstated as a reinforcer of desired behavior. Patients slowly recovering from posttraumatic encephalopathy and amnesia find themselves in a highly unstable, unfamiliar, and constricted world. Relationships with health professionals provide an indispensable link with reality and normalcy. Explicit, frequent approval can be a potent source of a subjective sense of well being and progress. Positive reinforcers also can be used to improve communication in abulic patients, attention to specified task in distractible patients, and tolerance of painful physical therapy procedures by confused patients with poor insight into their medical condition. The absence of consistent praise can be a potent negative reinforcer of undesired behavior. These simple behavior modification techniques can be highly effective, especially when patients and their families are taught to identify the antecedents of negative behaviors and utilize them to regain control.[32]

The interpersonal psychodynamic approach to behavioral management requires patients to be active participants in the setting of their rehabilitation goals.[33,34] Impaired insight often limits the extent of active involvement and decision making. Passive, negativistic, or overtly hostile behavior can result from organic denial of illness (anosognosia), leading to failure to engage in rehabilitation treatment. Patient feedback, repeated often in a supportive manner, is helpful in improving compliance in some. Others may need to "try and fail" before seeing the need for and submitting to a structured rehabilitation program.

Psychodynamic approaches to behavioral disturbances early in the rehabilitation process are of limited use, primarily because of impaired memory and limited recall for the content of therapeutic interactions. The empathetic identification of functional (and often financial and personal) losses, the gentle management of regressive behavior, and the assessment and mobilization of premorbid adaptive psychologic resources can help minimize maladaptive behaviors.[35-38] Recognition and treatment of alcohol and substance abuse should begin as soon as possible.[39]

Intermittent aggressive behavior can be managed with propanolol.[40] Valproic acid and carbamezipine have also been reported to be useful.[41,42] Tricyclic antidepressants, selective serotonin reuptake inhibitors, and buspirone are also described as helpful.[43-46] Carefully controlled trials will be needed in the future to determine which agent is most effective. At the present time, medication for rage and aggression is given on an empiric basis.

REFERENCES

1. Levin HS, Grossman RG: Behavioral sequelae of closed head injury. *Arch Neurol* 1978; 35:720–727.
2. Rosenthal M, Bond MR: Behavioral and psychiatric sequelae, in Rosenthal M, Griffith ER, Bond MR, Miller JD (eds): *Rehabilitation of the Adult and Child With Traumatic Brain Injury.* Philadelphia: F.A. Davis, 1990.
3. Teasedale G, Mendelow D: Pathophysiology of head injuries, in Brooks N (ed): *Closed Head Injury: Psychological, Social, and Family Consequences.* Oxford: Oxford University Press, 1984.
4. Hayes RL, Lyeth BG, Jenkins LW: Neurochemical mechanisms of mild and moderate head injury: Implications for treatment, in Levin HS, Eisenberg HM, Benton AL (eds): *Mild Head Injury.* New York: Oxford University Press, 1989.
5. Feeney DM, Sutton RL: Pharmacotherapy for recovery of function after injury. *CRC Crit Rev Neurobiol* 1987; 3:135–197.
6. Hornstein A, Lennihan L, Seliger G, Lichtman S, Schroeder K: Amphetamine in recovery from brain injury. *Brain Injury* 1996; 10(2):145–148.
7. Brooke MM, Questad KA, Patterson DR, Bashak KJ: Agitation and restlessness after closed head injury: A prospective study of 100 consecutive admissions. *Arch Phys Med Rehab* 1992; 73:320–323.
8. Gualtieri CT: *Neuropsychiatry and Behavioral Pharmacology.* New York: Springer-Verlag, 1991, p. 17ff.
9. Reyes RL, Bhattacharyya AK, Heller D: Traumatic head injury: Restlessness and agitation as prognosticators of physical and psychological improvement in patients. *Arch Phys Med Rehab* 1981; 62:20–23.
10. Trzepacz PT: Delirium, in Silver JM, Yudofsky SC, Hales RE (eds): *Neuropsychiatry of Traumatic Brain Injury.* Washington, DC: American Psychiatric Press, 1994.
11. Chaney RH, Olmstead CE: Hypothalamic dysthermia in persons with brain damage. *Brain Injury* 1994; 8(5): 475–481.
12. Edlund MJ, Goldberg RJ, Morris PLP: The use of physical restraints in patients with cerebral contusion. *Int J Psychiatr Med* 1991; 21(2):173–182.
13. Berrol S: Risk of restraints in head injury. *Arch Phys Med Rehab* 1988; 69:537–538.
14. Goldstein K: *The Organism.* New York: Zone Books, 1995.
15. DeChancie H, Walsh JM, Kessler LA: An enclosure for the disoriented head-injured patient. *J Neurosci Nurs* 1987; 19;341.
16. Silver JM, Yudofsky SC: Aggressive disorders, in Silver JM, Yudofsky SC, Hales RE (eds): Neuropsychiatry of Traumatic Brain Injury. Washington, DC: American Psychiatric Press, 1994.
17. Gualtieri CT: *Neuropsychiatry and Behavioral Pharmacology.* New York: Springer-Verlag, 1991, p. 19.
18. Schatzberg AF, Nemeroff CB: *The American Psychiatric Press Textbook of Psychopharmacology.* Washington, DC: American Psychiatric Press, Inc., 1995.
19. Professional Staff Association of the Rancho los Amigos Hospital: *Rehabilitation of the Head Injured Adult.* Palm Springs, CA: Professional Staff Association of the Rancho los Amigos Hospital, Inc., 1980.
20. Eames P: Behavior disorders after severe head injury: Their nature and causes and strategies for management. *J Head Trauma Rehab* 1988; 3(3):1–6.
21. Cassidy JW: Neuropathology, in Silver JM, Yudofsky SC, Hales RE (eds): *Neuropsychiatry of Traumatic Brain Injury.* Washington, DC: American Psychiatric Press, Inc., 1994.
22. Mesulam MM, Mufson EJ: Insula of the old world monkey: Architectonics in the insulo-orbito-temporal component of the paralimbic brain. *J Comp Neurol* 1982; 212: 1–22.
23. Zald DH, Kim SW: Anatomy and function of the orbital frontal cortex, I: Anatomy, neurocircuitry, and obsessive-

compulsive disorder. *J Neuropsychiatr Clin Neurosci* 1996; 8:125–138.

24. Smith GS, Kraus JF: Alcohol and residential, recreational, and occupational injuries: A review of the epidemiological evidence. *Am J Public Health* 1988; 79:99–121.

25. Oakley DA: Learning capacity outside neocortex in animals and man: Implications for therapy after brain injury, in Davey GCL (ed): *Animal Models of Human Behavior.* London: John Wiley & Sons, 1983.

26. Lloyd LF, Cuvo AJ: Maintenance and generalization of behaviours after treatment of persons with traumatic brain injury. *Brain Injury* 1994; 8(6):529–540.

27. Fussey I, Cumberpatch J, Grant C: The application of a behavioral model in rehabilitation, in Fussey I, Giles, GM (eds): *Rehabilitation of the Severely Brain Injured Adult.* London, Croom Helm, 1988.

28. Wood RL, Burgess PW: The psychological management of behaviour disorders following brain injury, in Fussey I, Giles GM: *Rehabilitation of the Severely Brain Injured Adult.* London: Croom Helm, 1988.

29. Corrigan PW, Jakus MR: Behavioral treatment, in Silver JM, Yudofsky SC, Hales RE (eds): *Neuropsychiatry of Traumatic Brain Injury.* Washington, DC: American Psychiatric Association Press, 1994.

30. Eames P, Wood R: Rehabilitation after severe brain injury: A follow-up study of a behaviour modification approach. *J Neurol Neurosurg Psychi* 1985; 48:613–619.

31. Eames P, Haffey WJ, Cope DN: Treatment of behavioral disorders, in Rosenthal M, Griffith ER, Bond MR, Miller JD (eds): *Rehabilitation of the Adult and Child With Traumatic Brain Injury.* Philadelphia: F.A. Davis Co., 1990.

32. Uomoto JM, Brockway JA: Anger management training for brain injured patients and their family members. *Arch Phys Med Rehabil* 1992; 73:674–679.

33. Bergquist TF, Jacket MP: Awareness and goal setting with the traumatically brain injured. *Brain Injury* 1993; 7(3):275–282.

34. McGann W, Werven G: Social competence and head injury: A new emphasis. *Brain Injury* 1995; 9(1):93–102.

35. Lewis L: A framework for developing a psychotherapy treatment plan with brain-injured patients. *J Head Trauma Rehabil* 1991; 6(4):22–29.

36. Drubach D, McAlaster R, Hartman P: The use of a psychoanalytic framework in the rehabilitation of patients with traumatic brain injury. *Am J Psychoanalysis* 1994; 54(3):255–263.

37. Prigatano GP: Psychotherapy after brain injury, in Prigatano GP (ed): *Neuropsychological Rehabilitation after Brain Injury.* Baltimore: The Johns Hopkins University Press, 1986.

38. Pollack IW: Individual psychotherapy, in Silver JM, Yudofsky SC, Hales RE (eds): *Neuropsychiatry of Traumatic Brain Injury.* Washington, DC: American Psychiatric Association Press, 1994.

39. Kramer TH, Hoisington D: Use of AA and NA in the treatment of chemical dependencies of traumatic brain injury survivors. *Brain Injury* 1992; 6(1):81–88.

40. Yudofsky SC, Silver JM, Schneider SE: Pharmacologic treatment of aggression. *Psychiatr Ann* 1987; 17:397–407.

41. Giakas WJ, Seibyl JP, Mazure CM: Valproate in the treatment of temper outbursts. *J Clin Psychiatry* 1990; 51:525.

42. Folks DG, King LD, Dowdy SB, et al: Carbamazepine treatment of selective affectively disordered inpatients. *Am J Psychiatry* 1982; 139:115–117.

43. Szlabowicz JW, Stewart JT: Amitriptyline treatment of agitation associated with anoxic encephalopathy. *Arch Phys Med Rehab* 1990; 71:612–613.

44. Coccaro EF, Astill JL, Herbert JL, et al: Fluoxetine treatment of impulsive aggression in DSM-III-R personality disorder patients. *J Clin Psychopharmacol* 1990; 10:373–375.

45. Gualtieri CT: Buspirone for the behavior problems of patients with organic brain disorders. *J Clin Psychopharmacol* 1991; 11:280–281.

46. Hass JF, Cope N: Neuropharmacologic management of behavior sequelae in head injury: A case report. *Arch Phys Med Rehab* 1985; 66:474–474.

Chapter 35

DIAGNOSIS AND TREATMENT OF SPATIAL NEGLECT

Anjan Chatterjee
Mark Mennemeier

Unilateral spatial neglect is one of the most striking disorders of cognition. Patients with neglect are profoundly impaired, and the presence of neglect bodes ill for functional recovery. In this chapter we review the phenomenology, assessment, neural and theoretical underpinnings, recovery, and rehabilitation of neglect. Recognizing the multifaceted nature of neglect is necessary to appreciate the complexity of neglect rehabilitation. A clear understanding of the disorder will help guide rehabilitation interventions.

PHENOMENOLOGY

Patients with spatial neglect act as though entire regions of space contralateral to their brain lesions have vanished from existence. These patients do not orient toward, respond to, or act on meaningful stimuli in contralateral space.[1] They may also neglect stimuli in ipsilateral space, but contralateral neglect is more pronounced. It is common for these patients to appear lethargic in the first few days after brain damage. They often lie in bed with their head and eyes deviated ipsilaterally. They seem unaware of objects on the contralateral side of their environment. They may only eat food on the ipsilateral side of their plate. Despite being able to hear sound emanating from contralateral space, they may search ipsilaterally for its source. When ambulating, or navigating a wheelchair, they may hit contralateral objects, or take circuitous routes to their destination.

In the early stages, patients may neglect parts of their own body and deny ownership of their contralateral limb. When dressing, they may not clothe the contralateral side. They may fail to groom (comb, shave, apply make-up to) their body contralateral to their brain lesion. Occasionally, rather than denying ownership of the contralateral side of their body, neglect patients may express an intense dislike of these affected side.[2] Despite being functionally devastated, these patients often appear unconcerned or peculiarly resigned to their condition.

Neglect is more common and severe after right- than left-hemisphere damage.[3–5] In this chapter, neglect will refer to left-sided neglect. Analogous right-sided symptoms sometimes occur after left-hemisphere damage. Neglect usually is a consequence of stroke, brain tumors, and head trauma. Lesions producing neglect may also result in other neurologic deficits, such as visual field defects, somatosensory loss, or hemiplegia. However, primary sensory or motor abnormalities do not produce neglect. The associated neurological deficits occur because primary sensory and motor cortices lie close to neural structures critical for spatial awareness.

Since most patients with neglect have relatively intact language abilities, they may be able to carry out reasonable conversations about their lives and current events. This preserved intellectual functioning presents a marked contrast to their poor insight into their own obvious disabilities and occasionally bizarre behavior. For example, Bisiach and Geminiani described a patient who thought that her left hand did not belong to her. She claimed that this hand had been left in the ambulance by a previous patient. She was unable to explain why her rings appeared on this alien hand. A few days later, when asked to pick up a series of cubes laid out horizontally in front of her, she started with the rightmost cube until arriving at her midsagittal plane. At that point she pushed the remainder of the cubes leftward, even as she verbally claimed there were no more cubes.[6] The fact that a discrete brain lesion can produce deep fissures within the very structure of our awareness and beliefs

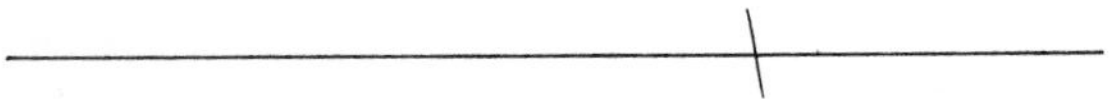

Figure 35-1

Line bisection performance by BT, a 33-year-old woman with left neglect after a stroke in the distribution of the right middle cerebral artery distribution. Reprinted with permission from Chatterjee.[102]

poses a serious challenge to designing remediation strategies.

ASSESSMENT

A number of bedside tasks are used to detect neglect and assess its severity. The more commonly used tasks are described in the following.

Line Bisection Tasks

Line bisection tasks are simple to administer. Patients are presented with horizontal lines, centered traditionally at their midsagittal plane. They are asked to place a mark at the midpoint of the line. The task generally is administered without restricting head or eye movements and without time limitations. Patients with left-sided neglect typically place their mark to the right of the true midposition (Figure 35-1).[7] Patients make larger errors with longer lines.[8–10] If stimuli are placed in space contralateral to the lesion, patients frequently make larger errors.[11] Thus, long lines (generally, 20 cm) placed in left space will provide the most sensitive measure of left-sided neglect.

Cancellation Tasks

In cancellation tasks, sheets with arrays of targets are placed before patients. Patients are asked to place a mark on, or "cancel," each of the targets. Similar to line bisection tasks, cancellation tasks usually are administered without restricting head or eye movements and without time limitations. Patients with left-sided neglect cancel targets on the right side of arrays and neglect targets on the left (Figure 35-2).[12] Sometimes patients cancel the same right-sided targets repeatedly. Increasing the number of targets may uncover neglect not evi-

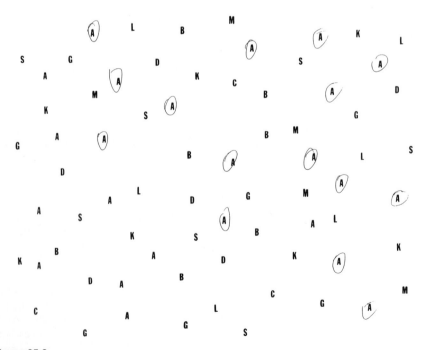

Figure 35-2

Cancellation performance by BT. She was asked to circle all the "A"s. Reprinted with permission from Chatterjee.[102]

dent on arrays with fewer targets.[13] Arrays may also be constructed with distractor stimuli interspersed among targets. The sensitivity of cancellation tasks may be increased by presenting arrays in which targets are difficult to discriminate from distractor stimuli.[14] Thus, the most-sensitive cancellation tasks would contain a large number of stimuli (>80) with difficult-to-discriminate distractors embedded in the array.

Drawing Tasks

Neglect may be assessed by having patients copy drawings or draw from memory. Variations of two patterns may be observed.[15] When asked to copy stimulus arrays with multiple objects, or complex objects with multiple parts, patients may neglect left-sided objects in the array and/or neglect the left side of individual objects, regardless of where they appear in the array (Figure 35-3).

Occasionally, patients may draw left-sided features of the target item on the right side of their drawing.[16] Items commonly used in drawing from memory are clock faces or flowers. In clock drawings, when patients place numbers 1 to 6 on the right side of the clock face and nothing on the left, they are clearly demonstrating neglect. However, when they place all 12 numbers on the right or inaccurately space left-sided numbers, the correct interpretation is less obvious. Such behavior may represent poor strategic planning rather than neglect per se. When patients with neglect draw simple objects like a daisy, they may omit left-sided petals or leaves in their drawings (Figure 35-4), or depict left-sided features with less detail than right-sided features.

Reading

When patients with left-sided neglect read, they sometimes have trouble bringing their gaze to the left margin

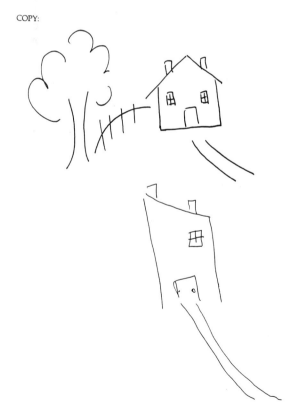

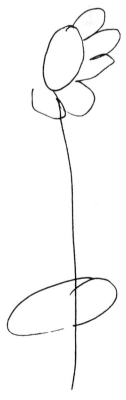

Figure 35-3
Drawing (top) copied by BT (bottom). Reprinted with permission from Chatterjee.[102]

Figure 35-4
Drawing of flower by BT. Reprinted with permission from Chatterjee.[102]

of the page. As a consequence they may read lines starting in the middle of the page, resulting in sequences of words or sentences that do not make sense. When reading single words, they may either omit left-sided letters or substitute confabulated letters.[17] Thus, the word "walnut" might be read as either "nut" or as "peanut." This reading disorder is called neglect dyslexia.[18]

Double Simultaneous Stimulation

Many patients with neglect also demonstrate extinction to double simultaneous stimulation. Extinction refers to the unawareness of stimuli, which are perceived if presented in isolation, when competing stimuli are simultaneously presented.[19,20] In left-sided neglect, right-sided stimuli preferentially penetrate consciousness at the expense of awareness of left-sided stimuli of equivalent intensity. Extinction may occur in visual, auditory, or tactile modalities.

At the bedside, extinction may be tested by asking patients to count fingers presented to one or both hemifields, snapping fingers at one and both ears, and touching one and both hands. When presented with stimuli on both sides, patients with neglect preferentially report only the right-sided stimulus. It is important to ensure that right-left confusion or perseverative responses do not contaminate patients' responses. Extinction cannot be tested adequately in the presence of a primary sensory disorder such as a visual field defect, unilateral hearing loss, or lateralized somatosensory loss. However, manifestations of neglect may occasionally masquerade as a primary sensory loss.[21–23]

Comment

Many patients with right-brain damage demonstrate neglect on the preceding tasks, but not all patients with neglect manifest a uniform array of deficits in all tasks.[24–27] Such observations have led some investigators to question the notion that neglect refers to a single coherent neuropsychological entity.[28] Rather, "neglect" may be more meaningfully viewed as referring to a family of symptoms, in the same sense in which "aphasia" refers to a family of language disorders.

For assessment purposes, it is important to recognize that a patient may demonstrate neglect on some but not other tasks. The Behavioral Inattention Test is a standardized neuropsychological test that can be used to assess neglect.[29] This test incorporates many of the conventional bedside tests mentioned, and provides quantitative scores that can be used to identify spatial neglect and monitor change, recovery, or response to treatment.

NEUROANATOMIC CORRELATES OF NEGLECT

Cortical Lesions

Neglect is more commonly associated with right- than left-hemisphere damage.[3–5,30] Within the right hemisphere neglect may occur with lesions to several different areas. The characteristic lesion involves the right inferior parietal lobe.[31–33] Neglect may also be observed after lesions of the dorsolateral frontal cortex, and cingulate cortex.[34–36] The cortical areas where lesions produce neglect are supramodal or polymodal areas into which unimodal association cortices project. This observation underscores the clinical recognition that neglect is not a primary sensory disorder.

Neurons in the inferior parietal lobe are selectively responsive to stimuli of importance.[37] The inferior parietal lobe and the dorsolateral prefrontal cortex and the cingulate are monosynaptically and reciprocally connected. Within the prefrontal cortex, Rizolatti has described multiple premotor circuits mediating actions to specific spatial locations.[38] The limbic connections to the anterior cingulate may provide an anatomic basis for the abnormal alerting or poor motivation in neglect patients.[36,39]

Subcortical Lesions

Subcortical lesions in the thalamus, putamen, and the midbrain are also reported to produce neglect.[40–42] In animal studies, lesions of the mesencephalic reticular formation produce severe neglect. These lesions are associated with abnormal states of arousal. Neglect in humans is also associated with decreased arousal, suggesting that interruptions of ascending monoaminergic or cholinergic projections may in part mediate clinical observations.[43,44] The thalamic extension of the reticular system, the nucleus reticularis (NR), is a thin shell of neurons encasing much of the thalamus. The NR inhibits sensory thalamic relays to the cortex. Both ascending mesencephalic reticular systems and polymodal association cortices project to and inhibit the NR. Therefore, damage to these systems may result in a release of the inhibitory action of the NR on thalamic relay nuclei, with the resultant impairment of sensory processing.[40]

Patients with basal ganglia lesions may also have neglect.[41,45,46] Such patients may manifest typical neglect symptoms, or primarily those of intentional neglect, or even just slowed reaction times.[46,47] The basal ganglia are tightly linked to the prefrontal and cingulate cortex, and may implicate the importance of dopaminergic systems in the clinical manifestations of the disorder.[48]

Distributed Neural Networks

The clinical observations that lesions to disparate cortical and subcortical structures produce neglect led Heilman and coworkers to propose that an anatomically distributed network mediates spatially directed attention.[33,34,40] Mesulam has also proposed a similar model, emphasizing that different regions within a large-scale network implement different aspects of an individual's interaction with his or her spatial environment.[39,49] The close anatomic interconnections among the different anatomic sites associated with neglect reflect the fact that spatial attention and intention are subserved by widely distributed neural networks.[39,40,50] The complexity of this network underscores the multifaceted nature of spatial representations. Damage to different parts of this network presumably underlies the observations that patients may fractionate into divergent clinical subtypes.[24,33,51]

THEORY

The phenomenology of neglect is puzzling and profoundly disturbing. These patients behave in ways that offend our commen sense intuitions of self and space. An understanding of the underlying mechanisms of the disorder would presumably guide rational remediation strategies. Contemporary explanations of the neglect syndrome focus on sensory attentional, premotor intentional, and representational mechanisms.

Sensory Attentional Theories

A major issue in neglect is explaining why neglect is more common and more severe after right- than after left-brain damage.[4] Kinsbourne postulates that each hemisphere generates a vector of spatial attention directed toward contralateral space, and that this attentional vector is inhibited by the opposite hemisphere.[52,53] He further posits that the left hemisphere's vector of spatial attention is powerfully directed, in contrast to the right hemisphere, which only produces a weak vec-

tor. As a consequence of this neural organization of spatially directed attention, after right-brain damage, the left hemisphere's unfettered vector of attention produces a powerful orientation bias to the right. Since the right hemisphere's intrinsic vector of attention is only weakly directed, after left-brain damage, there is not a powerful orientation bias to the left. Thus, right-sided neglect is less common and not as severe as left-sided neglect.

Heilman and coworkers, in contrast to Kinsbourne, propose that the right hemisphere is dominant for arousal and spatial attention.[54] Patients with right-brain damage have greater electroencephalographic slowing than those with left-brain damage.[55] They also demonstrate diminished galvanic skin responses compared to normal control subject or patients with left hemisphere damage.[43] Heilman and coworkers suggested that the right hemisphere is capable of directing attention into both hemispaces, whereas the left hemisphere directs attention only into contralateral space. Thus, after right-brain damage, the left hemisphere is ill equipped to direct attention into left hemispace. However, after left-brain damage, the right is capable of directing attention into both hemispaces, and neglect does not occur with the same severity as after right-brain damage. Positron emission tomographic studies confirm the notion that the right hemisphere is capable of attending to stimuli in both hemispaces.[56]

Posner and colleagues propose that spatially directed attention can be decomposed into elementary operations, such as "engage," "disengage," and "shift."[50] They reported that patients with right parietal damage are selectively impaired at disengaging attention from right-sided stimuli in order to shift and engage left-sided stimuli.[57] This "disengage deficit" underlies some aspects of the neglect syndrome, most likely the phenomenon of extinction to double simultaneous stimulation and some features of cancellation performance.[58]

Premotor Intentional Theories

Heilman, Watson, and colleagues also advanced the idea that premotor, or intentional, aspects of behavior contribute to the deficit observed in the neglect syndrome.[59] They argued that neglect patients may have a disinclination to initiate movements, or move toward or in contralateral hemispace.[11] Intentional disorders may present as akinesia, hypokinesia, motor extinction, or motor impersistence.[60]

In most situations, attention and intention are inextricably linked, since attention is usually directed to objects on which one acts. It is not always easy to dissect intentional from attentional contributions to the neglect syndrome. Coslett and coworkers had patients perform line bisections in right and left hemispace.[61] However, visual feedback for the task was limited to a video monitor that was placed in either right or left hemispace. Thus, by dissociating the locus of attention (location of the monitor) from the locus of intention (location of their movements), they were able to demonstrate that some patients' errors were primarily influenced by the intentional rather than attentional demands of the task. Bisiach and coworkers, using a set of pulleys, were able to dissociate the direction in which attention and intention were moved in a line bisection task, and also confirmed the intentional influences on the deficits in some patients.[62] Tegner and Levander, using mirrors set at right angles to each other, were also able to dissociate attentional from intentional variables in cancellation tasks.[63] Patients viewed targets directly or through mirrors. In the mirror condition, targets that were seen on the right (reflection in the mirror) actually lay on the left, and vice versa. Tegner and Levander demonstrated that some patients had attentional neglect, others intentional neglect, and some a combination of both. Intentional neglect tends to be associated with frontal lesions. However, there are exceptions to this trend, such as the recent report of a patient with relatively pure intentional neglect produced by a lesion confined to the parietal lobe.[64] Mattingley et al. have reported that slowness in the *initiation* of leftward movements is associated with right posterior lesions, whereas slowness in the *execution* of leftward movements is associated with right anterior and subcortical lesions.[65]

Representational Theories

Neglect can be demonstrated in the absence of external stimuli or movements in external space. Representational theories propose that the inability to form adequate contralateral mental representations of space underlies the behavioral deficits in neglect.[66,67] Denny-Brown had described a patient who, after discharge from the hospital, only recalled patients to her right and, when asked to describe the corridor from the ward, only reported right-sided structures.[20] The importance of this casual observation was not underscored, and it remained buried in the literature. A quarter of a century later, Bisiach and Luzzatti made similar observations in two patients asked to imagine the Piazza del Duomo in Milan, Italy from two perspectives: looking into the square toward the cathedral, and from the cathedral door looking into the square.[68] The patients only reported structures to the right of their imaginal space, resulting in the reporting of different structures, in both conditions. These observations have been replicated and even extend to the imaginal descriptions of routes that would be used by patients going from one point to another.[66–71] By preferentially reporting right turns, patients may describe circuitous and bizarre routes to locations that could be reached more directly if left turns were used.

Patients with neglect may also have difficulties forming contralateral representations in an anterograde manner. Bisiach and coworkers had neglect patients view pairs of abstract cloudlike shapes as they were moved through a narrow slit centered at the midsagittal plane. They were asked to decide if the two shapes were similar or different. In order to do the task patients had to imagine the form of the shape, since they never saw entire shapes at one time. Patients with neglect were inaccurate when these judgments depended on distinguishing features on the left side of these shapes.[72] Rapid eye movements in sleeping neglect patients also are restricted ipsilaterally, raising the intriguing possibility that these patients' dreams are spatially restricted.[73]

Representational theories of neglect are generally presented in opposition to attentional and intentional theories. This distinction may not be warranted. Farah, and colleagues point out that attention is not allocated to stimuli, but rather to representations.[74] In vision, elementary features such as edges, orientation, and color are processed preattentively at different locations within visual cortex.[75] Representations are formed by the binding of these elementary features into percepts. This means that attention is allocated to nascent topographic representations, derived from stimuli in space rather than the stimuli themselves. Bisiach, in recent writings, has suggested that attentional processes are linked to the intrinsic dynamic activity of circuits dedicated to spatial representations.[67] Attentional (and intentional) and representational accounts of neglect may be theoretical accounts of neglect aimed at different levels of analysis.

Recent Theoretical Issues

Neglect and Coordinate Systems   Neglect usually is described along the horizontal (left/right) axis. Recent reports have expanded the concept of spatial neglect to multiple coordinate systems. Our spatial environment also encompasses altitudinal (up-down) and radial (near-far) coordinates. Patients have been described that have neglect of either upper or lower space, and of either near or far peripersonal space.[76-78] Left neglect may also vary depending on whether the stimuli are in near peripersonal space, or in far space.[25,79]

Neglect and Reference Frames We represent objects in space along different reference frames.[80,81] These frames generally are divided into viewer-centered, object-centered, and environment-centered coordinate systems. For example, imagine a chair in an office. The *viewer, centered* reference frame locates the chair with respect to the viewer: left–right, near–far, and above–below. Viewer-centered coordinates change with movement of either the viewer or the object. *Environment-centered* reference frames refer to an object's relationship to the environment, such as the chair's location in relation to its surrounding topography: where in the room, relationship to other stable objects, or relationship to geographic coordinates. This reference frame is unaffected by changes in the viewer's location, but is altered by changes in the object's location, such as if the chair is moved in the room. *Object-centered* reference frames refer to the intrinsic spatial coordinates of the object itself, such as the chair's top–bottom, left–right, and front–back. Object-centered reference frames remain stable irrespectively of movements of the viewer or object. Changing positions of the viewer or the chair within the office does not alter the chair's object-centered coordinates. Our ability to construct object-centered references allows us to recognize familiar objects even when viewed from unfamiliar vantage points. Recent reports demonstrate that neglect may occur in any of these reference frames.[15,82-87]

Quantification of Neglect Patients with neglect respond to stimuli in ways systematically influenced by the quantity of stimuli presented. Bisiach et al. first reported that line bisection performances of patients with neglect are affected by the length of target lines.[8] Marshall and Halligan suggested that this behavior could be ascribed to psychophysical principles.[9] Chatterjee et al. have shown that patients' performance on line bisection, cancellation, and reading tasks can be described by power functions ($\psi = K\phi^\beta$).[10,13,17,88] In this formulation, the subjective psychological (ψ) value is systematically related to the physical (ϕ) value. The constant and exponent of the power function are empirically derived. In general, neglect patients have decreased exponents (β), demonstrating that their performance is continuous with but deviates from normal psychophysical laws. The diminished exponent suggests a decreasing capacity to be aware of increasing quantity of stimuli. The ability to precisely describe performance as a power function provides a potentially valuable tool with which to probe issues of recovery and rehabilitation in neglect.

Implicit Processing of Neglected Stimuli One implication of the kinds of psychophysical relationships described earlier is that patients' performances are influenced by stimuli of which they are unaware, or that they are implicitly processing neglected stimuli. Volpe et al. initially reported that neglect patients were able to make same-different judgments when presented with two pictures simultaneously, despite extinguishing the contralateral picture.[89] These patients were sure they were guessing, and yet responded more accurately than predicted by chance. Since then, other investigators have reported related phenomena. Pictures in neglected fields can facilitate processing of ipsilateral pictures if both belong to the same semantic category.[90] Lexical decisions on ipsilateral stimuli can be influenced by neglected stimuli.[91,92] Whether implicit processing of neglect stimuli can be used to improve functional rehabilitation is not known.

RECOVERY

The presence of neglect or just extinction is associated with poor functional recovery.[93-95] Stone et al. found that degree of paralysis, severity of neglect, and patients' age at 2 or 3 days poststroke significantly impeded functional recovery to independence at 3 and 6 months after the stroke.[96]

The severity of neglect and patterns of recovery are highly variable. Hier and coworkers found that after right-hemisphere stroke visual inattention and neglect recovered much more quickly (median 8–9 weeks) than hemianopia (median 32 weeks) or hemiparesis (median 64 weeks). More-subtle symptoms associated with neglect, such as extinction (median 19 weeks) and motor impersistence (median 26 weeks), lasted longer.[97] These findings were interpreted as indicating that elementary neural functions recover more slowly because local neural structures implement these functions. In contrast, functions mediated through more widely distributed neural networks recover more rapidly. Recovery was also related to size of lesion, and hemorrhagic strokes recovered more quickly than ischemic strokes. Levine and coworkers reported that neglect severity and rate of recovery were adversely affected by premorbid cortical atrophy, suggesting that the integrity of undamaged structures plays a role in the recovery of neglect.[98] By contrast, Chatterjee et al. did not find a clear relationship between lesion size and neglect severity in neglect patients in the subacute poststroke period.[88]

Primate studies suggest that both interhemispheric and intrahemispheric mechanisms are involved in recovery. Monkeys with neglect from frontal ablations have more-severe neglect if their corpus callosi are sectioned, suggesting that compensatory mechanisms are mediated through the contralateral hemisphere.[99,100] However, the rate of recovery after callosal sectioning remains relatively unchanged, implicating intrahemispheric factors in recovery.[100] Consistent with these findings, recovery of severe left-sided neglect in humans is associated with remission of metabolic abnormalities in the left and undamaged right hemisphere on positron emission tomographic studies.[101]

REHABILITATION

Unfortunately, no treatment protocols have been demonstrated to be unequivocally efficacious in neglect.[102] The complexity and heterogeneity of the neglect syndrome defies straightforward treatment strategies. Symptoms associated with right-brain damage other than neglect are also complicating factors.[103] Unawareness of deficits, poor motivation, and abnormalities of emotional processing all contribute to difficulties in rehabilitation. The research program initiated at the Institute of Rehabilitation Medicine, New York University (NYU) Medical Center, is the largest systematic effort to treat neglect.[104] In the following we review their approach to rehabilitation and then more-recent therapeutic options currently being considered.

Behavioral Strategies

The NYU behavioral approach is structured around three training modules, which are administered in sequential order: scanning, somatosensory awareness and size estimation, and perceptual organization.[104] Patients progress through the modules after meeting established criteria. The appropriate starting point for each patient is determined by his or her neglect severity in comparison with normative samples. The program recommends a minimum of 20 hours of training, although these recommendations were made when the average inpatient rehabilitation hospital stay was 34 days.

Training Modules   Patients with neglect tend to scan from the right, and frequently move vertically rather than horizontally.[105–107] The NYU scanning module is designed to train patients to scan stimuli in a systematic and orderly fashion. Patients view a black oval board (78 in. long and 8 in. wide) with two rows of 10 colored lights and a target that moves around the periphery. Patients are trained to track the target, scan the board from left to right for illuminated lights, and then simultaneously track the target and report illuminated lights as the target moves by. Scanning also is trained using structured cancellation tasks, reading, copying, and arithmetic tasks. A large red line is used as an "anchor" on the left side of the page, and each row of stimuli is numbered on both ends. With improving performance, cues such as the anchor line, row number, and experimenter instructions gradually are eliminated.

Somatosensory awareness and size estimation modules are designed to remediate neglect, patients' perceptual distortions of personal body space, and extrapersonal visual size estimation. Somatosensory awareness training consists of touching a patient's back and having him or her touch the same location on the back of a manikin. The patient's unimpaired side, impaired side, lateral borders, spine, shoulder blades, and combinations of unimpaired and impaired sides are sequentially stimulated. Size estimation training involves making judgments of stimulus rods of varying lengths by placing pegs on a board. Patients estimate the midpoint of the board and are trained to locate the midline, right, and left ends of the rod.

Perceptual organization training is designed to increase awareness of the organization of visual stimuli and the interrelationship of component parts. Patients are trained to point to circled words in a paragraph and then find the same word in an identical but unmarked paragraph. They also examine dot configurations within a frame and try to reproduce them from memory. Finally, they scan schematic drawings in a counterclockwise fashion, and compare them to details in target schematics.

Treatment Efficacy   Weinberg et al. reported the efficacy of training in the first module.[108] They classified 59 patients as having severe or mild neglect and entered them into experimental and control groups. Response to treatment was assessed on tests similar to the training tasks, and tasks diverging from the training tasks. Improvement was most evident in the experimental groups, particularly the severely impaired group. After 1 year, the experimental group still maintained their benefits. Benefits were most evident on tasks related to scanning such as reading and cancellation tasks.

Weinberg et al. followed the above study with a report of the efficacy of training a combination of the first (15 hours) and the second (5 hours) module in 53 right-brain–damaged patients grouped similarly to those in previous study.[109] Control subjects received extra occupational and physical therapy. The experimental group again showed improvement, which was most evident in the severely impaired group. Additionally, greater improvements were observed for treatment with both modules, rather than with just the first module alone.

Gordon et al. assessed the efficacy of training in all three modules at time of discharge and after 4 months.[110] Mood and activities of daily living (ADL) measures were included in the study, which was carried out at two institutions. Experimental and control patients were not further divided into severely and mildly impaired groups. At time of discharge, experimental patients differed from controls on scanning and perceptual organization tasks, but not on somatosensory awareness tasks. At 4 months there were no differences between the experimental and control groups. Minimal differences were observed in mood measures and no differences in ADLs. Further attempts at replication of these behavioral techniques suggest that improvement either does not generalize beyond the specific tasks being trained or is difficult to maintain.[111–114]

Orienting Attention

Since a major manifestation of left neglect is thought to be due to a vector of spatial attention being driven to the right, one treatment strategy is to have patients orient towards the left.[53] In some studies, cueing to the left has been shown to improve line bisection performance.[115] The strategic question is how best to get patients to orient to the left.

The superior colliculus is a sensory integrative center involved in mediating contralateral attention and orientation.[116,117] Butter and coworkers postulated that dynamic visual stimulation would activate superior collicular neurons and serve as an attentional cue, prompting patients to orient to the left side. They created a line bisection task on a computer screen in which small squares on the top and bottom of the left end of lines appeared to jump back and forth.[118] They found that patients' performances improved when patients were required to point to the middle of the line with the dynamic visual stimulation at the left. Following this lead, they placed light-emitting diodes on the left edge of patients' spectacles. Unfortunately, the improvements in task performance did not generalize to everyday activities.

Each superior colliculus receives input from the contralateral eye and also inhibits the contralateral superior colliculus; that is, the left superior colliculus receives input from the right eye and also inhibits the left superior colliculus. In animal models, neglect is reduced by damaging the ipsilesional superior colliculus, or transecting the intracollicular commissure.[119] Posner and Rafal suggested that patching the right eye in left-sided neglect would decrease left collicular activation and mitigate the rightward orientational bias by altering the balance of collicular activation.[120] Butter and Kirsh showed that 11 of 13 neglect patients benefitted during the time their contralesional eye was patched.[121] They found further improvement in patients with a combination of right eye patching and left-sided visual stimulation, particularly patients with more-severe neglect. Benefits, unfortunately, did not generalize to activities of daily living.

Using a similar line of reasoning, Ladavas et al. drew a distinction between automatic and voluntary orienting of attention.[122] The Butter et al. treatment strategies might be viewed as manipulating automatic orientation. Ladavas et al. manipulated voluntary attention by having 12 neglect patients look at a computer screen in which a central arrow cued them to the left or right. After 30 1-hour sessions, these patients' performance improved on other tasks assessing neglect. The improvement was restricted to visual tasks, without any cross-modal generalization to tactile extinction.[123] The authors suggest that these results occurred because of the modular structure of spatial attention.

Finally, if part of patients' deficits are due to a premotor intentional deficit, can motor cueing be used to improve neglect? Patients perform better on line bisection tasks if they use their left hand.[124] These improvements are matched if the right hand is first brought to the left end of the line (motor cueing) before patients bisect the lines. Robertson and coworkers similarly showed that some patients with neglect improved after being trained to use their left hand, by placing it at the left margin of the area in which an activity was to take place. Further analysis suggested that it was the movement of the arm, or the motor activation, rather than perceptual anchoring of the limb, that contributed to the improvement. These improvements also generalized to activities of daily living.[125] These results suggest that maximizing intention in left hemispace improves left-sided neglect.

Fresnel Prisms

Rossi and coworkers randomized 39 stroke patients with either visual field defects or neglect into groups wearing fresnel prisms on their spectacles for 4 weeks or untreated controls.[126] After the first day or two, patients had no difficulty tolerating the prisms, which displace images from the contralateral retinal field toward the center. Patients with neglect were not separated from the others for purposes of analysis. After 4 weeks, patients wearing the prisms performed better on visuoperceptual tasks than the stroke control subjects. No theoretical reasons for the improvements were offered, but improvement may have come about by the manipulation of viewer-centered reference frames. The fact that steady improvement was observed over the 4 weeks of treatment suggests that the response was more than simple adaptation to the prisms. Whether the improvement on task performance in these patients persisted after the prisms were removed was not reported. These neuropsychological improvements did not generalize to activities of daily living.

Music

Music preferentially arouses the right hemisphere, particularly in individuals musically untrained.[127] Since decreased arousal is thought to be a critical factor in the manifestations of the neglect syndrome, increasing right-hemisphere arousal might ameliorate neglect. Hommel et al. presented a number of passive and tactile stimuli to 14 patients with left neglect.[128] They were assessed on drawing tasks only. The patients did not improve with either tactile stimulation or verbal auditory stimuli. Their performance did improve with either background music or ambient white noise. Whether such improvements can be sustained, or if patients would habituate to the nonverbal auditory stimuli, is not known. The generalizability of effects to other tasks or functional activities also is not known. Tromp et al. reported improvements in reaction times with ambient music in a patient with neglect.[129] However, she was unable to replicate this finding or those of Hommel et al. in a group study of 9 neglect patients.[130]

Vestibular Stimulation

The vestibular system plays an important role in the mediation of attention in space, and may be critical to the formation and maintenance of spatial representations.[87] Cortical vestibular regions are closely linked to regions in the brain associated with neglect. The inferior parietal lobule and the superior temporal sulcus have been implicated as vestibular regions in anatomic studies, and vestibular stimulation activates these regions in blood flow studies.[131,132]

Irrigation of the external auditory canal with cold water induces nystagmus with the fast component away from the irrigated ear. Cold water caloric stimulation of the ear contralateral to the brain lesion stimulates the vestibular system and ameliorates neglect. Side effects of vestibular stimulation, such as nausea and vomiting, are not reported in neglect patients. Rubens reported improvement in tests of midline pointing, cancellation reading, and counting tasks in 17 of 18 patients with left neglect after stimulation of the left ear with cold water or the right ear with warm water.[133] Improvement was relatively short-lived. Since cold caloric stimulation drives eye movements to the side of stimulation, the orientational bias may have been minimized, resulting in improvement. A similar change in the orientation bias is produced by inducing optokinetic nystagmus to the left with a moving background. This change also produces improvements on line bisection performance.[134] Cappa et al. replicated and extended Rubens' findings.[135] Four neglect patients demonstrated improvement on tasks even with their eyes closed. Thus, the effects of stimulation could not be ascribed solely to effects of vestibular stimulation on eye movements. Two of the patients also became more aware of their hemiplegia, an observation not easily explained by a shifting of eye movements. Geminiani and Bottini replicated the caloric effects of remission of patients' unawareness of their hemiplegia in five patients with neglect.[136] They further showed an improvement in these patients' recollections of left-sided landmarks when imagining the Piazza del Duomo. Caloric stimulation may also improve hemianesthesia as well as hemiplegia, logorrhea, and delusions about affected limbs.[23,137] Long-term therapeutic effects of repeated caloric stimulation in neglect patients have not been reported.

The mechanism of action of vestibular stimulation is not known. Increase in arousal is one possibility. However, since cold water in the ipsilateral ear (which would presumably also be arousing) worsens neglect, increasing arousal cannot be the sole mechanism of beneficial action. Shifting the orientation of attention via eye movements may be partly responsible for the improvement, but it is not clear how eye movements could affect awareness and beliefs or deficits mimicking anaesthesia or hemiplegia. In a patient with neglect from a right frontal stroke, Mennemeier et al. found that contralateral cold water stimulation improved performance on cancellation tasks and increased activation of the basal ganglia, thalamus, and brain stem bilaterally.[138] Cortical activation was not observed. A control subject demonstrated bilateral subcortical and cortical activation. The specific mechanism by which activation of subcortical structures in neglect might mediate improvement remains to be elucidated.

Pharmacological Treatment

Lesions to the ascending mesencephalic reticular formation in animal studies produce neglectlike syndrome and are associated with diminished arousal. This observation raises the possibility that pharmacologic manipulation of widely projecting neurotransmitter systems might ameliorate neglect.

The mesolimbic and mesocortical dopaminergic pathways project from the ventral tegmental midbrain to the basal forebrain and frontal and cingulate cortices. In rats lateral hypothalamic lesions that interrupt ascending dopaminergic pathways produce an akinetic mute state if bilateral and a spatial neglect syndrome if unilateral.[139,140] Selective damage of dopaminergic fibers with 6-hydroxydopamine lesions also produces neglect.[141] After unilateral frontal lesions in rats, neglect can be ameliorated by the dopamine agonist apomorphine.[142] The beneficial effects of apomorphine are blocked by prior administration of the dopamine blocker spiroperidol.[141,143]

These observations led to a small open trial of the dopamine agonist bromocriptine in two patients with neglect.[144] Both patients' performances improved on neuropsychological testing measures. One patient was noted to have improvement in her activities of daily living. Bromocriptine has also been reported to help in cases of akinetic mutism, which might be considered a syndrome of severe bilateral intentional neglect.[145,146] Despite these promising preliminary clinical results, dopaminergic treatment in neglect remains virtually unexplored.

The role of central nervous system stimulants in the treatment of neglect is in the early stages of investigation. Methylphenidate, which is structurally related to amphetamine, releases catecholamines, and possibly dopamine, from nerve terminal storage sites. It has been used in poststroke depression and appears to be quite safe in this patient population.[147,148] We have observed individual patients improve in their arousal and engagement with their environment on low doses (10–20 mg/day) of methylphenidate.

The cholinergic system may also have ascending influences on arousal.[33] Cholinergic agonists produce electrophysiologic signs of arousal. Acetylcholine also makes some neurons more responsive to sensory input.[149] The recent commercial availability of cholinesterase inhibitors makes it possible for such medications also to be tried as a pharmacologic treatment of neglect.

CONCLUSION

The rehabilitation of neglect is still in its infancy. The fact that the clinical syndrome is common and significantly impairs functional recovery after stroke underscores the importance of developing treatments for this disorder.[102] We have reviewed the complexity of spatial neglect to make clear that any useful treatment is unlikely to be simple or straightforward. A firm grounding in the assessment, mechanisms, and manifestations of neglect will help in the design of rational rehabilitation strategies.

The burgeoning interest in theoretically motivated studies of neglect is beginning to result in innovative rehabilitation attempts. Several considerations apply to all of these studies. Does the treatment improve neglect symptoms? Does the treatment offer advantages over spontaneous recovery? Does improvement generalize to a wide range of tasks on which neglect might be evident? Can the improvement be maintained? Does the improvement translate into a difference in the functional abilities of the patients, or improve the quality of their lives? Finally, in the current climate of financial restraint, are the interventions cost-effective?

The experience with the NYU behavioral approach has been the most extensive. This treatment program is labor-intensive, but does seem to help some patients, especially those with most-severe impairment. However, the treatment has limited generalizability, and the time required for this treatment may make it impractical in many rehabilitation settings. All the other treatments reviewed have not been studied in sufficient detail to permit recommendation for general use.

If a treatment is to work, its effects must cross modalities and be manifest in patients' functional abilities. Vestibular stimulation and pharmacological interventions offer the most promise. Vestibular stimulation has been reported to ameliorate a wide range of symptoms, from apparent hemianesthesia to delusional beliefs. Currently, we do not know if repeated stimulation would confer long-lasting benefits, or if patients would habituate to treatment. Similarly, we do not know what kind of stimulation schedule would maximize benefit. Although the mechanism of action remains mysterious, the fact that the effects cut across widely different cognitive domains makes vestibular stimulation appealing. Similarly, pharmacological interventions have the advantage of modulating widely distributed neurotransmitter systems, and therefore influencing cognition broadly. Unfortunately, pharmacologic interventions in neglect have been barely studied. Controlled group studies of the efficacy of these recent theoretically driven rehabilitation approaches to spatial neglect are urgently needed.

ACKNOWLEDGMENTS

We thank Britt Anderson, M.D., for reviewing this chapter critically. This work was supported by an NIH-NINDS grant KO8 NS01702-03 to AC.

REFERENCES

1. Heilman KM, Watson RT, Valenstein E: Neglect and related disorders, in Heilman KM, Valenstein E (eds): *Clinical Neuropsychology,* 2nd ed. New York: Oxford University Press, 1985, pp. 243–293.
2. Critchley M: Misoplegia or hatred of hemiplegia. *Mt Sinai J Med* 1974; 41:82–87.
3. Costa LD, Vaughan HG, Horowitz M, Ritter W: Patterns of behavior deficit associated with visual spatial neglect. *Cortex* 1969; 5:242–263.
4. Gainotti G, Messerli P, Tissot R: Qualitative analysis of unilateral and spatial neglect in relation to laterality of cerebral lesions. *J Neurol Neurosurg Psychiatr* 1972; 35:545–550.
5. Halligan PW, Marshall JC, Wade DT: Visuospatial neglect: Underlying factors and test sensitivity. *Lancet* 1989; 2:908–911.
6. Bisiach E, Geminiani G: Anosagnosia related to hemiplegia and hemianopia, in Prigatano GP, Schacter DL (eds): *Awareness of Deficit after Brain Injury.* New York: Oxford University Press, 1991, pp. 17–39.
7. Schenkenberg T, Bradford DC, Ajax ET: Line bisection and unilateral visual neglect in patients with neurologic impairment. *Neurology* 1980; 30:509–517.
8. Bisiach E, Bulgarelli C, Sterzi R, Vallar G: Line bisection and cognitive plasticity of unilateral neglect of space. *Brain Cog* 1983; 2:32–38.

9. Marshall JC, Halligan PW: Line bisection in a case of visual neglect: Psychophysical studies with implications for theory. *Cog Neuropsychol* 1990; 7(2):107–130.
10. Chatterjee A, Mennemeier M, Heilman KM: The psychophysical power law and unilateral spatial neglect. *Brain Cog* 1994; 25:92–107.
11. Heilman KM, Valenstein E: Mechanisms underlying hemispatial neglect. *Ann Neurol* 1979; 5:166–170.
12. Albert ML: A simple test of visual neglect. *Neurology* 1973; 23:658–664.
13. Chatterjee A, Mennemeier M, Heilman KM: A stimulus-response relationship in unilateral neglect: The power function. *Neuropsychologia* 1992; 30:1101–1108.
14. Rapcsak S, Verfaellie M, Fleet W, Heilman K: Selective attention in hemispatial neglect. *Arch Neurol* 1989; 46:172–178.
15. Marshall JC, Halligan PW: Visuo-spatial neglect: A new copying test to assess perceptual parsing. *J Neurol* 1993; 240:37–40.
16. Halligan PW, Marshall JC, Wade DT: Left on the right: Allochiria in a case of left visuo-spatial neglect. *J Neurol Neurosurg Psychiatr* 1992; 55:717–719.
17. Chatterjee A: Cross over, completion and confabulation in unilateral spatial neglect. *Brain* 1995; 118:455–465.
18. Kinsbourne M, Warrington EK: Variety of reading disability associated with right hemisphere lesions. *J Neurol Neurosurg Psychiatr* 1962; 25:339–344.
19. Bender MB, Furlow CT: Phenomenon of visual extinction and homonomous fields and psychological principles involved. *Arch Neurol Psychiatr* 1945; 53:29–33.
20. Denny-Brown D, Meyer J, Horenstein S: The significance of perceptual rivalry resulting from parietal lesion. *Brain* 1952; 75:433–471.
21. Kooistra CA, Heilaman KM: Hemispatial visual inattention masquerading as hemianopsia. *Neurology* 1989; 39:1125–1127.
22. Nadeau SE, Heilman KM: Gaze-dependent hemianopia without hemispatial neglect. *Neurology* 1991; 41:1244–1250.
23. Vallar G, Bottini G, Rusconi ML, Sterzi R: Exploring somatosensory hemineglect by vestibular stimulation. *Brain* 1993; 116:71–86.
24. Binder J, Marshall R, Lazar R, Benjamin J, Mohr J: Distinct syndromes of hemineglect. *Arch Neurol* 1992; 49:1187–1194.
25. Halligan PW, Marshall JC: Left neglect for near but not for far space in man. *Nature* 1991; 350:498–500.
26. Anderson B: Spared awareness for the left side of internal visual images in patients with left-sided extrapersonal neglect. *Neurology* 1993; 43:213–216.
27. Guariglia C, Padovani A, Pantano P, Pizzamiglio L: Unilateral neglect restricted to visual imagery. *Nature* 1993; 364:235–237.
28. Halligan PW, Marshall JC: Left visuo-spatial neglect: A meaningless entity? *Cortex* 1992; 28:525–535.
29. Wilson B, Cockburn J, Halligan PW: *Behavioral Inatten-*

tion Test. Titchfield, Hants: Thames Valley Test Company, 1987.

30. Brain WR: Visual disorientation with special reference to lesions of the right hemisphere. *Brain* 1941; 64:224–272.

31. Critchley M: *The Parietal Lobes.* New York: Hafner, 1966.

32. Vallar G, Perani D: The anatomy of spatial neglect in humans, in Jeannerod M (ed): *Neurophysiological and Neuropsychological Aspects of Spatial Neglect.* Amsterdam: North-Holland, 1987; pp. 235–258.

33. Heilman KM, Watson RT, Valenstein E: Localization of lesions in neglect and related disorders, in Kertesz A (ed): *Localization and Neuroimaging in Neuropsychology.* New York: Academic Press, 1994; pp. 495–524.

34. Heilman KM, Valenstein E: Frontal lobe neglect in man. *Neurology* 1972; 22:660–664.

35. Maeshima S, Funahashi K, Ogura M, Itakura T, Komai N: Unilateral spatial neglect due to right frontal lobe haematoma. *J. Neurol Neurosurg Psychiatr* 1994; 57:89–93.

36. Watson RT, Heilman KM, Cauthen JC, King FA: Neglect after cingulectomy. *Neurology* 1973; 23:1003–1007.

37. Motter BC, Mountcastle VB: The functional properties of the light sensitive neurons of the posterior parietal cortex studies in waking monkeys: Foveal sparing and opponent vector organization. *J Neurosci* 1981; 1:3–26.

38. Rizolatti G, Berti A: Neural mechanisms in spatial neglect, in Robertson IH, Marshall JC (eds): *Unilateral Neglect: Clinical and Experimental Studies.* Hillsdale, NJ: LEA, 1993; pp. 87–105.

39. Mesulam M-M: A cortical network for directed attention and unilateral neglect. *Ann Neurol* 1981; 10:309–325.

40. Watson RT, Valenstein E, Heilman KM: Thalamic neglect. *Arch Neurol* 1981; 38:501–506.

41. Hier DB, Davis KR, Richardson EP, Mohr JP: Hypertensive putaminal hemorrhage. *Ann Neurol* 1977; 1:152–159.

42. Watson RT, Heilman KM, Miller BD, King FA: Neglect after mesencephalic reticular formation lesions. *Neurology* 1974; 24:294–298.

43. Heilman KM, Schwartz HD, Watson RT: Hypoarousal in patients with the neglect syndrome and emotional indifference. *Neurology* 1978; 28:229–232.

44. Yokoyama K, Jennings R, Ackles P, Hood P, Boller F: Lack of heart rate changes during an attention demanding task after right hemisphere lesions. *Neurology* 1987; 37:624–630.

45. Damasio AR, Damasio H, Chang CH: Neglect following damage to frontal lobe or basal ganglia. *Neuropsychologia* 1980; 18:123–132.

46. Valenstein E, Heilman K: Unilateral hypokinesia and motor extinction. *Neurology* 1981; 31:445–448.

47. Sakashita Y: Visual attentional disturbance with unilateral lesions of the basal ganglia and deep white matter. *Ann Neurol* 1991; 30:673–677.

48. Alexander GE, DeLong MR, Strick PL: Parallel organization of functionally segregated circuits linking basal ganglia and cortex. *Annu Rev Neurosci* 1986; 9:357–381.

49. Mesulam M-M: Large-scale neurocognitive networks and distributed processing for attention, language and memory. *Ann Neurol* 1990; 28:597–613.

50. Posner MI, Dehaene S: Attentional networks. *Trends Neurosci* 1994; 17:75–79.

51. D'Esposito M, McGlinchey-Berroth R, Alexander MP, Verfaellie M, Milberg WP: Dissociable cognitive and neural mechanisms of unilateral visual neglect. *Neurology* 1993; 43:2638–2644.

52. Kinsbourne M: The cerebral basis of lateral asymmetries in attention. *Acta Psychologica* 1970; 33:193–201.

53. Kinsbourne M: Mechanisms of unilateral neglect, in Jeannerod M (ed): *Neurophysiological and Neuropsychological Aspects of Spatial Neglect.* New York: North Holland, 1987, pp. 69–86.

54. Heilman KM, Van Den Abell T: Right hemisphere dominance for attention: The mechanisms underlying hemispheric asymmetries of inattention (neglect). *Neurology* 1980; 30:327–330.

55. Watson RT, Andriola M, Heilman KM: The electroencephalogram in neglect. *J Neurol Sci* 1977; 34:343–348.

56. Corbetta M, Miezen FM, Shulman GL, Peterson SE: A PET study of visuospatial attention. *J Neurosci* 1993; 11:1202–1226.

57. Posner M, Walker J, Friedrich F, Rafal R: Effects of parietal injury on covert orienting of attention. *J Neurosci* 1984; 4:1863–1874.

58. Mark VW, Kooistra CA, Heilman KM: Hemispatial neglect affected by non-neglected stimuli. *Neurology* 1988; 38:1207–1211.

59. Watson RT, Valenstein E, Heilman KM: Nonsensory neglect. *Ann Neurol* 1978; 3:505–508.

60. Heilman KM, Watson RT, Valenstein E: Neglect and related disorders, in Heilman KM, Valenstein E (eds): *Clinical Neuropsychology,* 3rd ed. New York: Oxford University Press, 1993, pp. 279–336.

61. Coslett HB, Bowers D, Fitzpatrick E, Haws B, Heilman KM: Directional hypokinesia and hemispatial inattention in neglect. *Brain* 1990; 113:475–486.

62. Bisiach E, Geminiani G, Berti A, Rusconi ML: Perceptual and premotor factors of unilateral neglect. *Neurology* 1990; 40:1278–1281.

63. Tegner R, Levander M: Through the looking glass: A new technique to demonstrate directional hypokinesia in unilateral neglect. *Brain* 1991; 114:1943–1951.

64. Triggs WJ, Gold M, Gerstle G, Adair J, Heilman KM: Motor neglect associated with a discrete parietal lesion. *Neurology* 1994; 44:1164–1166.

65. Mattingley JB, Bradshaw JL, Phillips JG: Impairments of movement initiation and execution in unilateral neglect. *Brain* 1992; 115:1849–1874.

66. Bisiach E, Capitani E, Luzzatti C, Perani D: Brain and conscious representation of outside reality. *Neuropsychologia* 1981; 19:543–551.

67. Bisiach E: Mental representation in unilateral neglect and

related disorders: The twentieth Bartlett Memorial lecture. *Q J Exp Psychol* 1993; 46A:435–461.

68. Bisiach E, Luzzatti C: Unilateral neglect of representational space. *Cortex* 1978; 14:129–133.

69. Meador KJ, Loring DW, Bowers D, Heilman KM: Remote memory and the neglect syndrome. *Neurology* 1987; 37:522–526.

70. Bartolomeo P, D'Erme P, Gainotti G: The relationship between visuospatial and representational neglect. *Neurology* 1994; 44:1710–1714.

71. Bisiach E, Brouchon M, Poncet M, Rusconi ML: Unilateral neglect in route description. *Neuropsychologia* 1993; 31:1255–1262.

72. Bisiach E, Luzzatti C, Perani D: Unilateral neglect, representational schema and consciousness. *Brain* 1979; 102:609–618.

73. Doricchi F, Guariglia C, Paolucci S, Pizzamiglio L: Disturbance of the rapid eye movements (REM) of REM sleep in patients with unilateral attentional neglect: Clue for the understanding of the functional meaning of REMs. *Electroencephalogr Clin Neurophysiol* 1993; 87:105–116.

74. Farah MJ, Wallace MA, Vecera SP: "What" and "where" in visual attention: Evidence from the neglect syndrome, in Robertson IH, Marshall JC (eds): *Unilateral Neglect: Clinical and Experimental Studies*. Hillsdale, NJ: LEA, 1993, pp. 123–137.

75. Van Essen DC, Feleman DJ, DeYoe EA, Ollavaria J, Knierman J: Modular and hierarchical organization of extrastriate visual cortex in the macaque monkey. *Cold Springs Harbor Symp Quant Biol* 1990; 55:679–696.

76. Rapcsak SZ, Fleet WS, Verfaellie M, Heilman KM: Altitudinal neglect. *Neurology* 1988; 38:277–281.

77. Shelton PA, Bowers D, Heilman KM: Peripersonal and vertical neglect. *Brain* 1990; 113:191–205.

78. Mennemeier M, Wertman E, Heilman KM: Neglect of near peripersonal space: Evidence for multidirectional attentional systems in humans. *Brain* 1992; 115:37–50.

79. Cowey A, Small M, Ellis S: Left visuo-spatial neglect can be worse in far than in near space. *Neuropsychologia* 1994; 32:1059–1066.

80. Marr D: *Vision: A Computational Investigation into the Human Representation and Processing of Visual Information*. New York: WH Freeman and Company, 1982, p. 397.

81. Feldman JA: Four frames suffice: A provisional model of vision and space. *Behavior Brain Sci* 1985; 8:265–289.

82. Ladavas E: Is the hemispatial damage produced by right parietal lobe damage associated with retinal or gravitational coordinates? *Brain* 1987; 110:167–180.

83. Farah MJ, Brun JL, Wong AB, Wallace MA, Carpenter PA: Frames of reference for allocating attention to space: Evidence from the neglect syndrome. *Neuropsychologia* 1990; 28(4):335–347.

84. Driver J, Halligan PW: Can visual neglect operate in object-centered coordinates? An affirmative single-case study. *Cog Neuropsychol* 1991; 8:475–496.

85. Caramazza A, Hillis AE: Levels of representation, co-ordinate frames, and unilateral neglect. *Cog Neuropsychol* 1990; 7:391–445.

86. Chatterjee A: Picturing unilateral spatial neglect: Viewer versus object centered reference frames. *J Neurol Neurosurg Psychiatr* 1994; 57:1236–1240.

87. Mennemeier M, Chatterjee A, Heilman KM: A comparison of the influences of body and environment centered references on neglect. *Brain* 1994; 117:1013–1021.

88. Chatterjee A, Dajani BM, Gage RJ: Psychophysical constraints on behavior in unilateral spatial neglect. *Neuropsychiatr Neuropsychol Behav Neurol* 1994; 7:267–274.

89. Volpe BT, Ledoux JE, Gazzaniga MS: Information processing of visual stimuli in an "extinguished" field. *Nature* 1979; 282:722–724.

90. Berti A, Rizzolatti G: Visual processing without awareness: Evidence from unilateral neglect. *J Cog Neurosci* 1992; 4:345–351.

91. McGlinchey-Berroth R, Milberg WP, Verfaelli M, Alexander M, Kilduff PT: Semantic processing in the neglected field: Evidence from a lexical decision task. *Cog Neuropsychol* 1993; 10:79–108.

92. Ladavas E, Paladini R, Cubelli R: Implicit associative priming in a patient with left visual neglect. *Neuropsychologia* 1993; 31:1307–1320.

93. Denes G, Semenza C, Stoppa E, Lis A: Unilateral spatial neglect and recovery from hemiplegia: A follow up study. *Brain* 1982; 105:543–552.

94. Henley S, Pettit P, Todd-Pokropek L, Tupper J: Who goes home? Predictive factors in stroke recovery. *J Neurol Neurosurg Psychiatr* 1985; 48:1–6.

95. Rose L, Bakal DA, Fung TS, Farn P, Weaver LE: Tactile extinction and functional status after stroke: A preliminary investigation. *Stroke* 1994; 25:1973–1976.

96. Stone SP, Patel P, Greenwood RJ: Selection of acute stroke patients for treatment of visual neglect. *J Neurol Neurosurg Psychiatr* 1993; 56:463–466.

97. Hier D, Mondlock J, Caplan L: Recovery of behavioral abnormalities after right hemisphere stroke. *Neurology* 1983; 33:345–350.

98. Levine DN, Warach JD, Benowitz L, Calvanio R: Left spatial neglect: Effects of lesion size and premorbid brain atrophy on severity and recovery following right cerebral infarction. *Neurology* 1986; 36:362–366.

99. Crowne DP, Yeo CH, Russell IS: The effects of unilateral frontal eye field lesions in the monkey: Visual-motor guidance and avoidance behavior. *Behav Brain Res* 1981; 2:165–185.

100. Watson RT, Valenstein E, Heilman KM: The effect of corpus callosum section on unilateral neglect in monkeys. *Neurology* 1984; 34:812–815.

101. Perani D, Vallar G, Paulesi E, Alberoni M, Fazio F: Left and right hemisphere contributions to recovery from neglect after right hemisphere damage—an [^{18}F]FDG PET study of two cases. *Neuropsychologia* 1993; 40:1278–1281.

102. Chatterjee A: Unilateral spatial neglect: Assessment

and rehabilitation studies. *NeuroRehabilitation* 1995; 5:115–128.

103. Heilman KM, Bowers D, Valenstein E: Emotional disorders associated with neurological disease, in Heilman KM, Valenstein E (eds): *Clinical Neuropsychology*. New York: Oxford University Press, 1993, pp. 461–497.

104. Diller L, Riley E: The behavioral management of neglect, in Robertson IH, Marshall JC (eds): *Unilateral Neglect: Clinical and Experimental Studies*. Hillsdale, NJ: LEA, 1993, pp. 293–308.

105. Chedru F, Leblanc M, Lhermitte F: Visual searching in normal and brain-damaged subjects (contributions to the study of unilateral inattention). *Cortex* 1973; 9:94–111.

106. Ishiai S, Furukawa T, Tsukagoshi H: Visuospatial processes of line bisection and the mechanisms underlying unilateral spacial neglect. *Brain* 1989; 112:1485–1502.

107. Chatterjee A, Mennemeier M, Heilman KM: Search patterns and neglect: A case study. *Neuropsychologia* 1992; 30(7):657–672.

108. Weinberg M, Diller L, Gordon W, et al: Visual scanning training effects on reading-related tasks in acquired right brain damage. *Arch Phys Med Rehab* 1977; 58:479–486.

109. Weinberg M, Diller L, Goedon W, et al: Training sensory awareness and spatial organization in people with right brain damage. *Arch Phys Med Rehab* 1979; 60:491–496.

110. Gordon WA, Ruckdeschel-Hibbard M, Egelko S, et al: Perceptual remediation in patients with right brain damage: A comprehensive program. *Arch Phys Med Rehab* 1985; 66:353–359.

111. Webster J, Jones S, Blanton P, Gross R, Beissel G, Wofford J: Visual scanning training with stroke patients. *Behav Ther* 1984; 15:129–143.

112. Gouvier W, Boa B, Blanton P, Urey J: Behavioral interventions with stroke patients for improving wheelchair navigation. *Int J Clin Neuropsychol* 1984; 1:186–190.

113. Gouvier W, Bua B, Blanton P, Urey J: Behavioral changes following visual scanning training: Observation of five cases. *Int J Clin Neuropsycholog* 1987; 9:74–80.

114. Robertson IH, Halligan PW, Marshall JC: Prospects for the rehabilitation of unilateral neglect, in Robertson IH, Marshall JC (eds): *Unilateral Neglect: Clinical and Experimental Studies*. Hillsdale, NJ: LEA, 1993, pp. 279–292.

115. Riddoch MJ, Humphreys GW: The effects of cueing on unilateral neglect. *Neuropsychologia* 1983; 21(6):589–599.

116. Sprague JM, Meikle TH: The role of the superior colliculus in visually guided behavior. *Exp Neurol* 1965; 11:115–146.

117. Stein BE, Meredith MA: *The Merging of the Senses*. Cambridge, MA: The MIT Press, 1993.

118. Butter CM, Kirsch NL, Reeves G: The effect of dynamic stimuli on unilateral spatial neglect following right hemisphere lesions. *Rest Neurol Neurosci* 1990; 2:39–46.

119. Sprague J: Interaction of cortex and superior colliculus in visually guided behavior. *Science* 1966; 153:1544–1547.

120. Posner MI, Rafal RD: Cognitive theories of attention and the rehabilitation of attentional deficits, in Meier MJ,

Benton A, Diller L (eds): *Neuropsychological Rehabilitation*. New York: Guilford, 1987, pp. 182–201.

121. Butter CM, Kirsch N: Combined and separate effects of eye patching and visual stimulation on unilateral neglect following stroke. *Arch Phys Med Rehab* 1992; 73:1133–1139.

122. Ladavas E, Carletti M, Gori G: Automatic and voluntary orienting of attention in patients with visual neglect: Horizontal and vertical dimensions. *Neuropsychologia* 1994; 32:1195–1208.

123. Ladavas E, Menghini G, Umilta C: A rehabilitation study of hemispatial neglect. *Cog Neuropsychol* 1994; 11:75–95.

124. Halligan PW, Manning L, Manning JC: Hemispheric activation versus spatio-motor cueing in visual neglect: A case study. *Neuropsychologia* 1991; 29:165–176.

125. Robertson I, North N, Geggie C: Spatiomotor cueing in unilateral left neglect: Three case studies in its therapeutic effects. *J Neurol Neurosurg Psychiatr* 1992; 55:799–805.

126. Rossi PW, Kheyfets S, Reding MJ: Fresnel prisms improve visual perception in stroke patients with homonymous hemianopia or unilateral neglect. *Neurology* 1990; 40:1597–1599.

127. Mazziotta JC, Phelps ME, Carson RE, Kuhl DE: Tomographic mapping of human cerebral metabolism: Auditory stimulation. *Neurology* 1982; 32:921–937.

128. Hommel M, Peres B, Pollack P, et al: Effects of passive tactile and auditory stimuli on left visual neglect. *Arch Neurol* 1990; 47:573–576.

129. Tromp E, Michels M, Mulder T: What music can do for a patient with visuo-spatial neglect. *J Clin Exp Neuropsychol* 1993; 15:414.

130. Tromp E: *Neglect in action: A neuropsychological exploration of some behavioural aspects of neglect* (PhD dissertation). Nijmegen Institute for Cognition and Information, 1995.

131. Fredrickson J, Rubin A: Vestibular cortex, in Jones E, Peters A (eds): *Sensory-Motor Areas and Aspects of Cortical Connectivity*. New York: Plenum Press, 1986; pp. 99–112.

132. Friberg L, Olson T, Roland P, Paulson O, Lassen N: Focal increase of blood flow in the cerebral cortex of man during vestibular stimulation. *Brain* 1985; 108:609–623.

133. Rubens A: Caloric stimulation and unilateral neglect. *Neurology* 1985; 35:1019–1024.

134. Pizzamiglio L, Frasca R, Guariglia C, Incoccia C, Antonucci G: Effect of optokinetic stimulation in patients with neglect. *Cortex* 1990; 26:535–540.

135. Cappa S, Sterzi R, Guiseppe V, Bisiach E: Remission of hemineglect and anosagnosia during vestibular stimulation. *Neuropsychologia* 1987; 25:775–782.

136. Geminiani G, Bottini G: Mental representations and temporary recovery from unilateral neglect after vestibular stimulation. *J Neurol Neurosurg Psychiatr* 1992; 55:332–333.

137. Rode G, Charles N, Perenin M, Vighetto A, Trillet M,

Aimard G: Partial remission of hemiplegia and somato-paraphrenia through vestibular stimulation in a case of unilateral neglect. *Cortex* 1992; 28:203–208.

138. Mennemeier M, Kazniak AW, Patton D, Rubens AB: Brain activation following caloric stimulation in neglect. *J Int Neuropsychol* 1995; 1:366.

139. Teitelbaum P, Epstein AN: The lateral hypothalamic syndrome. *Psychol Rev* 1962; 69:74–90.

140. Marshall JF, Turner BH, Teitelbaum P: Sensory neglect produced by lateral hypothalamic damage. *Science* 1971; 174:523–525.

141. Marshall JF, Gotthelf T: Sensory inattention in rats with 6-hydroxydopamine-induced degeneration of ascending dopaminergic neurons: Apomorphine-induced reversal of deficits. *Exp Neurol* 1979; 1986:683–689.

142. Ungerstedt U: Brain dopamine neurons and behavior, in Schmidt FO, Woren FG (eds): *The Neurosciences.* Cambridge, MA: MIT Press, 1974, pp. 695–703.

143. Corwin JV, Kanter S, Watson RT, Heilman KM, Valenstein E, Hashimoto A: Apomorphine has a therapeutic effect on neglect produced by unilateral dorsomedial prefrontal cortex lesions in rats. *Exp Neurol* 1986; 36:683–698.

144. Fleet WS, Valenstein E, Watson RT, Heilman KM: Dopamine agonist therapy for neglect in humans. *Neurology* 1987; 37:1765–1770.

145. Ross ED, Stewart RM: Akinetic mutism from hypothalamic damage: Successful treatment with dopamine agonists. *Neurology* 1981; 31:1435–1439.

146. Anderson B: Relief of akinetic mutism from obstructive hydrocephalus using bromocriptine and ephedrine. *J Neurosurg* 1992; 76:152–155.

147. Lazarus LW, Winemiller DR, Lingham VR, et al: Efficacy and side effects of methylphenidate for poststroke depression. *J Clin Psychiatr* 1992; 53:447–449.

148. Lazarus LW, Moberg PJ, Langsley PR, Lingam VR: Methylphenidate and nortriptyline in the treatment of poststroke depression: A retrospective comparison. *Arch Phys Med Rehab* 1994; 75:403–406.

149. McCormick DA: Cholinergic and noradrenergic modulation of thalamocortical processing. *Trends Neurosci* 1989; 12:215–221.

Chapter 36

FUNCTIONAL ELECTRICAL STIMULATION

Robert J. Jaeger
Jochen Quintern

In 1757 Benjamin Franklin wrote to a friend an account of the effects of applying electrical stimulation to paralyzed individuals.

> *I never knew any advantage from electricity in palsies that was permanent. And how far the temporary advantage might arise from the exercise in the patients' journey and coming daily to my house, or from the spirits given by the hope of success, enabling them to exert more strength in moving their limbs, I will not pretend to say.*[1]

The exact nature of Franklin's patient population and electrical stimulation protocol are difficult to verify today. He was, nevertheless, one of the first to speculate on the possible application of electrical current to remediate neurologic paralysis.

Functional Electrical Stimulation (FES) is, in the most general case, taken to mean the delivery of electrical impulses near excitable lower motor neurons to cause contraction of the upper motor neuron paralyzed muscles they innervate, as schematized in Figure 36-1. A synonymous term is Functional Neuromuscular Stimulation (FNS). The emphasis is on the word "functional" to distinguish the purpose of stimulation from related applications, such as therapeutic use as a modality in wound healing. The purpose of this chapter is to summarize several fundamental issues in neurophysiology that are relevant to FES focusing on spinal cord injury, and review some of the medically prescribable FES systems available in the world today. A brief overview of the status of applied research and future applications is also given.

NEUROPHYSIOLOGY RELEVANT TO APPLICATIONS OF FES

There are several basic neurophysiological issues that, in addition to describing the fundamental mechanisms

by which FES works, illustrate the limitations encountered in the clinical application of FES. It is important for physicians to convey a simple explanation of these principles to patients who may desperately want a particular FES device to work for them. This may be a physical and physiological impossibility. In the absence of an understandable explanation, some patients may take this predicament as a personal failure, attributing it to lack of effort or intelligence. The psychological issues related to FES have, unfortunately, received only minimal attention.[2–4]

Production of an Action Potential by Electrical Stimulation

The ability of a nerve (both cell body and axon) to be activated by FES depends on the physical properties of the membrane, sizes and relative position of the nerves and electrodes, and the parameters of the stimulus (such as current amplitude and pulse width). Consider a single pulse of current (negative charge) passing into the membrane close to one electrode (cathode), which returns to the source via a more distant electrode (anode). If the current is subthreshold, the membrane near the cathode is only slightly depolarized from its resting levels, and no action potential results. If the current is increased to (or above) threshold an action potential results.[5] This is an "all-or-none" event. A single action potential so initiated by a single pulse of stimulation is indistinguishable from a naturally occurring action potential. In neuromuscular applications, a single pulse of stimulation will typically generate a single action potential in a number of individual nerve fibers near the stimulating electrode. In motor nerves, these action potentials are all propagated toward the neuromuscular junction, and a single muscle twitch results. How to utilize a combination of such individual twitches to restore lost motor

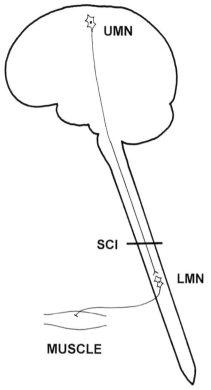

Figure 36-1
Schematic diagram illustrating upper and lower motor neurons in relation to conventional application of FES. If a given muscle is to be made to contract by FES, it must be innervated by an intact lower motor neuron. Typically, that lower motor neuron does not receive neural signals from a corresponding upper motor neuron because an injury to the spinal cord has permanently disrupted the transmission.

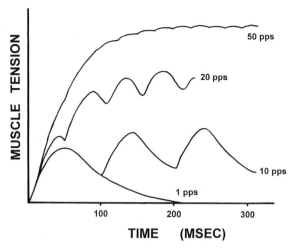

Figure 36-2
Strength–duration curves for innervated and denervated muscle. The curves define the stimulus parameters (for a single pulse) needed to produce a threshold twitch. An infinite variety of combinations of pulse width (horizontal axis) and pulse amplitude (vertical axis) may be used to produce the threshold twitch. Redrawn Benton et al.[7]

function is the challenge faced by FES. For completeness, it must be noted that sensory nerves are concomitantly stimulated when delivering FES. In most cases, this is inconsequential, but a more detailed treatment of this topic is beyond the scope of this chapter.

Upper Motor Neuron/Lower Motor Neuron Paralysis

Paralyzed muscle can be divided into two distinct categories, depending on whether the bulk of the lower motor neurons innervating a particular muscle are intact or destroyed by injury or disease process. It is generally agreed that FES applied to lower motor neuron paralyzed muscles of the limbs to produce functional move-

ment is not presently workable. At least one group of investigators is searching for applications of FES technology for lower motor neuron paralyzed muscle.[6] FES often is mistakenly referred to as muscle stimulation when actually it is nerve fibers innervating muscles that are stimulated. Activation of denervated muscle by electric current requires a much more potent stimulus, with a long pulse width (>5 ms), and high current amplitude. Such stimulation is technologically much more difficult to deliver than the stimulation that can cause contraction of upper motor neuron paralyzed muscle. This is seen schematically in Figure 36-2, which shows threshold curves for innervated and denervated muscles. Note the curve for denervated muscle is above and to the right of the innervated muscle curve, indicating that a stronger stimulus is required to produce a threshold response.[7] The high threshold requirement of denervated muscle is not the only obstacle in the attempts to produce functional movement by electrical stimulation. After denervation, muscle undergoes fundamental morphological and histochemical changes, resulting in a decline of contractile properties.

Figure 36-2 also shows that there are a variety of combinations of stimulus amplitude and pulse width that will produce an identical threshold response. The stimulus parameters that have evolved in clinical prac-

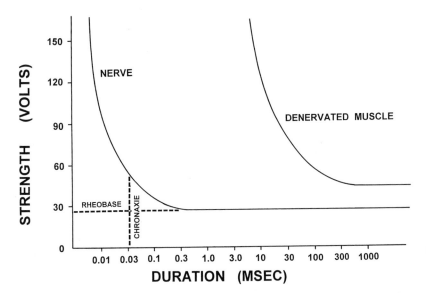

Figure 36-3
Schematic diagram indicating how muscle force in response to FES (vertical axis) as a function of time (horizontal axis) depends on the frequency of the stimulation. At low stimulation frequencies, the response is composed of essentially individual twitches. As the stimulation frequency is increased, the response gradually becomes a smooth, fused contraction. Redrawn Benton et al.

Twitch–Tetanus Relationships

Given that a single pulse of stimulation can produce a single muscle twitch, the next question is how to use twitches to obtain a useful muscle contraction. This is most typically done by applying a series of individual stimulus pulses (sometimes referred to as a "train") at a constant frequency (or interpulse interval). If trains of pulses are repetitively applied, with each train at a higher frequency, the resulting muscle tensions are similar to the schematic shown in Figure 36-3. At low frequencies, the muscle contraction is a series of individual twitches. As the frequency increases, the twitches summate and begin to form a smooth contraction, in which muscle force gradually builds up to a constant value.[7] One might think that high stimulation frequencies would be desirable in FES. Unfortunately, owing to fatigue induced by high stimulation frequencies, this is not the case (see the following).

Fatigue

All muscle contractions, whether volitional, reflex, or electrically stimulated, are subject to fatigue. Fatigue of electrically stimulated muscle contractions can be an

important limiting factor in FES, particularly lower extremity applications in which standing is important. Whereas the dynamics of fatigue may differ from muscle to muscle, electrically stimulated muscle contractions cannot be sustained continuously, and if the duty cycle is too severe, even alternating periods of rest and contraction cannot be sustained at a constant force level.

For example, during standing, postures can be observed in which constant stimulation of the quadriceps is required to maintain stance.[8] Even though resistance to muscle fatigue may be improved by electrical stimulation, fatigue will ultimately occur, and the knees will buckle.[8]

It can be seen also by referring to Figures 36-4 and 36-5 that there is a trade-off involved in selecting the frequency of stimulation. Fatigue considerations require as low a frequency as possible. However, the need for a smooth contraction makes higher frequencies preferable.[7] A protocol for establishing the lowest possible frequency for a particular muscle should be followed if minimization of fatigue is a concern.[9] Fatigue can be reduced by varying the duty cycle (if possible): this is the ratio of the time a muscle is stimulated to the time it is not stimulated and allowed to rest.

Fatigue also can be minimized by cyclically stimulating multiple heads of a muscle group or by periodically changing postures.[10] This brings the ground reaction vector in front of the knees, thus causing relaxation of the quadriceps to allow muscle groups periods of rest.[11] Mechanisms of fatigue for normally innervated

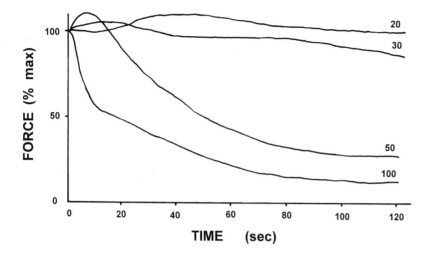

Figure 36-4
Schematic diagram illustrating how relative muscle force (as percent of initial force, on vertical axis) declines over time (horizontal axis) in response to constant delivery of stimulation at several values of stimulus frequency. Note that at lower frequencies, the force is maintained at relatively higher levels for longer periods than at higher stimulation frequencies. Redrawn Benton et al.

muscle are not yet fully understood.[12,13] Most studies of fatigue require determination of maximum voluntary contraction (MVC).[12] It is not advisable to attempt to elicit MVCs by FES because of potential damage to muscle, tendon, or bone from the high forces that can be developed. The exact nature of fatigue is highly specific to the past history of the individual muscle and individual. Efforts to better understand the fatigue of muscles subjected to FES are ongoing.[14–17]

Recruitment in FES

Recruitment means the activation of a certain number of motor units at a specific time. As each motor unit contributes to the total force of the muscle, the contraction force can be modulated or controlled by recruiting more or fewer motor units. Force also can be modulated by increasing or decreasing motor unit firing rates. Neurologically intact individuals are able to accurately con-

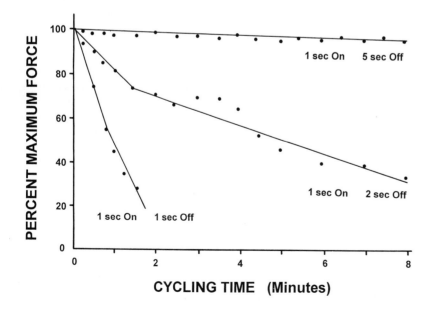

Figure 36-5
Schematic diagram illustrating the effect of duty cycle (period of stimulation versus period of rest) on muscle force production (vertical axis) over time (horizontal axis). Note that the longer the period of rest, the higher the level of force maintained over time. Redrawn Benton et al.

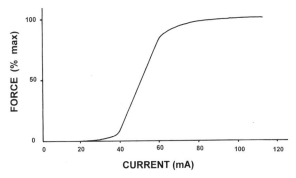

Figure 36-6
Schematic diagram of a typical FES recruitment curve. This curve describes the amount of torque developed at a joint in response to a given intensity of stimulation. The threshold and slope are likely to vary over time, making control difficult. Redrawn Benton et al.

trol muscle force production over a very wide range. This natural recruitment process does not apply when FES is used. In FES, the number of recruited motor units depends on amplitude, pulse width, and electrode configuration. It is not possible to determine the exact number of motor units recruited at a specific level of stimulation; therefore, an input–output relationship, known as the FES recruitment curve, is used to describe this process.

In the typical case, one stimulus parameter, usually amplitude or pulse width, is modulated in an attempt to control muscle-force output. When the amplitude or pulse width is low, the muscle force should be low. When the amplitude or pulse width is high, muscle force should be high. Ideally, there should be a smooth linear transition from zero force to maximum force, and the relationship between amplitude or pulse width applied and resulting muscle force should be constant over time. In the actual situation, the recruitment curve is typically like the one shown in Figure 36-6.[7] For completeness, it is also possible to modulate FES-induced contractile forces by varying the interpulse interval, or stimulation frequency. However, this technique is not widely used.

In Figure 36-6, the amplitude of the stimulating pulse train is shown on the horizontal axis. Keeping all other stimulating parameters (pulse width and frequency) constant, the resulting steady-state torque developed at a joint in response to the stimulus is plotted on the vertical axis. At amplitudes of 20 mA and below, no torque is produced. As the amplitude is increased above 20 mA, torque is produced. The slope of the recruitment curve in this example is steepest between

40 and 60 mA. Above 60 mA, the increment in torque obtained for each increment in pulse amplitude is reduced. This non-linear relationship may cause difficulty when attempting to control FES-induced contractions. This is further complicated by the fact that the threshold (here 20 mA) and slope in the steep part of the recruitment curve are not constant over time. Slight movement of a surface electrode, or the slow formation of scar tissue around an implanted electrode can cause the curve to change. This represents a serious problem for automatic computer-control of FES-induced contractions.

Electrode Systems

Many different stimulation systems and electrode types have been proposed for lower-extremity applications. Several are illustrated schematically in Figure 36-7. Each has advantages and disadvantages. The three broad categories are external systems that are noninvasive (entirely outside the body), percutaneous systems (stimulator and controls outside the body, electrodes inside the body), and implanted systems (stimulator and electrodes inside the body, controls outside the body). Important clinical consideration must be given to the possibility of tissue damage, skin burns from surface electrodes, and infection and nerve damage caused by implants.

Surface Electrodes The most commonly used electrodes have been those that are applied to the surface of the skin.[7,8] These include electrodes and coupling media such as conductive carbon rubber, karaya, water-soaked pads, and conductive polymers. Surface electrodes have a major advantage in clinical application in that they can be easily applied and removed without an invasive procedure. Major disadvantages include variation in electrode recruitment characteristics, lack of selectivity in obtaining a discrete response from a given muscle, inability to stimulate deep muscles (especially hip extensors in lower-extremity applications), external wire connections, skin reactions, and donning/doffing times when daily application is required. One system has been proposed in which surface electrodes are incorporated into a tight-fitting garment that greatly minimizes problems associated with donning and doffing surface electrodes.[18] Surface electrodes concomitantly deliver sensory stimulation that can provoke undesirable reflex responses or spasticity. If sensation is at least partially intact, comfort may also be an issue. This can be partially addressed by choice of stimulus waveform.[19,20]

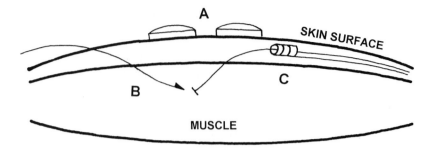

Figure 36-7
Schematic diagram illustrating several varieties of electrodes for delivering FES: noninvasive (A), percutaneous (B), and implanted (C).

Percutaneous Electrodes The Caldwell-Reswick electrode was originally designed for short-term research use, but has been refined over the years for more permanent use.[21,22] The electrodes have a failure rate of approximately 4 percent per month (after 6 months). The need to periodically replace electrodes and maintain the electrode entry site are major disadvantages of this system. Newer designs may reduce failure rate.[23] The difficulty in removing broken electrodes, should the need arise, remains a difficult problem. Advantages are comparable to the implanted systems described in the following.

Implanted Electrodes Implantable systems pose a host of technological problems.[24] At first glance, it would seem that implanted systems should offer user convenience and ease of operation compared to surface electrode systems, because the electrodes are permanently in place. Once stabilized, electrode recruitment characteristics are likely to remain essentially constant.[25] The nerve cuff electrode often has been proposed for use in this regard.[25–28] The only major long-term follow-up study using an implanted system with a cuff electrode is the "Neuromuscular Assist Device" for use in hemiplegia.[26] The epineural electrode has been used in some human studies.[29] This consists of a small electrode that is sewn on the epineurium. The epimysial electrode is sewn on the muscle sheath in the vicinity of the motor point.[30] Several variations of an intraneural electrode have been proposed, but these are still in early stages of development. They consist of a very fine wire inserted into the nerve fascicle.[31,32]

Safety and Waveform Considerations

There are a number of safety issues that relate to electrical stimulation of paralyzed muscle. Intermittent stimulation using surface electrodes with commonly accepted protocols appears to be safe. Skin burns are always

a potential complication with surface electrodes, and proper protocols should be followed to avoid them.[33]

Two major potential sources of damage to peripheral nerves from implantable devices are the delivery of the electrical stimulation itself and the mechanical attachment of the electrode to the tissue to be stimulated.[34] Adverse mechanical tension can damage nerves. It is also possible to irreversibly damage nerve by continuous stimulation at frequencies of 50 Hz for constant periods of between 8 and 16 hours. It may be difficult to ascribe any damage that might occur to one of these sources, since one cannot deliver stimulation without a mechanical attachment. The site of implantation and the routing of the cable must also be taken into account. Extensive previous experience and research indicate that it is highly unlikely that a commercially available, properly placed FES device can cause damage to the underlying neural structures in the course of normal operation of the device.

CURRENT FES SYSTEMS

A number of medically prescribable FES systems are commercially available today. Several representative examples have been chosen for illustrative purposes. Each section will give a brief description of indications and contraindications, a technical description of the system, and a scenario of how the device can be used by the patient on a daily basis. Following the description of what is commercially available, a brief summary of current research in the area will be given. Because of space limitations, a fully complete and definitive description of each device cannot be provided in this chapter, nor can all available devices be covered. Physicians must read all literature and instructions supplied by the manufacturer prior to prescribing the devices, described in overview form in the following.

Phrenic Pacing Systems

Medically Prescribable System Since 1966, when Glenn and coworkers developed the first implantable phrenic pacemaker, more than 1,000 phrenic pacing systems have been implanted in patients ranging in age from 2.5 months to over 80.[35–37] Most of these phrenic pacing system have been produced by the Avery Laboratories, Glen Cove, New York. The purpose of this and all other phrenic pacing systems is to provide part-time or full-time ventilation in patients with respiratory dysfunction caused by lesions in the central nervous system. Periodically applied electrical pulses to the phrenic nerves cause each hemidiaphragm to contract and the lungs to expand (inspiration). When the electrical pulses cease, the diaphragm relaxes, resulting in expiration. Inspiration by phrenic pacing is achieved by generation of negative pressure in the thorax, a more physiological approach to respiration than mechanical positive-pressure ventilation.

Phrenic pacing is indicated in patients with paralysis of the diaphragm after high cervical cord injury or lesions in the brain stem.[36,37] Only those patients with stable chronic ventilatory failure are candidates for phrenic pacing. Phrenic pacing also may be considered in patients with central alveolar hypoventilation (CAH) associated with central apnea, especially during sleep. CAH may be either idiopathic (Ondine's Curse) or secondary to organic lesions in the brain stem. In patients with suspected CAH, the central nature of nocturnal apnea must be proven by sleep studies. There is a risk of about 5 percent of damage to the phrenic nerve during implantation.[38,36] Therefore, the indications and therapeutic goals for implantation of a phrenic pacemaker should be considered carefully in all patients with preserved spontaneous breathing during the majority of the time during the day, and especially in children.

The most important contraindication for phrenic pacing is a lower motor neuron lesion of the phrenic nerves. Lower motor neuron lesions can be expected in patients with poliomyelitis, severe polyneuropathy, or advancing neurofibromas in von Recklinghausen's disease. The same is true for spinal lesions between the C3 and C5 levels, as many cell bodies of phrenic nerve fibers in the anterior horn of the spinal cord may be damaged. Phrenic pacing also is contraindicated if the diaphragm is affected by neuromuscular disorders or mitochondrial myopathy. Further contraindications for phrenic pacing include abnormal respiratory mechanics, such as in chronic obstructive pulmonary disease (COPD), or in kyphoscoliosis, with severe rib cage deformity. Also, phrenic pacing is not indicated in unconscious patients.

In order to assure the proper function of the phrenic nerve and the diaphragm, preoperative radiological neurophysiologic tests must be performed. In those with some preserved spontaneous breathing, voluntary contractions of the diaphragm are checked by radiographic screening or by ultrasound. If voluntary contractions of the diaphragm are not visible, transcutaneous electrical or magnetic stimulation of the phrenic nerve at the neck is used to evoke contractions of each hemidiaphragm.[40] In addition to the mechanical response, electromyographic (EMG) recordings of the electrical response can be performed with surface electrodes. In the literature a latency of the electrical response of less than 12.0 ms (normal range after magnetic stimulation of the phrenic nerve: 6.5–9.8 ms) has been proposed as an indicator for successful pacing.[36] The mechanical effectiveness of phrenic nerve stimulation can be assessed by measuring transdiaphragmatic pressure with balloon catheters placed in the mid-esophagus and in the stomach, by recording the pressure difference between them.

Unilateral phrenic pacing is only sufficient in selected adult patients with CAH who need part-time ventilatory support, who have good lung compliance and no airflow obstruction. Especially in children and quadriplegics, unilateral phrenic pacing leads to paradoxical excursions of the rib cage and the contralateral diaphragm, thus reducing the effectiveness of ventilation.[36] Therefore, synchronous bilateral phrenic pacing is superior with more efficient ventilation of both lungs and less charge required to effect the same ventilation. The risk of muscle fiber damage of the diaphragm is reduced in bilateral pacing, since bilateral pacing is possible with lower stimulation frequencies.[41]

A typical arrangement of the internal and external components of a bilateral system for phrenic pacing is pictured in Figure 36-8. An external battery-driven radio frequency transmitter sends signals and power through ring antennae, taped to the skin over the implanted receivers. The receivers generate the stimulation impulses delivered by the implanted electrodes. There is a wire connector between each receiver and the corresponding electrode to enable independent exchange of either component in the case of implant failure. The Avery Laboratories phrenic pacemaker uses monopolar electrodes with the anode integrated in the case of the receiver. Bipolar cuff electrodes are potentially available for patients who already have cardiac pacemakers or other electrical stimulation devices implanted, in order to avoid cross-currents. The new, improved version

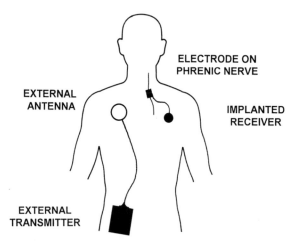

ELECTRODE ON
PHRENIC NERVE

EXTERNAL
ANTENNA

IMPLANTED
RECEIVER

EXTERNAL
TRANSMITTER

Figure 36-8
Schematic diagram illustrating the placement of an implantable phrenic pacing system.

of the Avery phrenic pacing system with the I-110A receiver (30 mm diameter, 8 mm thick) and the portable, battery-powered S-232G transmitter obtained approval from the U.S. Food and Drug Administration (FDA) in 1991. In contrast to older versions, thermal stabilization allows full outdoor activities while pacing. Transtelephonic monitoring provides remote assessment of stimulation effectiveness and problem troubleshootings from any telephone. A newer Mark IV transmitter system with redundant bilateral transmitters is available in countries outside the United States.

Prior to a successful application of phrenic pacing a period of conditioning of the diaphragm by part-time stimulation is necessary to increase the fatigue-resistance of the diaphragm.[41] This is especially true in those with central paralysis of the diaphragm, where a predominance of fast-fatiguing type II muscle fibers and a disuse atrophy of the diaphragm can be expected. It can take several weeks, and even a few months to achieve full-time pacing in quadriplegics. Reconditioning can often be done at home, if appropriate support by an instructed caregiver is provided. Overstimulation of the phrenic nerve can lead to lasting nerve damage. Therefore, monitoring blood gases by noninvasive pulse oximetry, capnography, and transtelephonic monitoring of the diaphragm electromyogram are indicated to detect the development of fatigue.[42] In those with sleep apnea, little or no reconditioning is usually necessary.

A mechanical ventilator is required as a backup for those who are fully ventilatory dependent, as the

S-232G transmitters' bilateral stimulus outputs are not redundant, and rely solely on a single battery power source. To maintain a patent airway for mechanical positive pressure ventilation, usually a tracheostomy is necessary prior to implantation of a phrenic pacemaker. Phrenic pacing is not synchronized with the activation of upper airway muscles, and therefore a tracheostomy may also be necessary to prevent upper airway obstruction, especially during sleep. Patients with brain-stem lesions have a high risk of aspiration, and sometimes require not only tracheostomy but also closure of the larynx.[43] Patients with a lesion confined to the upper spinal cord with preservation of the brain stem, who are able to control their upper airways, may be provided with a plug instead of a tracheostomy tube, that can be opened to suction secretions. This plug also facilitates phonation. Permanent closure of the tracheostomy can be considered in some patients, provided there is residual spontaneous ventilation or the patient is able to perform emergency ventilation using accessory muscles or glossopharyngeal ("frog") breathing using the tongue and pharyngeal muscles for 10 minutes or more. In those who do not require a tracheostomy tube, upper airway obstruction during phrenic pacing may also be prevented by nasal CPAP (Continuous Positive Airway Pressure).[44]

A successful application of the Avery phrenic pacing system provides a person with high-level spinal cord injury full-time ventilatory support. A full-time caregiver is required for positioning of the external antennas over the implanted receivers and for system setup in quadriplegics. After the system is correctly mounted, a quadriplegic is able to comfortably sit in a chair, and move around with a power-driven wheelchair indoors and outdoors. A successful user is able to carry on essentially normal conversation. The small battery-driven external S-232G transmitter of the Avery phrenic pacing system is less intrusive than a mechanical ventilator with respect to size and sound, which has important social ramifications.

Mechanical positive-pressure ventilation is the most important alternative to phrenic pacing.[45] In one retrospective clinical study of quadriplegic, ventilatory-dependent patients, those who were mechanical-ventilator-dependent expired earlier than those with phrenic pacemakers, but the difference in mortality rates did not reach statistical significance.[46] More recent studies reported several medical advantages of phrenic pacing compared to long-term mechanical positive-pressure ventilation, including reduced secretions, lower rate of pulmonary infections and atelectasis, reduced barotrauma of the lungs, and reduced risk of cor pulmonale.[47,48] The number of patients involved in these studies was rather small, and there is still the need to demonstrate a more favorable outcome with phrenic pacing compared to mechanical positive-pressure ventilation in a controlled prospective multi-center study. The price for the basic equipment for phrenic pacemakers, not including costs for surgery, is nearly twice that of a portable mechanical ventilator. However, in a recent comparative study between phrenic pacing and mechanical ventilation in quadriplegic patients, long-term treatment costs, including materials and nursing care in the phrenic pacing group, were reduced.[47] If both kinds of treatment are compared, not only relative to cost, but quality of life, phrenic pacing is favored by most patients. Long-term savings in health care costs, increased productivity, and patient satisfaction may justify differences in initial costs.

Another alternative or supplement to phrenic pacing is the pneumobelt, a corset-type device that is placed around the abdomen and allows for ventilation without the need for a tracheostomy.[49] Cyclic inflation of the pneumobelt is provided by a positive-pressure ventilator pump. In contrast to phrenic pacing or conventional positive-pressure ventilators, the pneumobelt produces ventilation by assisting expiration, rather than inspiration. Some patients with paralysis of the diaphragm of different etiologies with relative preservation of brain-stem function have achieved part-time or full-time ventilation with the pneumobelt for periods up to 10 years.[49,50]

Although reports in the literature are preliminarily positive, clinical experience with pneumobelts is limited to a few centers. Other techniques used successfully to achieve artificial mechanical ventilation include rocking beds and negative pressure ventilators, such as the original iron lung, the wrap ventilator, or the cuirass. This equipment, however, is cumbersome and eliminates or reduces mobility. Pharmacologic therapy to increase the respiratory drive has not proven effective in completely ventilatory-dependent patients. Drugs that prevent bronchospasm or reduce the amount and viscosity of secretions can be useful. Efforts to improve ventilatory insufficiency by increasing the strength and endurance of accessory respiratory muscles that remain functional (neck-muscle breathing, glossopharyngeal breathing) should be taught and encouraged for a few minutes to several hours per day.

Other commercially available phrenic pacing systems include the Atrotech OY (Tampere, Finland) and Medimplant Inc. (Vienna, Austria). These systems differ from the Avery unit primarily by their multipolar electrode arrangement and the stimulation patterns used. Systems with monopolar or bipolar electrodes (as the Avery system described earlier) always stimulate the same motor units during each inspiration, with the potential to cause earlier fatigue than systems using the multipolar electrode arrangement of the Atrotech and Medimplant. The Atrotech OY phrenic nerve stimulator model Jukka has one receiver for each side and a quadripolar electrode attached to each phrenic nerve. Two Teflon strip carriers with two pairs of electrode poles each are affixed to perineural tissue without the need for microsurgery. Four-pole sequential stimulation is used by selecting different combinations of the four electrodes for successive stimulation pulses. The firing frequency of the single motor units must be lower than the overall stimulation frequency, usually one fourth of the total stimulation frequency in the ideal case. This adjustment reduces the risk of muscle fatigue.[51] Because a certain proportion of motor units in the diaphragm are always producing force, a smooth fused contraction of the diaphragm still occurs.[52] Despite the more complex design of the Atrotech system compared to the Avery system, the size of the external controller (stimulator/transmitter) is reduced. Experience with implantation of the multipolar systems is growing considerably.[53]

The phrenic pacing system, developed in Vienna by Medimplant Inc., has one multichannel receiver that serves both sides that can be implanted with a single sternotomy approach. Four (epineural) wire loop electrodes are attached by microsurgical techniques to each phrenic nerve.[54] This multichannel system uses "carousel" stimulation, selecting different combinations of electrodes for successive pulse trains. This system has enjoyed early popularity in Germany and Austria, but has not yet been approved for the United States.

Current Research All presently available commercial implants for phrenic pacing need an external power supply and continuous telemetry control. A prototype of a fully implantable, battery-driven, microcontroller-based, eight-channel stimulator has recently been developed.[54] Research into the development of demand-type ventilatory pacemakers with synchronization to the upper-airway muscles is also ongoing.

As previously discussed, phrenic pacing is not possible after lower motor neuron lesions of the phrenic nerve. One possible solution is an anastomosis of a viable intercostal nerve to the damaged phrenic nerve. Once successful axonal regeneration and diaphragmatic reinnervation have occurred, the distal phrenic nerve can be paced.[55] The long-term success rate and viability of this procedure has not yet been determined.

Stimulation of intercostal accessory muscles for assisted ventilation is currently under investigation.[56] Similarly, abdominal muscle stimulation for ventilation, analogous to the pneumobelt, also has been explored.[57] Both of these techniques are new and will require substantial additional clinical investigation prior to their use.

In addition to the loss of ventilatory function in the high-level tetraplegic, many individuals with SCI in the cervical and upper thoracic levels have impaired cough. As a result, pulmonary complications are now the leading cause of death in this population.[58] The feasibility of using abdominal muscle stimulation to restore cough has been demonstrated in two laboratories.[59,60] Again, further research will be required to bring this technique into clinical practice.

Bladder-Micturition

Medically Prescribable System Today, the Finetech-Brindley sacral anterior nerve-root stimulator is the most successful FES system for assisted bladder control.[61–63] Its main purposes are to improve bladder emptying and to achieve continence in those with neurogenic bladder-voiding dysfunctions. In some, this device can be used to assist in defecation and to enable male patients to have sustained full penile erections. In 1992, over 500 of these systems have been implanted in Europe and Australia, most of them in patients with spinal cord lesions.[64–66] A clinical study under an Investigational Device Exemption (IDE) from the FDA, is now underway to approve this system for use in the United States.

This system is useful for patients with neurogenic voiding disorders, especially after spinal-cord lesions.[67] Implantation of a sacral anterior root stimulator is an invasive measure, and should be reserved only for patients with recurrent urinary infections or vesico-uretero-renal reflux despite conventional treatment. Another, less compelling indication for implantation is reflex incontinence, especially in women with spinal-cord lesions since no external collecting device is possible. The most important prerequisites for successful sacral anterior root stimulation are an intact sacral reflex arc, with at least an intact lower motor neuron function, and a detrusor that can generate a physiologic contraction. The integrity of the sacral reflex arc can be demonstrated on a cystometragram, by reflex erections of the

penis, and the presence of the bulbocavernosus reflex, the anal skin reflex, and the ankle jerk. These pathways can be studied by transrectal electrostimulation of the pelvic splanchnic nerves, normally used for electroejaculation, or by direct stimulation of the sacral nerve roots with needle electrodes in the sacral foramina.[68,69] Preserved pain sensitivity of the sacral segments in those with incomplete spinal lesions may limit successful application of this device. In order to assess patient tolerance for sacral stimulation, the "electroejaculation" procedure has been proposed as a preoperative screening test. Paraplegic patients, who are able to transfer to a toilet seat without help, usually gain more than tetraplegic patients. Sacral stimulators may interfere with sexual function, and therefore men with poor or absent reflex erections have less to lose than those with reflex erections useful for coitus. Patients with traumatic spinal cord injury, multiple sclerosis and other spinal dosorders may benefit from sacral anterior root stimulation.

The implantation of a sacral anterior root stimulator is contraindicated if a majority of the lower motor neurons innervating the detrusor are damaged. Implantation is also not recommended when a clinical recovery is anticipated, as in the first year after spinal cord injury. In those with incomplete spinal injuries, implantation of a sacral stimulator should be deferred until 2 years after injury.[66] Several patients with neurogenic bladder dysfunction owing to myelomeningocele, with preserved sacral anterior horn cells, have received sacral anterior root stimulators, but electromicturition could not be induced successfully.[67] Although a small subset of adult or adolescent patients with myelomeningocele may benefit from sacral anterior root stimulation, alternative stimulation sites are considered more promising.[70] The Finetech-Brindley sacral anterior root stimulator is designed for adults only. Therefore this device is not currently suitable for implantation in growing children.

The Finetech-Brindley system consists of an external control unit with a radio-frequency transmitter for three independent channels and a set of three receivers, that are implanted subcutaneously over the lower ribs. For special purposes, systems with two or four channels are available. The receivers are connected by platinum-iridium helical cables to a set of U-shaped platinum foil electrodes. The electrodes are mounted in a symmetrical tripolar arrangement, with two anodes and one cathode in the middle, in slots of silicone-rubber structures called "books."[62]. In the original surgical procedure proposed by Brindley and coworkers, the books are implanted intradurally at about the level of the last intervertebral disc, and the S2 to S5 anterior roots are trapped in different slots of the books. Usually three different groups of roots can be stimulated independently by paired excitation of both S2, S3, and S4 roots.

The sacral anterior roots S2–S4 innervate the detrusor by preganglionic parasympathetic nerve fibers as well as the external sphincter of the bladder and pelvic floor muscles by somatic nerve fibers through the pudendal nerve. During stimulation of these roots, detrusor contraction results in increased intravesical pressure. However, bladder emptying is prevented by simultaneously occurring contraction of the external sphincter. When stimulation is interrupted, the external sphincter (composed of striated muscle) relaxes faster than the detrusor (consisting of smooth muscle), resulting in voiding of a portion of the bladder contents. Therefore, repetitive bursts of stimulation pulses must be used for effective micturition.

The co-contraction of detrusor and external sphincter, referred to as detrusor-sphincter dyssynergia (DSD), is not only dependent on the electrical stimulation, but also spinal reflexes. DSD during bladder voiding can be diminished by dorsal sacral rhizotomy of roots S2–S5 for, in effect, interrupting the afferent part of the reflex arc to the bladder. Dorsal sacral rhizotomy serves to lower intravesical pressure in the intervals between stimulator-driven micturitions, and increase bladder capacity and bladder compliance, thereby preventing unintended reflex voiding of the bladder.[62,67,71,72] Autonomic dysreflexia also can be eliminated by dorsal rhizotomy.[65] Adverse consequences of dorsal rhizotomy include loss of reflex erection, reflex ejaculation, reflex micturition, and reflex defecation, in addition to loss of perineal sensation. Under most circumstances, the benefits outweigh potential disadvantages, and therefore dorsal sacral rhizotomy is strongly recommended during implantation of the sacral anterior root stimulator.[64]

Sacral anterior root stimulation combined with dorsal rhizotomy leads to excellent results in nearly 90 percent of patients; with restoration of full urinary continence, significant increase in bladder capacity and voluntary micturition with residual urine below 30 mL.[65] The frequency of urinary tract infections is reduced for many, but not all. Most patients who show dilatation of the upper urinary tract or reflux improve considerably after the combined surgery. Few patients with sacral anterior root stimulators require additional therapies to promote interstimulation continence and complete bladder voiding, if dorsal sacral rhizotomy is performed. Persistent bladder hyperreflexia can be treated with anticholinergic agents, but excessive use of these drugs may have an adverse effect on bladder contractility.[73] In cases of striated sphincter hyperactivity during micturition, parasphincteral infiltrations with Lidocaine 1 percent and intravenous or orally administered alpha-blockers may be applied. Transurethral sphincterotomy should only be considered, if dorsal rhizotomy and adjuvant drug therapy have failed. Five to ten percent of patients with sacral anterior root stimulators suffer from stress incontinence, probably owing to incompetence of the bladder neck.[65,74] Autonomic dysreflexia, heralded by a significant rise of blood pressure or headache during reflex micturition, improves in most cases after implantation of a sacral anterior root stimulator and dorsal rhizotomy.[65] However, in some patients generally with spinal lesions above T5, severe autonomic dysreflexia may limit this procedure's application.[62]

Sacral roots S2–S5, which are stimulated by the Finetech-Brindley system, innervate not only the bladder, but also the anal sphincter, the smooth muscles in the distal colon and anorectum through parasympathetic ganglia at S3 and S4. Therefore, sacral anterior root stimulation can also be used to assist defecation.[62,75] In a small prospective study, nearly half of those with complete spinal-cord injury achieved complete evacuation of faeces using the stimulator alone.[76] The mean frequency of defecation was significantly higher after implantation of the stimulator combined with dorsal rhizotomy than before, and the mean time spent defecating each week was significantly less. Patients who were not able to defecate using the stimulator alone and required rhizotomy had to perform manual evacuation of feces.

About two-thirds of male patients achieve adequate penile erections by sacral anterior root stimulation. This is especially relevant for males who lose their reflex erections after posterior rhizotomy. About one third of male patients with sacral anterior root stimulators can use electrically induced erections for intercourse successfully.[65] Lower limb spasms triggered by the stimulation may prevent some from having intercourse despite sufficient erectile function.[77]

The standard surgical procedure for implantation of the Finetech-Brindley stimulator is a laminectomy from L4–S2, with intradural implantation of electrode books combined with posterior rhizotomy in a single operation. Some centers prefer to implant the stimulating electrodes extradurally, to avoid a permanent connection between the intradural and extradural space, and to prevent CSF leakage and myelomeningitis. The best access to all posterior roots for rhizotomy is at their entry into the conus medullaris, making a laminectomy at T12–L1 necessary. Hohenfellner has proposed separating the ventral roots intradurally into their rootlets, so that individual rootlets can be tested by electrical stimulation to determine whether they innervate the external sphincter rather than the detrusor.[78] This technique enables a selective anterior rhizotomy of the rootlets innervating the sphincter to be performed.[78]

The optimum result from the combined rhizotomy sacral anterior root stimulator is complete voluntary bladder control. In order to apply stimulation, the patient holds an external transmitter immediately over the implanted receiver and switches on the small hand held unit. Bursts of stimulation cause micturition to occur in successive, small portions. After 1 to 2 minutes, the bladder is almost empty, with a residual of less than 20 mL. Frequently, a patient can remain completely continent between implant-driven micturitions.

Another stimulator for bladder voiding being implanted in the United States not only promotes effective bladder emptying, but also therapeutically reduces detrusor instability. This technique is called neuromodulation.[69,79] By enhancing tone within the urethral sphincter through chronic stimulation of the sacral roots of the pudendal nerve, a suppressive effect on the irritable detrusor muscle occurs. It is not clear whether the successful use of this technique in children with bladder and bowel incontinence due to myelomeningocele can be mainly attributed to tonic contraction of the striated urinary sphincter, or to inhibition of detrusor reflex activity by afferent stimulation of the pudendal nerve.[70]

Current Research To overcome detrusor-sphincter dyssynergia (DSD) during sacral anterior root stimulation, usually posterior rhizotomy or neurotomy of the pudendal nerve must be performed.[78] The major disadvantage of these measures is the elimination of reflex erections in males. An alternative method under investigation is high-frequency stimulation of the pudendal nerve, designed to fatigue the external sphincter prior to micturition. This method preserves reflex erections, and has been successfully tested in animal experiments.[80]

Another method to activate the detrusor without activating the sphincter is the use of anodal block to prevent propagation of action potentials in the large somatic axons of the external sphincter. In animal experiments, this technique has been developed to the point that contraction of the bladder and rectum can be produced without contraction of the external sphincters.[66]

In a pilot study, an artificial sphincter by surgical transposition and electrical stimulation of the gracilis muscle was successfully tested in three patients.[81]

Sacral anterior root stimulation fails when most lower motor neurons innervating the bladder are damaged. When this happens, direct stimulation of the bladder wall may still be possible. Some studies have demonstrated bladder voiding induced by stimulation via electrodes sutured to the bladder wall.[82,83] However, the failure rate was high, mainly owing to breakage and erosion of lead wires into the bladder wall or into the abdominal wall. Recently, only a handful of investigators have attempted to develop improved systems for direct bladder-wall stimulation.[84]

Lower Extremity Systems

Medically Prescribable Systems The Parastep (R) is the only FDA-approved lower-extremity FES system in commercial distribution in the United States.[85] The purpose of this FES system is to provide limited periods of standing and walking for either exercise or functional purposes, typically in the vicinity of the wheelchair. This FES system does not appear to be intended as a complete replacement for the wheelchair. The basic principle of operation is to provide constant tetanic stimulation to the knee extensors during stance, and transient stimulation to the common peroneal nerve to obtain a flexion-withdrawal reflex that produces the swing phase of gait.

It is most useful in certain individuals who are spinal-cord-injured, with complete lesions in the mid- to lower thoracic region, and some tetraplegics with incomplete lesions in the C5–C8 region with absence of sensation in the legs, strong upper extremities, manual dexterity to operate the controller, good sense of balance, and the ability to understand and operate the system. This system should not be used by patients who are suspected of having osteoporosis or diseases of the joints, autonomic dysreflexia, deconditioned cardiopulmonary systems, obesity, lower motor neuron paralysis of the quadriceps, hip flexors, and ankle dorsiflexors, skin problems that preclude use of surface electrodes, severe spasticity, severe joint contracture of the hip, knee, or ankle, severe scoliosis, pregnancy, or vision or hearing impairments that could interfere with training and use.

The system works as follows. To initiate standing, the knee extensors (quadriceps) are bilaterally stimulated with a waveform that provides for a gradual onset of muscle contraction. One pair of surface electrodes is used on each thigh. This assists the user in moving from a sitting to a standing position. The importance of the upper extremities in providing balance and additional vertical lifting force cannot be overemphasized. Once the user is standing, constant stimulation is used to maintain quadriceps contraction and knee stability. When the user is ready to take a step, weight is shifted to the control leg, and the step button in the walker is depressed. This switches stimulation to the quadriceps of the swing leg off, and triggers delivery of stimulation to the peroneal nerve to elicit a flexion withdrawal reflex. Surface electrodes are used. This reflex causes both ankle dorsiflexion and hip flexion. When the hip flexion occurs, the user releases the step button. Stimulation for flexion withdrawal is switched off, and quadriceps stimulation is switched on to extend the knee. The upper body is used to move forward and complete the step. Since each step must be carefully controlled by the user, gait velocity is slower than normal.

A precise and careful biomechanical analysis of the user's standing posture is essential to determine what the FES is actually accomplishing during stance. In this system, the hip joints are stabilized in a manner identical to that used with long-leg braces (the so-called c-curve posture) in which the net ground reaction vector (GRV) is kept behind the hip center of rotation. In this way, the hip is passively stabilized without the need for active hip extensor or flexor muscle activity. The knee is stabilized by the FES-induced contraction of the quadriceps. However, the net ground reaction vector typically fluctuates, moving both in front of and behind center of rotation of the knee. When the net ground reaction vector is in front of the knee, the knee can be passively stabilized against its anatomical extension constraint by gravity. In this situation, stability can be maintained without FES. As the net ground reaction vector moves behind the knee, the stabilization requirements for the FES-induced contraction increase. If a posture is assumed in which the net GRV moves farther behind the center of rotation of the knee then the FES-induced contraction is able to stabilize, then the knee will buckle. If the user always assumes standing postures in which the net GRV is always in front of the knee, then the FES-induced contraction becomes unnecessary during quiet standing.

The ankle joint is never stimulated with the Parastep System. The hip and knee are stabilized as described, essentially held against an anatomical constraint by an electrically stimulated muscle force or by gravity, whereas the ankle is free to rotate within its range of motion. Stability at the ankle essentially is regulated by upper-extremity function in conjunction with the balance aid. No method has yet been developed for stimulating ankle plantaflexors and dorsiflexors in a controlled way during FES-assisted standing.

An individual using the system is pictured in Figure 36-9. The system consists of the following components: a microcomputer-controlled stimulator, a battery pack with recharger, a testing unit for evaluation system operation and integrity electrode cables, surface electrodes, electrode power cables, and walker-attached control switches (activate by fingers).

Potential fault modes of the device include electronic failure or cable disconnection. If the stimulator fails, and the quadriceps is relaxed during weight bearing, this could lead to falling. Each patient must have risks and preventions clearly explained.

The optimum goal for Parastep use is independent ambulations for short distances without using long leg braces. This can be done at home or the workplace. Under optimum circumstances, some activities of daily living that require standing that is impossible from the wheelchair can be performed. Examples of activities of daily living that can be successfully performed using Parastep include filling and emptying a dishwasher, taking a drink from a water fountain, operating a photocopier, removing and placing books on a shelf, and obtaining a soft drink from a vending machine. The level of functional outcome that is actually achieved with this system is largely a function of individual motivation and ability to apply the system to activities of daily living. Most individuals can walk approximately 100 to 150 feet at a time. Walking and standing can last up to 20–45 minutes per session. The advantage of FES technology for assistance in walking and standing must always be compared to non-FES technologies, including standard bracing, hybrid systems, passive or powered standing aids, and Rizzoli Boots.[86]

Current Research

Recent applied research has focused on using multi-channel implantable systems to assist tetraplegic individuals with transfer.[87] Implantable systems with higher numbers of channels continue to be used in feasibility studies for restoration of lower-limb movements in paraplegia.[88] The flexion-withdrawal reflex has been an integral part of the four-channel surface electrode-based system, beginning with its introduction in the early 1970s to the present-day Parastep system.[8] Habituation of the flexion-withdrawal reflex has been problematic in some

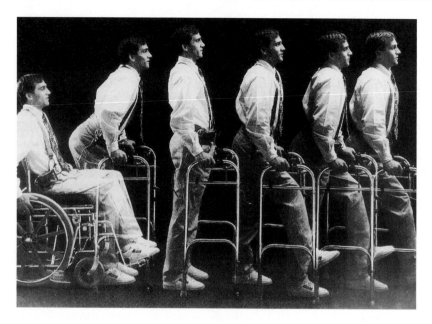

Figure 36-9
A paraplegic individual using the Parastep ® system. (Photo reproduced with permission of Krieger Publishing.)

subjects. Recent studies have suggested that multiplexing flexion-withdrawal reflex stimulation between two sites can sometimes reduce habituation.[89] Many researchers worldwide continue to explore variants of the original four-channel surface-electrode system.[8,90,91]

All of the lower-extremity FES Systems with clinical applications, typified by Parastep, have been open-loop systems. This means that, after being turned on or triggered by the patient, stimulation is applied in a pre-programmed sequence, delivered to achieve a predetermined functional goal. In standing, for example, if the patient decided not to stand after turning the stimulator on, the legs would continue to be stimulated to stand until the stimulator is switched off. Considerable interest is developing in the design and production of a closed-loop system, where sensors modify the stimulus output based on the movement that is generated. Extensive efforts are underway to convert computer models and simulations and rule-based systems into electrically based, functionally useful assisted devices.[92,93] At this point most researchers have employed ad hoc methods, such as the propositional-integral-derivation controller, non-numerical or finite state control schemes, cycle-to-cycle controller, and rule-based machine learning techniques.[94–97] Neural networks also are under investigation as possible controllers.[98] Technology that provides sensory feedback to the subject by vibrotactile stimulation and extended physiological proprioception also is under investigation.[99,100] Extensive analytical work will

be required to measure and quantify the actual movement patterns observed in FES-induced standing and walking.[96,101,102]

In FES systems that do not rely on bracing, such as hybrid systems, fatigue remains a problem, particularly for the quadriceps. Understanding the physiologic basis for fatigue by modeling is now underway.[103] The energy cost of FES-induced locomotion continues to be a limiting factor for many in achieving widespread patient acceptance and use.[104] The physiological cost index has been found to vary widely among those who use FES systems.[105]

In addition to standard lower-extremity FES systems, some FES-based orthotic systems incorporate lower-extremity bracing as the primary antigravity support and supplement the forces needed for locomotion with FES-evoked muscle contractors.[104,106–109] These are commonly referred to as hybrid systems. Recently, magnetic particle friction brakes have been incorporated into the joints of some devices to obtain additional control of FES-stimulated movements.[110]

Upper Extremity

Medically Prescribable System   FES systems designed to restore basic grip function, including gross and pincer grasp, now are available. Recently, these upper-extremity devices have been incorporated into thera-

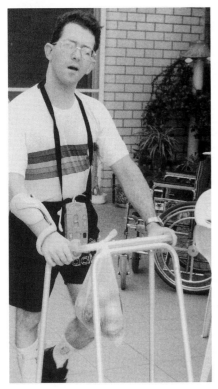

Figure 36-10
*An individual using the Handmaster system to grip his walker.
(Photo reproduced with permission of NESS, Inc.)*

peutic exercise programs in some patients after stroke, brain injury, cerebral palsy, and cervical spinal cord injury.[111–113] One such system is the Handmaster®.[111] This consists of a control unit housing the electronics and batteries, a splint worn on the forearm that contains the electrodes, and a cable connecting the control unit and splint. The electrodes are integrated into the splint, so that donning and doffing the orthosis is facilitated. The electrodes are covered with cloth pads that are dampened with tapwater, which provides the conductive interface. The device is operated by touch buttons on the control unit, and on the splint itself. The intensity of stimulation, function mode, and thumb position during the functional activity are easily controlled by the patient. (An individual using this system is shown in Fig. 36-10.)

Current Research Several upper-extremity FES-based systems are now in development and trial investigation that deliver the electrical stimulation through either percutaneous wire electrodes or implantable systems.[112–116] One of the more challenging research prob-

lems in upper extremity FES research is how to compose trains of stimulation sequences of a number of muscles that lead to kinesiologic function.[117] Experimental research to date has been hampered by variability in electrode-recruitment properties, both within and between subjects.[118,119] If these systems are to become clinically practical, computer-controlled and modulated-stimulation sequences will be required.[120] Although the vast majority of investigative efforts have focused on hand function, FES control of elbow flexion and forearm supination also under development.[121,122]

Signals for command and control of FES systems in the upper extremity have typically arisen from the contralateral side. Most units descend on contralateral shoulder movement, with different shoulder movements corresponding to different grasp/release functions in the stimulated hand.[123] EMG and joystick controls are also in development.[113,114] Sensory-feedback loops that modulate force and function in the fingertips are now available on an experimental basis.[124]

Exercise

Medically Prescribable Systems In addition to orthotic devices designed to produce functional movements, FES has been used for many years in therapeutic exercise. In cases of incomplete SCI (either tetraplegia or paraplegia) in which the major muscle groups of the legs have upper motor neuron paralysis, commercially available bicycle ergometers can be an appropriate method for exercise. The system consists of an adjustable seating module, bicycle, special pedal attachments, force and position sensors, a six-channel stimulator using surface electrodes, and a keyboard unit for therapist control.[125,126]

Surface electrodes are applied bilaterally over the quadriceps, hamstring, and gluteal muscle groups. Based on measurements of the pedal position, cranking velocity, and force, stimulation sequences are applied to these muscle groups by a computer-controlled electrical probe. As with any exercise program, exercise tolerance must be increased slowly. Numerous physiological studies confirm that response to FES-induced exercise is comparable to that of volitional exercise in neurologically normal individuals.[127]

Comparison with Competing Technologies

It is extremely important for physicians considering prescription of FES systems to consider competing technologies. Sometimes the patient, in addition to physical injury, may also be a victim of, for lack of a better phrase, the "high technology syndrome." The fact that a small box exists with a modern computer inside that delivers stimulation to paralyzed muscle may compel the patient to think that it must be better than some simple, perhaps mechanical, device that has been around for a number of years.

The first question to ask is not what FES device is appropriate for a patient, but what it is that a patient wants to do. The next question is what type of device will allow the patient to do this.

RECOMMENDED FURTHER READINGS

An enormous amount of additional information is available about FES, including a clinical guide,[7] a user's guide,[128] general reference texts,[34,129–135] specific application texts,[8,85] and a chapter in the *Handbook of Physiology*.[5] Several review articles also exist.[136–142] There have been several journals that have devoted entire issues to the topic.[143] The *Medical Device Register* lists 49 manufacturers of electrically powered muscle stimulators that are FDA-approved for various purposes and available in the United States.[144]

An important reference text not directly related to FES, Stover and Fine's *Spinal Cord Injury,* details the statistical distributions of characteristics of the spinal cord-injured population.[58] Such information is vital when assessing the size of potential user populations of specific lower-extremity FES.[145]

REFERENCES

1. Van Doren CC: *Benjamin Franklin*. New York: Viking Press, 1938.
2. Heinemann AW, Magiera-Planey R, Gimenes MG, Geist CS: Evaluating the special needs of functional neuromuscular stimulation research candidates. *J Med Eng Technol* 1985; 9(4):167–173.
3. Heinemann AW, Magiera-Planey R, Schiro-Geist C, Gimines G: Mobility for persons with spinal cord injury: An evaluation of two systems. *Arch Phys Med Rehab* 1987; 68:90–93.
4. Bradley MB: The effect of participating in a functional electrical stimulation exercise program on affect in people with spinal cord injuries. *Arch Phys Med Rehab* 1994; 75(6):676–679.
5. Mortimer JT: Motor Prostheses, in *The Handbook of Physiology: The Nervous System,* vol III. Bethesda, MD: American Physiological Society, 1981, pp. 155–187.

6. Eichhorn KF, Schubert W, David E: Maintenance, training and functional use of denervated muscle. *J Biomed Eng* 1984; 6:205–211.
7. Benton AB, Baker LL, Bowman BR, Waters RL: *Functional Electrical Stimulation: A Practical Guide,* 2nd ed. Downey, CA: Rancho Los Amigos Hospital, 1981, pp. 11–52.
8. Kralj A, Bajd T: *Functional Electrical Stimulation: Standing and Walking after Spinal Cord Injury*. Boca Raton, FL: CRC Press, 1989, p. 198.
9. Jaeger RJ, Yarkony GM, Smith RM: Standing the spinal cord injured patient by electrical stimulation: Refinement of a protocol for clinical use. *IEEE Trans Biomed Eng* 1989; 36:720–728.
10. Pournezam M, Andrews BJ, Baxendale RH, Phillips GF, Paul JP: Reduction of muscle fatigue in man by cyclical stimulation. *J Biomed Eng* 1988; 10(2):196–200.
11. Kralj A, Bajd T, Turk R, Benko H: Posture switching for prolonging functional electrical stimulation standing in paraplegic patients. *Paraplegia* 1986; 24:221–230.
12. Bigland-Ritchie B, Jones DA, Woods JJ: Excitation frequency and muscle fatigue: electrical responses during human voluntary and stimulated contractions. *Exp Neurol* 1979; 64:414–427.
13. Edwards RHT: Physiological analysis of skeletal muscle weakness and fatigue. *Clin Sci Mol Med* 1978; 54:463–470.
14. Boom HB, Mulder AJ, Veltink PH: Fatigue during functional neuromuscular stimulation. *Prog Brain Res* 1993; 97:409–418.
15. Rabischong E, Guiraud D: Determination of fatigue in the electrically stimulated quadriceps muscle and relative effect of ischaemia. *J Biomed Eng* 1993; 15(6):443–450.
16. Levy M, Mizrahi J, Susak Z: Recruitment, force and fatigue characteristics of quadriceps muscles of paraplegics isometrically activated by surface functional electrical stimulation. *J Biomed Eng* 1990; 12(2):150–156.
17. Rabischong E, Ohanna F: Effects of functional electrical stimulation (FES) on evoked muscular output in paraplegic quadriceps muscle. *Paraplegia* 1992; 30(7):467–473.
18. Patterson RP, Lockwood JS, Dykstra DD: A functional electric stimulation system using an electrode garment. *Arch Phys Med Rehab* 1990; 71:340–342.
19. Bowman BR, Baker LL: Effects of waveform parameters on comfort during transcutaneous neuromuscular electrical stimulation. *Ann Biomed Eng* 1985; 13(1):59–74.
20. Baker LL, Bowman BR, McNeal DR: Effects of waveform on comfort during neuromuscular electrical. *Clin Orthop* 1988; 233:75–85.
21. Caldwell CW, Reswick JB: A percutaneous wire electrode for chronic research use. *IEEE Trans Biomed Eng* 1974; 21:429–432.
22. Marsolais EB, Kobetic R: Implantation techniques and experience with percutaneous intramuscular electrodes in the lower extremities. *J Rehab Res Dev* 1986; 23(3):1–8.
23. Prochazka A, Davis LA: Clinical experience with reinforced, anchored intramuscular electrodes for functional

neuromuscular stimulation. *J Neurosci Meth* 1992; 42(3):175–184.

24. Donaldson PEK: Twenty years of neurological prosthesis making. *J Biomed Eng* 1987; 9:291–298.

25. McNeal DR, Baker LL, Symons JT: Recruitment data for nerve cuff electrodes: Implications for design of implantable stimulators. *IEEE Trans Biomed Eng* 1989; 36(3):301–308.

26. Waters RL, McNeal DR, Faloon W, Clifford B: Functional electrical stimulation of the peroneal nerve for hemiplegia: Long-term clinical follow-up. *J Bone Joint Surg Am* 1985; 67(5):792–793.

27. Sweeney JD, Ksienski DA, Mortimer JT: A nerve cuff technique for selective excitation of peripheral nerve trunk regions. *IEEE Trans Biomed Eng* 1990; 37(7):706–715.

28. Mortimer JT, Agnew WF, Horch K, Citron P, Creasey G, Kantor C: Perspectives on new electrode technology for stimulating peripheral nerves with implantable motor prostheses. *IEEE Trans Rehab Eng* 1995; 3(2):145–154.

29. Thoma H, Girsch W, Holle J, Mayr, W: Technology and long-term application of an epineural electrode. *ASAIO Trans* 1989; 35(3):490–494.

30. Waters RL, Campbell JM, Nakai R: Therapeutic stimulation of the lower limb by epimysial electrodes. *Clin Orthop* 1988; 233:44–52.

31. Rabischong P, Woloszko J: Intrafasicular nerve stimulation to restore locomotion in paraplegics. First Vienna International Workshop on Functional Electrostimulation, Vienna, Austria, 1983.

32. Bowman BR, Erickson RC: Acute and chronic implantation of coiled wire intraneural electrodes during cyclical electrical stimulation. *Ann Biomed Eng* 1985; 13:75–93

33. Balmaseda MT, Fatehi MT, Koozekanani SH, Sheppard JS: Burns in functional electric stimulation: Two case reports. *Arch Phys Rehab* 1987; 68:452–453.

34. Agnew WF, McCreery DB: *Neural Prostheses: Fundamental Studies.* Englewood Cliffs, NJ: Prentice-Hall, 1990.

35. Ilbawi MN, Idriss FS, Hunt CE, Brouillette RT, DeLeon SY: Diaphragm pacing in infants: Techniques and results. *Ann Thorac Surg* 1985; 40:323–329.

36. Moxham J, Shneerson JM: Diaphragmatic pacing. *Am Rev Respir Dis* 1993; 148:533–536.

37. Glenn WWL, Phelps ML: Diaphragm pacing by electrical stimulation of the phrenic nerve. *Neurosurgery* 1985; 17:974–984.

38. Chervin RD, Guilleminault C: Diaphragm pacing: Review and reassessment. *Sleep* 1994; 17:176–187.

39. Weese-Mayer DE, Morrow AS, Brouillette T, Ilbawi MN, Hunt CE: Diaphragm pacing in infants and children. A life-table analysis of implanted components. *Am Rev Respir Dis* 1989; 139:974–979.

40. Mueller-Felber W, Riepl R, Reimers CD, Wagner S, Pongratz D: Combined ultrasonographic and neurographic examination: A new technique to evaluate phrenic nerve function. *Electromyogr Clin Neurophysiol* 1993; 33:335–340.

41. Glenn WWL, Hogen JF, Loke JSO, Ciesielski TE, Phelps ML, Rowedder R: Ventilatory support by pacing of the conditioned diaphragm in quadriplegia. *New Engl J Med* 1984; 310:1150–1155.

42. Dobelle WMH, D'Angelo MS, Goetz BF, Kiefer DG, Lallier TJ, Lamb JI, Yazwinsky JS: 200 cases with a new breathing pacemaker dispel myths about diaphragm pacing. *ASAIO J* 1994; 40:M244–M252.

43. Glenn WWL, Brouillette RT, Dentz B, Fodstad H, Hunt CE, Keens TG, Marsh HM, Pande S, Piepgras DG, Vanderlinkden RG: Fundamental considerations in pacing of the diaphragm for chronic ventilatory insufficiency: A multi-center study. *PACE* 1988; 11:2121–2127.

44. Moue Y, Kamio K, Tanigaki T, Hayashi Y, Kuwahira I, Takasaki Y, Ohta Y, Yamabayashi H: [Successful treatment of diaphragm pacing-induced obstructive sleep apnea syndrome with nasal CPAP]. *Nippon Kyobu Shikkan Gakkai Zasshi* 1993; 31:990–993.

45. Tobin JM (ed): *Principles and Practice of Mechanical Ventilation.* New York: McGraw-Hill, 1994.

46. Carter RE, Donovan WH, Halstead L, Wilkerson MA: Comparative study of electrophrenic nerve stimulation and mechanical ventilatory support in traumatic spinal cord injury. *Paraplegia* 1987; 25:86–91.

47. Esclarin A, Bravo P, Arroyo O, Mazaira J, Garrido H, Alcaraz MA: Tracheostomy ventilation versus diaphragmatic pacemaker ventilation in high spinal cord injury. *Paraplegia* 1994; 32(10):687–693.

48. Ishii K, Kurosawa H, Koyanagi H, Nakano K, Sakakibara N, Sato I, Noshiro M, Ohsawa M: Effects of bilateral transvenous diaphragm pacing on hemodynamic function in patients after cardiac operations. *J Thorac Cardiovasc Surg* 1990; 100:108–114.

49. Miller HJ, Thomas E, Wilmot CB: Pneumobelt use among high quadriplegic population. *Arch Phys Med Rehab* 1988; 69:369–372.

50. Yang GFW, Alba A, Lee M, Khan A: Pneumobelt for sleep in the ventilator user: clinical experience. *Arch Phys Med Rehab* 1989; 70:707–711.

51. Baer GA, Talonen PP, Hakkinen V, Exner G, Yrjola H: Phrenic nerve stimulation in tetraplegia. A new regimen to condition the diaphragm for full-time respiration. *Scand J Rehab Med* 1990; 22(2):107–111.

52. Baer GA, Talonen PP, Shneerson JM, Markkula H, Exner G, Wells FC: Phrenic nerve stimulation for central ventilatory failure with bipolar and four-pole electrode systems. *PACE* 1990; 13:1061–1072.

53. Baer GA: Personal communication, 1994.

54. Mayr W, Bijak M, Girsch W, Holle J, Lanmuller H, Thoma H, Zrunek M: Multichannel stimulation of phrenic nerves by epineural electrodes. Clinical experience and future developments. *ASAIO J* 1993; 39(3):M729–M735.

55. Krieger AJ, Gropper MR, Adler RJ: Electrophrenic respiration after intercostal to phrenic nerve anastomosis in a

patient with anterior spinal artery syndrome: technical case report. *Neurosurgery* 1994; 35:760–764.

56. DiMarco AF, Supinski GS, Petro JA, Takaoka Y: Evaluation of intercostal pacing to provide artificial ventilation in quadriplegics. *Am J Respir Crit Care Med* 1994; 150:934–940.

57. Šorli J, Kandare F, Jaeger R, Stanič U: Ventilatory assistance using electrical stimulation of abdominal muscles. *IEEE Trans Rehab Eng* 1996; 4(1):1–6.

58. Stover SL, Fine PR: *Spinal Cord Injury: The Facts and Figures.* Birmingham, Alabama: University of Alabama, Birmingham Press, 1986.

59. Jaeger RJ, Turba RM, Yarkony GM, Roth EJ: Cough and spinal cord injured patients: comparison of three methods of cough production. *Arch Phys Med Rehab* 1993; 74:1358–1361.

60. Linder SH: Functional electrical stimulation to enhance cough in quadriplegia. *Chest* 1993; 103:166–169.

61. Brindley GS: An implant to empty the bladder or close the urethra. *J Neurol Neurosurg Psychiatr* 1977; 40:358–360.

62. Brindley GS, Polkey CE, Rushton DN, Cardozo L: Sacral anterior root stimulators for bladder control in paraplegia: The first 50 cases. *J Neurol Neurosurg Psychiatr* 1986; 49:1104–1114.

63. Brindley GS, Polkey CE, Rushton DN: The Finetech-Brindley bladder controller: Notes for surgeons and physicians. Maudsley Hospital, London, 1988, or Fineteh, Welsyn Garden City, 1994.

64. Brindley GS: The first 500 patients with sacral anterior root stimulator implants: general description. *Paraplegia* 1994; 32:795–805.

65. Van Kerrebroeck PEV, Koldewijn EL, Debruyne FMJ: Worldwide experience with the Finetech-Brindley sacral anterior root stimulator. *Neurourol Urodynam* 1993; 12:497–503.

66. Creasey GH: Electrical stimulation of sacral roots for micturition after spinal cord injury. *Urol Clin No Am* 1993; 20: 505–515.

67. Marsbach H, Fischer J: Sacral anterior root stimulation: prerequisites and indications. *Neurourol Urodynam* 1993; 12:489–494.

68. Brindley GS: Electroejaculation: its technique, neurological implications and uses. *J Neurol Neurosurg Psychol* 1981; 44:9–18.

69. Tanagho EA, Schmidt RA, Orvis BR: Neural stimulation for control of voiding dysfunction: a preliminary report in 22 patients with serious neuropathic voiding disorders. *J Urol* 1989; 142:340–345.

70. Schmidt RA, Kogan BA, Tanagho EA: Neuroprostheses in the management of incontinence in myelomeningocele patients. *J Urol* 1990; 143:779–782.

71. Robinson LQ, Grant A, Weston P, Stephenson TP, Lucas M, Thomas DG: Experience with the Brindley anterior sacral root stimulator. *Br J Urol* 1988; 62:553–557.

72. Koldewijn EL, van Kerrebroeck PEV, Rosier PFWM, Wijkstra H, Debruyne FMJ: Bladder compliance after

posterior sacral root rhizotomies and anterior sacral root stimulation. *J Urol* 1994; 151:955–960.

73. Isambert JL, Egon G, Colombel P: Adjuvant drug therapy: a review of 30 cases of sacral anterior root stimulator. *Neurourol Urodyn* 1993; 12:512–515.

74. Barat M, Egon G, Daverat P, Colombel P, Guerin J: Why does continence fail after sacral anterior root stimulator? *Neurourol Urodynam* 1993; 12:507–508.

75. Binnie NR, Smith AN, Creasey GH, Edmond P: Constipation associated with chronic spinal cord injury: the effect of pelvic parasympathetic stimulation by the Brindley stimulator. *Paraplegia* 1991; 29:463–469.

76. MacDonagh RP, Sun WM, Smallwood R, Forster D, Read NW: Control of defecation in patients with spinal injuries by stimulation of sacral anterior nerve roots. *Br Med J* 1990; 300:1494–1497.

77. Blaivas JG: Bladder function in the SCI patient. *J Neurol Rehab* 1994; 8:47–53.

78. Hohenfellner M, Paick JS, Trigo-Rocha F, Schmidt RA, Kaula NF, Thueroff JW, Tanagho EA: Site of deafferentation and electrode placement for bladder stimulation: clinical implications. *J Urol* 1992; 147:1665–1670.

79. Tanagho EA: Concepts of neuromodulation. *Neurourol Urodynam* 1993; 12:487–488.

80. Li JS, Hassouna M, Sawan M, Duval F, Elhilali MM: Long-term effect of sphincteric fatigue during bladder neurostimulation. *J Urol* 1995; 153:238–242.

81. Janknegt RA, Baeten CG, Weil EH, Spaans F: Electrically stimulated gracilis sphincter for treatment of bladder sphincter incontinence. *Lancet* 1992; 340:1129–1130.

82. Merrill DC, Conway CJ: Clinical experience with the mentor bladder stimulator. I. Patients with upper motor neuron lesions. *J Urol* 1974; 112:52–56.

83. Halverstadt DB, Parry WL: Electronic stimulation of the human bladder: 9 years later. *J Urol* 1975; 113:341–344.

84. Walter JS, Wheeler JS, Cogan SF, Plishka M, Riedy LW, Wurster RD: Evaluation of direct bladder stimulation with stainless steel woven eye electrodes. *J Urol* 1993; 150:1990–1996.

85. Graupe D, Kohn KH:. *Functional Electrical Stimulation for Ambulation by Paraplegics.* Malabar, FL: Krieger Publishing Co., 1994.

86. Jaeger RJ, Yarkony GM, Roth EJ: Rehabilitation technology for standing and walking after spinal cord injury. *Am J Phys Med Rehab* 1989; 68:128–133.

87. Marsolais EB, Miller PC, Kobetic R, Daly JJ: Augmentation of transfers for a quadriplegic patient using an implanted FNS system. Case report. *Paraplegia* 1994; 32(8):573–579.

88. Davis R, MacFarland WC, Emmons SE: Initial results of the nucleus FES-22-implanted system for limb movement in paraplegia. *Stereotact Funct Neurosurg* 1994; 63(1–4):192–197.

89. Granat MH, Heller BW, Nicol DJ, Baxendale RH, Andrews BJ: Improving limb flexion in FES gait using the

flexion withdrawal response for the spinal cord injured person. *J Biomed Eng* 1993; 15(1):51–56.

90. Malezic M, Hesse S: Restoration of gait by functional electrical stimulation in paraplegic patients: A modified programme of treatment. *Paraplegia* 1995; 33(3):126–131.

91. Franken HM, Veltink PH, Baardman G, Redmeyer RA, Boom HB: Cycle-to-cycle control of swing phase of para-plegic gait induced by surface electrical stimulation *Med Biol Eng Comput* 1995; 33:440–51.

92. Yamaguchi G, Zajac F: Restoring unassisted natural gait to paraplegics via functional neuromuscular stimulation: A computer simulation study. *IEEE Trans Biomed Eng* 1990; 37(9):886–902.

93. Quevedo AA, Cliquet Junior A: A paradigm for design of closed loop neuromuscular electrical stimulator control systems. *Artif Org* 1995; 19(3):280–284.

94. Abbas JJ, Chizeck HJ: Feedback control of coronal plane hip angle in paraplegic subjects using functional neuro-muscular stimulation. *IEEE Trans Biomed Eng* 1991; 38(7):687–698.

95. Mulder AJ, Boom HB, Hermens HJ, Zilvold G: Artificial-reflex stimulation for FES-induced standing with mini-mum quadriceps force. *Med Biol Eng Comput* 1990; 28(5):483–488.

96. Franken HM, Veltink PH, Baardman G, Redmeyer RA, Boom HB: Cycle-to-cycle control of swing phase of para-plegic gait induced by surface electrical stimulation. *Med Biol Eng Comput* 1995; 33(3):440–451.

97. Kostov A, Andrews BJ, Popovic DB, Stein RB, Arm-strong WW: Machine learning in control of functional electrical stimulation systems for locomotion. *IEEE Trans Biomed Eng* 1995; 42(6):541–545.

98. Graupe D, Kordylewski H: Artificial neural network con-trol of FES in paraplegics for patient responsive ambula-tion. *IEEE Trans Biomed Eng* 1991; 42(7):699–707.

99. Phillips CA, Koubek RJ, Hendershot DM: Walking while using a sensory tactile feedback system: potential use with a functional electrical stimulation orthosis. *J Biomed Eng* 1991; 13(2):91–96.

100. Kirtley C, Andrews BJ: Control of functional electrical stimulation with extended physiological proprioception. *J Biomed Eng* 1990; 12(3):183–188.

101. Bajd T, Kralj A, Turk R, Benko H: Symmetry of FES responses in the lower extremities of paraplegic patients. *J Biomed Eng* 1990; 12(5):415–418.

102. Oderkerk BJ, Inbar GF: Walking cycle recording and analysis for FNS-assisted paraplegic walking. *Med Biol Eng Comput* 1991; 29(1):79–83.

103. Giat Y, Mizrahi J, Levy M: A musculotendon model of the fatigue profiles of paralyzed quadriceps muscle under FES. *IEEE Trans Biomed Eng* 1993; 40(7):664–674.

104. Hjeltnes N, Lannem A: Functional neuromuscular stimu-lation in four patients with complete paraplegia. *Paraple-gia* 1990; 28(4):235–243.

105. Winchester P, Carollo JJ, Habasevich R: Physiologic costs

106. Phillips CA, Hendershot DM: A systems approach to medically prescribed functional electrical stimulation: Ambulation after spinal cord injury. *Paraplegia* 1991; 29(8):505–513.

107. Isakov E, Douglas R, Berns P: Ambulation using the reciprocating gait orthosis and functional electrical stimu-lation. *Paraplegia* 1992; 30(4):239–245.

108. Nene AV, Patrick JH: Energy cost of paraplegic loco-motion using the ParaWalker—electrical stimulation "hybrid" orthosis. *Arch Phys Med Rehab* 1990; 71(2):116–120.

109. Phillips CA, Hendershot DM: Functional electrical stimu-lation and reciprocating gait orthosis for ambulation exer-cise in a tetraplegic patient: A case study. *Paraplegia* 1991; 29(4):268–276.

110. Durfee WK, Hausdorff JM: Regulating knee joint position by combining electrical stimulation with a controllable friction brake. *Ann Biomed Eng* 1990; 18(6):575–596.

111. Mulcahey MJ, Betz RR, Smith BT, Weiss AA: Results of the functional electrical stimulation hand grasp system in adolescents with tetraplegia. *Am Parapleg Soc, Abs* 1995; 3–4.

112. Keith MW, Peckham PH, Thrope GB, Buckett JR, Stroh KC, Menger V: Functional neuromuscular stimulation neuroprostheses for the tetraplegic hand. *Clin Orthop Rel Res* 1988; 233:25–33.

113. Perkins TA, Brindley GS, Donaldson ND, Polkey CE, Rushton DN: Implant provision of key, pinch and power grips in a C6 tetraplegic. *Med Biol Eng Comput* 1994; 32(4):367–372.

114. Saxena S, Nikolic S, Popovic D: An EMG-controlled grasping system for tetraplegics. *J Rehab Res Dev* 1995; 32(1):17–24.

115. Nathan RH: FNS of the upper limb: Targeting the forearm muscles for surface stimulation. *Med Biol Eng Comput* 1990; 28(3):249–256.

116. Handa Y, Handa T, Ichie M, Murakami H, Hoshimiya N, Ishikawa S, Ohkubo K: Functional electrical stimulation (FES) systems for restoration of motor function of para-lyzed muscles: Versatile systems and a portable system. *Front. Med. Biol. Eng. (Netherlands)* 1992; 4:241–255.

117. Kilgore KL, Peckham PH: Grasp synthesis for upper-extremity FNS. Part 1. Automated method for synthe-sising the stimulus map. *Med Biol Eng Comput* 1993; 31(6):607–614.

118. Kilgore KL, Peckham PH: Grasp synthesis for upper-extremity FNS. Part 2. Evaluation of the influence of electrode recruitment properties. *Med Biol Eng Comput* 1993; 31(6):615–622.

119. Kilgore KL, Peckham PH, Keith MW, Thrope GB: Elec-trode characterization for functional application to upper extremity FNS. *IEEE Trans Biomed Eng* 1990; 37(1):12–21.

120. Lemay MA, Crago PE, Katorgi M, Chapman GJ: Auto-

mated tuning of a closed-loop hand grasp neuroprosthesis. *IEEE Trans Biomed Eng* 1993; 40(7):675–685.

121. Betz RR, Mulcahey MJ, Smith BT, Triolo RJ, Weiss AA, Moynahan M, Keith MW, Peckham PH: Bipolar latissimus dorsi transposition and functional neuromuscular stimulation to restore elbow flexion in an individual with C4 quadriplegia and C5 denervation. *J Am Paraplegia Soc* 1992; 15(4):220–228.

122. Naito A, Yajima M, Fukamachi H, Ushikoshi K, Handa Y, Hoshimiya N, Shimizu Y: Functional electrical stimulation (FES) to the biceps brachii for controlling forearm supination in the paralyzed upper extremity. *Tohoku J Exp Med* 1994; 173(2):269–273.

123. Durfee WK, Mariano TR, Zahradnik JL: Simulator for evaluating shoulder motion as a command source for FES grasp restoration systems. *Arch Phys Med Rehab* 1991; 72(13):1088–1094.

124. Riso RR, Ignagni AR, Keith MW: Cognitive feedback for use with FES upper extremity neuroprostheses. *IEEE Trans Biomed Eng* 1991; 38(1):29–38.

125. Ragnarsson KT, Pollack S, O'Daniel W, Edgar R, Petrofsky J, Nash MS: Clinical evaluation of computerized functional electrical stimulation after spinal cord injury: A multicenter pilot study. *Arch Phys Med Rehab* 1988; 69:672–677.

126. Pollack SF, Axen K, Spielholz N, Levin N, Haas F, Ragnarsson KT: Aerobic training effects of electrically induced lower extremity exercises in spinal cord injured people. *Arch Phys Med Rehab* 1989; 70(3):214–219.

127. Glaser RM: Physiologic aspects of spinal cord injury and functional neuromuscular stimulation. *Cent Nerv Syst Trauma* 1986; 3(1):49–62.

128. Teeter JO, Kantor C, Brown DL: *Functional Electrical Stimulation (FES) Resource Guide.* Cleveland: FES Information Center, 1995.

129. Fields WS, Leavit LA: *Neural Organization and Its Relevance to Prosthetics.* Miami: Symposia Specialists, 1973.

130. Hambrecht FT, Reswick JB: *Functional Electrical Stimulation: Application in Neural Prostheses.* New York: Marcel Dekker, 1977.

131. Lazorthes Y, Upton ARM: *Neurostimulation: An Overview.* Mt. Kisco, NY: Futura Publishing Co, 1985.

132. Mykelbust JB, Cusick JF, Sances A, Larson SJ: *Neural Stimulation,* vol 1. Boca Raton, FL: CRC Press, Inc., 1985.

133. Mykelbust JB, Cusick JF, Sances A, Larson SJ: *Neural Stimulation,* vol 2. Boca Raton, FL: CRC Press, Inc., 1985.

134. Rose FC, Jones R, Vrbova G: *Neuromuscular Stimulation: Basic Concepts and Clinical Implications.* New York: Demos, 1989.

135. Peckham PH, Popović DP: Replacing motor function after disease or disability. In: Stein RB (ed), *Neural Prostheses.* Oxford: Oxford University Press, 1992, p. 345.

136. Cybulski GR, Penn RD, Jaeger RJ: Lower extremity functional neuromuscular stimulation in cases of spinal cord injury. *Neurosurgery* 1984; 15(1):132–146.

137. Vodovnik L, Bajd T, Trnkoczy A, Kralj A, Gracanin F, Strojnik P: Functional electrical stimulation for control of locomotor systems. *CRC Crit Rev Bioeng* 1981; 6(2):63–131.

138. Yarkony GM, Roth EJ, Cybulski G, Jaeger RJ: Neuromuscular stimulation in spinal cord injury I: Restoration of functional movement of the extremities. *Arch Phys Med Rehab* 1992; 73:78–86.

139. Yarkony GM, Roth EJ, Cybulski GR, Jaeger RJ: Neuromuscular stimulation in spinal cord injury II: Prevention of secondary complications. *Arch Phys Med Rehab* 1992; 73:195–200.

140. Phillips C: Sensory feedback control of upper- and lower-extremity motor prostheses. *CRC Crit Rev Biomed Eng* 1988; 16:105–140.

141. Petrofsky JS, Phillips CA: Closed-loop control of movement of skeletal muscle. *CRC Crit Rev Biomed Eng* 1985; 13(1):35–96.

142. Heetderks WJ, Hambrecht FT: Applied neural control in the 1990s. *Proc IEEE* 1988; 76(9):1115–1121.

143. Peckham PH, Gray DB: Single topic issue: Functional neuromuscular stimulation (FNS). *J Rehab Res Dev* 1996; 33(2).

144. Medical Device Register, Inc. *Medical Device Register.* Stamford, CT: Directory Systems, Inc., 1992, pp. III–895.

145. Jaeger RJ, Yarkony GM, Roth EJ, Lovell L: Estimating the user population of a simple electrical system for standing. *Paraplegia* 1990; 28:505–511.

Chapter 37

MOTOR SPEECH DISORDERS: EVALUATION AND TREATMENT

Kathryn M. Yorkston
Edythe A. Strand

Motor speech disorders comprise a group of disorders arising from damage to the central or peripheral nervous system. They are impairments in the planning (apraxia of speech) and execution (the dysarthrias) of the movements of speech production. Apraxia of speech (AOS) is a motor speech disorder caused by a disturbance in motor planning or programming of sequential movement for volitional speech production. In AOS, the speech musculature itself is not impaired, yet the patient will have difficulty completing sequences of movements for sound production. In contrast, dysarthria is a motor speech disorder caused by disturbances in neuromuscular control of the muscles of the speech mechanism. Weakness, paralysis, or incoordination of the muscles owing to damage to the central or peripheral nervous system will cause difficulty in execution of movement during speech. The picture that will emerge in this chapter is one of wide variability in types, pattern, and severity of motor speech disorders. These disorders may be congenital or acquired, temporary or persistent, mild or severe, and may or may not be accompanied by other language and cognitive disorders.

Perspectives on Dysarthria and Apraxia of Speech

Like every complex phenomenon, motor speech disorders may be viewed from a variety of perspectives. Neurologists may see them as symptoms of neurologic disease. For example, the gradual onset of flaccid or spastic dysarthria may contribute to the diagnosis of amyotrophic lateral sclerosis. Speech physiologists may view motor speech disorders as a means of understanding the speech production process. The rehabilitation community views these disorders as functional limitations and barriers to effective communication. In this chapter, we will view motor speech disorders from the perspective of rehabilitation. First, motor speech disorders will be defined within the frame of the model of chronic disease. Next, general approaches to assessment of the various aspects of the disorders will be reviewed. Finally, issues related to treatment techniques will be organized by etiology with review of congenital disorders (cerebral palsy and developmental apraxia of speech), adult onset nonprogressive disorders (stroke and traumatic brain injury), and degenerative disease (amyotrophic lateral sclerosis, Parkinson's disease, and multiple sclerosis).

Motor Speech Disorders and the Model of Chronic Disease

The World Health Organization has proposed a model of chronic disease that has been used as a framework for describing approaches to assessment and treatment of motor speech disorders.[1-3] The five parameters of the model are pathophysiology, impairment, functional limitation, disability, and societal limitation. Table 37-1 contains definitions of these parameters, examples of the levels of deficits, assessment targets, and approaches to intervention. The assessment and intervention examples are taken from multiple sclerosis, a neurological disease of young adults that frequently results in dysarthria. The pathophysiologic deficit in multiple sclerosis involves demyelination and scarring of nerve tissue. Currently, there is no treatment proven effective at this physiologic level. The impairment associated with dysarthria in multiple sclerosis results from deficits in respiration, phonation, and oral articulation. One target for assessment and treatment at the level of the impair-

Table 37-1

A conceptual framework for assessment and intervention in motor speech disorders

	Pathophysiology	Impairment	Functional limitation	Disability	Societal limitation
Definition	Interruption of normal physiological and developmental processes or structures	Abnormality of physiological function	Restriction in ability to perform an activity in the manner considered normal that results from impairment	Limitation in performing socially defined activities and roles within a social and physical environment	Restriction attributable to social policy or barriers that limit fulfillment of roles or deny access to services or opportunities
Level of deficit	Cells and tissues	Components of the speech production process, including respiration, phonation, velopharyngeal function, and oral articulatory structures	Speech performance will full range, speed, strength, and coordination	Speech performance in a physical and social context	Performance of roles by speakers in social context
Examples of assessment targets	Cerebellar involvement	Reduction in the coordination of speech breathing	Speech intelligibility and naturalness	Comprehensibility	Premature retirement
Examples of approaches to intervention	No intervention for the demylenation associated with multiple sclerosis	Respiratory pattern stabilization techniques	Phrasing of utterances with appropriate syntactic breath group units	Appropriate distance between speaker and listener Partner signals when messages are not understood so that repair strategies can be initiated	Scaffolding to support work-related activities

Adapted from work initially developed by the Institute of Medicine: *Disability in America: Toward a National Agenda for Prevention.* Washington, DC: National Academy Press, 1991.

ment may be respiratory patterning for speech. Functional limitations arise because of the underlying impairment. Poorly coordinated speech breathing may interfere with speech and cause reduced intelligibility. An example of intervention at this level of functional limitation is use of proper phrasing so that words are grouped in appropriate grammatical units. The goal of this training would be to enhance speech naturalness. At this level of disability, intervention is targeted to enhance the effectiveness of communication in everyday settings.[3] Finally, at the level of societal limitations, poor communication skills at work may result in difficulty maintaining employment. Intervention may focus on employment policies and adequate accommodation for disability in the workplace. The broad prespective provided by the model of chronic disease allows clinicians to understand the motor speech disorders at multiple levels and to plan treatment that targets several paramenters of the disorder.

ASSESSMENT

Understanding the Impairment

Understanding the level and severity of impairment is crucial to appropriate treatment planning. Level of impairment relates to understanding which cognitive, linguistic, or motor deficits contribute to the functional limitation, and how those deficits interact with each other. In motor speech disorders, assessment focuses on determining the degree to which motor planning or motor execution contributes to the speech problem. In order to make such a determination, the clinician must focus on examination of the general neuromuscular condition of the patient, especially cranial nerve function, the structure and function of the oral articulatory mechanism, and speech motor control across different contexts.

The examination of neuromuscular condition of the patient allows the clinician to make predictions regarding probable neural systems that may be impaired. For example, if flaccidity, atrophy, and fasciculations are noted in the tongue, a lower motor neuron deficit is probable. This finding is indicative of dysarthria, and leads to decisions about subsequent assessment tasks. In this examination, the clinician examines muscle function (looks for hypertonicity or hypotonicity, checks reflexes); notes the presence or absence of adventitious movements such as tremor, myoclonus, or dyskinesias; and examines coordination and sensory function.

The examination of structure and function involves noting any abnormality in relative size or position of the oral structures, especially the lips, tongue, jaw, velum, and oro-pharynx. Tissue characteristics, symmetry of structures at rest, structural restrictions, and malocclusion may impede speech production. Several parameters of function are examined for each of the oral articulatory structures: range of motion, strength, speed, coordination, and the ability to vary muscular tension. These parameters are all examined in nonspeech movement (e.g., smile to pucker movements for lip function, having the patient say "ah" for velar movement) for isolated movements and repeated movements and at different speed requirements. Coordination and symmetry of movement is noted in all tasks. Nasal air emission or hypernasality, abnormal gag reflex, and fatigue effects are all noted. A complete discussion of this examination can be found elsewhere.[4-6]

The examination of structure and function also involves assessment of the function of the respiratory muscles and respiratory/laryngeal interaction. Measures of vital capacity are taken as a measure of respiratory adequacy. Voluntary cough, quality and stability of sustained phonation, and diadochokinesis of laryngeal abduction/adduction are evaluated. Together, the examination of the neuromuscular status of the patient and the examination of structure and function allow the clinician to determine if central and/or peripheral nervous system deficits may be contributing to an execution problem (dysarthria) in speech production.

The motor speech examination consists of a spontaneous speech sample, and sampling the ability to produce imitative responses of progressively more difficult utterance types. It allows evaluation of movement parameters in the production of speech across varying contexts, and is important in the diagnosis of apraxia of speech. A spontaneous speech sample usually is obtained in three contexts: conversation, picture description, and narrative. Conversation provides a context in which the speaker has the most control over intended utterances. As a result, it allows the examiner to evaluate

Table 37-2

Example of a hierarchy of utterances that may be sampled during the motor speech examination

Utterance type	Examples
Isolated vowels	a; o; ee; ou;
Consonant—vowel (CV) or vowel—consonant	me; bye; no up; at; in;
CVC	cup; fat; mop
Bisyllabic words	baseball; cupcake; outdoors
Words of increasing length	please; pleasing; pleasingly
Multisyllabic words	volcano; harmonica; aluminum
Phrases of increasing length	I eat. I eat lunch. I eat lunch every day. I eat lunch in the cafeteria every day.

those voluntary utterances that are likely well practiced. In picture description, the linguistic load is increased, in that the speaker must describe specific elements that are known to the examiner. Therefore, some assessment about types of errors and severity may be made. Narrative samples (tell me the story of *Gone with the Wind*) are important in order to determine the effect of increased linguistic processing on motor speech output. For severely impaired patients, narrative discourse may be impossible, and cannot be sampled. After eliciting spontaneous connected speech in those contexts, the clinician must examine the patient's ability to sequence phonetic segments from very easy utterances (e.g., be, my, mom) to those that are progressively more difficult. Table 37-2 illustrates a hierarchy of utterances that may be sampled. Not all levels are sampled for all patients. The clinician will begin where the patient is likely to be successful, and advance the difficulty of challenges until impairments are uncovered.

Understanding the Functional Limitation and Disability

In order to understand the nature and severity of the functional limitation imposed by dysarthria or apraxia of speech, two constructs are important, intelligibility and comprehensibility. Both relate to the degree to which the speaker can be understood. The term *intelligibility* refers to the degree to which the acoustic signal alone is understood by a listener, without any other cues, such as seeing the speaker's face or knowing the topic. Measures of intelligibility usually are obtained by having naive listeners transcribe words or sentences that the speaker has recorded. An intelligibility score then is computed as the percentage of words understood. Together with rate, intelligibility is used as one index of severity of dysarthria. It reflects both the impairment itself, and any compensatory strategies the speaker may use to improve the acoustic signal. *Comprehensibility* is a term used to indicate the extent to which speech is understood in a communicative context. Thus, it takes into account information that is not directly related to the acoustic signal itself, such as semantics, syntax, the presence of environmental noise, and whether or not the listener knows the topic. Because most messages are conveyed with a variety of cues from the environment, measures of comprehensibility provide an estimate of the adequacy of communicative efficiency in a naturalistic setting.

TREATMENT

Congenital Motor Speech Disorders

Cerebral Palsy Cerebral palsy is a nonprogressive motor disorder that results from an insult to the central nervous system during the prenatal or perinatal period. The prevalence of cerebral palsy in school children is between 2 and 2.5 per 1,000.[7] Although prevalence statistics for adults are difficult to obtain, studies suggest that the majority of even those with severely affected speech survive to adulthood.[8] Reports of the prevalence of dysarthria vary greatly from 31 to 88 percent.[9,10]

There is no pattern of speech that is typical of all individuals with cerebral palsy. The severity and pattern of dysarthria are dependent on the underlying pathophysiology. Spastic cerebral palsy is by far the most frequent type and results in abnormalities of voluntary movement, including spasticity, weakness, limitation of range, and slowness of movement. The speech pattern associated with spastic cerebral palsy is characterized by low pitch, hypernasality, pitch breaks, breathy voice, and excess and equal stress.[11] Athetosis occurs in approximately 5 percent of individuals with cerebral palsy and results in a pattern of speech different from that of spastic cerebral palsy. Speech in athetoid cerebral palsy is characterized by irregular articulatory breakdowns, inappropriate silences, prolonged interval and speech sounds, excessive loudness variation, and voice stop-

page. There also appear to be differences between the two groups in the severity and natural course of the dysarthria. Workinger and Kent summarize these differences[11]:

The youngsters with spasticity tend to develop speech relatively early and have comparatively good articulation skills. As they grow, they spend increasing amounts of time in flexed positions, and tend to develop contractures that lead to flexed postures. Respiratory support for speech becomes increasingly impaired, and they experience increased difficulty with voice quality and intensity. Youngsters with athetosis experience considerable difficulty with control of the oral mechanism from birth. They are late to speak and are frequently unintelligible. Communication boards are frequently used to augment communication. As they grow and gain stability, their speech improves and may become intelligible in their teens or early adulthood.

Speech abnormalities in respiration, laryngeal function, velopharyngeal function, and oral articulation occur in both spastic and athetoid dysarthria. These abnormalities are summarized in Table 37-3.

EMG techniques have been used to study the pathophysiology of dysarthria in cerebral palsy.[12–14] Results indicate that the temprospatial patterns of voluntary muscles activity in individuals with athetoid cerebral palsy were grossly abnormal.[15] Furthermore, speakers with cerebral palsy displayed idiosyncratic patterns of abnormal muscle activity that were reproducible across repetitions of the same phrase, thus indicating a consistent defect in motor programming. Barlow and Abbs found that individuals with spasticity were able to generate specific target levels for force and position but had difficulty controlling finer levels of isometric force in the articulators.[16–17]

Intervention Techniques Unfortunately, published reports of the effectiveness of speech treatment for individuals with cerebral palsy are largely lacking. However, there is evidence suggesting that some speakers with cerebral palsy are able to modify speech behaviors when faced with communication failure.[18] Other techniques also have been found to be effective, including chunking speech into appropriate breath groups and initial letter cueing.[19,20] As in other types of dysarthria, a component-by-component assessment of the speech mechanism is helpful in selecting and sequencing treat-

Table 37-3
Abnormalities in speech components for speakers with spastic and athetoid cerebral palsy

	Spastic cerebral palsy	Athetoid cerebral palsy
Respiration	Reduce respiratory reserve	Paradoxical or reverse breathing
Laryngeal function	Monopitch Monoloudness Harsh voice	Low pitch Weak intensity
Velopharyngeal function	Inappropriate timing of velar movement Hypernasality Nasal emission	Instability of velar elevation Slow velar movements
Oral articulation	Development delayed Motorically complex sounds more difficult Slow movement rates	Inappropriate posture of tongue Large ranges of jaw movements Prolonged transitions Retrusion of lower lip

Adapted from Love RJ: *Childhood Motor Speech Disability.* New York: Macmillan Publishing Co, 1992.

ment procedures.[21] For example, assessment of the respiratory support for speech may lead to a recommendation for adaptive seating devices that optimize posture for speech.[22] In the last decade, the field of augmentative communication has developed tremendously in its ability to enhance the communication of individuals with severe dysarthria. This type of intervention is reviewed elsewhere in this text.

Intervention Issues Individuals with cerebral palsy form a heterogeneous group, both in terms of severity and pattern of motor deficits. The speech problems frequently associated with cerebral palsy are diverse. Approximately 75 percent of the children studied by Murphy and colleagues had at least one of the following disorders: mental retardation, epilepsy, visual impairment, and hearing impairment. These comorbid conditions often have an impact on communication, and therefore must be accounted for in planning intervention. Long-term intervention must also take into account possible regression in the functional status of individuals with cerebral palsy. Although cerebral palsy is defined as a nonprogressive disorder, periods of rapid growth, such as infancy or adolescence, or aging may bring an exacerbation of symptoms and a change in function.

Developmental Apraxia of Speech Developmental apraxia of speech (DAS) is a diagnosis given to children who have articulatory speech problems that are owing to difficulty carrying out purposeful voluntary movement sequences for speech production in the absence of weak-

ness or paralysis of the speech musculature. This is in contrast to both dysarthria, where the innervation of the oral motor apparatus itself is abnormal, and phonological deficits, where articulatory problems result from delayed or deviant learning of the rules that govern phonology. Phonological disorders are considered linguistically based, and error patterns will consist of sound substitutions and omissions. DAS is believed to be caused by motor planning deficits and is considered a motor speech disorder. This distinction is tenuous, however, because children with DAS still develop linguistic rules, and motor planning development will influence language development.[24]

Frequency and Characteristics of the Speech Disorder Speech characteristics of children with DAS include consonant and vowel distortions, difficulty initiating sound sequences, and difficulty with sequencing sounds.[25,26] Some sound substitutions may be present, but are thought to be the result of the child's attempt to simplify a phonetic string. Errors increase with incremental length or phonetic complexity.

Intervention Issues Treatment of motor speech disorders in children is similar to that for adults. The goal is to improve execution of movement for sequential production of sounds. Issues in the treatment of developmental motor speech disorders can be complicated by the process of child language and motor control system development. Treatment cannot be approached from the perspective of motor planning alone. The clinician must pay attention to the interaction of language and motor skills in planning treatment strategies to improve articulatory production.[27] Because treatment will be focused on developing motor skills, the principles of motor learning must be considered. The therapist must insure adequate motor practice by maximizing the number of responses the child produces per session. Feedback about performance is essential. Speed may need to be sacrificed in order to improve accuracy.

Several basic principles are important in the treatment of DAS. First, pairing of auditory and visual stimuli is included in most approaches, and intensive, frequent, and systematic practice toward habituation of movement patterns is important. This is in direct contrast to teaching individual sounds that are produced in isolation. Several factors facilitate improvement during the treatment of DAS. These include using a slightly slower rate of speech, emphasizing stress and rhythm, and using gestures.

Common Treatment Techniques There is no single treatment approach or technique recognized as most appropriate for DAS. Most approaches utilize integral stimulation in which the therapist provides auditory and visual models of target utterances that the child can imitate.[28] A hierarchy of target utterances is used, starting with easier phonetic combinations, and progressing systematically to more-complex utterances. A child's functional communication needs should not be ignored. Often, a set of target utterances, such as bisyllabic words and short phrases (e.g., mom, daddy, help me, want more) can be used in combination.

Several specific treatment approaches have been described in the literature.[29] Many of these methods emphasize tactile or gestural components such as the Touch-Cue method, Prompt, and the Adapted Cueing Technique. (See Square for review.[30]) Methods based on prosodic factors, such as Melodic Intonation Therapy, have been proposed, as have techniques that incorporate linguistic components.[26,31]

Adult Onset Nonprogressive Motor Speech Disorders

Stroke

Apraxia of Speech FREQUENCY AND CHARACTERISTICS Epidemiologic figures on the incidence of pure AOS are difficult to identify, as it often goes hand in hand with aphasia and dysarthria. In a survey completed at the Mayo Clinic from 1987 to 1990, the primary diagnosis of AOS accounted for 9 percent of the motor speech disorders seen in the Section of Speech Pathology.[32] Because AOS is a frequent secondary diagnosis in those with aphasia due to left hemisphere lesions, it is certain that AOS occurs in a large percentage of patients who suffer stroke. The perceptual characteristics of AOS include disturbances in articulation, rate, and prosody, as well as the rhythm of spoken utterances.[33] Articulatory errors consist primarily of vowel and consonant distortions, although sound substitutions, additions, and omissions of sounds are also observed by listeners. Apraxic speakers have great difficulty initiating speech, owing to inability to achieve initial articulatory configurations. Transitions of movement out of one sound and into the next are also difficult, and add to the perception of dysprosody. In addition to the slower rate of speech output, prosody is affected by the tendency to equalize stress across syllables and words.

Articulatory errors are often perceived as approximations of target sounds, as the patient produces effortful groping for correct movement of articulators into a particular position. Errors will increase as the length or phonetic complexity of the utterance increases. Apraxic speakers exhibit more accuracy in well-practiced habituated utterances, such as counting. The apraxic speaker often is aware of his or her errors and often will attempt to correct error productions. Oral apraxia (difficulty planning volitional movement of oral structures for nonspeech movement tasks) may or may not be present with verbal apraxia.

INTERVENTION ISSUES Treatment goals for AOS are usually focused on maximizing the potential of the patient to use functional verbal communication. For those patients with very severe apraxia of speech, when the prognosis for improvement in speech is poor, treatment may be directed toward augmentative communication. One of the most crucial issues in planning treatment for apraxia of speech is the severity of a concomitant aphasia. The therapist must decide how much treatment should be focused on the language component in relation to motor speech. In some cases, language is only mildly affected, and treatment is most strategically focused on the motor planning deficit. In other cases, treatment for apraxia is a second-order goal, especially when language deficits are predominant. Under these circumstances, facilitating motor execution for speech production may be futile if the linguistic content of the message cannot be constructed. For many patients, a combination of treatment approaches, directed both at language and motor speech planning, is appropriate. This discussion will focus on treatment techniques specific to remediating apraxia of speech.

COMMON TREATMENT TECHNIQUES Most treatment approaches suggested for apraxia of speech focus on improving articulatory and prosodic factors in connected speech. Techniques involve intensive systematic drill of carefully selected utterances. Most approaches utilize visual and auditory stimulation with direct and repeated production of target words or phrases that have been selected based on that patient's assessment data and organized into hierarchies from easiest to most difficult. A few examples of approaches will be discussed briefly. For any technique chosen, however, effectiveness of treatment is dependent primarily on choosing appropriate targets for treatment and paying attention to the principles of motor learning. These principles include providing sufficient motor practice, providing feedback, and reducing speed to increase accuracy, then working toward more functional rate.

For those who are severely apraxic, initial treatment might begin using automatic speech tasks such as counting and repeating well-practiced social phrases (e.g., hi, bye), or completing well-practiced sentences (e.g., I'd like a cup of _____). Some patients exhibit apraxia for phonation in the first days after stroke, resulting in mutism. This usually resolves within the first couple of weeks of recovery, but may require intervention, such as moving from coughing or laughter into a prolonged vowel sound or providing a quick push against the diaphragm to initiate vocal fold abduction/adduction.

Integral stimulation is a technique in which a task continuum is created by systematically varying the time between the therapist's model and the patient's response.[28] Initially, the patient watches the therapist's face for visual cues, while listening to the target utterance. Later cues are gradually faded. Melodic Intonation Therapy is another technique used for remediation of apraxia of speech.[34] This is a structured approach similar in many ways to integral stimulation, but uses phrases intoned with familiar melody, accompanied by hand-tapped rhythms. The singing used in this approach does not rely on familiar tunes, but rather emphasizes patterns of stress in a spoken model. Again, efficacy of treatment depends on choosing appropriate treatment targets, and utilizing principles of motor learning.

Dysarthria Unfortunately, the prevalence of dysarthria following stroke is not well documented. Although the most debilitating dysarthrias occur with bilateral cortical lesions or lesions in the areas of vertebrobasilar circulation, dysarthria may also be associated with unilateral cerebral lesions.[35] Dysarthria associated with unilateral stroke is typically not as severe. However, cases of severe dysarthria have also been reported, often unilateral supratentorial cerebral insult.[36]

CHARACTERISTICS OF DYSARTHRIA The features of dysarthria associated with stroke are dependent on the size and site of the vascular lesion.

Duffy suggests that little attention has been paid to dysarthria in unilateral stroke because the motor speech problem is typically mild and temporary.[32] Further, it may coexist with and be masked by other neurological communication disorders, such as apraxia of speech or aphasia. In a retrospective study of 56 individuals with dysarthria associated with unilateral upper motor neuron lesions, imprecise consonant production was by far the most common deviant speech feature.[32] Slow speaking and oral movement rates were also found. These changes in articulation are consistent with the physical findings of unilateral lower facial weakness and unilateral lingual weakness. Although much less common than changes in articulation, changes in phonation (vocal harshness) and velopharyngeal function (hypernasality) are also noted on occasion. The neurologic bases of the phonatory and velopharyngeal dysfunction are unclear.

The perceptual characteristics of speakers with pseudobulbar dysarthria were studied as part of a classic study performed at the Mayo Clinic.[37] Bilateral upper motor neuron lesions result in a number of motor problems including spasticity, weakness, reduced range of movement, and bradykinesia. These motor problems may affect all components of speech production. The strained-strangled voice quality is associated with hyperadduction of the true and false vocal cords and is characterized aerodynamically by elevated laryngeal airway resistance and subglottal pressure, and by reduced laryngeal airflow.[38] Velopharyngeal dysfunction includes increased pharyngeal constriction; slow, sluggish velopharyngeal movement; and incomplete velopharyngeal closure.[32] Articulatory impairments result in imprecise consonant production and slowed speaking rates.

Brain-stem strokes are characterized by two major muscular abnormalities, weakness and hypotonia. These are associated with flaccid dysarthria. Darley and colleagues[37] summarized the perceptual speech characteristics of a group of 30 individuals with bulbar palsy as follows:

[T]he combination of auditory characteristics that best distinguishes flaccid dysarthria from other types consists of marked hypernasality often coupled with nasal emission of air, continuous breathiness during phonation, and audible inspiration (stridor on inhalation).

As with many types of dysarthria, imprecise consonant production is also associated with a flaccid condition.

COMMON TREATMENT TECHNIQUES A careful assessment of impairment of the various components of the speech production mechanism is necessary in order to develop a treatment plan. As was suggested earlier in this chapter, this includes assessment of respiratory, phonatory, velopharyngeal, and oral articulatory function. The following are some treatment approaches that have proven useful in individuals with dysarthria following stroke.

In individuals with flaccid dysarthria, weakness is an overriding feature. Techniques such as respiratory paddles, abdominal binders or belts, and proper positioning have been employed to increase respiratory support for speech.[2] Pushing exercises to increase vocal fold adduction also may be beneficial in this patient group. The respiratory/phonatory characteristics of individuals with spastic or pseudobulbar dysarthria are different from those of flaccid dysarthria. In pseudobulbar dysarthria, spasticity is the predominant feature, and stenosis of the laryngeal valve may reduce what may appear to be strained-strangled voice quality. Patients are taught to generate more-normal translaryngeal airflow by producing relaxed phonation in an effort to maintain adequate levels of respiratory support.[39]

Velopharyngeal dysfunction may occur in both flaccid and spastic dysarthria. Palatal lifts have been demonstrated to be effective in both populations.[40,41] This prosthodontic appliance consists of a retentive portion covering the hard palate and fastening to the maxillary teeth by means of wire and a lift portion that extends along the oral surface of the soft palate. The purpose of the lift is to allow the speaker to generate adequate air pressure in the mouth during production of pressure consonants. Speech sounds such as /t/, /s/, /p/, and others can be produced with more precision when the lift is in place. This lift may be difficult to fit in edentulous speakers, or those with excessive spasticity in the soft palate, or in individuals with severe swallowing problems.

In individuals with flaccid dysarthria, exercises to improve tongue and lip strength may be helpful in improving oral articulation. For individuals with weakness and spasticity, a slow speaking rate should be maintained so that articulatory targets can be achieved. Excessive effort levels may result in an overflow of movements and tightness. Speakers for whom this is a problem should be encouraged to produce relaxed movements that are under control.

INTERVENTION ISSUES Among of the most challenging aspects of management of dysarthria in stroke patients is timing of speech treatment and the need for long-term follow-up. For example, individuals with brain-stem stroke may initially need to rely on augmentative communication systems. Only later does natural speech become a potentially functional means of communication. This period when behavioral intervention is appropriate may occur long after discharge from the acute rehabilitation setting. Thus, long-term management may involve treatment delivery in more than one clinical service unit, by more than one clinician, and for extended periods of time.[40] Small but important changes in speech function may occur over periods of several years in the stroke population.

Traumatic Brain Injury (TBI) Individuals with TBI are becoming an increasingly important part of the caseloads of many speech/language pathologists. Because of the diffuse and variable neuropathology associated with this type of injury, a number of communication problems are common. Language frequently is disrupted as part of a complex constellation of memory and cognitive deficits. The focus of this chapter will not be on the cognitive-communication problems, but rather on the dysarthria, one of the motor speech disorders commonly associated with TBI.

Frequency and Characteristics of the Speech Disorder Overall dysarthria is present as a sequel to TBI in approximately one-third of cases.[42] However, the prevalence varies depending on the time after onset, with estimates of 60 percent of individuals acutely exhibiting dysarthria and 10 percent exhibiting the disorder at long-term follow-up.[43] A growing number of case reports document the diversity in the pattern of dysarthria associated with TBI. Most dysarthrias are characterized as mixed, either spastic-ataxic or flaccid-spastic. However, case reports also exist of predominately ataxic and flaccid types.[44] Instrumental measures of the physiologic aspects of speech production in dysarthric speakers with TBI have recently been reported for the respiratory, laryngeal, velopharyngeal, and articulation systems.[45-49] These studies suggest that the physiologic impairment is not restricted to a single subsystem. Multiple aspects of speech production are impaired.

Common Treatment Techniques Physiologic approaches that reduce the level of impairment in components of the speech production mechanism have been reported to be effective.[40-57] With the respiratory system, the goal of intervention is to help the speaker achieve a consistent subglottal air pressure during speech. This can be accomplished with breathing exercises, with postural adjustments, or by elimination of abnormal respiratory behaviors.[44] Intervention for laryngeal dysfunction may include techniques for establishing voluntary phonation, for increasing voice loudness, and for improving vocal quality. For some, behavioral interventions that focus on the velopharyngeal impairment are appropriate. These may include rate reduction so that articulatory targets can be achieved or articulatory exercises that focus on the production of pressure consonants. When the velopharyngeal impairment is severe, prosthetic management or palatal lift fitting may be appropriate.[40,41,58-60]

Numerous case reports suggest that important changes in speech can be obtained many years after onset of traumatic brain injury.[57,61,62] Together, these reports suggest that long-term follow-up is necessary for brain-injured individuals with severe dysarthria.

Intervention Issues A number of features distinguish the management of dysarthria in TBI from other dysarthrias. Not until very recently has the fund of information about dysarthria and TBI begun to evolve. The cognitive deficits experienced by individuals with TBI interact with the dysarthria in ways that are both complex and poorly understood. Finally, like those with dysarthria after stroke, those with dysarthria and TBI face the need for long-term management of a disorder that may change over extended periods of time. The timing of speech intervention must be focused during those critical periods where intervention is most likely to succeed.

Degenerative Disease

Amyotrophic Lateral Sclerosis (ALS) Amyotrophic lateral sclerosis is a rapidly progressive degenerative disease of unknown etiology. Because it frequently involves upper and lower motor neurons of the brain stem, dysarthria and dysphagia are frequently seen together.

Frequency and Characteristics of the Speech Disorder The dysarthria associated with ALS is classified as a mixed spastic/flaccid type. Initially, either spasticity or flaccidity may predominate. As bulbar symptoms become more severe, dysarthria is characterized by grossly defective consonant and vowel articulation, a laboriously slow speaking rate, marked hypernasality, and harsh or strained-strangled voice quality.[37] Severe dysarthria in ALS is marked by profound weakness, lack of oral movement, and reduced phonation. Although all of the components of the speech mechanism may be affected, tongue impairment may be the most pronounced.[63-66] Changes in phonatory function associated with laryngeal involvement have also been reported.

The presence and rate of progression of speech symptoms vary considerably from case to case. The vast majority of potentiator ALS will experience motor speech disorder that significantly imparts functional communication skills, 30 percent of which are on initial presentation.[71]

Common Treatment Techniques The management of dysarthria associated with ALS progresses through a number of stages (see Table 37-4).[73] In the early stages of management when bulbar symptoms are not apparent, speech may be normal. At this stage, the role of the speech-language pathologist is to confirm speech normalcy and to answer any questions the patient or family may have. When changes in speech become noticeable and worsen with fatigue, treatment focuses on maintaining comprehensibility. Counseling regarding environmental factors that may make communication difficult is essential. Practical strategies, such as noise reduction, or moving close to the listener so that visual and gestural cues can be transmitted, help enormously. Speech comprehensibility can also be enhanced by improving the hearing of frequent communication partners. Even mild hearing loss may compound speech intelligibility problems. If there is any suggestion of hearing impairment, referral for audiologic evaluation and management should be made. A more complete listing of suggestions for enhancing functional communication can be found elsewhere.[3]

When dysarthria progresses to the point where reduction in speech intelligibility is apparent, other intervention approaches become appropriate. Maintaining a slow rate of speech is essential so that articulatory targets can be achieved. At this stage, energy conservation techniques can be useful in preventing fatigue. Techniques that control lung volume levels and coordinate breath and speech can be especially helpful.

Table 37-4
Summary of speech intervention in ALS

	Normal speech process	Detectable speech disturbance	Behavioral modifications	Use of augmentative loss of useful	
				Communication	Speech
Presenting features	No changes or minimal changes are detected	Changes are noticed by unfamiliar partners	Some reduction in speech intelligibility	Needs augmentative communication systems as primary or secondary system	No functional natural speech
		Symptoms worsen with fatigue	Need for frequent repetition		
Intervention	Confirm normalcy	Minimize environmental adversity	Maintain slow speaking rate	Begin alphabet supplementation	Develop adequate yes/no system
	Answer questions	Establish context of messages	Conserve energy	Suggest changing mode in different situations	Develop eye-gaze systems
		Maximize hearing of partners	Fit with palatal life	Set up alerting systems	Enable communication for patients with ventilators
		Teach strategies for coping with groups	Develop breakdown resolution strategies	Teach strategies for telephone communication	
			Increase the precision of speech production	Introduce portable writing systems Introduce multipurpose communication systems	

Used with permission from Yorkston KM, Miller RM, Strand EA: *Management of Speech and Swallowing Disorders in Degenerative Disease.* Tucson, AZ: Communication Skill Builders, 1995.

In some cases, portable amplifiers may be used to compensate for the presence of reduced respiratory support. For those individuals with slowly progressive dysarthria and with adequate oral articulatory movement, palatal lifts may be considered to compensate for inadequate velopharyngeal valving. Strategies to resolve communication breakdowns also are important, and may ease frustration. Finally, techniques for increasing the precision of speech also can be useful. These include maintaining a slow rate of speech, exaggerating oral articulatory movements, inclusion of final consonants, and increasing the overall forcefulness with which speech is delivered. Techniques that supplement or replace natural speech when it is no longer functional are reviewed elsewhere in this text.

Intervention Issues The classic picture of ALS is one of preserved sensation, cognition, and language function in the face of increasing motor impairment. These preserved functions have implications for intervention. First, extended periods of behavioral intervention are typically not needed because the ability to im-

plement compensatory strategies is preserved. It may not be necessary to teach those with ALS to maintain a slow speaking rate in order to achieve target speech sounds. Compensatory techniques may be "automatically" adopted, such as exaggerated articulatory gestures. If some direct behavioral intervention is necessary, it is typically brief.

Early intervention is critical. Dysarthria need not be severe in order to affect many aspects of daily living. Even mild dysarthria may affect employment and cause difficulty in maintaining social closeness. The focus of intervention is on communication function rather than on speech impairment. Because of the relentless nature of ALS, interventions must be continuously reevaluated over a lifetime.

Parkinson's Disease Parkinson's disease, a relatively common, slowly progressive degenerative disorder, is characterized by the classic triad resting tremor, bradykinesia, and rigidity. Although typically not among the initial symptoms of the disease, voice and speech changes are common as progression occurs.

Frequency and Characteristics of the Speech Disorder Seventy percent of individuals with Parkinson's disease report deterioration in speech.[74] The dysarthria associated with Parkinson's disease is classified as hypokinetic, with characteristic features of monopitch, reduced stress, monoloudness, imprecise consonants, inappropriate silences, and short rushes of speech.[37] Reduced range of oral mandibular motion is implicated in the development of monotony and articulatory imprecision, and bradykinesia is reflected in inappropriate silences and short rushes of speech. Rigidity may be responsible for many speech characteristics, including breathiness, harsh vocal quality, and low pitch.

Multiple components of the speech production mechanism may be involved in Parkinson's disease. Recently, attention has been focused on respiratory aspects of parkinsonian speech.[75] Individuals with hypokinetic dysarthria have been described as having an inflexible respiratory pattern during speech.[76] This inflexibility may be the result of reduced compliance of the rib cage.[77] Because changes in vocal quality are typically the first speech symptoms in Parkinson's disease, laryngeal aspects of hypokinetic dysarthria have received considerable attention. Physically, adductor and abductor movements of the vocal folds are bilaterally symmetrical, but incomplete closure may lead to a breathy voice quality.[78,79] Velopharyngeal dysfunction is not a major aspect of parkinsonian dysarthria. Rigidity of oral muscles has been associated with articulatory undershoot, leveling to the failure of articulators to achieve intended targets. This unique oral articulatory disorder may be associated with consonants that require more constriction.[80] Speech rates vary considerably in those with Parkinson's disease, with some slower than normal, and others more rapid than normal. Parkinsonian speech is the only type of dysarthria where speaking rates may be in excess of normal.

Common Treatment Techniques There is a long history of attempts to document the effectiveness of speech intervention for individuals with Parkinson's disease.[73] Early studies lead to the impression that broad-based speech improvement programs brought about changes during the treatment session, but that these changes were not maintained outside treatment.[81,82] Later a more positive trend developed both with specific techniques and with more general speech improvement programs.[83,86–88] Most recently, the success of intensive treatment focusing on phonation has been reported and will be described in more detail below.[87–88]

As with other types of dysarthria, appropriate treatment is based on the severity of the disorder. Table 37-5 summarizes the presenting features and intervention for individuals with mild, moderate, or severe hypokinetic dysarthria. Individuals with mild hypokinetic dysarthria typically exhibit disorders that are predominantly phonatory. Treatment of these individuals may be appropriate for several reasons. Even mild dysarthria may be a functional limitation in people for whom quality of speech is critical. Further, recent studies have suggested that phonatory function is amenable to change in this population. The treatment of phonatory disorders involves tasks where speakers are encouraged to use maximum phonatory effort in order to bring the vocal folds together and thus improve vocal quality.[89] Individuals undergo an intensive, but brief, period of treatment where they learn to "calibrate" their speech. In other words, they learn to know and accept the amount of effect needed to consistently increase vocal loudness to normal levels. Ideal candidates for this type of treatment are highly motivated individuals who are able to produce louder phonation when asked to do so. Normal cognition enhances the likelihood of success in this type of intervention.

In addition to exhibiting phonatory dysfunction, individuals with moderate hypokinetic dysarthria experience oral articulatory problems that are characterized by blurred consonant contrasts. They may have difficulty initiating speech or may pause at inappropriate locations. Their speaking rate may be abnormal and intelligibility reduced. Behavioral intervention such as the type described by Ramig and colleagues may also be useful for individuals with moderate dysarthria.[89] Other treatment techniques may also be useful. Because articulatory undershooting and excessive speaking rate frequently occur, the treatment approaches may require slowing the rate of speech by either behavioral training or by a biofeedback technique known as delayed auditory feedback (DAF).[2] The DAF device consists of a microphone, a pocket-sized delay unit/battery, and earphones. Because speech is heard with a fraction-of-a-second delay, rates are slowed.[83,90,91] Little training is needed to learn to use the device, and it can be used for extended periods of time. Portable vocal amplifiers may also be useful for some patients with low-volume speech.

Intervention Issues Management of communication problems in individuals with Parkinson's disease is challenging for a number of reasons. First, dysarthria severe enough to pose functional limitations typically occurs late in the course of the disease. At this stage of

Table 37-5
Summary of speech intervention in Parkinson's disease

	Mild	*Moderate*	*Severe*
Presenting features	Little or no reduction in speech intelligibility Symptoms include reduced loudness, monotony, and breathiness	Some reduction in speech intelligibility Symptoms include reduced loudness, monotony, breathiness, and consonant imprecision	Natural speech is no longer functional Symptoms include severe difficulty initiating voice and short rushes of poorly articulated speech
Intervention	Increased vocal fold adduction Increased maximum duration of phonation Increased respiratory support Patient and family education Home practice drills	Rate-control drills Delayed auditory feedback Voice amplification Patient and family education	Pacing boards or alphabet supplementation Portable typing devices Development of partner-supported communication techniques Patient and family education

Used with permission from Yorkston KM, Miller RM, Strand EA: *Management of Speech and Swallowing Disorders in Degenerative Disease.* Tucson, AZ: Communication Skill Builders, 1995.

the disease, factors such as cognitive deficits or depression may complicate management. Individuals with Parkinson's disease and dysarthria typically have been on drug regimes for extended periods of time. Speech capabilities may fluctuate dramatically depending on the drug cycle; peak-dose dyskinesias when severe may interfere with speech production. Finally, management of dysarthria is complicated by the fact that many individuals with Parkinson's disease are not aware of the extent of their speech difficulties, and thus are not highly motivated to pursue treatment. Regardless of these challenges, functional communication skills can be enhanced by timely assessment and appropriate intervention.

Multiple Sclerosis (MS)　Multiple sclerosis, a disease of the white matter, is most frequently diagnosed in young to middle-aged adults. The scattered lesions in the central nervous system produce a variety of combinations of motor, sensory, and cognitive impairments. In addition to dysarthria, communication problems associated with the disorder include auditory deficits, dysfluency, and cognitively based disorders.[92]

Frequency and Characteristics of the Speech Disorder　Although early descriptions of MS included the feature of "scanning speech" (slow, drawling

speech), more-recent studies suggest that dysarthria is by no means a universal characteristic of MS.[37] When dysarthria is present, it may be solely attributable to cerebellar involvement (scanning speech). More commonly, the motor speech disorder in MS is characterized by features of both ataxic and spastic dysarthria. The prevalence of dysarthria in MS varies, depending on how dysarthria is defined and measured. The classical Mayo Clinic studies suggest that nearly 80 percent of those with MS exhibit speech deficits, most frequently impaired modulation of amplitude. Self-report studies on prevalence suggest that 44 percent report changes in speech or voice after the onset of the disease.[74] Speech adequacy is related to the number of neural systems involved. The most severe dysarthria is associated with a lesion load that involves the cerebral hemispheres, brain stem, and cerebellum.[37] The most-characteristic speech features in MS include impaired control of loudness, vocal harshness, and defective articulation.

Common Treatment Techniques　As with other dysarthrias, speech intervention in MS depends on the characteristics and severity of the impairment. If brain-stem involvement predominates, treatment techniques such as those used with flaccid dysarthria

Table 37-6
Summary of speech intervention in multiple sclerosis

	Mild	Moderate	Severe
Presenting features	Vocal tremor	Harsh voice	Natural speech no longer functional
	Harsh voice	Reduced speaking rate	
	Symptoms worsen with fatigue	Decreased speech naturalness	
Intervention	Teach energy-conservation techniques	Encourage maintenance of appropriate speaking rate	Compensate for severe visual/motor problems
	Teach loudness-regulation techniques	Teach appropriate respiratory patterning	Select appropriate vocabulary
		Supplement speech with alphabet board	

Used with permission from Yorkston KM, Miller RM, Strand EA: *Management of Speech and Swallowing Disorders in Degenerative Disease.* Tucson, AZ: Communication Skill Builders, 1995.

associated with brain-stem stroke may be appropriate. If upper motor neuron involvement predominates, appropriate techniques include those used with spastic dysarthria, similar to that associated with bilateral cortical stroke (see the preceding). Treatment approaches commonly used for individuals with the mixed spastic/ataxic dysarthria associated with MS are listed in Table 37-6.

In mild dysarthria, vocal quality changes may not interfere with normal speaking rate or intelligibility. Treatment techniques for energy conservation and for regulation of vocal tone usually focus on respiratory control. When ataxic motor speech is present, uncoordinated rather than weak respiratory movements produce subglottal air pressures far in excess of normal, leading to difficulty generating the stable pressures needed for normal speech. For these individuals, respiratory pattern stabilization techniques are especially helpful.[2] This intervention focuses on the establishment of appropriate lung volume levels for speech, use of appropriate chest wall shapes for breathing during speech, and the elimination of abnormal respiratory behaviors.

In moderately severe dysarthria, vocal changes are accompanied by changes in other aspects of speech, including a slow speaking rate and a pseudonormalized pattern of articulatory and phonemic stressing. When intelligibility is severely compromised, augmentative communication procedures are recommended.[93] Information about augmentative communication applica-

tions for individuals with severe dysarthria and MS is presented elsewhere in this text.

Intervention Issues Management of dysarthria associated with MS is unique in a number of respects. The typical age of onset is in early adulthood. For most this is a critical time for career and educational development. Even mild communication deficits may cause substantial disability. The protean and unpredictable course of MS makes long-term management of motor speech disorders especially challenging. Finally, cognition decline may limit goals in speech intervention.

REFERENCES

1. Institute of Medicine: *Disability in America: Toward a National Agenda for Prevention.* Washington, DC: National Academy Press, 1991.
2. Yorkston KM, Beukelman DR, Bell KR: *Clinical Management of Dysarthric Speakers.* Austin, TX: ProEd, 1988.
3. Yorkston KM, Strand EA, Kennedy MRT: Comprehensibility of dysarthric speech: Implications for assessment and treatment planning. *Am J Speech-Lang Pathol* 1996; 5:55–66.
4. Hodge M: Speech mechanism assessment, in Yoder D, Kent R (eds): *Decision Making in Speech-Language Pathology.* Toronto: B.C. Decker, 1988, pp. 104–109.
5. Kent R, Kent J, Rosenbek J: Maximum performance tests

of speech production. *J Speech Hearing Dis* 1987; 52:367–387.

6. Robbins J, Klee T: Clinical assessment of oropharyngeal motor development in young children. *J Speech Hearing Dis* 1987; 52:271–277.

7. Erenberg G: Cerebral palsy. *Postgrad Med* 1984; 75:87–93.

8. Evans PM, Evans SJ, Alberman E: Cerebral palsy: Why we must plan for survival. *Arch Dis Child* 1990; 65:1329–1333.

9. Wolfe W: A comprehensive evaluation of fifty cases of cerebral palsy. *J Speech Hear Dis* 1950; 15:234–251.

10. Achilles R: Communication anomalies of individuals with cerebral palsy: I. Analysis of communication processes in 151 cases of cerebral palsy. *Cer Palsy Rev* 1955; 16: 15–24.

11. Workinger MS, Kent RD: Perceptual analysis of the dysarthria in children with athetoid and spastic cerebral palsy, in Moore CA, Yorkston KM, Beukelman DR (eds): *Dysarthria and Apraxia of Speech: Perspectives on Management.* Baltimore: ProEd, 1991, pp. 109–126.

12. O'Dwyer N, Neilson P, Guitar BE, Quinn PT, Andrews G: Control of upper airway structures during nonspeech tasks in normal and cerebral-palsied subjects: EMG findings. *J Speech Hear Res* 1983; 26:162–170.

13. Neilson P, O'Dwyer N: Reproducibility and variability of speech muscle activity in athetoid dysarthria of cerebral palsy. *J Speech Hear Res* 1984; 27:502–517.

14. Vaughan CW, Neilson PD, O'Dwyer NJ: Motor control deficits of orfacila muscles in cerebral palsy. *J Neurol Neurosurg Psychiatr* 1988; 51(4):534–539.

15. O'Dwyer NJ, Neilson PD: Voluntary muscle control in normal and athetoid dysarthric speakers. *Brain* 1988; 111:877–899.

16. Barlow SM, Abbs JH: Orofacial fine-motor control impairments in congenital spasticity: Evidence against hypertonius-related performance deficits. *Neurology* 1984; 34: 145–150.

17. Barlow SM, Abbs JH: Fine force and position control of select orofacial structure in the upper motor neuron syndrome. *Exp Neurol* 1986; 94:699–713.

18. Ansel BM, McNeil MR, Hunker CJ, Bless DM: The frequency of verbal and acoustic adjustments used by cerebral palsied dysarthric adults when faced with communicative failure, in Berry W (ed): *Clinical Dysarthria.* Austin, TX: ProEd, 1983, pp. 85–108.

19. Tjaden K, Liss JM: The influence of familiarity on judgments of treated speech. *Am J Speech-Lang Pathol* 1995; 4(1):38–39.

20. Hunter L, Pring T, Martin S: The use of strategies to increase speech intelligibility in cerebral palsy: An experimental evaluation. *Br J Dis Commun* 1991; 26:163–174.

21. Love RJ: *Childhood Motor Speech Disability.* New York: Macmillan Publishing Co, 1992.

22. Hulme JB, Bain B, Hardin M, McKinnon A, Waldron D: The influence of adaptive seating devices on vocalization. *J Commun Dis* 1989; 22(2):137–145.

23. Murphy CC, Yeargin-Allsopp M, Decoufl'e P, Drews CD: Prevalence of cerebral palsy among ten-year-old children in metroplitan Atlanta, 1985 through 1987. *J Pediatr* 1993; 123:S13–20.

24. Crary MA: Phonological characteristics of developmental verbal dyspraxia. *Seminars in Speech and Language* 1984; 5:71–83.

25. Crary MA: *Developmental Motor Speech Disorders.* San Diego, Singular Publishing Group, 1993.

26. Hall P, Jordan L, Robin D: *Developmental Apraxia of Speech: Theory and Clinical Practice.* Austin, TX: ProEd, 1993.

27. Strand EA: Treatment of motor speech disorders in children. *Semin Speech Lang* 1995; 16(2):126–139.

28. Rosenbek J, Lemme M, Ahern M, Harris E, Wertz R: A treatment for apraxia of speech in adults. *J Speech Hear Dis* 1973; 38(4):462–472.

29. Haynes S: Developmental apraxia of speech: Symptoms and treatment, in Johns D (ed): *Clinical Management of Neurogenic Communication Disorders.* Boston: Little, Brown & Co., 1985, pp. 257–266.

30. Square P: Treatment approaches for developmental apraxia of speech. *Clin Commun Dis* 1994; 4(3):151–161.

31. Helfrich-Miller K: A clinical perspective: Melodic Intonation Therapy for developmental apraxia. *Clin Commun Dis* 1994; 4(3):175–182.

32. Duffy JR: *Motor Speech Disorders: Substrates, Differential Diagnosis, and Management.* St. Louis: Mosby, 1995.

33. Wertz R, LaPointe L, Rosenbek J: *Apraxia of Speech in Adults: The Disorder and Its Management.* Orlando, FL: Grune & Stratton, 1984.

34. Sparks RW, Helm N, Albert, M: Aphasia rehabilitation resulting from melodic intonation therapy. *Cortex* 1974; 10:303–316.

35. Hartman DE, Abbs JH: Dysarthria associated with focal unilateral upper motor neuron lesion. *Eur J Dis Commun* 1992; 27(3):187–196.

36. Ropper AH: Severe dysarthria with right hemisphere stroke. *Neurology* 1987; 37(6):1061–1063.

37. Darley FL, Aronson AE, Brown JR: *Motor Speech Disorders.* Philadelphia: WB Saunders, 1975.

38. Murdoch BE, Thompson EC, Stokes PD: Phonatory and laryngeal dysfunction following upper motor neuron vascular lesions. *J Med Speech-Lang Pathol* 1994; 2(3):177–190.

39. Aten JL: Treatment of spastic dysarthria, in Perkins WH (ed): *Dysarthria and Apraxia.* New York: Thieme-Stratton, 1983, pp. 69–77.

40. Simpson MB, Till JA, Goff AM: Long-term treatment of severe dysarthria: A case study. *J Speech Hear Dis* 1988; 53:433–440.

41. Aten J, McDonald A, Simpson M, Gutierrez R: Efficacy of modified palatal lifts for improved resonance, in McNeil M, Rosenbek J, Aronson A (eds): *The Dysarthria: Physiology, Acoustics, Perception, Management.* Boston: College-Hill Press, 1984, pp. 231–242.

42. Sarno MT, Buonaguro A, Levita E: Characteristics of ver-

bal impairment in closed head injured patients. *Arch Phys Med Rehab* 1986; 67:400–405.

43. Yorkston KM, Honsinger MJ, Mitsuda PM, Hammen V: The relationship between speech and swallowing disorders in head-injured patients. *J Head Trauma Rehab* 1989; 4:1–16.

44. Yorkston KM, Beukelman DR: Motor speech disorders, in Beukelman DR, Yorkston KM (eds): *Communication Disorders Following Traumatic Brain Injury: Management of Cognitive, Language, and Motor Impairment*. Boston: College-Hill Press, 1991, pp. 251–317.

45. Murdoch BE, Theodoros DG, Stokes PD, Chenery HJ: Abnormal patterns of speech breathing in dysarthric speakers following severe closed head injury. *Brain Injury* 1993; 7:295–308.

46. Theodoros DG, Murdoch BE: Laryngeal dysfunction in dysarthric speakers following severe closed-head injury. *Brain Injury* 1994; 8:667–684.

47. Theodoros DG, Murdoch BE, Stokes PD, Chenery HJ: Hypernasality in dysarthric speakers following severe closed head injury: A perceptual and instrumental analysis. *Brain Injury* 1993; 7:59–69.

48. Barlow SM, Burton MS: Ramp-and-hold force control in the upper and lower lips: Developing new neuromotor assessment applications in traumatic brain injured adults. *J Speech Hear Res* 1990; 33:660–675.

49. Theodoros DG, Murdoch BE, Chenery HJ: Perceptual speech characteristics of dysarthric speakers. *Brain Injury* 1994; 8:101–124.

50. Coelho CA, Gracco VL, Fourakis M, Rossetti M, Oshima K: Application of instrumental techniques in the assessment of dysarthria: A case study, in Till JA, Yorkston KM, Beukelman DR (eds): *Motor Speech Disorders: Advances in Assessment and Treatment*. Baltimore: Paul H. Brookes Publishing, 1994, pp. 103–118.

51. Enderby P, Crow E: Long-term recovery patterns of severe dysarthria following head injury. *Br J Dis Commun* 1990; 25:341–354.

52. Harris B, Murry T: Dysarthria and aphagia: A case study of neuromuscluar treatment. *Arch Phys Med Rehab* 1984; 65:408–412.

53. Hartman DE, Day M, Pecora R: Treatment of dysarthria: A case report. *J Commun Dis* 1979; 12:167–173.

54. McHenry M, Wilson R: The challenge of unintelligible speech following traumatic brain injury. *Brain Injury* 1994; 8: 363–375.

55. Netsell R, Daniel B: Dysarthria in adults: Physiologic approach to rehabilitation. *Arch Phys Med Rehab* 1979; 60:502.

56. Theodoros DG, Murdoch BE, Stokes P: A physiological analysis of articulatory dysfunction in dysarthric speakers following severe closed-head injury. *Brain Injury* 1995; 9: 237–254.

57. Workinger MS, Netsell R: Restoration of intelligible speech 13 years post-head injury. *Brain Injury* 1992; 6:183–187.

58. Bedwinek AP, O'Brian RL: A patient selection profile for the use of speech prosthesis in adult disorders. *J Commun Dis* 1985; 18:169–182.

59. Gonzalez J, Aronson A: Palatal lift prosthesis for treatment of anatomic and neurologic palatopharyngeal insufficiency. *Cleft Palatal J* 1970; 7:91–104.

60. Yorkston KM, Honsinger MJ, Beukelman DR, Taylor T: The effects of palatal lift fitting on the perceived articulatory adequacy of dysarthric speakers, in Yorkston KM, Beukelman DR (eds): *Recent Adv Clin Dysarthria*. Boston: College-Hill Press, 1989, pp. 85–98.

61. Keenan JE, Barnhart KS: Development of yes/no systems in individuals with severe traumatic brain injuries. *Augment Alt Commun* 1993; 9:184–190.

62. Light J, Beesley M, Collier B: Transition through multiple augmentative and alternative communication systems: A three-year case study of a head injury adolescent. *Augment Alt Commun* 1988; 4:2–14.

63. Hirose H, Kiritani S, Ushijima T, Sawashima M: Analysis of abnormal articulatory dynamics in two dysarthric patients. *J Speech Hear Dis* 1978; 43:96.

64. Dworkin JP: Tongue strength measurement in patients with amyotrophic lateral sclerosis: Qualitative vs. quantitative procedures. *Arch Phys Med Rehab* 1980; 61:422–424.

65. DePaul R, Abbs JH, Caligiuri MP, Gracco VL, Brooks BR: Hypoglossal, trigeminal, and facial motoneuron involvement in amyotrophic lateral sclerosis. *Neurology* 1988; 38:281–283.

66. Cha CH, Patten BM: Amyotrophic lateral sclerosis: Abnormalities of the tongue on magnetic resonance imaging. *Ann Neurol* 1989; 25:468–472.

67. Ramig LO, Scherer RC, Klasner ER, Titze IR, Horii Y: Acoustic analysis of voice in Amyotrophic Lateral Sclerosis: A longitudinal case study. *J Speech Hear Dis* 1990; 55:2–14.

68. Aronson AE, Ramig LO, Winholtz WS, Silber SR: Rapid voice tremor, or "flutter," in amyotrophic lateral sclerosis. *Ann Otolaryngol Rhinol Laryngol* 1992; 101:511–518.

69. Strand EA, Buder EH, Yorkston KM, Ramig LO: Differential phonatory characteristics of four women with amyotrophic lateral sclerosis. *J Voice* 1994; 8:327–339.

70. Kent RD, Kim H, Weismer G, Kent JF, Rosebek JC, Brooks BR, Workinger M: Laryngeal dysfunction in neurological disease: Amyotrophic lateral sclerosis, Parkinson disease, and stroke. *J Med Speech-Lang Pathol* 1994; 2:157–176.

71. Bonduelle M: Amyotrophic lateral sclerosis, in Vinten PJ, Bruyn GW (eds): *Handbook of Clinical Neurology*. Amsterdam: North-Holland, 1975, pp. 281–338.

72. Yorkston KM, Strand EA, Miller R, Hillel A, Smith K: Speech deterioration in amyotrophic lateral sclerosis: Implications for the timing of intervention. *J Med Speech-Lang Path* 1993; 1:35–46.

73. Yorkston KM, Miller RM, Strand EA: *Management of Speech and Swallowing Disorders in Degenerative Disease*. Tucson, AZ: Communication Skill Builders, 1995.

74. Hartelius L, Svensson P: Speech and swallowing symptoms associated with Parkinson's disease and multiple sclerosis: A survey. *Folia Phoniatrica et Logopaedica* 1994; 46:9–17.

75. Murdoch BE, Chenery HJ, Bowler S, Ingram JCL: Respiratory function in Parkinson's subjects exhibiting a perceptible speech deficit: A kinematic and spirometric analysis. *J Speech Hear Dis* 1989; 54:610–626.

76. Kim R: The chronic residual respiratory disorder in postencephalitic parkinsonism. *J Neurol Neurosurg Psychiatr* 1968; 31:393–398.

77. Solomon NP, Hixon TJ: Speech breathing in Parkinson's disease. *J Speech Hear Res* 1993; 36:294–310.

78. Aronson AE: *Clinical Voice Disorder: An Interdisciplinary Approach,* 2nd ed. New York: Thieme, 1985.

79. Hanson D, Gerratt BR, Ward PH: Cinegraphic observations of laryngeal function in Parkinson's disease. *Laryngoscope* 1984; 94:348–353.

80. Logemann J, Fischer H: Vocal tract control in Parkinson's disease: Phonetic feature analyses of misarticulations. *J Speech Hear Dis* 1981; 46:348.

81. Sarno M: Speech impairment in Parkinson's disease. *Arch Phys Med Rehab* 1968; 49:269–275.

82. Allan CM: Treatment of non-fluent speech resulting from neurological diseases: Treatment of dysarthria. *Br J Dis Commun* 1970; 5:3–5.

83. Downie AW, Low JM, Lindsay DD: Speech disorders in parkinsonism: Usefulness of delayed auditory feedback in selected cases. *Br J Dis Commun* 1981; 16:135–139.

84. Scott S, Caird FI: Speech therapy for Parkinson's disease. *J Neurol Neurosurg Psychiatr* 1983; 46:140–144.

85. Robertson SJ, Thomson F: Speech therapy in Parkinson's disease: A study of the efficacy and long term effects of intensive treatment. *Br J Dis Commun* 1984; 19:213–224.

86. LeDorze G, Dioone L, Ryalls J, Julien M, Ouellet L: The effects of speech and language therapy for a case of dysarthria associated with Parkinson's disease. *Eur J Dis Commun* 1992; 27:313–324.

87. Ramig LO, Countryman S, O'Brien C, Hoehn M, Thompson L: Intensive speech treatment for patients with Parkinson disease: Short and long-term comparison of two techniques. *Neurology* 1996; 47:1496–1503

88. Ramig LO, Countryman S, Thompson LL, Horii Y: A comparison of two forms of intensive speech treatment in Parkinson disease. *J Speech Hear Res* 1995; 38:1232–1251

89. Ramig LO, Pawlas AA, Countryman S: *The Lee Silverman Voice Treatment.* Iowa City, IA: National Center for Voice and Speech, 1995.

90. Hanson W, Metter E: DAF speech rate modification in Parkinson's disease: A report of two cases, in Berry W (ed): *Clinical Dysarthria.* Austin, TX: ProEd, 1983, pp. 231–254.

91. Adams SG: Accelerating speech in a case of hypokinetic dysarthria: Descriptions and treatment, in Till JA, Yorkston KM, Beukelman DR (eds): *Motor speech disorders: Advances in Assessment and Treatment.* Baltimore: Paul H. Brookes Publishing, 1994, pp. 213–228.

92. Sorensen P, Brown S, Logemann J, Wilson K: Communication disorders and dysphagia. Special focus issues: Comprehensive care in multiple sclerosis. *J Neurol Rehab* 1994; 8:137–143.

93. Beukelman DR, Yorkston KM: A communication system for the severely dysarthric speaker with an intact language system. *J Speech Hear Dis* 1977; 42:265–270.

Chapter 38

AUDIOLOGIC EVALUATION AND HEARING AIDS

Chris Halpin

Communication among the caregiver, the patient, and the patient's family is essential to effective neurorehabilitation. There are considerable obstacles to communication in some cases, including grief, reduced mental capacity, unresolved family issues, and language and cultural barriers. Neurorehabilitation professionals develop particular skills and techniques to overcome these obstacles and proceed with effective care. Some cases present the additional communication barrier of hearing loss, and audiologists are trained to provide evaluation, hearing aids, and specific communication strategies in order to allow rehabilitation to proceed optimally. Hearing evaluation, hearing aids, and communication strategies are not only adjunct forms of therapy, but may also serve as the initial gateway to communication.

OVERVIEW OF HEARING LOSS

Figure 38-1 shows the major features of the anatomy of the ear, including the outer, middle, and inner ear, the VIIIth nerve, and surrounding structures in the temporal bone. Conductive hearing loss results from a physical blockage somewhere in the sound transmission path through the outer and middle ear. Sound, in the form of oscillating compression waves traveling in air, passes into the external auditory meatus (ear canal) of the outer ear. If this canal is absent owing to facial anomaly, or is blocked by skin, cerumen (ear wax), or a foreign object, the amount of sound that can pass is reduced, and a conductive hearing loss will result.

If the outer ear is clear, the sound waves next reach the tympanic membrane (ear drum). This structure is light, stiff, and air-tight, and acts to collect the sound energy and refocus its force to produce motion in the tiny lever-action bones of the ossicular chain (malleus, incus, stapes). The tympanic membrane, ossicular chain, and surrounding space form the middle ear. If the tympanic membrane is punctured or its mass is changed by disease, it will lose effectiveness in the transmission of sound energy, and a conductive hearing loss will result. If the bones of the ossicular chain are broken or disjointed, sound will not pass effectively. A common disease known as otosclerosis presents with unwanted bone growing onto the stapes. This causes a conductive hearing loss by fixing the tiny stapes footplate so that its movement is impeded. The space surrounding the ossicular chain is naturally air filled, but may become filled with serous fluid, pus, or tumors, all of which act to reduce the sound transmission and result in a conductive hearing loss.

Sensorineural hearing loss results from a failure of the transduction/transmission mechanisms of the inner ear. The peripheral sensory organ is known as the cochlea and is filled with fluids (perilymph, endolymph) resembling cerebrospinal fluid. If all outer and middle ear structures are functioning, the pistonlike movement of the stapes creates a fluid wave motion inside the cochlea. The snail-shell turns of the cochlea contain a membrane (the basilar membrane) whose vibration characteristics progress from high frequency at the near (basal) end to low frequency at the far (apical) end. The sound is broken up into a spectrum along this membrane much as a prism divides the colors of light. Along the basilar membrane are approximately 15,500 hair cells.[1] The inner row of these cells synapse on the afferent fibers of the VIIIth nerve. The inner hair cells chemically transduce the local cochlear fluid motion into action potentials that are transmitted to the higher centers. There are also three rows of outer hair cells, connected predominantly to the efferent pathway. The full activity of these cells is not known, but it has been shown that they act to amplify incoming sounds.[2]

Unlike the outer and middle ear structures, the tiny size and deep location of the cochlea in the temporal bone precludes most forms of surgical exploration and treatment. Much less is known concerning the disease processes that cause sensorineural hearing loss than is

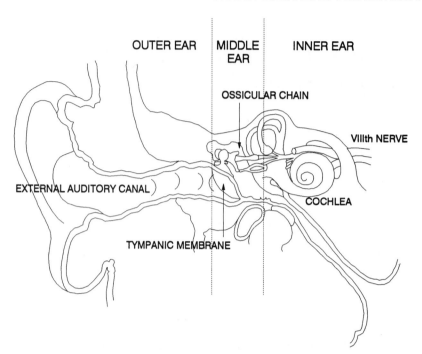

OUTER EAR   MIDDLE   INNER EAR
             EAR

OSSICULAR CHAIN

VIIIth NERVE

EXTERNAL AUDITORY CANAL

COCHLEA

TYMPANIC MEMBRANE

Figure 38-1
*Diagram of the anatomical struc-
tures related to conductive and
sensorineural hearing loss.*

known about conductive hearing loss. What is apparent
is that the cochlea grows less sensitive and less able to
separate the rapidly changing sounds of speech. Temporal bone histopathology from cases with sensorineural
hearing loss reveals a number of different possible disease mechanisms including loss of hair cells, loss of
nerve fibers, altered chemical environment, and disrupted vascular supply.[3]

INDICATIONS FOR THE
AUDIOLOGIC EVALUATION

Rationale: Rule Out or Evaluate
Hearing Loss

To Rule Out Hearing Loss   The audiologic evaluation, with its special booth and electronic technology,
may appear to be a major evaluation effort to be reserved for cases showing serious symptoms. In fact,
there are a number of factors relating to hearing loss
that combine to make this evaluation very valuable
when used to rule out hidden difficulties. Patients may
have serious problems affecting rehabilitation that are
not apparent to clinicians without audiological evalua-

tion. The human brain generally acts to fill in or smooth
over missing information in the sensory systems, giving
the patient the illusion that he or she is hearing well
enough to avoid medical intervention.[4] When the patient does recognize the problem, he or she typically
will avoid identifying him- or herself as hearing impaired
to others. Hearing loss, and especially hearing aids, are
viewed unsympathetically and negatively in our society,
and the patient will typically avoid medical intervention
if at all possible.[5] Although such a patient may use a
number of techniques to pass as hearing and understanding in social settings, the effect of the loss on learning and communicating in rehabilitation is more difficult
to avoid. The neurorehabilitation caregiver should be
made aware of both the extent of loss and the appropriate response, in order to succeed with therapy.

The special environment of the audiologic evaluation will reveal medically important symptoms that are
not otherwise apparent. For example, the patient may
communicate effectively with one good ear. Asymmetries in performance are medically significant and should
be investigated until an adequate cause is determined.
The sound booth is the only environment where the
limits of normal human hearing can be assessed. For
example, a measurable low-frequency sensorineural

hearing loss associated with Menieres disease may go unnoticed as the patient uses the mid- and high-frequency areas to communicate. In addition, the effects of a regimen of potentially ototoxic medication will be revealed by audiologic evaluation before it is apparent to patients or their caregivers. In short, a patient in need of neurorehabilitation should have hearing loss ruled out before embarking on therapy.

To Evaluate Hearing Loss Every patient with known hearing loss should have its type, severity, and site of lesion defined. The audiologic evaluation will reveal middle-ear and cochlear dysfunction separately. Lesions attributable to the VIIIth cranial nerve can also be discovered. A great deal is known concerning the relation of patterns of hearing loss with specific diseases, and findings may lead to effective treatment with medicine, surgery, or hearing aids.[6]

To Recommend Hearing Aids and Aural Rehabilitation Expectation of benefit from hearing aids is not tightly correlated with the simple presence of hearing loss. Benefit is best thought of in terms of realistic expectation of improvement in speech understanding when sounds are made louder. There may be no expectation of improvement with certain losses, and the optimization of improvement involves trade-offs in every case. Output power, frequency response, electronic processing, physical fit, and appearance mutually interact, with each trading off against the other. Simply put, it is not possible to optimize a single variable without reducing another.[7] The audiologist will evaluate these trade-offs and report whether a hearing aid is indicated.

The audiologist will evaluate the expectations for benefit from a set of techniques for optimizing communication known as aural rehabilitation.[8] Aural rehabilitation includes the use of assistive devices, along with hearing aids, for optimizing listening. These devices include special telephones and individual listening devices for entertainment. Other devices may be indicated that make use of vision or tactile stimulation, such as flashing-light doorbells and vibrating alarm clocks. Aural rehabilitation also includes training to change the communication habits of the patient, as well as his or her family and friends. Good communication habits include awareness of the effects of the communication environment and use of more-effective strategies to elicit meaning. Even with optimal application of hearing aids and good learning and cooperation by all concerned, the limiting factors imposed by the damaged ear prompt audiologists to include counseling regarding realistic expectations and grieving.

To Evaluate Communication Ability Neurorehabilitation care and therapy depend on communication. Audiologic care is best viewed not as one of many therapies, but as a gateway to all forms of care. Caregivers must be informed of the optimal method(s) for communicating with a patient. Communication difficulties will reduce the accuracy of history taking, effectiveness of psychological counseling, and the transmission of instructions during speech-language, physical, and occupational therapy. Nursing care is particularly dependent on the communication of needs and instructions. Hearing aids and communication strategies should be applied before attempting to work with the patient. The audiologist will address these issues during the audiologic evaluation.

Given the specifics of hearing loss type, severity, site of lesion, prognosis, and the expectations for benefit from hearing aids and aural rehabilitation, what is the best way to establish communication with this patient? What is the best performance that we can reasonably expect? Hearing loss and related problems are only two of several factors affecting communication in the rehabilitation of neurologically impaired patients. Are communication problems attributable to hearing loss, language and culture, development, or brain insult? The audiologist will address those aspects related to hearing, leaving a clearer path for other caregivers to address problems relating to other areas.

When to Refer

Age and Health Considerations There is no patient too old or too young to be referred for audiologic evaluation. Extremely young or old patients require more effort, and the expectation of exhaustive results is reduced. On the other hand, the most important questions regarding communication can be evaluated in any age group, from neonates to centenarians, using special techniques. In addition, the expectation for hearing ability is essentially the same; that is, normal hearing in all groups. Infants do not develop significant hearing sensitivity after birth, so any established hearing loss should be viewed as a disease process.[9] In the same way, some elderly patients hear normally, and the prevalence of hearing loss in this population should be viewed as a prevalent disease symptom and not a normal process of aging.[10] In the same manner, there is no patient too sick or too retarded to be tested. Some patients in serious medical condition present a case where hearing is not a high priority, and audiologic evaluation is only indicated if a clear benefit to the patient is expected. Audiologic evaluation and hearing aids often solve a host of problems for the patient and the rehabilitation team and should not be put off until other health goals are achieved or personal problems are resolved.

Requirements for Communication-Based Management	As discussed, audiologic evaluation may be indicated to rule out hearing loss and communication difficulties prior to embarking on a course of care or therapy requiring effective communication. These include medical care requiring history and symptom reporting, nursing care, psychologic testing and counseling, speech-language pathology, occupational and physical therapy, and social work. The patient's family often functions effectively to enhance rehabilitation, and this effort is also based on effective communication. Audiologic intervention is not needed when the patient hears normally, but the experienced clinician will not rely strictly on the patient's report nor on his or her own ability to elicit simple responses. Any report of difficulty coming from the family should be considered a more sensitive indicator.

Communication Signs and Symptoms	Difficulty in communication is not treated sympathetically.[11] Mishearing and mis-speaking are sources of derision rather than concern. If related to hearing loss, inability to communicate at high levels of competence constitutes an invisible condition that many patients will attempt to hide rather than remediate. Therefore, many symptoms of communication difficulty involve invisible adaptation, rather than visible failure or demands for intervention. Progressive social isolation is a common symptom of hearing loss.

Just as the absence of perceivable "blind spots" in the field of vision is an illusion, the typical patient will not actually perceive significant gaps or changes in tone, especially if hearing loss progresses slowly.[12] In addition, sensorineural hearing loss acts in a manner counterintuitive to most observers. Soft sounds are not heard, whereas loud sounds are perceived just as loud as if no loss were present. This phenomenon is known as recruitment.[13] This means that the patient will share some similar sound experiences with his or her normal-hearing associates. Finally, the normal-hearing person is provided by nature with much more hearing ability than is required to communicate. This redundancy acts as a buffer when the sound environment changes, and the healthy person does not notice any increase in difficulty. On the other hand, a hearing-impaired person lacks this redundancy and may communicate well in one situation and poorly in another. In general, the hearing loss may be difficult for the patient to accept based on self-perception, and those around him or her may experience wide swings in communication effectiveness with no apparent reason.

Because of the described phenomena, there are several common communication symptoms that can be useful in selecting patients for audiologic evaluation (Table 38-1). The patient may report that other people mumble and do not speak clearly as they were taught to do in the past. The patient may report that people, especially TV announcers, speak too fast for comprehension. The family may report that the patient has selective hearing or only hears when he or she wants to. In fact, there are changes in the environment that the family does not detect that greatly reduce the patient's ability to communicate. For example, a good view of the person's face will greatly increase communication. The patient may report that he or she cannot hear without glasses. This phenomenon extends to the exam room. Often, the exam room is a good face-to-face situation and communication success alone cannot be used to rule out significant hearing loss. Finally, one of the few ear-specific communication tasks in our lives is the use of the telephone, and any change in telephone ability in an ear should indicate the need for evaluation.

Table 38-1

Indications for audiologic evaluation: a brief listing of some common indications for audiologic evaluation

Communication indications
    Progressive social isolation
    Complaints that others mumble or speak too fast
    Complaints regarding television, radio, or the telephone
    Family reports of "selective hearing"
    "I can hear but I can't understand"

Medical indications
    Report of hearing loss
    Tinnitus
    Blocked sensation in ears
    Recreational or workplace noise exposure
    Hypoxic events
    Reduced kidney function
    Family history of hearing loss
    Unsteadiness/vestibular symptoms
    Ototoxic medication

Medical Signs and Symptoms   There are a large number of symptoms not strictly related to communication ability that should prompt a referral for audiologic evaluation and/or otolaryngology consult. These symptoms are exhaustively treated in other texts, and only a few are presented.[14] Tinnitus, or ringing in the ears, is a common symptom that may not impair communication, but that should prompt an audiologic evaluation. Exposure to loud steady noise, gunshots, or pressure trauma can cause hearing loss, and head trauma or temporal bone fractures should be investigated. Impaired function of other organ systems, especially the brain and kidneys, can be indicators for hearing loss. Unsteadiness, dizziness, and a host of related complaints may result from disorders of the vestibular system and also make an audiologic evaluation imperative. A history of hearing loss in parents or siblings, especially in early or midlife, may indicate a genetically transmitted mutation. A baseline hearing evaluation and regular monitoring evaluations should accompany any regimen of ototoxic medication.[15]

Follow-up Considerations   Once an audiologic evaluation is performed, it need only be repeated when there is an expectation of benefit to the patient. The validity of hearing tests does not decay over time, especially in the absence of reports of changes. On the other hand, any clear change in hearing or other related symptoms may prompt a reevaluation. For example, if the nursing staff reports a noticeable new behavior problem, the patient now wears his or her hearing aid at higher volume, or a child being followed for hearing loss has a drop in grades, hearing loss should be reevaluated. Regular retests are indicated when there is reason to suspect a progressive disease. Progressive hearing loss may be suspected because of the history of other members of the family, or because of the nature of a disease such as Meniere's disease, where a progressive loss is expected.[16]

A Special Case: Audiologic Evaluation Not Linked to Hearing Loss Per Se

Referrals for audiologic evaluation include a significant number not directly related to hearing loss, which will not be explored in this chapter. Audiologists have developed tests of neurologic function that are valuable, whether hearing loss is present or not. The best-known of these is the Auditory Evoked Response (AER) evaluation (also called ABR or BAER). This test measures far-field bio-electric potentials recorded from the scalp that arise from early brain-stem activity in response to brief auditory stimuli. This test is extraordinarily effective in detecting acoustic neuromas.[17] Similar potentials arising from higher brain regions are measured to address questions of function in those specific regions. These are known as Middle Latency Response (MLR), Late Potentials, and Contingent Negative Variation (CNV). Evaluation of the bio-electric potentials within the cochlea is known as Electrocochleography (ECoG). Audiologists also evaluate the vestibular system by measuring bio-electric potentials related to nystagmus. This evaluation is generally referred to as Electronystagmography (ENG). Electrical responses of facial function, known as Electroneuronography (ENoG), in cases of facial weakness or paralysis are also useful. When quantification of auditory processing ability is required, Central Auditory Processing (CAP) tests are useful.

HOW TO REFER AND WHAT TO EXPECT

Who to Refer to

Audiologists are the only professionals who are trained to administer, interpret, and evaluate the validity of electronic tests of hearing. Referral for evaluation should be made to certified audiologists.[18] Otolaryngologists are trained to interpret clinical hearing tests. For this reason, a common referral to an otolaryngologist can be made with the assumption that an audiologic evaluation from a certified audiologist can be expected when appropriate.

Expectations of the Referring Clinician

The referral for audiologic evaluation should be made with the assumption that the audiologist will perform the fewest tests necessary to allow a complete report on the specific medical questions, the need for hearing aids or other intervention, and the patient's general communication ability. It is generally counterproductive to ask for a specific list of tests, since this often results in more testing and less information than a flexible approach by the audiologist. On the other hand, a clear statement of the medical question is important and helpful. Should this patient have hearing aids before starting therapy? Is there a middle ear or a sensory problem, or both? Is the known hearing loss getting worse? Can this patient's communication difficulties be explained by hearing loss?

One medical prerequisite is an examination of the patient's external ear canals and removal of cerumen and debris. Audiologists have recently begun performing this task in some clinics, but if cleaning is done by the referring clinician before the arrival of the patient, the likelihood of an efficiently completed audiologic evaluation is increased.[19] Practically any patient can be tested by adjusting the technique to the difficulties imposed by age or health. It is helpful for the referring physician to provide information so that proper preparations may be made. For example, because hearing loss cannot be seen, individuals routinely attempt to obtain monetary compensation by refusing to respond honestly. Audiologists can take measures to discover the great majority of these individuals when told ahead of time that secondary gains are at stake.

Expectations of Patient Competence

The standard audiologic evaluation takes place in a specialized sound-treated room. Audiology sound booths will accommodate seated patients, wheelchairs, and stretchers (Figure 38-2). The transport status of the patient should be transmitted along with the referral to ensure that a proper-size booth is available.

The standard audiologic evaluation will take from 30 to 50 minutes, during which the patient will typically raise his or her hand or press a button to indicate detection of a low-intensity sound, and he or she will also be asked to repeat words delivered by a recording or by the audiologist's voice. The fact that a patient cannot easily accomplish these tasks should not prevent or delay referral. There are many ways in which the audiologist will adjust the evaluation technique to the abilities of the patient. If the patient has no function in his or her hands, another response will be agreed on. If the patient cannot speak, a picture-pointing task will be used to test speech intelligibility. The patient need not speak or understand the language used in speech tests. The ability to repeat sounds is at issue, not the ability to understand spoken language. Infants are evaluated using specialized conditioning and game-playing tasks.[20] Children over the age of four typically can be tested by the same means as adults. If no response is expected owing to extreme incapacitation, electrophysiologic techniques, such as ABR Threshold, are used.

A Special Case: The Bedside Evaluation

There are instances where the validity and accuracy provided by testing in a sound booth are outweighed

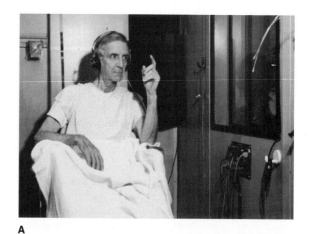

A

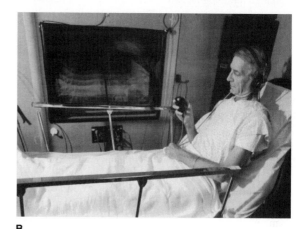

B

Figure 38-2
Patient undergoing audiologic evaluation while confined to wheelchair and stretcher.

by the need to determine gross hearing ability in a patient who cannot be transported. In such cases, a portable audiometer can be used at the bedside. Reports from such evaluations have limitations on validity, and further testing in a sound booth is often done when the patient's condition permits.

Standard audiologic evaluations involve no invasive or painful procedures, but often are dreaded because of the social stigma of hearing loss and hearing aids. During the evaluation, many patients feel as if they were on trial and may fail to perform properly. Given that the test centers on very soft stimuli that can only be detected 50 to 75 percent of the time, it is common to find that the expected uncertainties in responses worry the patient. The sound-booth environment is unusual as well. Physiologic noises and tinnitus are more easily audible without the constant noise background found in normal rooms. Certain patients will show varying degrees of aversion to an unusual enclosed space, but serious psychotic incidents related to claustrophobia are rare.

Expectations for Interpretation by the Referring Clinician

A written report containing the interpretation of the test results will be returned along with the graphical and numerical data. Issues regarding hearing loss, communication, and hearing aids can be reported definitively by the audiologist. Medical diagnoses typically require additional information, such as otoscopic results, radiologic investigation, and serology. Raw data from the audiogram must be provided, as well as a legend for symbols. If a clinician routinely refers for audiologic evaluation, learning to read the symbols is recommended.

INTERPRETATION OF THE AUDIOLOGIC EVALUATION

Evaluating the Evaluator

Audiograms may arrive in a patient's record from a number of sources. Those bearing a signature followed by "CCC-A" come from certified audiologists, and these reports adhere to national guidelines as reviewed in this chapter. Audiograms are also done by school nurses, hearing aid dealers, and medical office personnel. None of these tests should be considered, on the face of it, unlawful or improper. The assurance and validity provided by a trained audiologist are advantageous. The assumption of completeness and proper interpretation cannot be simply implied, and the clinician must be able to carefully evaluate the meaning and coherence of the results in order for them to be considered useful.

General Features of the Report

Figure 38-3 shows an example of a report returned after referral for audiologic evaluation. The information identifying the patient is found in the upper left corner. The large graph on the upper right contains threshold information for this patient and is known as the audiogram. Because this is generally the most distinctive

feature of the report, the entire evaluation and report are often referred to as the "audiogram." The center of the page contains the legend for interpretation of symbols. On the left side across from the audiogram is a graphic display of the results of word-testing versus threshold sensitivity, marked "Speech Intelligibility," and a table of numerical word test results marked "Word Recognition." The boxes on the lower left marked "Tympanometry" and "Reflex Decay" report the results of acoustic tests of the stiffness of the middle ear system. On the lower right, the boxes marked "Asymmetry" and "Air-Bone Gap" are graphic depictions of specific diagnostic features of the threshold data above. Finally, the bottom of the page is devoted to the text containing background, facts related to testing technique and validity, general impressions, and recommendations for further care. Although the aspect ratio and symbols of the audiogram itself are standardized, the overall report content and layout differ from clinic to clinic.

The Audiogram

The Technique Each vertical line on the audiogram form represents the frequency of a pure tone presented to the patient. Sounds in nature are almost always composed of many tones at once, and the patient might respond to detection of any one element of such a combination. In the cochlea, the basilar membrane acts to spread out the low and high frequency components of sound, and therefore pure tones are used to restrict the location being evaluated. Thresholds typically are found at successive octaves from the low range of a trombone (125 Hz) up through the squeak of the smallest bird (8000 Hz). Each frequency contributes to speech understanding, with the central octaves of the audiogram contributing the most-useful speech information.

A symbol is placed on the vertical line at the horizontal position corresponding to the intensity of the softest sound of that frequency that the patient can detect. The "0 dB HL" level, depicted with a double line, shows the expected human normal response. This is a case where human normal should be interpreted as the mean performance of young, healthy ears rather than as average performance across the population.[21] Louder sounds and greater hearing loss is expressed in log-ratio units (decibels or dB) of intensity, with the denominator as the human normal level. Therefore, the vertical axis units are decibels re: Hearing Threshold Level (or dB HL). More-intense sounds (and therefore

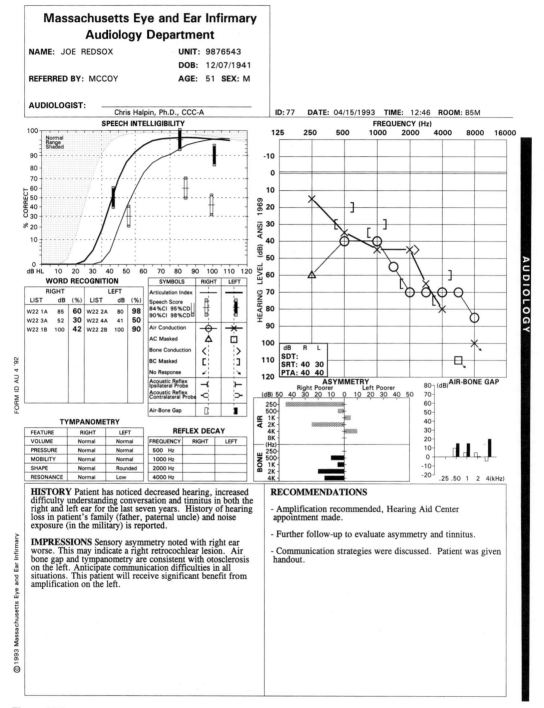

Figure 38-3
Example of a report returned after audiologic evaluation.

increasingly abnormal insensitivity) are found toward the bottom of the graph.

The audiologist will first take a brief history, then position the patient and instruct the patient to respond when the tones are detected. Headphones are placed, and as the testing begins, the audiologist establishes and evaluates the response profile of each patient. Does he or she respond as the stimulus comes on, or wait till it goes off? What is the expected latency of the response, and how does the response strengthen as the stimulus exceeds threshold? Does this patient give false responses, and how often? What sort of instruction or encouragement, if any, will enhance the speed and accuracy of this test? With a model of the patient's response characteristics in mind, the audiologist proceeds to find threshold, using 5-dB steps, for each tone by both air conduction (through headphones) and bone conduction (a bone vibrator on the skull). As each threshold is found, the symbol indicating the ear and the test method is placed on the audiogram.[22] As results accumulate, lines are drawn between the air-conduction symbols.

Figure 38-4 shows the legend for interpretation of standard audiogram symbols. There is a separate symbol for each presentation method for each ear. Note that the air-conduction (headphone) symbols are plotted directly on the vertical line, whereas the bone-conducted stimuli associated with the same frequency are plotted to the side. Paradoxically, the right bone conduction result appears on the left side of the line, and the left appears on the right side. This placement reflects the practice of facing the patient through the sound booth window such that the sides are reversed. The symbols marked "Masked" indicate that noise was presented to the ear not being tested in order to guarantee that the response arose from the test ear. The small arrow may be found attached to any one of the threshold symbols (in the case in Figure 38-3, left air results at 6 and 8 KHz). This indicates that the patient did not respond when presented with that sound level and that no further testing could be done, usually because the maximum output limit of the audiometer had been reached. In audiograms presented in color, the right ear results appear in red, and the left ear results appear in blue.[23]

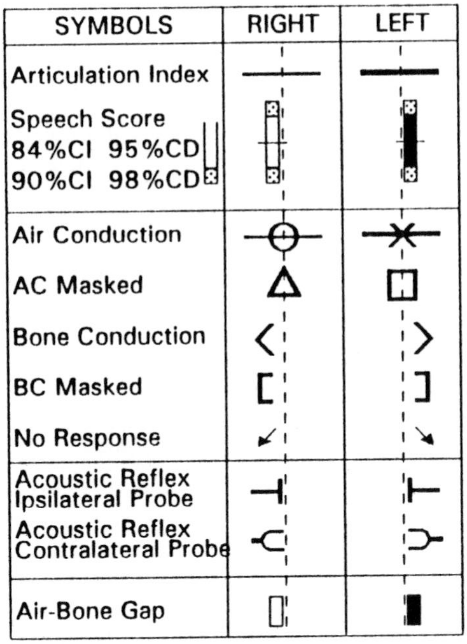

Validity of Audiogram Results The equipment used during routine audiometric evaluation includes standard headphones fitting over or into the patient's ear canals, a standard bone vibrator held in place on the mastoid bone by means of a headband, and loudspeakers. Each

Figure 38-4

Legend for audiologic symbols. The top panel refers to the speech intelligibility graph on the top left of Figure 38-2. CI refers to Confidence Interval for evaluating the variability of the percent correct score itself (hatched: p < .10). CD refers to Critical Difference (solid: p < .05) between two scores. The next panel contains the standard audiometric threshold symbols. The addition of the small arrow to any symbol indicates that no response was obtained at the intensity indicated, and that no higher intensity could be tested. The next panel contains the standard symbols for the threshold of the acoustic reflex.

of the transducers is calibrated to physical standards set by the American National Standards Institute (ANSI).[24] Simply put, the meters used to measure the loudness of each tone are themselves calibrated by a physical device (known as a piston phone) that has been certified as accurate (within 0.1 dB) compared to a national standard device. Electronic calibrations are performed quarterly, or whenever a new device is installed. National audiology practice guidelines limit the tolerance for calibration to 2.5 dB, which is half the smallest step size of the test. The result is that physical variability of the machines is smaller than the psychophysical variability of the normal patient, which has been shown to be approximately one (5-dB) step size.

The technique for arriving at the patient's threshold for each tone is standardized.[25] The patient must make at least two responses on an ascending run (getting louder) before the response is reported. It is important to note that the audiologist will quickly achieve stimulus control of the patient's response so that the patient is responding in a conditioned fashion and not making conscious decisions as to whether to respond or not. The typical, well-meaning patient will find it hard to separate extremely soft sounds from his or her own imagination. Audiologists learn to present tones without establishing a rhythm of presentation so that the patient cannot appear to be hearing by responding at a regular interval.

The validity of hearing-test results depends on certainty as to which ear is the source of the response. During a test, a stimulus can be intense enough to be heard by the other ear. To counteract this possibility, masking noise is presented to the nontest ear to prevent that ear from allowing the patient to respond. Unmasked bone-conducted stimuli stimulate both cochleae approximately equally, and so masking is required in every case where the right and left results could differ. Air-conducted stimuli must be more intense, and large difference between ears (>40 dB) must be present before invalid responses are suspected.[26] Figure 38-5 shows a matrix involving two cases that were not complete until masking was applied. In Panel 1, the unmasked bone symbols on the right could have arisen from stimulation of either (or both) cochleae, and so the testing is considered incomplete. Panel 2 shows that by adding masking, the right cochlea is shown to be the more sensitive ear responding, and the left will not respond on its own until higher levels are reached. In the second case, there is a large difference between the air-conducted stimuli between ears. This may be the true left ear sensitivity, or it may be the right ear responding, and so testing is not complete. In the next panel, masking has been applied and reveals a completely dead ear on the left side.

Interpretation of the Audiogram   *Normal Results*
Hearing thresholds of 20 dB HL or better are considered to be within normal limits. These limits work very well for most clinical judgments. On the other hand, Figure 38-6 shows an example of a case in which all thresholds in both ears are better than or equal to 20 dB HL. Despite this fact, there are significant sensorineural differences between ears, and a clinically significant air-bone gap in the low frequencies on the left side.

Results with No Hearing   Figure 38-7 shows typical results and rationale for the audiogram configura-

tion when no hearing is present (in this case, on the right side). Notice that repeatable thresholds are found and reported for high-intensity, low-frequency sound stimuli. This is due to vibrotactile stimulation of the patient and will be noted as such by the audiologist. At 500 Hz., there may appear to be a large air-bone gap. These findings actually reflect the different vibrotactile sensitivity, with the skin more responsive to bone conduction than air conduction. Note that the upper limits of bone conduction are reached at audiometric levels much lower than air conduction. A matrix of cases is presented in Figure 38-8 to provide a simplified rationale for interpretation of the audiogram by site of lesion. A case with normal function in both the middle ear and the cochlea appears as Panel 1.

Middle Ear Effects   Middle ear deficits may be present separately, or in conjunction with cochlear deficits. Effects of dysfunction of the middle ear can be seen in Panels 2 and 4. In Panel 2, the right cochlea is normal, since all bone-conducted stimuli are within the normal range. There is a large air-bone gap that is due to the reduction of the efficiency of the air pathway in the transmission of sound. This particular case is one characteristic of otosclerosis, but similar effects are seen in otitis media and Q-tip trauma. In Panel 4, the right middle ear deficit still appears as an air-bone gap even though, in this case, there is also a cochlear loss that has reduced the bone-conduction results to abnormal levels. The information revealed concerning the middle ear is essentially the same in both cases.

Cochlear Effects   Panel 3 shows a case where the middle ear is normal (e.g., there is no air-bone gap), but sensitivity falls below normal levels. This is interpreted as a deficit of the cochlea. Here, sound is carried properly into the cochlea, but the organ is insensitive. This may be seen, for example, in cases of ototoxicity or Meniere's disease. Panel 4 shows the same bone-conduction results as Panel 3. These two cases, then, have the same amount of cochlear deficit. In addition, Panel 4 shows poor function by the middle ear in transmitting the sound. The patient hears using air conduction in daily life, and so complaints by patients two and three may be similar, whereas those of patient four will be worse.

A Special Case: Auditory Evoked Response Thresholds

As mentioned in the preceding, there are a number of adaptations that can be made to achieve test results

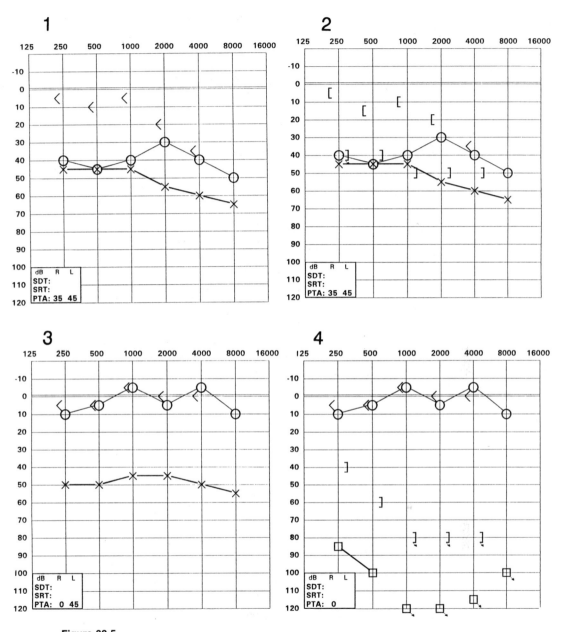

Figure 38-5

Masking. Panels 1 and 2 represent a single case. In Panel 1 unmasked bone and air-conduction scores are shown. Panel 2 shows the completed evaluation after performing masked bone-conduction testing on both sides. A clear air-bone gap on the right is shown. The right side is also revealed as the source of the original unmasked thresholds. The left side is shown to have a sensorineural loss. Panels 3 and 4 also represent a single case. Panel 3 shows initial unmasked air and bone results. The left air results could arise from crossover hearing on the right, and the left bone sensitivity remains unknown. Panel 4 shows the result after masking is applied during left air and bone conduction.

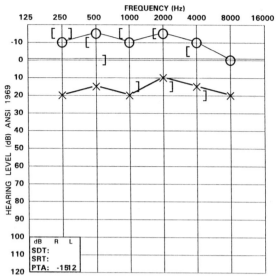

Figure 38-6

All thresholds within normal limits (20 dB HL). Nonetheless, there are both significant air-bone gaps and sensory asymmetries.

in young or disabled patients. Certain patients cannot perform any behavioral task that allows threshold information to be gathered reliably. Under these circumstances, audiologists use the presence of the auditory brain stem evoked potentials as the measurable response. Once this response is established, it can be used to evaluate the same parameters as those of a standard audiogram. Stimuli are delivered by both air and bone conduction, and masking is applied by the same principles. The test does require stimuli that are much more brief than the behavioral pure tone counterpart. Care must be taken to use sophisticated methods for turning the stimulus on and off (the "window" or "envelope") in order to assure that the tone energy is still restricted to the area of the test frequency. The response is hidden in the ongoing bioelectric noise of the brain, and the patient must remain very quiet (asleep if possible) throughout the evaluation. This may require an order for mild sedation from the referring physician.[27]

Speech Intelligibility Tests

The Technique Examination of most patients' complaint of hearing loss will show that they actually detect most words, but cannot recognize them. The ability to recognize words depends on the ability to resolve complex time-varying signals. Very small differences in the fine structure of sound intensity, frequency, and timing separate one speech sound from another. Many mechanisms in the cochlea must work together in order to recognize these small acoustic changes. The decreased sensitivity shown on the audiogram does not correlate tightly with the ability to recognize speech, and so speech intelligibility must be evaluated by focusing on the selectivity, rather than the sensitivity, of the cochlea. In order to achieve this, the patient is asked to repeat words presented at a level loud enough that they should achieve maximum performance (sometimes known as PB-MAX).[28] The cochlea is given every chance to succeed at the word task, and so deficits reducing the quality of the information of speech can be seen. The upper limit of possible performance given the audiogram may be predicted across intensity from a formula known as the Articulation Index (AI).[29] The panels in Figure 38-9 show such predictions for a patient's right ear. The AI has been used to plot the best predicted percent correct/intensity curve in the boxes marked "Speech Intelligibility." When speech is presented at a level on the asymptote of the curve, maximum scores are predicted. Also, it is useful in some cases to evaluate word recognition abilities at lower levels. For example, a model of hearing aid performance may be made by using speech tests at low levels.[30]

In the typical speech intelligibility test, the patient is instructed that he or she will hear a carrier phrase (e.g., "You will say . . .") before each item to prepare him or her to respond. Then the patient is asked to repeat the item (the last word of the phrase) and to guess if he or she is not sure. The standard words are 50-item lists of monosyllables. The lists are considered equally difficult and are used interchangeably. The audiologist records the patient's response as correct or incorrect and reports the results as a percent correct for each ear.[31]

Validity of Speech Intelligibility Results Speech varies rapidly between different frequencies and intensities, and its intensity cannot be modeled as simply as the steady pure tone. The intensity of audiometric speech tests is monitored by use of a standardized V.U. (volume unit) meter that is kept in view by the audiologist throughout the test. Before recorded materials were common, the audiologist used his or her own voice, being careful to peak the speech energy at the "0" line of the V.U. meter. This is known as monitored live

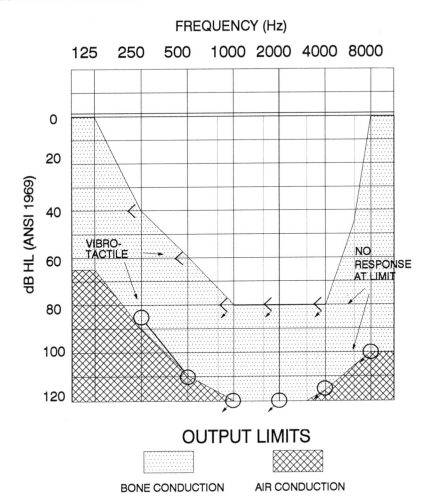

Figure 38-7

Expected results with no hearing. The different output limits for air- and bone-conduction devices appear as shaded areas. When these limits are reached, an arrow is added to the audiometric symbol. Typical response levels for low-frequency vibrotactile thresholds are shown using audiometric symbols. Differences arising from vibrotactile phenomena or output limits should not be interpreted as air-bone gaps.

voice testing (MLV). Recorded materials come with an intensity-reference steady pure tone used to set the intensity to 0 V.U. Once set, the materials will remain at the standard level.[32] Monitored live voice methods may be employed by audiologists whose patients cannot keep up with the recording. Recorded results are more valid, less variable, and more easily comparable to other tests. The application of CD-ROM technology allows both flexibility and validity in advanced audiometers.[33]

Patients routinely get 100 percent correct on word tests without knowing the language and vocabulary from which the words are drawn. The only requirement is to repeat the sound accurately. Articulation errors made by the patient may not imply impaired hearing, but may make scoring more difficult. In such cases, a picture-pointing task may be used to resolve exactly which word

the patient perceived.[34] Such tasks use a set of picture items, and so the probability of guessing correctly must be factored in. It is practically impossible to guess correctly in the standard word-list method.

Interpretation of word recognition results also depends on the ability to specify when differences between scores actually are significant, or when they merely reflect the inherent variability of the test itself. Although the variability of pure tone results reflects the psychophysical variability in patient responses, the most important sources of variability in speech intelligibility testing are the test parameters: the number of items, the type of response, and the range in which the score is found. Since the audiologist scores in binary fashion (correct vs. incorrect), the test results are best interpreted as being binomially distributed.[35] The variability of

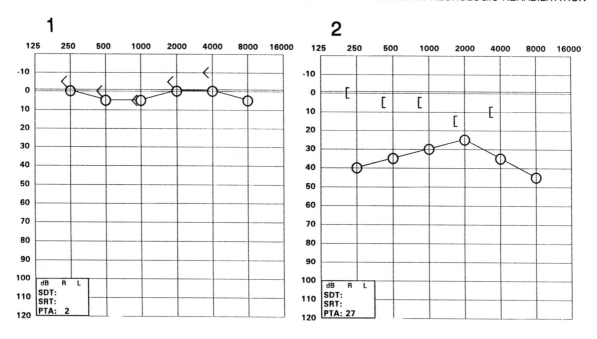

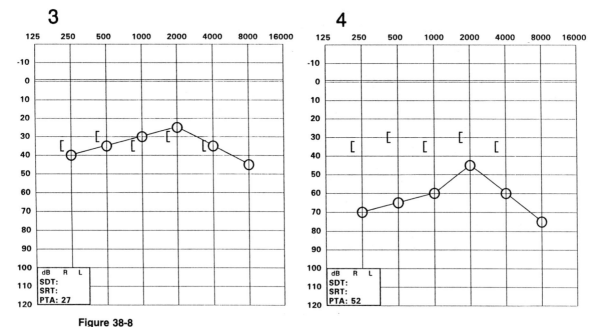

Figure 38-8

Middle ear versus cochlear effects. Panel 1 shows a normal audiogram. Panel 2 shows middle ear effects only. The cochlear sensitivity is normal as shown by the bone thresholds, whereas the air conduction is reduced by dysfunction of the middle ear. Panel 3 shows sensorineural (cochlear) effects only. The bone conduction is reduced, but there is no additional reduction of air conduction that would indicate a middle ear problem. Panel 4 shows both effects.

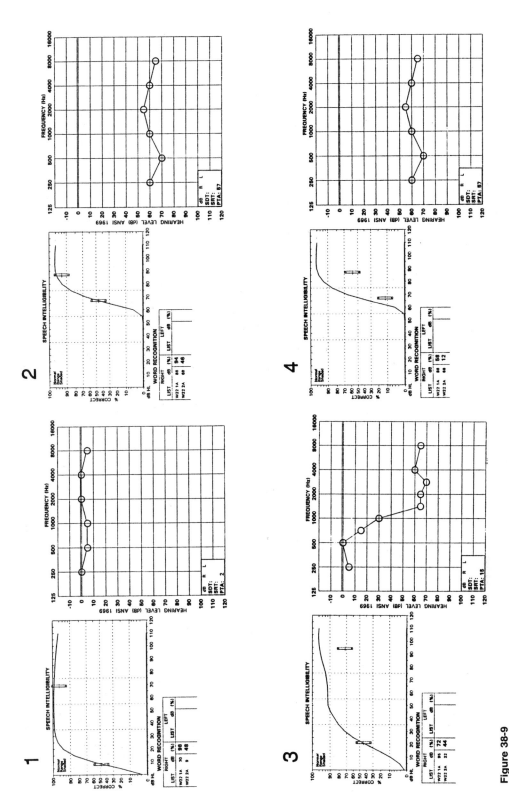

Figure 38-9

Speech intelligibility. Panel 1 shows normal audiogram and speech intelligibility results. The speech intelligibility graph appears on the left. The horizontal axis is intensity of sound. The vertical axis is percent correct. The curves are the predicted percent correct performance given the audiogram. The bars are the measured scores for this patient. (The center of the bar is the score, the extent of the bar is the 95 percent confidence interval.) Panel 2 shows a case where hearing loss has shifted the audible speech range, but scores remain good. Panel 3 shows a case where speech scores do not grow as predicted. Although the low level test shows good agreement, the optimal level test (PB-MAX) does not. Panel 4 shows a case where a deficit is seen at both low and high levels.

such a test decreases with the number of items presented. The standard tests were designed as 50-item lists, but both 50- and 25-item tests are used commonly. Another feature of binomial distributions is that of score variability: the center of the range (50 percent) is greater than that at either extreme. The determination of significant difference between scores is dependent on these factors. The vertical axes of the graphs marked "Speech Intelligibility" in Figure 38-9 reflect the transformation of percent scores to keep variability (shown by the extent of the speech score bars) constant. On these graphs, if the solid portions of the score bars do not overlap, the scores are significantly different at the ($p <$ .05) level.

Interpretation of Speech Intelligibility Results   The normal and expected value of word-recognition tests is 100 percent, as long as the speech can be made loud enough for the patient. Any score significantly less than this indicates some reduction in the quality of information imposed by a disease process in the cochlea; that is, even though sufficient information was made available by presenting the words loudly enough, the cochlea was only able to use some part of the information to recognize words. This might be owing to depopulation of the sensory elements (i.e., hair cells), leaving enough cells to allow simple detection, but not for the more difficult task of recognition.[36]

Figure 38-9 shows a matrix providing a simplified rationale for interpretation of word-recognition results. Panel 1 shows the normal case, in which speech is presented at maximum performance level and the patient scored 98 percent correct, which is not significantly less than the normally predicted 100 percent. An additional test was done at a very soft level (9 dBHL), where performance was predicted to drop to 50 percent. The patient performed as expected at this level as well. Panel 2 shows a severe hearing loss on the right that has not reduced the patient's word-recognition ability. The loudness of presentation is much higher than in the normal case, but once these levels are achieved, the patient's cochlea is able to process the speech as expected. In Panel 3, speech was tested at a low level (22 dB HL), where only the low-frequency regions of the ear were sensitive enough to hear it. The patient performed as expected at this low level. At a higher level, where performance should rise to 100 percent, the score is significantly less (72 percent). This asymptotic pattern may reflect the inability of the more damaged high-frequency cochlear regions to add information, even when it is loud enough to detect. Panel 4 shows the

same audiogram as Panel 2. In this case, the cochlear (or higher) disease process imposes a fairly constant deficit, causing the patient to fail to achieve predicted performance at both low and high intensities.

Functional Tests for Fictitious Hearing Loss

The Techniques   Patients wishing to exaggerate their hearing loss generally believe that it is possible to simply refuse to respond at low intensity levels. Audiologists are familiar with this attempt and have developed a series of countermeasures, generally known as functional testing. The most sensitive of these involves recognizing the unusual nature of the response pattern of the patient. If responses are slow and variable and the pattern of the loss reflects loudness curves rather than common diseases, malingering (pseudohypoacusis) is suspected. The patient is then reinstructed and/or confronted, and in most cases the true levels are found. For the more challenging cases where secondary gain is suspected, special tests based on psychophysical or electrophysiological phenomena are necessary.

Speech Reception Threshold (SRT)   The ability to maintain hearing loss exaggeration while repeating words is difficult, and patient's threshold for two-syllable words (known as spondees) may show sensitivity below that admitted for tones.

The Stenger Test   Sounds arriving at both ears simultaneously will appear to have originated exclusively on the side where the sound is louder. This phenomenon can be used to challenge a claim of unilateral hearing loss, since a response in the good ear will suddenly stop when the stimulus becomes louder in the (purportedly) bad ear, even when the original stimulus is not changed.

Auditory Brain-Stem Response Thresholds   When all else fails, thresholds can be evaluated without a behavioral response from the patient using the ABR. This is an expensive test, and the nervous faker will often present very noisy data and make the evaluation difficult. Even without actually performing ABR, the nature of this technique provides a very effective talking point that may be used to help resolve the situation.

Validity of Functional Test Results   It is very difficult for even the practiced listener to misrepresent hearing loss if the audiologist is alerted to this possibility.

The psychophysical bases of the Stenger and SRT tests are inescapable by all except the most sophisticated listeners.[37] In some cases, it is possible that statements of believability coming from the referral source, or from previous tests, may reduce the likelihood that functional testing need be applied.

Interpretation of Functional Test Results   The results of functional tests most often will be reported in the text of the report. General impressions of hearing loss exaggeration may be referred to as a "functional overlay." The report of SRT results inconsistent with tone thresholds is a functional finding. The Stenger test is reported positive when the patient is exaggerating. The method(s) used to find the true results usually are given. If credible results are not achieved, recommendations for additional testing (such as ABR) will be given. Not all cases of pseudohypoacusis are related to compensation. Patients, notably adolescents, will be using the process to indirectly express what are sometimes quite-serious psychological problems. Extreme detach-

ment from external stimuli is seen in psychotic patients and also may be the source of pseudohypoacusis.

Tympanometry

The Technique   These tests are very different from those discussed up to this point in that these do not evaluate auditory perception. Tympanometry and other tests of acoustic immittance (also known as impedance or admittance testing) are direct measures of the physical properties of the middle ear. Figure 38-10 shows a schematic diagram of the basic technique. A probe is inserted at the entrance of the external auditory canal. This probe contains a sound source, a microphone, and a pressure manometer. The sound source emits a tone, and the microphone measures the amount of sound pressure that is present after the middle ear absorbs (admits) as much as possible. If the middle ear does not admit sound easily, the microphone will detect a higher sound pressure. The pressure manometer is used to change the ear from its normal state to one that is less

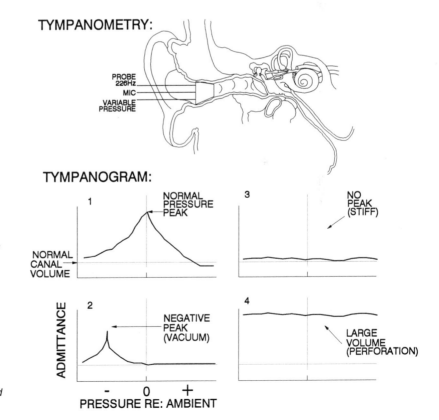

Figure 38-10
Tympanometry. The top panel is a diagram of the test probe as placed in the ear. The center panel shows four possible results. Case 1 shows normal results. Case 2 shows normal volume, but maximal admittance at a negative pressure. Case 3 shows normal volume but a stiff ear at all pressures. Case 4 shows an abnormally large, stiff ear space indicating a perforated tympanic membrane.

compliant by adding a small amount of air pressure until the tympanic membrane is tight. The pressure is then swept from the positive-tight condition to the corresponding negative-tight condition, passing through room ambient pressure (0 mm/H_2O) on the way. The admittance of the middle ear should be low when the ear is tight, and maximal at ambient pressure. In normal ears, this gives rise to results as shown in Figure 38-10 in the panel marked 1.[38]

Validity of Tympanometry Results The validity of tympanometry is assured by regular (typically quarterly) electronic calibration of the probe, microphone, and pressure manometer versus nationally established standards.[39] In addition, most units are supplied with a series of cavities of known size and admittance. Accuracy should be checked daily by the audiologist in the clinic. During the test, the change in pressure assumes that the audiologist can achieve an air-tight seal at the entrance of the ear canal, something achieved with great difficulty, for example, in active young children.

Interpretation of Tympanometry Results A matrix for simplified interpretation of the tympanogram is shown in the panel in the center of Figure 38-10. A normal tympanogram is diagramed in Panel 1. A normal result will have the characteristic peaked shape, with the peak near 0 for ambient air pressure. When the peak is found at a lower pressure, as in Panel 2, it is a sign that there is a vacuum in the middle ear, a common finding in cases of otitis media. When there is no peak, as in Panel 3, the ear does not admit sound normally at any pressure. This finding is often associated with an ear full of serous fluid. The baseline measurement of the ear stiffened by pressure is directly related to its size (volume). In Panels 1, 2, and 3 the test reveals a normal-size ear, even though other aspects are abnormal. In Panel 4, the test shows a stiff system that is larger than normal, indicating a perforated tympanic membrane. The results of tympanometry are found on the example report in Figure 38-3, in emphasizing the significant features of the tympanogram. A variety of classification schemes for organizing tympanographic data are now in use across the country.[40]

Otoacoustic Emissions

The Technique Otoacoustic emissions are very soft sounds produced in the cochleae of healthy ears in order to amplify sounds at the extreme low range of intensity.[41]

These sounds can be measured in the clinic in the course of an audiologic evaluation, using an instrument diagramed in Figure 38-11. Two sound sources are used to elicit a third sound (known as the distortion product) that arises from their interaction. This sound is detected by a microphone in the probe assembly, and the results are known as the distortion-product otoacoustic emission (DPOAE). The same sounds created by the ear in response to click stimuli are also measured in the same way and are known as transient evoked otoacoustic emissions (TEOAE).

Validity of OAE Results The OAE is a sound resulting from the movement of tiny structures within the cochlea. As a result, the level of other noise detected by the microphone must be small enough so that the presence of the response is clear. Commercial OAE units provide graphical indicators as to the level of noise that may render the results invalid. Distortion products are pervasive acoustic phenomena that do not require living tissue to be present. The validity of the OAE hinges on the assurance that the level of the response measured must have been amplified by the cochlea and exceeds that which would be present by acoustic interaction alone.

Interpretation of OAE Results Figure 38-11 shows a diagram of the results of a DPOAE test. Both the response at the test frequencies and the level of the noise floor are presented to show that the amplitude of the response is distinct from the noise. If the noise floor is low enough to allow an accurate measurement and the response is close to the level of the noise, as is the case at 4000 Hz, the OAE is judged to be absent at that frequency. The strength of otoacoustic emissions has little clinical significance because of the large variability of normal subjects relative to the full range of observed amplitudes. The response is present only in healthy ears and is not seen with even a mild (>30 dB HL) hearing loss.[42]

Conductive Hearing Loss Conductive hearing losses reflect a physical blockage or discontinuity in the anatomy of the outer and middle ear. Such patients should be referred to otolaryngologists in order to establish a diagnosis of the cause of the loss. For example, a patient with a small conductive hearing loss may not feel his or her hearing is a problem but, if the cause is an infection, failure to treat could have serious adverse consequences.[43] Conductive hearing loss does not imply any loss of function in the cochlea, and these patients

OTOACOUSTIC EMISSIONS

DISTORTION PRODUCT MEASUREMENT

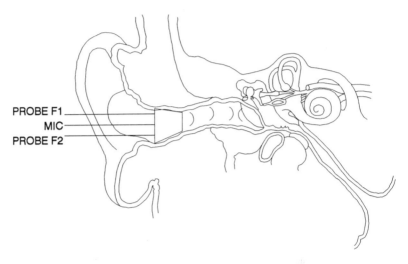

DISTORTION PRODUCT RESULTS

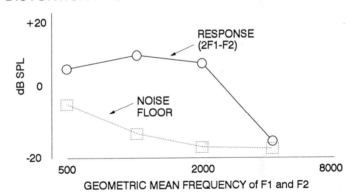

Figure 38-11
Distortion product otoacoustic emissions. The top panel shows a diagram of the probe as placed in the ear. The bottom panel shows results. The amplitude of the response at each frequency is significantly greater than the noise floor, and so the DPOAE is judged to be present.

respond very well to hearing aids because louder sound is all they need to regain function. On the other hand, conductive hearing loss may be remediable by surgery, and many patients prefer this approach if both options are available.

Sensorineural Hearing Loss Sensorineural hearing loss usually is due to reduced sensitivity of the cochlea (and in rare cases, higher structures). This sort of loss generally is not remediable. However, some progressive sensorineural hearing losses related to autoim-

mune disease may be improved by the use of steroid medication, and sensorineural losses due to cochlear fistulae may be improved by surgery.[44] Regardless, of course, most patients with sensorineural loss lose their ability to hear soft sounds, without a corresponding reduction in the perceived loudness of more-intense sounds (recruitment). Communication difficulties and misunderstandings during simple conversation are common. Since there is usually no management option except hearing aids, referral to an audiologist for evaluation and fitting of a hearing aid is essential.

Reduced Speech Intelligibility Deficits in speech intelligibility can limit the quality of information passing through the cochlea and higher centers, even when sufficient volume is attained. Speech intelligibility results may be characterized by standard nomenclature, but the referring clinician should bear in mind the basic expectation of 100 percent correct responses at the optimal test intensity.[45] When describing hearing loss, most patients focus on difficulty understanding speech or discriminating language from ambient noise.

Asymmetry in Hearing The audiologist should evaluate the significance of asymmetry in hearing. A sensorineural asymmetry in either tone sensitivity or speech intelligibility (or both) can be a sign of acoustic neuroma, and should be evaluated by an otolaryngologist.[46] Patients with side-to-side variability in hearing threshold also have difficulty discerning the origin or direction of sounds, since binaural hearing is required for this ability.[47]

Changes in Hearing If a previous evaluation is available, comparison of previous results is essential in order to determine whether hearing has significantly changed. When hearing deteriorates, a search for potentially ototoxic medication is mandatory in order to prevent further damage. Absent an identifiable and treatable medical cause, a simple adjustment in hearing aids may be all that is needed.

MECHANICAL CONSIDERATIONS FOR HEARING AIDS

How Hearing Aids Work

Figure 38-12 shows a simple diagram of a hearing aid. Sound waves in the air move the diaphragm of the microphone within an electrostatic field, producing electric current fluctuations analogous to sound. The next, or input stage, is used by circuit designers to condition the sound before amplification. For example, the dynamic range from soft to loud may be altered at this stage. This is known as input compression. The input stage may analyze the sound to determine its further processing. For example, a popular amplifier circuit acts primarily on soft sounds and not on loud sounds.[48] The input stage determines the loudness of the sound in order to guide this process. The intermediate stage may contain tone controls (filters). These controls may be set either by manual tone controls on the hearing aid

or, in programmable hearing aids, by computer commands.[49] The output stage contains the final amplifier, which increases the amplitude of the electric waves. The amplifier may be adjusted to reduce the ceiling of its power capacity (peak clipping), or to produce less output when sound is loud (output compression). Finally, in the reverse of the microphone mechanism, the amplified electric waves cause an electromagnetic field to fluctuate, which moves a diaphragm in a unit called the receiver. The air is pushed in the same pattern as the incoming sound, but with more force, resulting in a louder output to the ear.

The nature of sound processing by the hearing aid is dynamic, shifting constantly with the input sound, the control settings, and the placement in the ear canal. This is a very important point to remember when evaluating patient and staff reactions to the introduction of such an instrument. Most patients and staff assume that a proper hearing aid will act as a completely stable reliable solution to communication difficulties. A small, but constant, amount of attention is required to keep a hearing aid working optimally in a changing environment.

When sound escapes from the receiver and is picked up by the microphone, the result is a high-pitched squeal known as feedback. This phenomenon may be reported as "static" or "noise," and may lead some patients to believe that the hearing aid is malfunctioning. In fact, this is an inevitable result of any such circuit. Feedback may also result from the presence of a surface, such as a hand or a pillow, which is reflecting sound into the microphone. Patient and staff must learn to manage feedback and restore function, rather than discontinue the use of the hearing aid.

Maintenance is also required routinely to keep the prosthesis in working order. The hearing aid uses a small battery (1.5 V) and typically will exhaust a new battery in 10 days of daylong use. Hearing aids are exposed to dirt, moisture, and cerumen and require cleaning. Small parts, such as plastic tubing, will lose compliance or split after a year or two, and will require replacement. Finally, the typical hearing aid has a life expectancy of 5 years in normal use. Hearing aids may require physical and electronic repair but, as with any mechanical device, this will begin to be required sufficiently often at 5 years to necessitate a replacement.

How Well Do Hearing Aids Work?

Even though hearing aids produce excellent sound quality, patient acceptance can be low. Although hearing

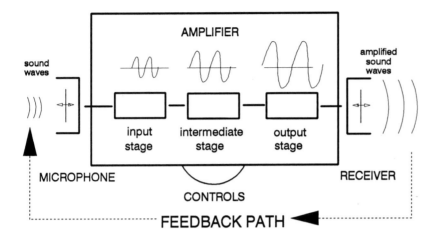

Figure 38-12
Diagram of a hearing aid. Note the unwanted feedback path from the receiver output back to the input microphone. Sound must be prevented from following this path by establishing a tight acoustic seal in the ear, and by removing reflective surfaces from the microphone area.

aids are very small, they produce sound within the quality range of expensive stereo units. Hearing aids have reached a mature and innovative level of engineering technology that has successfully balanced size, output, and power-consumption requirements. The limiting factor frequently is not the hearing aid, but the damaged auditory processing pathway of the patient.[50] Hearing aids amplify sound, but do not improve clarity, leading to poor acceptance.[51]

Indications for Hearing Aids

Hearing loss per se is not a stand-alone indication for the use of a hearing aid. The expectation of benefit by increasing loudness is the fundamental clinical indication. Figure 38-13 represents an array of audiometric problems and solutions. Panel 1 shows the straightforward case. This patient has a significant sensorineural hearing loss and does not hear normal speech unless it is amplified by the hearing aid. Speech intelligibility scores are consistent with those predicted by the AI performance curves. At midlevels (70 dB HL), where very loud speech is just audible, the patient scores about 50 percent, the highest possible score given the level of auditory stimulus presented. When the sound stimulus is increased to 100 dB HL, the patient's performance rises to about 90 percent correct. Under these circumstances, only acoustic amplification is required to improve functional performance. Sensitivity is reduced, but enough neural elements remain to form an audible acoustic signal.[52] The hearing aid must be set so that the performance curve is shifted

to the left, to bring the high performance range, now in the 80 to 90 dB HL range, closer to that of normal speech (50–60 dB HL).

By contrast, Panel 2 shows the same left ear audiogram, with a normal ear on the right side. Note that the greater difference in sensitivity required masking, making the symbols, therefore, different. Since the normal ear perceives sounds at normal levels, acoustical amplitude need not be increased. In this case, the audiologist should not recommend a hearing aid, even though there is a clear hearing loss on the left side.

Panel 3 shows another application of this same principle in the case of a binaural hearing loss with two very different speech intelligibility results. In this case, the patient has the same thresholds and speech intelligibility on the right side as in Panel 1. The speech intelligibility on the left is much worse, indicating little growth in word recognition with increased loudness. In this case, unlike Panel 2, the audiologist will definitely recommend a hearing aid, but will likely fit the right ear only in order to make use of the better speech intelligibility on that side. Finally, in Panel 4, there is poor speech intelligibility on both sides. Here the recommendation would be to apply two hearing aids in order to maximize the much more limited (but equal) benefits from both ears. This very simple matrix does not encompass all of the audiometric possibilities, but it does serve to indicate a portion of the complexity of decisions involved in recommending hearing aids. To further complicate matters, a wide range of technical, environmental, and personal issues must be balanced in each case to arrive at a sensible recommendation.[53]

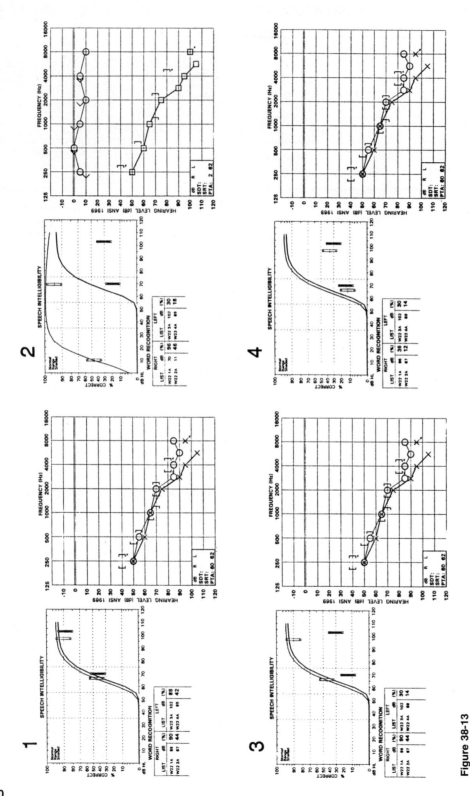

Figure 38-13

Four cases showing different hearing aid recommendations. Case 1 shows a straightforward case where sensitivity is reduced below normal, and the speech intelligibility results show improvement of scores with louder sound. Recommendation: two hearing aids. Case 2 shows one good ear. Recommendation: no hearing aid. Case 3 shows equal threshold sensitivity with one ear much better for speech. Recommendation: hearing aid on the right. Case four shows both ears with equal threshold and speech deficits. Recommendation: two hearing aids. This collection of cases does not represent all possibilities.

Expectations for Benefit

The most significant tangible benefit from a hearing aid is improvement in communication. Reports of family and caregivers are as important as those of the patient. Effort in communication must be reduced. Behaviors that suggest communication breakdown may indicate that the hearing aid is broken or the battery dead, or a deterioration in hearing.

Expectations Regarding Size Preference

All professionals encountering patients who depend on hearing aids should expect considerable pressure to use smaller in-the-ear (ITE) units.[54] Many patients will relate that they hear better with the smaller units, when they in fact, on objective testing, do not.

Larger (BTE and pocket) units have many acoustic and electronic advantages over smaller (ITE) units. The ITE units generally have less power output, and may be inadequate for severe hearing losses. The BTE unit, with its microphone at the top of the ear, has a much longer feedback path and generally is less susceptible to this particularly annoying problem. Larger BTE units also have broader low-frequency responses, which may be essential in some cases. If more high-frequency responses are needed, this can be accomplished best with the BTE unit by acoustically venting the earmold. Although ITE units can be vented, they will feed back more easily as a result. The ITE unit receiver is positioned in the ear canal, whereas the receiver of the BTE is behind the ear, safe from cerumen buildup. BTE units are superior by design, but there are cases of moderate loss where an ITE unit may be applied successfully.

Unwanted Sounds

The clinician should not be surprised to get reports of unwanted sound for two reasons. Some patients have slowly grown used to small amounts of sound, and may require time to adjust to normal amounts of sound input. Second, the tolerable range of loudness may be restricted in the damaged ear. Most patients requiring hearing aids have sensorineural hearing loss and experience abnormal recruitment, in which they perceive loud sounds as loudly as normal listeners. A basic hearing aid will make soft sounds louder and normal ambient noise louder as well. The audiologist should attempt to make the soft sounds louder without making the normal sounds too loud. Several electronic approaches are used to protect the patient from sounds at unwanted levels.[55]

Another category of unwanted sounds will be seen in patient reports of increased background, or competing, noises when the hearing aid is used. The most debilitating environmental factor for damaged ears is the presence of competing noise in amounts sufficient to reduce speech intelligibility.[56] The mathematical relation of wanted to unwanted input is known as the signal-to-noise ratio. The ability to separate signal from noise depends on two basic factors: the knowledge of the characteristics of both the signal and the noise, and the ability to integrate the results of a large number of receptors working independently to analyze the complex input. There is no way that the hearing aid circuit can determine which one of many voices the patient wishes to hear at a given moment. The hearing aid will not change the signal-to-noise ratio, especially when both signal and noise are voices and are therefore similar in character.

Hearing aids will make both signal and noise louder, and so the perception of the user may be that a significant amount of background competition (fans, footsteps, distant voices) are now a problem, where these sounds were inaudible before. Although there may be a net gain to the patient in terms of audibility of wanted sounds, most patients are very sensitive to the destructive effect of noise and will view any increase in background noise as unwanted, even if the signal-to-noise ratio is not actually changed.

Expectations for Hearing Aid Feedback

Clinicians caring for a patient with hearing aids should expect feedback from time to time. Properly working hearing aids will emit feedback if they are turned up in the open air. Hearing aid design assumes that the amplified sound is isolated in the ear canal, sealed away from the microphone. If the hearing aid is not firmly seated in the ear or if there is a hole in the tubing allowing sound to escape, feedback will result. Practically all hearing aids will feed back if a cupped hand is placed over the unit, reflecting amplified sound into the microphone port. Unfortunately, this situation is not very different from placing the hand on the hearing aid to adjust volume, and a patient may struggle to adjust the hearing aid to reduce feedback without evaluating the result with his or her hands down. When the hearing aid feeds back with the hands down, there is a true problem requiring adjustment. It is important to distinguish whether the upper limit of the hearing aid output is the point of feedback or the point where the patient feels it is loud enough. The optimal situation is the latter, where the patient can turn the hearing aid up to a level that is sufficiently loud. Hearing aids are not designed to be limited by feedback, and if this is the case with a patient, the hearing aid requires adjustment or replacement.

A Special Case: Assistive Listening Devices (ALDs)

Assistive listening devices (ALDs) are a class of devices designed for very specific uses. Figure 38-14 shows a patient making use of a device that allows him or her to place a microphone very close to his or her nurse during their discussion of the patient's care. This principle also is applied in similar devices that are used in theaters to send the stage sound directly to headphones.[57] In general, these units do not enjoy widespread popular use for two reasons. First, they are less powerful than hearing aids and will not be loud enough for many patients. Second, these devices require informed set-up, troubleshooting, and cooperation among several parties in order to work. These factors are not insurmountable, but they do add enough difficulty that the majority of patients will find that their hearing aids alone will suffice.

Another look at Figure 38-14 will reveal that the telephone in the room is designed for both the visually and the hearing impaired. This phone has larger touch-pad numbers to assist patients with vision

Figure 38-14
Assistive listening devices. The patient is using a device that allows him to place a microphone close to his nurse during a discussion. His telephone is also designed with larger numbers and a volume control.

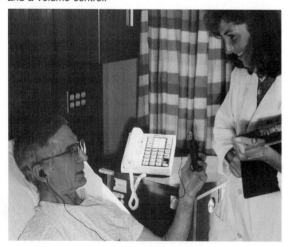

or dexterity problems. In addition, this phone has a volume control that allows the patient to boost the volume of the signal until it reaches the desired level. If the patient cannot distinguish speech adequately, this sort of telephone may be replaced with a Telephone Device for the Deaf (TDD) that allows typed communication. A wide range of other devices that use sight or touch now are available. These include vibrating alarm clocks, flashing doorbells, and lights indicating the crying of a baby. Specially trained hearing dogs can be used to alert the patient to the presence of specific warning sounds.

Cochlear Implants

Cochlear implants are devices applied in cases of very severe hearing loss in both ears. These units replace the natural sensory transducers in the cochlea with a surgically inserted electrode that delivers current to the auditory nerve in order to initiate action potentials. Complex strategies have been developed to relate the sound received at the microphone to the pattern of electrode activation, and the results have allowed some patients to receive and understand speech. Scores of 10 to 30 percent in the word recognition tests described earlier are common.[58] The indications for use of this device, rather than a hearing aid, are very severe hearing loss in both ears and speech reception (in the best ear) in the 10 percent range or less. It is likely that these parameters will be relaxed in the future when the microtechnology improves.

Surgical placement of a cochlear implant will still result in the patient having to wear a large, visible device, and many of the problems related to ordinary hearing aids, such as background noise, will still be present. The cochlear implant was developed to restore hearing to individuals who had some hearing during the critical developmental period for acoustical processing (birth to 2 years) and have since lost it. Deaf individuals, especially those deaf since birth, have often used sign language to achieve full function in society. Cochlear implants have shown very limited success in this population.

MANAGEMENT OF A PATIENT WITH HEARING AIDS

Obtaining a Hearing Aid

Once the recommendation for hearing aids is given by the evaluating audiologist, the selection process begins with testing, selection of specific hearing aids, and making an ear impression. An ear impression is made by injecting self-hardening material into the ear canal and outer ear. This impression is then removed and sent to the manufacturer as a model for construction of a hearing aid shell in the case of an in-the-ear unit, or a custom ear mold in the case of a behind-the-ear unit (Figures 38-16 and 38-17).

Regular Use and Maintenance

Putting on a hearing aid involves matching two complex surfaces, the ear mold and the ear, behind the plane of vision. It is an unusual but not difficult task, which is performed by very young and very old individuals every day. It will take several days to learn, and initial frustration must be overcome. The patient's manual dexterity may be a limiting factor, and some patients may never be able to accomplish this task without help from others (Figure 38-15).

The battery of most hearing aids will last approximately 10 days. When the battery is exhausted, the hearing aid will stop working, and the battery must be changed. Hearing aid batteries are very small, and the patient may require some assistance in manipulating

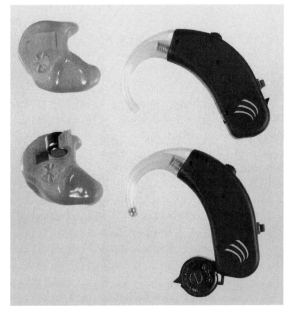

Figure 38-16
Hearing aid battery compartments. The batteries are placed in the swing-out door as shown above. The flat (+) surface of the battery faces up, whereas the ridged surface fits into the cup of the battery door. The door is then closed, positioning the battery for use. When stored at night, the battery door should be left open.

Figure 38-15
The patient's nurse is assisting in placing and adjusting the patient's hearing aid.

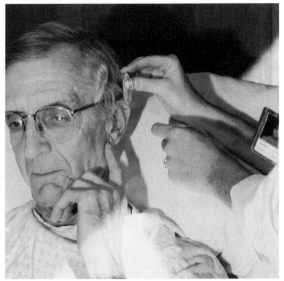

them. Figure 38-16 shows both common styles of hearing aids (ITE and BTE), showing the action of the battery doors. The battery itself has two distinct surfaces, flat on the top (positive) and a ridge on the bottom (negative). The ridged surface will drop easily into the cupped bottom of the battery door. The door then is shut, swinging the battery into place. Hearing aid batteries come in several sizes, and the size used by the patient's hearing aid will be specified in the owners' manual. These sizes are identified numerically. Manufacturers will add letters to their labels, but the sizes are the same. Hearing aid batteries are toxic if swallowed and should not be stored where they may be confused with food or medication.

Hearing aids will become soiled with cerumen and other substances and must be cleaned. Figure 38-17 shows the proper method for removing the ear mold section of a BTE hearing aid. Once this is done, the ear mold can be soaked in warm water, reamed with a pipe cleaner, or cleaned using a brush or wax loop that is typically provided for that purpose. The

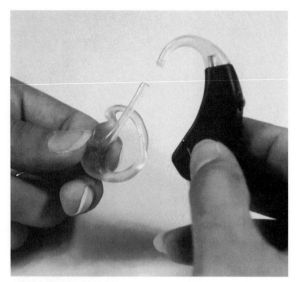

Figure 38-17
Removing the ear mold of a behind-the-ear (BTE) hearing aid for cleaning.

ear mold cleaned in this fashion must be allowed to dry very thoroughly before being reattached to the hearing aid. Small amounts of moisture may block the tube or corrode the electronic parts. The advantages of the BTE are clearly evident here since no equivalent cleaning can be done on an in-the-ear-unit. ITE units (Figure 38-16) do not have separable electronic components and must never be exposed to water or standard cleaning fluids. The ITE hearing aid may be wiped off or brushed off using special tools. Some form of wax guard is very important to prolong the life of ITE units. A wax guard is located at the output port of the hearing aid and acts as a filter that catches the cerumen before it seeps into the receiver mechanism. These filters should be cleaned, emptied, or changed as suggested in the owners' manual.

Normal Wear and Use

Interactions, discussions, and therapy sessions should not proceed unless the patient's hearing aid is on and functioning properly. Visits from family and friends should be preceded by putting on the hearing aid and adjusting it to the proper volume level. Watching television typically is enhanced by the extra volume provided by the hearing aid and allows the television to be operated at a volume that does not disturb others.

Hearing aids should not be worn while sleeping. Before the user goes to sleep, they should be placed in their carrying case with the battery doors open to prevent draining the battery. Hearing aids should never be allowed to get wet, and so care must be taken to prevent the patient from forgetting to remove them when showering, bathing, or swimming. Noisy situations, such as cafeterias, city traffic, and parties, may present particular difficulty to the patient, and the patient may elect not to wear the aids.

Troubleshooting and Repairs

The most common problem with hearing aids is that of feedback. If a high-pitched squeal begins, it is caused by sound leaking from the receiver to the microphone and being reamplified (Figure 38-12). The patient, or if necessary a staff member, should reseat the ear mold to form a tight seal. Feedback is also caused by a reflective surface, such as a pillow, being placed near the microphone. If feedback interferes with the patient's need for amplification, the vendor should be contacted to make a physical adjustment, reevaluate hearing levels, or suggest a different device.

Many complaints of hearing aid malfunction turn out to result from a dead battery. It is a simple matter to remove the hearing aid, turn the hearing aid all the way up, and listen for amplified sound or feedback. If this does not occur, the battery may be replaced and the aid turned up and listened to again. Another common source of trouble is occlusion of the ear mold (BTE) or receiver port (ITE) with cerumen. The hearing aid should be cleaned and cerumen cleared from the output port. The aid should then be retested by listening to see if the problem is resolved. If problems are not solved by such activities as cleaning or replacing the battery, evaluation and repair should be referred to the manufacturer. Several kinds of simple repairs can be performed in the audiologist's office. These generally involve grinding, drilling, or adding material to the ear mold or shell to enhance the fit and feel, or to tighten the seal to avoid feedback. Small parts such as battery doors or volume knobs may be replaced in the office, if parts are available.

REFERENCES

1. Schuknecht H: *Pathology of the Ear,* 2nd ed. Philadelphia: Lea & Febiger, 1993.

2. Brownell W: Outer hair cell electromotility and otoacoustic emissions. *Ear and Hearing* 1990; 11:82.

3. Schuknecht H: *Pathology of the Ear,* 2nd ed. Philadelphia: Lea & Febiger, 1993.

4. Becker G: Coping with stigma: Lifelong adaptation of deaf people. *Social Sci Med* 1981; 15:21.

5. Kandel E, Schwartz J (eds): *Principles of Neural Science.* New York: Elsevier, 1985.

6. Katz J (ed.): *Handbook of Clinical Audiology,* 4th ed. Baltimore: Williams & Wilkins, 1994.

7. Skinner M: *Hearing Aid Evaluation.* Englewood Cliffs, New Jersey: Prentice-Hall, 1988.

8. Schow R, Balsara N, Smedley T, Whitcom C: Aural rehabilitation by ASHA audiologists 1980–1990. *Am J Audiol* 1993; 2:28.

9. Olsho L, Koch E, Carter E, Halpin C, Spetner N: Pure-tone sensitivity of human infants. *J Acoust Soc Am* 1988; 84:1316.

10. Davis L: Hearing health care for the aging. *Curr Opin Otolaryngol* 1995; 3:337.

11. Mykelbust H: *Psychology of Deafness,* 2nd ed. New York: Grune & Stratton, 1964.

12. Stevens S: *Psychophysics: Introduction to Its Perceptual, Neural and Social Prospects.* New York: Wiley, 1975.

13. Reger S: Difference of loudness response of normal and hard-of-hearing ears at intensity levels slightly above threshold. *Ann Otol Rhinol Laryngol* 1936; 45:1029.

14. Nadol J Jr: Hearing loss. *N Engl J Med* 1994; 329:1092.

15. Hawke M, Jahn A: *Diseases of the Ear.* Philadelphia: Lea & Febiger, 1987.

16. Nadol J Jr (ed): *Second International Symposium on Menieres Disease.* Amsterdam: Kughler and Ghedini, 1989.

17. Selters W, Brackmann D: Acoustic tumor detection with brainstem electric response audiometry. *Arch Otolaryngol* 1977; 103:181.

18. American Speech-Language-Hearing Association: Implementation procedures for the standards for the certificates of clinical competence. *ASHA* 1993; 30:27.

19. American Speech-Language-Hearing Association: External auditory canal examination and cerumen management. *ASHA* 1992; 34:22.

20. Wilson W, Thompson G: Behavioral audiometry, in Jerger J (ed): *Pediatric Audiology,* vol 1. San Diego: College Press, 1984.

21. Goodman A: Reference zero levels for pure-tone audiometers. *ASHA* 1965; 7:262.

22. American Speech-Language-Hearing Association: Guidelines for audiometric symbols. *ASHA* 1988; 30:39.

23. American Speech-Language-Hearing Association: Guidelines for manual pure-tone audiometry. *ASHA* 1978; 20:297.

24. American National Standards Institute: Methods for manual pure-tone aduiometry S3.21-1978. New York: American National Standards Institute, 1989.

25. Carhart R, Jerger J: Preferred method for clinical determination of pure-tone thresholds. *J Speech Hear Dis* 1959; 24:330.

26. Linden G, Nilsson G, Anderson H: Minimum effective masking levels in threshold audiometry. *J Speech Hear Dis* 1974; 39:280.

27. Eggermont J, Herrmann B, Thornton A, Hyde M: Peer commentary on clinical usefulness of auditory evoked potentials. *J Speech Lang Pathol Audiol* (Canada) 1991; 15:19.

28. Hirsch I: *The Measurement of Hearing.* New York: McGraw-Hill, 1952.

29. American National Standards Institute: *Methods for Calculation of the Articulation Index S3.5.* New York: American National Standards Institute, 1969.

30. Halpin C, Thornton A, Hasso M: Low-frequency sensorineural loss: Clinical evaluation and implications for hearing aid fitting. *Ear Hear* 1994; 15:71.

31. Speaks C, Jerger J: Method for measurement of speech identification. *J Speech Hear Res* 1965; 8:185.

32. American National Standards Institute: American national standards for audiometers. New York: American National Standards Institute, 1989.

33. Thornton A, Halpin C, Han Y, Hou Z: Innovations in computer-assisted audiometry. *ASHA* 1992; 34:148.

34. Ross M, Lerman J: A picture identification test for the hearing impaired child. *J Speech Hear Res* 1970; 13:44.

35. Thornton AR, Raffin MJ: Speech discrimination scores modeled as a binomial variable. *J Speech Hear Res* 1978; 21:507.

36. Delgutte B: Peripheral processing of speech information: Implications from a physiological study of intensity discrimination, in Schouten M (ed): *The Psychophysics of Speech Perception,* vol 333. Dordrecht: Nijhof. 1987, p. 333.

37. Monro DA, Martin FN: The effects of sophistication on four tests for non-organic hearing loss. *J Speech Hear Dis* 1977; 42:528.

38. Shanks JE, Lilly DJ, Margolis RH, Wiley TH: Tympanometry. *J Speech Hear Dis* 1988; 53:354.

39. American National Standards Institute: S3.39 *Specifications for Instruments to Measure Aural Acoustic Impedance and Admittance.* New York, Author, 1987.

40. Feldman A: Tympanometry, procedures, interpretation and variables, in Feldman A, Wilber L (eds): *Acoustic Impedance and Admittance: The Measurement of Middle Ear Function.* Baltimore: Williams & Wilkins, 1976, p. 103.

41. Kemp D: Stimulated acoustic emissions from within the human auditory system. *J Acoust Soc Am* 1978; 64:1386.

42. Probst R, Lonsbury-Martin B, Martin G: A review of otoacoustic emissions. *J Acoust Soc Am* 1991; 89:2027.

43. American Academy of Opthamology and Otolaryngology Committee on Hearing and Equilibrium and the American Council of Otolaryngology Committee on the Medical Aspects of Noise: Guide for the evaluation of hearing handicap. *JAMA* 1979; 240:2055.

44. Mosicki R, San Martin J, Quintero C, Rauch S, Nadol J

Jr, Bloch K: Serum antibody to inner ear proteins in patients with progressive hearing loss. *JAMA* 1994; 272:611.

45. French M, Steinberg J: Factors governing the intelligibility of speech sounds. *J Acoust Soc Am* 1947; 19:90.

46. Johnson E: Auditory test results in 500 cases of acoustic neuroma. *Arch Otolaryngol* 1977; 103:152.

47. Gardner M: Some monaural and binaural facets of median plane localization. *J Acoust Soc Am* 1973; 54:1489.

48. Killion M: A high-fidelity hearing aid. *Hear Instr* 1990; 41:38.

49. Killion M, Staab W, Preves D: Classifying automatic signal processors. *Hear Instr* 1990; 41:24.

50. Killion M, Fikret-Pasa S: The three types of sensorineural hearing loss: Loudness and intelligibility considerations. *Hear Instr* 1994; 44:8.

51. Kochkin S: MarkeTrak III: Why 20 million in the U.S. don't use hearing aids for their hearing loss. *Hear J* 1993; 46:20.

52. Young E, Sachs M: Representation of steady-state vowels in the the temporal aspects of the discharge patterns of populations of auditory nerve fibers. *J Acoust Soc Am* 1979; 66:1381.

53. Pollack M (ed): *Amplification for the Hearing Impaired*. New York: Grune & Stratton, 1980.

54. Kochkin S: MarkeTrak III identifies key factors in consumer satisfaction. *Hear Instr* 1993; 45:1.

55. Plomp R: The negative effect of amplitude compression in multichannel hearing aids in the light of the modulation transfer function. *J Acoust Soc Am* 1988; 83:2322.

56. Plomp R: Auditory handicap of hearing impairment and the limited benefit of hearing aids. *J Acoust Soc Am* 1978; 63:533.

57. Vaughn G, Lightfoot R, Teter D: Assistive listening devices and systems enhance the lifestyles of hearing impaired persons. *Am J Otol* 1988; 9:101.

58. Tyler R. (ed): *Cochlear Implants: Audiological Foundations*. San Diego: Singular Publishing Group, 1993.

INDEX

INDEX

INDEX

Page numbers in *italics* refer to illustrations; those ending in the letter t refer to charts.

NOTES

NOTES

NOTES

NOTES

NOTES

NOTES

NOTES

NOTES

NOTES

NOTES

NOTES

NOTES

NOTES

NOTES

ISBN 0-07-036794-9